Plant Extracts

Plant Extracts: Biological and Pharmacological Activity

Editors

Raffaele Capasso
Lorenzo Di Cesare Mannelli

MDPI • Basel • Beijing • Wuhan • Barcelona • Belgrade • Manchester • Tokyo • Cluj • Tianjin

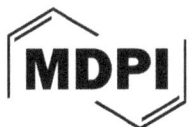

Editors
Raffaele Capasso
University of Naples Federico II
Italy

Lorenzo Di Cesare Mannelli
Universita degli Studi di Firenze
Italy

Editorial Office
MDPI
St. Alban-Anlage 66
4052 Basel, Switzerland

This is a reprint of articles from the Special Issue published online in the open access journal *Molecules* (ISSN 1420-3049) (available at: https://www.mdpi.com/journal/molecules/special_issues/Molecules_Plant_Extracts).

For citation purposes, cite each article independently as indicated on the article page online and as indicated below:

LastName, A.A.; LastName, B.B.; LastName, C.C. Article Title. *Journal Name* **Year**, *Volume Number*, Page Range.

ISBN 978-3-03943-987-4 (Hbk)
ISBN 978-3-03943-988-1 (PDF)

© 2021 by the authors. Articles in this book are Open Access and distributed under the Creative Commons Attribution (CC BY) license, which allows users to download, copy and build upon published articles, as long as the author and publisher are properly credited, which ensures maximum dissemination and a wider impact of our publications.

The book as a whole is distributed by MDPI under the terms and conditions of the Creative Commons license CC BY-NC-ND.

Contents

About the Editors ix

Raffaele Capasso and Lorenzo Di Cesare Mannelli
Special Issue "Plant Extracts: Biological and Pharmacological Activity"
Reprinted from: *Molecules* **2020**, *25*, 5131, doi:10.3390/molecules25215131 1

Fang-Rong Cheng, Hong-Xin Cui, Ji-Li Fang, Ke Yuan and Ying Guo
Ameliorative Effect and Mechanism of the Purified Anthraquinone-Glycoside Preparation from *Rheum Palmatum* L. on Type 2 Diabetes Mellitus
Reprinted from: *Molecules* **2019**, *24*, 1454, doi:10.3390/molecules24081454 7

Rosa Martha Pérez Gutierrez, Abraham Heriberto García Campoy, Silvia Patricia Paredes Carrera, Alethia Muñiz Ramirez, José Maria Mota Flores and Sergio Odin Flores Valle
3′-O-β-D-glucopyranosyl-α,4,2′,4′,6′-pentahydroxy- dihydrochalcone, from Bark of *Eysenhardtia polystachya* Prevents Diabetic Nephropathy via Inhibiting Protein Glycation in STZ-Nicotinamide Induced Diabetic Mice
Reprinted from: *Molecules* **2019**, *24*, 1214, doi:10.3390/molecules24071214 23

Thilina L. Gunathilaka, Kalpa W. Samarakoon, P. Ranasinghe and L. Dinithi C. Peiris
In-Vitro Antioxidant, Hypoglycemic Activity, and Identification of Bioactive Compounds in Phenol-Rich Extract from the Marine Red Algae *Gracilaria edulis* (Gmelin) Silva
Reprinted from: *Molecules* **2019**, *24*, 3708, doi:10.3390/molecules24203708 37

Truong Ngoc Minh, Truong Mai Van, Yusuf Andriana, Le The Vinh, Dang Viet Hau, Dang Hong Duyen and Chona de Guzman-Gelani
Antioxidant, Xanthine Oxidase, α-Amylase and α-Glucosidase Inhibitory Activities of Bioactive Compounds from *Rumex crispus* L. Root
Reprinted from: *Molecules* **2019**, *24*, 3899, doi:10.3390/molecules24213899 55

Nguyen Van Quan, Tran Dang Xuan, Hoang-Dung Tran, Nguyen Thi Dieu Thuy, Le Thu Trang, Can Thu Huong, Yusuf Andriana and Phung Thi Tuyen
Antioxidant, α-Amylase and α-Glucosidase Inhibitory Activities and Potential Constituents of *Canarium tramdenum* Bark
Reprinted from: *Molecules* **2019**, *24*, 605, doi:10.3390/molecules24030605 67

Thania Alejandra Urrutia-Hernández, Jorge Arturo Santos-López, Juana Benedí, Francisco Jose Sánchez-Muniz, Claudia Velázquez-González, Minarda De la O-Arciniega, Osmar Antonio Jaramillo-Morales and Mirandeli Bautista
Antioxidant and Hepatoprotective Effects of *Croton hypoleucus* Extract in an Induced-Necrosis Model in Rats
Reprinted from: *Molecules* **2019**, *24*, 2533, doi:10.3390/molecules24142533 81

Lucia Recinella, Annalisa Chiavaroli, Giustino Orlando, Luigi Menghini, Claudio Ferrante, Lorenzo Di Cesare Mannelli, Carla Ghelardini, Luigi Brunetti and Sheila Leone
Protective Effects Induced by Two Polyphenolic Liquid Complexes from Olive (*Olea europaea*, mainly *Cultivar Coratina*) Pressing Juice in Rat Isolated Tissues Challenged with LPS
Reprinted from: *Molecules* **2019**, *24*, 3002, doi:10.3390/molecules24163002 99

Jae Sung Lim, Sung Ho Lee, Sang Rok Lee, Hyung-Ju Lim, Yoon-Seok Roh, Eun Jeong Won, Namki Cho, Changju Chun and Young-Chang Cho
Inhibitory Effects of *Aucklandia lappa* Decne. Extract on Inflammatory and Oxidative Responses in LPS-Treated Macrophages
Reprinted from: *Molecules* **2020**, *25*, 1336, doi:10.3390/molecules25061336 113

Chukwuemeka R. Nwokocha, Isheba Warren, Javier Palacios, Mario Simirgiotis, Magdalene Nwokocha, Sharon Harrison, Rory Thompson, Adrian Paredes, Jorge Bórquez, Astrid Lavado and Fredi Cifuentes
Modulatory Effect of Guinep (*Melicoccus bijugatus* Jacq) Fruit Pulp Extract on Isoproterenol-Induced Myocardial Damage in Rats. Identification of Major Metabolites Using High Resolution UHPLC Q-Orbitrap Mass Spectrometry
Reprinted from: *Molecules* **2019**, *24*, 235, doi:10.3390/molecules24020235 127

Tianshuang Xia, Xin Dong, Yiping Jiang, Liuyue Lin, Zhimin Dong, Yi Shen, Hailiang Xin, Qiaoyan Zhang and Luping Qin
Metabolomics Profiling Reveals Rehmanniae Radix Preparata Extract Protects against Glucocorticoid-Induced Osteoporosis Mainly via Intervening Steroid Hormone Biosynthesis
Reprinted from: *Molecules* **2019**, *24*, 253, doi:10.3390/molecules24020253 141

Serena Silvestro, Santa Mammana, Eugenio Cavalli, Placido Bramanti and Emanuela Mazzon
Use of Cannabidiol in the Treatment of Epilepsy: Efficacy and Security in Clinical Trials
Reprinted from: *Molecules* **2019**, *24*, 1459, doi:10.3390/molecules24081459 157

Laura E. Ewing, Charles M. Skinner, Charles M. Quick, Stefanie Kennon-McGill, Mitchell R. McGill, Larry A. Walker, Mahmoud A. ElSohly, Bill J. Gurley and Igor Koturbash
Hepatotoxicity of a Cannabidiol-Rich Cannabis Extract in the Mouse Model
Reprinted from: *Molecules* **2019**, *24*, 1694, doi:10.3390/molecules24091694 183

Mario A. Tan, Mark Wilson D. Lagamayo, Grecebio Jonathan D. Alejandro and Seong Soo A. An
Anti-Amyloidogenic and Cyclooxygenase Inhibitory Activity of *Guettarda speciosa*
Reprinted from: *Molecules* **2019**, *24*, 4112, doi:10.3390/molecules24224112 201

Uthaiwan Suttisansanee, Somsri Charoenkiatkul, Butsara Jongruaysup, Somying Tabtimsri, Dalad Siriwan and Piya Temviriyanukul
Mulberry Fruit Cultivar 'Chiang Mai' Prevents Beta-Amyloid Toxicity in PC12 Neuronal Cells and in a *Drosophila* Model of Alzheimer's Disease
Reprinted from: *Molecules* **2020**, *25*, 1837, doi:10.3390/molecules25081837 213

Thais Biondino Sardella Giorno, Carlos Henrique Corrêa dos Santos, Mario Geraldo de Carvalho, Virgínia Cláudia da Silva, Paulo Teixeira de Sousa Jr., Patricia Dias Fernandes and Fabio Boylan
Study on the Antinociceptive Activity and Mechanism of Action of Isolated Saponins from *Siolmatra brasiliensis* (Cogn.) Baill
Reprinted from: *Molecules* **2019**, *24*, 4584, doi:10.3390/molecules24244584 227

Giustino Orlando, Gokhan Zengin, Claudio Ferrante, Maurizio Ronci, Lucia Recinella, Ismail Senkardes, Reneta Gevrenova, Dimitrina Zheleva-Dimitrova, Annalisa Chiavaroli, Sheila Leone, Simonetta Di Simone, Luigi Brunetti, Carene Marie Nancy Picot-Allain, Mohamad Fawzi Mahomoodally, Kouadio Ibrahime Sinan and Luigi Menghini
Comprehensive Chemical Profiling and Multidirectional Biological Investigation of Two Wild *Anthemis* Species (*Anthemis tinctoria* var. *Pallida* and *A. cretica* subsp. *tenuiloba*): Focus on Neuroprotective Effects
Reprinted from: *Molecules* **2019**, *24*, 2582, doi:10.3390/molecules24142582 239

Phyu Phyu Myint, Thien T. P. Dao and Yeong Shik Kim
Anticancer Activity of *Smallanthus sonchifolius* Methanol Extract against Human Hepatocellular Carcinoma Cells
Reprinted from: *Molecules* **2019**, *24*, 3054, doi:10.3390/molecules24173054 265

Weihui Deng, Ke Liu, Shan Cao, Jingyu Sun, Balian Zhong and Jiong Chun
Chemical Composition, Antimicrobial, Antioxidant, and Antiproliferative Properties of Grapefruit Essential Oil Prepared by Molecular Distillation
Reprinted from: *Molecules* **2020**, *25*, 217, doi:10.3390/molecules25010217 277

Seham Abdel-Shafi, Abdul-Raouf Al-Mohammadi, Mahmoud Sitohy, Basma Mosa, Ahmed Ismaiel, Gamal Enan and Ali Osman
Antimicrobial Activity and Chemical Constitution of the Crude, Phenolic-Rich Extracts of *Hibiscus sabdariffa*, *Brassica oleracea* and *Beta vulgaris*
Reprinted from: *Molecules* **2019**, *24*, 4280, doi:10.3390/molecules24234280 289

Cinzia Pagano, Maura Marinozzi, Claudio Baiocchi, Tommaso Beccari, Paola Calarco, Maria Rachele Ceccarini, Michela Chielli, Ciriana Orabona, Elena Orecchini, Roberta Ortenzi, Maurizio Ricci, Stefania Scuota, Maria Cristina Tiralti and Luana Perioli
Bioadhesive Polymeric Films Based on Red Onion Skins Extract for Wound Treatment: An Innovative and Eco-Friendly Formulation
Reprinted from: *Molecules* **2020**, *25*, 318, doi:10.3390/molecules25020318 307

Anna Kurek-Górecka, Michał Górecki, Anna Rzepecka-Stojko, Radosław Balwierz and Jerzy Stojko
Bee Products in Dermatology and Skin Care
Reprinted from: *Molecules* **2020**, *25*, 556, doi:10.3390/molecules25030556 325

Justine Bodin, Amandine Adrien, Pierre-Edouard Bodet, Delphine Dufour, Stanislas Baudouin, Thierry Maugard and Nicolas Bridiau
Ulva intestinalis Protein Extracts Promote In Vitro Collagen and Hyaluronic Acid Production by Human Dermal Fibroblasts
Reprinted from: *Molecules* **2020**, *25*, 2091, doi:10.3390/molecules25092091 343

Yeon-hee Kim, Amy Cho, Sang-Ah Kwon, Minju Kim, Mina Song, Hye won Han, Eun-Ji Shin, Eunju Park and Seung-Min Lee
Potential Photoprotective Effect of Dietary Corn Silk Extract on Ultraviolet B-Induced Skin Damage
Reprinted from: *Molecules* **2019**, *24*, 2587, doi:10.3390/molecules24142587 365

Md. Adnan, Md. Nazim Uddin Chy, A.T.M. Mostafa Kamal, Md Obyedul Kalam Azad, Arkajyoti Paul, Shaikh Bokhtear Uddin, James W. Barlow, Mohammad Omar Faruque, Cheol Ho Park and Dong Ha Cho
Investigation of the Biological Activities and Characterization of Bioactive Constituents of *Ophiorrhiza rugosa* var. *prostrata* (D.Don) & Mondal Leaves through In Vivo, In Vitro, and In Silico Approaches
Reprinted from: *Molecules* **2019**, *24*, 1367, doi:10.3390/molecules24071367 . . . . **387**

Muhammad Taher, Siti Syazwani Shaari, Deny Susanti, Dayar Arbain and Zainul Amiruddin Zakaria
Genus *Ophiorrhiza*: A Review of Its Distribution, Traditional Uses, Phytochemistry, Biological Activities and Propagation
Reprinted from: *Molecules* **2020**, *25*, 2611, doi:10.3390/molecules25112611 . . . . **411**

Bahare Salehi, Lorene Armstrong, Antonio Rescigno, Balakyz Yeskaliyeva, Gulnaz Seitimova, Ahmet Beyatli, Jugreet Sharmeen, Mohamad Fawzi Mahomoodally, Farukh Sharopov, Alessandra Durazzo, Massimo Lucarini, Antonello Santini, Ludovico Abenavoli, Raffaele Capasso and Javad Sharifi-Rad
Lamium Plants—A Comprehensive Review on Health Benefits and Biological Activities
Reprinted from: *Molecules* **10**, *24*, 1913, doi:10.3390/molecules24101913 . . . . **439**

Bahare Salehi, Esra Capanoglu, Nabil Adrar, Gizem Catalkaya, Shabnum Shaheen, Mehwish Jaffer, Lalit Giri, Renu Suyal, Arun K Jugran, Daniela Calina, Anca Oana Docea, Senem Kamiloglu, Dorota Kregiel, Hubert Antolak, Ewelina Pawlikowska, Surjit Sen, Krishnendu Acharya, Zeliha Selamoglu, Javad Sharifi-Rad, Miquel Martorell, Célia F. Rodrigues, Farukh Sharopov, Natália Martins and Raffaele Capasso
Cucurbits Plants: A Key Emphasis to Its Pharmacological Potential
Reprinted from: *Molecules* **2019**, *24*, 1854, doi:10.3390/molecules24101854 . . . . **463**

Radu Claudiu Fierascu, Georgeta Temocico, Irina Fierascu, Alina Ortan and Narcisa Elena Babeanu
Fragaria Genus: Chemical Composition and Biological Activities
Reprinted from: *Molecules* **2020**, *25*, 498, doi:10.3390/molecules25030498 . . . . **487**

Xu Zhang, Xiao Cheng, Yali Wu, Di Feng, Yifan Qian, Liping Chen, Bo Yang and Mancang Gu
In Vitro and In Situ Characterization of the Intestinal Absorption of Capilliposide B and Capilliposide C from *Lysimachia capillipes* Hemsl
Reprinted from: *Molecules* **2019**, *24*, 1227, doi:10.3390/molecules24071227 . . . . **509**

Lee Suan Chua, Cher Haan Lau, Chee Yung Chew and Dawood Ali Salim Dawood
Solvent Fractionation and Acetone Precipitation for Crude Saponins from *Eurycoma longifolia* Extract
Reprinted from: *Molecules* **2019**, *24*, 1416, doi:10.3390/molecules24071416 . . . . **523**

Ya-Han Chen, Dong-Sheng Guo, Mei-Huan Lu, Jian-Ying Yue, Yan Liu, Chun-Ming Shang, De-Rong An and Ming-Min Zhao
Inhibitory Effect of Osthole from *Cnidium monnieri* on Tobacco Mosaic Virus (TMV) Infection in *Nicotiana glutinosa*
Reprinted from: *Molecules* **2020**, *25*, 65, doi:10.3390/molecules25010065 . . . . **533**

About the Editors

Raffaele Capasso is Associate Professor at the Department of Agricultural Sciences of the University of Naples Federico II, Portici (Naples), Italy. He holds a degree in Pharmacy (1996), Master's in Medicinal Plants (2000), Master's in Pharmacology (2002), and Ph.D. in Drug Science (2005). He has taught at the University of Naples Federico II as Professor of Applied Pharmacognosy (starting from 2006) and Phytotherapy (starting from 2011). His main research interests are as follows: role of cannabinoid, vanilloid, and kappa-opioid receptors in the gastrointestinal tract, both in physiological (e.g., intestinal motility) and pathophysiological states (e.g., inflammation and cancer); ethnopharmacological studies on medicinal plants and their active ingredients used in traditional medicine; clinical pharmacology of herbal products; and nutritional pharmacology. He has published 150 articles in peer-reviewed international journals (cited in JCI). He is the recipient of the Farmindustria Prize (2006), from the Italian Society of Pharmacology, to the best article published by a researcher under 35 years as a first author.

Lorenzo Di Cesare Mannelli was born in Florence, Italy, on September 29th, 1975. He obtained his Degree in Pharmacy summa cum laude in 1999 (University of Florence), his Ph.D. in Pharmacology and Toxicology (2005; University of Florence), and his specialization in Applied Pharmacology (2006; University of Florence). He received postdoctoral fellowships in the years 2006–2017. He has been a researcher (RTD-B) in pharmacology at Dept. Neurofarba, University of Florence, since July 2017 (RTD-A till December 2018, then RTD-B). He became Associate Professor in Pharmacology in 2016 and Full Professor in Pharmacology in 2018. He received the following awards: Simpar, Study on multidisciplinary pain research, "Young against Pain" award (2016); "AlbericoBenedicenti" award (2015); award at the Congress of Pharmacognosy, Italy (2014); travel fellowship for Worldpharma (2010); award at 34° Nat Met Pharmacol (2009); travel fellowship for VI Summer School of Neuroscience (2008). He organized the meetings "The Pharmacological Basis of Novel Pain Therapeutics" (2017) and "Glial cells and therapeutic perspectives: from maladaptive plasticity to neurorestoration" (2018). He was invited to speak at several (30) international scientific meetings. He is a member of the editorial board or guest editor of the following journals: Frontiers in Pharmacology, Frontiers in Cell Neuroscience, Molecules, Neural Regeneration Research, Current Drug Targets, and Journal of Applied Pharmacology and Toxicology. He has received grants from the "Istituto Toscano Tumori" (2014), the Italian Foundation for Multiple Sclerosis (2017), and Fondazione Cassa di Risparmio di Firenze (2018); he also received a grant from the European Union for the project IMI2 "Neuroderisk" (2019). He has collaborated with and received grants from the following pharmaceutical companies: Apharm, Italy; MDM, Italy; Aboca, Italy, Metys Pharm, Switzerland; Bioiberica, Spain; Kineta, USA; Daya, USA. His research activity is focused on the physiopathological mechanisms of pain, cognitive functions, and memory and the relative pharmacological modulation. In particular, he studies the neurotoxicity of anticancer drugs widely in vitro and in vivo. His research activity is documented by about 200 full papers published in international peer-reviewed journals.

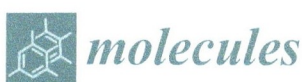

Editorial

Special Issue "Plant Extracts: Biological and Pharmacological Activity"

Raffaele Capasso [1],* and Lorenzo Di Cesare Mannelli [2],*

1. Department of Agricultural Sciences, University of Naples Federico II, 80055 Portici, Naples, Italy
2. Department of Neuroscience, Psychology, Drug Research and Child Health-Neurofarba-Section of Pharmacology and Toxicology, University of Florence, 50139 Florence, Italy
* Correspondence: rafcapas@unina.it (R.C.); lorenzo.mannelli@unifi.it (L.D.C.M.)

Academic Editor: Derek J. McPhee
Received: 30 October 2020; Accepted: 2 November 2020; Published: 4 November 2020

The use of plant extracts for therapeutic purposes knows a wide diffusion. The vegetal origin of these products intercepts people's desire to cure themselves with natural drugs; this aspect, together with effectiveness and regulatory opportunities, is the base of the modern broad use of medicinal plants. Traditional uses and novel biological effects allow for availability of an extraordinary high number of different compounds that may constitute a formidable therapeutic potential. Nevertheless, pitfalls are hidden behind poor pharmacological and toxicological knowledge of plant extracts, non-standardized methods of extraction, and undefined and not repeatable qualitative and quantitative composition.

In this context, novel experimental studies on plant products are necessary and appreciated to reinforce the scientific soundness of phytotherapy. This Special Issue aims to respond to this medical need, comprehensively highlighting the newest discoveries in vegetal resources with an emphasis on pharmacological activity. More than 30, highly cited, articles were collected.

Cheng et al. [1] showed the hypoglycemic and anti-dyslipidemic effect of purified anthraquinone-glycoside from *Rheum palmatum* L. in a rat model of type 2 diabetes mellitus. The anthraquinone can reduce oxidative stress and regulate Fas/FasL-mediated apoptosis signaling pathway improving β-cell function.

The dihydrochalcone 3'-O-β-D-glucopyranosyl α,4,2',4',6'-pentahydroxy–dihydrochalcone isolated from *Eysenhardtia polystachya* was able to protect mice against diabetic nephropathy. It improved renal dysfunction as well as it reduced glycated hemoglobin and advanced glycation end products in the presence of significant histological recovery of kidney [2].

Gunathilaka and coworkers [3] reported the hypoglycemic and antioxidant in vitro activities of the marine red algae *Gracilaria edulis*. A de-polysaccharide methanol extract of *G. edulis* was sequentially partitioned by different solvents. The ethyl acetate fraction exhibited the strongest hypoglycemic and antiglycation potential. Gas chromatography-mass spectrometry analysis of the ethyl acetate fraction revealed the presence of several candidate anti-diabetic compounds.

Chrysophanol and physcion, isolated from the root of *Rumex crispus* L. emerged as relevant in the medicinal properties of the plant against gout and diabetes. Compounds showed scavenging capacity, xanthine oxidase and α-glucosidase inhibitory activity [4].

Quan et al. [5] showed the result of a phytochemical and pharmacological study on the *Canarium tramdenum* bark. Five different extracts were chemically characterized, revealing that *C. tramdenum* fruit possesses phenols and terpenoids, which might contribute to reducing risks from diabetes. A high quantity of α- and β-amyrins highlighted the potentials of anti-inflammatory, anti-ulcer, anti-hyperlipidemic, anti-tumor, and hepatoprotective properties of *C. tramdenum* bark.

An ethanol extract of *Croton hypoleucus* showed antioxidant and hepatoprotective activity in rats with liver necrosis. Hepatic damage markers were reduced, whereas *SOD* and *Cat* gene expression were increased, suggesting a control of antioxidant defense levels [6].

Recinella et al. [7] described the antinflammatory effects of polyphenolic liquid complexes from olive pressing juice with high levels of hydroxytyrosol. In isolated rat colon, liver, heart, and prefrontal cortex samples, a tissue-dedicated molecular analysis revealed that the products exhibited protective effects on multiple inflammatory and oxidative stress pathways.

The Korean plant *Aucklandia lappa* Decne., known as "Mok-hyang" was investigated as ethanol extract for studying in vitro the anti-inflammatory and antioxidative effects. The extract reduced redox unbalance and proinflammatory mediators by decreasing the nuclear translocation of p65 and by the enhanced expression of hemeoxygenase 1 [8].

Nwokocha and collegues [9] reported the cardioprotective effects of the juice of *Melicoccus bijugatus* fruit pulp. Using a rat model of myocardial injury, the authors showed that a repeated treatment reduced blood pressure and heart rate as well as decreased heart to body weight ratio. Vitamin C and related compounds, phenolic acids, flavonoid, fatty acids and terpene derivatives were individuated as components.

In vivo and in vitro experiments, as well as a UHPLC-Q/TOF-MS-based metabolomics study, showed the effect of the dry rhizome of *Rehmannia glutinosa* Libosch. in preventing osteoporosis and its underlying mechanisms. *Rehmannia glutinosa* enhanced bone mineral density and improved the micro-architecture of trabecular bone via interfering with the steroid hormone biosynthesis [10].

Regarding the nervous system, Silvestro et al. [11] studied the effect of cannabidiol, one of the cannabinoids with non-psychotropic action extracted from *Cannabis sativa*, against the severe treatment-resistant epilepsy in addition to common anti-epileptic drugs. An overview of recent literature and clinical trials showed that the use of cannabidiol could represent hope for patients who are resistant to conventional anti-epileptic drugs.

Cannabidiol was also studied for toxicological aspects [12]. In mice, cannabidiol induced signs of hepatotoxicity, possibly of a cholestatic nature; hepatotoxicity gene expression arrays revealed that it differentially regulated more than 50 genes, many of which were linked to oxidative stress responses, lipid metabolism pathways and drug metabolizing enzymes.

Tan and coworkers [13] described the anti-inflammatory and neuroprotective properties of *Guettarda speciosa* (chloroform and methanol extracts). *G. speciosa* was able to inhibit cyclooxygenase assay (partial selectivity for COX-1), further it reduced amyloid-beta aggregates in the neuronal cell line, suggesting possible anti-neurodegenerative applications.

Beta-amyloid-induced neurotoxicity was also prevented by an aqueous extract of *Morus nigra* 'Chiang Mai' [14]. High amounts of cyanidin, keracyanin, and kuromanin as anthocyanidin and anthocyanins were found in the extract. *M. nigra* promoted neurite outgrowth and improved locomotory coordination of *Drosophila* co-expressing human amyloid precursor protein and BACE-1 specifically in the brain.

Siolmatra brasiliensis (Cogn.) Baill, ("taiuiá", "cipó-tauá") and its isolated substances (cayaponoside A1, cayaponoside B4, cayaponoside D, and siolmatroside I) were studied for relieving pain [15]. Hydroethanol extract, ethyl acetate fraction, and isolated saponins showed analgesic effects and reduced capsaicin- or glutamate-induced hypersensitivity by a mechanism involving muscarinic and opioid signaling.

Ethyl acetate, methanol, and aqueous extracts of aerial parts of *Anthemis tinctoria* var. *pallida* and *A. cretica* subsp. *tenuiloba* were investigated for their phenol and flavonoid content, antioxidant, and key enzyme (AChE, BChE. tyrosinase and α-glucosidase) inhibitory potentials [16]. Further, ex vivo studies highlighted neuroprotective properties after an excitotoxicstimulus promoting LDH level and 5-HT turnover normalization as well as the restoration of proteins involved in neuron morphology and neurotransmission.

Myint et al. [17] studied the activity of a methanol extract of *Smallanthus sonchifolius* leaf against a human hepatocellular carcinoma cell line. The extract reduced cell proliferation and cell migration, it also induced cell cycle arrest and necrosis in a concentration-dependent manner. Putative active components were melampolide-type sesquiterpenoids.

Antiproliferative properties were also depicted for the grape fruit essential oil [18]. Deng et al. detected by GC-MS twenty-four components (terpenes and oxygenated terpenes); the light phase oil displayed inhibitory effects on liver cancer cells proliferation, antimicrobial effects against *Bacillus subtilis*, *Escherichia coli*, *Staphylococcusaureus* and *Salmonella typhimurium* as well as antioxidant activity.

Antimicrobial activities were described for crude, phenolic-rich extracts of *Hibiscus sabdariffa Brassica oleracea* var. capitata f. rubra and *Beta vulgaris* [19]. Total anthocyanins, phenols, flavonoids contents were analyzed. Extracts and isolated compounds showed antimicrobial effects against pathogenic bacteria and fungi. Electron microscopy analysis revealed bacteria morphological alteration, indicating death and loss of cell content.

Pagano et al. [20] studied the non-edible outside layers of onion for wound healing. A hydroalcoholic extract was formulated in auto adhesive, biocompatible and pain-free hydrogel polymeric films, it showed antioxidant, radical scavenging, antibacterial and anti-inflammatory activities suggesting a potential dermal application for wound treatment.

Kurek-Gorecka and colleagues [21] reported the beneficial effects of bee products in dermatology and skin care. Honey, propolis, bee pollen, bee bread, royal jelly, beeswax and bee venom contain biologically active components, such as flavonoid schrysin, apigenin, kaempferol, quercetin, galangin, pinocembrin or naringenin. These components justify the use of bee products for medical or cosmetic skin treatment based on antibacterial, anti-inflammatory, antioxidant, disinfectant, antifungal and antiviral properties.

A protein fraction from *Ulva intestinalis* containing 51% of proteins and 22% of polysaccharides was analyzed and tested for the anti-aging potential, fibroblast proliferation and collagen and hyaluronic acid production on human fibroblast cell lines. A significant increase in collagen and hyaluronic acid production per cell, and a reduction in cell proliferation without increasing cell mortality were demonstrated [22].

UVB-induced skin damage in mice was reduced by dietary corn silk [23]. Oral administration decreased epidermal thickness, wrinkle formation, and positive staining for PCNA, Ki67, and 8-OHdG, and increased collagen staining. Pro-inflammatory NF-κB target genes and MMP-9 expressions were lowered, whereas TGF-β/Smad signaling increased. Low skin lipid peroxidation and blood DNA oxidation levels and high blood glutathione were detected in parallel with higher levels of catalase, SOD1 and glutaredoxin.

A wide description of *Ophiorrhiza rugosa* var. *prostrata* was performed by Adnan and coworkers [24]. The ethanolic extract of leaves, in three different vivo models, evoked antidiarrheal, anti-inflammatory, anthelmintic and antibacterial effects. Additionally, ADME and PASS analysis revealed a suitable profile for future medicinal development.

Almost 50 species of *Ophiorrhiza* plants were reviewed by Taher and colleagues [25]. The analysis revealed their wide distribution across Asia and the neighboring countries, whereby they were utilized as traditional medicine to treat various diseases. Biological activities encompass anti-cancer, antiviral, antimicrobial, and more. The genus propagation reported could produce a high quality and quantity of potent anticancer compound, namely camptothecin (CPT).

An updated snapshot of *Lamium* plants and their biological activities were provided by Salehi et al. [26]. Botanical, phytochemical and biological characteristics were described, highlighting antimicrobial, antiviral, anti-inflammatory, cytoprotective, anti-nociceptive properties.

Again, Salehi with an international team provided a deed analysis of the *Cucurbita* genus [27]. The traditional efficacy against gastrointestinal diseases and intestinal parasites were correlated with their nutritional and phytochemical composition. Among chemical constituents, carotenoids, tocopherols, phenols, terpenoids, saponins, sterols, fatty acids, and functional carbohydrates and polysaccharides were those occurring in higher abundance. More recently, a huge interest in a class of triterpenoids, cucurbitacins, has been stated.

A deep analysis of the *Fragaria* genus was presented by Fierascu and colleagues [28]. Strawberries possess biological properties, including antioxidant, antimicrobial and anti-inflammatory effects, but only a few species represent the subject of the last decade of scientific research. The main components identified in the *Fragaria* species were here described.

Zhang et al. [29] determined the processes and mechanisms of intestinal absorption of capilliposide B and C from *Lysimachia capillipes* Hemsl. Mechanisms involve processes such as facilitated passive diffusion, efflux transporters, and enzyme-mediated metabolism. Both capilliposides were suggested to be substrates of P-glycoprotein and multidrug resistance-associated protein 2. Capilliposide B may interact with the CYP3A4 system.

A phytochemical analysis on saccharide-containing compounds from *Eurycoma longifolia* was perfomed by Chua et al [30]. Non-toxic solvent fractionation increased the total saponin content, evoking anti-proliferative activity against human breast cancer cells.

Osthole was proposed for the treatment of tobacco mosaic virus [31]. Extracted from *Cnidium monnieri*, osthole showed comparable or stronger antiviral activity than eugenol and ningnanmycin. A direct effect on the viral particles was suggested.

A second edition of this Special Issue is in preparation.

References

1. Cheng, F.-R.; Cui, H.X.; Fang, J.L.; Yuan, K.; Guo, Y. Ameliorative Effect and Mechanism of the Purified Anthraquinone-Glycoside Preparation from *Rheum Palmatum* L. on Type 2 Diabetes Mellitus. *Molecules* **2019**, *24*, 1454. [CrossRef] [PubMed]
2. Rosa, M.P.G.; Abraham, H.G.C.; Silvia, P.P.C.; José, A.M.R.; Maria, M.F.; SergioOdin, F.V. 3′-O-β-D-glucopyranosyl-α,4,2′,4′,6′-pentahydroxy-dihydrochalcone, from Bark of Eysenhardtiapolystachya Prevents Diabetic Nephropathy via Inhibiting Protein Glycation in STZ-Nicotinamide Induced Diabetic Mice. *Molecules* **2019**, *24*, 1214.
3. Gunathilaka, T.L.; Samarakoon, K.W.; Ranasinghe, P.; Peiris, L.D.C. In-Vitro Antioxidant, Hypoglycemic Activity, and Identification of Bioactive Compounds in Phenol-Rich Extract from the Marine Red Algae *Gracilaria edulis* (Gmelin) Silva. *Molecules* **2019**, *24*, 3708. [CrossRef] [PubMed]
4. Truong, N.M.; Truong, M.V.; Yusuf, A.; Le, T.V.; Dang, V.H.; Dang, H.D.; Chona, D.G.-G. Antioxidant, XanthineOxidase, α-Amylase and α-Glucosidase Inhibitory Activities of Bioactive Compounds from *Rumexcrispus* L. Root. *Molecules* **2019**, *24*, 3899.
5. Nguyen, V.Q.; Tran, D.X.; Hoang-Dung, T.; Nguyen, T.D.T.; Le, T.T.; Can, T.H.; Yusuf, A.; Phung, T.T. Antioxidant, α-Amylase and α-Glucosidase Inhibitory Activities and Potential Constituents of *Canarium tramdenum* Bark. *Molecules* **2019**, *24*, 605.
6. Urrutia-Hernández, T.A.; Santos-López, J.A.; Benedí, J.; Sánchez-Muniz, F.J.; Velázquez-González, C.; De La O-Arciniega, M.; Jaramillo-Morales, O.A.; Bautista, M. Antioxidant and Hepatoprotective Effects of *Croton hypoleucus* Extract in an Induced-Necrosis Model in Rats. *Molecules* **2019**, *24*, 2533. [CrossRef]
7. Lucia, R.; Annalisa, C.; Giustino, O.; Luigi, M.; Claudio, F.; Lorenzo, D.C.; Mannelli, C.G.; Luigi, B.; Sheila, L. Protective Effects Induced by Two Polyphenolic Liquid Complexes from Olive (*Olea europaea*, mainly Cultivar Coratina) Pressing Juice in Rat Isolated Tissues Challenged with LPS. *Molecules* **2019**, *24*, 3002.
8. Jae, S.L.; Sung, H.L.; Sang, R.L.; Hyung, J.; Yoon-Seok, R.; Eun, J.W.; Namki, C.; Changju, C.; Young-Chang, C. Inhibitory Effects of *Aucklandia lappa* Decne. Extract on Inflammatory and Oxidative Responses in LPS-Treated Macrophages. *Molecules* **2020**, *25*, 1336.
9. Chukwuemeka, R.; Nwokocha, I.W.; Javier, P.; Mario, S.; Magdalene, N.; Sharon, H.; Rory, T.; Adrian, P.; Jorge, B.; Astrid, L.; et al. Modulatory Effect of Guinep (*Melicoccus bijugatus* Jacq) Fruit Pulp Extract on Isoproterenol-Induced Myocardial Damage in Rats. Identification of Major Metabolites using High Resolution UHPLC Q-Orbitrap Mass Spectrometry. *Molecules* **2019**, *24*, 235.
10. Xia, T.; Dong, X.; Jiang, Y.; Lin, L.; Dong, Z.; Shen, Y.; Xin, H.; Zhang, Q.; Qin, L. Metabolomics Profiling Reveals Rehmanniae Radix Preparata Extract Protectsagainst Glucocorticoid-Induced Osteoporosis Mainly via Intervening Steroid Hormone Biosynthesis. *Molecules* **2019**, *24*, 253. [CrossRef]
11. Silvestro, S.; Mammana, S.; Cavalli, E.; Bramanti, P.; Mazzon, E. Use of Cannabidiol in the Treatment of Epilepsy: Efficacy and Security in Clinical Trials. *Molecules* **2019**, *24*, 1459. [CrossRef] [PubMed]

12. Ewing, L.E.; Skinner, C.M.; Quick, C.M.; Kennon-McGill, S.; McGill, M.R.; Walker, L.A.; ElSohly, M.A.; Gurley, B.J.; Koturbash, I. Hepatotoxicity of a Cannabidiol-Rich Cannabis Extract in the Mouse Model. *Molecules* **2019**, *24*, 1694. [CrossRef]
13. Tan, M.A.; Lagamayo, M.W.D.; Alejandro, G.J.D.; An, S.S.A. Anti-Amyloidogenic and Cyclooxygenase Inhibitory Activity of *Guettarda speciosa*. *Molecules* **2019**, *24*, 4112. [CrossRef] [PubMed]
14. Suttisansanee, U.; Charoenkiatkul, S.; Jongruaysup, B.; Tabtimsri, S.; Siriwan, D.; Temviriyanukul, P. Mulberry Fruit Cultivar 'Chiang Mai' Prevents Beta-Amyloid Toxicity in PC12 Neuronal Cells and in a Drosophila Model of Alzheimer's Disease. *Molecules* **2020**, *25*, 1837. [CrossRef] [PubMed]
15. Thais, B.S.G.; Carlos, H.C.S.; Mario, G.d.C.; Virgínia, C.d.S.; Paulo, T.d.S., Jr.; Patricia, D.F.; Fabio, B. Study on the Antinociceptive Activity and Mechanism of Action of Isolated Saponins from *Siolmatra brasiliensis* (Cogn.) Baill. *Molecules* **2019**, *24*, 4584.
16. Giustino, O.; Gokhan, Z.; Claudio, F.; Maurizio, R.; Lucia, R.; Ismail, S.; Reneta, G.; Dimitrina, Z.-D.; Annalisa, C.; Sheila, L.; et al. Comprehensive Chemical Profiling and Multidirectional Biological Investigation of Two Wild Anthemis Species (*Anthemis tinctoria* var. *Pallida* and *A. cretica* subsp. tenuiloba): Focus on Neuroprotective Effects. *Molecules* **2019**, *24*, 2582.
17. Phyu, P.M.; Thien, T.P.D.; Yeong, S.K. Anticancer Activity of *Smallanthus sonchifolius* Methanol Extractagainst Human Hepatocellular Carcinoma Cells. *Molecules* **2019**, *24*, 3054.
18. Deng, W.; Liu, K.; Cao, S.; Sun, J.; Zhong, B.; Chun, J. Chemical Composition, Antimicrobial, Antioxidant, and Antiproliferative Properties of Grapefruit Essential Oil Prepared by Molecular Distillation. *Molecules* **2020**, *25*, 217. [CrossRef]
19. Abdel-Shafi, S.; Al-Mohammadi, A.-R.; Sitohy, M.; Mosa, B.; Ismaiel, A.; Enan, G.; Osman, A. Antimicrobial Activity and Chemical Constitution of the Crude, Phenolic-Rich Extracts of Hibiscus sabdariffa, *Brassica oleracea* and *Beta vulgaris*. *Molecules* **2019**, *24*, 4280. [CrossRef]
20. Pagano, C.; Marinozzi, M.; Baiocchi, C.; Beccari, T.; Calarco, P.; Ceccarini, M.; Chielli, M.; Orabona, C.; Orecchini, E.; Ortenzi, R.; et al. Bioadhesive Polymeric Films Based on Red Onion Skins Extract for Wound Treatment: An Innovative and Eco-Friendly Formulation. *Molecules* **2020**, *25*, 318. [CrossRef]
21. Kurek-Górecka, A.; Górecki, M.; Rzepecka-Stojko, A.; Balwierz, R.; Stojko, J. Bee Products in Dermatology and Skin Care. *Molecules* **2020**, *25*, 556. [CrossRef] [PubMed]
22. Bodin, J.; Adrien, A.; Bodet, P.-E.; Dufour, D.; Baudouin, S.; Maugard, T.; Bridiau, N. *Ulva intestinalis* Protein Extracts Promote In Vitro Collagen and Hyaluronic Acid Production by Human Dermal Fibroblasts. *Molecules* **2020**, *25*, 2091. [CrossRef]
23. Yeon-hee, K.; Amy, C.; Sang-Ah, K.; Minju, K.; Mina, S.; Hyewon, H.; Eun-Ji, S.; Eunju, P.; Seung-Min, L. Potential Photoprotective Effect of Dietary Corn Silk Extract on Ultraviolet B-Induced Skin Damage. *Molecules* **2019**, *24*, 2587.
24. Adnan, M.; Nazim Uddin Chy, M.; Mostafa Kamal, A.T.M.; Obyedul Kalam Azad, M.; Arkajyoti, P.; Shaikh, B.U.; James, W.; Mohammad, O.F.; Cheol, H.P.; Dong, H.C. Investigation of the Biological Activities and Characterization of Bioactive Constituents of *Ophiorrhiza rugosa* var. prostrata (D.Don) & Mondal Leaves through In Vivo, In Vitro, and In SilicoApproaches. *Molecules* **2019**, *24*, 1367.
25. Taher, M.; Shaari, S.S.; Susanti, D.; Arbain, D.; Zakaria, Z.A. Genus Ophiorrhiza: A Review of Its Distribution, Traditional Uses, Phytochemistry, Biological Activities and Propagation. *Molecules* **2020**, *25*, 2611. [CrossRef] [PubMed]
26. Salehi, B.; Armstrong, L.; Rescigno, A.; Yeskaliyeva, B.; Seitimova, G.; Beyatli, A.; Jugreet, S.; Mahomoodally, F.M.; Sharopov, F.; Durazzo, A.; et al. Lamium Plants—A Comprehensive Review on Health Benefits and Biological Activities. *Molecules* **2019**, *24*, 1913. [CrossRef] [PubMed]
27. Salehi, B.; Capanoglu, E.; Adrar, N.; Catalkaya, G.; Shaheen, S.; Jaffer, M.; Giri, L.; Suyal, R.; Jugran, A.K.; Calina, D.; et al. Cucurbits Plants: A Key Emphasis to Its Pharmacological Potential. *Molecules* **2019**, *24*, 1854. [CrossRef]
28. Fierascu, R.C.; Temocico, G.; Fierascu, I.; Ortan, A.; Babeanu, N.E. Fragaria Genus: Chemical Composition and Biological Activities. *Molecules* **2020**, *25*, 498. [CrossRef]
29. Xu, Z.; Xiao, C.; Yali, W.; Di, F.; Yifan, Q.; Liping, C.; Bo, Y.; Mancang, G. In Vitro and In Situ Characterization of the Intestinal Absorption of Capilliposide B and Capilliposide C from *Lysimachia capillipes* Hemsl. *Molecules* **2019**, *24*, 1227.

30. Lee, S.C.; Cher, H.L.; Chee, Y.C.; Dawood, A.S.D. Solvent Fractionation and Acetone Precipitation for Crude Saponins from *Eurycoma longifolia* Extract. *Molecules* **2019**, *24*, 1416.
31. Chen, Y.H.; Guo, D.S.; Lu, M.H.; Yue, J.Y.; Liu, Y.; Shang, C.M.; An, D.R.; Zhao, M.M. Inhibitory Effect of Osthole from *Cnidium monnieri* on Tobacco Mosaic Virus (TMV) Infection in *Nicotiana glutinosa*. *Molecules* **2020**, *25*, 65. [CrossRef]

Sample Availability: Samples of the compounds … … are available from the authors.

Publisher's Note: MDPI stays neutral with regard to jurisdictional claims in published maps and institutional affiliations.

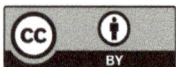

© 2020 by the authors. Licensee MDPI, Basel, Switzerland. This article is an open access article distributed under the terms and conditions of the Creative Commons Attribution (CC BY) license (http://creativecommons.org/licenses/by/4.0/).

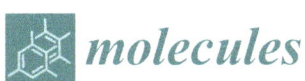

Article

Ameliorative Effect and Mechanism of the Purified Anthraquinone-Glycoside Preparation from *Rheum Palmatum* L. on Type 2 Diabetes Mellitus

Fang-Rong Cheng [1], Hong-Xin Cui [1,2], Ji-Li Fang [3], Ke Yuan [3,*] and Ying Guo [4]

[1] College of Pharmacy, Henan University of Chinese Medicine, Zhengzhou 450046, China; chengfr1963888@126.com (F.-R.C.); cuihongxin1974@163.com (H.-X.C.)
[2] Collaborative Innovation Center for Respiratory Disease Diagnosis and Treatment & Chinese Medicine Development of Henan Province, Zhengzhou 450046, China
[3] Jiyang College of Zhejiang Agriculture and Forestry University, Zhu'ji 311800, China; fang_qiao418@163.com
[4] Zhejiang Chinese Medical University, Zhejiang, Hangzhou 310053, China; littlegy@163.com
* Correspondence: keyuan@zafu.edu.cn; Tel.: +86-0575-87760143

Academic Editors: Raffaele Capasso and Lorenzo Di Cesare Mannelli
Received: 28 February 2019; Accepted: 4 April 2019; Published: 12 April 2019

Abstract: *Rheum palmatum* L. is a traditional Chinese medicine with various pharmacological properties, including anti-inflammatory, antibacterial, and detoxification effects. In this study, the mechanism of the hypoglycemic effect of purified anthraquinone-Glycoside from *Rheum palmatum* L. (PAGR) in streptozotocin (STZ) and high-fat diet induced type 2 diabetes mellitus (T2DM) in rats was investigated. The rats were randomly divided into normal (NC), T2DM, metformin (Met), low, middle (Mid), and high (Hig) does of PAGR groups. After six weeks of continuous administration of PAGR, the serum indices and tissue protein expression were determined, and the pathological changes in liver, kidney, and pancreas tissues were observed. The results showed that compared with the type 2 diabetes mellitus group, the fasting blood glucose (FBG), total cholesterol (TC), and triglyceride (TG) levels in the serum of rats in the PAGR treatment groups were significantly decreased, while superoxide dismutase (SOD) and glutathione peroxidase (GSH-PX) levels were noticeably increased. The expression of Fas ligand (FasL), cytochrome C (Cyt-c), and caspase-3 in pancreatic tissue was obviously decreased, and the pathological damage to the liver, kidney, and pancreas was improved. These indicate that PAGR can reduce oxidative stress in rats with diabetes mellitus by improving blood lipid metabolism and enhancing their antioxidant capacity, thereby regulating the mitochondrial apoptotic pathway to inhibit β-cell apoptosis and improve β-cell function. Furthermore, it can regulate Fas/FasL-mediated apoptosis signaling pathway to inhibit β-cell apoptosis, thereby lowering blood glucose levels and improving T2DM.

Keywords: *Rheum palmatum* L.; type 2 diabetes mellitus; oxidative stress; apoptosis

1. Introduction

Diabetes mellitus is an endocrine and metabolic disease characterized by hyperglycemia, often accompanied by a series of complications, including neuropathy, nephropathy, retinopathy, and cardiovascular and cerebrovascular disease [1,2]. It is a global disease affecting over 300 million people and is the fourth cause of death and disability in the world [3]. Notably, 90% of patients are type 2 diabetes mellitus (T2DM). The metabolic disorder of T2DM is associated with insulin resistance, which is linked to genetic, environmental interactions, and lifestyle [4]. Insulin resistance and insulin secretion defect are the two most recognized causes of T2DM [5]. Insulin resistance is caused by a decrease in the efficiency of insulin-induced glucose uptake and utilization, and insulin secretion defects are caused by insufficient insulin secretion due to apoptosis or dysfunction of β-cells of the pancreatic islets, resulting in the insulin which cannot meet normal physiological needs [6]. β-cell can regulate systemic metabolism by secreting insulin, the body's only hormone lowering glucose [7]. Studies have shown that the mass of β-cell is lowered in the pancreas when there is an imbalance of regeneration and apoptosis [8]. There are many mechanisms inducing apoptosis of β-cells, including hyperglycemia, hyperlipidemia, oxidative stress, and activation of proinflammatory factors [9,10]. Therefore, protecting β-cells in the pancreas, inhibiting β-cell apoptosis, and increasing insulin secretion are important for T2DM patients [11].

Rheum palmatum L., a traditional Chinese medicine, has antibacterial, heat-clearing, and detoxifying properties, and has been used for the treatment of constipation and gastrointestinal diseases for more than 2000 years [12,13]. Although its chemical composition is relatively complex [14], it is known that anthraquinone, forming 3–5% of its content, is the most important activity component [15]. Modern pharmacological studies have shown that rhubarb-derived anthraquinones have a variety of physiological functions, such as antioxidant, antiviral, and anti-tumor properties, and protect cerebral cortex neurons [16–18]. In this paper, we studied the glucose-lowering effect of purified anthraquinone-Glycoside from *Rheum palmatum* L. (PAGR) in T2DM rats and explored the potential mechanism in the context of lipid metabolism, oxidative stress, and apoptosis.

2. Results

2.1. Anthraquinone-Glycosides Content of PAGR

The prepared working solution was analyzed three times under 4.3.1 chromatographic conditions of high-performance liquid chromatography (HPLC), and the contents of the three anthraquinone-Glycosides were determined (Figure 1). The concentrations of emodin-8-*O*-β-D-glucoside, aloe-emodin-8-*O*-β-D-glucoside, and chrysophanol-8-*O*-β-D-glucoside were calculated using the previously determined standard curve and determined to be 6.36%, 8.13%, and 6.78%, respectively, while the relative standard deviation (RSD) was 1.87%, 2.02%, and 1.58% respectively. The results showed that these three anthraquinone-Glycosides make up more than 20% of the total anthraquinone-Glycosides, and aloe-emodin-8-*O*-β-D-glucoside was the major anthraquinone-Glycoside among them.

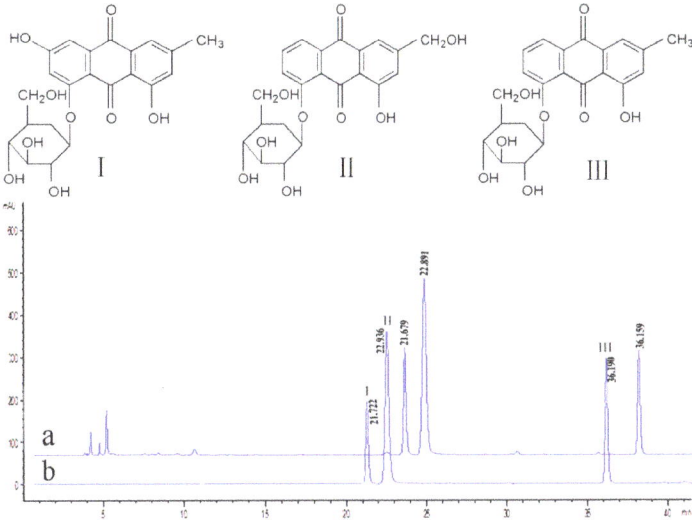

Figure 1. The structure of the emodin-8-*O*-β-D-glucoside (**I**), aloe-emodin-8-*O*-β-D-glucoside (**II**), and chrysophanol-8-*O*-β-D-glucoside (**III**) and HPLC chromatogram of purified anthraquinone-Glycoside from *Rheum palmatum* L. (PAGR) (**a**) and mixed Reference (**b**).

2.2. Acute Toxicity Study

The acute toxicity of PAGR was evaluated at a dose of 2000 mg/kg. There were no deaths or obvious symptoms of poisoning within the initial 24 h of close observation and no behavioral abnormalities over the following 14 days. Therefore, the doses of PAGR for the low, middle (Mid), and high (Hig) groups were selected as 100, 200, and 400 mg/kg, respectively.

2.3. Changes in Body Weight and Fasting Blood Glucose in Rats

Polydipsia, polyuria, polyphagia, weight loss, and hyperglycemia are the most typical symptoms of T2DM [19]. The changes in rats' body weight and fasting blood glucose (FBG) during the administration of streptozotocin (STZ) and PAGR are shown in Figure 2. The body weight of rats treated with STZ and a high-fat diet was obviously decreased, while FBG levels were markedly increased. After administration of metformin (Met) and PAGR, the body weight and FBG levels of rats began to recover. Notably, after six weeks of treatment, the body weight of the rats in the Met and PAGR treatment groups was significantly higher than that of the T2DM group ($p < 0.05$), and their FBG concentration was significantly lower than the T2DM group ($p < 0.05$). Furthermore, the Hig treatment group had returned to close to normal levels.

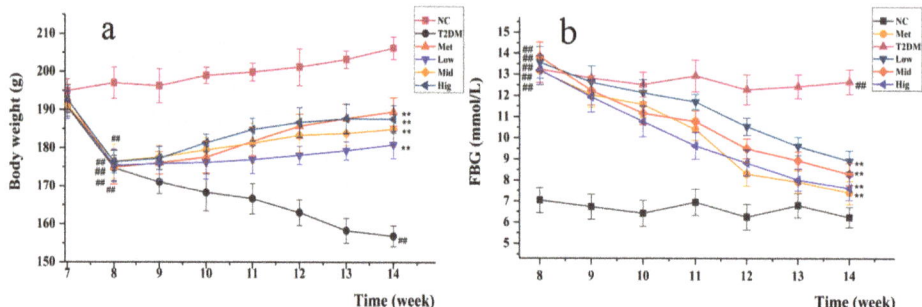

Figure 2. The changes in body weight (**a**) and fasting blood glucose (FBG) (**b**) of rats during the administration of Met and purified anthraquinone-Glycoside from *Rheum palmatum* L. (PAGR). NC, normal group; T2DM, type 2 diabetes mellitus; Met, metformin group; Low, low group (100 mg/kg); Mid, middle group (200 mg/kg); Hig, high group (400 mg/kg). The data were expressed as mean ± standard deviation (SD) ($n = 10$), $^{\#}$ $p < 0.05$ $^{\#\#}$ $p < 0.01$ vs.NC group; * $p < 0.05$ ** $p < 0.01$ vs. T2DM group.

2.4. Effect of PAGR on Lipid Metabolites and Antioxidant Enzyme Activities in Rats

The effect of PAGR on triglyceride (TG) and total cholesterol (TC) is shown in Figure 3a,b. Compared with the normal (NC) group, the TC and TG of the T2DM group were significantly increased ($p < 0.01$). However, compared with the T2DM group, the TC and TG of the Met and PAGR treatment groups were significantly decreased in a dose-dependent manner. The specific dates were shown in Table S.

By measuring the concentration of superoxide dismutase (SOD) and glutathione peroxidase (GSH-PX) in the serum of rats, it was found that the SOD and GSH-PX levels in the T2DM group were significantly decreased when compared with the NC group ($p < 0.05$), while those in the Met and PAGR treatment groups were markedly increased when compared with the T2DM group, with significant differences between the Met and PAGR Hig groups ($p < 0.05$) (Figure 3c,d).

In the course of the development of T2DM, the renal tissue is damaged, and its functions were altered due to long-term of dysglycemia [20]. It is shown as Figure 3e,f that the serum creatinine and blood urea nitrogen (BUN) in the T2DM group were significantly increased compared with the NC group ($p < 0.01$), while the serum creatinine and BUN in the Met and PAGR treatment groups were significantly decreased when compared with T2DM group, indicating that PAGR has a protective effect on the kidney.

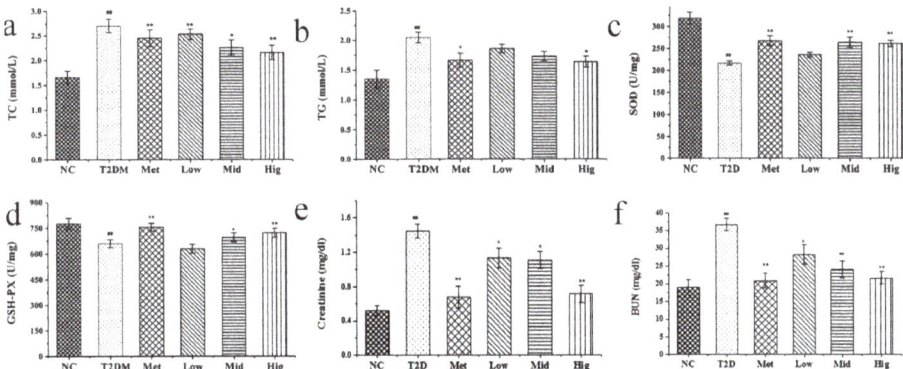

Figure 3. Effects of purified anthraquinone-Glycoside from *Rheum palmatum* L. (PAGR) on total cholesterol (TC) (**a**), triglyceride (TG) (**b**), superoxide dismutase (SOD) (**c**), glutathione peroxidase (GSH-PX) (**d**), creatinine (**e**), and BUN (**f**) in serum of rats. NC, normal group; T2DM, type 2 diabetes mellitus; Met, metformin group; Low, low group (100 mg/kg); Mid, middle group (200 mg/kg); Hig, high group (400 mg/kg). The data were expressed as mean ± SD ($n = 10$), [#] $p < 0.05$, [##] $p < 0.01$ vs. NC group. * $p < 0.05$, ** $p < 0.01$ vs. T2DM group.

2.5. The Effect of PAGR on Histopathological Changes

2.5.1. Effects of PAGR on Histopathological Changes in Liver

Hyperglycemia not only affects the transduction of apoptotic signals in islet cells but also damages tissues and organs [21]. As one of the major metabolic organs, the liver is the main organ damaged by diabetes. Steatosis, inflammatory cell infiltration, and necrosis are the main characteristics of hyperglycemia-induced liver injury [22]. As evident in Figure 4, the structure of liver tissue of rats in the NC group is intact, and the hepatocytes are arranged radially around the central vein. In contrast, compared with the NC group, the number of hepatocytes in the T2DM group is reduced, the hepatic cord is disordered, and hepatocytes show obvious degeneration and necrosis. The hepatocytes surrounding the central vein are filled with lipid droplets, and the infiltration of inflammatory cells is also evident. Notably, these histopathological changes in the livers of the Met and PAGR treatment groups were improved to varying degrees when compared with the T2DM group.

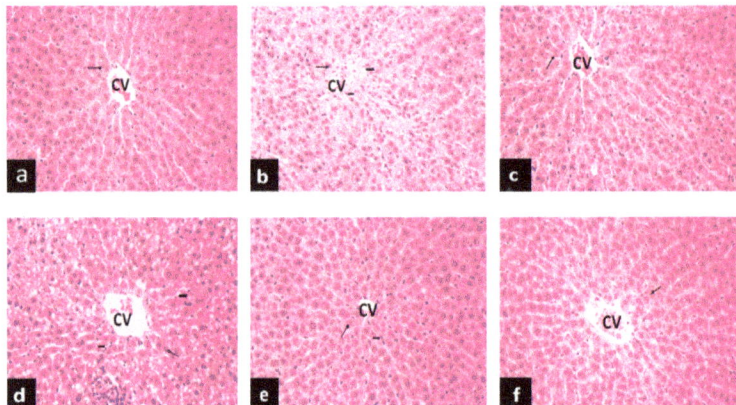

Figure 4. The effects of purified anthraquinone-Glycoside from *Rheum palmatum* L. (PAGR) on histopathological changes in the liver of rats. Histological observation, H&E, a–f×200; (**a**), normal (NC) group; (**b**), type 2 diabetes mellitus (T2DM) group; (**c**), metformin (Met) group; (**d**), Low group; (**e**), middle (Mid) group; (**f**), high (Hig) group; CV, central veins; →, hepatocyte; ➡, inflammatory cell; ➡, lipid droplet.

2.5.2. Effects of PAGR on Histopathological Changes in Kidney

Reduction of SOD and GSH-PX levels and an increase of lipid peroxide and free radicals in vivo can all increase the expression of transforming growth factor (TGF)-β1 [23]. TGF-β1 can inhibit cell proliferation, promote renal cell hypertrophy, and lead to glomerulosclerosis and tubule interstitial fibrosis [24]. It can be seen in Figure 5 that the renal tissue structure was distinct and clear and the glomerular structure was normal in the NC group. In contrast, the glomerular volume of the model group was enlarged, and the basement membrane was thickened when compared with the NC group. However, compared with the T2DM group, the glomerular volume of the Met and PAGR treatment groups was smaller, the mesangial matrix had slight hyperplasia, and the histopathological changes were obviously improved.

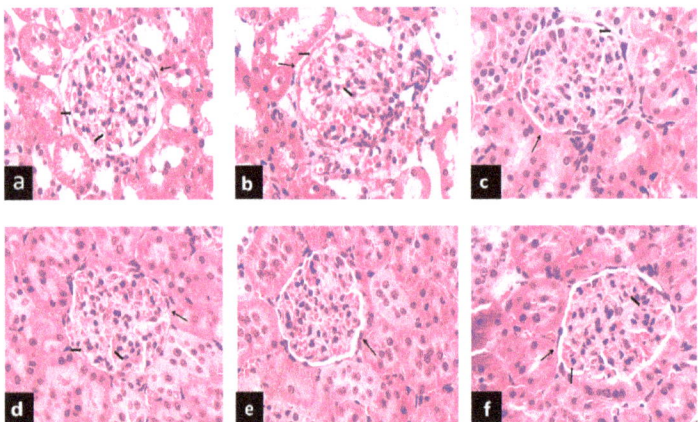

Figure 5. Effects of purified anthraquinone-Glycoside from *Rheum palmatum* L. (PAGR) on histopathological changes in the kidney of rats. Histological observation, H&E, a-f×400; (**a**), normal (NC) group; (**b**), type 2 diabetes mellitus (T2DM) group; (**c**), metformin (Met) group; (**d**), Low group; (**e**), middle (Mid) group; (**f**), high (Hig) group; →, glomerulus; ➡, base membrane; ➡, mesangial.

2.5.3. Effects of PAGR on Histopathological Changes in Pancreas

In addition to persistent hyperglycemia, patients with type 2 diabetes often have accompanying hyperlipidemia, and long-term exposure to high concentrations of glucose or lipids not only causes functional disorders of islet cells but also disrupts the islet structure [25]. It can be seen in Figure 6 that NC group rats showed normal histology. The islet shape was regular. Islet cells formed clumps and were distributed among the pancreas exocrine glands. Compared with the NC group, the islet structure in the T2DM group showed obvious deformation, fewer islet cells, blurred boundaries, and the structure was unclear. Compared with the T2DM group, the histopathological changes present in the islet tissue of the Met and PAGR treatment groups were attenuated to some degree.

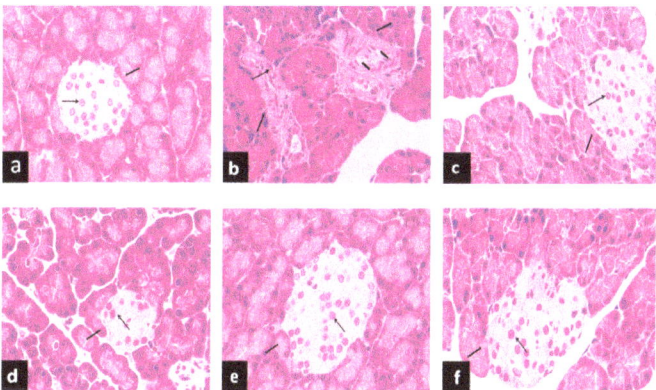

Figure 6. Effects of purified anthraquinone-Glycoside from *Rheum palmatum* L. (PAGR) on histopathological changes in the pancreas of rats. Histological observation, H&E, a–f×400; (**a**), normal (NC) group; (**b**), type 2 diabetes mellitus (T2DM) group; (**c**), metformin (Met) group; (**d**), Low group; (**e**), middle (Mid) group; (**f**), high (Hig) group; ➡, islet; ➡, islet cell; ➡, lipid droplet.

2.6. *Effect of PAGR on the Expression of Cytochrome C (Cyt-c), Caspase-3, and FasL in Pancreas*

As shown in Figure 7, the expression of FasL, Cyt-c, and caspase-3 in pancreatic tissue of rats after administration of PAGR and metformin was significantly reduced compared with the T2DM group.

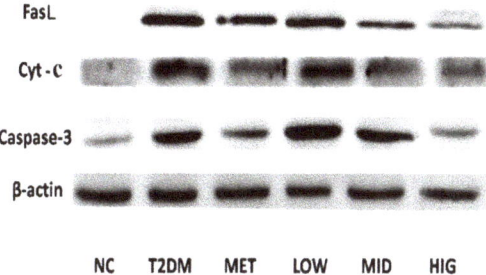

Figure 7. The effect of purified anthraquinone-Glycoside from *Rheum palmatum* L. (PAGR) on the protein expression of Fas ligand (FasL), cytochrome C (Cyt-c), and Caspase-3 in pancreatic tissue. NC, normal group; T2DM, type 2 diabetes mellitus; Met, metformin group; Low, low group (100 mg/kg); Mid, middle group (200 mg/kg); Hig, high group (400 mg/kg).

3. Discussions

STZ is the most commonly used hydrophilic compound for inducing T2DM. It can be transported into the cell membrane through the glutamine transaminase transporter to induce DNA alkylation. DNA alkylation can induce β-cell death [26], which consequently leads to hyperglycemia. Moreover, a high-fat diet plays an important role in insulin resistance [27]. The gradual natural progression and changes in the metabolism of human patients with T2DM are well mimicked by a high-fat diet and low-dose STZ in rats [28].

There is an inseparable relationship between glucose metabolism and lipid metabolism. Hyperglycemia can lead to dyslipidemia, while abnormal lipid metabolism is considered a major risk factor for diabetes and its multiple complications [29]. Lipid metabolites, such as TG and TC, directly antagonize insulin signaling and are considered the main cause of insulin resistance [30]. When TG remains high, heparin activates lipoprotein lipase, increasing intravascular lipolysis of TG, thereby increasing the exposure of tissues to free fatty acids, leading to insulin resistance and impairing β-cell function [31]. TC is the sum of cholesterol contained in all lipoproteins in the blood and is closely related to various diabetic complications, including cardio-cerebral vascular disease and neuropathy [32]. Therefore, improving lipid metabolism may ameliorate diabetes and its complications [33].

Hyperglycemia can also induce oxidative stress and lipid peroxidation. Importantly, oxidative stress can regulate insulin secretion in different ways and accelerate the development of diabetes mellitus [34]. For example, increased oxidative stress may have a negative effect on the regulation of blood glucose and cause dysfunction or apoptosis of glucose-regulating cells, such as β-cells, by stimulating the stress-responsive pathway for regulation [35]. Oxidative stress stimulates mitogen-activated protein kinase (MAPK) stress signals and causes inhibition of insulin signaling [36]. In addition, oxidative stress can promote the expression of many proinflammatory factors, including tumor necrosis factor (TNF)-α and interleukin (IL)-6, and significantly decrease insulin sensitivity [37]. Furthermore, studies have shown that there is a direct interaction between oxidative stress and insulin resistance, and the accumulation of oxidation products may damage critical macromolecules in insulin-sensitive tissues [38]. Therefore, from the perspective of treatment, reducing oxidative stress in the body may ameliorate diabetes. SOD and GSH-PX are two important enzymes in the antioxidant system, which can reflect the body's antioxidant capacity. It was found in our study that PAGR could improve glucose and lipid metabolism in diabetic rats and reduce oxidative stress. Therefore, it may act by improving the function of insulin secreting β cells.

Under normal physiological conditions, the number of β-cells in the pancreas is in a dynamic equilibrium due to the regulation of apoptosis, proliferation of pancreatic islet, and production of new insulin by secretory tube. However, diabetes can develop when β-cell apoptosis occurs in excess [29]. There are two main pathways of apoptosis, the intrinsic (mitochondrial driven) pathway and the extrinsic (receptor-mediated) pathway [39]. Both oxidative stress and abnormal lipid metabolism promote the production of reactive oxygen species (ROS) and reactive nitrogen species (RNS). ROS and RNS can change the membrane potential of mitochondria, leading to the release of Cyt-c [40]. The release of Cyt-c activates caspase-3 [41], which is the final effector caspase in the caspase cascade and is the common downstream effector of multiple apoptotic pathways [42]. Caspase-3 induces apoptosis and thereby drives the death of β-cells resulting in insufficient insulin secretion. Correspondingly, the process of apoptosis is accompanied by a change in mitochondrial function and structure, which will also lead to the leakage of Cyt-c. As a marker of mitochondrial damage, Cyt-c levels can reflect the degree of mitochondrial structural damage [43]. Mitochondria act as energy transducers for cells, and their destruction can result in the abnormal function of islet β-cells, as shown in Figure 8. The expression of Cyt-c and caspase-3 corresponded with the increased levels of SOD and GSH-PX in the serum. PAGR can improve the antioxidant capacity of rats with diabetes and thus reduce the level of oxidative stress, regulating the mitochondrial-induced apoptosis pathway and reducing the damage to the mitochondrial structure, thereby protecting the pancreatic β-cells from apoptosis and restoring the function of β-cells.

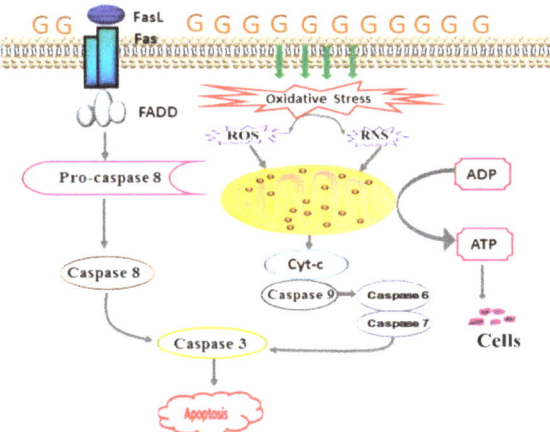

Figure 8. The signaling pathway of apoptosis. Hyperglycemia leads to the production of reactive oxygen species (ROS) and reactive nitrogen species (RNS) which change the membrane potential of mitochondria, leading to the release of cytochrome C (Cyt-c). It also leads to the expression of Fas ligand (FasL) and Fas, and they combine to form the Fas-associated death domain protein (FADD). The Cyt-c and FADD all activate caspase cascade reaction, leading to apoptosis.

High concentration of glucose also promotes the expression of Fas and FasL in pancreatic tissue [44]. FasL is an important ligand for inducing cell death and is a signaling factor of the extrinsic apoptosis pathway [45]. When it binds to Fas, which is the death receptor, it induces the assembly of a series of proteins that induce the death signaling complex in seconds. These proteins then activate procaspase-8, leading to activation of the caspase cascade, which finally induces the activation of caspase-3 [46]. When the caspase cascade is activated, it induces apoptosis swiftly [47], resulting in decreased islet β-cells, which is the basis for the decline of insulin secretion. The results of western blotting suggested that PAGR could inhibit apoptosis of β-cells and improve insulin secretion by regulating the Fas/FasL-mediated apoptotic signal pathway.

4. Material and Methods

4.1. Drugs and Chemicals

Rheum palmatum L. medicinal materials were purchased from Zhejiang University of Traditional Chinese Medicine Chinese Herbal Pieces Co., Ltd. (Zhejiang, China) and identified by the Professor Jiawei Huang who is from Zhejiang Chinese Medical University. STZ was purchased from Aladdin Bio-reagent (Shanghai, China). Glucose, Superoxide dismutase, Glutathione peroxidase, Triglyceride, Total cholesterol, Serum creatinine, Blood urea nitrogen Kits were purchased from Nanjing Jiancheng Biotechnology Co., LTD (Nanjing, China). The BCA Kit was purchased from Aidlab Biotechnologies Co., LTD (Beijing, China). The antibodies specific to FasL, Cyt-c, caspase-3 were purchased from Xinbosheng Technology Co., LTD (Shanghai, China). Emodin-8-O-β-D-glucoside, aloe-emodin-8-O-β-D-glucoside, chrysophanol-8-O-β-D-glucoside substances were prepared in the laboratory, the structure was identified by ^{1}H NMR, ^{13}C-NMR, and MS, and the purity was over 98% calibrated by HPLC peak area normalization method. All other reagents used were also chromatographically or analytically pure.

4.2. The Preparation and Determination of PAGR

Ten kg roots of *Rheum palmatum*. L. medicinal material was weighed and crushed and passed through a 60-mesh sieve. Then, it was extracted by reflux extraction three times for 1.5 h each, with a 1:7 ratio of plant material to 80% ethanol, followed by extraction filtration. The filtrate was combined and concentrated under reduced pressure at 60 °C bya rotary evaporator (RV3V, Staufen, Germany) until no alcohol could be smelled, and the appropriate amount of water was added for ultrasonic dissolution. A concentrate of 6000 mL was obtained. The concentrate was extracted three times with petroleum ether, ethyl acetate, and n-butanol at a volume ratio of 2 times, and the extraction liquid was combined. Then, it was concentrated under vacuum pressure to obtain the dry powder from each extracted fraction, in which the petroleum ether fraction was 158.4g, the ethyl acetate fraction was 212.7 g, the n-butanol fraction was 343.6 g, and the water was 425.9 g. The dry powder from the n-butanol fraction was dispersed in water by ultrasound and enriched and purified using a macroporous resin column (Diaion HP-20, Tokyo, Japan). First, it was eluted with distilled water, followed by 10%, 20%, 40%, and 60% methanol. Each eluted fraction was collected and concentrated under reduced pressure to dryness to obtain dry powder from each elution fraction. The total anthraquinone-Glycoside content in each elution fraction was determined by ultraviolet absorption spectrometry (UV-1801, Beijing, China) with emodin-8-O-β-D-glucoside as the standard substance, and the content was 4.63%, 8.84%, 21.91%, and 6.32%, respectively, determined by ultraviolet and visible spectrophotometer (UV-1801, Beijing, China). The anthraquinone-Glycoside was mainly concentrated in the 40% methanol elution fraction. Therefore, it was selected as the active fraction for the following experiments and is henceforth referred to as PAGR.

4.3. Determination of Three Anthraquinone-Glycosides in PAGR by HPLC

4.3.1. HPLC Chromatographic Conditions

Agilent 1200 (Santa Clara, CA, USA) High-Performance Liquid Chromatography consists of a quaternary pump, autosampler, column oven, and VWD detector. Column: Agilent Extend-C18 (4.6 mm × 250 mm, 5 μm). The column temperature was 30 °C, flow rate 1.0 mL/min, detection wavelength 280 nm. Mobile phase acetonitrile was 0.1% formic acid (A) and acetonitrile (B), 0–10 min, A: 90%, B: 10%, 10–25 min, A: 88%, B: 12%, 25–30 min, A: 78%, B: 22%, 30–40 min, A: 67%, B: 33%, and the injection volume was 5 μL.

4.3.2. Preparation of Working Solution and Standard Curve

A certain amount of PAGR was accurately weighed, dissolved by ultrasound, and a working solution was prepared in methanol at constant volume. Certain amounts of emodin-8-O-β-D-glucoside, aloe-emodin-8-O-β-D-glucoside, and chrysophanol-8-O-β-D-glucoside were dissolved in methanol to form a mixed reference solution, which was then diluted with methanol to prepare mixed standard solutions with concentrations of 0.5200, 0.2600, 0.1300, 0.0625, 0.0163, 0.0081, 0.0040, and 0.0020 mg/mL respectively. The peak area of the different concentrations of the mixed standard solution was determined by HPLC, and the standard curve was prepared with the peak area as the ordinate and the mixed standard solution concentration as the abscissa. It was determined that the regression equation of emodin-8-O-β-D-glucoside was y = 14932x + 1.496, R^2 = 0.999, aloe-emodin-8-O-β-D-glucoside was y = 96120x + 1.555, R^2 = 0.999, and chrysophanol-8-O-β-D-glucoside was y = 26804x − 1.231, R^2 = 0.999, indicating that the three anthraquinone-Glycosides had a good linear relationship in the concentration range of 0.0020–0.5200 mg/mL.

4.3.3. Stability and Precision

A certain concentration of the mixed reference solution was injected six times within a day according to the chromatographic conditions to determine the peak area. The RSD of the peak areas of emodin-8-O-β-D-glucoside, aloe-emodin-8-O-β-D-glucoside, and chrysophanol-8-O-β-D-glucoside was1.18%, 1.52%, and 2.06%, respectively, which indicated that the precision of the instrument was good. The reference solution was placed at room temperature and analyzed at 2, 4, 6, 8, and 10 h according to the chromatographic conditions, and the RSD of the peak area of emodin-8-O-β-D-glucoside, aloe-emodin-8-O-β-D-glucoside, and chrysophanol-8-O-β-D-glucoside was 2.30%, 1.26%, and 1.20%, respectively, indicating that the sample was stable within 10 h.

4.4. Acute Toxicity Test

A single dose of 2000 mg/kg of PAGR was intragastrically administered in rats. The death and poisoning symptoms of the rats were observed closely within the first 24 h after administration, and their behavior was monitored routinely over the next 14 days to evaluate the acute toxicity of PAGR.

4.5. AnimalsTreatment and Sample Collection

Male Sprague-Dawley (SD) rats (150 ± 10 g) were purchased from the Experimental Animal Center of Zhejiang Academy of Medical Sciences (SCXK, 2015-0033, Zhejiang, China). All experimental animals were housed in a standard animal room at a temperature of 23 °C ± 1 °C and humidity of 50–60%. Rats were adapted to the environment for one week before the experiment and were then randomly divided into six groups (n = 10): NC group, T2DM group, Met treated group, and Low, Mid, and Hig dose groups of PAGR treated. Except for the NC group, the rats in the other groups were fed with a high-fat diet (corn starch 60%, casein 20%, soybean oil 20%) [48] for 6 weeks and then injected intraperitoneally with STZ (30 mg/kg) two times every other day. FBG was measured after 72 h of the last injection and was >11.1 mol/L, indicating that the diabetes model was successful. Next, the NC and T2DM groups were intragastrically administered with normal saline, Met group was administered with 100 mg/kg metformin [49], and the Low, Mid, and Hig groups were treated with 100, 200, and 400 mg/kg of PAGR for 6 weeks. They all were injected once a day. Blood samples were drawn from the orbit to measure FBG every week. After fasting for 12 h after the last administration of PAGR, rats were anesthetized with 10% chloral hydrate, the blood was taken from the abdominal aorta, and the liver, kidneys, and pancreas were removed quickly and stored at -80°Cfor further study. All experimental procedures were in accordance with the Guide for the Care and Use of Laboratory Animals of Zhejiang and were approved by the Committee on the Ethics of Animal Experiments at Animal Center of Zhejiang Agriculture and Forestry University [Ethics Certificate No. 2014001812184].

4.6. Biochemical Measurements

The SOD, GSH-PX, TG, and TC of serum were measured by Superoxide dismutase, Glutathione peroxidase, Triglyceride, and Total cholesterol Kits of Nanjing Jiancheng, respectively, according to the commercial instruction.

4.7. Histopathological Examinations

The liver, pancreas, and kidneys were fixed in 10% formalin solution for 24 h and then paraffin-embedded. Paraffin sections of 5–7 μm thickness were carved up and stained with hematoxylin and eosin (H&E), and histopathological changes were observed under a BX20 optical microscope (Tokyo, Japan).

4.8. Western Blot Analysis

The pancreatic sample was lysed using RIPA lysis buffer on ice and centrifuged at 10,001× g (4 °C, 10min). The protein concentration of the supernatants was determined by the BCA Kit. For western blot analysis, the protein was separated by sodium dodecyl sulfate polypropylene gel electrophoresis (SDS-PAGE) and then electrotransferred to polyvinylidene difluoride (PVDF) membranes. All membranes were incubated with 50 g/L non-fat milk powder in triethanolamine buffer for 1 h at room temperature and then with primary antibodies against FasL, Cyt-c, caspase-3 (diluted 1:1000), and β-actin (diluted 1:1500) at 4 °C overnight. The following day membranes were washed with tris-buffered saline containing Tween-20 (TBST), then incubated with peroxidase-conjugated anti-rabbit secondary antibody for 1 h at room temperature. After washing with TBST three times, ECL reagent was added, and images were captured using a chemiluminescence detection system (Amersham Pharmacia, Piscataway, NJ, USA).

4.9. Statistical Analysis

All data were expressed as mean ± SD and analyzed by the SPSS statistical software (SPSS19.0 Inc., Chicago, IL, USA). One-way ANOVA with Duncan's test was used for inter-group comparison. *p*-values < 0.05 were considered statistically significant, and *p*-values < 0.01 were considered extremely significant.

5. Conclusion

In conclusion, PAGR has glucose-lowering properties and attenuates type 2 diabetes. The potential mechanism is that PAGR reduces the level of oxidative stress by improving lipid metabolism and enhancing antioxidant capacity, which reduces damage to mitochondrial structures and downregulates activation of mitochondrial-induced cell death pathways; thereby inhibiting β-cell apoptosis and improving β-cell function. It also downregulates Fas/FasL-mediated apoptosis in pancreatic tissue, further inhibiting apoptosis of β-cells.

Supplementary Materials: The following are available online, Table S: Data of Serum indicators (FBG, TC, TG, SOD, GSH-PX, creatinine and BUN) and body weight of rats.

Author Contributions: F.-R.C. and K.Y. conceived and designed the experiments, H.-X.C., J.-L.F. and Y.G. performed the experiments, F.-R.C. and H.-X.C. analyzed the data, J.-L.F. and K.Y. wrote the paper.

Funding: This project was supported by the Zhejiang Provincial Science Foundation of China (Grant No: LY16H280007).

Conflicts of Interest: The authors have no conflicts of interest to declare. All of the authors have approved the final article.

Data availability: The data used to support the findings of this study are included in the article.

Abbreviations

PAGR	purified anthraquinone-Glycoside from *Rheum palmatum* L.
STZ	streptozotocin
T2DM	type 2 diabetes mellitus
NC	normal
Met	metformin
Mid	medium
Hig	high
FBG	fasting blood glucose
TC	total cholesterol
TG	triglyceride
SOD	superoxide dismutase
GSH-PX	glutathione peroxidase
Cyt-c	cytochrome C
HPLC	High-Performance Liquid Chromatography
BUN	blood urea nitrogen
H&E	hematoxylin and eosin
SD	standard deviation
ROS	reactive oxygen species
RNS	reactive nitrogen species
MAPK	mitogen-activated protein kinase
SDS-PAGE	sodium dodecyl sulfate polypropylene gel electrophoresis
PVDF	polyvinylidene difluoride

References

1. Sharma, A.K.; Bharti, S.; Goyal, S.; Arora, S.; Nepal, S.; Kishore, K. Upregulation of PPARγ by Aegle marmelos Ameliorates Insulin Resistance and β-cell Dysfunction in High Fat Diet Fed-Streptozotocin Induced Type 2 Diabetic Rats. *Phytother. Res.* **2011**, *25*, 1457–1465. [CrossRef]
2. Orchard, T.J.; Olson, J.C.; Erbey, J.R.; Williams, K.; Forrest, K.Y. Insulin resistance-related factors, but not glycemia, predict coronary artery disease in type 1 diabetes: 10-year follow-up data from the Pittsburgh Epidemiology of Diabetes Complications Study. *Diabetes Care* **2003**, *26*, 1374–1379. [CrossRef]
3. Nishihama, K.; Yasuma, T.; Yano, Y.D.; Alessandro-Gabazza, C.N.; Toda, M.; Hinneh, J.A.; Baffour, T.P. Anti-apoptotic activity of human matrix metalloproteinase-2 at tenuates diabetes mellitus. *Metabolism* **2018**, *82*, 88–99. [CrossRef]
4. Manisha, J.O.; Yogesh, A.K. Biochanin A improves insulin sensitivity and controls hyperglycemia in type 2 diabetes. *Biomed. Pharmacother.* **2018**, *107*, 1119–1127.
5. Wing, R.R.; Rosen, R.C.; Fava, J.L.; Bahnson, J.; Brancati, F.; Gendrano, I.N.C.; Kitabchi, A.; Schneider, S.H.; Wadden, T.A. Effects of Weight Loss Intervention on Erectile Function in Older Men with Type 2 Diabetes in the Look AHEAD Trial. *J. Sex Med.* **2010**, *7*, 156–165.
6. Olson, J.C.; Erbey, J.R.; Forrest, K.Y.; Williams, K.; Becker, D.J. Glycemia (or, in women, estimated glucose disposal rate) predict lower extremity arterial disease events in type 1 diabetes. *Metabolism* **2002**, *51*, 248–254. [CrossRef]
7. Jakob, G.K.; Patrik, R. β-Cell Dysfunction in Type 2 Diabetes: Draned of Energy? *Cell Metabol.* **2019**, *29*, 1–2.
8. Tania, G.D.; Manuel, S.P.; Fernando, V.A.; Ángel, A.V.; Olga, D.L.; Eduardo, L.G.; Aurora, M.R. Apoptosis in pancreatic β-cells is induced by arsenic and atorvastatin in Wistar rats with diabetes mellitus type 2. *J. Trace Elem. Med. Biol.* **2018**, *46*, 146–199.
9. Tatsuo, T. Apoptosis in pancreaticβ-islet cells in Type 2 diabetes. *Bosanian J. Basic Med.* **2016**, *16*, 162–179.
10. Diana, C.; Minna, W. Executioners of apoptosis in pancreatic β-cells: Not just for cell death. *Am. J. Physiol. Endocrinol. Metab.* **2010**, *298*, 735–741.
11. Guariguata, L. Contribute data to the 6th edition of the IDF Diabetes Atlas. *Diabetes Res. Cli. PR.* **2013**, *100*, 280–281. [CrossRef]
12. Wang, Z.; Ma, P.; Xu, L.; He, C.; Peng, N.; Xiao, P. Evaluation of the content variation of anthraquinone glycosidesin rhubarb by UPLC-PDA. *Chem. Cent. J.* **2012**, *7*, 153–160.
13. Cirillo, C.; Capasso, R. Constipation and Botanical Medicines: An Overview. *Phytother. Res.* **2015**, *29*, 1488–1493. [CrossRef]
14. Ullah, H.; Kim, J.; Rehman, N.U.; Kim, H.J.; Ahn, M.J.; Chung, H.J. A Simple and Sensitive Liquid Chromatography with Tandem Mass Spectrometric Method for the Simultaneous Determination of Anthraquinone Glycosides and Their Aglycones in Rat Plasma: Application to a Pharmacokinetic Study of Rumex acetosa Extract. *Pharmaceutics* **2018**, *10*, 100. [CrossRef]
15. Wang, J.; Zhao, H.; Kong, W.; Jin, C.; Zhao, Y.; Qu, Y. Microcalorimetric assay on the antimicrobial property of five hydroxyanthraquinone derivatives in rhubarb (*Rheum palmatum* L.) to Bifidobacterium adolescentis. *Phytomedicine* **2010**, *7*, 684–689.
16. Agarwal, S.K.; Singh, S.S.; Verma, S.; Kumar, S. Antifungal activity of anthraquinone derivatives from Rheum emodi. *J. Ethnopharmacol.* **2000**, *72*, 43–46. [CrossRef]
17. Iizuka, A.; Iijima, O.T.; Kondo, K.; Itakura, H.; Yoshie, F.; Miyamoto, H. Evaluation of rhubarb using antioxidative activity as an index of pharmacological usefulness. *J. Ethnopharmacolo.* **2004**, *91*, 89–94. [CrossRef]
18. Liu, Y.F.; Yan, F.F.; Liu, Y.; Zhang, C.; Yu, H.M.; Zhang, Y. Aqueous extract of rhubarb stabilizes vulnerable atherosclerotic plaques due to depression of inflammation and lipid accumulation. *Phytother. Res.* **2008**, *22*, 935–942. [CrossRef]
19. Latcha, S.; Lubetzky, M.; Weinstein, A.M. Severe hyperosmolarity and hypernatremia in an adipsic young woman. *Clin. Nephrol.* **2011**, *76*, 407–411. [CrossRef]
20. Sharma, A.K.; Kanawat, D.S.; Mishr, A.; Dhakad, P.K.; Sharma, P.; Srivastava, V.; Joshi, S.; Joshi, M.; Raikwar, S.K.; Kurmi, M.K.; et al. Dual therapy of vildagliptin and telmisartan on diabetic nephropathy in experimentally induced type 2 diabetes mellitus rats. *J. Renin Angiotensin Aldosterone Syst.* **2013**, *15*, 410–418.

21. Li, J.P.; Yuan, Y.; Zhang, W.Y.; Jiang, Z.; Hu, T.J.; Feng, Y.T. Effect of Radix isatidis polysaccharide on alleviating insulin resistance in type 2 diabetes mellitus cells and rats. *J. Pharm. Pharmacol.* **2018**, *71*, 220–229. [CrossRef]
22. Tziomalos, K.; Athyros, V.G.; Karagiannis, A. Non-alcoholic fatty liver disease in type 2 diabetes: Pathogenesis and treatment options. *Curr. Vasc. Pharmacol.* **2012**, *10*, 162–172. [CrossRef]
23. Petersen, K.F.; Shulman, G.I. New insights into the pathogenesis of insulin resistance in humans using magnetic resonance spectroscopy. *Obesity (Silver Spring)* **2006**, *14* (Suppl. 1), 34S–40S.
24. Rerolle, J.P.; Hertig, A.; Nguyen, G.; SraerEric, J.D.; Rondeau, E.P. Plasminogen activator inhibitor type 1 is a potential target in renal fibrogenesis. *Kidney Int.* **2000**, *58*, 1841–1850. [CrossRef]
25. Graus, N.F.; Marinho, T.S.; Barbosa, S.S.; Aguila, M.B.; Mandarim, L.; Souza, M.V. Differential effects of angiotensin receptor blockers on pancreatic islet remodelling and glucose homeostasis in diet-induced obese mice. *Mol. Cell Endocrinol.* **2017**, *439*, 54–64.
26. Radenković, M.; Stojanović, M.; Prostran, M. Experimental diabetes induced by alloxan and streptozotocin: The current state of the art. *J. Pharm. Toxicolo. Methods.* **2016**, *78*, 13–31.
27. Zhu, C.F.; Peng, H.B.; Liu, G.Q.; Zhang, F.; Li, Y. Beneficial effects of oligopeptides from marine salmon skin in a rat model of type 2 diabetes. *Nutrition* **2010**, *26*, 1014–1020. [CrossRef]
28. Srinivasan, K.; Viswanad, B.; Lydiasrat, C.L.; Kaul, P.R. Combination of high-fat diet-fed and low-dose streptozotocin-treated rat: A model for type 2 diabetes and pharmacological screening. *Pharmacol. Res.* **2005**, *52*, 313–320. [CrossRef]
29. Pazdro, R.; Burgess, J.R. The role of vitamin E and oxidative stress in diabetes complications. *Mech. Ageing Dev.* **2017**, *131*, 276–286. [CrossRef]
30. Glass, C.K.; Olefsky, J.M. Inflammation and lipid signaling in the etiology of insulin resistance. *Cell Metab.* **2012**, *15*, 635–645. [CrossRef]
31. Unger, R.H.; Zhou, Y.T. Lipotoxicity of beta-cells in obesity and in other causes of fatty acid spillover. *Diabetes* **2001**, *50*, S118–S121. [CrossRef]
32. Khavandi, M.; Duarte, F.; Ginsberg, H.N.; Reyes, S.G. Treatment of Dyslipidemias to Prevent Cardiovascular Disease in Patients with Type 2 Diabetes. *Curr. Cardiol. Rep.* **2017**, *19*, 7–16. [CrossRef]
33. Ming, Z.; Zhou, J.M.; Liu, Y.; Sun, X.Z.; Luo, X.P.; Han, C.Y. Risk of type 2 diabetes mellitus associated with plasma lipid levels: The rural Chinese cohort study. *Diabetes Res. Clin. Pract.* **2018**, *35*, 150–157.
34. Styskal, J.; Van, R.H.; Richardson, A.; Salmon, A.B. Oxidative stress and diabetes: What can we learn about insulin resistance from antioxidant mutant mouse models? *Free Radic. Biol. Med.* **2012**, *52*, 46–58. [CrossRef]
35. Bravi, M.C.; Armiento, A.; Laurenti, O.; Cassone, F.M.; De, L.O. Insulin decreases intracellular oxidative stress in patients with type 2 diabetes mellitus. *Metabolism* **2006**, *55*, 691–695. [CrossRef]
36. Kamata, H.; Honda, S.; Maeda, S.; Chang, L.; Hirata, H. Reactive oxygen species promote TNF alpha-induced death and sustained JNK activation by inhibiting MAP kinase phosphatases. *Cell* **2005**, *120*, 649–661. [CrossRef]
37. Lumeng, C.N.; Bodzin, J.L.; Saltiel, A.R. Obesity induces a phenotypic switch in adipose tissue macrophage polarization. *J. Clin. Invest.* **2007**, *117*, 175–184. [CrossRef]
38. Grimsrud, P.A.; Xie, H.; Griffin, T.J.; Bernlohr, D.A. Oxidative stress and covalent modification of protein with bioactive aldehydes. *J. Biol. Chem.* **2008**, *283*, 21837–21841. [CrossRef]
39. Emamaullee, J.A.; Shapiro, A.M. Interventional strategies to prevent beta-cell apoptosis in islet transplantation. *Diabetes* **2006**, *55*, 1907–1914. [CrossRef]
40. Yang, R.Y.; Zhang, Z.F.; Pei, X.R.; Han, X.L.; Wang, J.B.; Wang, L.L. Immunomodulatory effects of marine oligopeptide preparation from Chum Salmon (Oncorhynchus keta) in mice. *Food Chem.* **2009**, *113*, 464–470. [CrossRef]
41. Zhang, T.; Chi, Y.Q.; Kang, Y.L.; Lu, H.; Niu, H.G.; Liu, W. Resveratrol ameliorates podocyte damage in diabetic mice via SIRT1/PGC-1α mediated attenuation of mitochondrial oxidative stress. *J. Cell Physiol.* **2018**, *28*, 1–11. [CrossRef]
42. Mohamad, N.; Buang, F.; Lazim, A.M.; Ahmad, N.; Martin, C.; Mohd Amin, M.C.I. Characterization and biocompatibility evaluation of bacterial cellulose-based wound dressing hydrogel: Effect of electron beam irradiation doses and concentration of acrylic acid. *J. Biomed. Mater. Res. B Appl. Biomater.* **2017**, *105*, 2553–2564.
43. Routray, I.; Ali, S. Boron inhibits apoptosis in hyperapoptosis condition: Acts by stabilizing the mitochondrial membrane and inhibiting matrix. *Biochim. Biophys. Acta-Gen. Subj.* **2019**, *1863*, 144–152.

44. Nolsøe, R.L.; Hamid, Y.H.; Pociot, F.; Paulsen, S.; Andersen, K.M.; Borch-Johnsen, K. Association of a microsatellite in FASL to type II diabetes and of the FAS-670G4A genotype to insulin resistance. *Genes Immun.* **2016**, *7*, 316–321. [CrossRef]
45. Loweth, A.C.; Williams, G.T.; James, R.F.L.; Scarpello, J.H.B.; Morgan, N.G. Human islets of Langerhans express fas ligand and undergo apoptosis in response to interleukin-1b and fas ligation. *Diabetes* **1998**, *47*, 727–732. [CrossRef]
46. Tian, C.; Chang, H.; La, X.; Li, J.A.; Ma, L. *Wushenziye* Formula Inhibits Pancreatic β Cell Apoptosis in Type 2 Diabetes Mellitus via MEK-ERK-Caspase-3 Signaling Pathway. *Evid. Based Complement Alternat Med.* **2018**, *25*, 259–298. [CrossRef]
47. Maedler, K.; Fontana, A.; Ris, F.; Sergeev, P.; Toso, C.; Oberholzer, J. FLIP switches Fas-mediated glucose signaling in human pancreatic beta cells from apoptosis to cell replication. *Proc. Natl. Acad. Sci. USA* **2002**, *99*, 8236–8241. [CrossRef]
48. Hong, S.C.; So, H.T.; Sonia, C.; Wen, P.; Joash, B.; Lee, T. Increased susceptibility of post-weaning rats on high-fat diet to metabolic syndrome. *J. Adv. Res.* **2017**, *8*, 30106–30116.
49. Arvindekar, A.; More, T.; Payghan, P.V.; Laddha, K.; Ghoshal, N.; Arvindekar, A. Evaluation of anti-diabetic and alpha glucosidase inhibitory action of anthraquinones from Rheum emodi. *Food Funct.* **2015**, *6*, 2693–2700. [CrossRef]

Sample Availability: Samples of the compounds are available from the authors.

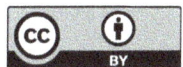

© 2019 by the authors. Licensee MDPI, Basel, Switzerland. This article is an open access article distributed under the terms and conditions of the Creative Commons Attribution (CC BY) license (http://creativecommons.org/licenses/by/4.0/).

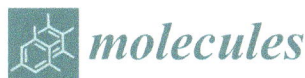

Article

3′-*O*-β-D-glucopyranosyl-α,4,2′,4′,6′-pentahydroxy-dihydrochalcone, from Bark of *Eysenhardtia polystachya* Prevents Diabetic Nephropathy via Inhibiting Protein Glycation in STZ-Nicotinamide Induced Diabetic Mice

Rosa Martha Pérez Gutierrez [1,*], Abraham Heriberto García Campoy [1], Silvia Patricia Paredes Carrera [2], Alethia Muñiz Ramirez [3], José Maria Mota Flores [1] and Sergio Odin Flores Valle [4]

[1] Natural Products Research Laboratory, Higher School of Chemical Engineering and Extractive Industries, National Polytechnic Institute, Av. Instituto Politécnico Nacional S/N,
Unidad Profesional Adolfo Lopez Mateos, Ciudad de México CP 07708, Mexico;
abrahamhgc27@hotmail.com (A.H.G.C.); josemariamota@yahoo.com.mx (J.M.M.F.)
[2] Sustainable Nanomaterials Laboratory, Higher School of Chemical Engineering and Extractive Industries, National Polytechnic Institute (IPN) Professional Unit Adolfo Lopez Mateos,
S/N Av. Instituto Politécnico Nacional, Ciudad de México CP 07708, Mexico; silviappcar@gmail.com
[3] CONACYT/IPICYT-CIIDZA, Camino a la Presa de San José 2055, Col. Lomas 4 Sección,
San Luis Potosí CP 78216, Mexico; alethiamura@gmail.com
[4] Green Chemistry Research Laboratory, School of Chemical Engineering and Extractive Industries, National Polytechnic Institute, Av. Instituto Politécnico Nacional S/N,
Unidad Profesional Adolfo Lopez Mateos, Ciudad de México CP 07708, Mexico; sergioodin@gmail.com
* Correspondence: rmpg@prodigy.net.mx; Tel.: +52-55-5729-6000

Academic Editor: Raffaele Capasso
Received: 5 February 2019; Accepted: 22 March 2019; Published: 28 March 2019

Abstract: Previous studies have shown that accumulation of advanced glycation end products (AGEs) can be the cause of diabetic nephropathy (DN) in diabetic patients. Dihydrochalcone 3′-*O*-β-D-glucopyranosyl α,4,2′,4′,6′-pentahydroxy–dihydrochalcone (**1**) is a powerful antiglycation compound previously isolated from *Eysenhardtia polystachya*. The aim was to investigate whether (**1**) was able to protect against diabetic nephropathy in streptozotocin (STZ)-induced diabetic mice, which displayed renal dysfunction markers such as body weight, creatinine, uric acid, serum urea, total urinary protein, and urea nitrogen in the blood (BUN). In addition, pathological changes were evaluated including glycated hemoglobin (HbA1c), advanced glycation end products (AGEs) in the kidney, as well as in circulation level and pro-inflammatory markers ICAM-1 levels in diabetic mice. After 5 weeks, these elevated markers of dihydrochalcone treatment (25, 50 and 100 mg/kg) were significantly ($p < 0.05$) attenuated. In addition, they ameliorate the indices of renal inflammation as indicated by ICAM-1 markers. The kidney and circulatory AGEs levels in diabetic mice were significantly ($p < 0.05$) attenuated by (**1**) treatment. Histological analysis of kidney tissues showed an important recovery in its structure compared with the diabetic group. It was found that the compound (**1**) attenuated the renal damage in diabetic mice by inhibiting AGEs formation.

Keywords: dihydrochalcone; advanced glycation end-product; *Eysenhardtia polystachya*; diabetic mice; renoprotective

1. Introduction

Type 2 diabetes mellitus is a cause of mortality due to complications such as diabetic nephropathy (DN), which is the main cause of end-stage renal failure [1]. DN is characterized by kidney structural changes, declining glomerular filtration rate, and mesangial sclerosis. Hyperglycemia, oxidative stress, and dyslipidemia are the main causes of increased advanced glycation end products (AGEs) and contribute to the development of DN in diabetes [2], which has been demonstrated in several studies with the treatment of anti-glycation compounds such as alagebrium chloride [3], benfotiamine [4], pyridoxamine [5], and aminoguanidine [6] attenuated development of diabetic nephropathy. The generation of AGEs promotes kidney damage by protein cross linking, leading to changes in structure and function of the proteins [7]; they also generate an increase of the expression of monocyte chemoattractant protein 1 (MCP-1). Previous studies indicated that endothelial cell exhibition to a uremic environment augment IL-8, vascular adhesion molecule-1 (VCAM-1) and MCP-1 expression indicating a relationship between systemic inflammation and vascular damage with a uremic toxicity [8]. Other studies indicated that reduction of AGEs production and accumulation in the tissues could be an effective strategy to improvement of diabetic complications [9].

In previous studies, we isolated several dihydrochalcones from the Bark of *Eysenhardtia polystachya* [10], which showed an efficient inhibition fluorescent and non-fluorescent AGE formation, reduced level of fructosamine, significantly suppressed oxidation of thiols and protein carbonyl content in a BSA/glucose system; in addition, inhibited generation of MGO, and the formation of amyloid cross-β structure. Dihydrochalcone demonstrated inhibition at multiple stages of glycation. The aim was to isolate a dihydrochalcone and study if it can be renoprotective in diabetic mice by inhibiting AGEs formation.

2. Results and Discussion

2.1. Identification of 3′-O-β-D-glucopyranosyl α,4,2′,4′,6′-pentahydroxy–dihydrochalcone (1)

Dihydrochalcone was first found in the methanol extract of *Eysenhardtia polystachya*, and its structure was elucidated by spectroscopic methods (IR, ^{1}H-NMR, ^{13}C-NMR, COSY, and HMBC). Compound **1** shows a molecular formula $C_{21}H_{24}O_{12}$, and this is suggested by using the positive HRMS that implied ten degrees of unsaturation. The IR spectrum indicates the presence of hydroxyl at 3448 cm^{-1}, carbonyl (1645 cm^{-1}) and benzene ring (3010, 1586, 1441 cm^{-1}) functionalities.

^{1}H, ^{13}C-NMR, and DEPT spectra show the presence of five aromatic signals at δ_H 7.49, δ_H 6.65, and δ_H 6.39, and also showed signals for 21 C-atoms, including two methylene (CH_2), eleven methylenes (CH) groups, and eight quaternary carbons. In the ^{1}H-NMR spectrum there are five aromatic signals at δ_H 7.49 (2H), δ_H 6.65 (2H) and δ_H 6.09 (1H). In the HMBC spectrum correlation of δ_H 7.49 with δ_C 131.6 (C-2, 6), 6.65 with δ_C 118.2 (C-3, C-5) suggested the presence of one monosubstituted aromatic ring with a hydroxyl group at C-4 (δ_C 160.7). The glucopyranosyl moiety was located at C-3′ which was further supported by the HMBC correlation of the anomeric proton resonating at δ_H 4.80 (1H, d, J = 7.3 Hz, H-1″) to C-3′ (102.6) together with the coupling constant of the anomeric proton (d, J = 7.3 Hz) indicated that was β-glucoside.

2′,4′,6′-trihydroxy substitution of the dihydrochalcone ring A was determined by evaluating the ^{1}H coupling pattern and the ^{13}C-NMR chemical shifts which showed the characteristic pattern of nethofagin dehydrochalcone skeleton [11] except that (**1**) differs from nethofagin by the presence of a hydroxyl group at C-8 (C-α). Aliphatic proton was assigned to ABX system at δ_H 2.75 (1H, dd, J = 16.5, 13.4 Hz, H-α), 2.36 (1H, dd, J = 16.5, 3.1 Hz, H-α), 5.25 (1H, dd, J = 13.4, 3.1 Hz, H-β), suggested a linked -CH (α)-CH$_{2}$(β)- moiety leading to the presence of a -CO-CH (OH)-CH$_2$- moiety. Therefore, compound **1** was assigned as 3′-O-β-D-glucopyranosyl-α,4,2′,4′,6′-pentahydroxy-dihydrochalcone (Figure 1).

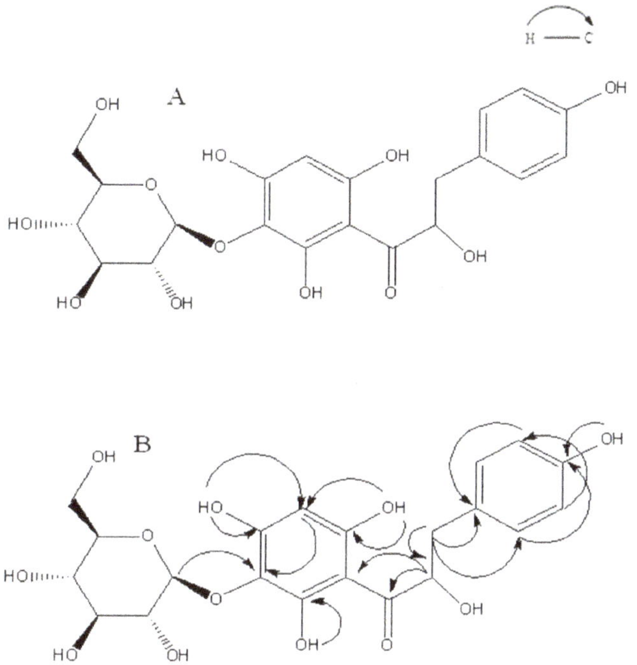

Figure 1. (**A**) Dihydrochalcone **1** isolated from bark of *Eysenhardtia polystachya*; (**B**) Heteronuclear Multiple Bond Connectivity (HMBC) of **1**.

2.2. Effect of Dihydrochalcone on Glucose, Water Intake, Body Weight, Kidney Weight, Food Consumption, Urine Volumen and Urine Protein

As shown in the Figure 2 urine volume (A), food consumptions (B), water intake (C), and body weight (D) were significantly higher when compared to that of the normal control mice. Treatment with compound (**1**) at a dose of 100 mg/kg during a period of 5 weeks significantly decrease the urine volume by 52.68% (Figure 2A; $p < 0.05$) and urine protein by 52.22% compared to that diabetic control group (Table 1). While treatment with (**1**) food consumptions and water intake decreased by 32.75% (Figure 2B; $p < 0.05$) and 53.84% (Figure 1C; $p < 0.05$), respectively, compared to that diabetic control group. However, using compound (**1**) during the 5 weeks of treatment did not significantly modify levels of blood glucose in STZ-induced diabetes mice, which developed a stable increase in the hyperglycemia. In addition, treatment with compound (**1**) or metformin did not show significant changes in body weight (Figure 2D). During the period of experimental treatment with compound (**1**), there was an improvement in urine volume, urine protein, food consumption, and water intake in different degrees when compared to metformin, which was used as standard (Figure 2A–D). Figure 3A shows kidney size during the experimental period; it was observed that a gain in kidney size in the diabetic control mice was in contrast to a reduction of kidney size when the diabetic mice were treated with compound (**1**) or metformin for 5 weeks.

Kidney weight was significantly increased ($p < 0.05$) in the diabetic group compared to the control group, while oral administration with compound **1** (100 mg/kg) and metformin (200 mg/kg) exhibited a significant reduction ($p < 0.05$) in kidney weight by 32% and 28.6%, respectively, as compared to diabetic-STZ mice (Figure 3B).

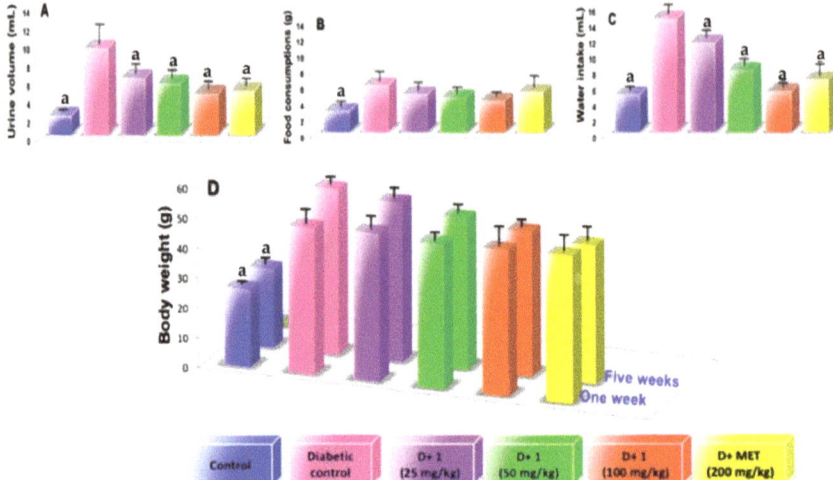

Figure 2. (**A**) examination of urine volume at the fifth weeks; (**B**) examination of food consumptions at the fifth weeks; (**C**) examination of water intake at the fifth weeks; (**D**) examination of body weigh at the fifth weeks; Results are expressed as mean ± SD; [a] $p < 0.05$ vs. diabetic control.

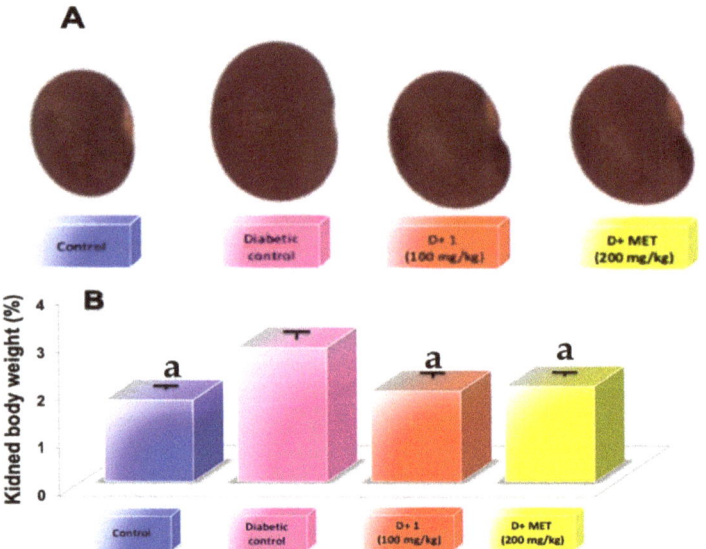

Figure 3. (**A**) Images of kidney representative of five weeks of the different treatments; (**B**) examination of kidney weight at the fifth weeks; Results are expressed as mean ± SD; [a] $p < 0.05$ vs. diabetic control.

It was observed that in the STZ-induced diabetic model that a selective destruction of pancreatic cells producing insulin led to hyperglycemia. Consequently, we have an experimental diabetic nephropathy model to study pathological changes in the kidney [12]. Hyperglycemia produces an increase in urine volume, urine protein, food consumption, water intake, blood glucose level, and reduction of body weight [13]. Treatment with compound (**1**) significantly enhances these pathological characteristics in the DN mice model. The finding indicated that the renoprotective effect of compound

1 on the DN model is related to the improvement of renal function, and avoids the proteinuria. However, its effect does not depend on changes in blood glucose levels.

Table 1. Effect of dihydrochalcone (1) on urine protein of diabetic-nephropathy mice.

Groups	Urine Protein (mg/dL)	
	0 Weeks	5 Weeks
NormaL ControL	0.45 ± 0.03 [a]	0.44 ± 0.08 [a]
Diabetic ControL	2.82 ± 0.7	3.61 ± 0.4
D + 1 (25 mg/dL)	2.81 ± 0.9	2.69 ± 0.5
D + 1 (50 mg/dL)	2.88 ± 0.6	2.16 ± 0.7
D + 1 (100 mg/dL)	2.89 ± 1.0	1.72 ± 0.9 [a]
D + Met (200 mg/dL)	2.80 ± 1.3	1.70 ± 0.6 [a]

Results are expressed as mean $\pm$ SD; [a] $p < 0.05$ vs. diabetic control (D).

2.3. Effect of Dihydrochalcone on Kidney Index, Creatinine, Uric Acid, Serum Urea, and Urea Nitrogen in the Blood (BUN)

The development of diabetic nephropathy can be detected by the elevated level of kidney index indicators such as uric acid, serum urea, BUN, and creatinine. These renal indexes were significantly higher in the STZ-induced diabetic mice group (DN) in comparison with normal control. Groups treated with 25, 50, and 100 mg/kg of the dihydrochalcone showed a significantly decreased ($p < 0.05$) in kidney index in comparison to DN control group such as BUN, creatinine, uric acid, urea and urine protein in a dependent dose manner (Tables 1 and 2). In addition, metformin used as a standard also significantly reduced ($p < 0.05$) the elevated level of these biomarkers. STZ-induced diabetic mice showed a significant increase in volume and kidney mass. However, treatment with compound 1 (25, 50 and 100 mg/kg) or metformin (200 mg/kg) significantly re-established ($p < 0.05$) both volume and renal mass look closer to the normal group (Figure 3A,B).

Atrophic changes in the renal tubules and glomeruli in the kidneys were observed in the DN mice model, producing elevated levels of blood urea nitrogen, urea, uric acid, and creatinine in blood. An important index of glomerular function is the creatinine generated as a metabolite in the muscle, excreted through glomerular filtration [14]. In the metabolic process, protein breakdown leads to the production of urea, which is excreted mainly through the kidneys [15]. Metabolism in humans serum urea nitrogen level is the main end-product of proteins causing a spike in serum, BUN level is commonly found in DN or glomerulonephritis patients with inhibition glomerular filtration rate. The accumulation of uric acid generates the production of monosodium urate crystals that can cause inflammatory and pain response, leading to renal and hepatic injuries. High levels of serum urea, BUN, uric acid, and creatinine suggest injuries in the kidney [16]. Thus, it could be used as markers for diagnosis in DN [17].

Table 2. Effect of dihydrochalcone (1) on biochemical parameters in serum of diabetic-nephropathy mice.

Groups	BUN (mg/dL)		Creatinine (mg/dL)		Uric Acid (mg/dL)		Urea (mg/dL)	
	0 Weeks	5 Weeks	0 Weeks	5 Weeks	0 Weeks	5 Weeks	0 Weeks	5 Weeks
NormaL ControL	15.89 ± 3.4 [a]	16.34 ± 2.8 [a]	0.73 ± 0.03 [a]	0.073 ± 0.03 [a]	5.12 ± 1.4 [a]	5.11 ± 1.0 [a]	35.06 ± 4.3 [a]	36.49 ± 1.0 [a]
Diabetic ControL	36.12 ± 4.1	42.51 ± 2.9	3.01 ± 0.9	3.90 ± 0.7	13.11 ± 3.7	16.20 ± 3.1	80.10 ± 5.9	90.38 ± 6.4
D + 1 (25 mg/dL)	38.24 ± 2.9	30.47 ± 3.5 [a]	3.25 ± 1.0	2.47 ± 0.5	13.30 ± 2.8	8.13 ± 2.5 [a]	82.12 ± 3.7	69.28 ± 5.3 [a]
D + 1 (50 mg/dL)	37.23 ± 5.3	25.48 ± 4.1 [a]	3.94 ± 0.8	2.10 ± 0.4 [a]	12.94 ± 1.7	6.24 ± 2.9 [a]	83.43 ± 4.2	58.19 ± 6.1 [a]
D + 1 (100 mg/dL)	38.48 ± 4.6	22.11 ± 3.9 [a]	3.76 ± 0.6	1.70 ± 0.08 [a]	13.84 ± 1.5	5.41 ± 1.6 [a]	81.71 ± 5.3	50.13 ± 3.7 [a]
D + Met (200 mg/dL)	38.40 ± 5.0	21.43 ± 4.2 [a]	3.83 ± 0.9	1.55 ± 0.6 [a]	12.67 ± 3.6	3.43 ± 2.3 [a]	82.84 ± 3.8	56.22 ± 4.6 [a]

Results are expressed as mean ± SD; [a] $p < 0.05$ vs. diabetic control (D).

2.4. Effect of Dihydrochalcone on MCP-1

Diabetic nephropathy is considered an inflammatory disease where progressive glomerular damage is related by infiltration to CD11b-positive macrophages [18] wherein MCP-1 is secreted from resident glomerular cells. In our study, the diabetic model is related to the increase in MCP-1 and simultaneously with accumulation of macrophages in the cortex. Treatment with compound (**1**) and metformin were able to significantly reduce ($p < 0.05$) the expression of the chemokine MCP-1 associated with diabetes (Figure 4). The finding suggested that the anti-inflammatory effect of compound (**1**) participates in DN attenuation. AGEs-induced chronic inflammation, and subsequently cells and tissues, were disabled and triggered an increasing inflammatory cytokines or oxidative stress via interaction between RAGE and AGEs [19].

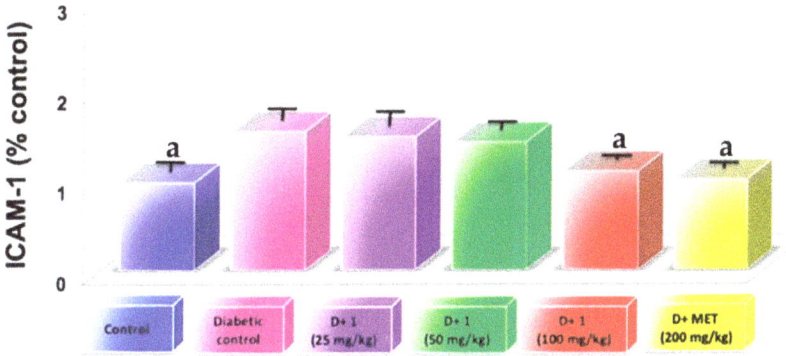

Figure 4. Examination of inflammation markers ICAM-1 in glomeruli of kidneys from diabetic mice at the fifth weeks; Results are expressed as mean ± SD; [a] $p < 0.05$ vs. diabetic control.

2.5. Effect of Dihydrochalcone on Glycosylated Haemoglobin Concentration (HbA1c)

The level of glycosylated hemoglobin in STZ-induced diabetes mice was significantly increased ($p < 0.05$) in comparison with normal control mice. However, HbA1C significantly decreased ($p < 0.05$) in groups treated with compound **1** in comparison with diabetic group (Table 3) at a dose of 25, 50, and 100 mg/kg by 19.47%, 33.65% and 54.49% respectively. Metformin also significantly reduced ($p < 0.05$) the elevated concentration of glycosylated hemoglobin by 48.14% (Table 3).

Table 3. Effect of dihydrochalcone (**1**) on glycosylated haemoglobin levels and AGEs in Kidney of diabetic mice.

Groups	Glycosylated Haemoglobin (%)	AGEs (RFU/mg Protein)
NormaL controL	3.52 ± 0.7 [a]	1.71 ± 0.9 [a]
Diabetic controL	9.45 ± 1.1 [a]	3.8 ± 0.8
D + 1 (25 mg/dL)	7.61 ± 1.8	3.0 ± 0.7
D + 1 (50 mg/dL)	6.27 ± 0.9 [a]	2.6 ± 0.9
D + 1 (100 mg/dL)	4.3 ± 0.8 [a]	2.0 ± 0.6
D + Met (200 mg/dL)	4.9 ± 0.6 [a]	1.9 ± 0.7

Results are expressed as mean ± SD of five mice in each group to five weeks of experimentation. Values [a] $p < 0.05$ vs. diabetic control (D).

In diabetes, the excess of glucose in blood reacts with hemoglobin to form HbA1C, which is an early glycosylation adduct, and with time undergoes complex and slow rearrangements to generate AGEs. Thus, glycosylated hemoglobin is used in diabetic patients mostly for prognosticate the developing of diabetic complications, mainly at long term [20].

2.6. Effect of Dihydrochalcone on AGEs Kidney

In diabetes hyperglycemic condition leads to excessive accumulation of AGEs participating in the pathogenesis of diabetic nephropathy, leading to structural abnormality [4]. In this study, treatment with STZ markedly increased AGEs formation in kidneys of diabetic mice in comparison to normal control. Groups treated with dihydrochalcone (100 mg/kg) or metformin (200 mg/kg) showed attenuation in AGEs formation in kidney in comparison to the diabetic control group by 47.73% and 50% respectively (Table 3). Results showed that compound (**1**) is able to block the accumulation and formation of AGEs in kidney in nephropathy model streptozotocin induced diabetic mice. Reduction of the formation of AGEs is considered a potential therapy in diabetic nephropathy.

2.7. AGEs Levels in Plasma

AGEs levels in plasma showed a significant increase in 5 weeks of diabetes induction. However, treatment of compound **1** to diabetic mice showed progressive decrease circulating AGEs in respect to diabetic control mice (Figure 5A,B). AF show that are better related to the time of illness than AGI. Plasma AGE levels circulation stopped incrementing, possibly because it is eliminated from blood by liver and renal filters. This study showed higher serum AGE level in diabetic mice and an increase in renal dysfunctions. Oral administration of compound (**1**) act as AGE-inhibitors near the normal levels as well as AGE-breakers, reducing the serum AGE level and delay the progression of DN. In addition, metformin treatment showed AGEs level near to normal levels compared to the diabetic group (Figure 5A,B); this effect is due to its interaction with dicarbonyl compounds formed throughout the glycation process [21].

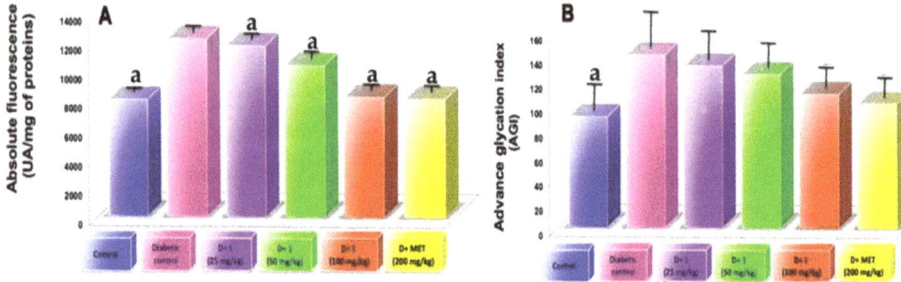

Figure 5. (**A**) Circulating AGE levels measured as absolute fluorescence at 5 weeks of experimental period; (**B**) Circulating AGE levels expressed as advanced glycation index. Results are expressed as mean ± SD; [a] $p < 0.05$ vs. diabetic control.

2.8. Histopathology on in Renal Tissues

The renal tissue of control mice revealed normal parenchyma, renal cortex, renal tubules, and glomeruli (Figure 6A). Sections of STZ-induced diabetic mice kidney showed perivascular lymphocytic aggregates, endotheliosis, inflammatory cell infiltration, degenerative changes, fibrotic, interstitial hemorrhage, and glomerular necrosis (Figure 6B). Administration of 100 mg/kg (Figure 6E) of dihydrochalcone, or 200 mg/kg of metformin (Figure 6F) to the experimental animals showed an important recovery in the structure of the kidney compared to the diabetic group. However, treatment a 25 and 50 mg/kg showed a moderate improvement on normal glomerulus compared to the diabetic group.

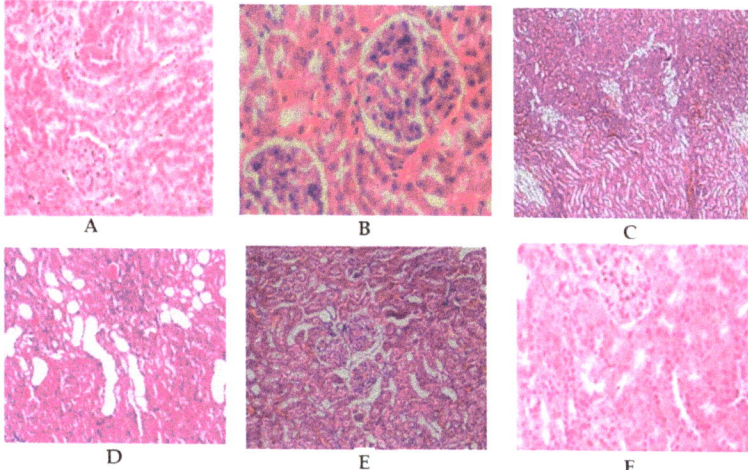

Figure 6. Kidney sections from mice by light microscopy (H and E stained). (**A**) Control group, (**B**) Diabetic control, (**C**) D + **1** (25 mg/kg), (**D**) D + **1** (50 mg/kg), (**E**) D + **1** (100 mg/kg), (**F**) D + MET (200 mg/kg).

3. Conclusions

Our findings suggest that the treatment with dihydrochalcone protects renal function and prevents kidney injury in STZ-nicotinamide induced diabetic nephropathy, ameliorated markers of DN, as well as inflammation, HbA1C, AGE-inhibition in kidneys and circulation.

The renoprotective effect of dihydrochalcone isolated from *Eysenhardtia polystachya* might be associated in part to its ability to react with reactive carbonyl species and cleavage of pre-formed AGEs within the kidney by a cross- link breaker inhibiting AGEs-formation.

4. Materials and Methods

4.1. Plant

The specimen was identified and authenticated by Biol. Aurora Chamal, Department of Botany, Universidad Autonoma Metropolitana-Xochimilco, where a voucher specimen (No. 53290) has been deposited for further reference.

*4.2. Extraction, Isolation and Characterization 3'-O-β-D-glucopyranosyl α,4,2',4',6'-pentahydroxy–dihydrochalcone (**1**)*

The extraction, isolation, and characterization of dihydrochalcone from the bark of *Eysenhardtia polystachya* was carried out as follows. Briefly, the bark (40 kg) was pulverized into powder and extracted with distilled water and methanol (1:1) two times at room temperature. Both extracts were combined and concentrated under reduced pressure. The extract was subjected to a silica gel column eluted with ethyl acetate/methylene chloride (2:9) to yield seven fractions (PA-1 to PA-7). Subfraction PA-5 was then separated by silica gel chromatography with methanol/acetone/ethyl acetate (1:3:6) and preparative chromatography eluted with methanol/acetone/ethyl acetate (0.5/3/1.5) to give 4 subfractions (PA5-1 to PA5-4). PA5-3 was purified in a sephadex LH-20 column with a gradient of water/methanol 1:1 increasing the ratio of water to 100% to obtain compound **1** (630 mg).

3'-O-β-D-glucopyranosyl-α,4,2',4',6'-pentahydroxy–dihydrochalcone: Is a pale yellow powder, m.p. 143–144 °C; HRMS [M$^+$] at m/z 468.4130, $C_{21}H_{24}O_{12}$ requires 468.4110; UV λ max (MeOH) nm 260, 303, 375; IR vmax (KBr) cm^{-1}: 3448, 2932, 1645, 1586, 1519, 1441, 1182, 1071; The ^{1}H-NMR espectra (300 MHz, DMSO-d6) showed the following data: δ_H 2.75 (1H, dd, J = 16.5, 13.4 Hz, H-α), 2.36 (1H, dd,

J = 16.5, 3.1 Hz, H-α), 5.25 (1H, dd, *J* = 13.4, 3.1 Hz, H-β), 7.49 (2H, d, *J* = 8.2 Hz, H-2, 6), 6.65 (2H, d, *J* = 8.2 Hz, H-3, 5), 9.10 (s, OH-4), 6.09 (1H, s, H-5'), 10.60 (s, OH-4'), 12.24 (s, OH-2'), 13.50 (s, OH-6'); Glu: δ_H 4.80 (1H, d, *J* = 7.3 Hz, H-1''), 3.87 (1H, d, *J* = 4.4 Hz, OH-2''), 3.54 (1H, d, *J* = 5.3 Hz, OH-3''), 3.28 (1H, dd, *J* = 12.2, 4.5 Hz, OH-4''), 3.20 (1H, d, *J* = 9.3 Hz, OH-5''), 3.76 (1H, dd, *J* = 11.6, 5.2 Hz, H-6''α), 3.45 (1H, dd, *J* = 11.6, 6.0 Hz, H-6''β); ^{13}C NMR (125 MHz, CDCl3) δ_C: 128.7 (C-1), 131.6 (C-2, C-6), 118.2 (C-3, C-5), 160.7 (C-4), 44.30 (C-α), 78.97 (C-β), 192.94 (C-9, C=O); 109.4 (C-1'), 164.2 (C-2'), 102.6 (C-3'), 166.2 (C-4'), 111.5 (C-5'), 165.7 (C-6'); Glu: δ_C 108.6 (C-1''), 72.3 (C-2''), 78.0 (C-3''), 69.7 (C-4''), 76.8 (C-5''), 60.4 (C-6'').

4.3. Animals

The study was conducted on healthy adult male C57BL/6J mice, weighing about 25–30 g. Before and during the experiment, animals were fed a standard laboratory diet (Mouse Chow 5015, Purina) with free access to water. Mice were procured from the bioterium of ENCB and were housed in microloan boxes cages in a controlled environment (temperature 25 ± 2 °C). Animals were allowed to acclimate for a period of three days in their new environment prior to the study. Before commencing the experiment, litter in cages was renewed three times a week to ensure hygiene and maximum comfort for the animals. The experiments reported in this study followed the guidelines stated in "Principles of Laboratory Animal Care" (NIH publication 85-23, revised 1985 and the Mexican Official Normativity (NOM-062-Z00-1999). All animal procedures were performed in accordance with the recommendations for the care and use of laboratory animals (756/lab/ENCB).

4.4. Induction of Mild Diabetes (Type 2)

After 15 min of administrating an intraperitoneal injection with 120 mg/kg nicotinamide (Sigma Chemical Company, St. Louis, MO, USA), mice were made diabetic by administering a single intraperitoneal injection of freshly prepared streptozotocin (STZ) (60 mg/kg b.w. i.p.) in 0.1 M citrate buffer at pH 4.5. The animals were allowed to drink 5% glucose solution overnight to overcome the drug-induced hypoglycaemia. After 10 days of diabetes development, moderately diabetic mice having persistent glycosuria and hyperglycaemia (blood glucose > 200 mg/dL) were used for further experimentation [22]. After the diabetic mice were randomly divided into five groups (eight mice per group) matched by body weight. Normal mice were administered with distilled water.

Forty-eight mice were divided into eight groups of six animals and had free access to water and food, and then animals were treated for five weeks as follows: Group 1: normal mice, Group 2: diabetic control mice, Group 3: Dihydrochalcone (25 mg/kg/day p.o) treated diabetic mice, Group 4: Dihydrochalcone (50 mg/kg/day p.o) treated diabetic mice, Group 5: Dihydrochalcone (100 mg/kg/day p.o) treated diabetic mice, Group 6: Mentformin (AG) (200 mg/kg/day p.o) treated diabetic mice as a standard drug.

4.5. Preparation of Urine, Serum, and Kidney Homogenate

After 5 weeks of treatment, diabetes mice were placed inside individual metabolic cages for 24 h and urine was collected. Body weight, kidney weight, food, and water intake were recorded; after 12 h fasting, the blood samples were collected from the tail vein. The animals were then sacrificed by asphyxiation using carbon dioxide. The serum was centrifuged for 20 min at 877× *g* and stored at −80 °C for further assays. After the kidneys were removed, weighed and washed with phosphate buffer saline (PBS pH 7.4). The right kidneys were homogenized in ice-cold PBS, and stored in liquid nitrogen for further biochemical and molecular assays. The left kidneys were removed and used for histopathological examination.

4.6. Measured of Biochemical Parameters in Diabetic Mice

The plasma glucose concentration was determined using an enzymatic colorimetric method using a commercial kit (Sigma Aldrich, San Luis, MO, USA). Total urinary protein levels were measured using a Rat Urinary Protein Assay Kit (Chondrex, Redmond, WA, USA). In serum, creatinine was evaluated using a QuantiChrom™ Protein Creatinine Ratio Assay Kit (BioAssay Systems, San Francisco, CA, USA), urea, uric acid and blood urea nitrogen test (BUN) were measured using Assay Kits (Abcam, Cambridge MA, USA) according to the manufacturer's instructions. Kidneys were dissected and weighed (wet weight).

4.7. Glycosylated Hemoglobin

Blood samples were obtained by ocular venipuncture into tubes with EDTA and centrifuged at $800 \times g$ at 4 °C for 10 min to remove packed cells and plasma. Using two volumes of water packed cells were lysed. Then was added one volume of carbon tetrachloride to the hemolysate, and refrigerated at 4 °C overnight. Lysate was centrifuged at $27,000 \times g$ at 4 °C, for 30 min supernatant removed and used to analysis. Colorimetric estimation was measured according to the procedure of Parker et al. [23]. One mLof diluted hemolysate (10 mg of hemoglobin or fructose standard) was mixed with 1 mL of oxalic acid reagent. The mixture was incubated for 60 min at 124 °C in sealed tubes. After incubation, the mixture was allowed to cool to room temperature and added 1 mL of the trichloroacetic acid to each tube, mixed, and filtered through a 15 cm × 0.5 (1.d) glass column with a glass wool plug in the bottom. To 1.5 mL of the filtering add thiobarbituric acid reagent (0.05 M) and measured the absorbance at 443 nm of glycated hemoglobin.

4.8. AGEs Levels in Kidney

The kidneys were homogenized in 2 mL of 0.25 M sucrose, followed by centrifugation at 5 °C with $900 \times g$ and the pellet obtained was resuspended in 2 mL sucrose and centrifuged again then both supernatant obtained were mixed. The proteins were precipitated by adding trichloroacetic acid (TCA) in equal volume and centrifugated at 5 °C at $900 \times g$, then protein pellet was added 1 mL methanol to eliminate the lipid fraction. Then, washing the insoluble protein using 10% cooled TCA and centrifuged: after the residue was solubilized in 1 mL of 1 N NaOH and the AGEs concentration was evaluated fluorometrically with an emission at 440 nm and excitation at 370 nm, and the results were indicated as relative fluorescence units (RFU)/mg protein [24].

4.9. AGEs Levels in Serum

Mouse plasma was centrifuged to collect supernatants. AGEs levels in plasma were used to determine Absolute Fluorescence (AF; 80 µL) and Advanced Glycation Index (AGI; 20, 40, 80 µL diluted in 1 mL of PBS) [25] using a Micro-plate Reader (Thermo Fisher Scientific, Voltam, MA, USA). AGE fluorescence was indicated at excitation wavelength of 350 nm and emission wavelengths of 450 nm in a spectrofluorometric detector (BIO-TEK, Synergy, Salt Lake City, UT, USA). AF was in arbitrary units (AU) with respect to protein concentrations. AGI was produced by the three points of dilution and expressed as the slope of the line.

4.10. Measure of the Expression of Intracellular Adhesion Molecule (ICAM)-1

After 5 weeks of treatment, frozen cortex was chopped on ice, then flushed through a disposable filter (100-mm; BioScientific Corp, Austin, TX, USA) with cold saline solution and collected. The solution was then flushed through filter (70-mm). The glomerular solution was obtained by inversion of the filter (70-mm), and afterward was flushed with a cold saline solution, followed by spinning at 6000 rpm at 4 °C for 15 min. The supernatant was eliminated and the pellets were suspended in 1 mL of Trizol. The presence of glomeruli was supported in a microscopy. Protein obtained from kidney cortex were used to evaluate the level of the expression of (ICAM)-1 (BioScientific Corp, Austin, TX, USA) according to ELISA kit instructions.

4.11. Histopathology

Kidney fragments were fixed in 10% neutral buffered formalin solution, dehydrated in ethanol, embedded in paraffin, and sectioned at 5 μm thickness using a rotary microtome. After dehydration, sections were stained with hematoxylin and eosin (HE). To evaluate the histopathological damage, each image of sections was examined for microscopic observations (400; Nikon, Tokyo, Japan).

4.12. Statistical Analyses

The data are presented as mean ± standard deviation. The significance of the differences was analyzed by one-way ANOVA with the Dunnett's test using GraphPad Prism 7.0 for Windows (GraphPad Software Inc., San Diego, CA, USA). The value of statistical significance was established at $p < 0.05$.

Author Contributions: Conceptualization of the study and design of the experiments, R.M.P.G.; performed the experiments A.H.G.C., S.O.F.V., and J.M.M.F.; analyzed the data, A.M.R. and S.P.P.C.; Writing of the manuscript R.M.P.G., A.M.R, and S.P.P.C.

Funding: This study received no external funding.

Conflicts of Interest: The authors claim no conflict of interest in this study.

References

1. Yan, H.D.; Li, X.Z.; Xie, J.M.; Li, M. Effects of advanced glycation end products on renal fibrosis and oxidative stress in cultured NRK-49F cells. *Chin. Med. J.* **2007**, *120*, 787–793. [CrossRef] [PubMed]
2. Barnett, A. Prevention of loss of renal function over time in patients with diabetic nephropathy. *Am. J. Med.* **2006**, *119*, S40–S47. [CrossRef]
3. Babaei-Jadidi, R.; Karachalias, N.; Ahmed, N.; Battah, S.; Thornalley, P. Prevention of incipient diabetic nephropathy by high-dose thiamine and benfotiamine. *Diabetes* **2003**, *52*, 2110–2120. [CrossRef]
4. Forbes, J.M.; Thallas, V.; Thomas, M.C. The breakdown of preexisting advanced glycation end products is associated with reduced renal fibrosis in experimental diabetes. *FASEB J.* **2003**, *17*, 1762–1764. [CrossRef] [PubMed]
5. Williams, M.E.; Bolton, W.K.; Khalifah, R.G.; Degenhardt, T.P.; Schotzinger, R.J.; McGill, J.B. Effects of pyridoxamine in combined phase 2 studies of patients with type 1 and type 2 diabetes and overt nephropathy. *Am. J. Nephrol.* **2007**, *27*, 605–614. [CrossRef]
6. Vlassara, H.; Uribarri, J.; Cai, W.; Striker, G. Advanced glycation end product homeostasis: Exogenous oxidants and innate defenses. *Ann. N. Y. Acad. Sci.* **2008**, *1126*, 46–52. [CrossRef]
7. Stinghen, A.E.; Goncalves, S.M.; Martines, E.G. Increased plasma and endothelial cell expression of chemokines and adhesion molecules in chronic kidney disease. *Nephron. Clin. Pract.* **2009**, *111*, 117–126. [CrossRef]
8. Sanajou, D.; Haghjo, A.G.; Argani, H.; Aslani, S. Age-rage axis blockade in diabetic nephropathy: Current status and future directions. *Eur. J. Pharmacol.* **2018**, *833*, 158–166. [CrossRef]
9. Perez, R.M.G.; Garcia, A.H.C.; Mota, J.M.F. Dihydrochalcones from the bark of *Eysenhardtia polystachya* inhibit formation of advanced glycation and products at multiple stages in vitro studies. *NESSA J. Pharm. Pharm.* **2017**, *1*, 3–23.
10. Madeline, J.; Simpson, I.; Hjelmqvist, D.; López-A, C.A.; Karamehmedovic, N.; Minehan, T.G.; Yepremyan, A.; Salehani, B.; Lissi, E.; Joubert, E.; et al. Anti-Peroxyl radical quality and antibacterial properties of rooibos infusions and their pure glycosylated polyphenolic constituents. *Molecules* **2013**, *18*, 11264–11280. [CrossRef]
11. Tesch, G.H.; Allen, T.J. Rodent models of streptozotocin-induced diabetic nephropathy. *Nephrology* **2007**, *12*, 261–266. [CrossRef] [PubMed]
12. Zheng, H.; Whitman, S.A.; Wu, W.; Wondrak, G.T.; Wong, P.K.; Fang, D.; Zhang, D.D. Therapeutic Potential of Nrf2 Activators in Streptozotocin-Induced Diabetic Nephropathy. *Diabetes* **2011**, *60*, 3055–3066. [CrossRef] [PubMed]
13. Eidi, A.; Eidi, M. Antidiabetic effects of sage (*Salvia officinalis* L.) leaves in normal and streptozotocin-induced diabetic rats. *Diabetes Metab. Syndr. Clin. Res. Rev.* **2009**, *3*, 40–44. [CrossRef]

14. Walmsley, S.J.; Broeckling, C.; Hess, A.; Prenni, J.; Curthoys, N.P. Proteomic Analisis of brush-border membrane vesicles isolated from purified proximal convoluted tubules. *Am. J. Physiol.-Ren. Physiol.* **2010**, *298*, F1323–F1331. [CrossRef]
15. Dollah, M.A.; Parhizkar, S.; Izwan, M. Effect of *Nigella sativa* on the kidney function in rats. *Avicenna J. Phytomed.* **2013**, *3*, 152–156.
16. Huang, M.; Liang, Q.; Li, P. Biomarkers for early diagnosis of type 2 diabetic nephropathy: A study based on an integrated biomarker system. *Mol. BioSyst.* **2013**, *9*, 2134–2141. [CrossRef]
17. Sassy-Prigent, C.; Heudes, D.; Mandet, C. Early glomerular macrophage recruitment in streptozotocin-induced diabetic rats. *Diabetes* **2000**, *49*, 466–475. [CrossRef]
18. Rani, N.; Bharti, S.; Bhatia, J.; Nag, T.; Ray, R.; Arya, D.S. Chrysin, a PPAR-γ agonist improves myocardial injury in diabetic rats through inhibiting AGE-RAGE mediated oxidative stress and inflammation. *Chem. Biol. Interact.* **2016**, *250*, 59–67. [CrossRef]
19. Gobbay, K.H. Glycosylated haemogobin and diabetic control. *N. Eng. J. Med.* **1976**, *295*, 443–444. [CrossRef]
20. Rahbar, S.; Figarola, J.L. Novel inhibitors of advanced glycation end products. *Arch. Biochem. Biophys.* **2003**, *419*, 63–79. [CrossRef]
21. Ahangarpour, A.; Heidari, H.; Oroojan, A.A.; Mirzavandi, F.; Nasr, K.E.; Dehghan, Z.M. Antidiabetic, hypolipidemic and hepatoprotective effects of Arctium lappa root's hydro-alcoholic extract on nicotinamide-streptozotocin induced type 2 model of diabetes in male mice. *Avicenna J. Phytomed.* **2017**, *7*, 169–179. [PubMed]
22. Parker, K.M.; England, J.K.; Da-Costa, J.; Hess, R.L.; Goldstein, D.E. Improved colorimetric assay for glycosylated hemoglobin. *Clin. Chem.* **1981**, *27*, 669–672. [PubMed]
23. Kalousova, M.; Skrha, J.; Zima, T. Advanced glycation end-products and advanced oxidation protein products in patients with diabetes mellitus. *Physiol. Res.* **2002**, *51*, 597–604. [PubMed]
24. Sampathkumar, R.; Balasubramanyam, M.; Rema, M.; Premanand, C.; Mohan, V. Novel advanced glycation index and its association with diabetes and microangiopathy. *Metabolism* **2005**, *54*, 1002–1007. [CrossRef] [PubMed]
25. Fiorentino, T.V.; Marini, M.A.; Succurro, E.; Sciacqua, A.; Andreozzi, F.; Perticone, F.; Sesti, G. Elevated hemoglobin glycation index identify non-diabetic individuals at increased risk of kidney dysfunction. *Oncotarget* **2017**, *8*, 79576–79586. [CrossRef] [PubMed]

Sample Availability: Samples of the compounds are not available from the authors.

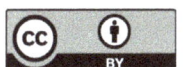

© 2019 by the authors. Licensee MDPI, Basel, Switzerland. This article is an open access article distributed under the terms and conditions of the Creative Commons Attribution (CC BY) license (http://creativecommons.org/licenses/by/4.0/).

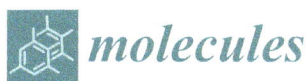

Article

In-Vitro Antioxidant, Hypoglycemic Activity, and Identification of Bioactive Compounds in Phenol-Rich Extract from the Marine Red Algae *Gracilaria edulis* (Gmelin) Silva

Thilina L. Gunathilaka [1], Kalpa W. Samarakoon [2], P. Ranasinghe [3] and L. Dinithi C. Peiris [1,*]

1. Department of Zoology, Faculty of Applied Sciences (Center for Instrumentation Facility & Center for Biotechnology), University of Sri Jayewardenepura, Nugegoda 10250, Sri Lanka; gunathilakathilina2@gmail.com
2. National Science and Technology Commission, Dudley Senanayake Mawatha, Colombo 8 00800, Sri Lanka; kalpa.samarakoon@gmail.com
3. Industrial Technology Institute, Halbarawa Gardens, Malabe 10115, Sri Lanka; pathmasiri@iti.lk
* Correspondence: dinithi@sci.sjp.ac.lk; Tel.:+94-714-018-537

Academic Editor: Lorenzo Di Cesare Mannelli
Received: 4 July 2019; Accepted: 3 October 2019; Published: 15 October 2019

Abstract: Obesity and diabetes are major metabolic disorders which are prevalent worldwide. Algae has played an important role in managing these disorders. In this study, *Gracilaria edulis*, a marine red algae, was investigated for antioxidant and hypoglycemic potential using in vitro models. De-polysaccharide methanol extract of *G. edulis* was sequentially partitioned with hexane, chloroform, ethyl acetate, and antioxidants, and hypoglycemic potentials were evaluated using multiple methods. High antioxidant potential was observed in the ethyl acetate fraction in terms of ferric reducing antioxidant power, iron chelating, and DPPH and ABTS radical scavenging activities, while the crude methanol extract exhibited potent oxygen radical-absorbance capacity. Potent α-amylase inhibitory activity was observed in the ethyl acetate fraction, while the ethyl acetate fraction was effective against α-glucosidase inhibition. Glucose diffusion was inhibited by the ethyl acetate fraction at 180 min, and the highest antiglycation activity was observed in both chloroform and ethyl acetate fractions. Additionally, gas chromatography-mass spectrometry analysis of the ethyl acetate fraction revealed the presence of several potent anti-diabetic compounds. In conclusion, *G. edulis* exhibited promising antidiabetic potential via multiple mechanisms. The ethyl acetate fraction exhibited the strongest hypoglycemic and antiglycation potential among the four fractions, and hence the isolation of active compounds is required to develop leads for new drugs to treat diabetes.

Keywords: *Gracillaria edulis*; methanol extract; fractionation; α-amylase; α-glucosidase; antiglycation; glucose diffusion

1. Introduction

The incidences of type 2 diabetes and obesity have increased globally due to rapid urbanization and unhealthy diets. More than 90% of patients with diabetes mellitus are either overweight or obese [1]. Diabetes mellitus is a chronic disorder that is linked with persistent hyperglycemia due to the deficiency of insulin secretion. The World Health Organization (WHO) has estimated that by 2035, the incidence of diabetes mellitus and impaired glucose tolerance will increase by up to 592 million and 471 million people, respectively [2]. Type 1 diabetes is widespread among Northern European countries, while type 2 diabetes is most common in African and South Asian countries. For instance, type 2 diabetes is prevalent among the Sri Lankan population [3]. According to recent statistics, one in every five Sri Lankan adults either suffers from diabetes or is in the prediabetes stage [4]. The consumption of more refined fast-release staple carbohydrate food is considered as the major cause for the progression of obesity. Carbohydrate-rich diets release glucose quickly into the bloodstream, thus increasing the levels of blood sugar and insulin [5]. High blood glucose level is linked with increased risk of hypertension, retinopathy, nephropathy, neuropathy, and macrovascular diseases. These health complications result in an increased risk of morbidity and mortality, and hence reduce the life expectancy of diabetic patients [4].

The inhibition of carbohydrate digestive enzymes—α-amylase and α-glucosidase—is one of the significant alternatives to the management of chronic hyperglycemia in diabetic patients [1]. Polyphenols purified from plants are good inhibitors of vital enzymes responsible for carbohydrate digestion. The enzymes alpha amylase and α-glucosidase are involved in carbohydrate metabolism, and act synergistically to digest starch [6]. Alpha amylase hydrolyzes the alpha bonds present in insoluble starch molecules, while α-glucosidase catalyzes the final step of carbohydrate digestion to convert disaccharides into glucose. The inhibition of such enzymes leads to a reduction of starch breakdown and an increase in postprandial blood glucose level; thus, enzyme inhibitors can be used as therapeutic agents for the development of novel drugs to treat diabetes [6].

Recent investigations have reported an association between obesity and chronic inflammation in adipose tissues. As a result of obesity, the amount of adipose tissue tends to increase and the tissue undergoes molecular and cellular alterations. Adipocytokines secreted by the adipocytes in adipose tissues can induce production of reactive oxygen species, thus leading to oxidative stress [7]. Oxidative stress is tightly linked with the pathophysiological process of chronic inflammatory conditions such as diabetes mellitus [8]. Therefore, researchers have primarily focused on natural products to discover novel preventive and regenerative therapies to combat oxidative stress and postprandial hyperglycemia with minimum side effects.

Marine seaweeds rich in bioactive metabolites play a significant role in the development of novel drugs and nutraceuticals. Due to the bioactive compounds they contain—namely polyphenols, sterols, alkaloids, flavonoids, tannins, proteins, essential fatty acids, enzymes, vitamins, and carotenoids—marine seaweeds are able to withstand harsh environments [9]. *Gracilaria edulis* (Gmelin) Silva is a red algae belonging to the family Gracilariaceae, and it has attracted widespread attention due to its biological and pharmacological properties and various therapeutic benefits such as antidiabetic, antioxidant, antimicrobial, anticoagulant, anti-inflammatory, and antiproliferative activities [10]. Shanura et al. [11] established the anti-inflammatory activity of methanol extract and fractions of *G. edulis* against lipopolysaccharide-induced inflammatory responses, while Koneri and Jha [12] documented the antidiabetic potential of methanol extracts of *G. edulis* against fructose-induced type 2 diabetes mellitus in male rats. Patra and Muthuraman [13] revealed the anticancer activity of ethanol extracts of *G. edulis* against ascites tumors in mice. Although past studies focused on several biological properties of *G. edulis*, this is the first study carried out in Sri Lanka to investigate the antioxidant and hypoglycemic activities of *G. edulis* using multiple in vitro mechanisms. The present study aimed to appraise the antidiabetic potential of *G. edulis* through inhibitory activities of carbohydrate digestive enzymes, glucose diffusion, and protein glycation. We also attempted to identify the bioactive compounds present in *G. edulis* that are responsible for the above pharmacological activities.

2. Results

2.1. Quantification of Total Phenolic, Flavonoid, and Alkaloid Contents of G. edulis

Results obtained for the crude methanol extract and four fractions of *G. edulis* with increasing polarity were used to evaluate the total phenolic, flavonoid, and alkaloid contents of *G. edulis*. These results are shown in Table 1. The alkaloid content in the crude methanol extract and in the hexane and chloroform fractions was higher than the phenol and flavonoid contents, whereas the phenol content in the ethyl acetate and aqueous fractions was higher than the flavonoid and alkaloid contents.

Table 1. Phenol, flavonoid, and alkaloid contents of crude methanol extract and fractions of *Gracillaria edulis*.

Extract/Fraction	TPC (μg GAE/g)	TFC (μg QE/g)	Total Alkaloids (μg PE/g)
Crude methanol extract	1007.81 ± 54.21 [a]	541.02 ± 51.84 [a]	7177.72 ± 63.04 [a]
Hexane fraction	760.85 ± 37.75 [b]	688.60 ± 9.55 [a]	1656.97 ± 45.80 [b]
Chloroform fraction	560.85 ± 55.08 [c]	289.39 ± 9.55 [b]	2875.54 ± 22.29 [c]
Ethyl acetate fraction	2414.51 ± 50.34 [d]	1461.49 ± 75.22 [c]	1073.75 ± 45.88 [b]
Aqueous fraction	1704.69 ± 43.16 [e]	786.95 ± 62.04 [d]	522.34 ± 67.13 [d]

TPC: total phenol content; TFC: total flavonoid content; GAE: gallic acid equivalent; QE: quercetin equivalent; PE: Piperine equivalent. Data presented as mean ± standard deviation ($n = 4$). Mean values in a column superscripted by different letters ([a–e]) are significantly different at $p < 0.05$.

The total phenolic content in the ethyl acetate fraction (2414.51 ± 50.34 μg GAE/g) was higher than that in the crude methanol extract and the hexane, chloroform, and aqueous fractions. The lowest total phenolic content was observed in the chloroform fraction. Similarly, a significant difference was observed in the phenolic content of the crude methanol extract and the four fractions ($p < 0.05$). The total flavonoid content of the crude methanol extract and all fractions increased in the order chloroform fraction < crude methanol extract < hexane fraction < aqueous fraction < ethyl acetate fraction, with respective contents of 289.39 ± 9.55, 541.02 ± 51.84, 688.60 ± 9.55, 786.95 ± 62.04, and 1461.49 ± 75.22 μg QE/g. Among the crude methanol extract and four fractions, total alkaloid content decreased in the order crude methanol extract > chloroform fraction > hexane fraction > ethyl acetate fraction > aqueous fraction, with respective values of 7177.72 ± 63.04, 2875.54 ± 22.29, 1656.97 ± 45.80, 1073.75 ± 45.88, and 522.34 ± 67.13 μg PE/g.

2.2. In Vitro Antioxidant Activity

The antioxidant capacity of crude methanol extract and fractions of *G. edulis* were determined using 1,1-diphenyl-2-picrylhydrazine (DPPH) and 2,2′-azino-bis (3-ethylbenzothiazoline-6-sulphonic acid) (ABTS) radical scavenging activities, ferrous ion chelating assay, ferric reducing antioxidant power, and oxygen radical-absorbance capacity. The results obtained for the antioxidant capacity are presented in Table 2.

The highest DPPH radical scavenging activity was observed in the ethyl acetate fraction (IC_{50}: 3.17 ± 0.04 mg/mL) and the crude methanol extract (IC_{50}: 3.19 ± 0.02 mg/mL). By comparison, the standard Trolox had free radical scavenging activity of IC_{50}: 0.011 mg/mL. In this study, the reduction of DPPH occurred in a concentration-dependent manner, as observed from the high reduction of DPPH (higher radical activity) at 3.75 mg/mL concentrations (Figure A1). The most potent ABTS radical scavenging activity was observed in the ethyl acetate fraction (IC_{50}: 0.41 ± 0.02 mg/mL), while the lowest activity was observed in the crude methanol extract (IC_{50}: 0.56 ± 0.01 mg/mL). Moreover, a significant positive correlation was observed between the radical scavenging activity of DPPH ($r = 0.91$) and that of ABTS ($r = 0.85$) with the total phenol content of the ethyl acetate fraction. The highest ferrous iron chelating activity (FICA) was observed in the ethyl acetate fraction (IC_{50}: 2.22 ± 0.01 mg/mL), while the lowest ferrous ion chelating activity was observed in the crude methanol extract (IC_{50}: 9.23 ± 0.19 mg/mL); the standard EDTA (ethylenediaminetetraacetic acid) exhibited a chelating activity of IC_{50}: 0.019 mg/mL. Ferric reducing antioxidant powder (FRAP) and oxygen radical absorbance capacity (ORAC) are the most frequent measures used to determine antioxidant activity, which is expressed as Trolox equivalent antioxidant capacity. The ethyl acetate fraction of *G. edulis* showed the highest reducing ability (8.51 ± 0.09 mg TE/g), while crude methanol extract (1.61 ± 0.19 mg TE/g) showed potent oxygen radical absorbance capacity.

Table 2. IC$_{50}$ values of methanol extract of *G. edulis* and fractions against antioxidant activity and activities equivalent to standards.

Extract/Fraction	IC$_{50}$ (mg/mL)			Activity Equivalent to Standard (mg TE/g)	
	DPPH	ABTS	FICA	FRAP	ORAC
Crude methanol extract	3.19 ± 0.02 [a]	0.56 ± 0.01 [a]	9.23 ± 0.19 [a]	0.26 ± 0.03 [a]	1.61 ± 0.19 [a]
Hexane fraction	6.22 ± 0.01 [b]	0.54 ± 0.01 [b]	2.58 ± 0.03 [bc]	1.93 ± 0.35 [b]	0.57 ± 0.07 [bc]
Chloroform fraction	3.29 ± 0.02 [c]	0.44 ± 0.01 [c]	2.43 ± 0.01 [c]	2.19 ± 0.23 [b]	0.77 ± 0.05 [b]
Ethyl acetate fraction	3.17 ± 0.04 [a]	0.41 ± 0.02 [d]	2.22 ± 0.01 [bc]	8.51 ± 0.09 [c]	1.44 ± 0.29 [a]
Aqueous fraction	3.91 ± 0.03 [d]	0.45 ± 0.03 [c]	2.71 ± 0.02 [b]	1.23 ± 0.21 [d]	0.44 ± 0.09 [c]
Trolox (standard)	0.011 ± 0.00 [e]	0.008 ± 0.00 [e]	-	-	-
EDTA (standard)	-	-	0.019 ± 00 [d]	-	-

Results are expressed as mean ± SD; $n = 4$. DPPH (1,1-diphenyl-2-picrylhydrazine); ABTS (2,2′-azino-bis (3-ethylbenzothiazoline-6-sulphonic acid)); FICA (ferrous iron chelating activity); FRAP (ferric reducing antioxidant powder); ORAC (oxygen radical absorbance capacity); EDTA (ethylenediaminetetraacetic acid); TE (Trolox equivalent). Mean values in a column superscripted by different letters ([a–e]) are significantly different at $p < 0.05$.

2.3. In Vitro α-Amylase Inhibitory Assay

The α-amylase inhibitory potential of *G. edulis* methanol extract and four fractions was evaluated using starch as the substrate and acarbose as the positive control. Acarbose, crude methanol extract, and the four fractions exhibited a dose-dependent enzyme inhibition (Figure A2).

The ethyl acetate fraction (IC$_{50}$: 279.48 ± 5.62 µg/mL) of *G. edulis* exhibited more potent α-amylase inhibitory activity, whereas the lowest activity was observed in the hexane fraction (IC$_{50}$: 393.04 ± 4.73 µg/mL) (Table 3) compared to the standard acarbose (IC$_{50}$: 87.43 µg/mL). The inhibition of the α-amylase enzyme exhibited by the ethyl acetate fraction varied from 10% at 12.5 µg/mL to 64% at 400 µg/mL assay concentration.

Table 3. IC$_{50}$ values exhibited by *G. edulis* methanol extract and methanol fractions against the inhibitory activity of the enzymes α-amylase and α-glucosidase and antiglycation activities.

Extract/Fraction	Alpha-Amylase (µg/mL)	Alpha-Glucosidase (µg/mL)	Anti-Glycation (µg/mL)
Crude methanol extract	349.59 ± 2.44 [a]	102.24 ± 0.89 [a]	702.33 ± 12.72 [a]
Hexane fraction	393.04 ± 4.73 [b]	163.90 ± 5.23 [b]	637.53 ± 6.21 [b]
Chloroform fraction	322.71 ± 4.80 [c]	122.65 ± 2.37 [c]	258.23 ± 3.24 [c]
Ethyl acetate fraction	279.48 ± 5.62 [d]	87.92 ± 1.62 [d]	586.54 ± 4.37 [b]
Aqueous fraction	376.49 ± 12.14 [e]	148.57 ± 1.87 [e]	723.78 ± 12.81 [d]
Acarbose (standard)	87.43 ± 0.59 [f]	0.38 ± 0.06 [f]	-
Rutin (standard)	-	-	11.55 ± 0.82 [e]

Results are expressed as mean ± SD ($n = 4$). *$p < 0.05$ compared with the respective standard. Mean values in a column superscripted by different letters ([a–f]) are significantly different at $p < 0.05$.

2.4. In Vitro α-Glucosidase Inhibitory Assay

All the fractions and the crude methanol extract of *G. edulis* exhibited a dose-dependent inhibition of the α-glucosidase enzyme with different degrees of potential (Figure A3). The inhibitory activity on α-glucosidase enzymes of the crude methanol extract and the fractions of *G. edulis* are presented in Table 3. The ethyl acetate fraction, which exhibited the lowest IC$_{50}$ of 87.92 ± 1.62 µg/mL, was considered to be a more potent α-glucosidase inhibitor than the crude methanol extract and the other three fractions. The inhibition of α-glucosidase exhibited by the ethyl acetate fraction varied from 6% (4.16 µg/mL) to 68% (133.3 µg/mL). The hexane fraction, which had the highest IC$_{50}$ of 163.90 ± 5.23 µg/mL, exhibited the weakest α-glucosidase inhibitory activity.

2.5. Glucose Diffusion Inhibitory Activity

The inhibitory activity of glucose diffusion was determined using a dialysis tube containing the sample and glucose that had been soaked in NaCl solution. The diffusion of glucose into the external solution was measured by glucose oxidase kit every 30 min for 3 h. The effects of the methanol extract and the four fractions of *G. edulis* (1000 µg/mL) on glucose diffusion are represented in Figure 1. The inhibitory activity of acarbose or the reference drug was considered as 100%, while the glucose diffusion of the control at 180 min was considered as 100% with a glucose concentration of 57.65 ± 1.67 µg/mL in the external solution, compared to the acarbose standard (22.79 ± 0.47 µg/mL). Among the tested fractions, the ethyl acetate fractions exhibited the maximum inhibition of glucose diffusion at 180 min, and the glucose concentration of the external solution was found to be 38.15 ± 1.11 µg/mL. The inhibition of glucose diffusion by the hexane fraction (52.01 ± 0.96 µg/mL) and aqueous fraction (52.69 ± 1.31 µg/mL) were similar compared to the glucose concentration in the external solution (Table A1).

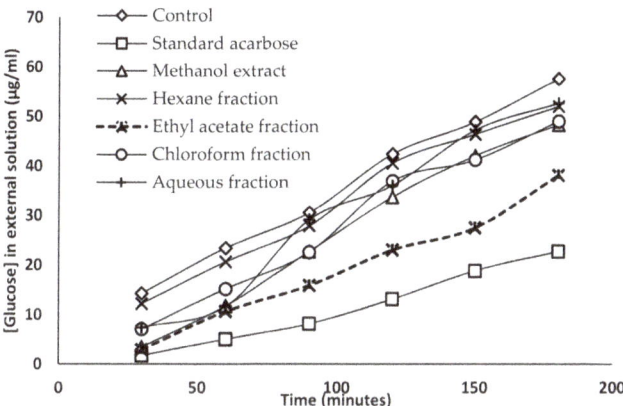

Figure 1. Effect of methanol extract and fractions of *G. edulis* (1000 µg/mL) on glucose diffusion through dialysis membrane compared to the standard acarbose and control. Data presented as means ± standard deviation ($n = 4$).

2.6. Antiglycation Activity

The anti-glycation activity of the crude methanol extract and fractions of *G. edulis* was determined using bovine serum albumin as a protein source. The crude methanol extract and all four fractions showed dose-dependent antiglycation activity (Figure 2). As shown in Table 3, among the tested fractions, the most potent antiglycation activity was observed with the chloroform fraction (IC_{50}: 258.23 ± 3.24 µg/mL), followed by the ethyl acetate fraction (IC_{50}: 586.54 ± 4.37 µg/mL), compared to the standard rutin (IC_{50}: 11.55 ± 0.82 µg/mL). The aqueous fraction, which had the highest IC_{50} value of 723.78 ± 12.81 µg/mL, exhibited the weakest antiglycation activity.

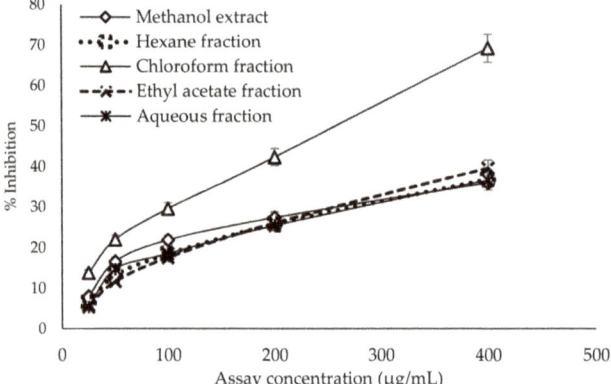

Figure 2. Dose–response relationship of methanol extract and its fractions of *G. edulis* for antiglycation activity determined by glucose-induced protein glycation and formation of protein-bound fluorescent advanced glycation end products. Data presented as mean ± standard deviation ($n = 4$).

2.7. GC-MS or Gas Chromatography-Mass Spectrometry Analysis of Extract and Solvent Fractions

The ethyl acetate fraction of *G. edulis*, which showed promising biological activities, was subjected to gas chromatography-mass spectrometry (GC-MS) analysis. The chromatogram obtained for the ethyl acetate fraction is presented in Figure 3.

Based on the retention time and molecular weights of the GC-MS chromatogram, six compounds were identified in the ethyl acetate fraction of *G. edulis*. As listed in Table 4, these compounds included 2,5-dimethylhexane-2,5-dihydroperoxide, phthalic acid-6-ethyloct-3-yl 2-ethylhexyl ester, 1H-Indole-2-carboxylic acid, 6-(4-ethoxyphenyl)-3-methyl-4-oxo-4,5,6,7-tetrahydro-isopropylester, 2,3,5-Trichlorobenzaldehyde, Benz(b)1,4-oxazepine-4 (5H)-thione, 2,3-dihydro-2,8-dimethyl, and 2-acetoxymethyl-3-(methoxycarbonyl) biphenylene.

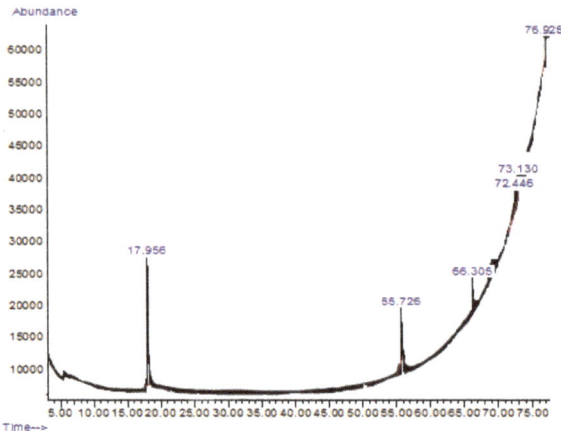

Figure 3. Chromatograms obtained from the gas chromatography-mass spectrometry (GC-MS) analysis of the ethyl acetate fraction of *G. edulis*.

Table 4. Active compounds identified in the ethyl acetate fraction of *G. edulis* by gas chromatography-mass spectrometry (GC-MS) analysis.

Retention Time and %	Name	Molecular Formula	Compound Class	Reported Biological Activity
17.956 (54.27%)	2,5-Dimethylhexane-2,5-dihydroperoxide	$C_8H_{18}O_4$	Organic compound	Anti-inflammatory Antioxidant [14,15]
55.726 (11.46%)	Phthalic acid-6-ethyloct-3-yl 2-ethylhexyl ester	$C_{26}H_{42}O_4$	Phthalic acid derivative	Anticancer Antimicrobial [16]
66.305 (15.39%)	1H-Indole-2-carboxylic acid,6-(4-ethoxyphenyl)-3-methyl-4-oxo-4,5,6,7-tetrahydro-isopropyl ester	$C_{19}H_{20}FNO_3$	Indole derivative	Antidiabetic [17,18]
72.446 (10.93%)	1,2-dimethoxy-4 (1,3-dimethoxy-1-propenyl) benzene	$C_{13}H_{18}O_4$	Benzene derivatives	Antifungal [19]
73.130 (1.52%)	Benz(b)1,4-oxazepine-4 (5H)-thione, 2,3-dihydro-2,8-dimethyl	$C_{11}H_{13}NOS$	Benzoxazepine derivatives	Anti-inflammatory Antimicrobial [20]
76.925 (6.49%)	2-acetoxymethyl-3-(methoxycarbonyl)biphenylene	$C_{17}H_{14}O_4$	Biphenyl derivatives	Antibacterial [21]

Among these active compounds, 1H-Indole-2-carboxylic acid,6-(4-ethoxyphenyl)-3-methyl-4-oxo-4,5,6,7-tetrahydro-isopropyl ester was identified as possessing antidiabetic activity through insulin sensitizing and glucose lowering effects [17]. In addition, most of the indole derivatives act as an activators of glycogen synthase enzyme, which involved in the glycogen synthesis pathway [18], while 2,5-dimethylhexane-2,5-dihydroperoxide has been identified to have antioxidant properties which help to prevent the development of oxidative stress related to diabetes [14,15].

3. Discussion

Recently, red marine algae has received significant attention due to its immense therapeutic benefits. However, only a limited number of studies have been performed on Sri Lankan marine algae. Therefore, to discover the therapeutic potential of tropical marine algae against diabetes and obesity, we studied *G. edulis*, a red algae from the northwestern coast of Sri Lanka to investigate its mechanisms of action.

Polyphenols, flavonoids, and alkaloids are secondary plant metabolites that have shown therapeutic benefits and are considered as potential sources of antioxidants. The polyphenol, flavonoid, and alkaloid contents of plants may vary depending on environmental factors, soil type, sun exposure, rainfall, etc. [22]. As determined by the present study, the ethyl acetate fraction of *G. edulis* contained the highest phenol and flavonoid content, whereas the highest alkaloid content was observed in the crude methanol extract of *G. edulis*. The present study found comparatively lower phenolic content compared to the results of Ganesan et al. [23], who reported 3.98 mg/mL phenolic content. This variation may be due to the different sample collection locations, temperature conditions, and stress tolerance [24].

Oxidative stress is linked with the development of diabetes, and increases in accumulated fat in obese individuals through the activation of nicotinamide adenine dinucleotide phosphate (NADPH) oxidase and the impaired production of adipocytokines [25]. The antioxidant activity determined by the DPPH assay revealed high free radical scavenging activities in the ethyl acetate fraction and crude methanol extract of *G. edulis*, which occurred in a concentration-dependent manner (Figure A1). In the present study, strong DPPH free-radical scavenging ability was observed at 950 µg/mL of the ethyl acetate fraction (21.06%) and crude methanol extract (19.52%). This result contradicts a previous report in India [23]; compared to the present study, [16] reported lower DPPH free radical scavenging activity of the ethyl acetate fraction (4.73%) and the crude methanol extract (5.20%). The higher antioxidant activity observed in the present study may be due to the use of different extraction procedures and the differences in the phenolic compounds responsible for antioxidant activity.

The highest ABTS radical scavenging activity was observed in the ethyl acetate fraction of *G. edulis*, with a significant positive correlation being observed with total phenol content (r = 85). The reducing power of the sample depends on the available phenol and flavonoid contents of the sample [26]. In the present study, the ethyl acetate fraction exhibited the highest FRAP activity, which can be attributed to the presence of phenolic or flavonoid compounds with functional groups such as hydroxyl and carbonyl, which leads to the reduction or inhibition of oxidation. In contrast, Francavilla et al. reported the highest ABTS radical scavenging activity and ferric reducing antioxidant power in ethyl acetate fraction (0.43 and 0.809 mmol TE/g) of *G.edulis* collected seasonally in the Lesina Lagoon in Italy during the period of July [27]. Similarly, the ethyl acetate fraction of the present study exhibited higher reducing power compared to the previous study, which was collected in February. Therefore, differences in reducing power might be due to the seasonal variation.

The chelating power of the sample was determined using ferrozine reagent. Ferrozine can chelate with Fe^{2+}, forming a red-colored ferrozine-Fe^{2+} complex [28]. According to the chelation activity, the highest FICA was observed in the ethyl acetate fraction. The ORAC assay determines the oxidative degradation of fluorescein in the presence of a free radical generator, such as an azo compound, for example, 2-azobis (2-amidinopropane) dihydrochloride [29]. The ORAC assay confirmed the high antioxidant capacity of the crude methanol extract of *G. edulis*. The high phenol and flavonoid contents of the ethyl acetate fraction are responsible for the potent antioxidant activity of *G. edulis*. Additionally, the presence of bioactive compounds such as 2,5-dimethylhexane-2,5-dihydroperoxide may also contribute to the antioxidant activity of *G. edulis*.

The inhibition of key metabolic carbohydrate-digesting enzymes is one of the main strategies to determine the antidiabetic activity of medicinal plants [30]. Therefore, natural bioactive compounds that reduce blood glucose levels by inhibiting the key metabolic enzymes (α-amylase, α-glucosidase) and glucose absorption can be considered to be useful for the management of diabetes [31]. From the results, it is evident that the ethyl acetate fraction of *G. edulis* showed potential inhibitory activities with an effective dose for inhibition of α-amylase (IC_{50}: 279.48 ± 5.62 µg/mL) and α-glucosidase (IC_{50}: 87.92 ± 1.62 µg/mL) enzymes that are comparable to the standard drug acarbose (Table 3). The potential enzyme-inhibiting activity of the ethyl acetate fraction of *G. edulis* can be attributed to the presence of phytochemicals such as phenolic and flavonoid compounds. Senthil and Sudha [32] reported potent effective doses of inhibitory activity of α-amylase (IC_{50}: 83 µg/mL) and α-glucosidase (IC_{50}: 46 µg/mL) in an aqueous extract of *G. edulis* collected from India. The difference between the results obtained in the present study may be due to the different solvents used for the extraction method; in the present study, polyphenol was initially used to extract methanol, while the study conducted by Senthil and Sudha used water as a solvent.

The glucose diffusion inhibition test was carried out to evaluate the effect of methanol extract and fractions of *G.edulis*, with respect to its glucose retardation activity across the dialysis tube. The glucose entrapment ability of the crude methanol extract and four fractions were found to be significantly different at different times. Among them, the ethyl acetate fraction of *G.edulis* exhibited a significant glucose entrapment ability, which decreased the glucose movement into the external solution at 180 min compared to the control. The fact that the ethyl acetate fraction exhibited the highest inhibition of glucose diffusion may be due to the presence of insoluble fiber particles which entrap glucose molecules [33,34]. The dialysis tube method is a simple technique, which only determines the potential effect of methanol extract and fractions of *G.edulis* to retard the glucose diffusion through the normal dialysis membrane, whereas in the intestinal tract, transportation of glucose is assisted by glucose transporters incorporated with other molecules, in addition to the intestinal contractions [35]. Therefore, further in vivo studies should be carried out to determine the real effect of methanol extract and fractions of *G. edulis* on glucose diffusion.

Chronic hyperglycemia in diabetic patients leads to the progression of microvascular and macrovascular complications. The high level of blood glucose leads to the formation of a complex between glucose and plasma proteins through non-enzymatic reactions and forms AGEs, which are associated with the pathogenesis of vascular complications in diabetes, renal failure, Alzheimer's disease, aging, and other chronic diseases [27]. The present study is the first to report the inhibitory activity of the methanol extract and four fractions of *G. edulis* on the formation of AGE products. The results of the study show that the lowest effective dose of inhibition of AGE formation was exhibited by chloroform (IC_{50}:258.23 ± 3.24 µg/mL) and ethyl acetate fractions (IC_{50}: 586.54 ± 4.37 µg/mL) of *G. edulis*, compared to the standard drug rutin. The antiglycation activity of the chloroform and ethyl acetate fractions may be due to the presence of phenolic and flavonoid compounds, which are significantly correlated with anti-glycation activity [36].

Furthermore, GC-MS analysis of the ethyl acetate fraction of *G. edulis* revealed the presence of active compounds with strong antioxidant and antidiabetic activity, including 1*H*-Indole-2-carboxylic acid,6-(4-ethoxyphenyl)-3-methyl-4-oxo-4,5,6,7-tetrahydro-isopropyl ester and 2,5-dimethylhexane-2,5-dihydroperoxide. 1*H*-Indole-2-carboxylicacid,6-(4-ethoxyphenyl)-3-methyl-4-oxo-4,5,6,7 tetrahydro-isopropyl ester is an indole derivative, which has insulin sensitizing and glucose lowering effects [17]. In addition, most of the indole derivatives act as an activator of the glycogen synthase enzyme, which is involved in the glycogen synthesis pathway [18], while 2,5-dimethylhexane-2,5-dihydroperoxide was identified to have antioxidant properties, which help to prevent the development of oxidative stress related to diabetes [14,15].

4. Materials and Methods

4.1. Chemicals and Reagents

Trolox, DPPH, trichloroacetic acid, ABTS, potassium persulpahte, 2,4,6-tripyridyl-s-triazine (TPTZ), soluble starch, Folin–Ciocalteu reagent, alpha glucosidase from *Saccharomyces cerevisiae*, gallic acid, acarbose, quercetin, aluminum chloride, *p*-nitrophenyl a-D-glucopyranoside, bovine serum albumin (BSA), and alpha-amylase were purchased from Sigma Aldrich (Allentown, PA, USA). The chemicals and reagents used for all experiments were of analytical grade.

4.2. Collection of Algae Sample

Permission to collect an algae sample was obtained from the Department of Wildlife Conservation (permit number WL/3/280/17). Marine red algae (*Gracillaria edulis*) was manually collected from Kalpitiya, Sri Lanka (6^0 4' 54.19" N; 80^0 8' 51.78" E). The samples were identified based on their morphological characteristics by Dr. Kalpa Samarakoon. The collected samples were cleaned and washed with fresh water to remove salt, sand, and other debris. The samples were freeze-dried using a LyoBeta freeze drying unit (Telstar), powdered, and stored at −20 °C until further use.

4.3. Preparation of Gracillaria edulis Extract and Its Solvent Fractions

The extraction procedure was conducted according to the method of Lakmal et al., [37] with some modifications. Homogenized *G. edulis* powder was extracted three times using 70% methanol, and was then subjected to sonication (Clifton, 91695) at 25 °C. Polyphenols were separated using 70% ethanol ($v/w\%$ = 1:25) and allowed to stand overnight. The supernatant was separated by centrifugation (Centurion K241R, Surrey, UK) at 12,000 rpm before being filtered to separate the polyphenol portion. A portion of the de-polysaccharide methanol extract was subjected to sequential solvent–solvent partition with hexane, chloroform, and ethyl acetate, respectively. Finally, the four fractions and crude methanol extract were dried under vacuum (BUCHI, Rotavapor, R-300, New Castle, DE, USA) and used to conduct the assays.

4.4. Quantification of Phenol, Flavonoid, and Alkaloid Contents

The total phenol content of the methanol extract and fractions was evaluated using the Folin–Ciocalteu method ($n = 4$). Different concentrations (5, 10, and 20 mg/mL) of methanol extract and the four fractions were prepared by diluting with distilled water. The sample (20 µL), diluted Folin–Ciocalteu reagent (110 µl), and 10% sodium carbonate solution (70 µL) were mixed and incubated at room temperature for 30 min. Absorbance was measured at 765 nm. Gallic acid was used as the standard, and results were expressed as mg gallic acid equivalent per 1 g of dry weight of the extract/fraction [38].

The total flavonoid content of the methanol extract and fractions ($n = 4$) of *G. edulis* were evaluated by the aluminium chloride method [39]. Different concentrations (5, 10, and 20 mg/mL) of the methanol extract and fractions were prepared by diluting with methanol. The absorbance before adding the 2% aluminum chloride was taken at 415 nm. A total of 100 µl of 2% aluminium chloride solution was added and incubated at room temperature for 10 min. A plate reading was recorded at 415 nm. Quercetin was used as a standard, and results was expressed as mg quercetin equivalent per 1 g of dry weight of the extract or reaction.

The total alkaloid content of the methanol extract and fractions ($n = 4$) of *G. edulis* was evaluated by the method described by Sreevidya et al. [40] with some modifications. Different concentrations (5, 10, and 20 mg/mL) of the methanol extract and fractions of *G. edulis* were prepared by diluting with 95% ethanol and pH was adjusted to 2–2.5. A total of 100 µL of sample was mixed with 200 µL of Dragendorff reagent and centrifuged at 5000 rpm for 5 min. The precipitate was separated and washed with 95% ethanol. A total of 200 µL of 1% disodium sulfide solution was added, and the resulting brownish-black precipitate was centrifuged at 5000 rpm for 5 min. The supernatant was discarded and the pellet was dissolved in concentrated HNO_3 and diluted up to 1 mL with distilled water. A total of 100 µL of the solution was pipetted and mixed with 500 µL of 3% thiourea. Absorbance was recorded at 460 nm. Piperine was used as the standard, and the results were expressed as mg piperine equivalent per 1 g of dry weight of extract or fraction.

4.5. In Vitro Antioxidant Activity

4.5.1. DPPH Radical Scavenging Activity

The DPPH scavenging activity of the extracts and fractions of *G. edulis* ($n = 4$) was determined using the method described by Blois [41]. A concentration series (3.75, 1.875, 0.938, 0.469, 0.234, 0.1170, and 0.058 mg/mL) of algal samples was prepared in methanol. A total of 50 µL of sample was mixed with methanol and absorbance before adding the DPPH solution was taken at 517 nm. Subsequently, DPPH solution was added and incubated in a dark area for 15 min at 25 °C. After incubation, a plate reading was taken at 517 nm. Trolox was used as the standard, and the DPPH scavenging activity was expressed as mg Trolox equivalent per 1 g of dry weight of extract or fraction.

4.5.2. $ABTS^+$ Radical Scavenging Activity

The $ABTS^+$ scavenging activity was measured using the method described by Re et al. [42]. Before conducting the experiment, $ABTS^+$ radical was produced by incubating ABTS tablet (10 mg) with 2.5 mM potassium persulpahte solution (2.5 mL). Five different concentrations (0.5, 0.25, 0.125, 0.063, and 0.031mg/mL) of the methanol extract and fractions ($n = 4$) were diluted in 50 mM PBS (pH 7.4) and absorbance before adding ABTS reagent was taken at 734 nm. A total of 40 µL of diluted ABTS+ reagent was added and incubated for 10 min at room temperature. After incubation, a plate recording was taken at 734 nm. Trolox was used as the standard antioxidant and the results were expressed as mg Trolox equivalent per 1 g of dry weight of extract or fraction.

4.5.3. Ferric Reducing Antioxidant Power (FRAP)

Ferric reducing antioxidant power was measured according to the method of Benzie and Szeto [43], with some modifications. Different concentrations (5, 2.5, 1, and 0.5 mg/mL) of the methanol extract and four fractions (n = 4) were diluted in 300 mM acetate butter (pH 3.6). Before conducting the experiment, FRAP reagent was prepared using 300 mM acetate buffer (pH 3.6), 10 mM of 2,4,6-tripyridyl-s-triazine (TPTZ), and 20 mM $FeCl_3$ solution mixed with a ratio of 10:1:1 and incubated at 37 °C for 10 min. The FRAP reagent (150 µL), acetate buffer (30 µL), and algae samples (20 µL) were mixed together and incubated for 8 min at room temperature. After incubation, a plate reading was made at 600 nm. Trolox was used as the standard and the results were expressed as mg Trolox equivalent per 1 g dry weight of extract or fraction.

4.5.4. Ferrous Iron Chelating Capacity (FICC)

The ferrous iron chelating capacity (FICC) was measured using the method of Carter [44], with some modifications. Five different concentrations (6.25, 5, 3.13, 2.5, and 1.56 mg/mL) of the methanol extract and fractions were diluted in distilled water, 1 mM ferrozine (4,4-disulfonic acid sodium salt) solution, and 1 mM ferrous sulphate solution (n = 4). Algal samples (100 µL), $FeSo_4$ solution (20 µL), and distilled water (40 µL) were mixed, and absorbance before adding ferrozine solution was taken at 562 nm. Ferrozine solution (40 µL) was mixed and incubated for 10 min at room temperature. A plate reading was recorded at 562 nm and the results were expressed as mg EDTA equivalent per 1 g of dry weight of the extract or fraction.

4.5.5. Oxygen Radical Absorbance Capacity (ORAC)

The ORAC was measured using the method of Ou et al. [45], with modifications. Different concentrations (5, 2.5, and 1.25 mg/mL) of the extract and fractions were diluted in phosphate buffer saline (75 mM, pH 7.4). Before conducting the experiment, flourcein (16 mg in 100 mL of phosphate buffer saline) and AAPH [2,2'-azobis (2-amidinopropane) dihydrochloride] solutions (40 mg in 1 mL of phosphate buffer saline) were prepared. The reaction mixture (200 µL), containing algal samples (10 µL), PBS (40 µL) and fluorescein solution (100 µL), was preincubated at 37 °C for 5 min. After incubation, AAPH solution was added and absorbance recordings were made at excitation and emission wavelengths of 494 nm and 535 nm, respectively, at 1 min intervals for 35 min. Trolox was used as the standard, and the results were expressed as mg Trolox equivalent per 1 g dry weight of the sample.

4.6. In Vitro α-amylase and α-glucosidase Inhibitory Assay

4.6.1. Alpha-Amylase Inhibitory Activity

The anti-amylase activity was measured using the method of Bernfeld [46], with modifications (n = 4). Various concentrations of the algal extract (400, 200, 100, 50, 25, and 12.5 µg/mL) and acarbose (200, 100, 50, 25, 12.5, and 6.25 µg/mL) were preincubated with starch (40 µL) and sodium acetate buffer (710 µL) at 40 °C in a shaking water bath (Wise Bath, WSB-30, Wertherim, Germany) for 10 min. The α-amylase enzyme solution (50 µl:1 mg/mL) was added and incubated again for 15 min. After incubation, 500 µL of 3,5-dinitrosalicylic acid (DNS) solution was added and boiled for 5 min until color developed and was then kept in an ice bath to cool. The absorbance was recorded at 540 nm using a SpectraMax Plus 384 instrument (Molecular Devices, San Jose, CA, USA). Another experiment was carried out in an identical way by replacing enzyme solution with acetate buffer to determine the absorbance produced by the sample itself. A control experiment was conducted by replacing extracts with 100 mM sodium acetate buffer. Acarbose was used as the standard and percentage α-amylase inhibition was calculated.

4.6.2. Alpha-Glucosidase Inhibitory Activity

The α-glucosidase inhibition assay was performed according to the method of Matsui et al. [47], with some modifications. Different concentrations of algal samples (133.3, 66.6, 33.3, 16.6, 8.3, and 4.16 µg/mL) or acarbose (2.5, 1.25, 0.625, 0.313, 0.156, 0.078, and 0.039 µg/mL) in acetate buffer, and p-nitrophenyl-a-D-glucopyranoside (PNPG) solution were incubated at 37 °C for 5 min. After measuring the absorbance, 25 mU/mL of α-glucosidase was added and incubated at 37 °C for 35 min. After incubation, 10% NaCO$_3$ solution was added to stop the reaction. The absorbance was then recorded at 400 nm. The reaction mixture without extract was used as the control and anti-glucosidase activity (% inhibition) was calculated.

4.6.3. Glucose Diffusion Inhibitory Activity

Glucose diffusion inhibitory activity was determined using a dialysis bag and a glucose oxidase kit [48]. Initially, a dialysis membrane (D9777) was activated according to the manufacturer's instructions. Briefly, 2 mL of the algae sample (1 mg/mL) was placed in a dialysis tube with 2 mL of 0.22 mM glucose solution. Subsequently, the dialysis tube was dipped in a beaker containing 80 mL of 0.15M NaCl and 20 mL of distilled water and was shaken constantly at 150 rpm at 37 °C. The glucose concentration (µg/mL) in the external solution was measured at 30 min intervals for 3 h using a GAGO-20 glucose oxidase kit (Sigma Aldrich). Acarbose and distilled water were used as the standard and the control, respectively.

4.6.4. Antiglycation Activity

Antiglycation activity was measured using the method of Matsuura et al. [49], with some modifications. Algal extracts were prepared by dissolving with phosphate buffer saline. Bovine serum albumin (80 µL), algae extract (80 µL), 400 mM glucose (360 µL), and 50 mM PBS (pH 7.4, 480 µL) was incubated at 60 °C for 50 h. After incubation, the solution was cooled and 200 µl of 50% trichloroacetic acid was added and centrifuged at 15,000 rpm at 4 °C for 4 min. The resulting precipitate was dissolved in PBS (pH 10) and absorbance values were recorded at an excitation wavelength of 370 nm and emission wavelength of 440 nm (Amino-Bowman Series 2, Thermo Spectronic, Fitchburd, WI, USA). A sample negative was carried out in the same way, however without adding glucose. A sample control was conducted by replacing algal extracts with 50 mM PBS. Rutin was used as the standard and antiglycation activity (% inhibition) was calculated.

4.7. GC-MS Analysis of Extract and Solvent Fractions

The GC-MS analysis was performed on active fraction (ethyl acetate fraction) using a 5975C gas chromatograph (Agilent Technologies, Palo Alto, CA, USA) and an HP-5MS capillary column (30 m × 25 µm with a film thickness of 0.25 µm). Briefly, the sample (1 µL) was injected into the HP-5MS capillary column and was exposed to a temperature of 70 °C for 2 min; then, the temperature was increased from 70 °C to 200 °C at a rate of 3 °C/min^{-1} and held at 200 °C for 15 min. Helium was used as the carrier gas with a flow rate of 1 mL/min. After obtaining the chromatogram, the mass spectrum of the unknown component was identified using the NIST (NIST 17) library [50].

4.8. Statistical Analysis

Statistical analysis of each experiment was carried out using the Minitab 17 software (Cubic Computing Pvt. Ltd., Bangalore, India) and Microsoft Excel 2016. All the experiments were performed using four replicates. Mean and standard deviation were calculated using standard equations. One-way ANOVA was used to determine the significant differences between the methanol extract and the fractions of G. edulis. p-values less than 0.05 were considered significant. The Pearson's correlation coefficient was used for the correlation analysis.

5. Conclusions

The present study found that *G. edulis* exhibited promising hypoglycemic activity by inhibiting key carbohydrate-digesting enzymes, glucose absorption, and the formation of antiglycation end products. Although antioxidant activity and enzyme inhibitory activity are stronger in commercial drugs than in *G. edulis* methanol extracts and its fractions, the hypoglycemic potential of *G. edulis* was evident in the present study. GC-MS analysis further confirmed the presence of bioactive compounds rich in antioxidants and antidiabetic properties. The ethyl acetate fraction exhibited promising antiglycation, and hypoglycemic potential. Hence, 3T3-L1 mature adipocytes and animal models are required to confirm anti-obesity and antidiabetic potentials of *G. edulis*. Isolation of active compounds for the development of new drugs is also warranted.

Author Contributions: Conceptualization, L.D.C.P., P.R. and K.W.S.; methodology, L.D.C.P., P.R., and K.W.S.; software, T.L.G.; formal analysis, T.L.G. and P.R.; investigation, T.L.G. and P.R.; data curation, T.L.G.; writing—original draft preparation, T.L.G.; writing—review and editing, L.D.C.P., and K.W,S.; supervision, L.D.C.P., P.R. and K.W.S.; project administration, L.D.C.P.; funding acquisition, L.D.C.P. All authors read and approved the final manuscript.

Funding: This research was funded by the University of Sri Jayewardenepura, Sri Lanka (ASP/01/RE/SCI/2017/50).

Conflicts of Interest: The authors declare no conflict of interest.

Appendix A

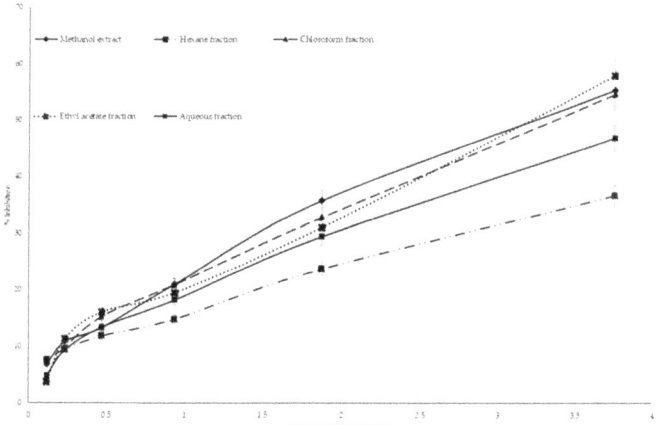

Figure A1. Dose dependent DPPH (1, 1-diphenyl-2-picrylhydrazine) radical scavenging activity of methanol extract and fractions of *Gracillaria edulis*. Data presented as mean ± standard deviation ($n = 4$).

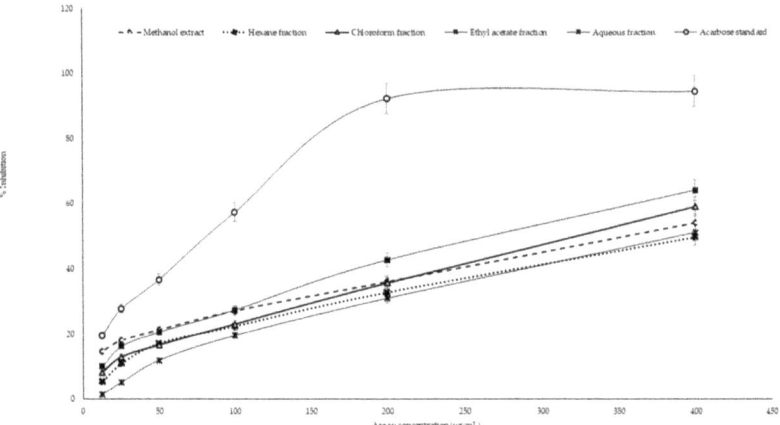

Figure A2. Percentage inhibition of α-amylase by *G. edulis* methanol extract and its fractions. Results are expressed as mean ± standard deviation ($n = 4$).

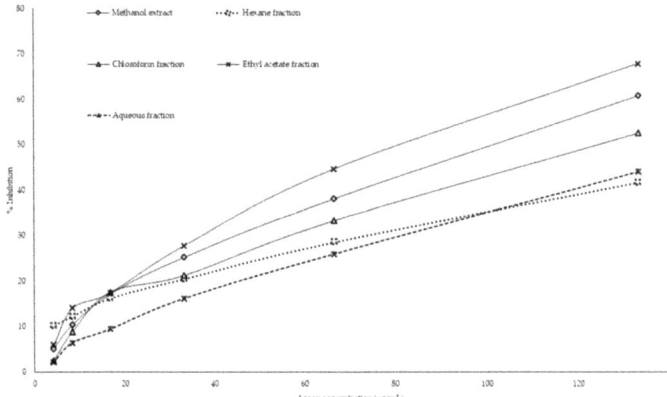

Figure A3. Dose–response relationship of methanol extract and its fractions of *G. edulis* for anti glucosidase activity. Results are expressed as mean ± standard deviation ($n = 4$).

Table A1. Effect of methanol extract and its fractions of *Gracillaria edulis* (1000 µg/mL) on glucose diffusion.

Time (min)	Glucose Concentration (µg/mL)						
	Control	Standard (Acarbose)	Methanol Extract	Hexane Fraction	Chloroform Fraction	Ethyl Acetate Fraction	Aqueous Fraction
30	14.32 ± 0.77 [a]	1.72 ± 0.34 [b]	3.51 ± 0.47 [b]	12.26 ± 1.96 [a]	7.09 ± 0.82 [c]	2.96 ± 0.47 [b]	7.43 ± 0.59 [c]
60	23.41 ± 1.01 [a]	5.09 ± 0.72 [b]	11.77 ± 0.47 [c]	20.66 ± 1.97 [a]	15.22 ± 1.13 [d]	10.67 ± 0.75 [c]	11.64 ± 1.62 [c]
90	30.58 ± 1.14 [a]	8.19 ± 0.47 [b]	22.73 ± 0.57 [c]	27.89 ± 1.13 [d]	22.59 ± 1.12 [c]	15.91 ± 0.61 [e]	29.13 ± 0.79 [a,d]
120	42.43 ± 1.54 [a]	13.15 ± 0.61 [b]	33.75 ± 0.79 [c]	40.57 ± 1.44 [a]	36.98 ± 1.19 [e]	23.07 ± 2.02 [d]	36.09 ± 1.54 [c,e]
150	48.90 ± 1.22 [a]	18.87 ± 0.57 [b]	42.08 ± 1.37 [c]	46.42 ± 0.91 [d]	41.25 ± 0.61 [c]	27.55 ± 0.59 [e]	47.25 ± 1.35 [a,d]
180	57.65 ± 1.67 [a]	22.79 ± 0.47 [b]	48.36 ± 1.04 [c]	52.01 ± 0.96 [d]	49.04 ± 0.67 [c]	38.15 ± 1.11 [e]	52.69 ± 1.31 [d]

Results are expressed as mean ± standard deviation ($n = 4$). Mean values in a column superscripted by different letters ([a–e]) are significantly different at $p < 0.05$.

References

1. American Diabetes Association. Diagnosis and classification of diabetes mellitus. *Diab. Care* **2013**, *36*, 67–74. [CrossRef] [PubMed]
2. World Health Organization. *Diabetes*. 2016. Available online: http://www.who.int/mediacentre/factsheets/fs312/en/ (accessed on 31 January 2019).
3. Jenum, A.K.; Diep, L.M.; Holmboe-Ottesen, G.; Holme, I.M.; Kumar, B.N.; Birkeland, K.I. Diabetes susceptibility in ethnic minority groups from Turkey, Vietnam, Sri Lanka and Pakistan compared with Norwegians - the association with adiposity is strongest for ethnic minority women. *BMC Pub. Heal.* **2012**, *12*, 1–50. [CrossRef] [PubMed]
4. Chawla, A.; Chawla, R.; Jaggi, S. Microvasular and macrovascular complications in diabetes mellitus: Distinct or continuum. *Indian J. Endocrinol. Metab.* **2016**, *20*, 546–551. [CrossRef] [PubMed]
5. Eleazu, C.O. The concept of low glycemic index and glycemic load foods as panacea for type 2 diabetes mellitus. *Afr. Health Sci.* **2016**, *16*, 468–479. [CrossRef] [PubMed]
6. Nair, S.S.; Kavrekar, V.; Mishra, A. In vitro studies on alpha amylase and alpha glucosidase inhibitory activities of selected plant extracts. *Eur. J. Exp. Biol.* **2013**, *3*, 128–132.
7. Ferná1ndez-Sánchez, A.; Madrigal-Santillán, E.; Bautista, M.; Esquivel-Soto, J.; Morales-González, A.; Esquivel-Chirino, C.; Durante-Montiel, I.; Sánchez-Rivera, G.; Valadez-Vega, C.; Morales-González, J.A. Inflammation, Oxidative Stress, and Obesity. *Int. J. Mol. Sci.* **2011**, *12*, 3117–3132. [CrossRef]
8. Wright, E., Jr.; Glass, L.C. Oxidative stress in type 2 diabetes: The role of fasting and postprandial glycaemia. *Int. J. Clin. Pract.* **2006**, *60*, 308–314.
9. Pal, A.; Kamthania, M.C.; Kumar, A. Bioactive Compounds and Properties of Seaweeds—A Review. *Biotechnol. Bioinform.* **2014**, *1*, 1–11.
10. De Souza, M.D.F.V.; Barbosa-filho, J.M.; Batista, L.M. Bioactivities from Marine Algae of the Genus Gracilaria. *Int. J. Mol. Sci.* **2011**, *12*, 4550–4573.
11. Fernando, S.; Sanjeewa, A. Preliminary screening of two marine algae and sea grass harvested from Sri Lankan waters against the LPS-induced inflammatory responses in RAW 264.7 macrophages and in vivo Zebra fish embryo model. *J. Natl. Sci. Found.* **2018**, *46*, 117–124. [CrossRef]
12. Koneri, R.; Jha, D.K. A Study on the Type II Antidiabetic Activity of Methanolic Extract of Marine Algae, *Gracilaria edulis* and *Sargassum polycystum*. *Int. J. Pharm. Sci. Rev. Res.* **2017**, *47*, 154–159.
13. Patra, S.; Muthuraman, M.S. *Gracilaria edulis* extract induces apoptosis and inhibits tumor in Ehrlich Ascites tumor cells in vivo. *BMC Complementary Altern. Med.* **2013**, *13*, 331–335. [CrossRef] [PubMed]
14. Al-Marzoqi, A.H.; Hameed, I.M.; Ali Idan, S. Analysis of bioactive chemical components of two medicinal plants (Coriandrum sativum and Melia azedarach) leaves using gas chromatography-mass spectrometry (GC-MS). *Afr. J. Biotchenol.* **2015**, *14*, 2812–2830.
15. Villalva, M.; Jaime, L.; Aguado, E.; Nieto, J.A.; Reglero, G.; Santoyo, S. Anti-Inflammatory and Antioxidant Activities from the Basolateral Fraction of Caco-2 Cells Exposed to a Rosmarinic Acid Enriched Extract. *J. Agric. Food Chem.* **2018**, *66*, 1167–1174. [CrossRef]
16. Jalill, A.; Dh, R.; Jalill, A. GC-MS analysis of Calendula officinalis and cytotoxic effects of its flower crude extract on human epidermoid larynx carcinoma (hep-2). *World J. Pharm. Pharm. Sci.* **2014**, *3*, 237–275.
17. Ali, N.; Dar, B.; Farooqui, M. Chemistry and Biology of Indoles and Indazoles: A Mini-Review. *Med. Chem.* **2012**, *13*, 1–16.
18. World Intellectual Property Organization. Indole and Indazole derivatives as glycogen synthase activators. *Int. Appl. Publ. Under Pat. Coop. Treaty* **2011**, *74*, 1–10.
19. Zeng, H.; Chen, X.; Liang, J. In vitro antifungal activity and mechanism of essential oil from fennel (Foeniculum vulgare L.) on dermatophyte species. *J. Med. Microbiol.* **2015**, *64*, 93–103. [CrossRef]
20. Agirbas, H.; Budak, F. Synthesis and structure-antibacterial activity relationship studies of 4-substituted phenyl -4, 5-dihydrobenzo [f] [1, 4] oxazepin-3 (2H)-thiones. *Med. Chem. Res.* **2011**, *20*, 1170–1180. [CrossRef]
21. Peng, W.; Li, D.; Ohkoshi, M. Characteristics of antibacterial molecular activities in poplar wood extractives. *Saudi J. Biol. Sci.* **2017**, *24*, 399–404. [CrossRef]
22. Pandey, K.B.; Rizvi, S.I. Plant polyphenols as dietary antioxidants in human health and disease. *J. Clin. Investig.* **2009**, *2*, 270–278. [CrossRef]

23. Ganesan, P.; Kumar, C.S.; Bhaskar, N. Antioxidant properties of methanol extract and its solvent fractions obtained from selected Indian red seaweeds. *Bioresour. Technol.* **2008**, *99*, 2717–2723. [CrossRef] [PubMed]
24. Fellah, F.; Louaileche, H.; Touati, N. Seasonal variations in the phenolic compound content and antioxidant activities of three selected species of seaweeds from Tiskerth islet, Bejaia, Algeria. *J. Mater. Environ. Sci.* **2017**, *8*, 4451–4456. [CrossRef]
25. Marseglia, L.; Manti, S.; Angelo, G.D.; Nicotera, A.; Parisi, E.; Rosa, G.D.; Gitto, E.; Arrigo, T. Oxidative Stress in Obesity: A Critical Component in Human Diseases. *Int. J. Mol. Sci.* **2015**, *16*, 378–400. [CrossRef] [PubMed]
26. Sampath, S.G.; Dheeba, K.P.; Sivakumar, R. In vitro anti-diabetic, antioxidant and anti-inflammatory activity of Clitoria Ternatea, L. *Artic. Int. J. Pharm. Pharm. Sci.* **2014**, *6*, 342–347.
27. Francavilla, M. The red seaweed *Gracilaria gracilis* as a multi products source. *Mar. Drugs* **2013**, *11*, 3754–3776. [CrossRef] [PubMed]
28. Ranasinghe, P. Antioxidant Activity of Caryota urens L. (Kithul) Sap. *Trop. Agric. Res.* **2012**, *23*, 117–125. [CrossRef]
29. Bernaert, N. Antioxidant capacity, total phenolic and ascorbate content as a function of the genetic diversity of leek (Allium ampeloprasum var porrum). *Food Chem.* **2012**, *134*, 669–677. [CrossRef]
30. Gulati, V.; Harding, I.H.; Palombo, E.A. Enzyme inhibitory and antioxidant activities of traditional medicinal plants: Potential application in the management of hyperglycemia. *Bmc Complementary Altern Med.* **2012**, *12*, 2–9.
31. Unnikrishnan, P.S.; Suthindhiran, K.; Jayasri, M.A. Antidiabetic potential of marine algae by inhibiting key metabolic enzymes. *J. Front. Life Sci.* **2015**, *8*, 148–159. [CrossRef]
32. Senthil Kumar, P.; Sudha, S. Evaluation of Alpha-Amylase and Alpha-Glucosidase Inhibitory Properties of Selected Seaweeds from Gulf of Mannar. *Irjponline. Com.* **2012**, *3*, 128–130.
33. Gallagher, A.M.; Flatt, P.R.; Duffy, G.; Abdel-Wahab, Y.H.A. The effects of traditional antidiabetic plants on in vitro glucose diffusion. *Nutr. Res.* **2003**, *23*, 413–424. [CrossRef]
34. Sudasinghe, H.P.; Peiris, D.C.P. Hypoglycemic and hypolipidemic activity of aqueous leaf extract of *Passiflora suberosa* L. *Peer J.* **2018**, *6*, e4389.
35. Navale, A.M.; Paranjape, A.N. Glucose transporters: physiological and pathological roles. *Biophys Rev.* **2016**, *8*, 5–9. [CrossRef] [PubMed]
36. Grzegorczyk-Karolak, I.; Goła, G.; Gburek, J.; Wysokin, H.; Matkowski, A. Inhibition of Advanced Glycation End-Product Formation and Antioxidant Activity by Extracts and Polyphenols from *Scutellaria alpina* L. and *S. altissima* L. *Molecules* **2016**, *21*, 739. [CrossRef] [PubMed]
37. Lakmal, H.; Samarakoon, K.; Lee, W.; Lee, J.; Abeytunga, D.; Lee, H.; Jeon, Y. Anticancer and antioxidant effects of selected Sri Lankan marine algae. *J. Natl. Sci. Found. Sri Lanka* **2014**, *42*, 117–124. [CrossRef]
38. Singleton, V.L.; Orthofer, R.; Lamuela-Raventos, R.M. Analysis of total phenols and other oxidation substrates and antioxidants by means of Folin-Ciocaltue reagent. *Methods Enzym.* **1999**, *299*, 152–178.
39. Chang, C.C.; Yang, M.H.; Ucen, H.M.; Chern, J.C. Estimation of total flavonoid content in propolis by complementary colorimetric method. *J. Food Drug Anal.* **2002**, *10*, 178–182.
40. Sreevidya, N.; Mehrotra, S. Spectrometric method for estimation of precipitable with Dragendorff's reagent in plant material. *J. Aoac Int.* **2003**, *36*, 1124–1127.
41. Blois, M.S. Antioxidant determination by use of stable free radical. *Nature* **1958**, *181*, 1199–1200. [CrossRef]
42. Re, R.; Pellegrini, N.; Proteggente, A.; Pannala, A.; Yang, M.; Rice-Evans, C. Antioxidant activity applying an improved ABTS radical cation decolorization Assay. *Free Rad. Biol. Med* **1999**, *26*, 1231–1237. [CrossRef]
43. Benzie, I.F.F.; Szeto, Y.T. Total antioxidant capacity of teas by the ferric reducing/antioxidant power assay. *J. Agric. Food Chem.* **1999**, *47*, 633–636. [CrossRef] [PubMed]
44. Carter, P. Spectrophotometric determination of serum iron at the sub-microgram level with a new reagent ferrozine. *Annu. Biochem.* **1971**, *40*, 450–458. [CrossRef]
45. Ou, B.; Hampsch-Woodill, M.; Prior, R.L. Development and validation of an improved oxygen radical absorbance capacity assay using fluorescein as the fluorescent probe. *J. Agric. Food Chem.* **2001**, *49*, 4619–4626. [CrossRef] [PubMed]
46. Bernfeld, P. Amylases, alpha and beta. In *Methods in Enzymology*; Colowick, S.P., Kaplan, N.O., Eds.; Academic Press: New York, NY, USA, 1955; Volume 1, pp. 149–158.

47. Matsui, T.; Ueda, T.; Oki, T.; Sugita, K.; Terahara, N.; Matsumoto, K. α-Glucosidase inhibitory action of natural acylated anthocyanins. *J. Agric. Food Chem.* **2001**, *49*, 1948–1951. [CrossRef]
48. Roy, A.; Mahalingam, M.G. The in-vitro antidiabetic activity of Phoenix roebelenii leaf extract. *Int. J. Green Pharm.* **2017**, *11*, 884–890.
49. Matsuura, N.; Aradate, T.; Sasaki, C.; Kojima, H.; Ohara, M.; Hasegawa, J.; Ubukata, M. Screening system for the Maillard reaction inhibitor from natural product extracts. *J. Health Sci.* **2002**, *48*, 520–526. [CrossRef]
50. Jerkovi, I. Phytochemical study of the headspace volatile organic compounds of fresh algae and sea grass from the Adriatic Sea (single point collection). *PLoS ONE* **2008**, *13*, e0196462.

Sample Availability: Samples of the compounds are available from the authors.

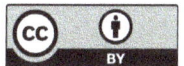

© 2019 by the authors. Licensee MDPI, Basel, Switzerland. This article is an open access article distributed under the terms and conditions of the Creative Commons Attribution (CC BY) license (http://creativecommons.org/licenses/by/4.0/).

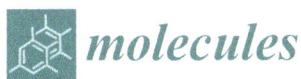

Article

Antioxidant, Xanthine Oxidase, α-Amylase and α-Glucosidase Inhibitory Activities of Bioactive Compounds from *Rumex crispus* L. Root

Truong Ngoc Minh [1,*], Truong Mai Van [2], Yusuf Andriana [2,3], Le The Vinh [1], Dang Viet Hau [1], Dang Hong Duyen [1] and Chona de Guzman-Gelani [4]

1. Center for Research and Technology Transfer (CRETECH), Vietnam Academy of Sciences and Technology, Hanoi 10072, Vietnam; thevinh3839@gmail.com (L.T.V.); hauhoahock20@gmail.com (D.V.H.); hongduyen1908@gmail.com (D.H.D.)
2. Graduate School for International Development and Cooperation (IDEC), Hiroshima University, Higashi-Hiroshima 739-8529, Japan; truongmaivan1991@gmail.com (T.M.V.); yusufandriana@yahoo.com (Y.A.)
3. Research Center for Appropriate Technology, Indonesian Institute of Sciences, Subang, 41213, Indonesia
4. Department of Chemistry, College of Science and Mathematics, Mindanao State University - Iligan Institute of Technology, Iligan 9200, Philippines; chona.gelani@g.msuiit.edu.ph
* Correspondence: minhtn689@gmail.com; Tel./Fax: +84-912-990-197

Academic Editors: Raffaele Capasso and Lorenzo Di Cesare Mannelli
Received: 19 September 2019; Accepted: 22 October 2019; Published: 31 October 2019

Abstract: The root of *Rumex crispus* L. has been shown to possess anti-gout and anti-diabetic properties, but the compounds responsible for these pharmaceutical effects have not yet been reported. In this study, we aimed to isolate and purify active components from the root of *R. crispus*, and to evaluate their anti-radical, anti-gout and anti-diabetic capacities. From the ethyl acetate (EtOAc) extract, two compounds, chrysophanol (**1**) and physcion (**2**), were isolated by column chromatography with an elution of hexane and EtOAc at a 9:1 ratio. Their structures were identified by spectrometric techniques including gas chromatography-mass spectrometry (GC-MS), electrospray ionization-mass spectrometry (ESI-MS), X-ray diffraction analyses and nuclear magnetic resonance (NMR). The results of bioassays indicated that (**1**) showed stronger activities than (**2**). For antioxidant activity, (**1**) and (**2**) exhibited remarkable DPPH radical scavenging capacity (IC_{50} = 9.8 and 12.1 µg/mL), which was about two times stronger than BHT (IC_{50} = 19.4 µg/mL). The anti-gout property of (**1**) and (**2**) were comparable to the positive control allopurinol, these compounds exerted strong inhibition against the activity of xanthine oxidase (IC_{50} = 36.4 and 45.0 µg/mL, respectively). In the anti-diabetic assay, (**1**) and (**2**) displayed considerable inhibitory ability on α-glucosidase, their IC_{50} values (IC_{50} = 20.1 and 18.9 µg/mL, respectively) were higher than that of standard acarbose (IC_{50} = 143.4 µg/mL). Findings of this study highlight that (**1**) and (**2**) may be promising agents to treat gout and diabetes, which may greatly contribute to the medicinal properties of *Rumex crispus* root.

Keywords: bioactive compound; anti-radical; anti-gout; anti-diabetic; *Rumex crispus*; chrysophanol; physcion

1. Introduction

Rumex crispus L. is known as the curly dock or yellow dock in most of Europe, North Africa, Turkey, Northern Iran, Central and East Asia, and North America [1]. The roots of this plant have been used in traditional medicine as a tonic, laxative, and for hemostasis medication. The fruits (seeds) are used for the treatment of dysentery. The young leaves of the plant are eaten as servings of mixed greens and soups. The plant has been utilized for treating the relevant disease, dermatology contaminations, gastrointestinal tract maladies, upper respiratory tract illnesses, and loose bowels [2,3]. The bioactive substances detected in this plant include flavonoids (isorientin, vitexin, orientin and isovitexin), lipids, vitamins, carotenoids, natural acids and minerals. The root of R. crispus may be a wealthy source of anthraquinones glycosides (chrysophanol and emodin) [4].

Antioxidant prevention agents are common or manufactured substances having the capacity to hinder or delay oxidation at relatively low concentrations [5]. Antioxidant compounds are known to combat oxidative stress. When oxidative stress is uncontrolled it is associated with several pathophysiological processes [6]. In a pharmacological examination of the ether, ethanol, and hot water extracts of R. crispus, the water extract showed the most elevated antioxidant activity. The most noteworthy amount of total phenolic compounds was found within the ethanol extract of the seeds. In regards to the reducing power and DPPH scavenging activity, the ethanol extract of the seeds was the foremost compelling [7]. The power to quench singlet oxygen and the protective effects of various extracts (hexane, chloroform, ethyl acetate and butanol) of R. crispus seeds against photodynamic damage were investigated in a biological system. A higher total phenolic content was observed for the ethyl acetate (EtOAc) and butanol extracts. The level of *in vitro* antioxidant action of the methanol concentrate of R. crispus was determined by measuring its ferric-lessening antioxidant activity, without DPPH radical searching movement and the ability to impact the lipid peroxidation in liposomes. It was seen that the methanol concentrate had direct antioxidant prevention agent movement. In view of the *in vivo* tests, it was inferred that the dose routine did not impact the degrees of lipid peroxidation. The methanol concentrate of R. crispus roots displayed DPPH radical searching (IC_{50} = 42.86 µg/mL) [7,8]. The ethereal piece of R. crispus can be utilized as a compelling and safe wellspring of antioxidant prevention agents. However, information on the anti-gout and anti-diabetic properties of the underground plant parts is still limited.

Xanthine oxidase (XOD) is an important enzyme responsible for hyperuricemia, and a predisposing factor for gout and oxidative stress-related diseases. This enzyme plays an important role in catalyzing the oxidation of hypoxanthine to xanthine and xanthine to uric acid [9,10]. Nowadays, few drugs are commonly used to treat gout including allopurinol and febuxostat. However, some serious and undesirable effects on skin caused by allopurinol and febuxostat may occur when taking the drug, including Steven-Johnson syndrome (SJS) and toxic epidermal necrolysis (TEN), causing death in up to 39% of cases. Lesions can occur on other organs such as the liver and kidney [11,12]. Many studies have reported that compounds possessing both antioxidant properties will be effective in gout treatment [13]. On the other hand, antioxidants are able to prevent or slow down oxidation by eliminating free radicals, which further help prevent oxidative disease and increase people's lifespan [14]. On the other hand, xanthine oxidase enzyme inhibitors can reduce the enzyme activity, preventing the formation of urate salts [15,16].

Diabetes has become a worldwide health problem in developed and developing countries. It is reported that about 425 million people are suffering from diabetes, which accounts for 12% of global health expenditure [17]. Among diabetic types, the pathogenesis of type 2 diabetes may launch from many factors such as genetic predisposition, environment, and pancreatic beta-cell dysfunction [18]. Therefore, one of the diabetes treatments is to inhibit the enzyme activity of α-amylase and α-glucosidase to minimize the formation of blood glucose [19]. On the other hand, oxidative tension in diabetes coexists with a reduction in antioxidant status [20], which can increase the deleterious effects of free radicals. It has also been known that alloxan induces diabetogenic activity mainly by inducing oxygen free base and thereby damaging the pancreas [21]. Supplementation with non-toxic antioxidants may have a chemoprotective role in diabetes [22]. Antioxidants as well as vitamins C and E, have been shown to reduce oxidative stress in experimental diabetes [23]. Supplementation of vitamin C has also been shown to lower berth glycosylated hemoglobin in diabetic patients [23]. Many industrial plant excerpts and plant products have been shown to have significant antioxidant activity [24–26].

This study aims to isolate compounds from R. crispus root that can scavenge free radicals and inhibit xanthine oxidase, α-amylase and α-glucosidase. The results of the study will contribute to a better understanding of the value of medicinal plants, as well as contribute to the database for the production of gout and diabetes medications. Biological properties of the isolated compounds were also examined for their efficacy and safety in antioxidant activity and inhibition of xanthine oxidase, α-amylase and α-glucosidase enzyme by *in vitro* methods. The obtained compounds were identified by gas chromatography-mass spectrometry (GC-MS), electrospray ionization (ESI), atmospheric pressure chemical ionization (APCI), nuclear magnetic resonance (NMR), and X-ray diffraction.

2. Results

2.1. Structure Elucidation of Isolated Fractions

Separation of bioactive compounds from *Rumex crispus* root (RCR) was conducted following the procedure illustrated in Figure 1.

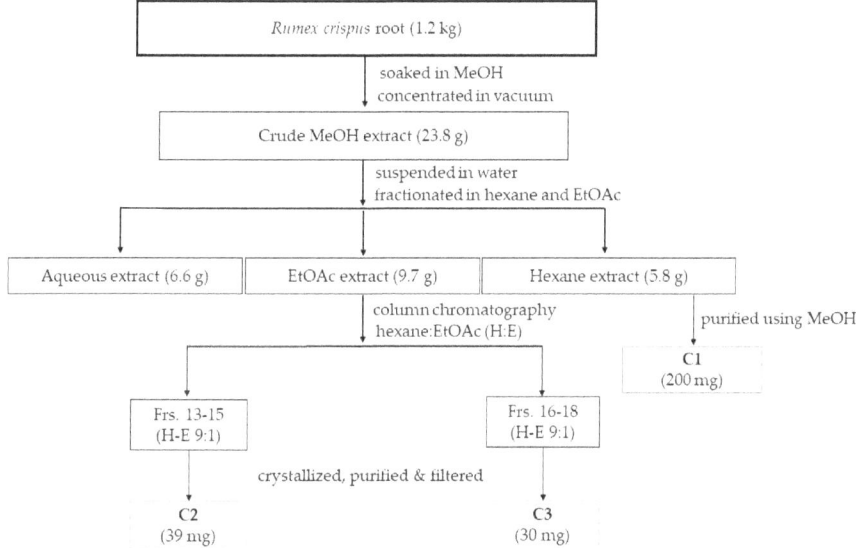

Figure 1. Isolation and purification of bioactive compounds from *Rumex crispus* root.

The isolated metabolites were characterized and identified by GC-MS, ESI-MS, APCI-MS, ^{1}H- and ^{13}C-NMR and X-ray analyses (Supplementary Figures S1–S21 and Tables S1–S3).

On the basis of GC-MS data (Table 1), isolated fractions were identified. The structure and formula of compounds were further confirmed by ESI-MS. Two fractions, **C2** and **C3**, were elucidated by ^{1}H NMR and ^{13}C NMR. Chemical structures of the identified compounds are illustrated in Figures 2 and 3.

Table 1. Bioactive compounds identified in EtOAc extract of *Rumex crispus* root by GC-MS.

Fractions	Retention Time	Peak Area (%)	Compounds	Chemical Formula	Molecular Weight	Similarity
C1	20.70	73.39	Chrysophanol	$C_{15}H_{10}O_4$	254	90.8
	22.98	24.82	Physcion	$C_{16}H_{12}O_5$	284	91.8
C2	20.71	98.10	Chrysophanol	$C_{15}H_{10}O_4$	254	98.1
C3	22.99	97.79	Physcion	$C_{16}H_{12}O_5$	284	97.8

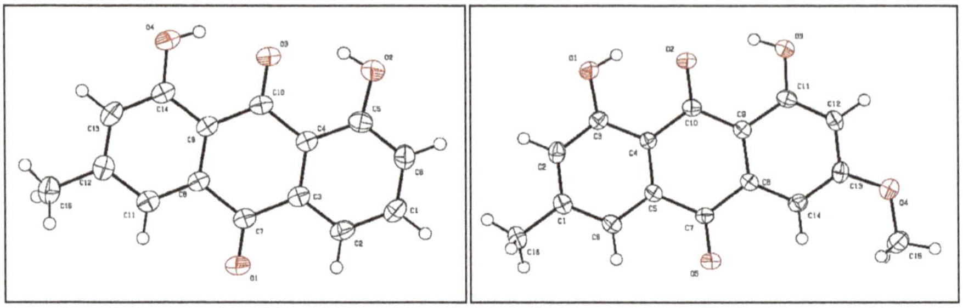

Chrysophanol (**C1, C2**)　　　　　Physcion (**C1, C3**)

Figure 2. Chemical structures of bioactive constituents identified in EtOAc extract of *Rumex crispus* L. root by single-crystal X-ray.

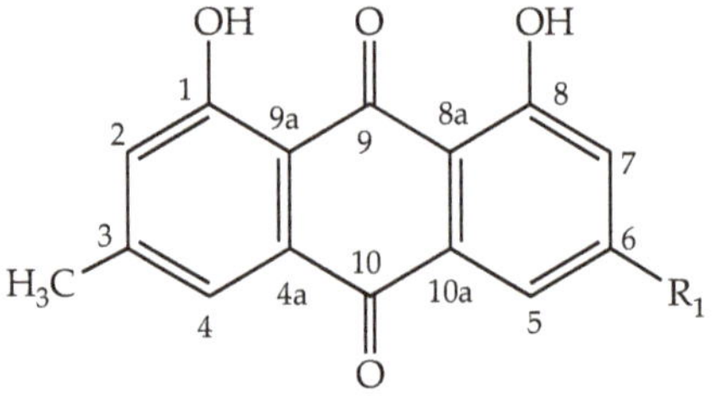

1: R_1 = H
2: R_1 = OCH_3

Figure 3. Structures of compounds **1** and **2** from *Rumex crispus* L. root.

2.2. NMR Structural Elucidation

Compound **1** was isolated as an orange needle from the EtOAc extract of RCR. Its molecular formula, $C_{15}H_{10}O_4$, was deduced from a combined analysis of the positive ESI MS at *m/z* 255.3 [M + H]$^+$ ($C_{15}H_{11}O_4$) and ^{1}H-, ^{13}C-NMR, HSQC, and HMBC spectra. The ^{1}H-NMR spectrum of **1** showed the presence of a methyl group at δ_H 2.46 (3H, s, H-11) and five protons of aromatic ring at δ_H 7.82 (1H, dd, *J* = 7.0, 1.0 Hz, H-5), 7.67 (1H, t, *J* = 8.0 Hz, H-6), 7.64 (1H, s, H-4), 7.30 (1H, dd, *J* = 8.5, 1.0 Hz, H-7), 7.09 (1H, d, *J* = 0.5 Hz, H-2) and two protons of hydroxyl groups at δ_H 12.1 (1H, s, OH-8), 11.99 (1H, s, OH-1). The ^{13}C NMR of **1** displayed 15 carbon signals including a methyl, two ketone groups, five methines, seven quaternary carbons (two of which are bonded to O atoms) (Table 2). Assignments of all ^{1}H and ^{13}C NMR signals were accomplished by interpretation of HSQC and HMBC spectra. The melting point of compound was 196 °C. The above spectral data were diagnostic of an anthraquinone having two hydroxyl groups at C-1, C-8 position, and a methyl group. Moreover, methyl group and two hydroxyl group positions were determined by the HMBC spectral correlation between the proton of methyl group H-11 (δ_H 2.46) with C-2 (δ_C 124.4)/C-4 (δ_C 121.4); OH-1 (δ_H 11.99) with C-2 (δ_C 124.4)/C-9a (δ_C 113.8) and OH-8 (δ_H 12.1) with C-7 (δ_C 124.6)/C-8a (δ_C 115.9). By means of its spectrometric analysis and comparison with previously published data [27], compound **1** was determined as chrysophanol or 1,8-dihydroxy-3-methylanthraquinone.

Compound **2** was obtained as orange-yellow needles. The ^{1}H and ^{13}C NMR spectra of **2** closely resembled those of **1**, except for the appearance of one methoxy group (δ_H 3.93, (3H, s), δ_C 56.0) and the chemical shift of C-6 (Table 2). This suggested that **2** also has an anthraquinone of **1** and **2** was the result of replacing the aromatic ring proton at C-6 in **1** by a methoxy group. This was confirmed by comparison of the NMR data of **2** with those of a known anthraquinone in Reference [28]. Thus **2** was determined to be 1,8-dihydroxy-3-methoxy-6-methylanthraquinone or physcion.

Table 2. ^{13}C-NMR data for compounds **1** and **2**.

Position	1		2	
	$\delta_C{}^*$	δ_C	$\delta_C{}^{**}$	δ_C
1	161.1	162.7	162.5	162.5
2	124.2	124.4	124.5	124.5
3	149.0	149.3	148.4	148.4
4	120.4	121.4	121.3	121.3
5	119.2	119.9	108.2	108.2
6	137.2	136.9	166.5	166.5
7	123.9	124.6	106.8	106.8
8	161.4	162.4	165.2	165.2
9	191.4	192.6	190.8	190.7
10	181.3	182.0	181.5	181.9
4a	132.8	133.3	133.2	133.2
8a	115.7	115.9	110.3	110.3
9a	113.6	113.8	113.7	113.7
10a	133.2	133.7	135.3	135.2
CH$_3$	21.6	22.2	22.1	22.1
OCH$_3$			56.0	56.0

$\delta_C{}^*$ Chrysophanol in DMSO; $\delta_C{}^{**}$ Physcion in CDCl$_3$.

2.3. Quantitative Analysis of Fraxetin from Rumex Crispus Root

The content of two pure compounds chrysophanol and physcion in RCR is presented in Table 3. The quantity of these compounds was determined by the instrumentation used in this study.

Table 3. Quantity of pure compounds from *R. crispus* root.

Fractions	Retention Time	Compounds	Concentration (µg/g DW)
C2	20.70 ± 0.02	Chrysophanol	32.50 ± 0.11
C3	22.99 ± 0.05	Physcion	25.04 ± 0.08

Data express means ± SD (standard deviation).

2.4. Antioxidant Activities of the Isolated Fractions

Antioxidant activities of the isolated fractions were determined using three assays namely DPPH, ABTS free radical scavenging, and reducing power. BHT was used as a standard for all methods. The results are summarized in Table 4.

Table 4 summarizes the antioxidant activities of the EtOAc *R. crispus* root extract. For the DPPH scavenging assay, the antioxidant activity of **C2** was the highest as its IC$_{50}$ value was the lowest (10.0 µg/mL), followed by **C3** (IC$_{50}$ = 12.0 µg/mL). Statistically, the DPPH radical scavenging properties of **C2** and **C3** were stronger than BHT (IC$_{50}$ = 19.2 µg/mL). The fraction **C1** (IC$_{50}$ = 35.0 µg/mL) exhibited intermediate antioxidant capacities. For ABTS (2,2′-azinobis-(3-ethylbenzothiazoline-6-sulfonic acid)), **C2** exhibited the maximum scavenging activity with IC$_{50}$ value of 34.3 µg/mL, followed by **C3** and BHT (IC$_{50}$ = 44.8 and 46.9 µg/mL). The lowest antioxidant property was fraction **C1** (IC$_{50}$ = 194.7 µg/mL). For the reducing power ability, **C2** displayed the maximum reducing power with IC$_{50}$ value of 312.6 µg/mL. Generally, the antioxidant properties of the pure compounds **C2** and **C3** were higher than standard BHT.

Table 4. Antioxidant activities measured by DPPH, ABTS (2,2'-azinobis-(3-ethylbenzothiazoline-6-sulfonic acid)) and ferric reducing antioxidant power test (FRAP) of EtOAc extract fractions from *R. crispus* root in term of IC_{50} values.

Fractions	IC_{50} (µg/mL)		
	DPPH	ABTS	FRAP
C1	35.0 ± 1.6^a	194.7 ± 2.0^a	1366.5 ± 8.4^a
C2	10.0 ± 0.3^c (39.4 µM)	34.3 ± 0.7^c (135.0 µM)	312.6 ± 6.3^c (1230.7 µM)
C3	12.0 ± 0.2^c (42.3 µM)	44.8 ± 0.8^b (157.7 µM)	408.6 ± 6.8^b (1438.7 µM)
BHT*	19.2 ± 0.3^b (87.1 µM)	46.9 ± 0.9^b (212.8 µM)	422.1 ± 1.1^b (1915.8 µM)

* Positive control. Values are means ± SD (standard deviation); ^{a,b,c} indicate significant differences at $p < 0.05$.

2.5. In Vitro Inhibition of Xanthine Oxidase (XOD), α-Amylase (AAI) and α-Glucosidase (AGI)

The inhibitory effect of the isolated fractions on xanthine oxidase is presented in Table 5. The results showed that **C1–C3** exhibited a considerable activity against xanthine oxidase (IC_{50} = 36.4–88.8 µg/mL). Furthermore, **C2** manifested the highest inhibitory activity (IC_{50} = 36.4 µg/mL) followed by **C3** (IC_{50} = 36.4 µg/mL) while **C1** exhibited the least (IC_{50} = 88.8 µg/mL).

Table 5. Xanthine oxidase, α-amylase and α-glucosidase inhibitory activities of isolated fractions from *Rumex crispus* root in term of IC_{50} values.

Fractions	IC_{50} (µg/mL)		
	XOD	AAI	AGI
C1	88.8 ± 0.9^a	199.1 ± 1.4^a	91.6 ± 1.4^b
C2	36.4 ± 0.6^c (143.3 µM)	117.3 ± 1.0^b (461.8 µM)	20.1 ± 0.6^c (79.1 µM)
C3	45.0 ± 0.7^b (158.5 µM)	113.3 ± 1.3^c (398.9 µM)	18.9 ± 0.4^c (66.5 µM)
Allopurinol*	20.5 ± 0.5^d (150.6 µM)	-	-
Acarbose*	-	90.9 ± 0.8^d (140.8 µM)	143.8 ± 2.6^a (222.7 µM)

* Positive control. Values are means ± SD (standard deviation); ^{a,b,c,d} indicate significant differences at $p < 0.05$.

A starch-iodine method was applied to examine the inhibitory effect of isolated fractions on porcine pancreatic α-amylase. Among isolated compounds, **C3** displayed the maximum α-amylase inhibition with IC_{50} value of 113.3 µg/mL, followed by **C2** (IC_{50} = 117.3 µg/mL). The α-amylase inhibition is as follows: acarbose > **C3** > **C2** > **C1** corresponding to IC_{50} values 90.9, 113.3, 117.3, and 199.1 µg/mL, respectively.

The α-glucosidase inhibitory activity of isolated fractions was assayed using a synthetic substrate *p*-nitrophenyl-α-D-glucopyranoside (pNPG). All isolated fractions expressed higher α-glucosidase activity than that of standard acarbose. (Table 5). Of which, the activity of all isolated fractions was significantly higher than that of standard acarbose. **C3** showed the highest inhibitory activity (IC_{50} = 18.9 µg/mL) followed by **C2** (IC_{50} = 20.1 µg/mL). Fraction **C1** (IC_{50} = 91.6 µg/mL) exhibited intermediate α-glucosidase inhibition.

3. Discussion

In this study, two compounds were isolated and identified from the EtOAc extract of *R. crispus* root, namely chrysophanol (**1**) (fraction **C2**) and physcion (**2**) (fraction **C3**). They are biologically active compounds belonging to the flavonoid group. The radical scavenging activity of the isolated fractions was examined using DPPH, which is a frequently used method in natural product antioxidant evaluation [27], and ABTS assays. The results of this present study serve as an additional scientific finding with regards to the radical scavenging activity of the EtOAc extract of *R. crispus* root. The IC_{50} values of (**1**) (10.0 ± 0.3 µg/mL) and (**2**) (12.0 ± 0.2 µg/mL) are comparable to the value reported by a previous study on the acetone extract of the *R. crispus* root with IC_{50} of 14.0 µg/mL [28]. Moreover, a study reported that methanol extract of the fruits of *R. crispus* exhibited antioxidant activity with IC_{50} value of 3.7 µg/mL [29]. These findings strengthen the antioxidant potential of the roots of *R. crispus* over its fruits. Furthermore, this results shows that the antioxidant activities of the pure compounds (**1**) and (**2**) are higher than the standard BHT (Table 4). The results also show a strong correlation between the concentration of the pure compound (Table 3) and its antioxidant activity. Compound (**1**) (32.50 ± 0.11 µg/g DW) exhibits a stronger radical scavenging activity as seen in both DPPH and ABTS assays (IC_{50} = 10.0 ± 0.3 and 34.3 ± 0.7 µg/mL, respectively) than (**2**) (25.04 ± 0.08 µg/g DW, 12.0 ± 0.2 and 44.8 ± 0.8 µg/mL, respectively). This result is in agreement with the findings of Elzaawely et al. [30] who reported the correlation between the phenolic content and DPPH assay of the EtOAc extract of the aerial parts of *R. japonicus*. The same correlation is observed between the concentration of the pure compound and its reducing power, in that the higher the concentration, the stronger its reducing power.

Xanthine oxidase (XO) plays a role in gout formation since it catalyzes the oxidation of xanthine to uric acid. Compounds that inhibit the activity of XO, therefore, can be used to treat gout [31,32]. Dietary flavonoids have been reported to possess inhibitory activity against free radicals and xanthine oxidase. The antioxidant property is mainly characterized by flavonoid contents that can effortlessly release hydrogen donors to naturalize free radicals. Therefore, flavonoids could be a promising remedy for human gout and ischemia by decreasing both uric acid and superoxide concentrations in human tissues [13]. According to Mohamed Isa et al. [15], *Plumeria rubra* contains a high amount of flavonoids and could be used as a new alternative to allopurinol with increased therapeutic activity and fewer side effects. The XO inhibitory activity *in vitro* assay of methanol extract of *Plumeria rubra* flowers possesses the highest inhibition effects at IC_{50} = 23.91 µg/mL. Baicalein, baicalin and wogonin, isolated from *Scutellaria rivularis*, have been reported to exhibit a strong xanthine oxidase inhibition as evaluated by modified xanthine oxidase inhibition methods. The results showed that the order was baicalein > wogonin > baicalin, IC_{50} = 3.12, 157.38 and 215.19 µM, respectively [33]. From this present study, (**1**) (IC_{50} = 143.3 µM) exhibited a higher inhibitory effect on XO than wogonin and baicalin, whereas (**2**) (IC_{50} = 158.5 µM) inhibited XO stronger than baicalin and showed comparable inhibitory activity as wogonin. The XO inhibition activity of (**1**) and (**2**) is directly related to their concentration as extracted from the root of *R. crispus* (Table 3). Allopurinol showed a much lower IC_{50} value of 20.5 ± 0.5 µg/mL, which is why allopurinol is the preferred treatment for gout.

Both α-amylase (AA) (responsible for starch digestion) and α-glucosidase (AG) (produces glucose in the final step of the digestive process of carbohydrates) are related to type 2 diabetes since these enzymes are responsible for postprandial blood glucose levels [34]. AA and AG inhibitors are therefore widely used in the treatment of patients with type 2 diabetes, which is related to elevated postprandial blood glucose levels. Results of this present study showed consistent inhibition activities of (**1**) and (**2**) in both AA and AG in that (**2**) exhibited a stronger inhibition than (**1**) (Table 5). However, in terms of AGI, (**1**) and (**2**) turned out to be much better inhibitors compared to acarbose (Table 5). Both terpenoids and flavonoids might play crucial roles in α-amylase and α-glucosidase inhibition [35,36]. The pure compounds (**1**) and (**2**) registered a stronger anti-diabetic activity than the mixture **C3**. Moreover, the synergic effect of the two pure compounds, **C3** exerted stronger inhibition against α-glucosidase than acarbose (IC_{50} = 143.8 µg/mL). Although this study to isolate and purify active components from the root of R. crispus, as well as test their biological activities, was successful, *in vivo* tests should be considered in order to ascertain the anti-gout and anti-diabetic properties of this prospective plant.

4. Materials and Methods

4.1. Materials

Rumex crispus root (RCR) was collected (34°23′28.3″ N 132°43′06.0″ E) in October 2017. The specimen with voucher number RCR-M2017 was deposited at the Plant Physiology and Biochemistry Laboratory (IDEC, Hiroshima University, Japan). The samples were cleaned by 1% NaOCl. After blotting with tissues, samples were dried at 45 °C in the oven for one week then ground to a fine powder [37].

4.2. Extraction of Rumex Crispus Root

The RCR powder (1.2 kg) was soaked in MeOH (2 L) to produce 23.8 g of MeOH crude extract. The crude extract was suspended in water (300 mL), then fractionated in hexane and EtOAc to obtain 6.6, 5.8, and 9.7 g water, hexane and EtOAc extracts, respectively.

4.3. Isolation of Pure Compounds

The hexane extract was dried at room temperature, then was purified by MeOH to obtain fraction **C1** (200 mg).

The EtOAc extract was subjected to normal phase column chromatography (CC) using silica gel (200 g) of 70–230 mesh ASTM and LiChroprep RP-18 (40–63 mm). All fractions were examined by thin-layer chromatography (TLC) (Merck, Darmstadt, Germany). Fraction 13–15 (**C2**) (39 mg), and fraction 16–18 (**C3**) (30 mg) were crystallized after separation by CC (Figure 1). Compound **C2** (**1**) and **C3** (**2**) were obtained as pure compounds, the purity levels were confirmed by GC-MS of 98.10% and 97.79%, respectively.

4.4. Antioxidants Activity

Antioxidant activity of the isolated compounds was determined using DPPH (2,2-diphenyl-1-picrylhydrazyl) radical scavenging assay, ABTS (2,2′-azinobis-(3-ethylbenzothiazoline-6-sulfonic acid)) radical cation decolorization assay, ferric reducing antioxidant power test (FRAP) following previous study [37–39] with slight modifications.

4.5. Identification and Quantification of Isolated Compounds

Identification and quantification of isolated compounds was by GC-MS following previous study [40,41]. Therefore, the GC-MS system was equipped with a DB-5MS column (30 m × 0.25 mm internal diameter × 0.25 μm in thickness (Agilent Technologies, J & W Scientific Products, Folsom, CA, USA). The carrier gas was Helium and the split ratio was 5:1. GC oven temperatures operated with the initial temperature of 50 °C without hold time, followed by an increase of 10 °C/min up to a final temperature of 300 °C and holding time of 20 min. The injector and detector temperature were programmed at 300 °C and 320 °C, respectively. The MS ranged from 29 to 800 amu. JEOL's GC-MS Mass Center System Version 2.65a was used to control the GC-MS system and process the data peak.

ESI-MS analysis was conducted on negative/positive ion mode [42]. APCI-MS analysis was implemented using a mass spectrometer with an electrospray ion source [43].

X-ray diffraction measurement was conducted with a Bruker APEX-II ULTRA diffractometer (Bruker Corporation, Billerica, MA, USA). The crystals were irradiated using Mo-Kα radiation at −100 °C. Cell parameters and intensities for the reflection were estimated using the APEX2 crystallographic software package, in which data reduction and absorption corrections were carried out with SAINT and SADABS, respectively. The structures were solved and refined with the aid of the program SHELXL. The refined structures of crystals were reported as a crystallographic information file (CIF) [44].

4.6. Nuclear Magnetic Resonance (NMR) Data of Chrysophanol and Physcion

Chrysophanol: ^{1}H-NMR (500 MHz, CDCl$_3$), δ (ppm), J (Hz): 12.1 (1H, s, OH-8), 11.99 (1H, s, OH-1), 7.82 (1H, dd, J = 7.0, 1.0 Hz, H-5), 7.67 (1H, d, J = 8.0 Hz, H-6), 7.64 (1H, d, J = 1.5 Hz, H-4), 7.30 (1H, dd, J = 8.5, 1.0 Hz, H-7), 7.09 (1H, d, J = 0.5 Hz, H-2), 2.46 (3H, s, H-11). ^{13}C-NMR (125 MHz, CDCl3), δ (ppm): 192.6 (C-9), 182.0 (C-10), 162.7 (C-1), 162.4 (C-8), 149.3 (C-3), 136.9 (C-6), 133.7 (C-10a), 133.3 (C-4a), 124.6 (C-7), 124.4 (C-2), 121.4 (C-4), 119.9 (C-5), 115.9 (C-8a), 113.8 (C-9a), 22.2 (CH$_3$).

Physcion: ^{1}H-NMR (500 MHz, CDCl$_3$), δ (ppm), J (Hz): 12.28 (1H, s, OH-8), 12.08 (1H, s, OH-1), 7.60 (1H, d, J = 1.0 Hz, H-4), 7.34 (1H, d, J = 2.5 Hz, H-5), 7.06 (1H, d, J = 0.5 Hz, H-2), 6.67 (1H, d, J = 2.5 Hz, H-7), 3.93 (3H, s, OCH3), 2.44 (3H, s, H-11). ^{13}C-NMR (125 MHz, CDCl3), δ (ppm): 190.7 (C-9), 181.9 (C-10), 166.5 (C-6), 165.2 (C-8), 162.5 (C-1), 148.4 (C-3), 135.2 (C-10a), 133.2 (C-4a), 124.5 (C-2), 121.3 (C-4), 113.7 (C-9a), 110.3 (C-8a), 108.2 (C-5), 106.8 (C-7), 56.0 (OCH$_3$), 22.1 (C-11).

4.7. Xanthine Oxidase Inhibition (XOD) Activity

The inhibitory effect on xanthine oxidase (XO) of isolated compounds (**C1**–**C3**) was measured spectrophotometrically according to the method reported previously [10] with minor modifications.

4.8. α-Amylase Inhibition (AAI) Assay

The inhibitory effect of **C1**–**C3** on α-amylase was assessed by a starch-iodine method [34] with modification as follows: in each well of a microplate (U-shape, Greiner Bio-one, NC, USA), 20 μL of each isolated compound was pre-incubated with 20 μL of 1 U/mL α-amylase solution (from *Aspergillus oryzae*, Sigma-Aldrich, St. Louis, MO, USA) at 37 °C for 10 min. The reaction was initiated by pipetting 30 μL of soluble starch (0.5% in deionized water). After 6 min of incubation at 37 °C, an aliquot of 20 μL of hydrochloric acid (1 M) was added to stop reaction, followed by 120 μL of 0.25 mM iodine solution. The absorbance at 565 nm was read by a microplate reader (Multiskan^{TM} Microplate Spectrophotometer, Thermo Fisher Scientific, Osaka, Japan). The inhibitory activity of **C1**–**C3** on α-amylase was performed as the inhibition percentage calculated using the formula:

$$\% \text{ inhibition} = (A - C)/(B - C) \times 100$$

where A is the absorbance of the compound, B is the absorbance of reaction without enzyme, C is the absorbance of the negative control. A commercial diabetes inhibitor acarbose was used as a positive reference. Dilutions of test samples and dissolutions of enzyme used 20 mM sodium phosphate buffer (pH 6.9 comprising of 6 mM sodium chloride). α-Amylase solution and soluble starch solution were prepared and used on the day of the experiment. The IC$_{50}$ value was calculated to exhibit 50% inhibitory activity of **C1**–**C3** against α-amylase.

4.9. α-Glucosidase Inhibition (AGI) Assay

The anti-α-glucosidase activity of **C1**–**C3** was evaluated using a method described previously [35] with some modifications. In brief, an amount of 20 μL methanolic stock solution of isolated compounds was pre-mixed with an equal volume of 0.1 M potassium phosphate buffer (pH 7) and 40 μL of α-glucosidase (from *Saccharomyces cerevisiae*, Sigma-Aldrich, St. Louis, MO, USA) enzyme solution (0.5 U/mL in 0.1 M potassium phosphate buffer, pH 7). After 6 min incubation at 25 °C, a 20 μL aliquot of 5 mM p-nitrophenyl-α-D-glucopyranoside (pNPG) substrate (in 0.1 M potassium phosphate buffer, pH 7) was added to each reaction and the mixture was incubated for another 8 min. The reaction was terminated by adding 100 μL of 0.2 M Na$_2$CO$_3$, and absorbance was recorded at 405 nm. The inhibition percentage was calculated by the following equation:

$$\% \text{ inhibition} = (1 - A_{sample}/A_{control}) \times 100$$

where A$_{sample}$ is absorbance of isolated compound, A$_{control}$ is the abosrbance of positive controls (acarbose or quercetin).

4.10. Statistical Analysis

All obtained data were analyzed by Minitab Software (version 16.0, copyright 2015, Minitab Inc., State College, PA, USA). One-way analysis of variance (ANOVA) and Tukey's post hoc test were used to identify the significant difference among mean values with $p < 0.05$. All trials were designed randomly in triplicate.

5. Conclusions

This study documented that the root of *Rumex crispus* possessed potent antioxidant, xanthine oxidase, α-amylase and α-glucosidase inhibitory activity in *in vitro* assays. More specifically, the compounds isolated from the EtOAc extracts emerged as a promising source of natural antioxidants, xanthine oxidase, α-amylase, and α-glucosidase inhibitors. *In vivo* tests should be conducted to affirm the bioactivity of the isolated compounds from the root of *Rumex crispus* for the development of food additives and supplements to reduce the risks type 2 diabetes and gout. The isolation of novel constituents, as well as investigations on the potent pharmaceutical properties of the root of *Rumex crispus* need to be considered.

Supplementary Materials: The following are available online at http://www.mdpi.com/1420-3049/24/21/3899/s1, Figures S1–S21 and Tables S1–S3 are provided.

Author Contributions: T.N.M., Y.A., and T.M.V. conceived of the idea and implemented the experiments. T.N.M., D.V.H., D.H.D., and T.M.V. analyzed data and wrote the manuscripts. D.V.H. interpreted NMR data. C.d.G.-G., L.T.V., T.N.M., and T.M.V. gave advice and revised the manuscript. All authors agreed with the final version of the manuscript.

Funding: No funding was provided in support of this study.

Acknowledgments: Center for Research and Technology Transfer, Vietnam is appreciated for partly supporting to this research. We thank Tran Dang Xuan and Nobukazu Nakagoshi for helpful advice on this research.

Conflicts of Interest: All authors have no conflicts of interest.

References

1. Cavers, P.B.; Harper, J.L. *Rumex obtusifolius* L. and *R. crispus* L. *J. Ecol.* **1964**, *52*, 737–766. [CrossRef]
2. Orbán-Gyapai, O.; Liktor-Busa, E.; Kúsz, N.; Stefkó, D.; Urbán, E.; Hohmann, J.; Vasas, A. Antibacterial Screening of *Rumex* Species Native to the Carpathian Basin and Bioactivity-Guided Isolation of Compounds from *Rumex aquaticus*. *Fitoterapia*. **2017**, *118*, 101–106. [CrossRef] [PubMed]
3. Idris, O.A.; Wintola, O.A.; Afolayan, A.J. Comparison of the Proximate Composition, Vitamins (Ascorbic Acid, α-Tocopherol and Retinol), Anti-Nutrients (Phytate and Oxalate) and the GC-MS Analysis of the Essential Oil of the Root and Leaf of *Rumex crispus* L. *Plants* **2019**, *8*, 51. [CrossRef] [PubMed]
4. Mostafa, H.A.M.; Elbakry, A.A.; Eman, A.A. Evaluation of Antibacterial and Antioxidant Activities of Different Plant Parts of *Rumex vesicarius* L. (polygonaceae). *Int. J. Pharm. Pharm. Sci.* **2011**, *3*, 109–118.
5. Kulczyński, B.; Sidor, A.; Gramza-Michałowska, A. Characteristics of Selected Antioxidative and Bioactive Compounds in Meat and Animal Origin Products. *Antioxidants* **2019**, *8*, 335. [CrossRef]
6. Tan, B.L.; Norhaizan, M.E.; Liew, W.P.; Sulaiman Rahman, H. Antioxidant and Oxidative Stress: A Mutual Interplay in Age-Related Diseases. Antioxidant and Oxidative Stress: A Mutual Interplay in Age-Related Diseases. *Front Pharmacol.* **2018**, *9*, 1162. [CrossRef]
7. Wegiera, M.; Kosikowska, U.; Malm, A.; Smolarz, H. Antimicrobial Activity of the Extracts from Fruits of *Rumex*, L. Species. *Open Life Sci.* **2011**, *6*, 1036–1043. [CrossRef]
8. Feduraev, P.; Chupakhina, G.; Maslennikov, P.; Tacenko, N.; Skrypnik, L. Variation in Phenolic Compounds Content and Antioxidant Activity of Different Plant Organs from *Rumex crispus* L. and *Rumex obtusifolius* L. at Different Growth Stages. *Antioxidants* **2019**, *8*, 237. [CrossRef]

9. Kapoor, N.; Saxena, S. Potential Xanthine Oxidase Inhibitory Activity of Endophytic *Lasiodiplodia pseudotheobromae*. *App. Biochem. Biotech.* **2014**, *173*, 1360–1374. [CrossRef]
10. Nguyen, M.T.T.; Awale, S.; Tezuka, Y.; Tran, Q.L.; Watanabe, H.; Kadota, S. Xanthine Oxidase Inhibitory Activity of Vietnamese Medicinal Plants. *Biol. Pharm. Bull.* **2004**, *27*, 1414–1421. [CrossRef]
11. Lien, Y.H.; Logan, J.L. Cross-reactions between Allopurinol and Febuxostat. *Am. J. Med.* **2017**, *130*, e67–e68. [CrossRef] [PubMed]
12. Chohan, S. Safety and Efficacy of Febuxostat Treatment in Subjects with Gout and Severe Allopurinol Adverse Reactions. *J. Rheumatol.* **2011**, *38*, 1957–1959. [CrossRef] [PubMed]
13. Cos, P.; Ying, L.; Calomme, M.; Hu, J.P.; Cimanga, K.; Van, P.B.; Pieters, L.; Vlietinck, A.J.; Berghe, D.V. Structure−Activity Relationship and Classification of Flavonoids as Inhibitors of Xanthine Oxidase and Superoxide Scavengers. *J. Nat. Prod.* **1998**, *61*, 71–76. [CrossRef] [PubMed]
14. Pacher, P.; Nivorozhkin, A.; Szabó, C. Therapeutic Effects of Xanthine Oxidase Inhibitors: Renaissance Half a Century After the Discovery of Allopurinol. *Pharmacol. Rev.* **2006**, *58*, 87–114. [CrossRef]
15. Mohamed Isa, S.S.P.; Ablat, A.; Mohamad, J. The Antioxidant and Xanthine Oxidase Inhibitory Activity of *Plumeria rubra* Flowers. *Molecules* **2018**, *23*, 400. [CrossRef]
16. Cotelle, N.; Bernier, J.L.; Henichart, J.P.; Catteau, J.P.; Gaydou, E.; Wallet, J.C. Scavenger and Antioxidant Properties of Ten Synthetic Flavones. *Free Radical Bio. Med.* **1992**, *13*, 211–219. [CrossRef]
17. International Diabetes Federation. IDF Diabetes Atlas, 8th ed. Available online: http://diabetesatlas.org/key-messages.html (accessed on 1 August 2018).
18. Leahy, J.L. Pathogenesis of Type 2 Diabetes Mellitus. *Arch. Med. Res.* **2005**, *36*, 197–209. [CrossRef]
19. Abesundara, K.J.M.; Matsui, T.; Matsumoto, K. α-Glucosidase Inhibitory Activity of some Sri Lanka Plant Extracts, one of which, *Cassia auriculata*, Exerts a Strong Antihyperglycemic Effect in Rats Comparable to the Therapeutic Drug Acarbose. *J. Agric. Food Chem.* **2004**, *52*, 2541–2545. [CrossRef]
20. Collier, A.; Wilson, R.; Bradley, H.; Thomson, J.A.; Small, M. Free Radical Activity is type 2 Diabetes. *Diabetic Med.* **1990**, *7*, 27–30. [CrossRef]
21. Halliwell, B.; Gutteridge, J.M.C. *Free radicals in Biology and Medicine*, 4th ed.; Clarendon: Oxford, UK, 2007.
22. Logani, M.K.; Davis, R.E. Lipid Peroxidation in Biologic Effects and Antioxidants: A Review. *Lipids* **1979**, *15*, 485–493. [CrossRef]
23. Madhu, C.G.; Devi, D.B. Protective Antioxidant Effect of Vitamins C and E in Streptozotocin Induced Diabetic Rats. *Ind. J. Exp. Biol.* **2000**, *38*, 101–104.
24. Nagarajan, S.; Jain, H.C.; Aulakh, G.S. *Indigenous Plants Used in the Control of Diabetes*; Publication and Information Directorate CSIR: New Delhi, India, 1987; p. 586.
25. Jain, S.R.; Sharma, S.N. Hypoglycemic Drugs of Indian Indigenous Origin. *Planta Medica* **1967**, *15*, 439–442. [CrossRef] [PubMed]
26. Anjali, P.; Manoj, K.M. Same Comments on Diabetes and Herbal Therapy. *Ancient Sci. Life* **1995**, *15*, 27–29.
27. Idris, O.A.; Wintola, O.A.; Afolayan, A.J. Phytochemical and Antioxidant Activities of *Rumex crispus* L. in Treatment of Gastrointestinal Helminths in Eastern Cape Province, South Africa. *Asian Pac. J. Trop. Bio.* **2017**, *12*, 1071–1078. [CrossRef]
28. Maksimović, Z.; Kovacević, N.; Lakusić, B.; Cebović, T. Antioxidant Activity of Yellow Dock (Rumex crispus L., Polygonaceae) Fruit Extract. *Phytother Res.* **2011**, *25*, 101–105. [CrossRef]
29. Huang, D.; Ou, B.; Prior, R.L. The Chemistry Behind Antioxidant Capacity Assays. *J. Agric. Food Chem.* **2005**, *53*, 1841–1856. [CrossRef]
30. Elzaawely, A.A.; Xuan, T.D.; Tawasta, S. Antioxidant and Antibacterial Activities of *Rumex japonicus* Houtt. Aerial Parts. *Biol. Pharm. Bull.* **2005**, *28*, 2225–2230. [CrossRef]
31. Andriana, Y.; Xuan, T.D.; Quy, T.N.; Minh, T.N.; Van, T.M.; Viet, T.D. Antihyperuricemia, Antioxidant, and Antibacterial Activities of *Tridax procumbens* L. *Foods* **2019**, *8*, 21. [CrossRef]
32. Nagao, A.; Seki, M.; Kobayashi, H. Inhibition of Xanthine Oxidase by Flavonoids. *Biosci. Biotechnol. Biochem.* **1999**, *63*, 10. [CrossRef]
33. Shieh, D.E.; Liu, L.T.; Lin, C.C. Antioxidant and Free Radical Scavenging Effects of Baicalein, Baicalin and Wogonin. *Anticancer Res.* **2000**, *20*, 2861–2865.
34. Agarwal, P.; Gupta, R. Alpha-amylase Inhibition can Treat Diabetes Mellitus. *RRJMHS.* **2016**, *5*, 1–8.
35. Yin, Z.; Zhang, W.; Feng, F.; Zhang, Y.; Kang, W. α-Glucosidase Inhibitors Isolated from Medicinal Plants. *Food Sci. Hum. Wellness.* **2014**, *3*, 136–174. [CrossRef]

36. Rana, Z.H.; Alam, M.K.; Akhtaruzzaman, M. Nutritional Composition, Total Phenolic Content, Antioxidant and α-Amylase Inhibitory Activities of Different Fractions of Selected Wild Edible Plants. *Antioxidants* **2019**, *8*, 203. [CrossRef] [PubMed]
37. Minh, T.N.; Xuan, T.D.; Ahmad, A.; Elzaawely, A.A.; Teschke, R.; Van, T.M. Efficacy from Different Extractions for Chemical Profile and Biological Activities of Rice Husk. *Sustainability* **2018**, *10*, 1356. [CrossRef]
38. Minh, T.N.; Tuyen, P.T.; Khang, D.T.; Quan, N.V.; Ha, P.T.T.; Quan, N.T.; Yusuf, A.; Fan, X.; Van, T.M.; Khanh, T.D.; et al. Potential Use of Plant Wastes of Moth Orchid (*Phalaenopsis* Sogo Yukidian 'V3') as an Antioxidant Source. *Foods* **2017**, *6*, 85. [CrossRef]
39. Minh, T.N.; Khang, D.T.; Tuyen, P.T.; Minh, L.T.; Anh, L.H.; Quan, N.V.; Ha, P.T.T.; Quan, N.T.; Toan, N.P.; Elzaawely, A.A.; et al. Phenolic Compounds and Antioxidant Activity of *Phalaenopsis* Orchid Hybrids. *Antioxidants* **2016**, *5*, 31. [CrossRef]
40. Van, T.M.; Xuan, T.D.; Minh, T.N.; Quan, N.V. Isolation and Purification of Potent Growth Inhibitors from *Piper methysticum* Root. *Molecules* **2018**, *23*, 1907. [CrossRef]
41. Minh, T.N.; Xuan, T.D.; Tran, H.-D.; Van, T.M.; Andriana, Y.; Khanh, T.D.; Quan, N.V.; Ahmad, A. Isolation and Purification of Bioactive Compounds from the Stem Bark of *Jatropha podagrica*. *Molecules* **2019**, *24*, 889. [CrossRef]
42. Viet, T.D.; Xuan, T.D.; Van, T.M.; Andriana, Y.; Rayee, R.; Tran, H.-D. Comprehensive Fractionation of Antioxidants and GC-MS and ESI-MS Fingerprints of *Celastrus hindsii* Leaves. *Medicines* **2019**, *6*, 64. [CrossRef]
43. Minh, T.N.; Xuan, T.D.; Van, T.M.; Andriana, Y.; Viet, T.D.; Khanh, T.D.; Tran, H.-D. Phytochemical Analysis and Potential Biological Activities of Essential Oil from Rice Leaf. *Molecules* **2019**, *24*, 546. [CrossRef]
44. He, C.; Liu, X.; Jiang, Z.; Geng, S.; Ma, H.; Liu, B. Interaction Mechanism of Flavonoids and α-Glucosidase: Experimental and Molecular Modelling Studies. *Foods* **2019**, *8*, 355. [CrossRef] [PubMed]

Sample Availability: Samples of the compounds are available from the authors.

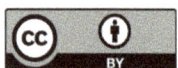

© 2019 by the authors. Licensee MDPI, Basel, Switzerland. This article is an open access article distributed under the terms and conditions of the Creative Commons Attribution (CC BY) license (http://creativecommons.org/licenses/by/4.0/).

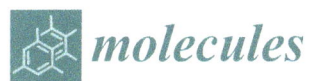

Article

Antioxidant, α-Amylase and α-Glucosidase Inhibitory Activities and Potential Constituents of *Canarium tramdenum* Bark

Nguyen Van Quan [1], Tran Dang Xuan [1,*], Hoang-Dung Tran [2,*], Nguyen Thi Dieu Thuy [1], Le Thu Trang [1], Can Thu Huong [1], Yusuf Andriana [1] and Phung Thi Tuyen [3]

[1] Division of Development Technology, Graduate School for International Development and Cooperation (IDEC), Hiroshima University, Higashi Hiroshima 739-8529, Japan; nguyenquan26@gmail.com (N.V.Q.); dieuthuykttb@gmail.com (N.T.D.T.); trangle9872@gmail.com (L.T.T.); cth1412@gmail.com (C.T.H.); yusufandriana@yahoo.com (Y.A.)

[2] Department of Biotechnology, NTT Institute of Hi-Technology, Nguyen Tat Thanh University, 298A-300A Nguyen Tat Thanh Street, Ward 13, District 4, Ho Chi Minh 72820, Vietnam

[3] Faculty of Forest Resources and Environmental Management, Vietnam National University of Forestry, Xuan Mai, Hanoi 156200 Vietnam; phungtuyen@gmail.com

* Correspondence: tdxuan@hiroshima-u.ac.jp (T.D.X.); thdung@ntt.edu.vn (H.-D.T.); Tel./Fax: +81-82-424-6927 (T.D.X.)

Academic Editors: Raffaele Capasso and Lorenzo Di Cesare Mannelli
Received: 13 January 2019; Accepted: 7 February 2019; Published: 9 February 2019

Abstract: The fruits of *Canarium tramdenum* are commonly used as foods and cooking ingredients in Vietnam, Laos, and the southeast region of China, whilst the leaves are traditionally used for treating diarrhea and rheumatism. This study was conducted to investigate the potential use of this plant bark as antioxidants, and α-amylase and α-glucosidase inhibitors. Five different extracts of *C. tramdenum* bark (TDB) consisting of the extract (TDBS) and factional extracts hexane (TDBH), ethyl acetate (TDBE), butanol (TDBB), and water (TDBW) were evaluated. The TDBS extract contained the highest amount of total phenolic (112.14 mg gallic acid equivalent per g dry weight), while the TDBB extract had the most effective antioxidant capacity compared to other extracts. Its IC_{50} values were 12.33, 47.87, 33.25, and 103.74 µg/mL in 2,2-diphenyl-1-picrylhydrazyl (DPPH), 2,2′-azino-bis (ABTS), reducing power (RP), and nitric oxide (NO) assays, respectively. Meanwhile, the lipid peroxidation inhibition of the four above extracts was proximate to that of butylated hydroxytoluene (BHT) as a standard antioxidant. The result of porcine pancreatic α-amylase inhibition showed that TDB extracts have promising effects which are in line with the commercial diabetic inhibitor acarbose. Interestingly, the inhibitory ability on α-glucosidase of all the extracts was higher than that of acarbose. Among the extracts, the TDBB extract expressed the strongest activity on the enzymatic reaction (IC_{50} = 18.93 µg/mL) followed by the TDBW extract (IC_{50} = 25.27 µg/mL), TDBS (IC_{50} = 28.17 µg/mL), and TDBE extract (IC_{50} = 141.37 µg/mL). The phytochemical constituents of the TDB extract were identified by gas chromatography–mass spectrometry (GC-MS). The principal constituents included nine phenolics, eight terpenoids, two steroids, and five compounds belonging to other chemical classes, which were the first reported in this plant. Among them, the presence of α- and β-amyrins were identified by GC-MS and appeared as the most dominant constituents in TDB extracts (1.52 mg/g). The results of this study revealed that *C. tramdenum* bark possessed rich phenolics and terpenoids, which might confer on reducing risks from diabetes. A high quantity of α- and β-amyrins highlighted the potentials of anti-inflammatory, anti-ulcer, anti-hyperlipidemic, anti-tumor, and hepatoprotective properties of *C. tramdenum* bark.

Keywords: *Canarium tramdenum*; bark; antioxidants; α-glucosidase inhibitors; diabetes; phenolics; terpenoids; biological activity

1. Introduction

Diabetes or diabetes mellitus has become a burden for the global economy in recent decades. According to the World Health Organization's report, this disease and its complications cause substantial economic loss through direct medical costs and loss of work and wages [1]. Among diabetes cases, type 2 diabetes is much more common and chiefly occurs in adults; however, it is being increasingly noted in adolescents [2]. The pathogenesis of type 2 diabetes is currently attributed to endogenous factors such as genetics and metabolic abnormalities and exogenous factors such as behavior and environment [3]. The type 2 diabetes increases blood sugar level which is considered as a typical symptom in diabetic patients. Monitoring and control of hyperglycemia are the most prevalent methods in the treatment of type 2 diabetes nowadays.

As an endogenous toxin, oxidative stress is considered to be an important determinant of type 2 diabetes complications [4]. The causal relation between oxidative stress and type 2 diabetes has been elucidated through molecular mechanisms [5], whereby the overproduction of reactive oxygen species related to hyperglycemia likely leads to an imbalance of the quantity of antioxidants inside the body and eventually, to oxidative stress. On the other hand, the blood sugar level is crucially determined by the act of digestive enzymes such as α-amylase and α-glucosidase. While α-amylase is responsible for breaking down long-chain carbohydrates, α-glucosidase directly converts carbohydrate to glucose in the small intestine. The inhibition of α-glucosidase has been acknowledged as a therapeutic target for the control of postprandial hyperglycemia, as well as type 2 diabetes [6,7]. Therefore, simultaneously providing antioxidants and α-amylase and α-glucosidase inhibitors through nutriments is a potential and feasible method for the management of type 2 diabetes. However, the origin and dose of ingredients should be scrupulously studied before application and production. Additionally, natural products are recommended owing to their long history of medicinal and beneficial effects on human health [8].

Among natural sources, plants have been the most thoroughly scrutinized thanks to their vast diversity and wide distribution across the Earth. It is easy to derive antioxidant and nutrient components from every part of plants as fruits, leaves, stems, and roots which exhibit a wide range of biological effects such as anti-inflammatory, antibacterial, antiviral, anti-aging, and anticancer [9]. Nonetheless, this is also a reason why the potential of plants in treating certain diseases has not yet been fully exploited. *Canarium tramdenanum* Dai & Yakovlev, a synonym of *Canarium pimela* Koenig, a woody tree belonging to Burseraceae family, is not an exception. This plant is widely distributed in subtropical and tropical regions of China and Indochina [10]. In Vietnam, ripe fruits of *C. tramdenum* are commonly used as foods and cooking ingredients, whilst leaves are traditionally used for treating diarrhea and rheumatism [10,11]. In China, *C. tramdenum* or "Chinese black olive" is used in folk medicine as an anti-bacterial, anti-viral, anti-inflammatory, and detoxifying substance [3]. Recently, vasorelaxant and antioxidant activities of the fruits and leaves of this plant have been reported [3,12]. The nutritional compositions of *C. tramdenum* kernels were also documented [13]; however, their biological activities were not investigated. To date, no study on the anti-diabetic property of this plant has been reported. Hence, in this research, we investigated the antioxidant and potential diabetic inhibitory properties of *C. tramdenum* bark extracts through in vitro assays of α-amylase and α-glucosidase suppression.

2. Results

2.1. Extraction Yield and Total Phenolic Contents

From 30 g dry TDB, five extracts with different yields were obtained by using an extraction method based on various polarity solvents. The yield of TDBS was 20% (6 g), followed by TDBW (6.67%, 2 g), TDBE (5%, 1.5 g), TDBB (5%, 1.5 g), and TDBH (0.42%, 0.13 g).

The total phenolic contents (TPC) of TDB extracts were shown in Table 1. It is noteworthy that there was a variation in TPC among extracts which ranged from 20.5 to 112.14 mg GAE/g DW. The total extract TDBS was found to have the highest TPC (112.14 mg GAE/g DW) compared with fractional extracts. The lowest TPC was determined in TDBE extract which accounted for 20.5 mg GAE/g DW. TPC of three fractional extracts TDBE, TDBB, and TDBW (90.62 mg GAE/g DW) were not equal to that of the total extract TDBS. This could be explained by the loss in fractionation and filtration steps (around 21.52 mg GAE/g DW). However, TPC in extracts by higher polar solvents (TDBB and TDBW) were significantly greater than those of extracts by lower polar solvents (TDBE).

Table 1. Total phenolic contents and antioxidant activities of TDB extracts.

Samples	TPC (mg GAE/g DW)	DPPH Assay IC$_{50}$ (µg/mL)	ABTS Assay IC$_{50}$ (µg/mL)	RP Assay IC$_{50}$ (µg/mL)	βC Assay LPI (%)
TDBS	112.14 ± 1.19 [a]	15.41 ± 0.10 [c]	62.21 ± 1.78 [b]	33.25 ± 0.04 [b]	86.12 ± 0.98 [ab]
TDBE	20.50 ± 0.60 [c]	22.23 ± 0.09 [e]	76.96 ± 1.04 [c]	41.60 ± 0.03 [d]	87.52 ± 0.73 [a]
TDBB	36.57 ± 0.36 [b]	12.33 ± 0.02 [a]	47.87 ± 0.12 [a]	26.24 ± 0.02 [a]	86.75 ± 0.84 [ab]
TDBW	33.55 ± 0.48 [b]	16.45 ± 0.07 [d]	45.25 ± 0.17 [a]	33.25 ± 0.06 [b]	84.09 ± 0.56 [b]
BHT	-	14.99 ± 0.06 [b]	80.26 ± 1.11 [c]	38.34 ± 0.01 [c]	86.67 ± 0.33 [ab]

Data express means ± SE (standard error); Different superscript letters ([a,b,c,d,e]) in a column indicate significant differences at $p < 0.05$; -: not measured; TPC, total phenolic contents; GAE, gallic acid equivalent; DW, dry weight; DPPH, 2,2-diphenyl-1-picrylhydrazyl; ABTS, 2,2'-azino-bis; RP, reducing power; NO, nitric oxide; βC, β-carotene bleaching; TDBS, *C. tramdenum* total extract; TDBE, ethyl acetate extract; TDBB, butanol extract; TDBW, water extract; BHT: butylated hydroxytoluene.

2.2. Antioxidant Activities

The antioxidant capacities of TDB extracts by DPPH, ABTS, reducing power and β-carotene bleaching assays are displayed in Table 1.

DPPH is a stable reagent and widely used in most antioxidant tests. The principle of this sensitive assay is based on the reaction of samples with the organic radical DPPH [14]. The antioxidant ability of samples can be observed visually by the discoloration of DPPH (from purple to yellow or colorless) or be determined by the reduced absorbance of the final reaction at 517 nm wavelength. In this study, TDBB extract showed the strongest anti-DPPH radical activity (IC$_{50}$=12.33 µg/mL) which was significantly higher than standard BHT (IC$_{50}$=14.99 µg/mL) and other extracts, see Table 1.

In the case of the ABTS assay, antioxidants in samples reacting with an organic cation radical named ABTS$^{•+}$ are the basis for this test. In the mixture, with the presence of antioxidants, the nitrogen atom of ABTS$^{•+}$ quenches the hydrogen atom of antioxidants yielding the solution decolorization [15]. The decolorization of ABTS$^{•+}$ solution illustrates the antioxidant capacity of samples. As shown in Table 2, except for TDBE extract, all TDB extracts presented more powerful activity on ABTS assay than the standard BHT. Of which, IC$_{50}$ values of TDBB and TDBW were 1.7-times higher than that of BHT. Additionally, the TDBS extract was 1.3-times the antioxidant activity of BHT.

Table 2. α-Amylase and α-glucosidase inhibitory activities of *C. tramdenum* bark (TDB) extracts.

Sample	α-Amylase Inhibition IC$_{50}$ (µg/mL)	α-Glucosidase Inhibition IC$_{50}$ (µg/mL)
TDBS	359.32 ± 6.73 [c]	28.17 ± 0.12 [c]
TDBE	491.23 ± 2.49 [d]	141.37 ± 0.86 [b]
TDBB	257.20 ± 1.15 [b]	18.93 ± 0.07 [e]
TDBW	555.02 ± 9.10 [e]	25.27 ± 0.12 [d]
Acarbose	80.26 ± 0.24 [a]	145.35 ± 0.62 [a]

Data express means ± SE (standard error); Different superscript letters ([a,b,c,d,e]) in a column indicate significant difference at $p < 0.05$; TDBS, *C. tramdenum* total extract; TDBE, ethyl acetate extract; TDBB, butanol extract; TDBW, water extract.

Reducing power assay or potassium ferricyanide reducing power is based on the competence of antioxidants in converting potassium ferricyanide (Fe^{3+}) to potassium ferrocyanide (Fe^{2+}). The final reaction with ferric trichloride results in a mixture of Fe^{3+} and Fe^{2+}, a blue solution which can be spectrophotometrically determined at 700 nm [14]. An increase in the absorbance (high content of

Fe^{2+} in the final reaction) indicates a strong antioxidant activity. By comparing IC$_{50}$ values, see Table 1, the order of the antioxidant capacity of TDB extracts was TDBB (26.24 µg/mL) > TDBS and TDBW (33.25 µg/mL for both) > TDBE (41.60 µg/mL) whilst the IC$_{50}$ value of BHT was 38.34 µg/mL.

In the β-carotene bleaching assay using linoleic acid, the oxidized product (linoleate-free radical and other free radicals) of the linoleic acid peroxidation process can gradually decolorize the β-carotene color by time. The process can be delayed by the presence of antioxidants and the reaction can be recorded at 492 nm. It is apparent that, at the same concentration of 1000 µg/mL, all total extract and fractional extracts of TDB exhibit a similar inhibitory level of lipid peroxidation to the standard BHT, see Table 1. These results demonstrated that antioxidants involved in TDB extracts could negate the free radicals in the system, thereby they could protect β-carotene color from the bleaching process [16].

Sodium nitroprusside in phosphate buffer saline (pH 7.2) generate nitric oxide (NO) which can be spontaneously converted into the more stable forms of nitrate and nitrite ions under the aerobic reaction with oxygen [15,17]. The Griess reagent is used to detect these ions in the mixture by forming the conspicuous pink solution that can be measured at 546 nm. Antioxidants can prevent the formation of nitrate and nitrite ions and, therefore, reduce the absorbance of the reaction. Figure 1 shows that all TDB extracts possess potential NO scavenging activities which are comparable to the standard gallic acid. Among fractional extracts, TDBB expressed the highest antioxidant activity (IC$_{50}$ = 103.74 µg/mL), followed by TDBW (IC$_{50}$ = 112.54 µg/mL), and TDBE (IC$_{50}$ = 131.43 µg/mL). The activity of the total extract TDBS (IC$_{50}$ = 116.80 µg/mL) was significantly higher than that of TDBE but lower than those of TDBB and TDBW. In the body, NO associates with many biological systems including neuronal messenger, vasodilatation, and antimicrobial and antitumor activities [17]. Additionally, the complex interplay between NO production and the pathogenesis of diabetic nephropathy and angiopathy has been interpreted [18,19]. Hence, a nitric oxide scavenging assay is indispensable in the research on the antioxidant and antidiabetic properties of natural products.

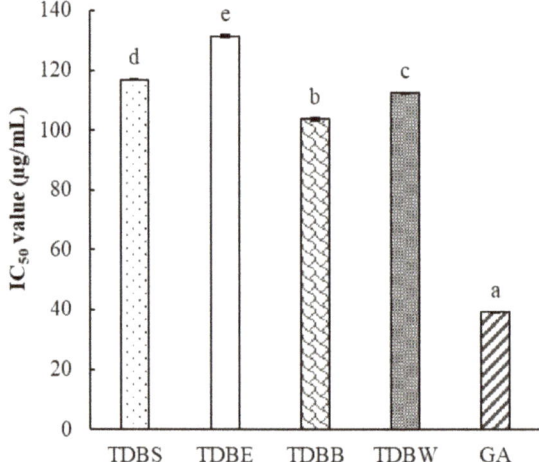

Figure 1. Nitric oxide scavenging activity of TDB extracts. Values are means ± SE (standard error) (n = 3); Different letters indicate significant difference at $p < 0.05$; TDBS, *C. tramdenum* total extract; TDBE, ethyl acetate extract; TDBB, butanol extract; TDBW, water extract; BHT: butylated hydroxytoluene; GA: gallic acid.

2.3. α-Amylase and α-Glucosidase Inhibitory Activities

In this study, starch-iodine method was applied to examine the inhibitory effect of TDB extracts on porcine pancreatic α-amylase. The degradation of starch by enzyme activity was visually observed or spectrophotometrically measured at 565 nm based on changing dark-blue color to yellow color of reaction solution. Accordingly, in mixtures with inhibitors, the solution with higher absorption (darker color) signifies the higher inhibitory activity. As shown in Table 2, the anti-α-amylase activity was recorded at all TDB extracts and comparable with the standard acarbose. Among extracts, TDBB extract manifested the highest inhibitory activity (IC_{50} = 257.20 µg/mL) while TDBW represented the lowest one (IC_{50} = 555.02 µg/mL).

The α-glucosidase inhibitory activity of TDB extracts was assayed using a synthetic substrate pNPG. In physiological buffer (pH 7), α-glucosidase hydrolyzes pNPG to release *p*-nitrophenol, a yellow product that can be measured at wavelength 405 nm [20]. The lower absorbance indicates the stronger suppression on enzymatic activity. All TDB extracts expressed a remarkable inhibition on α-glucosidase activity (Table 2). Of which, the activity of TDBS, TDBB and TDBW extracts were extraordinarily higher than that of standard acarbose. The order of α-glucosidase inhibition is TDBB > TDBW > TDBS > TDBE > acarbose corresponding to IC_{50} values 18.93, 27.27, 28.17, 141.37, and 145.35 µg/mL, respectively.

2.4. Correlations between Total Phenolics and Biological Activities

According to Table 3, there was no significant correlation between the total phenolic contents and biological activities of TDB extracts. These results indicated that TPC might not be the main contributor to the antioxidant, anti-α-amylase, and anti-α-glucosidase activities of TDB extracts. On the other hand, except for the β-carotene bleaching assay, all methods showed a strong correlation with each other, regardless of whether they were based on different methods ($p < 0.05$). Especially, antioxidant assays including DPPH, ABTS, reducing power, and nitric oxide were strongly correlated with the α-glucosidase inhibitory assay at $p < 0.05$. Meanwhile, ABTS assay was not significantly associated with the α-amylase inhibitory assay.

Table 3. Pearson's correlation coefficients between total phenolics and biological activities.

	TPC	DPPH	ABTS	RP	NO	βC	AG
DPPH	0.24	-	-	-	-	-	-
ABTS	−0.15	0.68*	-	-	-	-	-
RP	0.10	0.99*	0.72 *	-	-	-	-
NO	0.08	0.96*	0.86 *	0.97 *	-	-	-
βC	−0.08	−0.10	−0.52	−0.10	−0.26	-	-
AG	0.23	0.95*	0.85 *	0.94 *	0.98 *	−0.33	-
AA	0.20	0.85*	0.25	0.84 *	0.70 *	0.30	0.65 *

* a significance at $p < 0.05$; TPC, total phenolic contents; DPPH, 2,2-diphenyl-1-picrylhydrazyl assay; ABTS, 2,2′-azino-bis assay; RP, reducing power assay; NO, nitric oxide scavenging assay; βC, β-carotene bleaching assay; AG, α-glucosidase inhibitory assay; AA, α-amylase inhibitory assay.

2.5. GC-MS Results

Phytochemical compositions of TDB extracts analyzed by GC-MS were listed in Table 3. Twenty-four compounds were identified and classified which might be regarded as antioxidants and α-glucosidase inhibitors of TDB extracts.

To the best of our knowledge, except for α-cubebene and (-)-spathulenol that were previously identified in the essential oil of TDB [21], the remaining 22 compounds were the first reported as the principal component of TDB extracts by this study.

Among the identified compounds, phenolics accounted for the highest amount with nine compounds, followed by terpenoids (eight compounds), steroids (two compounds), carbohydrates (glycerol), monosaccharides (levoglucosan), phenylpropanoic acids (ibuprofen methyl ester), carboxylic acids (acetyltributyl citrate) and one unidentified compound. All phenolic compounds were detected in fractional extracts TDBB and TDBW while all terpenoids were identified in the TDBE extract. Although the phenolic components were scant in the total extract TDBS, they were accompanied with greater amounts in the fractional extracts of TDBB and TDBW. This is reasonable when lower polar components have been eliminated through hexane and ethyl acetate solvents. Whereas, 2-propylphenol and acetyltributyl citrate were only detected in fractional extracts TDBB and TDBE, respectively, but were not recognized in the total extract TDBS. Significantly, β-amyrin and α-amyrin were the most dominant compositions in the TDB extract, which showed the highest contents in TDBS (41.45% and 19.17%, respectively) and TDBE (29.51% and 20.18%, respectively) extracts.

2.6. Identification of α- and β-Amyrins by GC-MS

The GC-MS analysis on the crystal mixture isolated from F15–F18 of TDBE extract confirmed the presence of α- and β-amyrins (with a 3:4 ratio) as the dominant components. MS data showed that the relative intensity corresponding to the main fragments of α-amyrin were 27, 25, 100, and 13 for peaks at m/z 189, 203, 218, and 426, respectively. Meanwhile, β-amyrin data were 15, 52, 100, and 5, respectively at m/z values similar to the peaks described above, see Supplementary Materials, Figure S1. The result was coincident with the results of [22,23].

There has been extensive research that validated the diverse pharmacological activity of α- and β-amyrins, including anti-inflammatory, anti-ulcer, anti-hyperlipidemic, anti-tumor, and hepatoprotective actions [24,25]. Also, natural sources of α- and β-amyrins are available which can be easily extracted and isolated in various plants. The most important sources of α- and β-amyrins are Mexican copal (5 mg/g) and *Nelumbo nucifera* (3 mg/g), respectively [25]. Apart from the reported list of plants containing α- and β-amyrins [25], in this study, we supplemented some other sources together with their contents and biological activities, see Table 4. Accordingly, the content of isolated α- and β-amyrins in our study (1.52 mg/g) showed substantial potential in comparison with other plants. Noticeably, *C. tramdenum* bark involves a greater amount of these terpenoids than *C. subulatum* (0.03 mg/g of β-amyrin), a species that belongs to the same *Canarium* genus (Table 4).

Table 4. Natural sources of α-amyrin and β-amyrin and their principal biological activities.

Plant Species	Plant Parts	Quantity	Biological Activities	References
Protium kleinii	Resin	Mixture of α-,β-amyrins (1:1) 2.4 mg/g	Antinociception against the visceral pain in mice	[26]
Protium heptaphyllum	Trunk wood resin	Mixture of α-,β-Amyrins	Gastroprotective, anti-inflammatory and hepatoprotective properties	[24,27,28]
Symplocos cochinchinensis	Leaves	β-Amyrin 0.17 mg/g	Antioxidant and free-radical scavenging effects	[29]
Alstonia boonei	Stem barks	β-Amyrin 0.08 mg/g	Anti-inflammatory activity	[30]
Memecylon umbellatum	nm	nm	α-Glucosidase inhibitory activities	[31]
Melastoma malabathricum	Leaves	α-Amyrin 0.06 mg/g	nm	[32]
Maesobotrya barteri	Aerial parts	β-Amyrin	Antimicrobial activity	[33]
Swertia longifolia	Aerial parts	α-Amyrin 0.01 mg/g; β-Amyrin 0.02 mg/g	α-Amylaseinhibitory activity	[34]
Canarium subulatum	Stem bark	β-Amyrin 0.03 mg/g	Anti-herpetic activity	[35]
Canarium tramdenum	Barks	Mixture of α-,β-amyrins (3:4) 1.52 mg/g	nm	This study

nm, not mentioned

3. Discussion

Canarium is a genus of approximately 100 species in the Burseraceae family [36]. However, very few studies on antioxidant and anti-diabetic potentials were conducted on the species of this genus. Most of them focused on exploiting pharmaceutical and medicinal properties of several species possessing edible fruits. The extracts of *C. album* fruits had potent antioxidants as tannins [37] and phenolics [38] and exhibited effective anti-diabetic properties through antiglycation [39]. The leaf and fruit extracts of *C. odontophyllum* exerted inhibitory effects on diabetic and obese rats [40,41]. The information regarding antioxidant and antidiabetic effects of other inedible parts as stem barks of *Canarium* plants was fragmented and scant. Only stem bark extract of *C. schweinfurthii* was proved to acquire anti-diabetic effects [42]; however, bioactive components of this object were not described. By this study, for the first time, we comprehensively assessed the antioxidant and potential anti-diabetic activities and identified the phytochemicals of *C. tramdenum* bark's extracts. All extracts presented a similar antioxidant level to BHT, see Table 1, a well-known antioxidant compound and also commonly used in food additives [43]. The TDBB extract was even more active than BHT in DPPH, ABTS, and reducing power assays, see Table 1. Furthermore, TDB extracts showed a potential effect on the restraint of α-amylase activity and exerted much more powerful α-glucosidase inhibition than acarbose—a standard inhibitor that is ordinarily used in the clinical practice of diabetes treatment [44].

The antioxidant property is mainly characterized by phenolic contents [45] which can effortlessly release hydrogen donors to naturalize free radicals. Meanwhile, in α-amylase and α-glucosidase inhibition, both terpenoids and phenolics might play crucial roles [46]. In this study, we found that although the total extract of TDBS showed the highest phenolic content, its biological activities were not stronger than others, see Tables 1 and 2 and Figure 1. We assumed that phenolics might not be the only contributors toward the antioxidant and antidiabetic properties of TDB extracts. The examination of correlations between phenolics and biological activities of TDB extracts, see Table 3, revealed that the total amount of phenolics might not be the determinant of the biological activities of TDB extracts. The other factors such as functional groups of individual compounds may play more important roles in this case. In particular, the number of free hydrogen donors determines the antioxidant activity, the position of hydroxyl groups, methoxy groups, and lactone rings in the structure of compounds induce inhibitions of α-amylase and α-glucosidase and even the interaction among compounds in an extract may result in differences in biological activities. In this study, we hypothesized that the synergistic interaction between phenolic and terpenoid components might result in the greater biological activities for TDB extracts. However, the composition of phenolics seemed to be more essential when TDBB and TDBW extracts contained a high content of phenolics but not terpenoids and presented stronger antioxidant and anti-α-glucosidase activities than other extracts, see Table 5. Integrating with correlation results, we suggested that the presence of some phenolics, apart from other components, might be the major factor that determines the biological activity of TDB extracts. On the other hand, a previous study demonstrated the potential antihyperglycemic and hypolipidemic effects of α- and β-amyrins [47]. However, the successful isolation of α- and β-amyrins should be further approached to investigate the role of the two compounds in the TDB extracts, see Table 3. Moreover, the high yield of the isolation of these bioactive compounds in this study suggested the potential practical use of TDB extracts, see Table 5. Therefore, although the GC-MS results showed most of the major components of TDB extract, more sensitive methods such as the ultra-high performance liquid chromatography integrated with tandem mass spectrometry (UPLC-MS-MS) should be conducted to affirm and quantify phenolic compounds and other active components. Additionally, the subsequent in vivo tests and clinical trials should be implemented in order to certify the antidiabetic property of this prospective plant.

Table 5. Major phytochemical components of TDB extracts analyzed by GC-MS.

No.	Identified Compounds	RT (min)	Chemical Classification	Peak Area in Extracts (%)			
				TDBS	TDBE	TDBB	TDBW
1	Glycerol	4.62	Carbohydrates	<	-	-	37.73
2	2-Methoxyphenol	6.39	Phenolics	1.19	-	1.57	3.63
3	Pyrocatechol	7.88	Phenolics	1.28	-	19.31	6.66
4	4-Methylcatechol	9.21	Phenolics	<	-	1.67	1.38
5	2,6-Dimethoxyphenol	10.08	Phenolics	<	-	-	1.43
6	2-Propylphenol	10.35	Phenolics	-	-	3.54	-
7	α-Cubebene	10.58	Terpenoids	0.67	<	-	-
8	3,4-Dimethoxyphenol	11.05	Phenolics	<	-	-	5.22
9	Levoglucosan	11.82	Monosaccharides	<	-	4.30	1.92
10	3,7(11)-Eudesmadiene	12.37	Terpenoids	1.10	<	-	-
11	Ibuprofen methyl ester	12.55	Phenylpropanoic acids	1.20	<	-	-
12	4-Propylresorcinol	13.18	Phenolics	<	-	13.90	1.75
13	3,4,5-Trimethoxyphenol	13.24	Phenolics	0.71	-	1.99	5.24
14	β-Guaiene	13.69	Terpenoids	0.78	2.22	-	-
15	Homovanillic acid	13.79	Phenolics	1.06	-	13.39	3.26
16	(−)-Spathulenol	15.30	Terpenoids	<	0.92	-	-
17	Methyl hinokiate	16.62	Terpenoids	<	2.05	-	-
18	Ylangenol	17.07	Terpenoids	<	1.00	-	-
19	Acetyltributyl citrate	19.78	Carboxylic acids	-	1.89	-	-
20	Stigmasterol	27.86	Steroids	<	2.41	-	-
21	γ-Sitosterol	28.56	Steroids	0.89	6.52	-	-
22	β-Amyrin	29.12	Terpenoids	41.45	29.51	-	-
23	Not identified	29.32	Not identified	7.41	9.49	-	-
24	α-Amyrin	29.72	Terpenoids	19.17	20.18	-	-

RT, retention time; -, not detected; <, trace of peak area that was lower than 0.5%.

4. Materials and Methods

4.1. Materials and Instrumentations

Stem bark of *C. tramdenum* (TDB) was collected at 21.07°N, 106.10°E, Bac Ninh province, Vietnam in 2016. The species was identified at a study field based on Vietnam Plant Data Center (http://www.botanyvn.com) and Plants Database Missouri Botanical Garden, United States (TROPICOS—http://www.tropicos.org). The specimen with voucher number TDB-J2016 was deposited at the Plant Physiology and Biochemistry Laboratory, IDEC, Hiroshima University, Japan.

All extraction solvents including methanol, hexane, ethyl acetate, and butanol were purchased from Junsei Chemical Co., Ltd., Tokyo, Japan. The analytical reagents for antioxidant assays were acquired from Kanto Chemical Co., Inc., Tokyo, Japan while those of enzymatic assays were procured from Sigma-Aldrich, St. Louis, MO, USA.

A vacuum evaporator (Rotavapor® R-300, Nihon Buchi K.K., Tokyo, Japan), a microplate reader (Multiskan™ Microplate Spectrophotometer, Thermo Fisher Scientific, Osaka, Japan), and GC-MS system (JMS-T100 GCV, JEOL Ltd., Tokyo, Japan) were the main instruments used in this study.

4.2. Sample Preparation and Extraction

After air-drying for 2 days, the outer layer of TDB was scraped to remove all fungi and lichen. Then, the sample was washed with 1% sodium hypochlorite (NaOCl) and water. After blotting with tissues, bark samples were dried at 45 °C for 1 week by an oven, then ground to make the powder.

The TDB sample (30 g) was extracted using 1 L of methanol in one week. Afterwards, dry methanol crude extract (TDBS) was blended with distilled water (200 mL), then successively fractionated by an equal volume of hexane, ethyl acetate, and butanol. Each fractionation step was conducted three times. After filtrations, they were separately dried under vacuum by an evaporator at 50 °C. Eventually, five dried extracts including TDBS (total extract), hexane (TDBH), ethyl acetate (TDBE), butanol (TDBB), and water (TDBW) extracts were obtained as fractional extracts. They were preserved in sterilized vials and kept in a refrigerator (−20 °C) for further tests on the physical properties, biological activities, and identification of phytochemical components.

4.3. Determination of Total Phenolic Content

The total phenolic content (TPC) was calculated according to the Folin-Ciocalteu method described previously [48]. Specifically, 20 µL of extract was homogenized with 100µL of Folin-Ciocalteu's reagent (10%) and 80µL of 7.5% Na_2CO_3 (w/v), respectively. The mixture was then shaken and incubated at room temperature for 30 min. The absorbance was measured at 765 nm using a microplate reader. TPC was expressed as mg gallic acid equivalent per g dry weight of sample (mg GAE/g DW).

4.4. DPPH Radical Scavenging Assay

DPPH assay was evaluated following Elzaawely et al. [49] with a slight modification. Fifty microliters of extract were mixed with 50 µL of DPPH solution (0.2 mg/mL) and 100 µL of 0.1 M acetate buffer (pH 5.5). Thereafter, the combination was incubated for 20 min in darkness at room temperature. The absorbance was recorded at 517 nm using a microplate reader. BHT was used as a standard reference while pure methanol was used as a negative control. The IC_{50} value was calculated as the concentration required to reach a 50% reduction of DPPH.

4.5. ABTS Radical Cation Decolorization Assay

2,2′-Azino-bis radical cation ($ABTS^{\bullet +}$) decolorization was measured as described by Pellegrini et al. [50] with minor modifications. $ABTS^{\bullet +}$ solution was prepared by mixing aqueous ABTS (7 mM) solution with 2.45 mM potassium persulfate (1:1 v/v) and incubating in darkness at room temperature for 16 h. The working solution was then obtained by diluting $ABTS^{\bullet +}$ solution in methanol to an absorbance of 0.70 ± 0.05 at 734 nm. In each well of a 96 well-plate, 25 µL of TDB sample was added to 200 µL of the working solution. After a slight shake, the plate was covered by an aluminum foil and kept at room temperature for 30 min. Subsequently, the absorbance was recorded by a Multiskan™ Microplate Spectrophotometer (Thermo Fisher Scientific, Osaka, Japan). The ABTS radical decolorizing activity was calculated by the following formula

$$\text{ABTS radical decolorizing activity (\%)} = (1 - A_{sample}/A_{control}) \times 100$$

where A_{sample} is the absorbance of reaction with momilactones or positive control (BHT) and $A_{control}$ is the absorbance of reaction without momilactone or positive control. The IC_{50} value was determined as the concentration needed to bleach 50% of $ABTS^{\bullet +}$.

4.6. Reducing Power Assay

The reducing capacity was carried out referring to the modified method of Minh et al. [51] with a 10-times reduction in the volume of each reaction component. Initially, 100 µL of sample, 250 µL of 0.2 M phosphate buffer (pH 6.6), and 250 µL of potassium ferricyanide (1%, w/v) were combined and incubated at 50 °C for 30 min. Subsequently, the reaction mixture was stopped by 500µL of trichloroacetic acid (10%, v/v) and centrifuged for 10 min at 4000 rpm. Eventually, 100µL of the supernatant was double diluted with distilled water (100 µL) followed by adding 20 µL of ferric chloride solution (0.1%, w/v). After shaking, the absorbance of the resulting mixture was read at 700 nm by a microplate reader. BHT was used as a standard reference. The IC_{50} value was calculated as mentioned above.

4.7. β-Carotene Bleaching Assay

The β-Carotene bleaching activity of TDB extracts was assayed using a β-carotene linoleate bleaching system [52] with trivial adjustments. Briefly, a mixture of 1mL β-carotene (200 µg/mL in chloroform), 20 µL linoleic acid, and 200 mg Tween 40 was evaporated at 40 °C. Afterwards, a volume of 50 mL of oxygenated water was slowly added and the mixture which was then vigorously shaken to form a stable emulsion. The emulsion was freshly prepared before each experiment. In each well of a 96 well-plate, 25 µL of sample or control (1000 µg/mL in methanol) and 200 µL of the emulsion solution were blended. The reaction was incubated at 45 °C and the absorbance was recorded at 492 nm every 15 min up to 180 min. The lipid peroxidation inhibition (LPI) was calculated as:

$$\text{LPI inhibition (\%)} = A_{180}/A_0 \times 100$$

where A_0 is the absorbance of reaction at the zero-minute time and A_{180} is the absorbance of reaction at the 180-min time. Methanol was used as negative control, whilst BHT was the positive control.

4.8. Nitric Oxide Scavenging Assay

Nitric oxide scavenging was measured following the method of Govindarajan et al. [53] with some modifications. At the beginning, 100 µL of sample and 100 µL of 5 mM sodium nitroprusside in 0.1 M phosphate buffer saline (pH 7.2) were assimilated and incubated for 30 min at 25 °C. In the next step, 100 µL of the above mixture was blended with 100 µL of Griess reagent (1% sulfanilamide, and 0.1% naphthyl ethylenediamine dihydrochloride in 2% phosphoric acid). The absorbance decrease of the resulting purple solution was recorded at 546 nm by a microplate reader. Pure methanol was used as a negative control while gallic acid was used as a positive reference. The IC_{50} value was obtained in the same way as described above.

4.9. Porcine Pancreatic α-Amylase Inhibition Assay

The α-amylase inhibitory activity was assayed based on the starch-iodine method [54]. α-Amylase solution (2 mg/mL) from porcine pancreas (type VI-B, Sigma-Aldrich, St. Louis, MO, USA) and TDB extracts were dissolved in 0.2 M phosphate buffer saline (pH 6.9). Iodine (0.25 mM) and soluble starch (0.5%) solutions were prepared in deionized water. Firstly, 20 µL of α-amylase was mixed and incubated with 20 µL of the test sample at 37 °C in 10 min. After that, 30 µL of starch solution was added and then incubated for 8 min. The reaction was suspended by adding 20 µL of 1 M HCl, followed by 100 µL of iodine solution. The resulting mixture was measured at a wavelength of 565 nm by a microplate reader. The inhibition percentage and IC_{50} value were calculated as described previously [54]. Acarbose was used as a positive reference.

4.10. α-Glucosidase Inhibition Assay

The anti-α-glucosidase activity of TDB extracts was measured using a modified version of the method described by Johnson et al. [55]. In brief, 40 µL of TDB extract in 0.1 M potassium phosphate buffer (pH 7) were pre-mixed with 40 µL of 0.5 U/mL α-glucosidase (from *Saccharomyces cerevisiae*, Sigma-Aldrich, St. Louis, MO, USA). After 6 min of incubation at 25 °C, a 20 µL aliquot of 5 mM p-nitrophenyl-α-D-glucopyranoside (pNPG) substrate in the buffer was added and the mixture was incubated for another 8 min. Finally, the reaction was terminated by adding 100 µL of 0.1 M Na_2CO_3, and absorbance was recorded at 405 nm. Inhibition percentage was calculated by:

$$\% \text{ inhibition} = (1 - A_{sample}/A_{control}) \times 100$$

where A_{sample} is absorbance of the reaction with samples or positive controls (acarbose) and $A_{control}$ is absorbance of reaction with 10% methanol. The enzymatic inhibitory activity of TDB extracts was expressed as IC_{50} value as well.

4.11. Identification of Phytochemical Component by GC-MS

The phytochemical components of TDB extracts were identified by GC-MS analysis. The GC-MS system (JMS-T100 GCV, JEOL Ltd., Tokyo, Japan) with an autosampler coupled with a 30 m x 0.25 mm I.D. x 0.25 μm film thickness DB-5MS column (Agilent Technologies, J & W Scientific Products, Folsom, CA, USA). A concentration of 1000 μg/mL of each TDB extract was used for the initial injection. Helium was used as a carrier gas at split ratio 5:1. The GC oven conditions were as follows: The initial temperature was 50 °C without hold time, the boosted temperature was up to 300 °C at 10 °C/min, and held for 20 min. The injection port and detector temperature were set at 300 °C and 320 °C, respectively. The mass range scanned from 29 to 800 amu. The control of the GC-MS system and the confirmation of analytes were conducted using JEOL's GC-MS Mass Center System Version 2.65a [56].

4.12. Isolation of Bioactive Compounds α-Amyrin and β-Amyrin from TDBE Extract

By preliminarily screening the GC-MS results, we found that two major compounds in TDB extracts were tentatively the pentacyclic triterpenes α-amyrin and β-amyrin. Therefore, we implemented an isolation of these two compounds by column chromatography. In brief, The TDBE extract (1.2 g) was premixed with 5 g silica gel (70-230 mesh, Merck, Darmstadt, Germany). The mixture was then loaded onto a normal phase silica gel (40 g) column (2 × 50 cm). The mobile phase was 100% hexane and hexane:ethyl acetate (98:2, v/v) which yielded 8 fractions (F1–F8) and 12 fractions (F9–F20), respectively. The elution step for every fraction was 100 mL. Fractions F15–F18 afforded a mixture of colorless crystal (45.6 mg) which was subsequently identified as α-amyrin and β-amyrin (75% purity) by GC-MS, see Supplementary Material, Figure S1.

4.13. Statistical Analysis

Data were elaborated on the Minitab 16.0 software (Minitab Inc., State College, PA, USA). All assays were thrice implemented, and results were displayed as means ± standard errors (SE). Significant differences among tests were determined by one-way ANOVA using Tukey's test at $p < 0.05$. Pearson's correlation coefficients among total phenolics, antioxidant, anti-alpha amylase, and glucosidase activities of TDB extracts ($n = 3$ for each extract) were calculated by using the same software.

5. Conclusions

This study documented that *Canarium tramdenum* bark possessed potent antioxidant and α-glucosidase inhibitory activity in in vitro trials. It was found that the fractions of ethyl acetate, butanol, and water extracts enriched with terpenoids and phenolics appeared as a promising source of natural antioxidants, α-amylase, and α-glucosidase inhibitors. In vivo tests and clinical trials should be elaborated to affirm the bioavailability of *C. tramdenum* bark for the development of food additives and supplements to reduce the risks from type 2 diabetes. The isolation of novel constituents, as well as investigations on potent pharmaceutical properties of *C. tramdenum* bark, should also be conducted. The contribution of α- and β-amyrins to biological activities of *C. tramdenum* bark should be further investigated.

Supplementary Materials: The following are available online, Figure S1: GC-MS chromatography of crystal from fractions F15–F18.

Author Contributions: N.V.Q. designed the experiments and wrote the manuscript. N.T.D.T., L.T.T and C.T.H. conducted biological assays. N.V.Q. and Y.A. implemented GC-MS analysis and measured total phenolic contents. P.T.T. assisted in collection and identification of the species and extraction of samples. T.D.X. and H-D.T. revised and approved the final submission of the manuscript.

Funding: Nguyen Tat Thanh University Vietnam has partly funded to this research.

Acknowledgments: The authors thank Do Tan Khang, Truong Ngoc Minh and Truong Mai Van for their support to this research. The Japanese government (Monbukagakusho) is appreciated for providing Nguyen Van Quan a scholarship.

Conflicts of Interest: The authors declare no conflict of interest.

References

1. World Health Organization. *Global report on diabetes*; World Health Organization: Geneva, Switzerland, 2016; pp. 1–88.
2. Diabetes mellitus. Available online: https://www.who.int/mediacentre/factsheets/fs138/en/ (accessed on 18 December 2018).
3. Wu, J.; Fang, X.; Yuan, Y.; Dong, Y.; Liang, Y.; Xie, Q.; Ban, J.; Chen, Y.; Zhufen, L. UPLC/Q-TOF-MS profiling of phenolics from *Canarium pimela* leaves and its vasorelaxant and antioxidant activities. *Braz. J. Pharmacog.* **2017**, *27*, 716–723. [CrossRef]
4. Wright, E.; Scism-Bacon, J.L.; Glass, L.C. Oxidative stress in type 2 diabetes: The role of fasting and postprandial glycaemia. *Int. J. Clin. Pract.* **2006**, *60*, 308–314. [CrossRef] [PubMed]
5. Folli, F.; Corradi, D.; Fanti, P.; Davalli, A.; Paez, A.; Giaccari, A.; Perego, C.; Muscogiuri, G. The role of oxidative stress in the pathogenesis of type 2 diabetes mellitus micro- and macrovascular complications: Avenues for a mechanistic-based therapeutic approach. *Curr. Diabetes Rev.* **2011**, *7*, 313–324. [CrossRef] [PubMed]
6. Yao, Y.; Sang, W.; Zhou, M.; Ren, G. Antioxidant and α-glucosidase inhibitory activity of colored grains in China. *J. Agric. Food Chem.* **2010**, *58*, 770–774. [CrossRef] [PubMed]
7. Tundis, R.; Marrelli, M.; Conforti, F.; Tenuta, M.; Bonesi, M.; Menichini, F.; Loizzo, M. *Trifolium pratense* and *T. repens* (Leguminosae): Edible flower extracts as functional ingredients. *Foods* **2015**, *4*, 338–348. [CrossRef] [PubMed]
8. Dias, D.A.; Urban, S.; Roessner, U. A historical overview of natural products in drug discovery. *Metabolites* **2012**, *2*, 303–336. [CrossRef] [PubMed]
9. Xu, D.P.; Li, Y.; Meng, X.; Zhou, T.; Zhou, Y.; Zheng, J.; Zhang, J.J.; Li, H.B. Natural antioxidants in foods and medicinal plants: Extraction, assessment and resources. *Int. J. Mol. Sci.* **2017**, *18*, 96. [CrossRef]
10. Hoang, V.S.; Nanthavong, K.; Keßler, P.J.A. Trees of Laos and Vietnam: A field guide to 100 economically or ecologically important species. *Blumea: J. Plant Taxo. Plant Geo.* **2004**, *49*, 201–349.
11. Hoang, V.S.; Baas, P.; Keßler, P.J.A. Uses and conservation of plant species in a national park—A case study of Ben En, Vietnam. *Econ. Bot.* **2008**, *62*, 574–593. [CrossRef]
12. Liang, Y.L.; Luo, Y.; Li, Y.L.; Dong, Y.F. Effect of fruit of *Canarium pimela* Koening on vascular tension in rats. *Chin. J. Gerontol.* **2011**, *31*, 3099–3100.
13. Zhen-Cheng, L.; Chen, K.; Zeng, Y.W.; Peng, Y.H. Nutritional composition of *Canarium pimela* L. kernels. *Food Chem.* **2011**, *125*, 692–695.
14. Pisoschi, A.M.; Negulescu, G.P. Methods for total antioxidant activity determination: A review. *Biochem. Anal. Biochem.* **2011**, *1*, 106. [CrossRef]
15. Alam, M.N.; Bristi, N.J.; Rafiquzzaman, M. Review on in vivo and in vitro methods evaluation of antioxidant activity. *Saudi Pharm. J.* **2013**, *21*, 143–152. [CrossRef] [PubMed]
16. Jayaprakasha, G.K.; Singh, R.P.; Sakariah, K.K. Antioxidant activity of grape seed (*Vitis vinifera*) extracts on peroxidation models in vitro. *Food Chem.* **2001**, *73*, 285–290. [CrossRef]
17. Boora, F.; Chirisa, E.; Mukanganyama, S. Evaluation of nitrite radical scavenging properties of selected Zimbabwean plant extracts and their phytoconstituents. *J. Food Process.* **2014**, *2014*, 1–7. [CrossRef]
18. Ki, C.C.; Seong, D.L.; Soo, W.K.; Nam, H.K.; Jong-Un, L.; Young, J.K. Role of nitric oxide in the pathogenesis of diabetic nephropathy in streptozotocin-induced diabetic rats. *Korean J. Intern. Med.* **1999**, *14*, 32–41.
19. Santilli, F.; Cipollone, F.; Mezzetti, A.; Chiarelli, F. The role of nitric oxide in the development of diabetic angiopathy. *Horm. Metab. Res.* **2004**, *36*, 319–335.
20. Hogan, S.; Zhang, L.; Li, J.; Sun, S.; Canning, C.; Zhou, K. Antioxidant rich grape pomace extract suppresses postprandial hyperglycemia in diabetic mice by specifically inhibiting alpha-glucosidase. *Nutr. Metab.* **2010**, *7*, 71. [CrossRef]
21. Thang, T.D.; Dai, D.N.; Luong, N.X.; Ogunwande, I.A. Constituents of essential oils from the leaves, stem barks and resins of *Canarium parvum* Leen., and *Canarium tramdenanum* Dai et Yakovl. (Burseracea) grown in Vietnam. *Nat. Prod. Res.* **2014**, *28*, 461–466. [CrossRef]

22. Fingolo, C.E.; Santos, T.D.S.; Filho, M.D.M.V.; Kaplan, M.A.C. Triterpene esters: Natural products from *Dorstenia arifolia* (Moraceae). *Molecules* **2013**, *18*, 4247–4256. [CrossRef]
23. Zheng, X.; Luo, X.; Ye, G.; Chen, Y.; Ji, X.; Wen, L.; Xu, Y.; Xu, H.; Zhan, R.; Chen, W. Characterisation of Two Oxidosqualene Cyclases Responsible for Triterpenoid Biosynthesis in *Ilex asprella*. *Int. J. Mol. Sci.* **2015**, *16*, 3564–3578. [CrossRef] [PubMed]
24. Oliveira, F.A.; Chaves, M.H.; Almeida, F.R.C.; Lima, R.C.P.; Silva, R.M.; Maia, J.L.; Brito, G.A.A.C.; Santos, F.A.; Rao, V.S. Protective effect of α- and β-amyrin, a triterpene mixture from *Protium heptaphyllum* (Aubl.) March. trunk wood resin, against acetaminophen-induced liver injury in mice. *J. Ethnopharmacol.* **2005**, *98*, 103–108. [CrossRef] [PubMed]
25. Vázquez, L.H.; Palazon, J.; Navarro-Ocaña, A. The pentacyclic triterpenes α, β-amyrins: A review of sources and biological activities. In *Phytochemicals—A Global Perspective of Their Role in Nutrition and Health*; Venketeshwer, R., Ed.; InTech: Rijeka, Croatia, 2012; pp. 487–502.
26. Otuki, M.F.; Ferreira, J.; Lima, F.V.; Meyre-silva, C.; Muller, L.A.; Cani, G.S.; Santos, A.R.S.; Yunes, R.A. Antinociceptive properties of mixture of α-amyrin and β-amyrin triterpenes: Evidence for participation of protein kinase C and protein kinase A pathways. *Pharmacology* **2005**, *313*, 310–318. [CrossRef] [PubMed]
27. Oliveira, F.A.; Vieira-Júnior, G.M.; Chaves, M.H.; Almeida, F.R.C.; Florêncio, M.G.; Lima, R.C.P.; Silva, R.M.; Santos, F.A.; Rao, V.S.N. Gastroprotective and anti-inflammatory effects of resin from *Protium heptaphyllum* in mice and rats. *Pharmacol. Res.* **2004**, *49*, 105–111. [CrossRef] [PubMed]
28. Oliveira, F.A.; Vieira, G.M.; Chaves, M.H.; Almeida, F.R.C.; Santos, K.A.; Martins, F.S.; Silva, R.M.; Santos, F.A.; Rao, V.S.N. Gastroprotective effect of the mixture of α- and β-amyrin from *Protium heptaphyllum*: Role of capsaicin-sensitive primary afferent neurons. *Planta Med.* **2004**, *70*, 780–782. [CrossRef] [PubMed]
29. Sunil, C.; Irudayaraj, S.S.; Duraipandiyan, V.; Al-Dhabi, N.A.; Agastian, P.; Ignacimuthu, S. Antioxidant and free radical scavenging effects of β-amyrin isolated from *S. cochinchinensis* Moore. leaves. *Ind. Crops Prod.* **2014**, *61*, 510–516. [CrossRef]
30. Okoye, N.N.; Ajaghaku, D.L.; Okeke, H.N.; Ilodigwe, E.E.; Nworu, C.S.; Okoye, F.B.C. Beta-amyrin and alpha-amyrin acetate isolated from the stem bark of *Alstonia boonei* display profound anti-inflammatory activity. *Pharm. Biol.* **2014**, *52*, 1478–1486. [CrossRef]
31. Sridevi, H.; Jayaraman, P.; Pachaiyappan, P. Evaluation of α-glucosidase inhibitory action of isolated compound beta amyrin from Memecylon umbellatum Burm. F. *Int. J. Pharmacogn. Phytochem. Res.* **2015**, *7*, 1033–1038.
32. Sirat, H.M.; Susanti, D.; Ahmad, F.; Takayama, H.; Kitajima, M. Amides, triterpene and flavonoids from the leaves of *Melastoma malabathricum* L. *J. Nat. Med.* **2010**, *64*, 492–495. [CrossRef]
33. Ogwuche, C.E.; Amupitan, J.O.; Ayo, R.G. Isolation and biological activity of the triterpene β-amyrin from the aerial plant parts of *Maesobotrya barteri* (Baill). *Med. Chem.* **2014**, *4*, 729–733.
34. Saeidnia, S.; Ara, L.; Hajimehdipoor, H.; Read, R.W.; Arshadi, S.; Nikan, M. Chemical constituents of *Swertia longifolia* Boiss. with α-amylase inhibitory activity. *Res. Pharm. Sci.* **2016**, *11*, 23–32. [PubMed]
35. Sritularak, B.; Boonplod, N.; Lipipun, V.; Likhitwitayawuid, K. Chemical constituents of *Canarium subulatum* and their anti-herpetic and DPPH free radical scavenging properties. *Rec. Nat. Prod.* **2013**, *7*, 129–132.
36. Canarium. Available online: http://www.theplantlist.org/1.1/browse/A/Burseraceae/Canarium/ (accessed on 20 December 2018).
37. Zhang, L.; Lin, Y. Tannins from *Canarium album* with potent antioxidant activity. *J. Zhejiang Univ. Sci. B* **2008**, *9*, 407–415. [CrossRef] [PubMed]
38. He, Z.; Xia, W. Preparative separation and purification of phenolic compounds from *Canarium album* L. by macroporous resins. *J. Sci. Food Agric.* **2008**, *88*, 493–498. [CrossRef]
39. Kuo, C.T.; Liu, T.H.; Hsu, T.H.; Lin, F.Y.; Chen, H.Y. Antioxidant and antiglycation properties of different solvent extracts from Chinese olive (*Canarium album* L.) fruit. *Asian Pac. J. Trop. Med.* **2015**, *8*, 1013–1021. [CrossRef] [PubMed]
40. Balkis Budin, S.; Kumar, S.; Warif, M.A.; Saari, S.M.; Fredalina Basri, D. Protective effect of aqueous extracts from *Canarium odontophyllum* Miq. leaf on liver in streptozotocin-induced diabetic rats. *Life Sci. Med. Biomed.* **2018**, *2*, 1–5.
41. Mokiran, N.N.; Ismail, A.; Azlan, A.; Hamid, M.; Hassan, F.A. Effect of dabai (*Canarium odontophyllum*) fruit extract on biochemical parameters of induced obese-diabetic rats. *J. Funct. Foods* **2014**, *8*, 139–149. [CrossRef]

42. Kamtchouing, P.; Kahpui, S.M.; Dzeufiet, P.D.D.; Tédong, L.; Asongalem, E.A.; Dimo, T. Anti-diabetic activity of methanol/methylene chloride stem bark extracts of *Terminalia superba* and *Canarium schweinfurthii* on streptozotocin-induced diabetic rats. *J. Ethnopharmacol.* **2006**, *104*, 306–309. [CrossRef]
43. Yehye, W.A.; Rahman, N.A.; Ariffin, A.; Abd Hamid, S.B.; Alhadi, A.A.; Kadir, F.A.; Yaeghoobi, M. Understanding the chemistry behind the antioxidant activities of butylated hydroxytoluene (BHT): A review. *Eur. J. Med. Chem.* **2015**, *101*, 295–312. [CrossRef]
44. DiNicolantonio, J.J.; Bhutani, J.; O'Keefe, J.H. Acarbose: Safe and effective for lowering postprandial hyperglycaemia and improving cardiovascular outcomes. *Open Heart* **2015**, *2*, e000327. [CrossRef]
45. Soong, Y.Y.; Barlow, P.J. Antioxidant activity and phenolic content of selected fruit seeds. *Food Chem.* **2004**, *88*, 411–417. [CrossRef]
46. Yin, Z.; Zhang, W.; Feng, F.; Zhang, Y.; Kang, W. α-Glucosidase inhibitors isolated from medicinal plants. *Food Sci. Hum. Wellness* **2014**, *3*, 136–174. [CrossRef]
47. Santos, F.A.; Frota, J.T.; Arruda, B.R.; De Melo, T.S.; Da Silva, A.A.D.C.A.; Brito, G.A.D.C.; Chaves, M.H.; Rao, V.S. Antihyperglycemic and hypolipidemic effects of α, β-amyrin, a triterpenoid mixture from *Protium heptaphyllum* in mice. *Lipids Health Dis.* **2012**, *11*, 98. [CrossRef] [PubMed]
48. Quan, N.V.; Khang, D.T.; Dep, L.T.; Minh, T.N.; Nobukazu, N.; Xuan, T.D. The Potential use of a food-dyeing plant *Peristrophe bivalvis* (L.) Merr. in northern Vietnam. *Int. J. Pharmacol. Phytochem. Ethnomed.* **2016**, *4*, 14–26. [CrossRef]
49. Elzaawely, A.A.; Tawata, S. Antioxidant activity of phenolic rich fraction obtained from *Convolvulus arvensis* L. leaves grown in Egypt. *Asian J. Crop Sci.* **2012**, *4*, 32–40. [CrossRef]
50. Pellegrini, N.; Serafini, M.; Colombi, B.; Del Rio, D.; Salvatore, S.; Bianchi, M.; Brighenti, F. Total antioxidant capacity of plant foods, beverages and oils consumed in Italy assessed by three different in vitro assays. *J. Nutri.* **2003**, *133*, 2812–281. [CrossRef] [PubMed]
51. Minh, T.N.; Tuyen, P.T.; Khang, D.T.; Quan, N.V.; Ha, P.T.T.; Quan, N.T.; Xuan, T.D. Potential use of plant waste from the moth orchid (*Phalaenopsis* Sogo Yukidian "V3") as an antioxidant source. *Foods* **2017**, *6*, 85. [CrossRef] [PubMed]
52. Tuyen, P.T.; Xuan, T.D.; Khang, D.T.; Ahmad, A.; Quan, N.V.; Tu Anh, T.; Minh, T.N. Phenolic compositions and antioxidant properties in bark, flower, inner skin, kernel and leaf extracts of *Castanea crenata* Sieb. et Zucc. *Antioxidants* **2017**, *6*, 31. [CrossRef] [PubMed]
53. Govindarajan, R.; Rastogi, S.; Vijayakumar, M.; Shirwaikar, A.; Rawat, A.K.S.; Mehrotra, S.; Pushpangadan, P. Studies on the antioxidant activities of *Desmodium gangeticum*. *Biol. Pharm. Bull.* **2003**, *26*, 1424–1427. [CrossRef] [PubMed]
54. Quan, N.V.; Hoang-Dung, T.; Xuan, T.D.; Ahmad, A.; Dat, T.D.; Khanh, T.D.; Teschke, R. Momilactones A and B are α-amylase and α-glucosidase inhibitors. *Molecules* **2019**, *24*, 482. [CrossRef] [PubMed]
55. Johnson, M.H.; Lucius, A.; Meyer, T.; Gonzalez De Mejia, E. Cultivar evaluation and effect of fermentation on antioxidant capacity and in vitro inhibition of α-amylase and α-glucosidase by highbush blueberry (*Vaccinium corombosum*). *J. Agric. Food Chem.* **2011**, *59*, 8923–8930. [CrossRef] [PubMed]
56. Andriana, Y.; Xuan, T.D.; Quan, N.V.; Quy, T.N. Allelopathic potential of *Tridax procumbens* L. on radish and identification of allelochemicals. *Allelopathy J.* **2018**, *43*, 223–237. [CrossRef]

Sample Availability: Samples of *Canarium tramdenum* bark extracts and the mixture of α and β-amyrins are available from the authors.

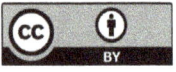

© 2019 by the authors. Licensee MDPI, Basel, Switzerland. This article is an open access article distributed under the terms and conditions of the Creative Commons Attribution (CC BY) license (http://creativecommons.org/licenses/by/4.0/).

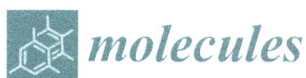

Article

Antioxidant and Hepatoprotective Effects of *Croton hypoleucus* Extract in an Induced-Necrosis Model in Rats

Thania Alejandra Urrutia-Hernández [1], Jorge Arturo Santos-López [2], Juana Benedí [2], Francisco Jose Sánchez-Muniz [3], Claudia Velázquez-González [1], Minarda De la O-Arciniega [1], Osmar Antonio Jaramillo-Morales [1] and Mirandeli Bautista [1]

[1] Área Académica de Farmacia, Universidad Autónoma del Estado de Hidalgo, Mariano Abasolo 600, Colonia Centro, Pachuca, Hidalgo CP 42000, Mexico
[2] Departamento de Farmacología, Farmacognosia y Botánica, Facultad de Farmacia, Universidad Complutense de Madrid, Plaza Ramón y Cajal S/N, 28040 Madrid, Espana
[3] Departamento de Nutrición y Ciencia de los Alimentos, Facultad de Farmacia, Universidad Complutense de Madrid, Plaza Ramón y Cajal S/N, 28040 Madrid, Espana
* Correspondence: mibautista@uaeh.edu.mx; Tel.: +52-(771)-72000 (ext. 4327)

Received: 14 June 2019; Accepted: 9 July 2019; Published: 11 July 2019

Abstract: The aim of this study was to evaluate the antioxidant and hepatoprotective activity of *Croton hypoleucus* (EC). The present work reports the first pharmacological, toxicological, and antioxidant studies of EC extract on liver injury. Liver necrosis was induced by thioacetamide (TAA). Five groups were established: *Croton* Extract (EC), thioacetamide (TAA), *Croton* extract with thioacetamide (EC + TAA), vitamin E with thioacetamide (VE + TAA) and the positive control and vehicle (CT). For EC and EC + TAA, Wistar rats (n = 8) were intragastrically pre-administered for 4 days with EC (300 mg/kg.day) and on the last day, EC + TAA received a single dose of TAA (400 mg/kg). At 24 h after damage induction, animals were sacrificed. In vitro activity and gene expression of superoxide dismutase (SOD), catalase (*Cat*), and Nrf2 nuclear factor were measured. The results show that EC has medium antioxidant properties, with an IC_{50} of 0.63 mg/mL and a ferric-reducing power of 279.8 μM/mg. Additionally, EC reduced hepatic damage markers at 24 h after TAA intoxication; also, it increased *SOD* and *Cat* gene expression against TAA by controlling antioxidant defense levels. Our findings demonstrated the hepatoprotective effect of EC by reducing hepatic damage markers and controlling antioxidant defense levels. Further studies are necessary to identify the mechanism of this protection.

Keywords: antioxidant activity; hepatoprotective effect; *Croton hypoleucus*; oxidative stress

1. Introduction

Medicinal plants play a key role in the human health care system [1]. According to the World Health Organization, between 65% and 80% of the populations of developing countries currently use medicinal plants [2], as extracts, infusions, or bioactive compounds to treat primary conditions [3,4]. Several pharmacology studies have shown the role of medicinal plants on the treatment and prevention of liver diseases [5]. The biological and hepatoprotective activity of plant extracts defends hepatocytes against lipid peroxidation and other oxidative effects [6] as free radicals, toxic, viral, and bacterial agents [7]. The hepatoprotective activity of plants has been related to several compounds, like flavonoids (isoflavones, anthocyanins, catechins, quercetins), saponins, coumarins, alkaloids, and terpenes [5]. In the complementary traditional medicine, some *Croton* species are highlighted due to their anti-inflammatory, antiseptic, antinociceptive, antiplasmodic, antiproliferative, antiviral, and antibacterial properties, and some compounds, like terpenes, steroids, and flavonoids, have been identified in the *Croton* species. These compounds have important biological activities with therapeutic and medicinal value [3], as anethol from *C. zehtneri* [8]; triterpenes from *C. oblongifolius* [9]; and alkaloids, flavonoids, and glycosides in *C. sparciflorus* [10]. *Croton hypoleucus*, known as Palo blanco and Soliman Liso, is a native shrub of Hidalgo, Mexico. An infusion of its aerial parts is used in treatments of stomachache and pain. In a preliminary phytochemical screening of EC, we found the presence of saponins, alkaloids, tannins, flavonoids, sterols, terpenoids, and carbohydrates as they have been reported before in *Croton* species [3]. To our knowledge, biological studies of *C. hypoleucus* have not been previously reported, but some of its metabolites have been identified in hexane extract, such as three epoxy-clerodane bearing furan rings, named hypoleins A–C and the Crotonpenes A–B [11].

Liver is the main metabolic and detoxifying organ that first contacts and neutralizes xenobiotic [12] due to a cellular system of detoxification (cytochrome P_{450}, flavin-containing monooxygenase, glutathione transferase), which provides biotransformation of some xenobiotics to toxic intermediates, leading to liver toxic injury [13]. Acute toxic liver injury is characterized by membrane damage, massive necrosis of hepatocytes, infiltration of parenchyma by neutrophils, and activation of hepatic stellate cells, followed by a release of proinflammatory cytokines and the formation of reactive oxygen species (ROS) as the main factors that damage liver cells [14]. ROS are oxygen-containing molecules, including superoxide, hydrogen peroxide, and hydroxyl radical, that are highly reactive with other complex molecules in the cells, such as protein, DNA, and lipids. Endogenous radical scavengers, like antioxidant enzymes, including superoxide dismutase (SOD) and catalase (Cat), can lead to ROS degradation [15]. Nuclear factor erythroid 2-related factor 2 (*Nrf2*) functions as a xenobiotic-activated receptor to regulate the adaptive response to oxidants and electrophiles [16], and the repair and removal of damaged proteins [17]. Activation of *Nrf2* enhances the levels of antioxidant enzymes and phase-2- detoxifying enzymes by complex mechanisms, and this may be one of the ways to reduce oxidative/nitrosative stress and chronic inflammation [18].

Thioacetamide (TAA) is known as a hepatotoxicant, and is used to induce acute and chronic liver injury due to its effects on protein synthesis, RNA, and DNA [19]. TAA hepatotoxicity requires metabolic activation by CYP2E1 with the formation of the reactive metabolites, S-oxide (TASO) and S, S-dioxide ($TASO_2$) [20,21]. These active intermediates lead to the formation of adducts of proteins, lipids, and nucleic acids, as well as the formation of ROS, which promote lipid and protein peroxidation and mitochondrial damage [22]. The selective destruction of perivenous hepatocytes and proliferative liver cells allows the TAA model to be used in experimental tests to study the hepatic response against aggressive attack from xenobiotics and to identify the molecular, biochemical, and physiopathological mechanisms though which the hepatic lesion develops [5]. Due to taxonomy characteristics and the pharmacological and chemistry nature of the *Croton* genus, *Croton hypoleucus* could be a source of hepatoprotective compounds. In this sense, the aim of the present work was to evaluate the antioxidant and hepatoprotective effect of EC in thioacetamide-induced liver damage in a rat model.

2. Results

2.1. Purification of Main Compounds in Dichloromethane Fraction

Two clerodane-type diterpenoids were isolated from the dichloromethane fraction of EC. According to ^{1}H and ^{13}C NMR shifts, they were identified as hypolein B (35 mg) and Crotonpene B (21 mg) (Figure 1). The ^{1}H and ^{13}C NMR shifts are presented.

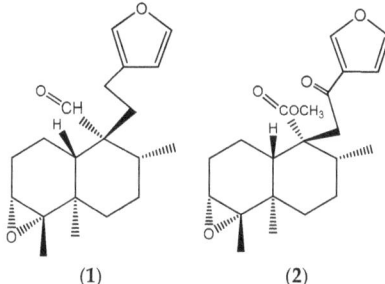

Figure 1. Clerodane-type diterpenoids identified in the dichloromethane fraction of EC: hypolein B (**1**) and Crotonpene B (**2**).

Hypolein B: Yellow oil. ^{1}H NMR (400 MHz) CDCl$_3$: δ 9.92 (s, H-20), 7.96 (s, H-16), 7.37 (dd, J = 1.6, 1.6, H-15), 6.24 (dd, J = 1.6, 0.4, H-14), β2.30, α2.17 (H-12), α1.63 (H-8), α1.66, β1.65 (H-7), α1.77, β1.46 (H-6), α0.95 (H-19), β1.20 (H-18), α1.90, β2.15 (m, H-2), α1.37, β1.53b (m, H-1). ^{13}C NMR (100 MHz) CDCl$_3$: δ 146.75 (C-16), 138.58 (C-15), 124.72 (C-13), 110.86 (C-14), 60.15 (C-3), 53.27 (C-9), 37.27 (C-5, C-6), 35.29 (C-8), 29.70 (C-11), 27.79 (C-2, C-7), 19.78 (C-18), 17.56 (C-12), 17.45 (C-19), 17.82 (C-17), 15.86 (C-1).

Crotonpene B: Colorless oil. ^{1}H NMR (400 MHz) CDCl$_3$: δ 7.96 (s, H-16), 7.37 (dd, J = 1.6, 1.6, H-15), 6.24 (dd, J = 1.6, 0.4, H-14), 3.63 (br. S, H-20), α2.07, β2.17 (H-2), β1.84 (m, H-10), β1.81 (m, H-8), α1.70 (d, J = 1.2, H-6, H,7), β1.48, α1.58 (dd, J = 2, 1.6, H-1), β1.47 (m, H-6), β1.46 (m, H-7), 1.19 (s, H-18), 1.10 (s, H-17), 0.89 (s, H-19). ^{13}C NMR (100 MHz) CDCl$_3$: δ 195.21 (C-12), 173.88 (C-20), 146.75 (C-16), 144.03 (C-15). 128.28 (C-13), 108.87 (C-14), 51.43 (C-20), 43.12 (C-11), 38.40 (C-8). 37.27 (C-5, C-6), 27.97 (C-2), 19.78 (C-18), 18.63 (C-1), 17.98 (C-17), 14.11 (C-19).

2.2. Antioxidant Activity of EC

In this study, the tested doses (2 to 6 mg/mL) were antioxidant dose dependent. The inhibition percentages were 28.13% and 78.36% to 2 and 6 mg/mL, respectively. According to the dose-response results, we estimated the IC$_{50}$, as the extract concentration required to reduce the initial concentration of DPPH to 50%. In this case, the EC IC$_{50}$ was 0.6307 mg/mL. To the FRAP assay, EC had an Fe^{+3} ion reducing capacity of 279.8 ± 3.3 µM. Eq. Trolox/mg.

2.3. Acute Toxicity of EC

In the LD$_{50}$ assay, no animals died during the 14 experimental days after administration of 10, 100, and 1000 mg EC/kg in the first phase, and 1600, 2900, and 5000 mg EC/kg in the second phase (Table 1).

Table 1. LD$_{50}$ of EC.

EC	Intragastric Doses (mg/kg)		
Phase I	10	100	1000
Mortality	0/3	0/3	0/3
Phase II	1600	2900	5000
Mortality	0/3	0/3	0/3
LD$_{50}$	>5000		

2.4. Liver Damage Biomarkers

In order to assess the degree of liver injury, biochemical parameters were estimated. The TAA effect on transaminases enzymes is shown in Figure 2. Remarkably, the TAA group presented the highest levels of AST and ALT when they were contrasted with the rest of the treatments. EC and CT did not show significant differences ($p \leq 0.05$) with each other, as well as VE and EC (data not shown).

In the EC + TAA group, ALT and AST presented a decrease of 65.9% and 75.8%, respectively, against TAA, with significant differences between groups. A similar behavior was observed for the positive control (VE + TAA).

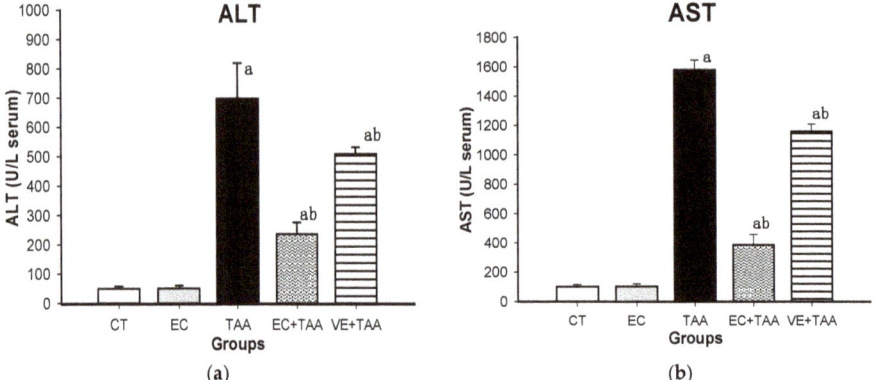

Figure 2. Effect of EC pretreatment on levels of (**A**) ALT and (**B**) AST analyzed by Wiener Lab equipment in the serum of rats intoxicated with a sublethal dose of thioacetamide (TAA). All data are expressed in U/L. Bars indicate the mean value with SE of two determinations (n = 8). The differences compared with the vehicle are expressed as "**a**"; while the differences due to TAA are expressed as "**b**", $p \leq 0.05$.

The EC + TAA group showed a significant reduction (38.75%) of ALP levels, which was comparable to the EC and CT groups. A similar tendency was observed in EC + TAA for the T-Bil and D-Bil plasma concentration, which showed a reduction of 58% and 73%, respectively (Figure 3). The TAA groups also presented elevated levels of GGT and LDH ($1.21 \pm 0.24 \times 10^{-4}$ and 7291 ± 907, respectively). While, EC + TAA exhibited a reduction of 99% and 68.9% to GGT and LDH, respectively (Figure 4).

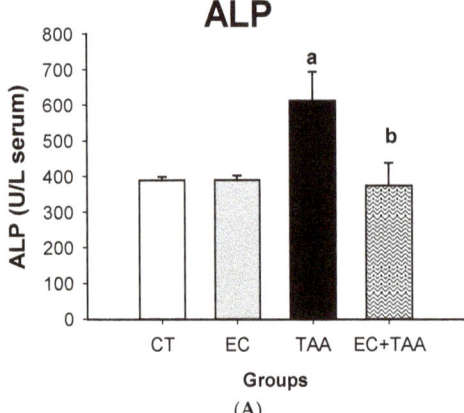

Figure 3. *Cont.*

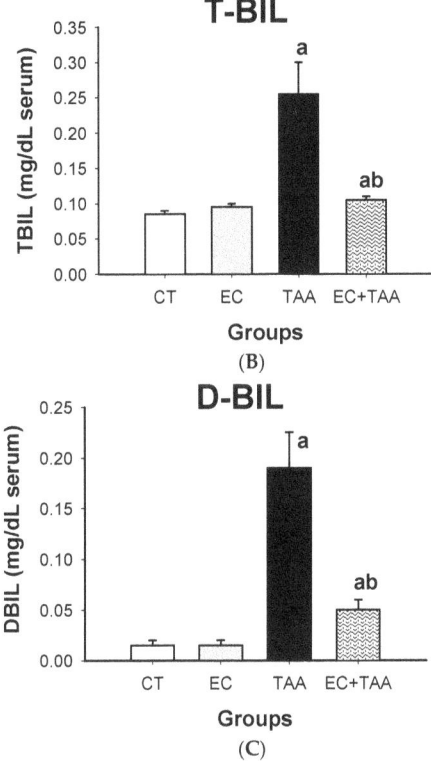

Figure 3. Effect of EC pretreatment on levels of (**A**) ALP, (**B**) T-Bil, and (**C**) D-Bil analyzed by Wiener Lab equipment in the serum of rats intoxicated with a sublethal dose of thioacetamide (TAA). In ALP, the results are expressed in U/L, while T-Bil and D-Bil are expressed in mg/dL of serum. Bars indicate the mean value with the SE of two determinations (n = 8). The differences compared with the vehicle are expressed as "**a**"; while the differences due to TAA are expressed as "**b**", $p \leq 0.05$.

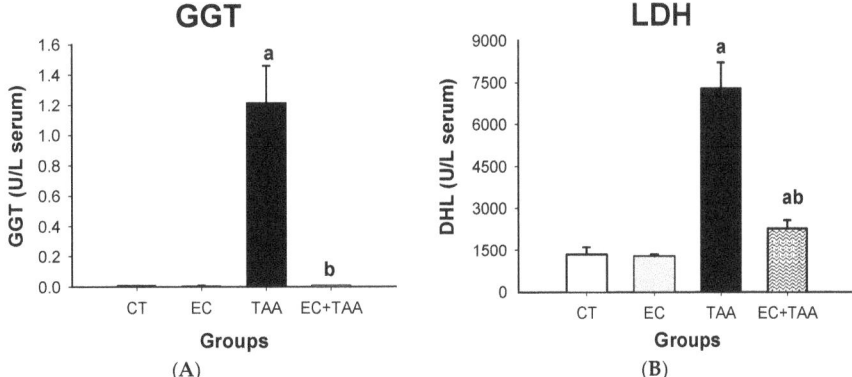

Figure 4. Effect of EC pretreatment on the levels of (**A**) GGT and (**B**) LDH analyzed by Wiener Lab equipment in the serum of rats intoxicated with a sublethal dose of thioacetamide (TAA). The results are expressed in U/L of serum. Bars indicate the mean value with the SE of two determinations (n = 8). The differences compared with the vehicle are expressed as "**a**"; while the differences due to TAA are expressed as "**b**", $p \leq 0.05$.

2.5. SOD and Cat Evaluation from Antioxidant Enzyme Activity

To assess the enzymatic antioxidant response of the liver, SOD and Cat activities were measured. The results showed that compared with the vehicle, the levels of both enzymes in EC + TAA (35.58 ± 1.7 and 9.09 ± 0.59 U/mg) decreased at 24 h after TAA administration, as TAA did (36.03 ± 1.56 and 8.52 ± 0.10 U/mg) for SOD and Cat, respectively (Figure 5). For Cat, no significant differences ($p \leq 0.05$) were reported between CT and EC + TAA.

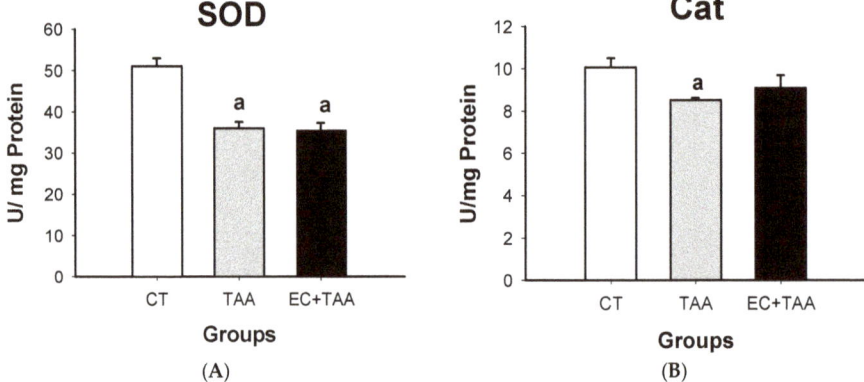

Figure 5. Effect of EC pretreatment on levels of (**A**) SOD and (**B**) Cat enzyme activities in rats' liver intoxicated by a sublethal dose of thioacetamide (TAA). The results are expressed in U/mg protein. Bars indicate the mean value with the SE of two determinations (n = 8). The differences compared with the vehicle are expressed as "**a**"; while the differences due to TAA are expressed as "**b**", $p \leq 0.05$.

2.6. MnSOD, CuZnSOD, Cat, and Nrf2 mRNA Expression

Results showed that TAA treatment led to a significant reduction of *MnSOD*, *CuZnSOD*, *Cat*, and *Nrf2* gene expression (Figure 6). On the other hand, the EC + TAA group stimulated relative mRNA expression of MnSOD, CuZnSOD, and Cat in comparison with its TAA counterparts, but without reaching similar values to the CT animals. In contrast, the *Nrf2* expression displayed a significant reduction in the EC + TAA group in comparison with both the CT and TAA groups.

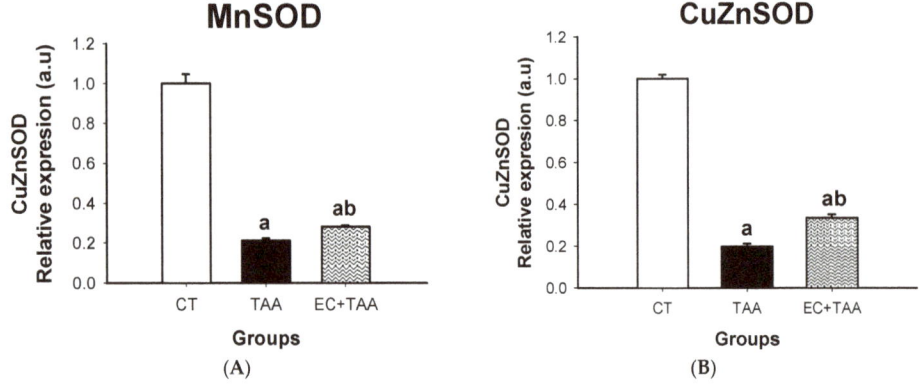

Figure 6. *Cont.*

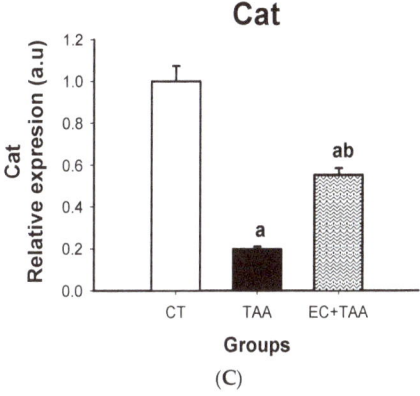
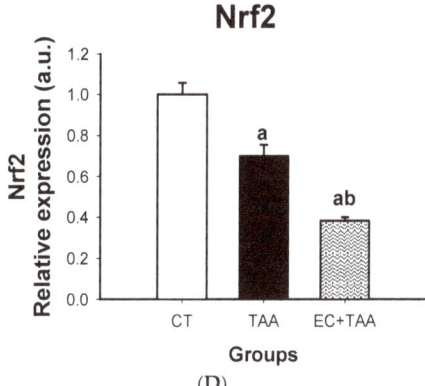

(C) (D)

Figure 6. Effect of EC on (**A**) MnSOD, (**B**) CuZnSOD, (**C**) Cat, and (**D**) *Nrf2* expression in homogenated liver of rats intoxicated with a sublethal dose of thioacetamide (TAA). The results are expressed in relative expression, arbitrary units (a.u.). Bars indicate the mean value with the SE of two determinations (n = 8). The differences compared with the vehicle are expressed as "**a**"; while the differences due to TAA are expressed as "**b**", $p \leq 0.05$.

3. Discussion

3.1. Main Compounds in Dichloromethane Fraction

Diterpenoids are characteristic components of the *Croton* species [3]. They represent 85% of terpenoid compounds identified in these species [23]. Apart from the Clerodane-type terpenoid, hypolein B and Crotonpene B have also been reported for *Croton hypoleucus* by Velazquez et al. [11] in the hexane extract of the aerial parts, as well as by Sun et al. [24] in the methanol extract of aerial parts of *Croton yanhuii*. Diterpenoids are well known as compounds with remarkable biological activities, such as anti-tumor, anti-malarial, anti-inflammatory, antimicrobial [25], hepatoprotective [26–29], and cytotoxic [30]. Some diterpenes may be toxic for humans, resulting in acute or chronic impacts on different tissues and organs. Kubo et al. [31] showed that the *nor*-diterpene *trans*dehydrocrotonin isolated from *C. cajucara* is responsible for its hepatotoxicity, while the extracts of the same plant showed hypolipidemic activity and an absence of hepatotoxicity in animal models [32]. Also, toxicity occurs when it is used long term or is taken at high doses [33].

3.2. Antioxidant Activity of EC

The in vitro antioxidant activity of the crude extract was evaluated through 2,2-diphenyl-1-picrylhydrazyl (DPPH) and the ferric reducing ability of plasma (FRAP) assays. The DPPH molecule can accept an electron from a hydrogen radical to become itself a stable molecule, and then it reacts with a reducing agent to form a new bind [21], so the DPPH assay determinates the EC capacity to scavenge free radicals as an antioxidant power measurement [34]. The percent of inhibition reported for EC is comparable with the ethanolic extract of *C. zambesicus*, which presented an inhibition of 72% [35]. On the other hand, IC_{50} is a widely used parameter to measure the antioxidant activity of extracts [36]. *Croton* species leave extracts of *C. argyrophyllus* and *C. heliotropiifolius* showed IC_{50} values of 0.22 and 0.352 mg/mL, respectively [34], while *C. leptstachyus* and *C. bonplandianum* have IC_{50} values of 11.6 and 416 µg/mL, respectively. The IC_{50} was 0.6307 mg/mL, which indicates that a higher EC concentration was needed to scavenge 50% of the DPPH free radical, as an antioxidant potential [37].

The FRAP assay is based on the reduction, at low pH, of a colorless ferric complex (Fe^{3+}-tripyridyltriazine) to a blue ferric complex (Fe^{2+}-tripiridyl-*s*-triazine) by the action of electron donating antioxidants [38]. The reduction is monitored by measuring the change in absorbance at

593 nm [39]. The extract composition is preponderant for the and the extract is rich in flavonoid-type phenolic compounds. Flavonoid compounds, such as quercetin, kaempferol, quercitrin, and 3-O-methyl ether [40], have been recognized in the *Croton* genus [3]. The participation and synergisms of flavonoid compounds could contribute to the EC antioxidant capacity [41], and their interactions with other compounds could potentiate or interfere with the EC antioxidant ability [42]. The antioxidant and inhibition of free radical production are important for the protection of cells from TAA-induced hepatotoxicity [43]. Different mechanisms, in which antioxidant compounds perform their scavenging properties, have been documented: They act as a physical barrier to prevent ROS generation, and they could access target biological sites, as a chemistry trap catching energy and chelating electrons; as a reactive species scavenging catalytic system and breaking redox chains, and scavenging radicals; or binding to targeted metal compounds and avoiding redox chain formation [44]. Most of them depend on the hydrogen atom transference rate from the compounds to the radicals [45]. The results of this experiment showed that EC may contain potential compounds able to donate hydrogen atoms to free radicals to become more stable molecules, and are responsible for the reported antioxidant activity. The EC capacity to the scavenging DPPH radical and reducing Fe^{3+} can contribute by reducing oxidative stress effects and liver damage. The discovery of antioxidant compounds is critical for new drug research and the treatment of diseases related to oxidative stress.

3.3. Acute Toxicity of EC

Acute toxicity testing is the defining and evaluating of a toxic syndrome produced by a single dose or a few doses of an extract or drug administered over the course of a day [46]. During the observation period, rats breathed, ate, and increased body weight normally. Conditions, such as difficulty to breath, loss of appetite, and death, are signs of toxicity [47]. During the post mortem examination, the macroscopic morphology of the liver, spleen, lungs, kidneys, and stomach showed normal color and morphology (data not showed) compared with the vehicle. A lot of *Euphorbiaceae* species are known in different countries as being toxic or medicinal plants. Given its therapeutic response, its chemical diversity can be hypothesized. Compounds, like alkaloids and forbol esters, have been reported in *Croton* species [3]. Different extracts and essential oils of *Croton* species, such as *C. membranaceus, C. sparsiflorus, C. bonplandianum*, and *C. zehntneri*, have been evaluated to find their toxicity level at different doses from 300 to 5000 mg/kg [10,48,49] and are considered safe. Nevertheless, a dose of 447.18 mg/kg of *C. polyandrus* essential oil produced the death of mice [50]. The extract toxicity depends on several factors, such as the chemistry composition, doses, and exposition time. In our study, the rat's survival in all evaluated doses during the two study weeks, and a higher 5000 mg/kg suggests that ethanolic *C. hypoleucus* extract is not toxic [51].

3.4. Liver Damage Biomarkers

The liver damage induced by xenobiotic agents as TAA is characterized by an increase of serum liver enzymes. TAA is a toxic agent that causes hepatocytes necrosis and it contributes to cirrhosis development through multiple action mechanisms, such as oxidative stress, decrease of the antioxidant system response, and lipid peroxidation [52]. Particularly, AST and ALT transaminases are used as biomarkers of hepatocellular necrosis. The serum transaminases concentration is referred as an indicator of the liver damage severity [53–56]. ALT is present in the liver at higher concentrations than other organs. AST is considered to have a lower specificity for liver damage than ALT due to it is presence in other organs [57]. Along with TAA metabolism, thioacetamide-s-oxide and reactive species are produced. The reactive species harm the cell by lipid peroxidation and produce a breakdown and loss of permeability of the cellular membrane [54]; this is a probable explanation of the increase in AST and ALT levels from the TAA group. These results are in accordance with several studies on TAA-induced liver necrosis in experimental animals [58–61]. The present results also demonstrated the protective role of vitamin E against TAA, and they were in line with a preliminary study [62]. EC + TAA showed a significant decrease in the serum levels of ALT and AST in relation with VE + TAA and TAA ($p \leq 0.05$). The results in EC + TAA are strongly related to the EC capacity to save the cell against necrotic damage produced by TAA to reduce the rate of transaminase release and cellular membrane stabilization [44].

ALP is a hydrolase enzyme, which is eliminated by bile. It is present in cells covering biliary conducts, as well as other organs, like bone, placenta, kidney, and intestine. Hepatotoxicity leads to an elevation of normal values due to the body´s excretion inability through bile due to the congestion or obstruction of the biliary tract, which may occur within the liver, such as was observed in the TAA group. The result showed for the EC + TAA indices that EC has the ability to reduce the effects of bile obstruction induced by TAA by decreasing ALP toward vehicle levels (Figure 3). A similar behavior was reported in bilirubin determination. The bilirubin is a product from regular hemoglobin breakdown, and it is released into the bile [54]. The T-Bil and D-Bil result to EC + TAA indicates that EC contributed to bilirubin metabolism after induced damage by TAA.

For D-Bil and T-Bil plasma concentrations, TAA lead to elevated levels of bilirubin. The induced liver damage by TAA caused the liver to lose its ability to conjugate to bilirubin; thereby, its excretions are affected, and it causes hyperbilirubinemia in serum. This alteration, along with higher transaminases levels, is a sign of acute or toxic injury [61] as the TAA group showed. GGT enzyme is localized in the liver, kidney, and pancreas. It catalyzes the conjugation of electrophilic species from TAA metabolism with GSH [53]. GGT levels tends to increase due to its release from the hepatocytes to the circulatory system by changing the membrane permeability. Although the mechanisms for GGT induction are uncertain, they have been associated with C-reactive protein, a general marker for increased oxidative stress, which leads to overconsumption of GSH with a compensatory increase in GGT synthesis [62,63].

On the other hand, GGT reflects a state of oxidative stress forward to chronic disease; while LDH increases its levels as a result of liver diseases [64]. The liver biomarker results describe the protective ability of EC against free radicals and electrophilic compounds from TAA biotransformation, which promotes cellular stability, serum transaminases and bilirubin depuration, as well as recovery competence, thus keeping biomarker levels closer to the vehicle, as *C. oblongifolius* ethanol extract [9], *C. zehnteneri* essential oil [8], *C. sparciflorus* [10], and *C. bonplandianus* methanol extract [21] have shown against necrotic effects of CCl_4, acetaminophen, and N-nitrosodietylamine. The liver biomarkers' regulation represents the liver's recovery to a normal state [65]. To date, the compounds responsible for the hepatoprotective activity of *C. hypoleucus* have not been revealed, however, several studies [8–10] report that flavones, terpenoids, alkaloids, tannins, and saponin may be responsible for this pharmacological effect.

3.5. SOD and Cat System

Defensive responses of organisms to oxidative stress include the utilization of endogenous antioxidant enzyme systems, lipid soluble and water-soluble antioxidant molecules, and phytochemicals, which can be detected through measurement of the total antioxidant capacity. Antioxidants, such as SOD, Cat enzymes, and GSH, are some of the most important elements that act as a defense against oxidative damage. They keep ROS at low levels and avoid excessive production [66]. For the purpose of this investigation, the effect of EC was evaluated on the levels of SOD and Cat as enzymes of the system of antioxidant defense. SOD is present in the cytoplasm and mitochondria of cells. The SOD molecule in the cytoplasm contains copper and zinc atoms, while mitochondrial SOD contains manganese. SOD catalyzes superoxide radical dismutation ($\cdot O_2$) into hydrogen peroxide (H_2O_2); even though H_2O_2 is not a radical, it is rapidly converted into hydroxyl radical, which is highly reactive, by means of the Fenton reaction and Cat enzymatic activity [67]. The regulatory activity of this enzyme enables mutual protection; when the superoxide radical is produced, it is disabled by Cat, while H_2O_2 inhibits SOD [68]. Hepatotoxicity by TAA requires metabolic activation with the formation of the reactive metabolites, S-oxide (TASO) and S, S-dioxide ($TASO_2$) [21], which bind to microsomal lipids, leading to is peroxidation, as well as ROS production, such as hydroxyl, peroxide, and superoxide radicals. ROS affect antioxidant defense mechanisms, and they decrease SOD, Cat, and GPx activity, leading to liver damage, cirrhosis, and hepatocellular carcinoma [54]. In our study, the acute liver injury by TAA was characterized by a reduction in the in vitro activity of SOD and Cat (Figure 5) due to the attack of superoxide and hydrogen peroxide radicals against the cell [68]. The TAA administration to rats may cause cellular structure changes, interfere with RNA movement from nuclei to the cytoplasm, and reduce the number of viable hepatocytes, as well as reduce the oxygen intake rate. TAA prolonged exposure leads to hyperplastic nodule formation, hepatocellular carcinoma, and cirrhosis. The induced cirrhosis by TAA in rats has been shown to be an experimental model of disease comparable with human ethology and pathology [69]. Higher Cat levels compared to SOD means that EC could promote the antioxidant defense system by increasing Cat activity against H_2O_2 and protecting cells against acute toxic liver damage at 24 h after TAA administration, as shown in Figure 5 shows.

3.6. MnSOD, CuZnSOD, Cat, and Nrf2 mRNA Gene Expression

Gene expression is a process by which DNA instructions are converted into functional products as proteins. In *MnSOD, CuZnSOD,* and *Cat*, the lower gene expression was derived from the process of TAA detoxification, which produces an attack of hydroxyl radicals and DNA damage. The results highlight a greater *Cat* gene expression due to EC + TAA toward basal stages, which means that EC has an inhibitory capacity against $·O_2$ and H_2O_2, avoiding peroxidation and DNA damage by activation of the defense antioxidant system [21]. These results are the opposite to the *Nrf2* gene expression, which was suppressed. *Nrf2* plays an important role in the activation of antioxidant enzymes by regulating their transcription. It is primarily regulated by *Keap1* (Kelch-like erythroid cell-derived protein with CNC homology-associated protein 1) dependent ubiquitination-proteasomal degradation and is activated by oxidants [70], so *Keap1* binds *Nrf2* in the cytoplasm and maintains *Nrf2* at a low steady state level [17]. Another mechanism for *Nrf2* degradation is phosphorylation by glycogen synthase kinase 3 (GSK3) via β-transducin repeats-containing protein (β-TrCP)-Cul1-based ubiquitin ligase [71]. As a consequence, *Nrf2* knockout means that the effect could also be mediated by inflammatory cells [68]. Although *Nrf2* activation is generally considered to have a beneficial effect in liver disease [72], we found that the antioxidant mechanism inducted by EC was independent of activation of *Nrf2* expression. The increase of levels of antioxidant enzymes by activating *Nrf2* may not be enough to decrease oxidative stress and chronic inflammation optimally due to antioxidants, which tend to decrease in an oxidative environment, and must also be elevated. Besides, the levels of antioxidant can be increased by supplementation or an *Nrf2* independent mechanism [18] as happened with the EC + TAA group.

4. Materials and Methods

4.1. Chemicals and Reagents

The main chemicals used in this study include: $CDCl_3$, 2,2-Diphenyl-1-picrylhydrazyl, thioacetamide, tween 80, 2,4,6-Tris(2-pyridyl)-s-triazine, TPTZ (2,4,6-tri (2-pyridyl-s-triazine) 6-hydroxy-2,5,7,8-tetramethil-chromal-2-carboxylic acid- Trolox, Chloride ferric, Tri-Reagent, and agarose were purchased from Sigma Chemical Co. (St. Louis, MO, USA); pentobarbital was provided by Pisa (Mexico City, Mexico). qPCR Master Mix (Nzytech, Portugal); SYBR Green (Biotools, Madrid, Spain); Silica gel 60, and other chemicals, such as ethanol, methanol, and hydrochloric acid, were reactive grade products from Merck (Darmstadt, Germany). DNase I RNase-free reagents were bought Thermo Fisher Scientific (Waltham, MA, USA).

4.2. Preparation of EC

Aerial parts of *C. hypoleucus* were collected on January 2016, from San Vidal, Tulancingo, Hidalgo State [20.116002, −98.305734]. The plant was identified by Manuel González Ledezma, taxonomist of Department of Botany, Autonomous University of Hidalgo State. The specimen, voucher number: DVM01, was deposited at the Herbarium of Biological Sciences Research Center. Aerial parts were dried for a period of 15 days in a light protected area and milled with a commercial grinder. Powdered plant (500 g) was extracted by maceration with 4 L of ethanol for a week in triplicate. The material was filtered and concentrated by a rotatory evaporator (Büchi, Switzerland) at 40 °C. The crude extract obtained was used for in vitro and in vivo analysis.

4.3. Purification of Main Compounds in Dichloromethane Fraction

A sample of 5 g of crude extract was fractionated through a flash column chromatography performed over silica gel 60 (230–400 mesh). The sample was eluted with 500 mL of hexane, dichloromethane, ethyl acetate, and methanol to yield 0.3, 1.8, 2.1, and 0.8 g, respectively. The dichloromethane fraction was dried and supported over silica gel 60 column chromatography and eluted with a hexane: Dichloromethane (6:4) mixture. In total, 64 fractions of 10 mL were collected and monitored by TLC on precoated silica gel aluminum sheets. The compounds were visualized through UV detection and by spraying with vanillin/H_2SO_4/EtOH solution, followed by heating. The fractions, 48–52, was selected and supported over a preparative layer chromatography with hexane: Dichlorometane (1:1) which lead to the isolation of two compounds (Figure 1), which were characterized by ^{1}H and ^{13}C NMR spectroscopy using a Spectrometer 400 MHz (Bruker Avance III, Billerica, MA, USA) and $CDCl_3$ as solvent. The NMR shifts were compared with literature data [11,24].

4.4. Antioxidant Capacity of EC

DPPH Free Radical Scavenging Activity. The DPPH radical scavenging was determined according to the method of Brand-Williams [73] with slight modifications. From a 50 mg/mL methanol solution of EC, 50 µL was mixed with 200 µL DPPH reactant (200 µM). The mix of 1 mL methanol and 1 mL DPPH solution was used as the control. The reaction was carried out in triplicate. The mixture was kept for 30 min in a 96-well plate. After incubation, the absorbance was measured at 517 nm using an absorbance plate reader (Fluostar Optima, BMG Labtech, Ortenberg, Germany). The percent of inhibition was calculated by the following equation:

$$\% \text{ inhibition} = \frac{\text{Abs Control} - \text{Abs CE}}{\text{Abs Control}} \times 100. \tag{1}$$

The IC_{50} or effective concentration values, representing the amount of extract required to decrease the absorbance of DPPH by 50%, were calculated from the percentage of radical scavenging activity.

Ferric-reducing power FRAP. The ferric-reducing power of the crude extract was determined according to a modified protocol of Benzie and Strain [74]. The working FRAP solution was prepared daily by mixing 25 mL of acetate buffer (0.3M pH 3.6), 2.5 mL of 10 mM TPTZ in HCl (40 µM), and 2.5 mL of ferric chloride in distilled water. The working solution was kept at 35 °C and in the dark. In the test, 30 µL of crude extract in methanol (10 mg/mL) was mixed in 90 µL of distilled water plus 900 µL of FRAP solution. The reaction mixture was incubated for 30 min at 37 °C. The absorbance was measured at 595 nm with a spectrophotometer (UVikon 930 spectrophotometer, Kontron Instruments S.A., Madrid, Spain). For the ferric-reducing power determination, ferrous sulfate heptahydrate solution (200–1000 µM) instead of extract was used as the calibration curve. The results (in triplicate) are expressed as µM Fe/mg crude extract.

4.5. Experimental Animals

Male Wistar rats weighing 180 to 200 g and aged 7 weeks were used in this study. The animals were obtained from the vivarium of the Autonomous University of Hidalgo State. They were adapted according to appropriate protocols prior to commencement of the experiment. The rats were maintained in clean polypropylene cages in a temperature controlled room and 12:12 h light/dark cycles with ad libitum access to pellet food and water. After 1 week of acclimation, rats were randomly assigned to experimental groups. Besides, all the experiments were conducted by approbation of the Internal and Ethical Committee for the care and use of experimental animals with the official certificate No. 5-12-2017 and according to the Official Mexican Norm (NOM 062-ZOO-1999) [75].

4.6. Acute Toxicity

The acute toxicity was evaluated using the Dietrich Lorke assay [52]. This study was conducted in two phases. In the first phase, three groups (n = 3) of rats were administered intragastrically with a homogeneous solution of EC in 1% tween 80 at the respective oral doses of 10, 100, and 1000 mg/kg body weight. The animals were observed frequently for 14 days and any adverse effects (mortality, body weight, water and food intake) were recorded for the 14 days. In the second phase, three new groups (n = 3) rats were administered respective oral doses of 1600, 2900, and 5000 mg/kg body weight of crude extract. In both phases, a vehicle was fed 1 mL of Tween 80.1% intragastrically. The possible number of deaths was recorded and the LD_{50} value was determined.

4.7. Thioacetamide-Induced Hepatotoxicity

The thioacetamide-induced damage was performed following a pre-established protocol [56]. Male Wistar rats were randomly distributed into 5 groups (n = 8). Groups EC and EC + TAA received a single dose intragastrically (i.g.) of crude extract (300 mg/kg body weight) every 24 h for four days of treatment. At the same time, VE + TAA was administered with 100 mg/kg (i.g.) and groups Thioacetamide (TAA) and vehicle (CT) were administered i.g. with a tween 80 solution (1% v/v). On the fourth day, group TAA, EC + TAA, and VE + TAA were administered one dose (400 mg/kg body weight) of TAA dissolved in 1 mL NaCl (0.9%) intraperitoneally (i.p.). Then, 24 h after TAA administration, all animals were sacrificed with intramuscular pentobarbital doses (50 mg/kg body weight) via the i.p. route. Then, through an abdominal dissection, samples of blood were obtained by portal vein puncture. Serum from blood was separated by centrifugation at 4000 rpm, 10 °C, and 15 min and analyzed for various biochemical parameters related to liver damage using well-established protocols. On the other hand, livers were rapidly dissected out and washed using 0.9% NaCl sterile solution and then immediately stored in a −80 °C freezer until tissue homogenate preparation.

4.7.1. Biochemical Parameters

Quantitative determination of the ALT, AST, ALP, GGT, and DHL enzymes and DB was carried out with WIENER-Lab optimized equipment (Rosario, Argentina). Quantitative determination of ALT enzyme was measured by diminution in absorbance to 340 nm at 25 °C, produced by the oxidation of NADH into NAD^+ while pyruvate reduction into lactate was done by lactate dehydrogenase [76]. The activity of AST was measured by the diminution in absorbance at 340 nm and 25 °C produced by NADH oxidation to NAD^+ in the paired reaction of the oxaloacetate reduction into malate by malate dehydrogenase activity [77]. ALP determination was done through pnitrophenylphosphate (pNPP) hydrolysis yielding phosphate and p-nitrophenol at alkaline pH and 405 nm. The *p*-nitrophenolate production is directly proportional to the enzymatic activity of the sample [78]. GGT was analyzed by the change in absorbance at 410 and 480 nm due to the formation of 5-amino-2-nitrobenzoate, a product from a glutamyl group transfer from the donor substrate, gamma-glutamyl-3-carboxy-4-nitroanilide, to the acceptor, glycylglycine, by GGT [79]. LDH catalytic activity was determined by measuring the NAD^+ formation rate from NADH oxidation in an alkaline pH at 340 nm and 37 °C [80]. The evaluation of bilirubin was performed through production of azobilirubin from the bilirubin reaction with diazotized sulfanilic acid photocolorimetrically measured at 530 nm [81].

4.7.2. SOD and Cat in Vitro Activity

Homogeneous samples of liver tissue were used for the SOD and Cat biochemical assays. Liver tissue was homogenized in phosphate-EDTA buffer (0.1 M sodium phosphate and 0.005 M EDTA, pH 8) at 100 mg/mL, with the addition of 10 μL/mL of perchloric acid. It was then centrifuged at 10,000 rpm for 10 min at 4 °C. Superoxide dismutase (SOD) activity was measured using the Nitroblue Tetrazolium reagent (NBT) method according to Neha and Mishra protocol [82] with modifications. This method is based on the generation of superoxide radical (O^{2-}) by autoxidation of hydroxylamine hydrochloride in the presence of NBT, which gets reduced to nitrite. Nitrite in the presence of EDTA gives a color measured at 560 nm. Cat activity was measured as described by the Aebi [83] method using hydrogen peroxide as a substrate. The decomposition of H_2O_2 was followed directly by a decrease in absorbance at 260nm. Enzyme activity was standardized to liver homogenate protein concentrations determined according to Bradford´s method [84]. Final enzyme activity results are expressed as IU/mg protein.

4.7.3. Extraction and Quantification of RNA by RT-PCR

RNA samples were isolated from 100 mg of liver using TRI-Reagent and treated with DNase I RNase-free reagents to avoid any contamination with genomic DNA. The yield and quality of RNA was assessed by measuring absorbance at 260, 280, and 310 nm and by electrophoresis on agarose gels (1%). Total RNA of sample was reverse-transcribed to first-strand complementary DNA (cDNA) using Nzytech qPCR Master Mixes. Relative Mn-SOD, CuZn-SOD, Cat, and Nrf2 mRNA levels were quantified with a LightCycler Real-Time PCR Detection System (Roche Diagnostics, Indianapolis, IN, USA), using SYBR Green as the fluorescent binding dye. Detection was monitored by measuring the increase in fluorescence throughout the cycles. The standardization was carried out to the β-actine value. The results are expressed as fold changes of the threshold cycle (Ct) value relative to the vehicle using the $2^{-\Delta\Delta Ct}$ method [85]. The PCR protocol was: Preincubation at 95 °C for 10 min followed by 45 cycles of denaturation at 95 °C for 10 s with an annealing temperature of 60 °C for each couple primer, extension at 72 °C for 15 s, and cooling at 40 °C for 30 s. Primer sequences were as indicated in Table 2.

Table 2. Primer sequences used in RT-PCR.

Mn-SOD	sense: 50-ACTGAAGTTCAATGGCGGG-30 and antisense: 50-TCCAGCAACTCTCCTTTGGG-30
CuZn-SOD	sense: 50-CTTCGAGCAGAAGGCAAGCG-30 and antisense: 50-GACATGGAACCCATGCTCGC-30
Cat	sense: 50-ATCAG**GGA**TGCCATGTTGTT-30 and antisense: 50-GGGTCCTTCAGGTGAGTTTG-30
Nrf2	sense: 50-TTGTAGATGACCATGAGTCGC-30 and antisense: 50-GAGCTATCGAGTGACTGAGCC-30

4.8. Statistical Analysis

Significant differences between the results were calculated by variance analysis (ANOVA). One-way ANOVA was determined by Statgraphics centurion XVII.II version (Statistical graphics Corporation, Inc., Rockville, MD, USA). A post-hoc Tukey test was performed to identify significant differences ($p \leq 0.05$) between treatments.

5. Conclusions

The current study reports the first antioxidant and hepatoprotective evaluation of ethanolic crude extract of *Croton hypoleucus* (EC) in a frame of a thioacetamide-induced (TAA) liver damage model in rats. The main mechanisms by which EC protects the liver from toxic damage are associated with its antioxidant properties and its ability to modulate Cat involved in the antioxidant defense system. Additionally, EC has the ability to recover cell mitochondria and regulate biomarkers of the liver after TAA injury, thus preventing the development of hepatotoxicity. Nrf2-no dependent catalase activation revealed the role of antioxidant mechanisms while biochemical parameters were the first sign of its hepatoprotective activity. *Croton hypoleucus* could offer a novel alternative to the limited therapeutic options that exist for the treatment of liver diseases.

Author Contributions: Conceptualization, M.B.; Data curation, O.A.J.-M.; Formal analysis, J.A.S.-L.; Investigation, M.D.l.O.-A.; Methodology, J.B.; Project administration, C.V.-G.; Supervision, F.J.S.-M.; Writing, review & editing, T.A.U.-H.

Funding: The present research received a scholarship number 236155 from CONACYT, Mexico.

Acknowledgments: We wish to thank the Pharmacology, Pharmacognosy and Botany Department of Pharmacy school from Complutense University of Madrid for their technical assistance during T.A.U.-H. internship.

Conflicts of Interest: The authors declare no conflicts of interest.

References

1. Bonini, S.A.; Premoli, M.; Tambaro, S.; Kumar, A.; Maccarinelli, G.; Memo, M.; Mastinu, A. *Cannabis sativa*: A comprehensive ethnopharmacological review of a medicinal plant with a long history. *J. Ethnopharmacol.* **2018**, *227*, 300–315. [CrossRef] [PubMed]
2. World Health Organization (WHO). *The World Medicines Situation, Traditional Medicines: Global Situation, Issues and Challenges*; WHO: Geneva, Switzerland, 2011; 12p.
3. Salatino, A.; Salatino, M.L.F.; Negri, G. Traditional uses, chemistry and pharmacology of Croton species (Euphorbiaceae). *J. Braz. Chem. Soc.* **2007**, *18*, 11–33. [CrossRef]
4. Kumar, A.; Premoli, M.; Bonini, S.A.; Maccarinelli, G.; Gianoncelli, A.; Memo, M.; Mastinu, A. Cannabimimetic plants: Are they new cannabbinoidergic modulators? *Planta* **2019**, *269*, 1681–1694. [CrossRef] [PubMed]
5. Adewusi, E.A.; Afolayan, A.J. A review of natural products with hepatoprotective activity. *JMPR* **2010**, *4*, 1318–1334. [CrossRef]
6. Govind, P. Medicinal plants against liver diseases. *Int. Res. J. Pharm.* **2011**, *2*, 115–151.
7. Jannu, V.; Baddam, P.G.; Boorgula, A.K.; Jambula, S.R. A Review on Hepatoprotective Plants. *Int. J. Drug Dev. Res.* **2012**, *4*, 1–8.
8. Lima, F.C.; Sousa, D.F.; Ferreira, J.M. *Croton zehntneri* essential oil prevents acetaminophen- induced acute hepatotoxicity in mice. *Rec. Nat. Prod.* **2008**, *2*, 135–140.
9. Ahmed, B.; Alam, T.; Varshney, M.; Khan, S.A. Hepatoprotective activity of two plants belonging to the Apiaceae and the Euphorbiaceae family. *J. Ethnopharmacol.* **2002**, *79*, 313–316. [CrossRef]
10. Jaya, S.E.; Beaulah, A.; Sadiq, A.M.; Chakkaravaarthy, M.V. Hepatoprotective activity of methanolic extract of *Croton sparciflorus* on DEN induced hepatotoxicity in wistar albino rats. *J. Pharm. Chem. Biol. Sci.* **2014**, *4*, 1002–1011.
11. Velázquez-Jiménez, R.; Vargas-Mendoza, D.; Gayosso-de-Lucio, J.A.; González-Montiel, S.; Villagómez-Ibarra, J.R. Three novel epoxy-clerodanes bearing a furan ring from *Croton hypoleucus*. *Phytochem. Lett.* **2018**, *24*, 21–26. [CrossRef]
12. Pandit, A.; Sachdeva, T.; Bafna, P. Drug-Induced Hepatotoxicity: A Review. *J. Appl. Pharm. Sci.* **2012**, *2*, 233–243. [CrossRef]
13. Robin, S.; Kumar, S.; Rana, A.C.; Sharma, N. Different models of hepatotoxicity and related liver diseases: A review. *Int. Res. J. Pharm.* **2012**, *3*, 86–95.
14. Luo, M.; Dong, L.; Li, J.; Wang, Y.; Shang, B. Protective effects of pentoxifylline on acute liver injury induced by thioacetamide in rats. *Int. J. Clin. Exp. Pathol.* **2015**, *8*, 8990–8996. [PubMed]
15. Zhang, W.; Wang, M.; Xie, H.Y.; Zhou, L.; Meng, X.Q.; Shi, J.; Zheng, S. Role of reactive oxygen species in mediating hepatic ischemia-reperfusion injury and its therapeutic applications in liver transplantation. *Transpl. Proc.* **2007**, *39*, 1332–1337. [CrossRef] [PubMed]
16. Ma, Q. Xenobiotic-activated receptors: From transcription to drug metabolism to disease. *Chem. Res. Toxicol.* **2008**, *21*, 1651–1671. [CrossRef] [PubMed]
17. Holmström, K.M.; Kostov, V.; Dinkova-Kostova, A.T. The multifaceted role of Nrf2 in mitochondrial function. *Curr. Opin. Toxicol.* **2016**, *1*, 80–91. [CrossRef] [PubMed]
18. Prasad, K.N. Simultaneous activation of Nrf2, elevation of antioxidants and reduction in glutamate level: An essential strategy for prevention and improved management of neurodegenerative Diseases. *J. Alzheimers Dis. Park.* **2016**, *6*, 6. [CrossRef]
19. Akhtar, T.; Sheikh, N. An overview of thioacetamide-induced hepatotoxicity. *Toxin Rev.* **2013**, *32*, 43–46. [CrossRef]
20. Ramahia, S.K.; Apte, U.; Mehendale, H.M. Cytochrome P4502E1 induction increases thioacetamide liver injury in diet-restricted rats. *Drug Metab. Diapos.* **2001**, *269*, 1088–1095.
21. Hajovsky, H.; Hu, G.; Koen, Y.; Sarma, D.; Cui, W.; Moore, D.S.; Staudinger, J.L.; Hanzlik, R.P. Metabolism and Toxicity of Thioacetamide and Thioacetamide S -Oxide in Rat Hepatocytes. *Chem. Res. Toxicol.* **2012**, *25*, 1955–1963. [CrossRef]

22. Chilakapati, J.; Shankar, K.; Korrapati, M.C.; Hill, R.A.; Mehendale, H.M. Saturation toxicokineticsof thioacetamide: Role in initiation of liver injury. *Drug Metab. Dispos.* **2005**, *33*, 2877–2885. [CrossRef]
23. Xu, W.H.; Liu, W.Y.; Lang, Q. Chemical constituents from Croton Species and their biological activities. *Molecules* **2018**, *23*, 2333. [CrossRef] [PubMed]
24. Sun, Y.; Wang, M.; Ren, Q.; Li, S.; Xu, J.; Ohizumi, Y.; Xie, C.; jing, D.-Q.; Guo, Y. Two novel clerodane diterpenes with NGF-potentiating activities from the twings of Croton yanhuii. *Fitorerapia* **2014**, *95*, 229–233. [CrossRef] [PubMed]
25. Shi, S.; Zhang, H.; Li, S.; Liu, Q.; Song, S. Review: Diterpenoids from croton genus (Euphorbiaceae) and their biological activity. *Asian J. Tradit. Med.* **2018**, *13*, 242–262.
26. Chao, W.-W.; Lin, B.-F. Hepatoprotective diterpenoids isolated from *Andrographis paniculate*. *Chin. Med. J.* **2011**, *3*, 136–143. [CrossRef]
27. Alqasoumi, S.I.; Farraj, A.I.; Abdel-Kader, M.S. Study of the hepatoprotective effect of *Janiperus phoenicea* constituents. *Pak. J. Pharm. Sci.* **2013**, *26*, 999–1008. [PubMed]
28. Park, E.J.; Zhao, Y.Z.; Young, H.K.; Jung, J.L.; Dong, H.S. Acanthoic acid from *Acanthopanax koreanum* protects against liver injury induced by tert-butyl hydroperoxide or carbon tetrachloride in vitro and in vivo. *Planta Med.* **2004**, *70*, 321–327.
29. Krishnamurthy, T.P.; Bajaj, J.; Sharma, A.; Maimaran, S.; Bommenahalli, R.P.K.; Pottkad, V. Hepatoprotective activity of terpenoids and terpenoid fractions of *Scoparia dulcis* L. *Orien. Pharm. Exp. Med.* **2010**, *10*, 263–270. [CrossRef]
30. Tian, J.-L.; Yao, G.-D.; Wang, Y.-X.; Gao, P.-Y.; Wang, D.; Li, L.-Z.; Lin, B.; Huang, X.-X.; Song, S.-J. Cytotoxic clerodane diterpenoids from *Croton crassifolius*. *Bioorg. Med. Chem. Lett.* **2017**, *27*, 1237–1242. [CrossRef]
31. Kubo, I.; Asaka, Y.; Shibata, K. Insect growth inhibitory nor-diterpenes, cisdehydrocrotonin and trans-dehydrocrotonin, from *Croton cajucara*. *Phytochemistry* **1991**, *30*, 2545–2546. [CrossRef]
32. Rodrígues, G.; Marcolin, E.; Bona, S.; Porawski, M.; Lehmann, M.; Possa, M.N. Hepatics alterations and genotoxic effects of *Croton cajucara* Beth (SACACA) in diabetic rats. *Arq. Gastroenterol.* **2010**, *47*, 301–305. [CrossRef] [PubMed]
33. Zhang, Y.; Liu, Z.; Zhang, R.; Hou, P.; Bi, K.; Chen, X. Nephrotoxicity evaluation of a new cembrane diterpene from *Euphorbiae pekinensis* Radix with HEK 293T cells and the toxicokinetics study in rats using a sensitive and reliable UFLC–MS/MS. *J. Pharm. Biomed. Anal.* **2016**, *119*, 159–165. [CrossRef] [PubMed]
34. da Silva Brito, S.S.; Silva, F.; Malheiro, R.; Baptista, P.; Pereira, J.A. *Croton argyrophyllus* Kunth and *Croton heliotropiifolius* Kunth: Phytochemical characterization and bioactive properties. *Ind. Crops Prod.* **2018**, *113*, 308–315. [CrossRef]
35. Abdalaziz, M.N.; Ali, A.; Kabbashi, A. In vitro antioxidant activity and phytochemical screening of *Croton zambesicus*. *J. Pharmacogn. Phytochem.* **2016**, *5*, 12–16.
36. Atoui, A.; Mansouri, A.; Boskou, G.; Kefalas, P. Tea and herbal infusions: Their antioxidant activity and phenolic profile. *Food Chem.* **2005**, *89*, 27–36. [CrossRef]
37. Teixeira, S.; Mendes, A.; Alves, A.; Santos, L. Simultaneous distillation–extraction of high-value volatile compounds from Cistus ladanifer L. *Anal. Chim. Acta* **2007**, *584*, 439–446. [CrossRef] [PubMed]
38. Min, B.; McClung, A.M.; Chen, M.-H. Phytochemicals and Antioxidant Capacities in Rice Brans of Different Color. *J. Food Sci.* **2011**, *76*, C117–C126. [CrossRef]
39. Dudonné, A.; Vitrac, X.; Woillez, M.; Mérillon, J.M. Comparative Study of Antioxidant Properties and Total Phenolic Content of 30 Plant Extracts of Industrial Interest Using DPPH, ABTS, FRAP, SOD, and ORAC Assays. *J. Agric. Food Chem.* **2009**, *57*, 1768–1774. [CrossRef]
40. Furlan, C.M.; Pereira, S.K.; Sedano-Partida, M.D.; Barbosa, D.L.; Santos, D.Y.A.C.; Salatino, M.L.F.; Negri, G.; Berry, P.E.; Van Ee, B.; Salatino, A. Flavonoids and antioxidant potential of nine Argentinian species of roton (Euphorbiaceae). *Braz. J. Bot.* **2015**, *38*, 693–702. [CrossRef]
41. Dos Santos, K.P.; Motta, L.B.; Santos, D.Y.; Salatino, M.L.; Salatino, A.; Ferreira, M.J.; Lago, J.H.; Ruíz, A.L.; Carvaho, J.E.; Furlan, C.M. Antiproliferative activity of flavonoids from *Croton sphaerogynus* Baill. (Euphorbiaccae). *BioMed Res. Int.* **2015**, *2015*, 212809. [CrossRef]
42. Letha, N.; Ganesan, K.; Nair, P.S.K.; Azalewor, H.G.; Gani, S.B. Evaluation of In Vitro Antioxidant Activity and Phytochemical Screening of *Croton macrostachyus* Hochst. by using Different Solvent Extracts. *Am. J. PharmTech Res.* **2016**, *6*, 73–85.
43. Lila, M.A.; Raskin, I. Health-related Interactions of Phytochemicals. *J. Food Sci.* **2005**, *70*, R20–R27. [CrossRef]

44. Marchyshak, T.; Yakovenko, T.; Shmarakov, I.; Tkachuk, Z. The potential protective effect of oligoribonucleotides-d-mannitol complexes against thioacetamide-induced hepatotoxicity in mice. *Pharmaceuticals* **2018**, *11*, 77. [CrossRef] [PubMed]
45. Mierziak, J.; Kostyn, K.; Kulma, A. Flavonoids as important molecules of plant interactions with the environment. *Molecules* **2014**, *19*, 16240–16265. [CrossRef] [PubMed]
46. Shon, M.-Y.; Lee, J.; Choi, J.-H.; Choi, S.-Y.; Nam, S.-H.; Seo, K.I.; Sang-Won, L.; Sung, N.J.; Park, S.K. Antioxidant and free radical scavenging activity of methanol extract of *chungkukjang*. *J. Food Compos. Anal.* **2007**, *20*, 113–118. [CrossRef]
47. Gad, S.C. Single-Dose (Acute) and Pilot (DRF) Toxicity Testing in Drug Safety Evaluation. In *Drug Safety Evaluation*; John Wiley & Sons, Inc.: Hoboken, NJ, USA, 2011; pp. 185–233. [CrossRef]
48. Bulus, T.; Atawodi, S.E.; Mamman, M. Acute toxicity effect on the aqueous extract of *Termelia* avicennioides on white albino rats. *Sci. World J.* **2011**, *6*, 1–4.
49. Asare, G.A.; Sittie, A.; Bugyei, K.; Gyan, B.A.; Adjei, S.; Addo, P.; Wiredu, E.K.; Nyarko, A.K.; Out-Nyarko, L.S.; Adjei, D.N. Acute toxicity studies of Croton membranaceus root extract. *J. Ethnopharmacol.* **2011**, *135*, 398–934. [CrossRef]
50. Sridhar, N. Comparative anti-inflammatory and anti-oxidant evaluation of *Jatropha gossypifolia* and *Croton bonplandianm*. *Int. J. Res. Pharm. Sci.* **2013**, *4*, 16–27.
51. Meireles, D.R.P.; Fernandes, H.M.B.; Rolim, T.L.; Batista, T.M.; Mangueira, V.M.; de Sousa, T.K.G.; Pita, J.C.L.R.; Xavier, A.L.; Beltrão, D.M.; Tavares, J.F.; et al. Toxicity and antitumor efficacy of *Croton polyandrus* oil against Ehrlich ascites carcinoma cells. *Rev. Bras. Farmacogn.* **2016**, *26*, 751–758. [CrossRef]
52. Lorke, D. A new approach to practical acute toxicity testing. *Arch. Toxicol.* **1983**, *54*, 275–287. [CrossRef]
53. Amin, K.A.; Mohamed, B.M.; El-wakil, M.A.M.; Ibrahem, S.O. Impact of Breast Cancer and Combination Chemotherapy on Oxidative Stress, Hepatic and Cardiac Markers. *J. Breast Cancer.* **2012**, *15*, 306–312. [CrossRef] [PubMed]
54. Singh, A.; Bhat, T.K.; Sharma, O.P. Clinical Biochemistry of Hepatotoxicity. *J. Clin. Toxicol.* **2011**, *S4*, 1–19. [CrossRef]
55. Ozer, J.; Ratner, M.; Shaw, M.; Bailer, W.; Schomaker, S. The current state of serum biomarkers of hepatotoxicity. *Toxicology* **2008**, *245*, 194–205. [CrossRef] [PubMed]
56. Bautista, M.; Velazquez-González, C.; De la O Arciniega, M.; Morales-González, J.; Benedí, J.; Gayosso-De-Lucio, J. Chemical composition and hepatotoxic effect of *Geranium schiedeanum* in a thioacetamide-induced liver injury model. *Pharmacogn. Mag.* **2014**, *10*, 574. [CrossRef] [PubMed]
57. Yang, X.; Schnackenberg, L.K.; Shi, Q.; Salminen, W.F. Hepatic toxicity biomarkers. In *Biomarkers*; Gupta, R.C., Ed.; Elsevier: Amsterdam, The Netherlands, 2011; pp. 241–260.
58. Aydin, A.F.; Kusku-Kiraz, S.Z.; Dogru-Abbasoglu, M.; Gulluoglu, M.U.; Kocak-Toker, N. Effect of carnosine against thioacetamide-induced liver cirrhosis in rat. *Peptides* **2010**, *31*, 67–71. [CrossRef] [PubMed]
59. Atef, M.A. Hepatoprotective influence of vitamin C on thioacetamide-induced liver cirrhosis in wistar male rats. *J. Toxicol. Pharmacol.* **2011**, *6*, 218–233. [CrossRef]
60. Miguel, F.M.; Schemitt, E.G.; Colares, J.R.; Hartmann, R.M.; Morgan-Martins, M.I.; Marroni, N.P. Actio of vitamin E on experimental severe acute liver failure. *Arq. Gastroenterol.* **2017**, *54*, 123–129. [CrossRef]
61. Braunwld, E.; Ghany, M.; Hoofnagle, J.; Berk, P.; Wolkoff, A.; Dienstag, J. *Harrison. Principios de Medicina Interna*, 17th ed.; Editorial Mc Graw-Hill Interamericana: México City, Mexico, 2009.
62. Everhart, J.E.; Wright, E.C. Association of γ-glutamyl transferase (GGT) activity with treatment and clinical outcomes in chronic hepatitis C (HCV). *Hepatology* **2013**, *57*, 1725–1733. [CrossRef]
63. Lee, D.-H.; Jacobs, D.R. Association between serum gamma-glutamyltransferase and C-reactive protein. *Atherosclerosis* **2005**, *178*, 327–330. [CrossRef]
64. Bigoniya, P.; Singh, C.S.; Shukla, A. A comprehensive review of different liver toxicants used in experimental pharmacology. *Int. J. Pharm. Sci. Drug Res.* **2009**, *1*, 124–135.
65. Zimmerman, H.J. Drug-induced liver disease. *Clin. Liver Dis.* **2000**, *4*, 79–96. [CrossRef]
66. Khalaf, N.A.; Shakya, A.K.; Al-Othman, A.; El-Agbar, Z.; Farah, H. Antioxidant Activity of Some Common Plants. *Turk. J. Biol.* **2008**, *32*, 51–55.
67. Pandey, K.B.; Rizvi, S.I. Markers of Oxidative Stress in Erythrocytes and Plasma During Aging in Humans. *Oxidative Med. Cell. Longev.* **2010**, *3*, 2–12. [CrossRef] [PubMed]

68. Li, J.; Gao, Y.; Chu, S.; Zhang, Z.; Xia, C.; Mou, Z.; Song, X.-Y.; He, W.-B.; Guo, X.-F.; Chen, N.-H. Nrf2 pathway activation contributes to anti-fibrosis effects of ginsenoside Rg1 in a rat model of alcohol- and CCl_4-induced hepatic fibrosis. *Acta Pharmacol. Sin.* **2014**, *35*, 1031–1044. [CrossRef] [PubMed]
69. Yeh, C.-N.; Maitra, A.; Lee, K.-F.; Jan, Y.-Y.; Chen, M.-F. Thioacetamide-induced intestinal-type cholangiocarcinoma in rat: An animal model recapitulating the multi-stage progression of human cholangiocarcinoma. *Carcinogenesis* **2003**, *25*, 631–636. [CrossRef] [PubMed]
70. Taguchi, K.; Motohashi, H.; Yamamoto, M. Molecular mechanisms of the Keap1-Nrf2 pathway in stress response and cancer evolution: Molecular mechanisms of the Keap1-Nrf2 pathway. *Genes Cells* **2011**, *16*, 123–140. [CrossRef] [PubMed]
71. Rada, P.; Rojo, A.I.; Chowdhry, S.; McMahon, M.; Hayer, J.D.; Cuadrado, A. SCF/b-TrCP Promotes Glycogen Synthase kinase 3-dependent degradation of the Nrf2 transcription factor in a keap1-independent manner. *Mol. Cell. Biol.* **2011**, *31*, 1121–1133. [CrossRef]
72. Bataille, A.M.; Manautou, J.E. Nrf2 a potential target to new therapeutics in liver disease. *Clin. Pharmacol. Ther.* **2012**, *92*, 340–348. [CrossRef]
73. Brand-Williams, W.; Cuvelier, M.E.; Berset, C. Use of a free radical method to evaluate antioxidant activity. *LWT—Food Sci. Technol.* **1995**, *28*, 25–30. [CrossRef]
74. Benzie, I.F.F.; Strain, J.J. The Ferric Reducing Ability of Plasma (FRAP) as a Measure of "Antioxidant Power": The FRAP Assay. *Anal. Biochem.* **1996**, *239*, 70–76. [CrossRef]
75. SAGARPA. Norma Oficial Mexicana NOM-062-ZOO-1999. Especificaciones técnicas para la producción, cuidado y manejo de animales de laboratorio. *Diario Oficial de la Federación* **2001**, 107–165.
76. Murray, R. Alanine aminotransferase. In *Clinical Chemistry: Theory, Analysis, and Correlation*, 2nd ed.; CV Mosby: St. Louis, MO, USA, 1989; pp. 898–989.
77. Rej, R.; Horder, M. Aspartate aminotransferase. L-aspartate: 2-oxoglutarate aminotranferase, EC 2.6.2.1. Routine, U.V. method. In *Methods of Enzymatic Analysis*; Verlag-CHemie: Weinheim, Germany, 1987; pp. 416–424.
78. Bessey, O.A.; Lowry, O.H.; Brock, M.J. A method for the rapid determination of alkaline phosphatase with five cubic millimeters of serum. *J. Biol. Chem.* **1946**, *164*, 321–329. [PubMed]
79. Theodorsen, L.; Strømme, J. Gamma-glutamyl-3-c arboxy4-nitroanilide: The substrate of choice for routine determinatinations of y-glutamyl-transferase activity in serum? *Clin. Chim. Acta* **1976**, *72*, 205–210. [CrossRef]
80. Vanderlinde, R.E. Measurement of total lactate dehydrogenase activity. *Ann. Clin. Lab. Sci.* **1985**, *15*, 13–31. [PubMed]
81. Martinek, R.G. Improved micro-method for determination of serum bilirubin. *Clin. Chim. Acta* **1966**, *13*, 161–170. [CrossRef]
82. Neha, J.; Mishra, R.N. Antioxidant activity of Trikatu megaExt. *Int. J. Res. Pharm. Biosci.* **2011**, *2*, 624–628.
83. Aebi, H. Catalase in Vitro. *Methods Enzymol.* **1984**, *105*, 121–126. [PubMed]
84. Bradford, M.M. A Rapid and Sensitive Method for the Quantitation of microgram quantities of protein utilizing the principle of protein-dye binding. *Anal. Biochem.* **1976**, *72*, 248–254. [CrossRef]
85. Livak, K.J.; Schimittgen, T.D. Analysis of relative gene expression data using real-time quantitative PCR and the $2^{-\Delta\Delta CT}$ Method. *Methods* **2001**, *25*, 402–408. [CrossRef]

Sample Availability: Samples of the compounds are available from the authors.

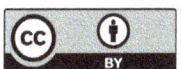

© 2019 by the authors. Licensee MDPI, Basel, Switzerland. This article is an open access article distributed under the terms and conditions of the Creative Commons Attribution (CC BY) license (http://creativecommons.org/licenses/by/4.0/).

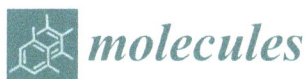

Article

Protective Effects Induced by Two Polyphenolic Liquid Complexes from Olive (*Olea europaea*, mainly *Cultivar Coratina*) Pressing Juice in Rat Isolated Tissues Challenged with LPS

Lucia Recinella [1,†], Annalisa Chiavaroli [1,†], Giustino Orlando [1], Luigi Menghini [1], Claudio Ferrante [1], Lorenzo Di Cesare Mannelli [2], Carla Ghelardini [2], Luigi Brunetti [1,*] and Sheila Leone [1]

1. Department of Pharmacy, "G. d'Annunzio" University, 66013 Chieti, Italy
2. Department of Neuroscience, Psychology, Drug Research and Child Health - NEUROFARBA - Pharmacology and Toxicology Section, University of Florence, 50139 Florence, Italy
* Correspondence: luigi.brunetti@unich.it; Tel.: +39 0871 3554758
† These authors contributed equally to the work.

Academic Editor: Derek J. McPhee
Received: 12 July 2019; Accepted: 15 August 2019; Published: 19 August 2019

Abstract: MOMAST(®) HY100 and MOMAST(®) HP30 are polyphenolic liquid complexes from olive pressing juice with a total polyphenolic content of 100 g/kg (at least 50% as hydroxytyrosol) and 36 g/kg (at least 30% as hydroxytyrosol), respectively. We investigated the potential protective role of MOMAST(®) HY100 and MOMAST(®) HP30 on isolated rat colon, liver, heart, and prefrontal cortex specimens treated with *Escherichia coli* lipopolysaccharide (LPS), a validated ex vivo model of inflammation, by measuring the production of prostaglandin (PG)E_2, 8-iso-PGF$_{2\alpha}$, lactate dehydrogenase (LDH), as well as cyclooxygenase (COX)-2, tumor necrosis factor α (TNFα), and inducible nitric oxide synthase (iNOS) mRNA levels. MOMAST(®) HY100 decreased LPS-stimulated PGE$_2$ and LDH levels in all tested tissues. Following treatment with MOMAST(®) HY100, we found a significant reduction in iNOS levels in prefrontal cortex and heart specimens, COX-2 and TNFα mRNA levels in heart specimens, and 8-iso-PGF$_{2\alpha}$ levels in liver specimens. On the other hand, MOMAST(®) HP30 was found to blunt COX-2, TNFα, and iNOS mRNA levels, as well as 8-iso-PGF$_{2\alpha}$ in cortex, liver, and colon specimens. MOMAST(®) HP30 was also found to decrease PGE$_2$ levels in liver specimens, while it decreased iNOS mRNA, LDH, and 8-iso-PGF$_{2\alpha}$ levels in heart specimens. Both MOMAST(®) HY100 and MOMAST(®) HP30 exhibited protective effects on multiple inflammatory and oxidative stress pathways.

Keywords: *Cultivar Coratina*; inflammation; oxidative stress; hydroxytyrosol

1. Introduction

It has been well established that olive tree (*Olea europaea*) polyphenols have healthy beneficial effects, including the prevention of several chronic diseases, such as cancer and aging-associated degenerative diseases [1,2]. These beneficial properties could be mainly related to the antioxidant activity of olive tree polyphenols, which were found able to both scavenge free radicals and reactive oxygen species and activate endogenous antioxidant enzymes, including glutathione peroxidase, glutathione reductase, and glutathione S-transferase [3–5]. Besides the antioxidant activity, anti-atherogenic, hepato-protective, hypoglycemic, anti-inflammatory, immunomodulatory, anticancer, and antimicrobic effects were also suggested for these compounds [5–7]. Hydroxytyrosol (HT) and the secoiridoid oleuropein (OE) are two abundant phenolic compounds in olives, virgin oil, and waste water from olive oil production [8–10]. Particularly, HT has antioxidant and scavenging activities comparable to oleuropein and catechol [11].

MOMAST® HY100 and MOMAST® HP30 (Bioenutra, Ginosa, TA, Italy) are polyphenolic liquid complexes from olive (*Olea europaea*, mainly *Cultivar Coratina*) pressing juice with a total polyphenolic content of 100 g/kg (at least 50% as HT) and 36 g/kg (at least 30% as HT), respectively (Tables 1 and 2). In addition to HT, both MOMAST® HY100 and MOMAST® HP30 are also characterized by the presence of tyrosol and oleuropein.

Table 1. Characteristics of the polyphenolic complex MOMAST® HY 100.

Name:	**MOMAST HY 100**
Description:	Polyphenolic active complex of hydroxytyrosol—Liquid, with total polyphenolic content of 100 g/kg
Source Type:	Mainly *Cultivar Coratina*
Physical State:	Liquid
Appearance:	Light brown to brown liquid
Moisture:	N.A.
Ash:	Less than 10% (600 °C)
Total heavy (as Pb):	Less than 10 ppm
Total Plate Count:	Less than 100 cfu/g
Pesticides:	Absence
Polyphenolic content measured through high performance liquid chromatography (HPLC)	
Hydroxytyrosol (HPLC):	50 g/Kg
Tyrosol (HPLC):	15 g/kg
Oleuropein (HPLC):	0.5 g/Kg
Total Polyphenols (HPLC):	100 g/Kg

Table 2. Characteristics of the Polyphenolic Complex MOMAST® HP 30.

Name:	**MOMAST HP 30**
Description:	Polyphenolic active complex from olives' pressing juice—Liquid, with total polyphenolic content of 30 g/kg
Source Type:	Mainly *Cultivar Coratina*
Fisic State:	Liquid
Appearance:	Brown liquid
Moisture:	N. A.
Ash:	Less than 10% (600 °C)
Total heavy (as Pb):	Less than 10 ppm
Total Plate Count:	Less than 100 cfu/g
Pesticides:	Absence
Polyphenolic Content	
Hydroxytyrosol (HPLC):	15 g/Kg
Tyrosol (HPLC):	3 g/kg
Oleuropein (HPLC):	0.2 g/Kg
Total Polyphenols (HPLC):	30 g/Kg

Considering the antioxidant effects displayed by both HT and oleuropein, the aim of the present study was to investigate the putative protective effects of MOMAST® HY100 and MOMAST® HP30, both including HT and oleuropein, on the burden of oxidative stress/inflammation occurring on various isolated rat tissue (i.e., colon, liver, heart, and prefrontal cortex) specimens exposed to *Escherichia coli* lipopolysaccharide (LPS), a well-established inflammatory stimulus. Specifically, we studied the effects of MOMAST® HY100 and MOMAST® HP30 on multiple inflammatory and oxidative stress pathways, by measuring the production of prostaglandin (PG)E_2, 8-iso-PGF$_{2\alpha}$, lactate dehydrogenase (LDH), as well as cyclooxygenase (COX)-2, tumor necrosis factor α (TNFα), and inducible nitric oxide synthase (iNOS) mRNA levels. The results support a rational use of these polyphenolic complexes in the prevention of tissue damage occurring during inflammation.

2. Results and Discussion

MOMAST® HY100 (10, 50, and 100 µg/mL) and MOMAST® HP30 (22, 110, and 220 µg/mL) were tested in vitro to evaluate their effects on cell viability. We observed that both polyphenolic liquid complexes were well tolerated by Hypo-E22 and C2C12 cell lines (Supplementary Figures S1–S2). Particularly, C2C12 and Hypo-E22 cell viability resulted in the limit of biocompatibility (>70 and <130% compared to the untreated control group) after exposition to polyphenolic extracts, in the respective tested concentration range, corresponding to identical concentrations of HT (5–50 µg/mL), which were in agreement with previous in vitro studies [11].

Considering these findings, we performed a second set of experiments aimed to evaluate the modulatory effects of MOMAST® HY100 (10, 50, and 100 µg/mL) and MOMAST® HP30 (22, 110, and 220 µg/mL) supplementation on oxidative stress and multiple inflammatory pathways in colon, liver, heart, and prefrontal cortex specimens challenged with LPS. As previously reported [12–14], isolated tissues challenged with LPS is a validated ex vivo experimental model to evaluate the modulatory effects of herbal extracts and drugs on inflammatory pathways and oxidative stress. The beneficial effects of plant polyphenols in humans have been confirmed by a large body of evidence [15–18]. A number of studies confirmed the antioxidant, anti-atherogenic, and protective effects of olive polyphenols, such as OLE and HT, against coronary artery disease [19–23]. In particular, HT, deacetoxy oleuropein aglycon, and oleuropein aglycon were classified as the strongest antioxidants in virgin olive oils [24]. Oxidative stress is defined as an imbalance in the pro-oxidant/antioxidant homeostasis, where increased production of reactive oxygen/nitrogen species (ROS/RNS) and free radicals can induce peroxidation reactions on biomolecules including proteins, lipids, and nucleic acids [25,26]. Oxidative damage is thought to play a key role in the pathogenesis of various chronic diseases, including cancer, atherosclerosis, cardiovascular diseases, chronic inflammation, and diabetes [27–29]. 8-Iso-PGF$_{2\alpha}$, an isomer of prostaglandins produced by free radical-catalyzed peroxidation of membrane arachidonic acid, is a stable marker of lipid peroxidation and oxidative stress [30]. We found that MOMAST® HP30 (110 and 220 µg/mL) was able to decrease 8-iso-PGF$_{2\alpha}$ levels on rat prefrontal cortex, colon, liver, and heart tissues, challenged with LPS inflammatory stimulus (Figures 1–4).

Molecules **2019**, *24*, 3002

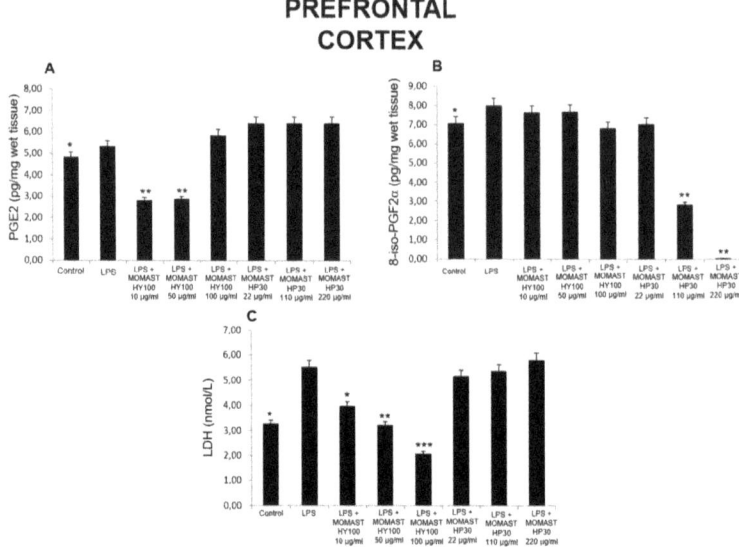

Figure 1. Effects of MOMAST(®) HY100 (10, 50, and 100 μg/mL) and MOMAST(®) HP30 (22, 110, and 220 μg/mL) on (**A**) PGE_2 levels (pg/mg wet tissue), (**B**) 8-iso-prostaglandin $F_{2\alpha}$ (8-iso-$PGF_{2\alpha}$) levels, and (**C**) lactate dehydrogenase (LDH) activity (nmol/L) in rat prefrontal cortex specimens. Data were reported as means ± SEM. ANOVA, $p < 0.01$; *post-hoc* test, * $p < 0.05$, ** $p < 0.01$, *** $p < 0.001$ vs. lipopolysaccharide (LPS)-treated group.

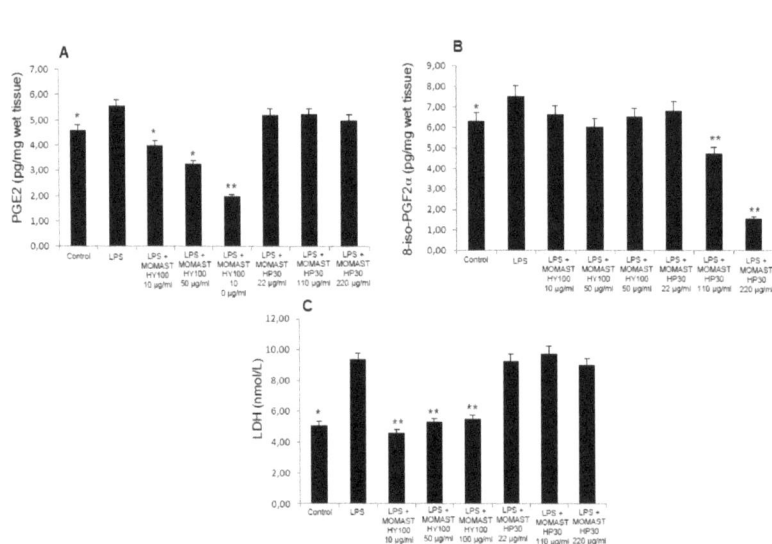

Figure 2. Effects of MOMAST(®) HY100 (10, 50, and 100 μg/mL) and MOMAST(®) HP30 (22, 110, and 220 μg/mL) on (**A**) PGE_2 levels (pg/mg wet tissue), (**B**) 8-iso-prostaglandin $F_{2\alpha}$ (8-iso-$PGF_{2\alpha}$) levels, and (**C**) lactate dehydrogenase (LDH) activity (nmol/L) in colon specimens. Data were reported as means ± SEM. ANOVA, $P < 0.01$; *post-hoc* test, * $p < 0.05$, ** $p < 0.01$ vs. LPS-treated group.

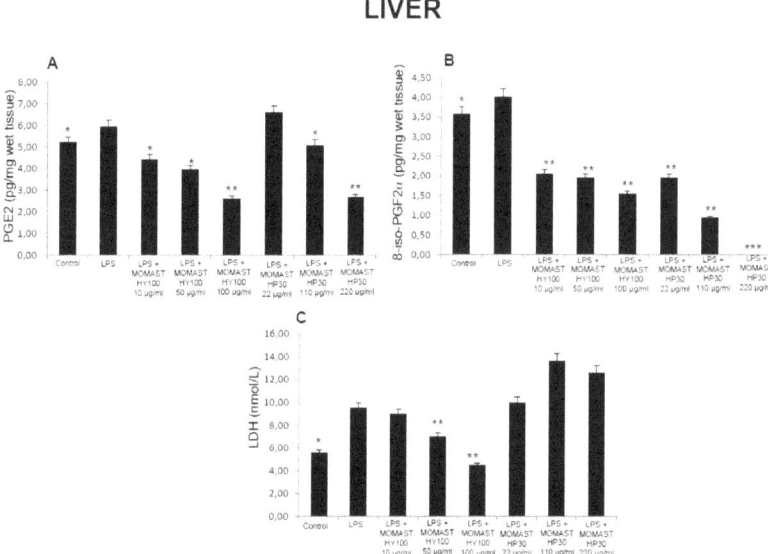

Figure 3. Effects of MOMAST(®) HY100 (10, 50, and 100 µg/mL) and MOMAST(®) HP30 (22, 110, and 220 µg/mL) on (**A**) PGE$_2$ levels (pg/mg wet tissue), (**B**) 8-iso-prostaglandin F$_{2\alpha}$ (8-iso-PGF$_{2\alpha}$) levels, and (**C**) lactate dehydrogenase (LDH) activity (nmol/L) in rat liver specimens. Data were reported as means ± SEM. ANOVA, $p < 0.01$; *post-hoc* test, * $p < 0.05$, ** $p < 0.01$, *** $p < 0.001$ vs. LPS-treated group.

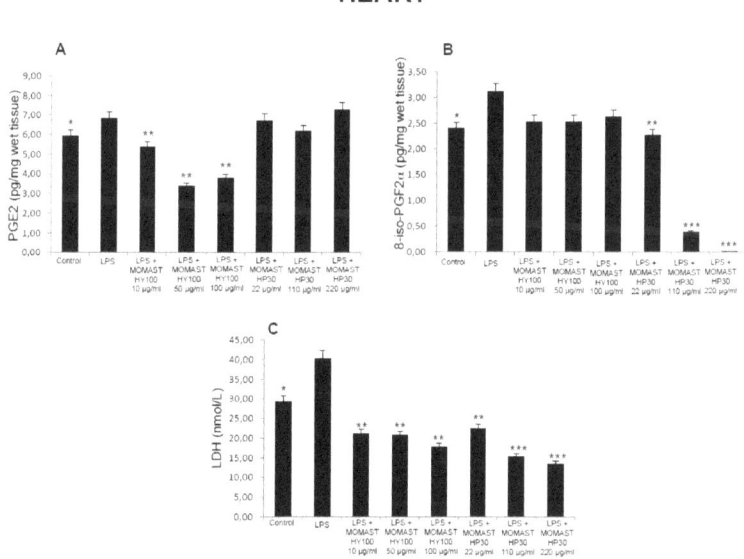

Figure 4. Effects of MOMAST(®) HY100 (10, 50, and 100 µg/mL) and MOMAST(®) HP30 (22, 110, and 220 µg/mL) on (**A**) PGE$_2$ levels (pg/mg wet tissue), (**B**) 8-iso-prostaglandin F$_{2\alpha}$ (8-iso-PGF$_{2\alpha}$) levels, and (**C**) lactate dehydrogenase (LDH) activity (nmol/L) in rat heart specimens. Data were reported as means ± SEM. ANOVA, $p < 0.01$; *post-hoc* test, * $p < 0.05$, ** $p < 0.01$, *** $p < 0.001$ vs. LPS-treated group.

Moreover, MOMAST® HY100 (10, 50, and 100 μg/mL) was effective in inhibiting LPS-induced 8-iso-PGF$_{2\alpha}$ in rat liver specimens (Figure 3B). These effects could be related, at least in part, to the free radical-reducing and -scavenging properties of HT [31,32], which is found in very high amounts in MOMAST® HY100 and MOMAST® HP30 (at least 50% and 30% of the phenolic fraction, respectively). HT was also shown to decrease low density lipoproteins oxidation [33], platelet aggregation [34], and 5- and 12-lipoxygenase activity [35] in vitro. However, we cannot exclude that our findings could also be related to other phenolic compounds which are present, even if in low content, in both liquid complexes. In this context, the antioxidant activity of OE has been widely confirmed both in vitro and in vivo [36]. We also investigated the activity of MOMAST® HY100 and MOMAST® HP30 on LDH level in inflamed tissues. LDH is a cytosolic enzyme, which can be considered a marker of tissue destruction [37,38]. Additionally, decreased LDH activity after treatment with herbal extracts has been related to protective effects in chronic inflammatory disorders such as inflammatory bowel disease (IBD) [39]. Following MOMAST® HY100 (10, 50, and 100 μg/mL) treatment, we found a significant inhibition of LPS-induced LDH level in all tested tissues (Figures 1–4). MOMAST® HP30 (22, 110, and 220 μg/mL) was also able to decrease LDH level induced by LPS in heart specimens (Figure 7C). Actually, the reduction of LDH level could be related to the presence of HT [40] in both extracts, and further supports the protective effects induced by MOMAST® HY100 and MOMAST® HP30. Finally, we evaluated the modulatory effects of MOMAST® HY100 and MOMAST® HP30 on pro-inflammatory markers, including PGE$_2$, COX-2, TNFα, and iNOS. LPS was found to induce macrophage production of inflammatory cytokines such as TNFα, interleukin-1β (IL-1β), and IL-6, along with inflammatory mediators including nitric oxide (NO) and PGE$_2$ [41,42]. COX-2, an inducible enzyme stimulated by mitogenic and inflammatory stimuli, including LPS and cytokines, is known to be mainly involved in the synthesis of pro-inflammatory PGE$_2$ in both neoplastic and inflamed tissues [43]. Similarly, iNOS, whose expression is induced by exposure to a number of stimuli, including LPS and TNFα, is involved in the generation of large amounts of NO, which plays a pivotal role in acute and chronic inflammation [44–46]. Following LPS inflammatory stimulus, we observed that MOMAST® HP30 was able to reduce COX-2, TNFα, and iNOS mRNA levels in prefrontal cortex, colon, and liver specimens (Figures 5–7).

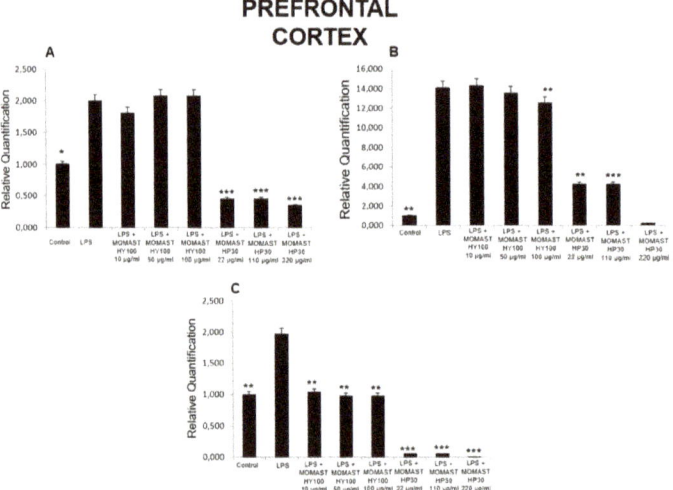

Figure 5. Effects of MOMAST® HY100 (10, 50, and 100 μg/mL) and MOMAST® HP30 (22, 110, and 220 μg/mL) on (**A**) cyclooxygenase (COX)-2, (**B**) tumor necrosis factor α (TNFα), and (**C**) inducible nitric oxide synthase (iNOS) in rat prefrontal cortex specimens. Data were reported as means ± SEM. ANOVA, $p < 0.01$; *post-hoc* test, * $p < 0.05$, ** $p < 0.01$, *** $p < 0.001$ vs. LPS-treated group.

COLON

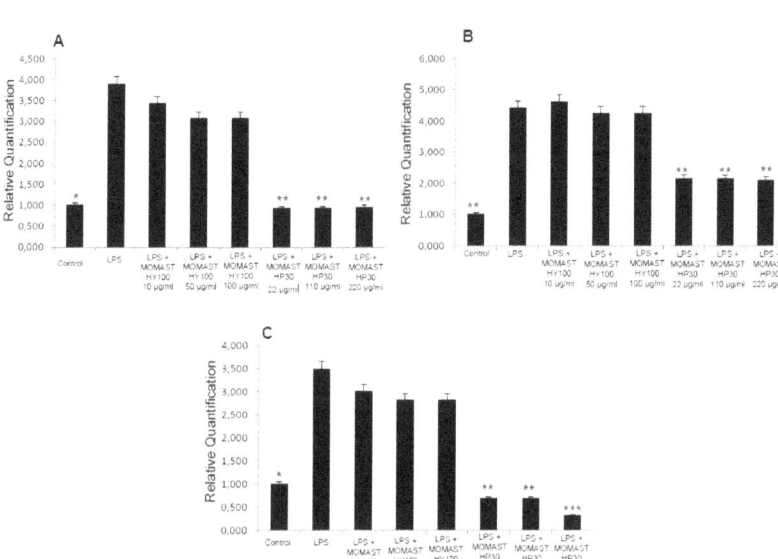

Figure 6. Effects of MOMAST(®) HY100 (10, 50, and 100 μg/mL) and MOMAST(®) HP30 (22, 110, and 220 μg/mL) on (**A**) cyclooxygenase (COX)-2, (**B**) tumor necrosis factor α (TNFα), and (**C**) inducible nitric oxide synthase (iNOS) in rat colon specimens. Data were reported as means ± SEM. ANOVA, $p < 0.01$; post-hoc test, * $p < 0.05$, ** $p < 0.01$, *** $p < 0.001$ vs. LPS-treated group.

LIVER

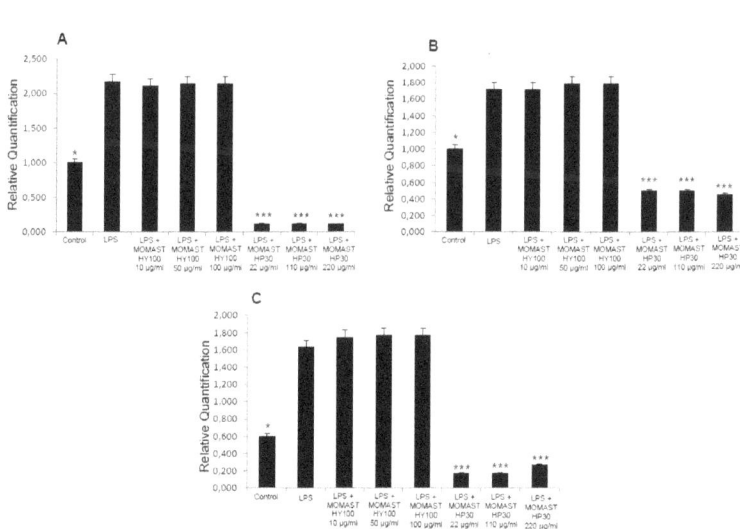

Figure 7. Effects of MOMAST(®) HY100 (10, 50, and 100 μg/mL) and MOMAST(®) HP30 (22, 110, and 220 μg/mL) on (**A**) cyclooxygenase (COX)-2, (**B**) tumor necrosis factor α (TNFα), and (**C**) inducible nitric oxide synthase (iNOS) in rat liver specimens. Data were reported as means ± SEM. ANOVA, $p < 0.01$; post-hoc test, * $p < 0.05$, *** $p < 0.001$ vs. LPS-treated group.

On the other hand, COX-2, TNFα, and iNOS mRNA levels were decreased by MOMAST(®) HY100 in heart tissue specimens (Figure 8). iNOS mRNA levels were also decreased by MOMAST(®) HY100 in prefrontal cortex specimens (Figure 5C) and by MOMAST(®) HP30 in heart tissue specimens (Figure 8C).

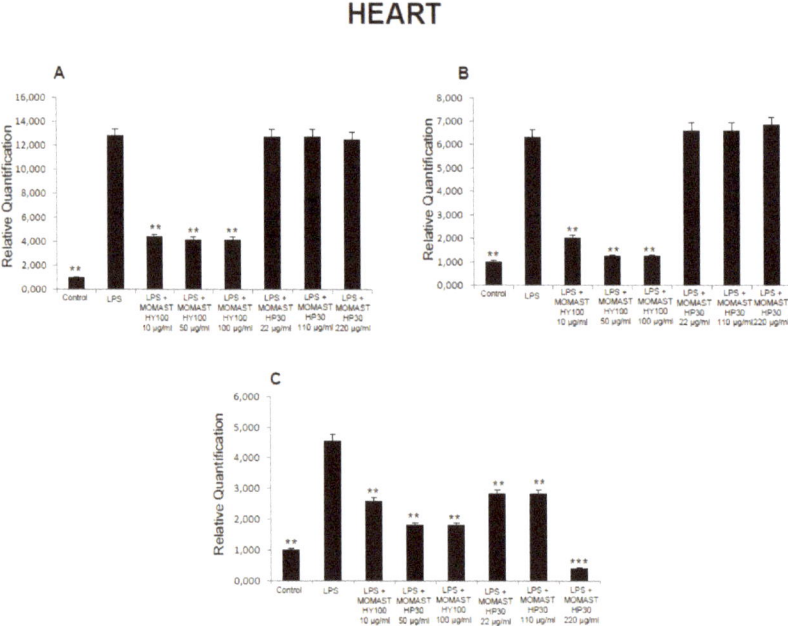

Figure 8. Effects of MOMAST(®) HY100 (10, 50, and 100 µg/mL) and MOMAST(®) HP30 (22, 110, and 220 µg/mL) on (**A**) cyclooxygenase (COX)-2, (**B**) tumor necrosis factor α (TNFα), (**C**) and inducible nitric oxide synthase (iNOS) in rat heart specimens. Data were reported as means ± SEM. ANOVA, $p < 0.01$; post-hoc test, ** $p < 0.01$, *** $p < 0.001$ vs. LPS-treated group.

As regards PGE$_2$, we found that while MOMAST(®) HY100 was effective in reducing LPS-induced PGE$_2$ levels in all tested tissues (Figures 1–4), MOMAST(®) HP30 was able to decrease PGE$_2$ levels only in liver tissue (Figure 5A). The inhibitory effects induced by MOMAST(®) HY100 and MOMAST(®) HP30 on PGE$_2$ levels, along with COX-2, TNFα, and iNOS mRNAs, support the protective effects of both polyphenolic liquid complexes in prefrontal cortex, colon, liver, and heart specimens. Accordingly, HT was shown to exert anti-inflammatory effects in LPS-stimulated RAW264.7 mouse macrophages by suppressing nuclear factor-kB (NF-κB) signaling and downregulating gene expression of iNOS, COX-2, TNFα, and IL-1β, and production of NO and PGE$_2$ [47]. We hypothesize that the protective effects induced by MOMAST(®) HY100 and MOMAST(®) HP30 could also be related to the presence of other phenolic compounds, including tyrosol and OE. In this context, tyrosol was found to significantly inhibit COX-2 gene and protein expression, as well as PGE$_2$ secretion in human glioblastoma cells [48]. Moreover, it has been found that OE significantly downregulated NO, COX-2, iNOS, and TNF-α in RAW264.7 macrophages following LPS treatment [49]. However, our findings indicate that MOMAST(®) HY100 and MOMAST(®) HP30 could display different effects in tissues. On one hand, Takeda et al. [50] reported that HT was able to suppress iNOS expression and NO production without any effect on NF-kB, COX-2, and TNFα expression in mouse peritoneal macrophages challenged with LPS; on the other hand, Maiuri et al. [51] and Zhang et al. [52] showed that HT was able to inhibit LPS-stimulated NFκB activation as well as COX-2 gene expression, in J774 murine macrophages and human monocytic THP-1 cells, respectively.

In conclusion, both MOMAST® HY100 and MOMAST® HP30 exhibited protective effects as indicated by the blunting effect on the tested pro-inflammatory mediators. On the basis of these results, HT seems to be the main extract component involved in the pharmacological effects. Nevertheless, considering the inherent limitations of the ex vivo experimental model, further investigations including oxidative stress and inflammation biomarkers in in vivo studies are needed for a more accurate evaluation of MOMAST® HY100 and MOMAST® HP30 efficacy.

3. Materials and Methods

3.1. In Vitro Studies

Rat Hypo-E22 cells (Cedarlane Cellution Biosystem) and mouse myoblast C2C12 cell lines (ATCC® CRL-1772™) were cultured in Dulbecco's modified eagle medium (DMEM) supplemented with 10% (v/v) heat-inactivated fetal bovine serum and 1.2% (v/v) penicillin G/streptomycin in 75 cm^2 tissue culture flask (n = 5 individual culture flasks for each condition). The cultured cells were maintained in a humidified incubator with 5% CO_2 at 37 °C. For cell differentiation, Hypo-E22 and C2C12 cell suspensions at a density of 1 × 10^6 cells/mL were treated with various concentrations (10, 50, and 100 ng/mL) of phorbol myristate acetate (PMA, Fluka) for 24 h or 48 h (induction phase). Thereafter, the PMA-treated cells were washed twice with ice-cold pH 7.4 phosphate buffer solution (PBS) to remove PMA and non-adherent cells, whereas the adherent cells were further maintained for 48 h (recovery phase). The morphology of the cells was examined under an inverted phase-contrast microscope. To assess the basal cytotoxicity of MOMAST® HY100 and MOMAST® HP30, a viability test was performed on 96-microwell plates, using a 3-(4,5-dimethylthiazol-2-yl)-2,5-diphenyltetrazolium bromide (MTT) test. Cells were incubated with MOMAST® HY100 (10, 50, and 100 μg/mL) and MOMAST® HP30 (22, 110, and 220 μg/mL), corresponding to HT (5, 25, and 50 μg/mL, respectively), for 24 h. Ten microliters of MTT (5 mg/mL) were added to each well and incubated for 3 h. The formazan dye formed was extracted with dimethyl sulfoxide and the absorbance was recorded as previously described [12,52]. The effects on cell viability were evaluated in comparison to the untreated control group.

3.2. Ex Vivo Studies

Male adult Sprague-Dawley rats (200–250 g) were housed in Plexiglass cages (40 cm × 25 cm × 15 cm), two rats per cage, in climatized colony rooms (22 ± 1 °C; 60% humidity), on a 12 h/12 h light/dark cycle (light phase: 07:00–19:00 h), with free access to tap water and food, 24 h/day throughout the study, with no fasting periods. Rats were fed a standard laboratory diet (3.5% fat, 63% carbohydrate, 14% protein, 19.5% other components without caloric value; 3.20 kcal/g).

Housing conditions and experimentation procedures were strictly in accordance with the European Union ethical regulations on the care of animals for scientific research.

According to the recognized ethical principles of "Replacement, Refinement, and Reduction of Animals in Research", colon, liver, heart, and prefrontal cortex specimens were obtained as residual material from vehicle-treated rats randomized in our previous experiments approved by the Local Ethical Committee of University "G. d'Annunzio" and the Italian Health Ministry (Italian Health Ministry authorization N. 880, delivered on 24th August 2015). Rats were sacrificed by CO_2 inhalation (100% CO_2 at a flow rate of 20% of the chamber volume per min) and colon, liver, heart, and prefrontal cortex specimens were immediately collected and maintained in a humidified incubator with 5% CO_2 at 37 °C for 4 h, in DMEM buffer with added bacterial LPS (10 μg/mL) (incubation period).

During the incubation period, tissues were treated with scalar concentrations of MOMAST(®) HY100 (10, 50, and 100 μg/mL) and MOMAST(®) HP30 (22, 110, and 220 μg/mL). Tissue supernatants were collected, and the PGE_2 and 8-iso-$PGF_{2\alpha}$ levels (ng/mg wet tissue) were measured by radioimmunoassay (RIA), as previously reported [13,53]. Briefly, specific anti-8-iso-$PGF_{2\alpha}$ and anti-PGE_2 were developed in the rabbit; the cross-reactivity against other prostanoids is <0.3%. One hundred microliters of prostaglandin standard or sample were incubated overnight at 4 °C with the 3H-prostaglandin (3000 cpm/tube; NEN) and antibody (final dilution: 1:120,000; kindly provided by Prof. G. Ciabattoni), in a volume of 1.5 mL of 0.025 M phosphate buffer. Free and antibody-bound prostaglandins were separated by the addition of 100 µL 5% bovine serum albumin and 100 µL 3% charcoal suspension, followed by centrifuging for 10 min at 4,000× g at 5 °C and decanting off the supernatants into scintillation fluid (Ultima Gold™, Perkin Elmer, Waltham, MA, USA) for β emission counting. The detection limit of the assay method was 0.6 pg/mL. Additionally, tissue supernatants were assayed for lactate dehydrogenase (LDH) activity [54]. LDH activity was measured by evaluating the consumption of nicotinamide adenine dinucleotide dehydrogenase (NADH) in 20 mM HEPES-K+ (pH 7.2), 0.05% bovine serum albumin, 20 µM NADH, and 2mM pyruvate using a microplate reader (excitation 340 nm, emission 460 nm) according to manufacturer's protocol (Sigma-Aldrich, St. Louis, MO). LDH activity was measured by evaluating the consumption of NADH in 20 mM HEPES-K+ (pH 7.2), 0.05% bovine serum albumin, 20 µM NADH and 2 mM pyruvate using a microplate reader (excitation 340 nm, emission 460 nm) according to manufacturer's protocol. In addition, individual prefrontal cortex, colon, liver, and heart specimens were quickly dissected to evaluate cyclooxygenase (COX)-2, tumor necrosis factor α (TNFα), and inducible nitric oxide synthase (iNOS) gene expression, as previously reported [55,56]. Tissue specimens were dissected and stored in RNAlater solution (Life Technologies, Carlsbad, CA, USA) at −20 °C until further processed. Total RNA was extracted from the tissues using TRI Reagent (Sigma-Aldrich, St. Louis, MO, USA) according to manufacturer's protocol. One microgram of total RNA extracted from each sample in a 20-µL reaction volume was reverse transcribed using a high capacity cDNA reverse transcription kit (Life Technologies, Carlsbad, CA, USA). Reactions were incubated in a 2720 thermal cycler (Life Technologies, Carlsbad, CA, USA) initially at 25 °C for 10 min, then at 37 °C for 120 min, and finally at 85 °C for 5 s. Gene expression was determined by quantitative real-time PCR using TaqMan probe-based chemistry (Life Technologies, Carlsbad, CA, USA). Reactions were performed in MicroAmp Fast Optic 96-well Reaction Plates (Life Technologies, Carlsbad, CA, USA) on an ABI PRISM 7900 HT fast real-time PCR system (Life Technologies, Carlsbad, CA, USA). PCR primers and TaqMan probes were obtained from Life Technologies (Assays-on-Demand Gene Expression Products, Rn01483828_m1 for COX-2 gene, Rn01525859_g1 for TNFα, Rn00561646_m1 for iNOS. β-actin (Life Technologies, Carlsbad, CA, USA, Part No. 4352340E) was used as the housekeeping gene. The real-time PCR was carried out in triplicate. Data were elaborated with the sequence detection system (SDS) software version 2.3 (Applied Biosystems, Foster City, CA, USA). The comparative $2^{-\Delta\Delta Ct}$ method was used to quantify the relative abundance of mRNA and then determine the relative changes in individual gene expression (relative quantification) [57].

3.3. Statistical Analysis

Statistical analysis was performed using GraphPad Prism version 5.01 for Windows (GraphPad Software, San Diego, CA, USA). Means ± S.E.M. were determined for each experimental group and analyzed by one-way analysis of variance (ANOVA), followed by Newman–Keuls comparison multiple test. As for gene expression analysis, 1.00 (calibrator sample) was considered the theoretical mean for the comparison [57]. Statistical significance was set at $p < 0.05$. The number of animals randomized for each experimental group was calculated on the basis of the "Resource Equation" N = (E + T)/T ($10 \leq E \leq 20$) [58–60], according to the guidelines suggested by the National Centre for the Replacement, Refinement, and Reduction of Animals in Research (NC3RS) and reported on the following web site: https://www.nc3rs.org.uk/experimental-designstatistics.

Supplementary Materials: The following are available on line: Supplementary Figure S1: Effects of MOMAST[®] HY100 (10, 50, and 100 µg/mL) and MOMAST[®] HP30 (22, 110, and 220 µg/mL) on HypoE22 cell line viability. Supplementary Figure S2: Effects of MOMAST[®] HY100 (10, 50, and 100 µg/mL) and MOMAST[®] HP30 (22, 110, and 220 µg/mL) on C2C12 cell line viability.

Author Contributions: Conceptualization, L.R. and L.B.; methodology, A.C., G.O., C.F., S.L.; software, G.O., L.M.; validation, L.M., C.F., and S.L.; formal analysis, L.D.C.M., C.G.; investigation, A.C., G.O., L.D.C.M., C.G.; resources,

A.C., L.D.C.M., C.G.; data curation, L.R., L.B., S.L.; writing—original draft preparation, L.R., S.L.; writing—review and editing, L.R., A.C., L.B., S.L.; visualization, C.F.; supervision, L.B.; project administration, L.R., A.C., L.B., S.L.; funding acquisition, L.B., S.L. and L.R.

Funding: This research was funded by Bioenutra S.r.l. (Ginosa, TA, Italy) and by grants from the Italian Ministry of University (FFABR 2017 to S. Leone).

Conflicts of Interest: The authors declare no conflict of interest.

References

1. Carrera-González, M.; Ramírez-Expósito, M.; Mayas, M.; Martínez-Martos, J. Protective role of oleuropein and its metabolite hydroxytyrosol on cancer. *Trends Food Sci. Technol.* **2013**, *31*, 92–99. [CrossRef]
2. Rahmani, H.A.; Albutti, S.A.; Aly, M.S. Therapeutics role of olive fruits/oil in the prevention of diseases via modulation of anti-oxidant, anti-tumour and genetic activity. *Int. J. Clin. Exp. Med.* **2014**, *7*, 799–808. [PubMed]
3. Masella, R.; Di Benedetto, R.; Varì, R.; Filesi, C.; Giovannini, C. Novel mechanisms of natural antioxidant compounds in biological systems: involvement of glutathione and glutathione-related enzymes. *J. Nutr. Biochem.* **2005**, *16*, 577–586. [CrossRef] [PubMed]
4. Tundis, R.; Loizzo, M.R.; Menichini, F.; Statti, G.A.; Menichini, F. Biological and pharmacological activities of iridoids: recent developments. *Mini Rev. Med. Chem.* **2008**, *8*, 399–420. [CrossRef] [PubMed]
5. Gorzynik-Debicka, M.; Przychodzen, P.; Cappello, F.; Kuban-Jankowska, A.; Marino Gammazza, A.; Knap, N.; Wozniak, M.; Gorska-Ponikowska, M. Potential Health Benefits of Olive Oil and Plant Polyphenols. *Int. J. Mol. Sci.* **2018**, *19*, E686. [CrossRef]
6. Tripoli, E.; Giammanco, M.; Tabacchi, G.; Di Majo, D.; Giammanco, S.; La Guardia, M. The phenolic compounds of olive oil: structure, biological activity and beneficial effects on human health. *Nutr. Res. Rev.* **2005**, *18*, 98–112. [CrossRef] [PubMed]
7. Fabiani, R.; de Bartolomeo, A.; Rosignoli, P.; Servili, M.; Selvaggini, R.; Montedoro, G.F.; di Saverio, C.; Morozzi, G. Virgin olive oil phenols inhibit proliferation of human promyelocytic leukemia cells (HL60) by inducing apoptosis and differentiation. *J. Nutr.* **2006**, *136*, 614–619. [CrossRef]
8. Angerosa, F.; d'Alessandro, N.; Corana, F.; Mellerio, G. Characterization of phenolic and secoiridoid aglycons present in virgin olive oil by gas chromatography-chemical ionization mass spectrometry. *J. Chromatogr.* **1996**, *736*, 195–203. [CrossRef]
9. Cinquanta, L.; Esti, M.; La Notte, E. Evolution of phenolic compounds in virgin olive oil during storage. *J. Am. Oil Chem. Soc.* **1997**, *74*, 1259–1264. [CrossRef]
10. El, S.N.; Karakaya, S. Olive tree (Olea europaea) leaves: Potential beneficial effects on human health. *Nutr. Rev.* **2009**, *67*, 632–638. [CrossRef]
11. Martínez, L.; Ros, G.; Nieto, G. Hydroxytyrosol: Health Benefits and Use as Functional Ingredient in Meat. *Medicines (Basel)* **2018**, *23*, 13. [CrossRef] [PubMed]
12. Ferrante, C.; Recinella, L.; Ronci, M.; Menghini, L.; Brunetti, L.; Chiavaroli, A.; Leone, S.; Di Iorio, L.; Carradori, S.; Tirillini, B.; et al. Multiple pharmacognostic characterization on hemp commercial cultivars: Focus on inflorescence water extract activity. *Food Chem. Toxicol.* **2019**, *125*, 452–461. [CrossRef] [PubMed]
13. Locatelli, M.; Macchione, N.; Ferrante, C.; Chiavaroli, A.; Recinella, L.; Carradori, S.; Zengin, G.; Cesa, S.; Leporini, L.; Leone, S.; et al. Graminex Pollen: Phenolic Pattern, Colorimetric Analysis and Protective Effects in Immortalized Prostate Cells (PC3) and Rat Prostate Challenged with LPS. *Molecules* **2018**, *23*, 1145. [CrossRef] [PubMed]
14. Mollica, A.; Stefanucci, A.; Zengin, G.; Locatelli, M.; Macedonio, G.; Orlando, G.; Ferrante, C.; Menghini, L.; Recinella, L.; Leone, S.; et al. Polyphenolic composition, enzyme inhibitory effects ex-vivo and in-vivo studies on two Brassicaceae of north-central Italy. *Biomed. Pharmacother.* **2018**, *107*, 129–138. [CrossRef] [PubMed]
15. Covas, M.I.; Nyyssönen, K.; Poulsen, H.E.; Kaikkonen, J.; Zunft, H.J.; Kiesewetter, H.; Gaddi, A.; de la Torre, R.; Mursu, J.; Bäumler, H.; et al. The effect of polyphenols in olive oil on heart disease risk factors: A randomized trial. *Ann. Intern. Med.* **2006**, *145*, 333–341. [CrossRef] [PubMed]

16. Camargo, A.; Ruano, J.; Fernandez, J.M.; Parnell, L.D.; Jimenez, A.; Santos-Gonzalez, M.; Marin, C.; Perez-Martinez, P.; Uceda, M.; Lopez-Miranda, J.; et al. Gene expression changes in mononuclear cells in patients with metabolic syndrome after acute intake of phenol-rich virgin olive oil. *BMC Genomics* **2010**, *11*, 253. [CrossRef] [PubMed]
17. de Bock, M.; Derraik, J.G.; Brennan, C.M.; Biggs, J.B.; Morgan, P.E.; Hodgkinson, S.C.; Hofman, P.L.; Cutfield, W.S. Olive (Olea europaea L.) leaf polyphenols improve insulin sensitivity in middle-aged overweight men: a randomized, placebo-controlled, crossover trial. *PLoS ONE* **2013**, *8*, e57622. [CrossRef] [PubMed]
18. Medina-Remón, A.; Tresserra-Rimbau, A.; Pons, A.; Tur, J.A.; Martorell, M.; Ros, E.; Buil-Cosiales, P.; Sacanella, E.; Covas, M.I.; Corella, D.; et al. Effects of total dietary polyphenols on plasma nitric oxide and blood pressure in a high cardiovascular risk cohort. The PREDIMED randomized trial. *Nutr. Metab. Cardiovasc. Dis.* **2015**, *25*, 60–67. [CrossRef] [PubMed]
19. Malik, N.S.; Bradford, J.M. Changes in oleuropein levels during differentiation and development of floral buds in 'Arbequina'olives. *Sci. Horticult.* **2006**, *110*, 274–278. [CrossRef]
20. Manna, C.; D'Angelo, S.; Migliardi, V.; Loffredi, E.; Mazzoni, O.; Morrica, P.; Galletti, P.; Zappia, V. Protective effect of the phenolic fraction from virgin olive oils against oxidative stress in human cells. *J. Agric. Food Chem.* **2002**, *50*, 6521–6526. [CrossRef]
21. Visioli, F.; Bellosta, S.; Galli, C. Oleuropein, the bitter principle of olives, enhances nitric oxide production by mouse macrophages. *Life Sci.* **1998**, *62*, 541–546. [CrossRef]
22. Carluccio, M.A.; Siculella, L.; Ancora, M.A.; Massaro, M.; Scoditti, E.; Storelli, C.; Visioli, F.; Distante, A.; de Caterina, R. Olive oil and red wine antioxidant polyphenols inhibit endothelial activation. *Arterioscler. Thromb. Vasc. Biol.* **2003**, *23*, 622–629. [CrossRef] [PubMed]
23. Edgecombe, S.C.; Stretch, G.L.; Hayball, P.J. Oleuropein, an antioxidant polyphenol from olive oil, is poorly absorbed from isolated perfused rat intestine. *J. Nutr.* **2000**, *130*, 2996–3002. [CrossRef] [PubMed]
24. Carrasco-Pancorbo, A.; Cerretani, L.; Bendini, A.; Segura-Carretero, A.; Del Carlo, M.; Gallina-Toschi, T.; Lercker, G.; Compagnone, D.; Fernández-Gutiérrez, A. Evaluation of the antioxidant capacity of individual phenolic compounds in virgin olive oil. *J. Agric. Food Chem.* **2005**, *53*, 8918–8925. [CrossRef] [PubMed]
25. Uttara, B.; Singh, A.V.; Zamboni, P.; Mahajan, R.T. Oxidative stress and neurodegenerative diseases: A review of upstream and downstream antioxidant therapeutic options. *Curr. Neuropharmacol.* **2009**, *7*, 65–74. [CrossRef] [PubMed]
26. Halliwell, B.; Whiteman, M. Measuring reactive species and oxidative damage in vivo and in cell culture: How should you do it and what do the results mean? *Br. J. Pharmacol.* **2004**, *142*, 231–255. [CrossRef] [PubMed]
27. Fridovich, I. Fundamental aspects of reactive oxygen species, or what's the matter with oxygen? *Ann. N. Y. Acad. Sci.* **1999**, *893*, 13–18. [CrossRef] [PubMed]
28. Fang, Y.Z.; Yang, S.; Wu, G. Free radicals, antioxidants, and nutrition. *Nutrition* **2002**, *18*, 872–879. [CrossRef]
29. Matsuda, M.; Shimomura, I. Increased oxidative stress in obesity: Implications for metabolic syndrome, diabetes, hypertension, dyslipidemia, atherosclerosis, and cancer. *Obes. Res. Clin. Pract.* **2013**, *7*, e330–e341. [CrossRef] [PubMed]
30. Praticò, D.; Lee, V.M.Y.; Trojanoswki, J.Q.; Rokach, J.; FitzGerald, G.A. Increased F2-isoprostanes in Alzheimer's disease: evidence for enhanced lipid peroxidation in vivo. *FASEB J.* **1998**, *12*, 1777–1783. [CrossRef]
31. Mateos, R.; Madrona, A.; Pereira-Caro, G.; Domínguez, V.; Cert, R.M.; Parrado, J.; Sarriá, B.; Bravo, L.; Espartero, J.L. Synthesis and antioxidant evaluation of isochroman-derivatives of hydroxytyrosol: Structure-activity relationship. *Food Chem.* **2015**, *173*, 313–320. [CrossRef]
32. Jemai, H.; El Feki, A.; Sayadi, S. Antidiabetic and antioxidant effects of hydroxytyrosol and oleuropein from olive leaves in alloxan-diabetic rats. *J. Agric. Food Chem.* **2009**, *57*, 8798–8804. [CrossRef] [PubMed]
33. Salami, M.; Galli, C.; De Angelis, L.; Visioli, F. Formation of F2-isoprostanes in oxidized low density lipoprotein: inhibitory effect of hydroxytyrosol. *Pharmacol. Res.* **1995**, *31*, 275–279. [CrossRef]
34. Petroni, A.; Blasevich, M.; Salami, M.; Papini, N.; Montedoro, G.F.; Galli, C. Inhibition of platelet aggregation and eicosanoid production by phenolic components of olive oil. *Thromb. Res.* **1995**, *78*, 151–160. [CrossRef]

35. Kohyama, N.; Nagata, T.; Fujimoto, S.; Sekiya, K. Inhibition of arachidonate lipoxygenase activities by 2-(3,4-dihydroxyphenyl)ethanol, a phenolic compound from olives. *Biosci. Biotechnol. Biochem.* **1997**, *61*, 347–350. [CrossRef] [PubMed]
36. Speroni, E.; Guerra, M.C.; Minghetti, A.; Crespi-Perellino, N.; Pasini, P.; Piazza, F.; Roda, A. Oleuropein evaluated in vitro and in vivo as an antioxidant. *Phytother. Res.* **1998**, *12*, 98–100. [CrossRef]
37. Manna, S.; Bhattacharyya, D.; Basak, D.K.; Mandal, T.K. Single oral dose toxicity study of a-cypermethrin in rats. *Indian J. Pharmacol.* **2004**, *36*, 25–28.
38. Nagarjun, S.; Dhadde, S.B.; Veerapur, V.P.; Thippeswamy, B.S.; Chandakavathe, B.N. Ameliorative effect of chromium-d-phenylalanine complex on indomethacin-induced inflammatory bowel disease in rats. *Biomed. Pharmacother.* **2017**, *89*, 1061–1066. [CrossRef] [PubMed]
39. Kannan, N.; Guruvayoorappan, C. Protective effect of Bauhinia tomentosa on acetic acid induced ulcerative colitis by regulating antioxidant and inflammatory mediators. *Int. Immunopharmacol.* **2013**, *16*, 57–66. [CrossRef]
40. Cabrerizo, S.; De La Cruz, J.P.; López-Villodres, J.A.; Muñoz-Marín, J.; Guerrero, A.; Reyes, J.J.; Labajos, M.T.; González-Correa, J.A. Role of the inhibition of oxidative stress and inflammatory mediators in the neuroprotective effects of hydroxytyrosol in rat brain slices subjected to hypoxia reoxygenation. *J. Nutr. Biochem.* **2013**, *24*, 2152–2157. [CrossRef] [PubMed]
41. Lee, J.D.; Kato, K.; Tobias, P.S.; Kirkland, T.N.; Ulevitch, R.J. Transfection of CD14 into 70Z/3 cells dramatically enhances the sensitivity to complexes of lipopolysaccharide (LPS) and LPS binding protein. *J. Exp. Med.* **1992**, *175*, 1697–1705. [CrossRef] [PubMed]
42. Yun, K.J.; Kim, J.Y.; Kim, J.B.; Lee, K.W.; Jeong, S.Y.; Park, H.J.; Jung, H.J.; Cho, Y.W.; Yun, K.; Lee, K.T. Inhibition of LPS-induced NO and PGE2 production by asiatic acid via NF-kappa B inactivation in RAW 264.7 macrophages: possible involvement of the IKK and MAPK pathways. *Int. Immunopharmacol.* **2008**, *8*, 431–441. [CrossRef] [PubMed]
43. Subbaramaiah, K.; Dannenberg, A.J. Cyclooxygenase 2: A molecular target for cancer prevention and treatment. *Trends Pharmacol. Sci.* **2003**, *24*, 96–102. [CrossRef]
44. Salvemini, D.; Ischiropoulos, H.; Cuzzocrea, S. Roles of nitric oxide and superoxide in inflammation. *Methods Mol. Biol.* **2003**, *225*, 291–303. [PubMed]
45. Denlinger, L.C.; Fisette, P.L.; Garis, K.A.; Kwon, G.; Vazquez-Torres, A.; Simon, A.D.; Nguyen, B.; Proctor, R.A.; Bertics, P.J.; Corbett, J.A. Regulation of inducible nitric oxide synthase expression by macrophage purinoreceptors and calcium. *J. Biol. Chem.* **1996**, *271*, 337–342. [CrossRef] [PubMed]
46. Weisz, A.; Cicatiello, L.; Esumi, H. Regulation of the mouse inducible-type nitric oxide synthase gene promoter by interferon-gamma, bacterial lipopolysaccharide and NG-monomethyl-L-arginine. *Biochem. J.* **1996**, *316*, 209–215. [CrossRef] [PubMed]
47. Yonezawa, Y.; Miyashita, T.; Nejishima, H.; Takeda, Y.; Imai, K.; Ogawa, H. Anti-inflammatory effects of olive-derived hydroxytyrosol on lipopolysaccharide-induced inflammation in RAW264.7 cells. *J. Vet. Med. Sci.* **2018**, *80*, 1801–1807. [CrossRef] [PubMed]
48. Lamy, S.; Ben Saad, A.; Zgheib, A.; Annabi, B. Olive oil compounds inhibit the paracrine regulation of TNF-α-induced endothelial cell migration through reduced glioblastoma cell cyclooxygenase-2 expression. *J. Nutr. Biochem.* **2016**, *27*, 136–145. [CrossRef]
49. Mao, X.; Xia, B.; Zheng, M.; Zhou, Z. Assessment of the anti-inflammatory, analgesic and sedative effects of oleuropein from Olea europaea L. *Cell. Mol. Biol. (Noisy-le-grand)* **2019**, *65*, 52–55. [CrossRef]
50. Takeda, Y.; Bui, V.N.; Iwasaki, K.; Kobayashi, T.; Ogawa, H.; Imai, K. Influence of olive-derived hydroxytyrosol on the toll-like receptor 4-dependent inflammatory response of mouse peritoneal macrophages. *Biochem. Biophys. Res. Commun.* **2014**, *446*, 1225–1230. [CrossRef]
51. Maiuri, M.C.; De Stefano, D.; Di Meglio, P.; Irace, C.; Savarese, M.; Sacchi, R.; Cinelli, M.P.; Carnuccio, R. Hydroxytyrosol, a phenolic compound from virgin olive oil, prevents macrophage activation. *Naunyn Schmiedebergs Arch. Pharmacol.* **2005**, *371*, 457–465. [CrossRef]
52. Zhang, X.; Cao, J.; Jiang, L.; Zhong, L. Suppressive effects of hydroxytyrosol on oxidative stress and nuclear Factor-kappaB activation in THP-1 cells. *Biol. Pharm. Bull.* **2009**, *32*, 578–582. [CrossRef] [PubMed]

53. Ferrante, C.; Recinella, L.; Locatelli, M.; Guglielmi, P.; Secci, D.; Leporini, L.; Chiavaroli, A.; Leone, S.; Martinotti, S.; Brunetti, L.; et al. Protective Effects Induced by Microwave-Assisted Aqueous Harpagophytum Extract on Rat Cortex Synaptosomes Challenged with Amyloid β-Peptide. *Phytother Res.* **2017**, *31*, 1257–1264. [CrossRef] [PubMed]
54. Chiavaroli, A.; Recinella, L.; Ferrante, C.; Locatelli, M.; Carradori, S.; Macchione, N.; Zengin, G.; Leporini, L.; Leone, S.; Martinotti, S.; et al. Crocus sativus, Serenoa repens and Pinus massoniana extracts modulate inflammatory response in isolated rat prostate challenged with LPS. *J. Biol. Regul. Homeost. Agents* **2017**, *31*, 531–541.
55. Menghini, L.; Leporini, L.; Vecchiotti, G.; Locatelli, M.; Carradori, S.; Ferrante, C.; Zengin, G.; Recinella, L.; Chiavaroli, A.; Leone, S.; et al. stigmas and byproducts: Qualitative fingerprint, antioxidant potentials and enzyme inhibitory activities. *Food Res. Int.* **2018**, *109*, 91–98. [CrossRef]
56. Ferrante, C.; Orlando, G.; Recinella, L.; Leone, S.; Chiavaroli, A.; Di Nisio, C.; Shohreh, R.; Manippa, F.; Ricciuti, A.; Vacca, M.; et al. Central apelin-13 administration modulates hypothalamic control of feeding. *J. Biol. Regul. Homeost. Agents* **2016**, *30*, 883–888. [PubMed]
57. Leone, S.; Chiavaroli, A.; Shohreh, R.; Ferrante, C.; Ricciuti, A.; Manippa, F.; Recinella, L.; Di Nisio, C.; Orlando, G.; Salvatori, R.; et al. Increased locomotor and thermogenic activity in mice with targeted ablation of the GHRH gene. *Growth Horm. IGF Res.* **2015**, *25*, 80–84. [CrossRef] [PubMed]
58. Livak, K.J.; Schmittgen, T.D. Analysis of relative gene expression data using real-time quantitative PCR and the 2(-Delta Delta C(T)). *Methods* **2001**, *25*, 402–408. [CrossRef]
59. Charan, J.; Kantharia, N.D. How to calculate sample size in animal studies? *J. Pharmacol. Pharmacother.* **2013**, *4*, 303–306. [CrossRef]
60. Recinella, L.; Leone, S.; Ferrante, C.; Chiavaroli, A.; Shohreh, R.; Di Nisio, C.; Vacca, M.; Orlando, G.; Salvatori, R.; Brunetti, L. Effects of growth hormone-releasing hormone gene targeted ablation on ghrelin-induced feeding. *Growth Horm. IGF Res.* **2017**, *37*, 40–46. [CrossRef]

Sample Availability: Samples of the compounds are not available from the authors.

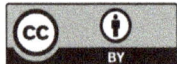

© 2019 by the authors. Licensee MDPI, Basel, Switzerland. This article is an open access article distributed under the terms and conditions of the Creative Commons Attribution (CC BY) license (http://creativecommons.org/licenses/by/4.0/).

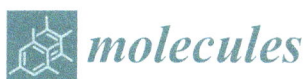

Article

Inhibitory Effects of *Aucklandia lappa* Decne. Extract on Inflammatory and Oxidative Responses in LPS-Treated Macrophages

Jae Sung Lim [1,2,†], Sung Ho Lee [3,†], Sang Rok Lee [4], Hyung-Ju Lim [2,5], Yoon-Seok Roh [6], Eun Jeong Won [7], Namki Cho [8], Changju Chun [8,*] and Young-Chang Cho [8,*]

1. Department of Biochemistry, Chonnam National University Medical School, Hwasun, Jeonnam-do 58128, Korea; dr.jslim7542@gmail.com
2. Combinatorial Tumor Immunotherapy Medical Research Center, Chonnam National University Medical School, Hwasun, Jeonnam-do 58128, Korea; akira0128@naver.com
3. Department of Molecular and Cellular Biology, Baylor College of Medicine, Houston, TX 77030, USA; puzim23@gmail.com
4. ROK-Biotech, Jeollanamdo Biopharmaceutical Research Center, Hwasun, Jeollanam-do 58141, Korea; rok94@hanmail.net
5. Department of Microbiology, Chonnam National University Medical School, Hwasun, Jeonnam-do 58128, Korea
6. College of Pharmacy and Medical Research Center, Chungbuk National University, Cheongju 28160, Korea; ysroh@cbnu.ac.kr
7. Department of Parasitology and Tropical Medicine, Chonnam National University Medical School, Hwasun, Jeonnam-do 58128, Korea; Parasite.woni@jnu.ac.kr
8. College of Pharmacy, Chonnam National University, Gwangju 61186, Korea; cnamki@jnu.ac.kr
* Correspondence: cchun1130@jnu.ac.kr (C.C.); yccho@jnu.ac.kr (Y.-C.C.); Tel.: +82-62-530-2944 (C.C.); +82-62-530-2925 (Y.-C.C.)
† These authors contributed equally to this paper.

Academic Editors: Raffaele Capasso and Lorenzo Di Cesare Mannelli
Received: 22 February 2020; Accepted: 13 March 2020; Published: 15 March 2020

Abstract: *Aucklandia lappa* Decne., known as "Mok-hyang" in Korea, has been used for the alleviation of abdominal pain, vomiting, diarrhea, and stress gastric ulcers in traditional oriental medicine. We investigated the anti-inflammatory and antioxidative effects of the ethanol extract of *Aucklandia lappa* Decne. (ALDE) in lipopolysaccharide (LPS)-stimulated RAW 264.7 cells. ALDE significantly inhibited the LPS-induced nitric oxide (NO) production and reduced inducible nitric oxide synthase (iNOS) expression in RAW 264.7 cells. The production of other proinflammatory mediators, including COX-2, interleukin (IL)-6, IL-1β, and tumor necrosis factor (TNF)-α, was reduced by ALDE in LPS-stimulated RAW 264.7 cells. The mechanism underlying the anti-inflammatory effects of ALDE was elucidated to be the suppression of LPS-induced nuclear translocation of p65, followed by the degradation of IκB and the inhibition of the phosphorylation of mitogen-activated protein kinases (MAPK). In addition, ALDE showed enhanced radical scavenging activity. The antioxidant effect of ALDE was caused by the enhanced expression of heme oxygenase (HO-1) via stabilization of the expression of the nuclear transcription factor E2-related factor 2 (Nrf2) pathway. Collectively, these results indicated that ALDE not only exerts anti-inflammatory effects via the suppression of the NF-κB and MAPK pathways but also has an antioxidative effect through the activation of the Nrf2/HO-1 pathway.

Keywords: *Aucklandia lappa* Decne. extract; lipopolysaccharide; nitric oxide; inducible nitric oxide; cyclooxygenase-2; nuclear factor-κB; mitogen-activated protein kinase; heme oxygenase-1; macrophage

1. Introduction

Inflammation is a central feature of various pathological conditions in the host defense against pathogens and in response to tissue injury. Macrophages are activated in response to various stimuli, such as LPS, and induce inflammation by producing inflammatory mediators, including nitric oxide (NO), prostaglandins (PGs), and proinflammatory cytokines, such as interleukin (IL)-1β, IL-6, and tumor necrosis factor (TNF)-α [1]. Although inflammation is important for the host defense against external stimuli, excess inflammation leads to severe immune disorders, such as septic shock, rheumatoid arthritis (RA), systemic lupus erythematosus (SLE), and inflammatory bowel disease (IBD) [2,3]. Thus, an agent that is able to alleviate the excessive inflammatory response may be a suitable candidate for the treatment of inflammatory disorders. Although a variety of anti-inflammatory drugs have been developed, including steroidal drugs and nonsteroidal anti-inflammatory drugs (NSAIDs), owing to the severe adverse effects of these drugs, natural products and their constituent compounds have been investigated for the development of new anti-inflammatory drugs.

Aucklandia lappa Decne., referred to as "Mok-hyang" in the 11th edition of the Korean Pharmacopoeia (KP11), is the root of Saussurea (Aucklandia) lappa Clarke (Chrysanthemum, Compositae). It contains approximately 1–2.5% of refined oils and has an abundance of sesquiterpenoid compounds (such as costunolide), which have many pharmacological effects, such as antibacterial [4] and anti-inflammatory [5] activity and an anti-inhibitory effect on vascular production [6]. Traditionally, "Mok-hyang" has been used for the treatment of vomiting, gastric pain, abdominal pain, anorexia, distension, and nausea [7]. Previously, it was reported that Aucklandia lappa Decne. has anti-ulcer [8], antiviral [9], and anticancer [10] effects. In addition, it has been reported that Aucklandia lappa Decne. extract (ALDE) inhibited inflammatory chemokine production in HaCaT cells [11] and exhibited anti-inflammatory effects in RAW 264.7 cells [12]. Thus, although the anti-inflammatory activity of ALDE has been reported, the mechanisms underlying these anti-inflammatory effects are not well elucidated. Herein, we investigated the anti-inflammatory and antioxidative effects of ALDE in LPS-stimulated macrophages and evaluated the associated molecular mechanism in vitro.

2. Materials and Methods

2.1. Extraction of ALDE

Aucklandia lappa Decne. was purchased from the Jeonnam Herb Medicine and Agriculture Cooperative (Hwasun, South Korea). Briefly, air-dried powdered (<0.2 mm) *Aucklandia lappa* Decne. (100 g) was extracted with 70% ethanol at approximately 70 °C for 9 h. The resultant ethanolic solution was filtered, evaporated, and freeze-dried to generate ALDE.

2.2. HPLC Chromatographic Analysis

Chromatographic analysis was performed on a reverse-phase Shimadzu HPLC system (Shimadzu Corp., Kyoto, Japan) with a Shimadzu LC-20AR solvent pump, coupled to a SPD-20A UV/VIS detector. Separation was performed on a Phenomenex C_{18} reverse-phase column (4.6 × 150 mm, 5 μm) using a gradient solvent system comprising acetonitrile (A) and water (B), with a composition by volume of 10% A at 0 min and 50% A at 40 min. The flow rate was 2 mL/min; the reaction was monitored spectrophotometrically at 254 nm.

2.3. Cell Culture

RAW 264.7 cells (ATCC, Manassas, VA, USA), a mouse monocytic cell line, were maintained in Dulbecco's modified Eagle's medium supplemented with 10% fetal bovine serum (both from GE Healthcare Bio-Sciences, Pittsburgh, PA, USA), 50 U/mL penicillin, and 50 μg/mL streptomycin (Gibco; Thermo Fisher Scientific, Inc., Waltham, MA, USA) at 37 °C in humidified air containing 5% CO_2.

2.4. Cell Viability Assay

RAW 264.7 cells (4×10^4/well) were plated in 96-well plates. The cells were treated with various concentrations (1, 3, 5, 7, 9, 11, and 13 µg/mL) of ALDE for 24 h. Following treatment, cell viability was measured using an EZ-Cytox Cell Viability Assay kit (Daeil Lab Services Co., Ltd., Seoul, Korea). Briefly, the cells were incubated with the EZ-Cytox solution (containing a water-soluble tetrazolium salt) for 2 h at 37 °C. The absorbance of the supernatant at 450 nm was measured using a Synergy H1 Microplate Reader (BioTek Instruments, Inc., Winooski, VT, USA).

2.5. Measurement of NO Production

RAW 264.7 cells (4.0×10^4 cells/well) were plated in 96-well plates. The cells were pretreated with various concentrations of ALDE (1, 2.5, 5, and 10 µg/mL) for 2 h and subsequently stimulated by LPS (0.5 µg/mL) for 24 h. The cell supernatants (100 µL) were transferred to new 96-well plates, and 100 µL Griess reagent (1% sulfanilamide, 0.1% N-1-naphthylethylenediamine dihydrochloride, and 2.5% phosphoric acid) was added. $NaNO_2$ solutions (2.5, 5, 10, 25, 50, and 100 M) were used to generate a standard curve to calculate the concentration of NO in the supernatant. The absorbance at 540 nm was measured using a Synergy H1 Microplate reader (BioTek Instruments, Winooski, VT, USA).

2.6. RNA Preparation and cDNA Synthesis

RAW 264.7 cells (8.0×10^5 cells/well) were seeded in 12-well plates. The cells were pretreated with various concentrations of ALDE (1, 2.5, 5, and 10 µg/mL) for 2 h and then stimulated with LPS (0.5 µg/mL) for 3 h. Total RNA was extracted using Accuzol (Bioneer Corporation, Daejeon, Korea) and synthesized into cDNA using a TOPscript cDNA synthesis kit in accordance with the manufacturer's instructions.

2.7. Semiquantitative Reverse Transcription (RT)-PCR

The mixture for PCR was subjected to the following thermal profile: 17–25 cycles at 94 °C for 30 s, 60 °C for 30 s, and 72 °C for 30 s using a Bioer thermal cycler (Bioer Technology Co., Hangzhou, China). Following amplification, the PCR products (10 µL) were separated on a 1.5% (w/v) agarose gel and stained with ethidium bromide. The following primers were used: Mouse iNOS (sense, 5'-GCA TGGAACAGTATAAGGCAAACA-3'; antisense, 5'-GTTTCTGGTCGATGTCATGAGCAA-3'), COX-2 (sense, 5'-GCATGGAACAGTATAAGGCAAACA-3'; antisense, 5'-GTTTCTGGT CGATGTCATGAGCAA-3'), TNF-α (sense, 5'-GTGCCAGCCGATGGGTTGTACC-3'; antisense, 5-'AGGCCCACAGTCCAGGTCACTG-3'), IL-6 (sense, 5'-TCTTGGGACTGATG CTGGTGAC-3'; antisense, 5'-CATAACGCACTAGGTTTGCCGA-3'), IL-1β (sense, 5'-AGC TGTGGCAGCTACCTGTG-3'; antisense, 5'-GCTCTGCTTGTGAGGTGCTG-3'), and GAPDH (sense, 5'-GTCTTCACCACCATGGAGAAGG-3'; antisense, 5'-CCTGCTTCACCA CCTTCTTGCC-3').

2.8. Western Blotting

The whole-cell lysate was prepared by incubating the cells in a RIPA buffer (50 mM Tris-HCl pH 8.0, 150 mM NaCl, 0.1% SDS, 0.5% deoxycholate, 1% NP-40, and 1 mM EDTA) with protease inhibitors (XXX) for 30 min at 4 °C followed by centrifugation (13,200 rpm for 15 min). The supernatant was denatured in 5× SDS sample buffer (200 mM Tris-HCl pH 6.8, 40% glycerol, 8% SDS, 200 mM dithiothreitol, and 0.08% bromophenol blue) at 95 °C for 5 min, separated by SDS-PAGE, and then transferred to nitrocellulose membranes. To block nonspecific binding, we incubated the membranes in 5% nonfat dry milk in Tris-buffered saline and Tween-20 (25 mM Tris-HCl pH 8.0, 125 mM NaCl, and 0.5% Tween-20) for 1 h at RT. The membranes were incubated with primary antibodies at 4 °C overnight and then incubated with horseradish peroxidase-conjugated (HRP)-conjugated secondary antibodies for 1 h at RT. Pierce ECL Western blotting substrate for enhanced chemiluminescence (Thermo Fisher Scientific, Inc.) was used to detect the HRP-conjugated secondary antibodies. Protein expression was analyzed and quantified using LabWorks software version 4.6 (UVP, LLC; Analytik Jena AG, Upland, CA, USA).

2.9. ELISA

RAW 264.7 cells (4.0×10^4 cells/well) were plated in 96-well plates. The cells were pretreated with various concentrations of ALDE (1, 2.5, 5, and 10 µg/mL) for 2 h and then stimulated with LPS (0.5 µg/mL) for 24 h. The expression of the indicated cytokines in the cell supernatant was measured using an ELISA kit in accordance with the manufacturer's instructions. Briefly, the culture plates were incubated overnight with a coating solution at 4 °C, washed three times with 1× PBS/0.05% Tween-20 (PBST), and then incubated with 1× assay diluent (from the ELISA kit) for 1 h at RT. The supernatants and standard solutions were incubated for 2 h at RT and then washed three times. Next, the plate was incubated with Ab Detection solution (also from the ELISA kit) for 1 h at RT and then washed three times. Subsequently, the plate was incubated with a horseradish peroxidase-streptavidin solution for 30 min at RT and then washed five times. Finally, the plate was incubated with a solution of 3,3′,5,5′-tetramethylbenzidine for 10 min in the dark; then, 1 N H_3PO_4 was added to stop the reaction. The absorbance at 450 nm was measured spectrophotometrically using a Synergy H1 Microplate reader.

2.10. Subcellular Fractionation

Subcellular fractionation was performed as described previously [13]. Briefly, the cells were washed twice with ice-cold PBS and lysed with 200 µL of cytoplasmic lysis buffer (10 mM HEPES, 60 mM KCl, 1 mM EDTA, 1 mM DTT, and 1 mM PMSF) on ice for 15 min; subsequently, 10 µL of 0.075% (v/v) IGEPAL CA-630 (Sigma-Aldrich, St. Louis, MO, USA) was added. After brief centrifugation (10 s), the supernatants were collected for the cytoplasmic fraction. Next, the pellet was resuspended in 25 µL of a nuclear extraction buffer (20 mM Tris Cl, 420 mM NaCl, 1.5 mM $MgCl_2$, 0.2 mM EDTA, 1 mM PMSF, and 25% (v/v) glycerol) on ice for 30 min and vortex mixed every 10 min. After centrifugation for 30 min at 4 °C, the supernatant was collected to obtain the nuclear fraction. Western blotting was performed using anti-α-tubulin (cytoplasm) and anti-lamin B1 (nucleus) antibodies to confirm the cytoplasmic and nuclear extracts, respectively.

2.11. DPPH Free Radical Scavenge Activity

ALDE ethanolic solution was mixed with the same volume of 0.4 mM DPPH ethanolic solution. The mixture was allowed to react at RT in the dark for 10 min. The absorbance at 517 nm was measured using a Synergy H1 Microplate reader. The free radical scavenging activity was calculated as a percentage using the following equation [14].

DPPH free radical scavenging activity (%) = $[1 - (A_{sample}/A_{blank})] \times 100$.

2.12. Statistical Analysis

The data are presented as the mean ± standard error of the mean. Multiple experimental groups were compared by one-way analysis of variance followed by Dunnett's post-hoc test calculated using GraphPad Prism (version 3.0; GraphPad Software, Inc., La Jolla, CA, USA); p-values < 0.05 were considered statistically significant.

3. Results

3.1. HPLC and Costunolide-Related Results

Before the investigation of the effects of ALDE on inflammation and oxidative stress, an evaluation of the major components that exhibit anti-inflammatory and antioxidative effects was required. Costunolide, a component of ALDE, has been known to inhibit the production of inflammatory mediators and enhance HO-1 expression [15]. HPLC analysis was performed to show that ALDE and costunolide exhibited the same retention time. As shown in Figure 1a,b, HPLC analysis of costunolide showed a single peak at 40.507 min. One of the major peaks of the ALDE HPLC data (40.587 and 41.626 min) has the same retention time as costunolide. As previously reported, costunolide inhibited LPS-induced NO production in RAW 264.7 cells and exhibited significant radical scavenging activity compared with BHA, a positive control (Figure 1c,d). These results indicated that costunolide was a major component of ALDE and led us to study the anti-inflammatory effects and underlying regulatory mechanism of action of ALDE in murine macrophages.

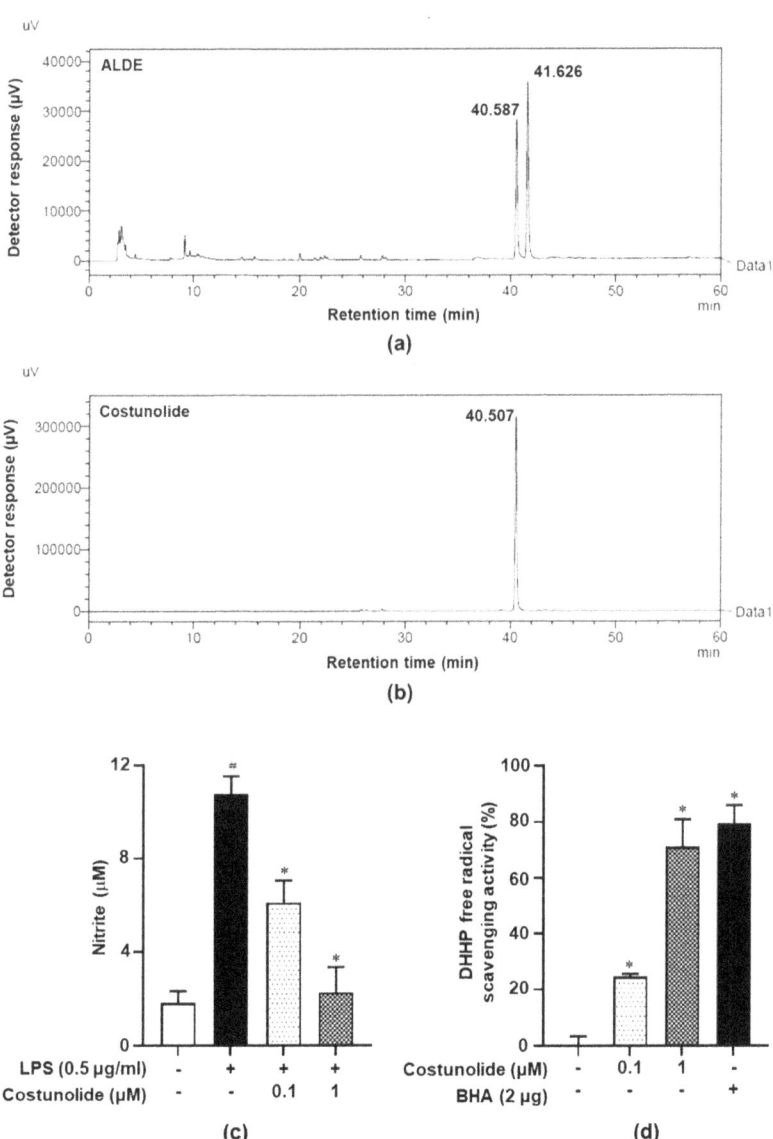

Figure 1. HPLC analysis of the ethanol extract of *Aucklandia lappa* Decne. (ALDE) and costunolide. The phytochemical characteristics of (a) ALDE and its major component, (b) costunolide, were analyzed using HPLC. (c,d) NO inhibitory effect of costunolide. Data represent the mean ± SEM of three independent experiments. $^{\#} p < 0.05$ vs. LPS-untreated control group; $* p < 0.05$ vs. LPS-treated group.

(**d**) DPPH radical scavenging activity of costunolide. Data represent the mean ± SEM of three independent experiments. * $p < 0.05$ vs. untreated group. ALDE: Ethanol extract of *Aucklandia lappa* Decne.; LPS: Lipopolysaccharide; NO: Nitric oxide.

3.2. ALDE Suppressed the Release of NO in LPS-Stimulated RAW 264.7 Cells

To investigate the effect of ALDE on the viability of RAW 264.7 cells, we treated the cells with the indicated concentrations of ALDE for 24 h and then quantified the metabolic conversion of a tetrazolium salt to a formazan dye to determine the percentage of viable cells. ALDE exerted no significant cytotoxicity in RAW 264.7 cells at concentrations below 13 µg/mL (Figure 2a). Therefore, subsequent experiments were performed at ALDE concentrations of 1, 2.5, 5, and 10 µg/mL, which were known to not exert cytotoxic effects. To investigate the anti-inflammatory effects of ALDE, we examined the effect of ALDE on the production of NO, a well-known proinflammatory mediator, in LPS-stimulated RAW 264.7 cells. The nitrite level in the culture medium of the RAW 264.7 cells was significantly increased upon LPS treatment. However, in the cells pretreated with ALDE, a considerable dose-dependent suppression of LPS-induced NO production was observed (Figure 2b). These results suggested that ALDE markedly reduced the NO production in LPS-stimulated RAW 264.7 cells.

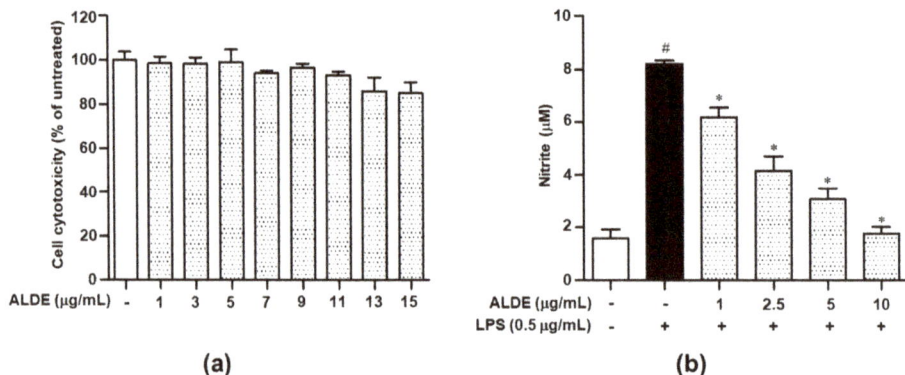

Figure 2. Effects of ALDE on cell viability and NO production in RAW 264.7 cells. (**a**) RAW 264.7 cells were treated with various concentrations of ALDE for 24 h. Subsequently, cell viability was measured using the EZ-Cytox reagent and compared with that in the untreated group. (**b**) RAW 264.7 cells were treated with LPS (0.5 µg/mL) in the presence of ALDE (1, 2.5, 5, and 10 µg/mL) for 24 h. Subsequently, NO production in the culture supernatant was measured using a Griess assay. NO secretion was calculated using a standard curve of concentrations of nitrite standard solution. The data presented are the mean ± SEM of three independent experiments. Differences between groups were analyzed using the Mann–Whitney *U* test. # $p < 0.05$ vs. LPS-untreated control groups; * $p < 0.05$ vs. LPS-treated groups. ALDE: Ethanol extract of *Aucklandia lappa* Decne.; LPS: Lipopolysaccharide; NO: Nitric oxide.

3.3. ALDE Inhibited the Expression of Proinflammatory Enzymes, iNOS and COX-2, in LPS-Stimulated RAW 264.7 Cells

The expression of proinflammatory enzymes, including COX-2 and iNOS, plays an important role in the immune response from activated macrophages through the production of NO and PGE2, respectively [16,17]. We investigated the effect of ALDE on the expression of iNOS and COX-2 in LPS-stimulated RAW 264.7 cells. As shown in Figure 3, the expression of iNOS and COX-2 was increased markedly in response to LPS treatment. When RAW 264.7 cells were treated with various concentrations of ALDE, the LPS-induced expression of iNOS and COX-2 was significantly decreased in a dose-dependent manner (Figure 3a,b). These results indicated that ALDE inhibited the production of proinflammatory mediators through the inhibition of the expression of their responsible enzymes, iNOS and COX-2.

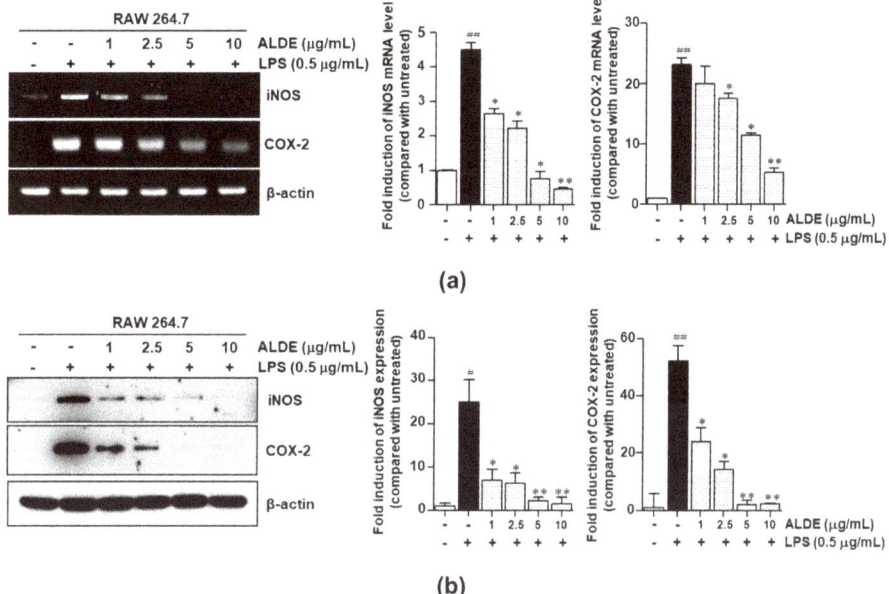

Figure 3. Effects of ALDE on the expression of iNOS and COX-2. RAW 264.7 cells were treated simultaneously with LPS and ALDE (1, 2.5, 5, and 10 μg/mL). (**a**) Following stimulation for 6 h, total RNA was extracted and reverse transcribed to cDNA. mRNA expression of *iNOS* and *COX-2* was analyzed by RT-PCR. (**b**) After stimulation for 24 h, the total protein was extracted. The protein expression of iNOS and COX-2 was detected by Western blotting. The protein β-actin was used as a loading control for both RT-PCR and Western blotting. The relative density of the mRNA or protein expression was normalized to that of β-actin and is presented in quantitative graphs. The data presented are the mean ± SEM of three independent experiments. Differences between groups were analyzed using the Mann–Whitney U test. $^{\#}\, p < 0.05$, $^{\#\#}\, p < 0.01$ vs. LPS-untreated control groups; $*\, p < 0.05$, $**\, p < 0.01$ vs. LPS-treated groups. COX-2: Cyclooxygenase-2; iNOS: Inducible nitric oxide synthase.

3.4. ALDE Inhibited the Production of Proinflammatory Cytokines in LPS-Stimulated Macrophages

To investigate whether ALDE affected the expression of proinflammatory cytokines, we performed Western blotting analysis and RT-PCR. The expression of IL-6, IL-1β, and TNF-α was significantly increased after treatment with LPS but markedly decreased in a dose-dependent manner after pretreatment with ALDE (Figure 4a,b). To confirm the inhibitory effect of ALDE on the cytokine production induced by LPS stimulation, we used ELISA. As shown in Figure 4c–e, LPS-stimulated RAW 264.7 cells treated with ALDE exhibited concentration-dependent inhibition of the proinflammatory cytokines, such as TNF-α, IL-6, and IL-1β. These results suggested that ALDE exerted anti-inflammatory effects through the inhibition of proinflammatory cytokines.

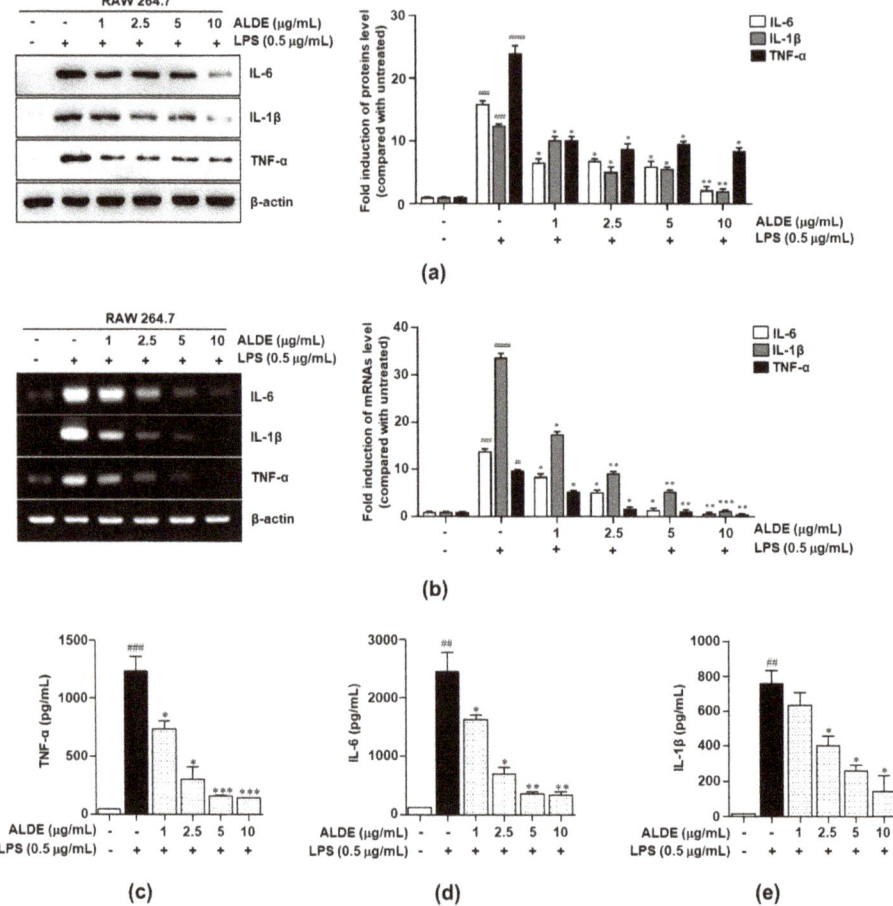

Figure 4. Inhibitory effects of ALDE on the production of proinflammatory cytokines. RAW 264.7 cells were treated with LPS in the presence of ALDE (1, 2.5, 5, and 10 µg/mL). (**a**) After stimulation for 24 h, the total cellular proteins were extracted. The expression of interleukin (IL)-6, IL-1β, and tumor necrosis factor (TNF)-α was detected by Western blotting. (**b**) After simulation for 6 h, total RNA was extracted. The mRNA expression of IL-6, IL-1β, and TNF-α was analyzed by RT-PCR. β-Actin was used as a loading control for both RT-PCR and Western blotting. The relative density of the mRNA or protein expression was normalized to that of β-actin and is presented in quantitative graphs. (**c–e**) After stimulation for 24 h, the culture supernatants were collected and analyzed for IL-6, IL-1β, and TNF-α production by ELISA. The data presented are the mean ± SEM of three independent experiments. Differences between groups were analyzed using the Mann–Whitney U test. $^{\#}\,p < 0.05$, $^{\#\#}\,p < 0.01$, $^{\#\#\#}\,p < 0.001$ vs. LPS-untreated control groups; $*\,p < 0.05$, $**\,p < 0.01$, $***\,p < 0.001$ vs. LPS-treated groups. IL: Interleukin; TNF: Tumor necrosis factor.

3.5. ALDE Suppressed Both NF-κB Activation and MAPK Phosphorylation in LPS-Stimulated Macrophages

The NF-κB and MAPK signaling pathways are the major regulators of the expression of inflammatory mediators [18,19]. To elucidate the mechanisms underlying the anti-inflammatory effects of ALDE, we examined the changes in NF-κB translocation into nucleus after treatment with ALDE. As shown in Figure 5a, the LPS-induced degradation of IκB was significantly suppressed by ALDE treatment in the cytosolic fraction. In contrast, the level of LPS-induced nuclear NF-κB/p65 protein, which is translocated into nucleus after IκB degradation, was decreased by ALDE treatment in RAW 264.7 cells (Figure 5a). Next, we investigated whether ALDE regulated the LPS-induced phosphorylation of MAPKs. As shown in Figure 5b, LPS treatment significantly induced the phosphorylation of p38, JNK, and ERK, although ALDE significantly suppressed the phosphorylation of these proteins in a dose-dependent manner. These results suggested that the anti-inflammatory effects of ALDE were mediated by the inhibition of the activation of both NF-κB and MAPK signaling.

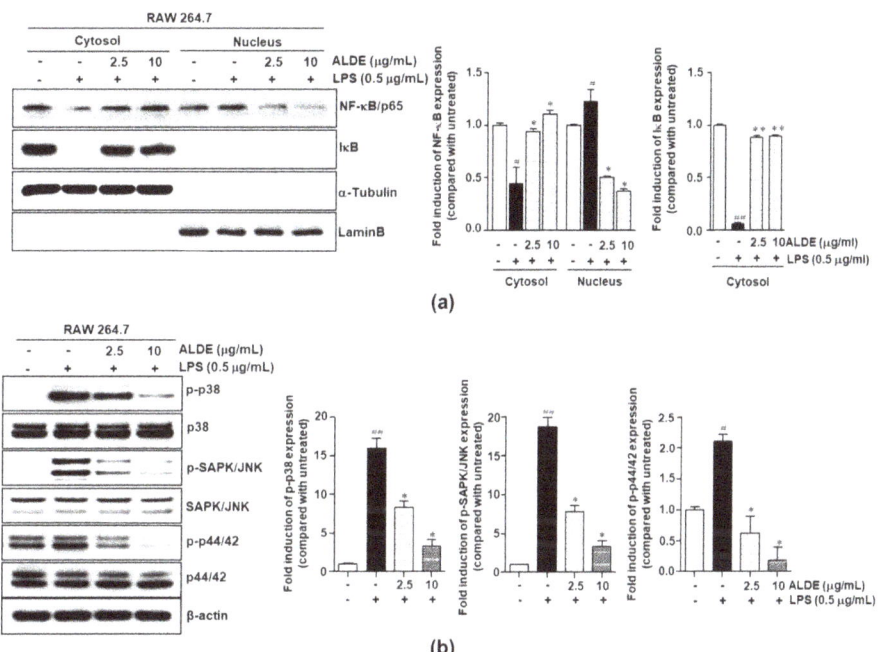

Figure 5. Inhibitory effects of ALDE on the nuclear translocation of NF-κB and the MAPK signaling pathway. RAW 264.7 cells were pretreated with ALDE (0, 2.5, and 10 μg/mL) for 2 h and then stimulated with LPS (0.5 μg/mL) for 15 min. Cytosolic extracts and nuclear extracts were prepared. (**a**) The expression of NF-κB/p65 and IκB was detected by Western blotting; α-tubulin was used as a cytosolic loading control and Lamin B was used as a nuclear loading control. (**b**) The expression of the proteins associated with the MAPK signaling pathway (p38, p44/42 ERK, and JNK) was detected by Western blotting, with β-actin used as a loading control. The relative density of the protein expression was normalized to each loading control and is presented in quantitative graphs. The data presented are the mean ± SEM of three independent experiments. Differences between groups were analyzed using the Mann–Whitney U test. $^{\#}$ $p < 0.05$, $^{\#\#}$ $p < 0.01$ vs. LPS-untreated control groups; * $p < 0.05$, ** $p < 0.01$ vs. LPS-treated groups. NF-κB: Nuclear-κB; IκB: Inhibitor of κB; MAPK: Mitogen-activated protein kinase; p-: Phosphorylated; SAPK/JNK: Stress-associated protein kinase/c-Jun N-terminal kinase; ERK: Extracellular signal-regulated kinase.

3.6. ALDE Increased the Expression of HO-1 and the Nuclear Translocation of Nrf2 in LPS-Stimulated Macrophages

To investigate whether ALDE exhibited antioxidative effects, we assayed the radical scavenging activity. As shown in Figure 6a, ALDE showed significant radical scavenging activity compared with BHA, a positive control. As the antioxidative effects were mediated by antioxidative regulators, such as HO-1, the profile of ALDE-mediated HO-1 expression was investigated in LPS-stimulated RAW 264.7 macrophages. Both mRNA expression and protein expression of HO-1 in LPS-stimulated RAW

264.7 cells were significantly increased by ALDE treatment in a dose-dependent manner (Figure 6b,c). As Nrf2 is a major regulator of the expression of HO-1 [20], we investigated whether ALDE enhanced the stability and, subsequently, the expression of Nrf2. We found that the expression of Nrf2 was increased by ALDE treatment (Figure 6d). These data suggested that ALDE exerts antioxidative effects through the activation of the Nrf2/HO-1 pathway.

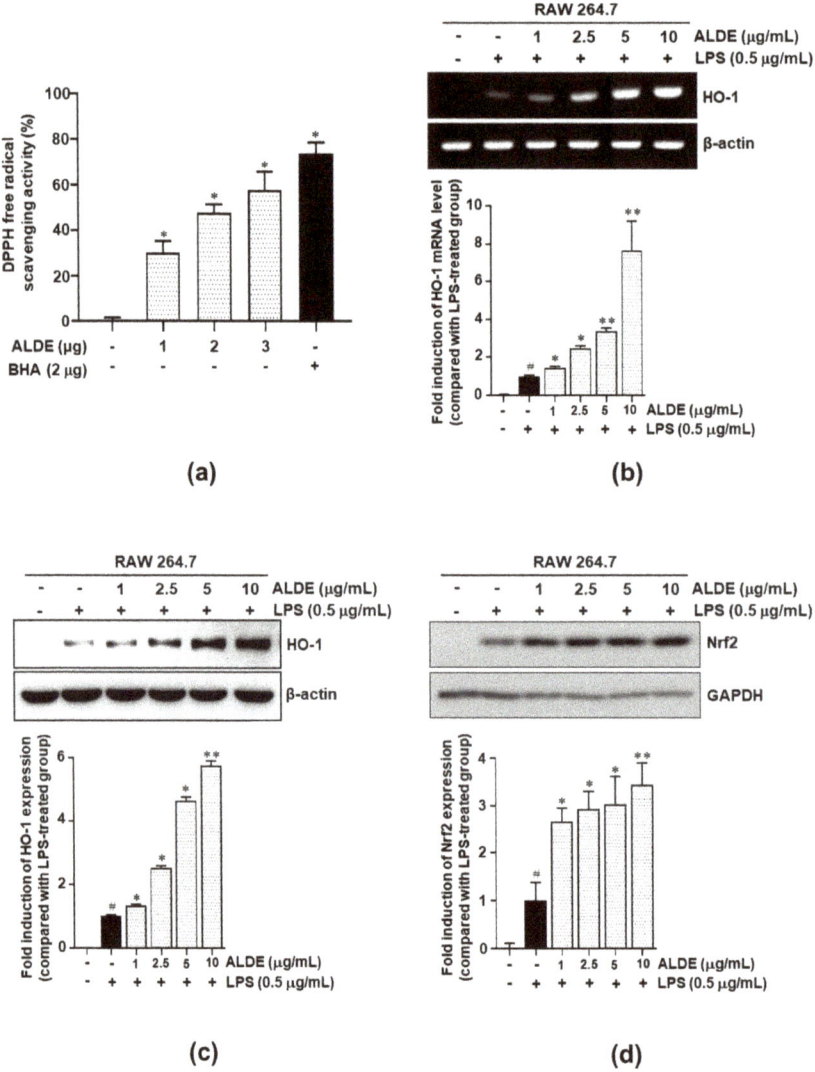

Figure 6. Antioxidative effects of ALDE. (**a**) DPPH free radical scavenging activity is represented as the mean ± SEM. * $p < 0.01$ relative to the MeOH-reacted group. BHA was used as a positive control. (**b**–**d**) RAW 264.7 cells were treated with LPS in the presence of ALDE (1, 2.5, 5, and 10 μg/mL). (**b**) After stimulation for 6 h, total RNA was extracted. HO-1 mRNA expression was analyzed by RT-PCR. (**c**,**d**) After stimulation for 24 h, total protein was extracted. The protein expression of HO-1 (**c**) and Nrf2 (**d**) was detected by Western blotting. The relative density of the mRNA and protein expression was

normalized to that of β-actin and is presented by quantitative graphs. The data presented are the mean ± SEM of three independent experiments. Differences between groups were analyzed using the Mann–Whitney U test. $^{\#} p < 0.05$ vs. LPS-untreated control groups; $^{*} p < 0.05$, $^{**} p < 0.01$ vs. LPS-treated groups. Nrf2: Nuclear factor erythroid 2-related factor; HO-1: Heme oxygenase-1.

4. Discussion

Recently, natural products have been considered important sources of drugs targeting a variety of diseases, such as cancer and inflammatory disorders [21–24]. In particular, many researchers have reported that the extracts of natural products, such as fruits, vegetables, plants, and their formulations have significant anti-inflammatory effects [25–30]. Similarly, as costunolide is a naturally occurring sesquiterpene lactone that has been extensively studied for its anti-inflammatory activity and is one of major components of ALDE, we investigated the anti-inflammatory effects of ALDE and the underlying mechanism of action [15,31,32].

The expression of iNOS is stimulated by not only proinflammatory cytokines, such as TNF-α, IL-1β, and IL-6 [33], but also bacterial products such as LPS [34]. Therefore, the inhibitory effects of natural products on NO production that occurs through the inhibition of iNOS expression, suggest that they may be potent drug candidates for the treatment of inflammatory diseases. TNF-α antagonists, including anti-TNF receptor antibodies and anti-IL-6 receptor antibodies, are currently used to inhibit the action of each proinflammatory cytokine for the treatment of RA and Crohn's disease [35,36]. Thus, agents that inhibit these proinflammatory cytokines have been suggested as therapeutic candidates for the treatment of immune diseases. In this study, we examined the inhibitory effects of ALDE on the production of various LPS-stimulated proinflammatory mediators in RAW 264.7 cells and found that ALDE significantly inhibited the production of these mediators (Figure 4). These results suggested that ALDE is a potent anti-inflammatory agent and exerts this action through the inhibition of proinflammatory responses.

HO-1 expression is enhanced by various proinflammatory stimulators, such as NO, LPS, cytokines, and other oxidants [17,20,37]. Previous studies have shown that the induction of HO-1 can represent an efficient antioxidant system and a potential pharmacological target in a variety of oxidant- and inflammatory-mediated diseases [38–40] and that this was involved in the inhibitory effects on LPS-induced NO production [41]. In this study, we observed that LPS itself caused a slight increase in HO-1 expression and that ALDE further enhanced HO-1 expression in LPS-stimulated RAW 264.7 macrophages. These results suggested that the increase in HO-1 expression induced by ALDE could inhibit NO production in LPS-stimulated RAW 264.7 cells.

The multifunctional regulator nuclear factor erythroid 2-related factor (Nrf2) is considered a cytoprotective factor that regulates the expression of genes coding for antioxidant, anti-inflammatory, and detoxifying proteins [20]. The major roles of Nrf2 are mediated by Nrf2-dependent genes and their encoded proteins, including HO-1, which have important roles in the removal of toxic heme, producing biliverdin, iron ions, and carbon monoxide. HO-1 and its products exert beneficial effects by protecting cells from oxidative injury, apoptosis, and inflammation [39]. Thus, the activation of the Nrf2 pathway is a possible explanation for the increase in HO-1 expression. As the nuclear translocation of Nrf2 allows the activation of the transcription of the HO-1 gene [20], we examined whether ALDE induced the nuclear translocation of Nrf2 in LPS-stimulated RAW 264.7 cells. We found that ALDE stabilized the Nrf2 protein expression (Figure 6d). These results suggested that the increase in HO-1 expression induced by ALDE may be mediated via the Nrf2 pathway.

In conclusion, we showed that ALDE significantly suppressed the production of NO and inhibited the expression of iNOS, COX-2, and proinflammatory cytokines in LPS-stimulated murine macrophages. The inhibitory effect was mediated by the inhibition of NF-κB translocation and MAPK phosphorylation. Moreover, we found that ALDE induced the expression of HO-1 and increased the nuclear translocation of Nrf2 in LPS-stimulated macrophages. Collectively, our results suggested that ALDE may exert potent therapeutic effects in various inflammatory diseases.

Author Contributions: Conceptualization, J.S.L., S.H.L., and Y.-C.C.; methodology, J.S.L. and H.-J.L.; validation, N.C.; resources, S.R.L.; data curation, Y.-S.R. and E.J.W.; writing—original draft preparation, J.S.L. and S.H.L.; writing—review and editing, C.C. and Y.-C.C.; visualization, Y.-S.R.; supervision, Y.-C.C.; project administration, C.C. and Y.-C.C.; funding acquisition, E.J.W. and Y.-C.C. All authors have read and agreed to the published version of the manuscript.

Funding: This study was financially supported by the Chonnam National University Hwasun Hospital Institute for Biomedical Science (HCRI 19026) and National Research Foundation of Korea, funded by the Ministry of Science and ICT (NRF-2019R1F1A1060688) and Ministry of Education (NRF- 2016R1A6A3A11931134; NRF-2018R1D1A1B07051207).

Conflicts of Interest: The authors declare no conflict of interest.

References

1. Hanada, T.; Yoshimura, A. Regulation of cytokine signaling and inflammation. *Cytokine Growth Factor Rev.* **2002**, *13*, 413–421. [CrossRef]
2. Cutolo, M. Macrophages as effectors of the immunoendocrinologic interactions in autoimmune rheumatic diseases. *Ann. N. Y. Acad. Sci.* **1999**, *876*, 32–41. [CrossRef] [PubMed]
3. Valledor, A.F.; Comalada, M.; Santamaría-Babi, L.F.; Lloberas, J.; Celada, A. Macrophage Proinflammatory Activation and Deactivation. A Question of Balance. *Adv. Immunol.* **2010**, *108*, 1–20. [PubMed]
4. Wedge, D.E.; Galindo, J.C.G.; Macías, F.A. Fungicidal activity of natural and synthetic sesquiterpene lactone analogs. *Phytochemistry* **2000**, *53*, 747–757. [CrossRef]
5. Kassuya, C.A.L.; Cremoneze, A.; Barros, L.F.L.; Simas, A.S.; da Rocha Lapa, F.; Mello-Silva, R.; Stefanello, M.É.A.; Zampronio, A.R. Antipyretic and anti-inflammatory properties of the ethanolic extract, dichloromethane fraction and costunolide from Magnolia ovata (Magnoliaceae). *J. Ethnopharmacol.* **2009**, *124*, 369–376. [CrossRef]
6. Jeong, S.J.; Itokawa, T.; Shibuya, M.; Kuwano, M.; Ono, M.; Higuchi, R.; Miyamoto, T. Costunolide, a sesquiterpene lactone from Saussurea lappa, inhibits the VEGFR KDR/Flk-1 signaling pathway. *Cancer Lett.* **2002**, *187*, 129–133. [CrossRef]
7. Choi, J.Y.; Na, M.; Hwang, I.H.; Lee, S.H.; Bae, E.Y.; Kim, B.Y.; Ahn, J.S. Isolation of betulinic acid, its methyl ester and guaiane sesquiterpenoids with protein tyrosine phosphatase 1B inhibitory activity from the roots of Saussurea lappa C.B.Clarke. *Molecules* **2009**, *14*, 266–272. [CrossRef]
8. Yoshikawa, M.; Hatakeyama, S.; Inoue, Y.; Yamahara, J. Saussureamines A, B, C, D, and E, New Anti-Ulcer Principles from Chinese Saussureae Radix. *Chem. Pharm. Bull.* **1993**, *41*, 214–216. [CrossRef]
9. Chen, H.C.; Chou, C.K.; Lee, S.D.; Wang, J.C.; Yeh, S.F. Active compounds from Saussurea lappa Clarks that suppress hepatitis B virus surface antigen gene expression in human hepatoma cells. *Antiviral Res.* **1995**, *27*, 99–109.
10. Kim, H.R.; Kim, J.M.; Kim, M.S.; Hwang, J.K.; Park, Y.J.; Yang, S.H.; Kim, H.J.; Ryu, D.G.; Lee, D.S.; Oh, H.; et al. Saussurea lappa extract suppresses TPA-induced cell invasion via inhibition of NF-κB-dependent MMP-9 expression in MCF-7 breast cancer cells. *BMC Complement. Altern. Med.* **2014**, *14*, 170. [CrossRef]
11. Seo, C.S.; Lim, H.S.; Jeong, S.J.; Shin, H.K. Anti-allergic effects of sesquiterpene lactones from the root of Aucklandia lappa Decne. *Mol. Med. Rep.* **2015**, *12*, 7789–7795. [PubMed]
12. Kim, M.S.; Kim, N.S.; Kwon, J.; Kim, H.R.; Lee, D.Y.; Oh, M.J.; Kim, H.J.; Lee, C.H.; Oh, C.H. Anti-inflammatory and Immune Regulatory Effects of Aucklandia lappa Decne 70% Ethanol Extract. *Korean J. Med. Crop Sci.* **2018**, *26*, 8–18.
13. Suzuki, K.; Bose, P.; Leong-Quong, R.Y.; Fujita, D.J.; Riabowol, K. REAP: A two minute cell fractionation method. *BMC Res. Notes* **2010**, *3*, 294.
14. Kim, M.H.; Park, D.H.; Bae, M.S.; Song, S.H.; Seo, H.J.; Han, D.G.; Oh, D.S.; Jung, S.T.; Cho, Y.C.; Park, K.M.; et al. Analysis of the Active Constituents and Evaluation of the Biological Effects of Quercus acuta Thunb. (Fagaceae) Extracts. *Molecules* **2018**, *23*, 1772.
15. Pae, H.O.; Jeong, G.S.; Kim, H.S.; Woo, W.H.; Rhew, H.Y.; Kim, H.S.; Sohn, D.H.; Kim, Y.C.; Chung, H.T. Costunolide inhibits production of tumor necrosis factor-α and interleukin-6 by inducing heme oxygenase-1 in RAW264.7 macrophages. *Inflamm. Res.* **2007**, *56*, 520–526.
16. Suh, G.Y.; Jin, Y.; Yi, A.K.; Wang, X.M.; Choi, A.M.K. CCAAT/enhancer-binding protein mediates carbon monoxide-induced suppression of cyclooxygenase-2. *Am. J. Respir. Cell Mol. Biol.* **2006**, *35*, 220–226.

17. Oh, G.S.; Pae, H.O.; Lee, B.S.; Kim, B.N.; Kim, J.M.; Kim, H.R.; Jeon, S.B.; Jeon, W.K.; Chae, H.J.; Chung, H.T. Hydrogen sulfide inhibits nitric oxide production and nuclear factor-κB via heme oxygenase-1 expression in RAW264.7 macrophages stimulated with lipopolysaccharide. *Free Radic. Biol. Med.* **2006**, *41*, 106–119.
18. Guha, M.; Mackman, N. LPS induction of gene expression in human monocytes. *Cell. Signal.* **2001**, *13*, 85–94.
19. Lawrence, T.; Willoughby, D.A.; Gilroy, D.W. Anti-inflammatory lipid mediators and insights into the resolution of inflammation. *Nat. Rev. Immunol.* **2002**, *2*, 787–795.
20. Loboda, A.; Damulewicz, M.; Pyza, E.; Jozkowicz, A.; Dulak, J. Role of Nrf2/HO-1 system in development, oxidative stress response and diseases: An evolutionarily conserved mechanism. *Cell. Mol. Life Sci.* **2016**, *73*, 3221–3247.
21. Yuan, G.; Wahlqvist, M.L.; He, G.; Yang, M.; Li, D. Natural products and anti-inflammatory activity. *Asia Pac. J. Clin. Nutr.* **2006**, *15*, 143–152. [PubMed]
22. Azab, A.; Nassar, A.; Azab, A.N. Anti-inflammatory activity of natural products. *Molecules* **2016**, *21*, 1321. [CrossRef] [PubMed]
23. Demain, A.L.; Vaishnav, P. Natural products for cancer chemotherapy. *Microb. Biotechnol.* **2011**, *4*, 687–699. [CrossRef] [PubMed]
24. Harvey, A.L. Natural products in drug discovery. *Drug Discov. Today* **2008**, *13*, 894–901. [CrossRef]
25. Yu, Y.; Li, X.; Qu, L.; Chen, Y.; Dai, Y.; Wang, M.; Zou, W. DXXK exerts anti-inflammatory effects by inhibiting the lipopolysaccharide-induced NF-κB/COX-2 signalling pathway and the expression of inflammatory mediators. *J. Ethnopharmacol.* **2016**, *178*, 199–208. [CrossRef]
26. Makchuchit, S.; Rattarom, R.; Itharat, A. The anti-allergic and anti-inflammatory effects of Benjakul extract (a Thai traditional medicine), its constituent plants and its some pure constituents using in vitro experiments. *Biomed. Pharmacother.* **2017**, *89*, 1018–1026. [CrossRef]
27. Noh, H.J.; Hwang, D.; Lee, E.S.; Hyun, J.W.; Yi, P.H.; Kim, G.S.; Lee, S.E.; Pang, C.; Park, Y.J.; Chung, K.H.; et al. Anti-inflammatory activity of a new cyclic peptide, citrusin XI, isolated from the fruits of Citrus unshiu. *J. Ethnopharmacol.* **2015**, *163*, 106–112. [CrossRef]
28. Hwang, K.A.; Hwang, Y.J.; Song, J. Aster yomena extract ameliorates pro-inflammatory immune response by suppressing NF-κB activation in RAW 264.7 cells. *J. Chin. Med. Assoc.* **2018**, *81*, 102–110. [CrossRef]
29. De Oliveira, R.G.; Mahon, C.P.A.N.; Ascêncio, P.G.M.; Ascêncio, S.D.; Balogun, S.O.; De Oliveira Martins, D.T. Evaluation of anti-inflammatory activity of hydroethanolic extract of Dilodendron bipinnatum Radlk. *J. Ethnopharmacol.* **2014**, *155*, 387–395. [CrossRef]
30. Kang, H.J.; Hong, S.H.; Kang, K.H.; Park, C.; Choi, Y.H. Anti-inflammatory effects of Hwang-Heuk-San, a traditional Korean herbal formulation, on lipopolysaccharide-stimulated murine macrophages. *BMC Complement. Altern. Med.* **2015**, *15*, 447. [CrossRef]
31. Kang, J.S.; Yoon, Y.D.; Lee, K.H.; Park, S.K.; Kim, H.M. Costunolide inhibits interleukin-1β expression by down-regulation of AP-1 and MAPK activity in LPS-stimulated RAW 264.7 cells. *Biochem. Biophys. Res. Commun.* **2004**, *313*, 171–177. [CrossRef] [PubMed]
32. Koo, T.H.; Lee, J.H.; Park, Y.J.; Hong, Y.S.; Kim, H.S.; Kim, K.W.; Lee, J.J. A sesquiterpene lactone, costunolide, from Magnolia grandiflora inhibits NF-κB by targeting IκB phosphorylation. *Planta Med.* **2001**, *67*, 103–107. [CrossRef] [PubMed]
33. Angeles Muñoz-Fernández, M.; Fresno, M. The role of tumour necrosis factor, interleukin 6, interferon-γ and inducible nitric oxide synthase in the development and pathology of the nervous system. *Prog. Neurobiol.* **1998**, *56*, 307–340. [CrossRef]
34. Aderem, A.; Ulevitch, R.J. Toll-like receptors in the induction of the innate immune response. *Nature* **2000**, *406*, 782–787. [CrossRef] [PubMed]
35. Ito, H.; Takazoe, M.; Fukuda, Y.; Hibi, T.; Kusugami, K.; Andoh, A.; Matsumoto, T.; Yamamura, T.; Azuma, J.; Nishimoto, N.; et al. A Pilot Randomized Trial of a Human Anti-Interleukin-6 Receptor Monoclonal Antibody in Active Crohn's Disease. *Gastroenterology* **2004**, *126*, 989–996. [CrossRef] [PubMed]
36. Choy, E.H.S.; Isenberg, D.A.; Garrood, T.; Farrow, S.; Ioannou, Y.; Bird, H.; Cheung, N.; Williams, B.; Hazleman, B.; Price, R.; et al. Therapeutic benefit of blocking interleukin-6 activity with an anti-interleukin-6 receptor monoclonal antibody in rheumatoid arthritis: A randomized, double-blind, placebo-controlled, dose-escalation trial. *Arthritis Rheum.* **2002**, *46*, 3143–3150. [CrossRef]

37. Chen, H.G.; Xie, K.L.; Han, H.Z.; Wang, W.N.; Liu, D.Q.; Wang, G.L.; Yu, Y.H. Heme oxygenase-1 mediates the anti-inflammatory effect of molecular hydrogen in LPS-stimulated RAW 264.7 macrophages. *Int. J. Surg.* **2013**, *11*, 1060–1066. [CrossRef]
38. Motterlini, R.; Foresti, R. Heme oxygenase-1 as a target for drug discovery. *Antioxidants Redox Signal.* **2014**, *20*, 1810–1826. [CrossRef]
39. Immenschuh, S.; Ramadori, G. Gene regulation of heme oxygenase-1 as a therapeutic target. *Biochem. Pharmacol.* **2000**, *60*, 1121–1128. [CrossRef]
40. Abraham, N.; Tsenovoy, P.; McClung, J.; Drummond, G. Heme Oxygenase: A Target Gene for Anti-Diabetic and Obesity. *Curr. Pharm. Des.* **2008**, *14*, 412–421. [CrossRef]
41. Oh, G.S.; Pae, H.O.; Choi, B.M.; Chae, S.C.; Lee, H.S.; Ryu, D.G.; Chung, H.T. 3-Hydroxyanthranilic acid, one of metabolites of tryptophan via indoleamine 2,3-dioxygenase pathway, suppresses inducible nitric oxide synthase expression by enhancing heme oxygenase-1 expression. *Biochem. Biophys. Res. Commun.* **2004**, *320*, 1156–1162. [CrossRef] [PubMed]

Sample Availability: Samples of the compounds are not available from the authors.

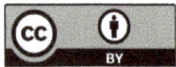

© 2020 by the authors. Licensee MDPI, Basel, Switzerland. This article is an open access article distributed under the terms and conditions of the Creative Commons Attribution (CC BY) license (http://creativecommons.org/licenses/by/4.0/).

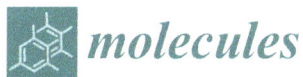

Article

Modulatory Effect of Guinep (*Melicoccus bijugatus* Jacq) Fruit Pulp Extract on Isoproterenol-Induced Myocardial Damage in Rats. Identification of Major Metabolites Using High Resolution UHPLC Q-Orbitrap Mass Spectrometry

Chukwuemeka R. Nwokocha [1,*], Isheba Warren [1], Javier Palacios [2,*], Mario Simirgiotis [3], Magdalene Nwokocha [4], Sharon Harrison [4], Rory Thompson [4], Adrian Paredes [5], Jorge Bórquez [6], Astrid Lavado [7] and Fredi Cifuentes [7]

[1] Department of Basic Medical Sciences Physiology Section, Faculty of Medical Sciences, The University of the West Indies, Mona, Kingston 7, KGN, Jamaica; Warren-Isheba.R@hotmail.com
[2] Facultad Ciencias de la Salud, Instituto de EtnoFarmacología (IDE), Universidad Arturo Prat, Iquique 1110939, Chile
[3] Instituto de Farmacia, Facultad de Ciencias, Universidad Austral de Chile, Valdivia 5110566, Chile; mario.simirgiotis@gmail.com
[4] Department of Pathology, Faculty of Medical Sciences, University of the West Indies, Mona Campus, Kingston 7, KGN, Jamaica; magdanwokocha@yahoo.com (M.N.); sharon.harrison@uwimona.edu.jm (S.H.); rorykthompson@gmail.com (R.T.)
[5] Laboratorio de Química Biológica, Instituto Antofagasta, Universidad de Antofagasta, Antofagasta 1270300, Chile; adrian.paredes@uantof.cl
[6] Departamento de Química, Facultad de Ciencias Básicas, Universidad de Antofagasta, Antofagasta 1270300, Chile; jorge.borquez@uantof.cl
[7] Laboratorio de Fisiología Experimental, Instituto Antofagasta, Universidad de Antofagasta, Antofagasta 1270300, Chile; astrid.lavado@uantof.cl (A.L.); fredi.cifuentes@uantof.cl (F.C.)
* Correspondence: chukwuemeka.nwokocha@uwimona.edu.jm (C.R.N.); clpalaci@unap.cl (J.P.); Tel.: +1-876-5895445 (C.R.N.); +56-57-2526910 (J.P.)

Academic Editors: Raffaele Capasso and Lorenzo Di Cesare Mannelli
Received: 25 December 2018; Accepted: 8 January 2019; Published: 10 January 2019

Abstract: Guinep is traditionally used in the management of cardiovascular ailments. This study aims to evaluate its medicinal constituents and effects in the management of myocardial injury in an experimental isoproterenol (ISO) rat model. Sprague-Dawley rats were randomly assigned to four groups: Group 1 was the control group; Group 2 received *M. bijugatus* extract (100 mg/Kg; MB) for six weeks; Group 3 was given ISO (85 mg/Kg) i.p. twice during a 24-hour period; and Group 4 was given ISO (85 mg/Kg) i.p. and MB extract (100 mg/Kg) for six weeks. The MB was administered orally by gavage, daily. The blood pressure of conscious animals was measured, while ECG was performed under anesthesia. Blood and serum were collected for biochemical and hematological analysis. The ISO group treated with MB showed a significant decrease ($p < 0.001$) in (SBP), diastolic (DBP), mean arterial (MAP) and heart rate (HR) compared to the ISO only group. Conversely, MB treated rats that were not induced with ISO displayed a significant decreases ($p < 0.001$) in SBP, DBP, MAP, and HR. ISO significantly elevated the ST segment ($p < 0.001$) and shortened the QTc interval ($p < 0.05$), which were recovered after treatment with 100 mg/Kg of MB. In addition, the results showed a significant decrease ($p < 0.001$) in the heart to body weight ratio of the ISO group treated with MB compared to the ISO only group. Furthermore, the extract normalized the hematological values depressed by the ISO while significantly elevating the platelet count. UHPLC high-resolution orbitrap mass spectrometry analysis results revealed the presence of several antioxidants like vitamin C and related compounds, phenolic acids, flavonoid, fatty acids (oxylipins), and terpene derivatives.

The results of this study indicated that *Melicoccus bijugatus* did display some cardio-protective effects in relation to myocardial injury.

Keywords: *Melicoccus bijugatus*; isoproterenol; myocardial infarction; high-resolution orbitrap mass spectrometry; rat

---

1. Introduction

Cardiovascular disease (CVD) like acute myocardial infarction (AMI) is one of the leading causes of death; causing prolonged ischemia of the heart muscle resulting in tissue death or infarction in the myocardium [1]. This results in edema, a reduction in cardiac output, abnormalities in cardiac rhythm and transmission blocks that can further impair cardiac function. A reduction in cardiac output and arterial pressure may stimulate baroreceptor reflexes that lead to the activation of compensatory mechanisms, such as those of the sympathetic nerves and the renin-angiotensin-aldosterone system [2], and to elevations in cardiac biomarkers [3].

ISO is a potent non-selective beta-adrenergic receptor ($\beta1$ and $\beta2$) agonist that causes severe stress to the myocardium, resulting in infarct-like necrosis of the heart muscle [4]. Its proposed mechanism of action is through the auto-oxidation and production of free cytotoxic radicals [5], as well as hyper-stimulation of beta adrenoceptors [6]. These actions lead to the peroxidation of the cellular membrane, a change in membrane permeability and possible derangement of calcium ion pathway signaling, hypertrophy and myocardial injury [7,8]. The net effect of these includes a fall in DBP and MAP while SBP may remain unchanged, rise or fall (depending on the dose). Similarly, cardiac output may increase because of the positive inotropic and chronotropic effects of the drug, due to a decrease in peripheral vascular resistance.

Melicoccus bijugatus, known colloquially in Jamaica as Guinep, is a minor member of the *Sapindaceae* family [9]. The therapeutic effects of these fruits, including the management of diarrhea, cardiovascular disease, asthma and constipation, and as an astringent [10], were attributed to the combination of phenolic compounds and sugars. The phenolic content of this fruit was previously reported [9,11]. In the seed embryo, flavonoids, epicatechin, catechin, epigallocatechin, B-type procyanidins, naringenin, naringenin derivatives, phloretin, phloridzin, quercetin, myricetin and resveratrol, were identified in high amounts. The pulp of the fruit contains phenolic acid derivatives such as coumaric and ferulic acid derivatives, and hydroxycinnamic and sinapic acid [10,12]. This study aims to scientifically examine the mechanism of action of *M. bijugatus* in the management of cardiovascular ailments like AMI via an experimental rat model.

2. Results

2.1. Blood Pressure Changes and Electrocardiogram (ECG)

Table 1 shows that the extract group displayed a significant decrease ($p < 0.001$) in the MAP, SBP, and DBP when compared to the control (normotensive rats). There was also a significant decrease in the MAP, SBP, and DBP of the ISO group treated with MB compared to the ISO only group ($p < 0.001$).

The MB group displayed a significantly decreased ($p < 0.01$) HR when compared to the normotensive animals (control). There was also a significant decrease ($p < 0.001$) in the HR of the ISO plus MB treatment group when compared to the ISO only treatment group (Figure 1, Table 1). In addition, there was an observable (24.5%) increase in the HR of the ISO only group when compared to the control group (normotensive). However, this increase was not statistically significant.

Although the PP significantly decreased in all groups, the causes in the MB group ($p < 0.001$), ISO group ($p < 0.01$) and ISO + MB group ($p < 0.01$) were different compared to that of the control. Table 1 shows that ISO significantly ($p < 0.05$) increased the DBP, did not increase the SBP, and decreased the

PP, consistent with decreased left ventricular compliance and increased myocardial stiffness [13]. MB significantly decreased the blood pressure (MAP, SBP, DBP), HR, and PP, which is proportional to the stroke volume [14].

Table 1. Effects of *Melicoccus bijugatus* (MB; 100 mg/Kg) on mean arterial blood pressure (MAP), systolic blood pressure (SBP), diastolic blood pressure (DBP), pulse pressure (PP), and heart rate (HR) of normotensive rats and those with myocardial damage with ISO.

	Normotensive		Myocardial Damage	
	Control	MB	ISO	ISO + MB
MAP, mmHg	101 ± 3	69 ± 2 ***	113 ± 5	83 ± 6 *,###
SBP, mmHg	131 ± 3	85 ± 2 ***	133 ± 4	106 ± 6 ***,###
DBP, mmHg	87 ± 5	60 ± 3 ***	108 ± 8 *	72 ± 8 ###
PP, mmHg	44 ± 5	27 ± 2 ***	28 ± 2 **	27 ± 3 **
HR, bpm	246 ± 25	146 ± 11 **	307 ± 20	181 ± 18 ###

Values are mean ±standard error of the mean of five experiments in mmHg. Statistically significant differences: * $p < 0.05$, ** $p < 0.01$, *** $p < 0.001$ vs. control; ### $p < 0.001$ vs. ISO.

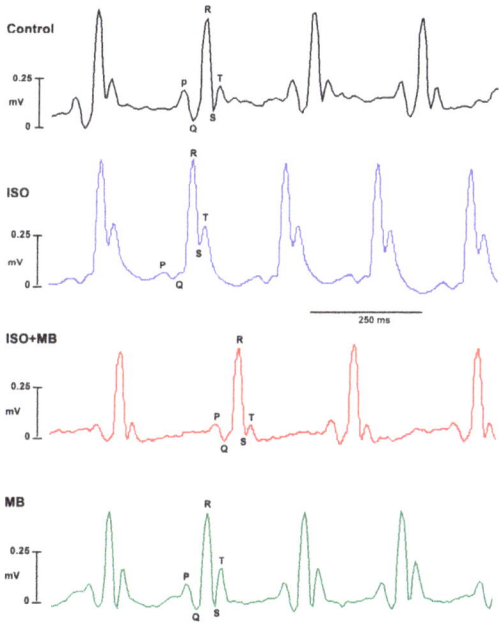

Figure 1. Electrocardiograms (ECG) showing the bradycardic effects of *M. bijugatus* extract (MB, 100 mg/Kg) in myocardial injury. Control shows the normal electrocardiograph. ISO (85 mg/Kg) shows an elevated ST segment; ISO + MB shows a restored ST segment.

In electrocardiograms from rats and mice, the beginning of the T-wave merges with the end of the QRS complex without an isoelectric ST segment. The changes, seen in the ECG, that affected the frequency of the waves can be seen to affect the HR also. ISO significantly elevated the ST segment ($p < 0.001$; Figures 1 and 2A) and shortened the QTc interval ($p < 0.05$; Figures 1 and 2B), which recovered after treatment with 100 mg/Kg of MB. The *M. bijugatus* of the plant did not, *per se*, cause any change.

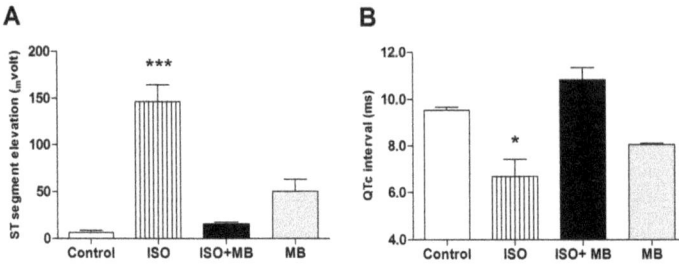

Figure 2. Treatment, with *M. bijugatus*, of a myocardial injury caused by ISO. The data shows the effects of MB and ISO on ST segment elevation (**A**) and the duration of the QTc interval of the ECG (**B**). ISO (85 mg/Kg) significantly elevated the ST segment ($p < 0.001$) and shortened the QTc interval ($p < 0.05$), which recovered after treatment with 100 mg/Kg of *M. bijugatus*. The extract did not, *per se*, cause any change. * $p < 0.05$, *** $p < 0.001$ vs. control; $n = 5$.

2.2. Hematological Parameters

There were significant differences ($p > 0.05$) in the hematological parameters of the treatment groups when compared to the control group (Tables 2 and 3). ISO significantly reduced the white blood count (WBC; $p < 0.05$), red blood count (RBC; $p < 0.01$), hematocrit (HCT; $p < 0.01$), mean cell volume (MCV; $p < 0.01$) and mean cell hemoglobin values (MCH; $p < 0.01$). *M. bijugatus* extract normalized the hematological values (WBC, RBC, HCT, MCV and MCH) depressed by ISO, while significantly ($p < 0.01$) elevating the platelet count.

Table 2. Effect of *M. bijugatus* on white cell parameters in ISO-induced cardiac injury.

	Control	MB	ISO	ISO + MB
WBC ($10^3/\mu L$)	9.5 ± 1.2	8.6 ± 1.3	4.1 ± 1.0 *	7.1 ± 1.2
LYM ($10^3/\mu L$)	5.8 ± 0.6	5.9 ± 1.0	3.0 ± 0.8	4.9 ± 0.8
MID ($10^3/\mu L$)	1.5 ± 0.2	1.1 ± 0.2	0.62 ± 0.2 *	1.1 ± 0.1
GRA ($10^3/\mu L$)	2.4 ± 0.5	1.5 ± 0.3	0.5 ± 0.1 **	1.2 ± 0.3
LYM (%)	61.4 ± 2.9	66.8 ± 2.7	73.9 ± 0.9 **	69.6 ± 1.1
MID (%)	14.5 ± 0.6	13.9 ± 1.0	14.5 ± 0.8	13.2 ± 1.5
GRA (%)	27.3 ± 0.9	19.3 ± 2.4	11.6 ± 1.0 ***	17.3 ± 1.4 *

WBC—White blood count, LYM—Lymphocyte, MID—Others white cells, GRA—Granulocyte. Values are mean ±standard error of the mean of five experiments in mmHg. Statistically significant differences: * $p < 0.05$, ** $p < 0.01$, *** $p < 0.001$ vs. control.

Table 3. Effect of *M. bijugatus* on red cell and trombocytes parameters in the ISO-induced cardiac injury.

	Control	MB	ISO	ISO + MB
RBC ($10^6/\mu L$)	6.8 ± 0.2	5.9 ± 0.4	5.2 ± 0.2 **	6.3 ± 0.42
HGB (g/dL)	14.8 ± 0.3	13.6 ± 0.6	12.5 ± 0.6	14.1 ± 1.0
HCT (%)	40.0 ± 0.8	36.2 ± 1.2	32.6 ± 1.5 **	34.8 ± 1.4
MCV (fL)	2.4 ± 0.5	1.5 ± 0.3	0.5 ± 0.1 **	1.2 ± 0.3
MCH (pg)	21.7 ± 0.2	22.2 ± 0.5	24 ± 0.6 **	22.2 ± 0.4
MCHC (g/dL)	37.1 ± 0.4	37.4 ± 0.6	38.6 ± 0.4	37.7 ± 0.2
RDW	15.0 ± 0.6	15.7 ± 0.5	15.3 ± 1.2	16.6 ± 0.9
PLT ($10^3/\mu L$)	680.3 ± 31.0	840.0 ± 21.1 *	668.8 ± 49.0	918.8 ± 42.7 **,##
MPV	6.6 ± 0.2	7.7 ± 0.4	7.0 ± 0.2	7.4 ± 0.5

RBC—Red blood count, HGB—Hemoglobin, HCT—Hematocrit, MCV—Mean corpuscular volume, MCH—Mean corpuscular hemoglobin, MCHC—Mean corpuscular hemoglobin concentration, RDW—Red cell distribution width, PLT—Platelets, MPV—Mean platelet volume. Values are mean ±standard error of the mean of five experiments in mmHg. Statistically significant differences: * $p < 0.05$, ** $p < 0.01$, *** $p < 0.001$ vs. control; ## $p < 0.01$ vs ISO.

2.3. Histo-Morphological Analysis

The microscopic changes in the muscle fibers of the heart were limited to the group that was exposed to both ISO and MB. The maximum dimension of the myocardial infarction was of 1.1 mm and appeared to be in the central region of the left ventricular muscle wall, which is the area furthest away from both endocardium and epicardium and is most susceptible to infarction from vascular compromise (Figure 3C).

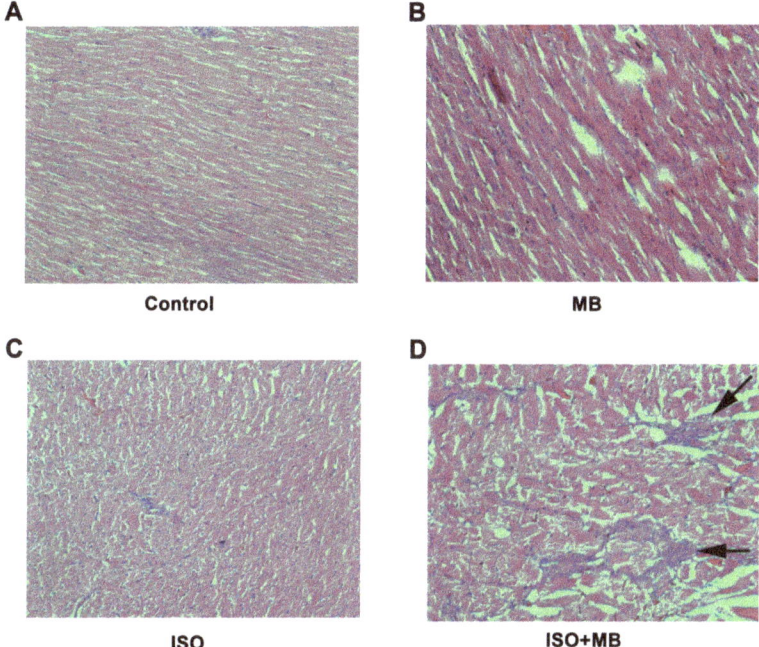

Figure 3. Histological analysis of myocardial injury. Histomicrograph of transverse sections of the heart [×200; hematoxylin and eosin stain] taken through the ventricles, just below the atrioventricular valves of control (**A**), 100 mg/Kg MB alone (**B**), ISO treatment alone (**C**), ISO + MB (**D**). The ISO group showed myocardial infarction in the central region of the left ventricular muscle wall (**C**). The Control (**A**) and MB only group (**B**) displayed no features of myocardial injury. The arrows demonstrated the area of fibrosis.

Longitudinal and/or transverse sections of the large caliber abdominal blood vessels, i.e., aorta and caudal vena cava revealed no changes in the intima, media or external layer. The adventitia was composed primarily of brown fat. No inflammation was appreciated (data not shown).

2.4. Ratio of Heart Weight to Body Weight

The data does not suggest that *M. bijugatus* is responsible for any significant changes in body weight that could not be accounted for in the natural growth pattern of the Sprague-Dawley rat. ISO caused an elevated heart weight/body weight ratio and treatment with MB (100 mg/Kg) caused a significant decrease (Figure 4).

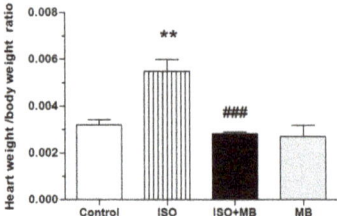

Figure 4. Effects of ISO and treatment with *M. bijugatus* extract on weight/body weight ratio. Depicts the ISO (85 mg/Kg) induced myocardial damage through an elevation of the heart weight to body weight ratio. This was significantly reduced in the MB (100 mg/Kg) treated groups. ** p <0.01 vs. control; ### p < 0.001 vs. ISO, n = 5.

2.5. Identification of the Compounds

Hyphenated UHPLC-MS experiments were employed for the identification of unknown compounds in the fruits of *M. bijugatus* since it provides high resolution and an accurate mass product ion spectra (Figure 5, Table 4 and Supplementary Material). Combining Q-orbitrap HRAM (high resolution accurate mass) full MS scans and MS^n experiments, all compounds were tentatively identified, including simple phenolic acids, terpenes, fatty acids, and one glycosylated flavonoid. As far as we know, some of the compounds, for this species, were reported for the first time. Below is a detailed explanation of the identification.

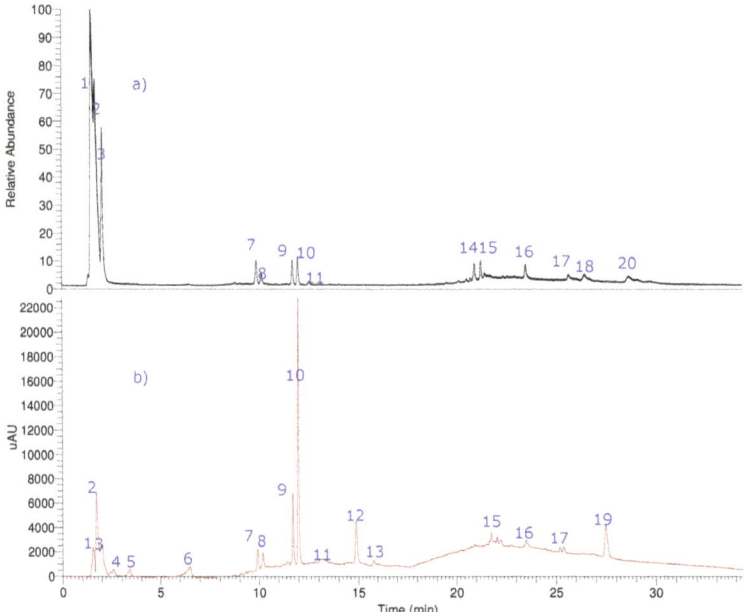

Figure 5. UHPLC chromatogram total ion current [total ion current (**a**), UV at 280 nm (**b**)] of aqueous extract of *M. bijugatus*. The details of metabolites are in the Supplementary Material S1.

Table 4. Identification of metabolites by UHPLC-PDA-OT-MS.

Peak	Retention Time (min)	UV Max	Tentative Identification	Elemental Composition [M − H]$^-$	Theoretical Mass (m/z)	Measured Mass (m/z)	Accuracy (dppm)	MSn Ions (dppm)
1	1.72	220	Citric acid	$C_6H_7O_7^-$	191.01863	191.01933	3.68	
2	1.82	222	Isocitric acid	$C_6H_7O_7^-$	191.01863	191.01955	3.04	
3	1.65	-	Saccharose	$C_{12}H_{21}O_{11}^-$	341.10784	341.10783	2.44	
4	2.55	-	Glucose	$C_6H_{11}O_6^-$	179.05501	179.05550	2.69	
5	3.37	230	Furoic acid	$C_5H_3O_3^-$	111.00767	111.00787	3.25	
6	6.35	245	Salicilic acid glucoside	$C_{13}H_{15}O_8^-$	299.07614	299.07712	3.25	137.02440
7	9.80	245–325	Aflavarin	$C_{24}H_{21}O_9^-$	453.11801	453.11703	−2.1	
8	10.24	-	Trihydroxyoctadecatrienoic acid	$C_{18}H_{29}O_5^-$	325.20205	325.18443	−54.2	
9	11.98	275–339	Coumaric acid glucoside	$C_{15}H_{17}O_8^-$	325.09179	325.09277	3.01	163.0291, 145.02870, 117.03368
10	12.24	275–339	Coumaric acid galactoside	$C_{15}H_{17}O_8^-$	325.09179	325.09271	2.82	163.0291, 145.02870, 117.03368
11	13.35	275–339	Feruloyl glucoside	$C_{16}H_{19}O_9^-$	355.10346	355.10336	3.34	147.04449, 193.05058
12	15.02	254–354	Isorhamnetin-3-O-gglucoside	$C_{22}H_{21}O_{11}^-$	477.11679	477.11670	−27.12	314.04370
13	15.83	275–339	Feruloyl galactoside	$C_{16}H_{19}O_9^-$	355.10346	355.10355	3.34	147.04449, 193.05056
14	21.57	236–329	3-O-Caffeoylquinic acid	$C_{16}H_{17}O_9^-$	353.0878	353.0878	0.53	191.05608
15	21.87	-	Rishitin	$C_{14}H_{22}O_2^-$	221.15488	221.15488	5.74	
16	23.54	300	Embelin	$C_{17}H_{26}O_4^-$	293.17474	293.17587	3.87	
17	25.38	235	Sedanenolide	$C_{12}H_{15}O_2^-$	191.10666	191.10741	3.92	
18	26.45	225	Valerenic acid	$C_{15}H_{21}O_2^-$	233.15470	233.15455	3.87	149.13301
19	27.78	214	Blumenol C	$C_{13}H_{22}O_2^-$	209.15631	209.15430	3.30	
20	28.32	220	Hydroxyheptadecatrienoic acid	$C_{17}H_{27}O_7^-$	311.18640	311.16876	−56.6	

2.5.1. Simple Organic Acids and Sugars

Peaks 1–5 and 8 were identified as simple organic acids such as vitamin C and sucrose. Peak 1, with an [M − H]$^-$ ion at m/z: 191.01933, was identified as citric acid ($C_6H_7O_7^-$) and Peak 2 as the isomer isocitric acid [4]. Peak 3 was identified as saccharose ($C_{12}H_{21}O_{11}^-$) and Peak 4 as glucose ($C_6H_{11}O_6^-$). Sucrose and glucose were already reported as important constituents of this fruit [10,12]. Peak 5, with an [M − H]$^-$ ion at m/z: 111.00787, was identified as furoic acid ($C_3H_3O_3^-$) and Peak 16, with an [M − H]$^-$ ion at m/z: 293.17587, was assigned to the bioactive, cell permeable, 1,4-benzoquinone embelin derivative ($C_{17}H_{26}O_4^-$) [15].

2.5.2. Flavonoids

Peak 12, with an [M − H]$^-$ ion at m/z: 477.11670, and the MS2 fragment at m/z: 314.04370 were identified as Isorhamnetin-3-O-Glucoside ($C_{22}H_{21}O_{11}^-$) [16].

2.5.3. Phenolic Compounds

Peak 6 was identified as salicilic acid glucoside ($C_{13}H_{15}O_8^-$), the parent ion 299.07712 delivered a diagnostic salicylic acid ion at m/z: 137.02440 [17], and Peak 7 was identified as the dicoumarin aflavarin ($C_{24}H_{21}O_9^-$). Peaks 9 and 10, with pseudomolecular ions at m/z: 325.09277 and dioagnostic MS2 fragments at m/z: 163.02910, 145.02870 and 117.03368, were identified as coumaric acid glucoside and coumaric acid galactoside, respectively ($C_{15}H_{17}O_8^-$). The presence of coumaric acid glucoside was already reported in this fruit pulp [10]. In the same manner, Peaks 11 and 13 were identified as the related compounds feruloyl glucoside and feruloyl galactoside ($C_{16}H_{19}O_9^-$) showing diagnostic MS2 ions at 147.04449 and 193.05056. Peak 14 was identified as chlorogenic acid: 3-O-caffeoylquinic acid (3-CQA, $C_{16}H_{17}O_9^-$), with a diagnostic quinic acid ion at 191.05608 [18].

2.5.4. Fatty Acids

Two peaks were tentatively identified as fatty acids known as oxylipins [19,20]. Peak 8, with a pseudomolecular ion at m/z: 325.18443, was identified as a trihydroxy-octadecatrienoic acid ($C_{18}H_{29}O_5^-$) and Peak 2, with a pseudomolecular ion at m/z: 311.16876, was identified as a hydroxyheptadecatrienoic acid ($C_{17}H_{27}O_7^-$) [21].

2.5.5. Terpenes and Related Compounds

Peak 17 was identified as the lactone sedanenolide ($C_{12}H_{12}O_2^-$) [22] and Peak 18 was assigned to the sesquiterpene valerenic acid ($C_{15}H_{21}O_2^-$) [23]. Peak 15, with a $[M - H]^-$ ion at m/z: 221.15488, was identified as the antifungic norsesquiterpene alcohol rishitin ($C_{14}H_{22}O_2^-$)[24]. Peak 19, with an $[M - H]^-$ ion at m/z: 209.15430, was identified as Blumenol C ($C_{13}H_{22}O_2^-$, 4-(3-hydroxybutyl)-3,5,5-trimethylcyclohex-2-en-1-one) [25].

3. Discussion

This study, for the first time, demonstrated the hypotensive effect of the *Melicoccus bijugatus* Jacq when it is administered orally in normotensive animals. This hypotensive effect was, in part, because of the decrease in HR. In addition, we demonstrated a partial recovery of ISO-induced myocardial infarction by the action of *M. bijugatus*.

ISO is an isopropyl analog of epinephrine that stimulates the α-1 adrenergic receptors [8], oxidative stress in cardiac myocytes, cell membrane destabilization and damage. It also increased intracellular adenylyl cyclase in the myocardium, increased lipid deposition in the myocardium, and increased the heart weight to body weight ratio and myocardial infarction [26]. ISO also significantly elevated the ST segment and shortened the QTc interval in the experimental animals; this was reversed by treatment with *M. bijugatus* extracts. The chronotropic and inotropic actions of ISO also caused an increase in the SBP. The sum of these cardiovascular changes is in an increase in HR and cardiac output and a decrease in the MAP, as observed in our study. Treatment of the animals exposed to ISO with *M. bijugatus* extracts caused decreases in HR, and MAP. This showed the cardioprotective role of the *M. bijugatus*.

This increase in the ratio of heart weight to body weight was thought to be a hypertrophic response, possibly due to an increase in the amount of protein synthesis that was occurring in the damaged tissue as it attempted to repair itself, as well as an increase the number of inflammatory cells to become mobilized in response to the damage [27]. Other possible mechanisms include increase in the glucose uptake in cardiac myocytes along with an increase in oxidative stress with ISO administration [28], accumulation of fluid in intracellular space of the tissue as well as an increase in the water content of the cells themselves [29]. Histo-morphological presentations of myocardial infarction to the ISO group were observed. There were no appreciable changes in the intima, media and adventitia layers of the aorta, caudal or vena cava (data not shown).

Using UHPLC high-resolution orbitrap mass spectrometry, (UHPLC-OT-HR-MS) we have identified 20 secondary metabolites in the aqueous extract of *M. bijugatus*, most of which, as far as we know, were reported here for the first time. Many of these compounds are simple organic acids, such as vitamin C, a flavonoid, several phenolic compounds, terpenoids, and two fatty acids. Furthermore, the results obtained in this study clearly show that the infusion can be a natural source of phenolic compounds with potential applications in the neutraceutical management of myocardial infarction.

A possible mechanism of action may be through the inhibition of the proliferation of cells of the vascular smooth muscle by caffeic acid, which is found in the fruit's pulp tissues [30]. The hypotensive properties displayed may also be due to the action of coumaric acid derivatives. A derivative of the sugar of coumaric acid was confirmed to be a major peak in the HPLC fingerprint profile at 280nm [12]. One such derivative of coumaric acid is p-coumaric which has been known to possess antioxidant effects as well as anti-platelet activity [31].

Increases in serum levels of troponin I, CK-MB, myoglobin, and high sensitivity C-reactive protein are often associated with myocardial damage [32,33], though with some limitations [3,34]. Our study showed no significant difference in the serum concentration of CK-MB in rats induced with ISO compared to the control group (data not shown), this could be due to the timeline of the analysis of these biomarkers. Our results are supported by Zhang et al. (2008), who reported a decline in these biomarkers, down to control levels, after 48 h [35].

Myocardial infarction is often associated with an increase in the white blood cell count as part of an inflammatory response to the damaged cells that are present due to the necrosis of the tissue [36]. Other hematological features associated with myocardial infarction include an increase in whole blood viscosity and plasma viscosity, an increase in the white blood cell, leukocyte and neutrophil count [1], an increase in the erythrocyte count and hemoglobin concentration [37], and an increase in red cell indices, such as mean corpuscular hemoglobin (MCH), mean corpuscular hemoglobin concentration (MCHC) and mean corpuscular volume (MCV) [4]. Sangeetha and Quine, (2008) reported increases in hemoglobin, RBC, hematocrit, WBC and platelet counts with ISO induced myocardial infarction in male Wister rats [37], while Lobo-Fiho et al., (2011) suggested no alterations in terms of the hemoglobin indices [1]. We observed significant alterations in the hematological parameters in the treatment groups when compared to the control group. This study showed that ISO significantly reduced the white blood count (WBC), red blood count (RBC), hematocrit (HTC), mean cell volume (MCV) and mean cell hemoglobin values (MCH). The extract normalized the hematological values (WBC, RBC, HCT and MCV) depressed by ISO while significantly elevating the platelet count. The increased production of platelets suggests that the extract did not present a toxic effect, such as that of *Colocasia esculenta* (L.) Schott [38], but presented an increase in platelets similar to *Carica papaya* Linn. [39].

4. Materials and Methods

4.1. Plant Material and Extraction

The fruit of the *M. bijugatus* tree was collected in September. Mr. Patrick Lewis, Department of Botany, University of the West Indies, Mona Campus (Kingston, Jamaica), made a botanical identification of the plant (voucher specimen AN 08, 10/11). The fruit pulp was separated from the seed by hand using a knife. The pulp was then blended and the juice was squeezed out through a strainer before being filtered to remove any remaining pulp fibers. Finally, the juice was placed inside a Freeze Dry machine (Freezone 4.5 L, Labconco, Kansas, MO, USA).

4.2. Experimental Animals

The study was conducted according to the Animal Scientific Procedures Act of 1986 following the receipt of approval from the UWI/FMS Ethics Committee (AN 06,15/16). Twenty male Sprague- Dawley rats (8–10 weeks old and 170 g to 230 g) were chosen, housed in plastic cages at the UWI Mona campus Animal House at room temperature (22–25 °C) with a humidity of 45–51%. Fresh tap water was available to the rats via a bottle and food was administered *ad libitum*. Four groups were identified, each of which consisted of five rats. The first group served as a control group and did not receive any drugs. Rats from the second group were administered, by gavage, 100 mg/Kg of *M. bijugatus* liquid extract only daily for six weeks. The third group of rats received only two doses of 85 mg/Kg b.w. ISO intraperitoneally within a 24-hour period. Finally, rats of Group 4 were injected intraperitoneally with two doses of 85 mg/Kg b.w. of ISO within a 24-hour period. Following this, they were given 100 mg/Kg b.w. *M. bijugatus* extract, by gavage, daily for six weeks. The animals were sacrificed under anesthesia seven days after the period of treatment. The heart and kidney tissues were harvested and weighed to obtain a ratio of the heart and kidney weights to body weight. In addition, a blood sample was collected to conduct biochemical and hematological assessments among the subject groups.

4.3. Blood Pressure Recordings and ECG

The tail cuff method (CODA) was used to measure the SBP and DBP of the rats once before the administration of ISO and once per week following the administration of ISO. The pulse pressure (PP) was calculated using the formula PP = (SBP − DBP). The MAP was calculated using the formula:

MAP = DBP + 1/3(SBP − DBP). For ECG recordings, rats were first anesthetized with ketamine (42 mg/Kg, i.p.) and xylazine (5 mg/Kg, i.p.). The ECG electrodes (BIOPAC System Inc, California, CA, USA) were placed subcutaneously in a bipolar configuration (DII). Measurements were done using the Electrocardiogram Amplifier equipment (ECG100C, BIOPAC System Inc, California, CA, USA) and tracings were recorded using the AcqKnowledge III computer software program (3.9.1., BIOPAC System Inc, California, CA, USA). The QT interval was taken as the time from the beginning of the QRS complex to the end of the T-wave. The RR interval was taken as the time elapsed between two consecutive maxima of the R-waves. The corrected QT interval (QTc) was calculated in accordance with the formula [40,41]:

$$QTc = QT/(RR)^{1/2}$$

4.4. Biochemical Estimation

Whole blood was collected and assessed using standardized ethylenediaminetetraacetic acid (EDTA) tubes to obtain a complete blood count (CBC). The Cell Dyn Emerald Hematology Analyzer (Abbott Laboratories, Chicago, IL, USA) was then used to assess hematological parameters.

4.5. Histo-Morphological Appraisal

Histo-morphologic analyses of the cardiac tissues of the Sprague-Dawley rats were done using a Nikon Eclipse C*i* research microscope (Nikon Instruments Inc., New York, NY, USA). Mirco-measurements were done via integrated mechanical stages with graduated locator margins and built in slide holders, as well as X-Y translator knobs. The tissues were harvested and immediately submerged in 10% neutral buffered formalin for preservation. They were subsequently processed, embedded in wax, and serial sectioned to a thickness of 4 microns then stained with haematoxylin and eosin (H and E) stain.

Twelve (12) full-thickness transverse sections from the heart, immediately subjacent to the atrioventricular valves (three from each group), were analyzed and evaluated for edema, mononuclear cell infiltration, fibrosis, interstitial hemorrhage and myocyte degeneration. The number of foci exhibiting degenerative features was recorded and the maximum diameter of the degenerated area was measured using a stage micrometer (Nikon Instruments Inc., New York, NY, USA).

Sixteen (16) longitudinal and/or transverse sections of the large caliber abdominal blood vessels, i.e., aorta (two from each group) and caudal vena cava (two from each group), were analyzed and evaluated for evidence of endothelial injury, degeneration of the intima or elastic lamina, atherosclerotic change, or any features of adventitial cellular injury.

The Ishak systems were employed to ascribe a stage of fibrosis and to grade the degree of inflammatory changes (1). In addition to these established, semi-objective parameters, subjective evaluation was performed for sinusoidal vascular congestion and the degree of nuclear chromatin density.

4.6. UHPLC-DAD-MS Instrument

The use of the Scientific Dionex Ultimate 3000 UHPLC system (Thermo Fisher Scientific, Bremen, Germany) hyphenated with a Q exactive focus machine (Thermo Fisher Scientific, Waltham, MA, USA) was already reported [42]. For the analysis, 5 mg of the lyophilized material were dissolved in 2 mL of methanol, filtered (PTFE filter) and 10 µL were injected in the instrument, with all specifications set as previously reported [42].

4.7. LC Parameters and MS Parameters

Liquid chromatography was performed using an UHPLC C18 column (Acclaim, 150 mm × 4.6 mm ID, 2.5 µm, Thermo Fisher Scientific, Bremen, Germany) operated at 25 °C. The detection wavelengths were 254, 280, 330 and 354 nm, and DAD was recorded from 200 to 800 nm for peak characterization. Mobile phases were 1% formic aqueous solution (A) and acetonitrile (B).

The gradient program time in minutes, % (B) was: (0.00, 5); (5.00, 5); (10.00, 30); (15.00, 30); (20.00, 70); (25.00, 70); (35.00, 5) and 12 min for column equilibration before each injection. The flow rate was 1.00 mL min^{-1}, and the injection volume was 10 µL. The standards and resin extract dissolved in methanol were kept at 10 °C during storage in the autosampler. The HESI II and Orbitrap spectrometer parameters were optimized as previously reported [42,43].

4.8. Statistical Analysis

The data collected were expressed as mean ±SEM (standard error of mean). The mean values from the different groups were analyzed using GraphPad Prism Version 6.0 Software (GraphPad Software, San Diego, CA, USA). One-way or two-way ANOVA were used to compare the means, followed by the Bonferroni test. A value of $p < 0.05$ was considered statistically significant [44].

5. Conclusions

In conclusion, we confirmed that *Melicoccus bijugatus* partially reversed myocardial damage and injury in an experimental ISO rat model. This was indicated by changes seen in the ECGs and in the reversal of the increased heart to body weight ratio in animals with ISO induced myocardial injury and blood pressure changes associated with a normalizing or reversal of symptoms associated with cardiac injury.

Supplementary Materials: The following are available online, Figure S1: Quadrupole Orbitrap full MS spectra and structures of all detected compounds in the fruits of *Melicoccus bijugatus*.

Author Contributions: C.R.N. was the author of the project design, conducted and designed the experiments, and drafted the manuscript; I.W. performed some experiments; J.P. participated in the design, performed some experiments, and wrote the manuscript; F.C., A.P. and A.L. participated in the design and conducted the pharmacological assays. J.B. and M.J.S. performed the isolation and structural elucidation of the pure compounds for UHPLC-MS; M.N., S.H. and R.T. participated in the design and performed the histopatological experiments.

Funding: This research was funded in part by the World Academy of Science/UNESCO (13–108 RG/BIO/LA) Grant and UWI Grants to C.R. Nwokocha. Mario Simirgiotis and Jorge Bórquez acknowledge funds from Fondecyt 1180059 Universidad Austral de Chile.

Acknowledgments: The authors wish to express their gratitude to the Rectoria y Vicerrectoria de Investigacion, Innovacion y Postgrado Universidad de Antofagasta for their financial and technical support.

Conflicts of Interest: The authors declare no conflicts of interest.

References

1. Lobo Filho, H.G.; Ferreira, N.L.; Sousa, R.B.; Carvalho, E.R.; Lobo, P.L.; Lobo Filho, J.G. Experimental model of myocardial infarction induced by isoproterenol in rats. *Rev. Bras. Cir. Cardiovasc.* **2011**, *26*, 469–476. [CrossRef] [PubMed]
2. Górecki, A.; Bednarz, B.; Jaxa-Chamiec, T.; Maciejewski, P.; Łukaszewicz, R.; Ceremużyński, L.; Dyduszyński, A. Lipid profile during the first 24 hours after myocardial infarction has significant prognostic value. *Kardiol. Pol.* **2004**, *60*, 229–236. [PubMed]
3. Thippeswamy, B.; Thakker, S.; Tubachi, S.; Kalyani, G.; Netra, M.; Patil, U.; Desai, S.; Gavimath, C.; Veerapur, V. Cardioprotective effect of Cucumis trigonus Roxb on Isoproterenol-induced myocardial infarction in rat. *Am. J. Pharmaco. Toxico.* **2009**, *4*, 29–37. [CrossRef]
4. Nwokocha, C.; Palacios, J.; Simirgiotis, M.J.; Thomas, J.; Nwokocha, M.; Young, L.; Thompson, R.; Cifuentes, F.; Paredes, A.; Delgoda, R. Aqueous extract from leaf of Artocarpus altilis provides cardio-protection from isoproterenol induced myocardial damage in rats: Negative chronotropic and inotropic effects. *J. Ethnopharmacol.* **2017**, *203*, 163–170. [CrossRef] [PubMed]
5. Singal, P.K.; Beamish, R.E.; Dhalla, N.S. Potential oxidative pathways of catecholamines in the formation of lipid peroxides and genesis of heart disease. *Adv. Exp. Med. Biol.* **1983**, *161*, 391–401. [PubMed]
6. Haenen, G.R.; Veerman, M.; Bast, A. Reduction of beta-adrenoceptor function by oxidative stress in the heart. *Free Radic Biol. Med.* **1990**, *9*, 279–288. [CrossRef]

7. Tappia, P.S.; Hata, T.; Hozaima, L.; Sandhu, M.S.; Panagia, V.; Dhalla, N.S. Role of oxidative stress in catecholamine-induced changes in cardiac sarcolemmal Ca^{2+} transport. *Arch. Biochem. Biophys.* **2001**, *387*, 85–92. [CrossRef]
8. Jagadeesh, G.S.; Nagoor Meeran, M.F.; Selvaraj, P. Activation of β1-adrenoceptor triggers oxidative stress mediated myocardial membrane destabilization in isoproterenol induced myocardial infarcted rats: 7-hydroxycoumarin and its counter action. *Eur. J. Pharmacol.* **2016**, *777*, 70–77. [CrossRef]
9. Bystrom, L.M.; Lewis, B.A.; Brown, D.L.; Rodriguez, E.; Obendorf, R.L. Phenolics, Sugars, Antimicrobial and Free-Radical-Scavenging Activities of Melicoccus bijugatus Jacq. Fruits from the Dominican Republic and Florida. *Plant Food. Hum. Nutr.* **2009**, *64*, 160–166. [CrossRef]
10. Bystrom, L.M. The potential health effects of Melicoccus bijugatus Jacq. fruits: Phytochemical, chemotaxonomic and ethnobotanical investigations. *Fitoterapia* **2012**, *83*, 266–271. [CrossRef]
11. Padilla, F.C.; Rincon, A.M.; Bou-Rached, L. Polyphenol content and antioxidant activity of several seeds and nuts. *Arch. Latinoam. Nutr.* **2008**, *58*, 303–308. [PubMed]
12. Bystrom, L.M.; Lewis, B.A.; Brown, D.L.; Rodriguez, E.; Obendorf, R.L. Characterisation of phenolics by LC–UV/Vis, LC–MS/MS and sugars by GC in Melicoccus bijugatus Jacq. 'Montgomery' fruits. *Food Chem.* **2008**, *111*, 1017–1024. [CrossRef] [PubMed]
13. Brooks, W.W.; Conrad, C.H. Isoproterenol-induced myocardial injury and diastolic dysfunction in mice: Structural and functional correlates. *Comp. Med.* **2009**, *59*, 339–343. [PubMed]
14. Cifuentes, F.; Bravo, J.; Norambuena, M.; Stegen, S.; Ayavire, A.; Palacios, J. Chronic exposure to arsenic in tap water reduces acetylcholine-induced relaxation in the aorta and increases oxidative stress in female rats. *Int. J. Toxicol.* **2009**, *28*, 534–541. [CrossRef] [PubMed]
15. Arora, R.; Deshmukh, R. Embelin Attenuates Intracerebroventricular Streptozotocin-Induced Behavioral, Biochemical, and Neurochemical Abnormalities in Rats. *Mol. Neurobiol.* **2017**, *54*, 6670–6680. [CrossRef] [PubMed]
16. Simirgiotis, M.J.; Quispe, C.; Mocan, A.; Villatoro, J.M.; Areche, C.; Bórquez, J.; Sepúlveda, B.; Echiburu-Chau, C. UHPLC high resolution orbitrap metabolomic fingerprinting of the unique species Ophryosporus triangularis Meyen from the Atacama Desert, Northern Chile. *Rev. Bras. Farmacogn.* **2017**. [CrossRef]
17. Vuong, Q.V.; Hirun, S.; Phillips, P.A.; Chuen, T.L.K.; Bowyer, M.C.; Goldsmith, C.D.; Scarlett, C.J. Fruit-derived phenolic compounds and pancreatic cancer: Perspectives from Australian native fruits. *J. Ethnopharmacol.* **2014**, *152*, 227–242. [CrossRef]
18. Simirgiotis, M.J.; Quispe, C.; Bórquez, J.; Areche, C.; Sepúlveda, B.X. Fast Detection of Phenolic Compounds in Extracts of Easter Pears (Pyrus communis) from the Atacama Desert by Ultrahigh-Performance Liquid Chromatography and Mass Spectrometry (UHPLC-Q/Orbitrap/MS/MS). *Molecules* **2016**, *21*, 92. [CrossRef]
19. Jiménez-Sánchez, C.; Lozano-Sánchez, J.; Rodríguez-Pérez, C.; Segura-Carretero, A.; Fernández-Gutiérrez, A. Comprehensive, untargeted, and qualitative RP-HPLC-ESI-QTOF/MS2 metabolite profiling of green asparagus (Asparagus officinalis). *J. Food Compos. Anal.* **2016**, *46*, 78–87. [CrossRef]
20. Simirgiotis, M.J.; Ramirez, J.E.; Hirschmann, G.S.; Kennelly, E.J. Bioactive coumarins and HPLC-PDA-ESI-ToF-MS metabolic profiling of edible queule fruits (Gomortega keule), an endangered endemic Chilean species. *Food Res. Int.* **2013**, *54*, 532–543. [CrossRef]
21. Dong, M.; Oda, Y.; Hirota, M. (10E,12Z,15Z)-9-hydroxy-10,12,15-octadecatrienoic acid methyl ester as an anti-inflammatory compound from Ehretia dicksonii. *Biosci. Biotechnol. Biochem.* **2000**, *64*, 882–886. [CrossRef]
22. Oguro, D.; Watanabe, H. Asymmetric Synthesis and Sensory Evaluation of Sedanenolide. *Biosci. Biotech. Bioch.* **2011**, *75*, 1502–1505. [CrossRef]
23. Torkamani, M.R.D.; Abbaspour, N.; Jafari, M.; Samadi, A. Elicitation of Valerenic Acid in the Hairy Root Cultures of Valeriana officinalis L (Valerianaceae). *Trop. J. Pharm. Res.* **2014**, *13*, 943–949. [CrossRef]
24. Ishizaka, N.; Tomiyama, K.; Katsui, N.; Murai, A.; Masamune, T. Biological activities of rishitin, an antifungal compound isolated from diseased potato tubers, and its derivatives1. *Plant Cell Physiol.* **1969**, *10*, 183–192. [CrossRef]
25. Zhang, H.Y.; Gao, Y.; Lai, P.X. Chemical Composition, Antioxidant, Antimicrobial and Cytotoxic Activities of Essential Oil from Premna microphylla Turczaninow. *Molecules* **2017**, *22*, 381. [CrossRef]

26. Subash, D.; Kapoor, N.; Nityanand, S. Effect of isoprenaline on lipid profil and cardiac enzymes in rats. *Ind. J. Exp. Biol.* **1978**, *16*, 376–378.
27. Nirmala, C.; Puvanakrishnan, R. Protective role of curcumin against isoproterenol induced myocardial infarction in rats. *Mol. Cell Biochem.* **1996**, *159*, 85–93. [CrossRef] [PubMed]
28. Montessuit, C.; Thorburn, A. Transcriptional activation of the glucose transporter GLUT1 in ventricular cardiac myocytes by hypertrophic agonists. *J. Biol. Chem.* **1999**, *274*, 9006–9012. [CrossRef]
29. Patel, V.; Upaganlawar, A.; Zalawadia, R.; Balaraman, R. Cardioprotective effect of melatonin against isoproterenol induced myocardial infarction in rats: A biochemical, electrocardiographic and histoarchitectural evaluation. *Eur. J. Pharmacol.* **2010**, *644*, 160–168. [CrossRef]
30. Li, P.G.; Xu, J.W.; Ikeda, K.; Kobayakawa, A.; Kayano, Y.; Mitani, T.; Ikami, T.; Yamori, Y. Caffeic acid inhibits vascular smooth muscle cell proliferation induced by angiotensin II in stroke-prone spontaneously hypertensive rats. *Hypertens. Res.* **2005**, *28*, 369–377. [CrossRef] [PubMed]
31. Luceri, C.; Giannini, L.; Lodovici, M.; Antonucci, E.; Abbate, R.; Masini, E.; Dolara, P. *p*-Coumaric acid, a common dietary phenol, inhibits platelet activity in vitro and in vivo. *Br. J. Nutr.* **2007**, *97*, 458–463. [CrossRef] [PubMed]
32. Ghoneim, M.A.; Hassan, A.I.; Mahmoud, M.G.; Asker, M.S. Protective Effect of Adansonia digitata against Isoproterenol-Induced Myocardial Injury in Rats. *Anim. Biotechnol.* **2016**, *27*, 84–95. [CrossRef] [PubMed]
33. Dianita, R.; Jantan, I.; Amran, A.Z.; Jalil, J. Protective effects of Labisia pumila var. alata on biochemical and histopathological alterations of cardiac muscle cells in isoproterenol-induced myocardial infarction rats. *Molecules* **2015**, *20*, 4746–4763. [CrossRef] [PubMed]
34. Sabeena Farvin, K.H.; Anandan, R.; Kumar, S.H.; Shiny, K.S.; Sankar, T.V.; Thankappan, T.K. Effect of squalene on tissue defense system in isoproterenol-induced myocardial infarction in rats. *Pharmacol. Res.* **2004**, *50*, 231–236. [CrossRef] [PubMed]
35. Zhang, J.; Knapton, A.; Lipshultz, S.E.; Weaver, J.L.; Herman, E.H. Isoproterenol-induced cardiotoxicity in sprague-dawley rats: Correlation of reversible and irreversible myocardial injury with release of cardiac troponin T and roles of iNOS in myocardial injury. *Toxicol. Pathol.* **2008**, *36*, 277–278. [CrossRef] [PubMed]
36. Ismail, Z.; Mahmoud, A.; Khaled, R.; Sami, A.; Karim, A.; Iyad, A.; Mohamed, K.; Samir, K.; Moaath, J.; Ahmad, A. Effects of experimental acute myocardial infarction on blood cell counts and plasma biochemical values in a nude rat model (Crl:NIH-Fox1RNU). *Comp. Clin. Pathol.* **2009**, *18*, 433–437. [CrossRef]
37. Sangeetha, T.; Quine, S.D. Protective effect of S-allyl cysteine sulphoxide (alliin) on glycoproteins and hematology in isoproterenol induced myocardial infarction in male Wistar rats. *J. Appl. Toxicol.* **2008**, *28*, 710–716. [CrossRef]
38. Nyonseu Nzebang, D.C.; Ngaha Njila, M.I.; Bend, E.F.; Oundoum Oundoum, P.C.; Koloko, B.L.; Bogning Zangueu, C.; Belle Ekedi, P.; Sameza, M.; Massoma Lembè, D. Evaluation of the toxicity of Colocasia esculenta (Araceae): Preliminary study of leaves infected by Phytophthora colocasiae on wistar albinos rats. *Biomed. Pharmacother.* **2018**, *99*, 1009–1013. [CrossRef] [PubMed]
39. Zunjar, V.; Dash, R.P.; Jivrajani, M.; Trivedi, B.; Nivsarkar, M. Antithrombocytopenic activity of carpaine and alkaloidal extract of Carica papaya Linn. leaves in busulfan induced thrombocytopenic Wistar rats. *J. Ethnopharmacol.* **2016**, *181*, 20–25. [CrossRef]
40. Cifuentes, F.; Paredes, A.; Palacios, J.; Muñoz, F.; Carvajal, L.; Nwokocha, C.R.; Morales, G. Hypotensive and antihypertensive effects of a hydroalcoholic extract from Senecio nutans Sch. Bip. (Compositae) in mice: Chronotropic and negative inotropic effect, a nifedipine-like action. *J. Ethnopharmacol.* **2016**, *179*, 367–374. [CrossRef]
41. Cifuentes, F.; Palacios, J.; Nwokocha, C.R. Synchronization in the Heart Rate and the Vasomotion in Rat Aorta: Effect of Arsenic Trioxide. *Cardiovasc. Toxicol.* **2016**, *16*, 79–88. [CrossRef] [PubMed]
42. Simirgiotis, M.J.; Quispe, C.; Bórquez, J.; Schmeda-Hirschmann, G.; Avendaño, M.; Sepúlveda, B.; Winterhalter, P. Fast high resolution Orbitrap MS fingerprinting of the resin of Heliotropium taltalense Phil. from the Atacama Desert. *Ind. Crops Prod.* **2016**, *85*, 159–166. [CrossRef]

43. Garneau, F.X.; Collin, G.J.; Jean, F.I.; Gagnon, H.; Lopez Arze, J.B. Essential oils from Bolivia. XII. Asteraceae: Ophryosporus piquerioides (DC) Benth. ex Baker. *J. Essent. Oil Res.* **2013**, *25*, 388–393. [CrossRef]
44. Cifuentes, F.; Palacios, J.; Paredes, A.; Nwokocha, C.R.; Paz, C. 8-Oxo-9-Dihydromakomakine Isolated from Aristotelia chilensis Induces Vasodilation in Rat Aorta: Role of the Extracellular Calcium Influx. *Molecules* **2018**, *23*, 3050. [CrossRef] [PubMed]

Sample Availability: Samples of *Melicoccus bijugatus* is available from the corresponding author.

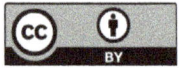

© 2019 by the authors. Licensee MDPI, Basel, Switzerland. This article is an open access article distributed under the terms and conditions of the Creative Commons Attribution (CC BY) license (http://creativecommons.org/licenses/by/4.0/).

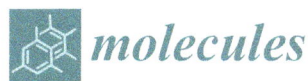

Article

Metabolomics Profiling Reveals Rehmanniae Radix Preparata Extract Protects against Glucocorticoid-Induced Osteoporosis Mainly via Intervening Steroid Hormone Biosynthesis

Tianshuang Xia [1,†], Xin Dong [1,†], Yiping Jiang [1,†], Liuyue Lin [1], Zhimin Dong [1], Yi Shen [1], Hailiang Xin [1,*], Qiaoyan Zhang [1,2,*] and Luping Qin [1,2,*]

[1] Department of Pharmacognosy, Second Military Medical University School of Pharmacy, Shanghai 200433, China; xiatianshuang@smmu.edu.cn (T.X.); dongxinsmmu@126.com (X.D.); msjyp@163.com (Y.J.); linliuyue2016@163.com (L.L.); dongzhiminedu@163.com (Z.D.); 18065148122@163.com (Y.S.)
[2] Zhejiang Chinese Medical University School of Pharmacy, Hangzhou 310053, China
* Correspondence: hailiangxin@163.com (H.X.); zqy1965@163.com (Q.Z.); qinsmmu@126.com (L.Q.); Tel.: +86-021-81871309 (L.Q.)
† These authors contributed equally to this work.

Received: 4 December 2018; Accepted: 5 January 2019; Published: 11 January 2019

Abstract: Rehmanniae Radix Preparata (RR), the dry rhizome of *Rehmannia glutinosa* Libosch., is a traditional herbal medicine for improving the liver and kidney function. Ample clinical and pharmacological experiments show that RR can prevent post-menopausal osteoporosis and senile osteoporosis. In the present study, in vivo and in vitro experiments, as well as a UHPLC-Q/TOF-MS-based metabolomics study, were used to explore the preventing effect of RR on glucocorticoid-induced osteoporosis (GIOP) and its underlying mechanisms. As a result, RR significantly enhanced bone mineral density (BMD), improved the micro-architecture of trabecular bone, and intervened in biochemical markers of bone metabolism in dexamethasone (DEX)-treated rats. For the in vitro experiment, RR increased the cell proliferation and alkaline phosphatase (ALP) activity, enhanced the extracellular matrix mineralization level, and improved the expression of runt-related transcription factor 2 (RUNX2) and osteopontin (OPN) in DEX-injured osteoblasts. For the metabolomics study, a total of 27 differential metabolites were detected in the DEX group vs. the control group, of which 10 were significantly reversed after RR treatment. These metabolites were majorly involved in steroid hormone biosynthesis, sex steroids regulation, and amino acid metabolism. By metabolic pathway and Western blotting analysis, it was further ascertained that RR protected against DEX-induced bone loss, mainly via interfering steroid hormone biosynthesis, as evidenced by the up-regulation of cytochrome P450 17A1 (CYP17A1) and aromatase (CYP19A1), and the down-regulation of 11β-hydroxysteroid dehydrogenase (HSD11B1). Collectively, these results indicated that RR had a notable preventing effect on GIOP, and the action mechanism might be related to steroid hormone biosynthesis.

Keywords: Rehmanniae Radix Preparata; glucocorticoid-induced osteoporosis; metabolomics; osteoblast; steroid hormone biosynthesis

1. Introduction

Glucocorticoids (GC) are widely used in clinics to treat rheumatoid arthritis, pulmonary, gastrointestinal, and autoimmune diseases for their excellent anti-inflammatory and immune-modulatory effects [1]. However, the life-time service of GC usually induces a series of complications, among which osteoporosis is the most devastating one. Currently, glucocorticoids-induced osteoporosis (GIOP) has become the third most-common etiology of pathological bone loss, only next to senile osteoporosis and postmenopausal osteoporosis. The underlying pathological mechanism of GIOP mainly lies in the direct inhibition of the osteoblastic cell cycle, differentiation, and function, and the stimulating action on endogenous gonadal steroids degeneration [2,3]. Clinical treatment for GIOP mainly includes calcium and active vitamin D supplementation and oral bisphosphonates, which is similar to that for postmenopausal osteoporosis and senile osteoporosis, and is incompatible with the pathological mechanism of GIOP. Besides, these therapeutic regimens may cause some potential adverse reactions, such as gastroesophageal irritation [4] and osteonecrosis of the jaw [5]. Thus, there is a desperate need to develop suitable therapeutic alternatives for GIOP with few adverse effects.

Rehmanniae Radix Preparata (RR), prepared from the dry rhizome of *Rehmannia glutinosa* Libosch., has traditionally been used for tonifying kidney essence in China [6]. This herb was first officially recorded in the Chinese Pharmacopoeia of 1963 version, and up to now, more than 140 compounds have been isolated and identified, including iridoid glycosides, phenylethanoid glycosides, monoterpenoids, and triterpenes. In traditional Chinese medicine (TCM), the kidney is in charge of bone, and bone loss is attributed to the kidney and liver deficiency. According to TCM theory, RR can promote the liver and kidney function. Hence, RR and TCM formulas containing RR are widely used to treat osteoporosis patients. In modern pharmacological studies, ample experiments have been used to understand the effect of RR on preventing osteoporosis. The water extract of RR was proved to improve BMD and increase the cortical bone thickness and trabeculation of the bone marrow spaces [7]. Liuwei Dihuang Pill, a traditional Chinese medicine formula mainly containing RR, was also proved to have remarkably preventive and therapeutic effects on primary osteoporosis through promoting bone formation [8,9]. In addition, it is noteworthy that RR can prevent the decrease of the splenic estrogen receptor and osteoblastic progestin receptor in aging female mice [10]. Inspired by these findings, we wonder if and how RR can alleviate bone loss induced by GC.

Metabolomics is a sensitive and unbiased analytical method that is used to comprehensively characterize the metabolite content of biological samples for understanding disease phenotypes. Metabolomics is characterized by "integrity and systematization", which is consistent with the "multi-component and multi-target" theory in TCM [11]. Analysis of metabolite profiling before and after treatment with TCM can help explore their comprehensive therapeutic efficacies and action mechanisms. In this study, an untargeted metabolomics strategy based on UHPLC-Q-TOF/MS was employed to analyze the metabolic profile of GIOP rats, intending to better understand the action mechanism of RR on preventing DEX-induced bone loss and provide more promising candidates for the prevention and treatment for GIOP.

2. Results

2.1. UHPLC-MS Analysis of RR Extract

The UHPLC-MS characteristics of RR extract were detected. As shown in Figure 1, RR extract contains catalpol, acteoside, and echinacoside.

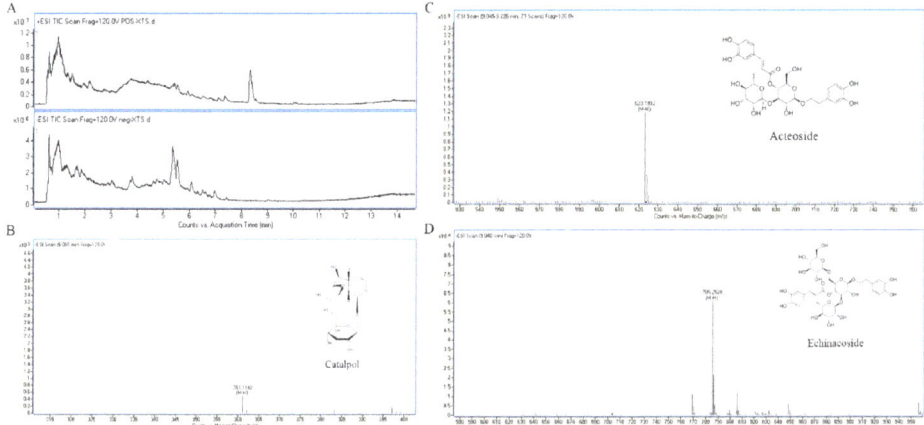

Figure 1. UHPLC-MS characteristics of RR extract. (**A**) The representative total ion chromatograms (TICs) in positive and negative ion mode; (**B**) catalpol in the RR extract sample; (**C**) acteoside in the RR extract sample; (**D**) echinacoside in the RR extract sample.

2.2. RR Improves the Micro-Architecture and BMD of the Femur in DEX-Treated Rats

As shown in Figure 2A–C, the micro-CT analysis showed a severe impairment of bone micro-architecture in the femur of DEX-treated rats, and the trabecular region exhibited a small, thin, and sparse morphology. RR could obviously improve the trabecular micro-architecture, with a slightly disordered trabecular arrangement and mild expanding medullary cavity. As shown in Figure 2D–G, the morphologic parameters of trabecular thickness (Tb.Th.) and bone volume fraction (BVF) decreased significantly, and trabecular separation (Tb.Sp.) and bone surface to bone volume (BS/BV) increased significantly in the femur of DEX-treated rats compared with those in the normal group ($p < 0.01$). RR treatment could significantly reverse the alterations of trabecular morphologic parameters, increase Tb.Th. and BVF, and decrease Tb.Sp. and BS/BV ($p < 0.01$). In addition, as shown in Figure 2K–H, DEX significantly reduced the BMD, bone mineral content (BMC), tissue mineral density (TMD), and tissue mineral content (TMC) compared with those in the normal group ($p < 0.01$), while RR administration significantly enhanced these indices ($p < 0.01$).

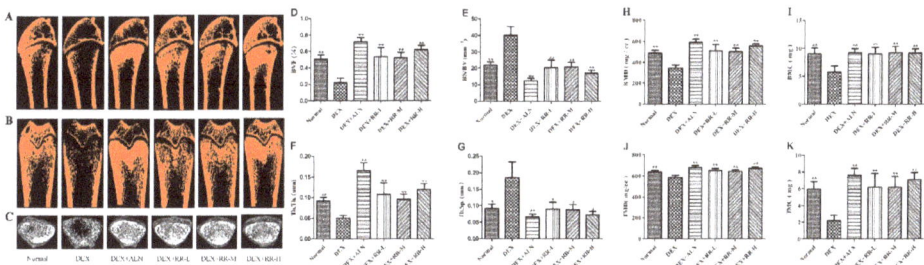

Figure 2. The region of interest (ROI) image and bone parameters analysis in the distal femur in DEX-treated rats. (**A–C**) Micro-CT images of ROI region in longitudinal section, transverse section, and 3-D architecture. (**D–K**) Trabecular bone parameters analysis of (**D**) BVF; (**E**) BS/BV; (**F**) Tb.Th.; (**G**) Tb.Sp.; (**H**) BMD; (**I**) BMC; (**J**) TMD; and (**K**) TMC in the distal femur region in DEX-treated rats. Values were expressed as the mean ± SD; $n = 7$. * $p < 0.05$, ** $p < 0.01$ compared with DEX group.

2.3. RR Regulates Bone Metabolism-Related Biochemical Markers in DEX-Treated Rats

As shown in Figure 3A–C, DEX significantly increased the urine calcium (U-Ca) level and decreased the serum phosphorus (S-P) level compared with those in the normal group ($p < 0.01$). RR at low- and medium-doses significantly reduced the U-Ca level, and increased the S-P level, in DEX-treated rats ($p < 0.05$). There was no significant difference in the serum calcium (S-Ca) level between the six groups. Alkaline phosphatase (ALP), bone gla-protein (BGP), deoxypyridinoline (DPD), and c-terminal telopeptides of type I collagen (CTX-I) are biochemical markers of bone turnover. As shown in Figure 3D–G, DEX significantly decreased the serum ALP level, and increased the urine DPD and serum CTX-I levels, compared with those in the normal group ($p < 0.01$ or $p < 0.05$). RR at medium- and high-dosages could significantly increase the ALP level and decrease the DPD level in DEX-treated rats ($p < 0.01$ or $p < 0.05$). RR also insignificantly decreased BGP and CTX-I levels in DEX-treated rats.

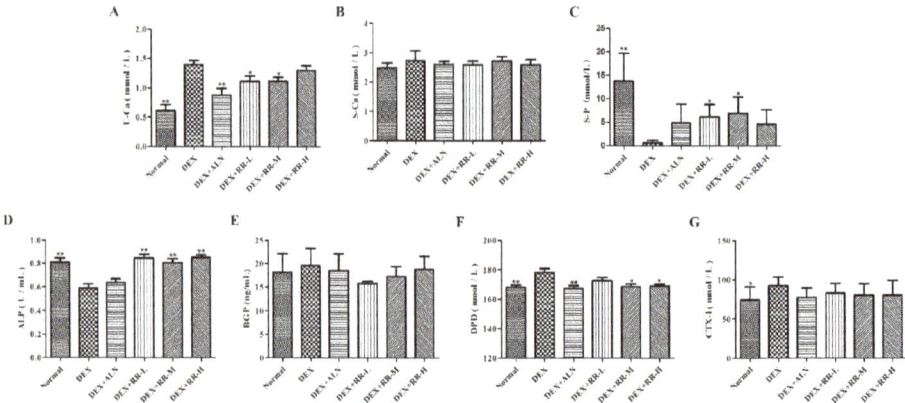

Figure 3. Effects of RR on biochemical markers levels of bone metabolism in DEX-treated rats. (**A**) U-Ca; (**B**) S-Ca; (**C**) S-P; (**D**) ALP; (**E**) BGP; (**F**) DPD; (**G**) CTX-I. Values were expressed as the mean ± SD; $n = 7$. * $p < 0.05$, ** $p < 0.01$ compared with DEX group.

2.4. RR Enhances the Proliferation, Differentiation, and Mineralization Levels of Osteoblasts Injured by DEX

To further validate the in vitro effect of RR on preventing bone loss, the activities of DEX-injured osteoblasts were assayed. The results showed that DEX significantly decreased the proliferation (Figure 4A), ALP activity (Figure 4B), and mineralization level (Figure 4C,D) of osteoblasts ($p < 0.01$). After treatment, RR at doses of 0.2 mg/L and 1 mg/L significantly increased the cells' proliferation compared with that of the DEX-treated control ($p < 0.05$). RR at all dosages prominently increased the ALP activity ($p < 0.01$ or $p < 0.05$), and the intensity and area of staining, as well as promoted the formation of mineralized nodules in DEX-treated osteoblasts ($p < 0.01$). In addition, DEX inhibited the expression of RUNX2 and OPN compared with that in the control group, while RR treatment improved the RUNX2 and OPN expression in DEX-injured osteoblasts to some extent (Figure 4E).

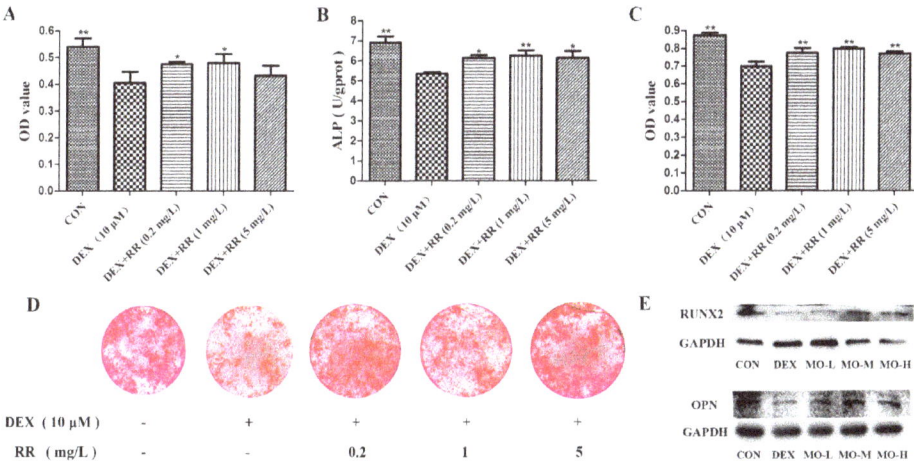

Figure 4. Effects of RR on the proliferation, differentiation, and mineralization levels of DEX-injured osteoblasts. (**A**) MTT assay; (**B**) ALP activity; (**C**) extracellular matrix mineralization; (**D**) representative images of osteoblastic bone mineralization nodule stained with alizarin red; (**E**) the protein expressions of RUNX2 and OPN. Values were expressed as the mean ± SD; (**A**) $n = 4$, (**B–F**) $n = 3$. * $p < 0.05$, ** $p < 0.01$ compared with DEX group.

2.5. Metabolomics Analysis

The TICs in both positive and negative ion modes of urine samples from three experimental groups are shown in Figure S1. The QC superposed graph is shown in Figure S2. To determine whether metabolite fingerprints in urine differed between the control, DEX, and DEX+RR-M groups in the metabolomics approach, the partial least squares discriminant analysis (PLS-DA) model was applied. The metabolic profiles showed that urine samples of the DEX group evidently separated from those of the normal group. Samples of the DEX+MO group were situated close to those of the control group and far away from those of the DEX group (Figure 5A,B). Validation of the PLS-DA model exhibited a good fitting degree (Figure 5C,D).

2.6. Identification of Potential Biomarkers in DEX-treated Rats

Variables far from the origin in the S-plot (Figure 5E,F) with a variable importance plot (VIP) > 1 and $p < 0.05$ were applied to select potential biomarkers. As a result, 27 differential metabolites between rats in the control group and DEX group were selected as potential biomarkers, 23 of which were the only ones for which the endogenous compound matched with the accurate mass via online database Metlin and Human Metabolome Database (HMDB), except for dipeptide. These differential metabolites were mainly involved in amino acid metabolism, fatty acid biosynthesis, steroid hormone biosynthesis, and arachidonic acid metabolism (Table 1).

Table 1. Screening of potential biomarkers in rat urine.

NO.	Metabolite Identification	Rt (min)	m/z	Adduct	VIP	Fold Change Value DEX/Control	Fold Change Value DEX+RR/DEX	p-Value DEX/Control	p-Value DEX+RR/DEX	Related Pathway	HMDB/MELIN ID
1	Glycine	3.818	76.0395	[M+H]⁺	1.78	0.491	1.280	0.025 *	0.845	Amino acid metabolism	HMDB0000123
2	Benzoic acid	2.449	140.0701	[M+NH₄]⁺	1.23	2.219	0.496	0.006 **	0.013 *	Amino acid metabolism	HMDB0001870
3	N-Acetylproline	2.450	158.0807	[M+H]⁺	2.29	2.155	0.492	0.008 **	0.012 *	Amino acid metabolism	HMDB0094701
4	Naphthol	0.842	162.0926	[M+NH₄]⁺	2.20	2.192	0.574	0.047 *	0.158	Metabolism of xenobiotics by cytochrome P450	HMDB0012138/ HMDB0012322
5	Indoleacetic acid	3.823	198.0513	[M+Na]⁺	1.30	0.467	1.280	0.013 *	0.848	Amino acid metabolism	HMDB0000197
6	4-Pyridoxic acid	1.156	201.0860	[M+H]⁺	1.05	0.373	2.167	0.000 **	0.014 *	Vitamin B6 metabolism	HMDB0000017
7	N-Hydroxy-L-tyrosine	1.563	215.1006	[M+NH₄]⁺	2.08	0.307	1.869	0.000 **	0.312	Amino acid metabolism	HMDB0038750
8	N-alpha-Acetylcitrulline	1.154	218.1137	[M+H]⁺	1.21	0.396	1.964	0.001 **	0.057	Amino acid metabolism	HMDB0000856
9	3-Oxododecanoic acid	6.690	232.1898	[M+NH₄]⁺	1.24	2.714	0.720	0.010 *	0.442	Fatty acid biosynthesis	HMDB0010727
10	Valerylcarnitine/Isovalerylcarnitine	5.306	246.1698	[M+H]⁺	1.15	2.136	0.725	0.042 *	0.479	Fatty acid biosynthesis	HMDB0013128/ HMDB0000688
11	N-Phenylacetylaspartic acid	4.080	252.0842	[M+H]⁺	1.53	2.064	0.551	0.007 **	0.022 *	Amino acid metabolism	HMDB0029355
12	Palmitic acid/Isopalmitic acid	9.939	274.2743	[M+NH₄]⁺	5.52	0.741	1.156	0.013 *	0.463	Fatty acid biosynthesis	HMDB0000220/ HMDB0031068
13	Androsterone/Epiandrosterone	8.665	313.2156	[M+Na]⁺	1.61	3.719	0.592	0.001 **	0.048 *	Steroid hormone biosynthesis	HMDB0000031/ HMDB0000365
14	Hydroxypregnenolone	10.545	333.2407	[M+H]⁺	1.01	0.414	1.438	0.029 *	0.795	Steroid hormone biosynthesis	—
15	Galactosylhydroxylysine	6.575	342.1904	[M+NH₄]⁺	1.01	6.878	0.867	0.006 **	0.942	Energy metabolism	HMDB0000600
16	11-Dehydrocorticosterone	9.011	345.2061	[M+H]⁺	1.90	0.325	3.389	0.003 **	0.001 **	Steroid hormone biosynthesis	HMDB0004029
17	Corticosterone	9.537	347.2219	[M+H]⁺	2.53	0.289	4.163	0.128	0.035 *	Steroid hormone biosynthesis	HMDB0001547
18	Arachidonic acid/Arachidonate	10.055	349.2378	[M+FA-H]⁻	1.87	0.306	0.853	0.014 *	0.989	Arachidonic acid metabolism	HMDB0011043/ HMDB0060102

Table 1. *Cont.*

NO.	Metabolite Identification	Rt (min)	m/z	Adduct	VIP	Fold Change Value		P-Value		Related Pathway	HMDB/ METLIN ID
						DEX/Control	DEX+RR/DEX	DEX/Control	DEX+RR/DEX		
19	Docosapentaenoic acid	9.795	353.2475	[M+Na]+	3.45	3.137	0.413	0.032 *	0.077	Fatty acid biosynthesis	HMDB0006528/ HMDB0001976
20	MG(t6:0/16:0/0:0)	13.949	353.2667	[M+Na]+	2.57	0.670	0.964	0.010 *	0.991	Fatty acid biosynthesis	—
21	**18-Hydroxycorticosterone**	9.008	361.2016	[M-H]-	1.59	0.215	4.840	0.001 **	0.000 **	Steroid hormone biosynthesis	HMDB0000319
22	HETE	8.666	365.2332	[M+FA-H]-	3.04	3.978	0.503	0.000 **	0.110	Arachidonic acid metabolism	—
23	**Cortolone**	8.667	367.2478	[M+H]+	1.40	4.327	0.553	0.000 **	0.042 *	Steroid hormone biosynthesis	HMDB0003128
24	Carbocyclic Thromboxane A2	9.793	371.2576	[M+Na]+	4.34	2.766	0.414	0.048 *	0.078	Arachidonic acid metabolism	METLIN-45632
25	α,α-Dimethyl anandamide	13.286	376.3186	[M+Na]+	1.34	1.694	1.017	0.026 *	0.999	Retrograde endocannabinoid signaling	METLIN-36748
26	LysoPA(i-14:0/0:0)	8.665	405.2038	[M+Na]+	2.41	7.529	0.452	0.000 **	0.027 *	Lysophosphatidic metabolism	HMDB0114765
27	O-Arachidonoyl Glycidol	9.789	405.2644	[M+FA-H]-	3.23	3.122	0.286	0.035 *	0.120	Retrograde endocannabinoid signaling	METLIN-44872

* $p < 0.05$, ** $p < 0.01$ compared with DEX group.

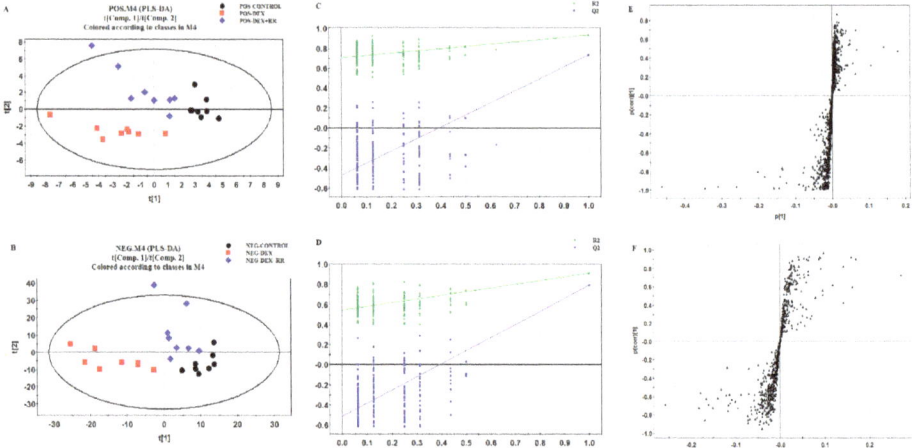

Figure 5. Multivariate analysis based on the UHPLC-Q/TOF-MS profiling data for samples in the control, DEX, and DEX+RR groups in positive and negative ion mode (*n* = 8). (**A**) PLS-DA score plot in positive ion mode; (**B**) validation of PLS-DA model in positive ion mode; (**C**) S-plot of PLS-DA model in positive ion mode; (**D**) PLS-DA score plot in negative ion mode; (**E**) validation of PLS-DA model in negative ion mode; (**F**) S-plot of PLS-DA model in negative ion mode.

2.7. RR Reverses Metabolic Dysregulation in DEX-Treated Rats

The metabolic changes after treatment with RR at 4 g/kg in GIOP rats were studied. Seen in Table 1, the levels of benzoic acid, N-acetylproline, 4-pyridoxic acid, androsterone, N-phenylacetylaspartic acid, 11-dehydrocorticosterone, 18-hydroxycorticosterone, cortolone, corticosterone, and lysoPA were significantly reversed after RR treatment, and these metabolites were majorly involved in steroid hormone biosynthesis, sex steroids regulation, and amino acid metabolism. The heat map was constructed based on the normalized data set of the reversed metabolites, and the results showed that the variation tendency of most metabolites after RR treatment was different from that in DEX group, while the same as that in the control group (Figure 6A). The ingenuity metabolic pathway analysis showed that the potential biomarkers were majorly involved in steroid hormone biosynthesis (Figure 6B). The metabolic pathway map associated with differential metabolites was depicted based on the Kyoto Encyclopedia of Genes and Genomes (KEGG) (Figure 6C). These results showed that RR reversed metabolic dysregulation in DEX-treated rats, mainly via intervening steroid hormone biosynthesis.

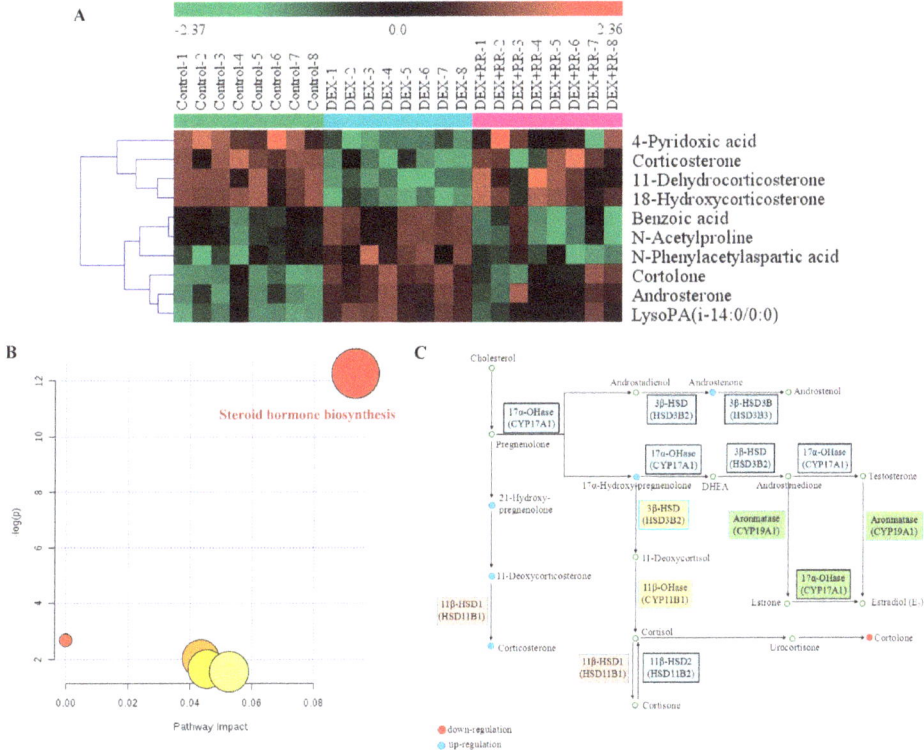

Figure 6. Heat map and metabolic pathway analysis based on the UHPLC-Q/TOF-MS profiling data for samples in the control, DEX, and DEX+RR groups. (**A**) Hierarchical clustering heat map of the differential metabolites before and after RR treatment in DEX-treated rats; (**B**) summary of ingenuity pathway analysis with MetPA. The size and color of each circle were based on pathway impact value and *p*-value, respectively; (**C**) construction of the metabolic pathway related to differential metabolites. The metabolites were labeled in blue (up-regulation after RR treatment) or red (down-regulation after RR treatment).

2.8. RR Regulates the Expressions of Key Proteins in Steroid Hormone Biosynthesis

To further validate the regulatory effect of RR on steroid hormone biosynthesis, the expression of key proteins related to steroid hormone biosynthesis was analyzed by Western blotting. As shown in Figure 7, DEX significantly disturbed the expression of CYP17A1, CYP19A1, HSD11B1, and HSD3B2 ($p < 0.01$ or $p < 0.05$). After treatment, RR at all doses prominently increased the expression of CYP19A1 compared with that in the DEX group ($p < 0.01$ or $p < 0.05$). RR at a dose of 0.2 mg/L prominently increased the expression of CYP17A1 ($p < 0.01$). RR at doses of 1 mg/L and 5 mg/L also significantly inhibited the HSD11B1 expression ($p < 0.05$). However, there was no effect of RR on HSD3B2 expression.

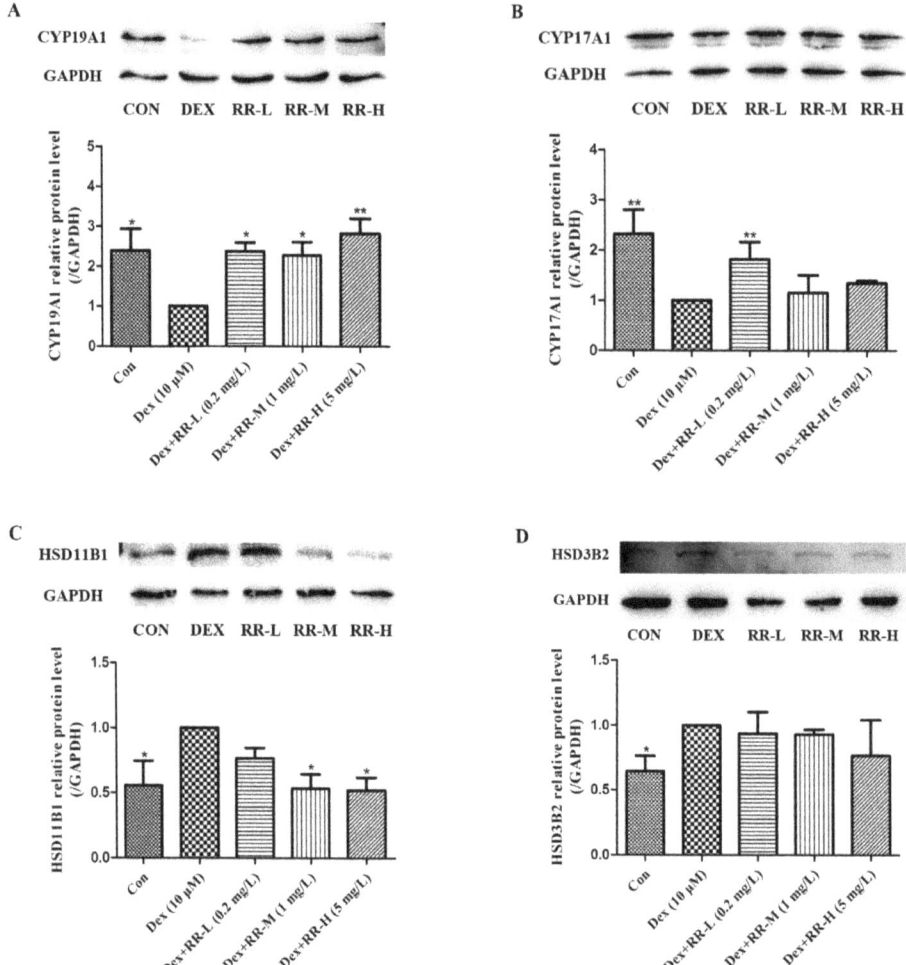

Figure 7. Effects of RR on the expression of key proteins related to steroid hormone biosynthesis. Protein expressions and relative levels of (**A**) CYP19A1; (**B**) CYP17A1; (**C**) HSD11B1; (**D**) HSD3B2 were analyzed by Western blotting. All values are expressed as the mean ± SD; $n = 3$. * $p < 0.05$, ** $p < 0.01$ compared with DEX group.

3. Discussion

GIOP, recognized as the most common iatrogenic cause of secondary osteoporosis, has imposed a serious threat to public health. The present investigation found that RR could prevent GIOP in both DEX-treated rats and DEX-injured osteoblasts. Our metabolomics analysis showed that DEX caused great metabolic disorders, while RR could rebalance the metabolic disruptions, mainly via regulating steroid hormone biosynthesis and amino acid metabolism. Through further pathway and Western blotting analysis, it was ascertained that RR preventing GIOP was related to intervening steroid hormone biosynthesis.

Both human and animal studies demonstrated deleterious skeletal effects within weeks of pharmacological GC administration, as evidenced by the alteration of BMD and the bone micro-architecture. The histomorphometric parameters of the trabecular bone could predict

GC-induced osteopenia and the deterioration of bone quality. The present study found that RR could improve the micro-architecture, enhance the BMD, and increase the trabecular parameters in the femur in DEX-treated rats, suggesting that administration with RR was effective in both preserving bone mass and rescuing the deterioration of bone micro-architecture. It is generally assumed that bone loss in the chronic state of GIOP is mostly attributable to the decrease of osteoblastic bone formation, and excessive GC can inhibit the osteoblastic proliferation, differentiation, and bone matrix mineralization [12]. In this study, RR was able to improve the osteoblastic proliferation, ALP activity, and bone matrix mineralization level, which further prove that RR has a potent anti-GIOP effect. RUNX2 is a regulator in osteoblast differentiation at an early stage, and plays a crucial role in skeletal morphogenesis, tooth development, chondrogenesis, and vasculogenesis [13]. It has been proved that RUNX2 can upregulate the expression of the PI3K-Akt pathway, and enhance its DNA binding ability in immature mesenchymal stem cells (MSCs) and immature osteoblasts [14]. The increased expression of bone matrix proteins, such as ALP, BGP, and OPN, also stimulates mineralization and leads to bone formation [15]. It was found in our study that RR could increase the ALP level in the serum of DEX-treated rats, and enhance the expression of RUNX2 and OPN in DEX-injured osteoblasts, further suggesting that RR was able to promote osteoblastic differentiation.

To delineate the mechanisms underlying the preventive effect of RR against GIOP, a metabolomics profiling of rat urine based on UHPLC-Q-TOF/MS analysis was applied. It is well-known that the deficiency of androgens or estrogens will induce bone loss [16]. Epiandrosterone is a metabolite of the most abundant adrenal androgenic steroid dehydroepiandrosterone (DHEA) [17], and androgens and estrogens are both made from DHEA [18]. It was found in our study that DEX decreased the epiandrosterone or androsterone level in GIOP rats, while RR could reverse its abnormal descent after eight-week treatment. It indicated that DEX might cause androgens and estrogens deficiency via suppressing DHEA secretion, whereas RR made a significant callback of these hormone levels, and further protected against glucocorticoid-induced bone loss. Pregnenolone is a well-known precursor for the biosynthesis of various sex hormones, such as estrogen, progesterone, and testosterone [19]. It has been proved that pregnenolone and its heterocyclic analogues have the potential to become novel anti-osteoporotic agents [20]. Hydroxypregnenolone is converted from pregnenolone by cytochrome P450, and is also involved in the biosynthesis of gonadal steroid hormones and adrenal corticosteroids [18,21]. In our study, a significant decrease of hydroxypregnenolone was found in GIOP rats, and compared with that, there was a rising tendency after RR treatment, indicating that RR could improve the pregnenolone level, and further sustain bone homeostasis.

Dehydrocorticosterone and corticosterone both belong to adrenocortical steroids. It was reported that corticosterone and 11-dehydrocorticosterone levels were decreased in GIOP model rats [22], which was consistent with the finding in the present study. Contrarily, elevated corticosterone, 18-hydroxycorticosterone, and 11-dehydrocorticosterone levels were detected after RR treatment. In addition, it was found in our study that the correlation coefficient of 18-hydroxycorticosterone and 11-dehydrocorticosterone vs. ALP and DPD levels was more than 0.6, suggesting that these two metabolites might be related to bone metabolism. The conversion of inactive 11-dehydrocorticosterone into active corticosterone is catalyzed by 11β-hydroxysteroid dehydrogenase (HSD11B1), which was confirmed to play a crucial role in metabolically relevant tissues, such as skeletal muscles [23]. Previous studies discovered a close relationship between HSD11B1 activity and osteoblast differentiation after continuous injury of human osteoblasts with DEX, and proved that DEX could induce an overexpression of HSD11B1 and decrease osteoblast differentiation [24]. In the present study, an elevated HSD11B1 level was found in DEX-injured osteoblasts, while RR treatment could depress its overexpression, further indicating that RR preventing bone loss might be related to regulating HSD11B1 activity and its conversion of inactive 11-dehydrocorticosterone into active corticosterone.

Except for HSD11B1, some other key proteins participating in steroid hormone biosynthesis also influence bone metabolism. Aromatase, known as cytochrome P450 19A1 (CYP19A1), is closely related to postmenopausal osteoporosis. The aromatase deficiency can result in estrogen deficiency [25], and the estrogen deficiency at menopause accelerated the age-dependent involution of the female skeleton and contributed to the loss of bone mass, architectural integrity, and strength [26]. CYP17A1 encodes an enzyme with both 17α-hydroxylase and 17,20-lyase activities, and 17α-hydroxylase is responsible for hydroxylating pregnelone and progesterone, which are then converted to C19 steroid precursors of testosterone and estrogen by 17,20-lyase activity [27]. The deficiency of CYP17A1 can result in reduced growth and osteoporosis. It was found in our study that RR could improve the CYP19A1 and CYP17A1 levels to some extent, further suggesting that RR preventing GIOP was related to intervening steroid hormone biosynthesis.

In conclusion, pharmacological experiments and UHPLC-Q/TOF-MS-based metabolomics analysis were used to evaluate the effects and underlying mechanisms of RR on protecting against GIOP. In GIOP model rats, RR was able to improve the cancellous bone structure, enhance BMD, and ameliorate bone metabolism homeostasis. In DEX-injured osteoblasts, RR could improve the cell proliferation, differentiation, and mineralization level, and increase the expression of RUNX2 and OPN. Metabolomics profiling indicated that RR might prevent DEX-induced bone loss through regulating sex steroids regulation, steroid hormone biosynthesis and amino acid metabolism. Metabolic pathway and Western blotting analysis further clarified that RR protected against GIOP, mainly via intervening steroid hormone biosynthesis. The above results demonstrated, for the first time, that RR helped protect against GIOP, and provided an excellent candidate for GIOP therapeutics.

4. Methods and Materials

4.1. Chemicals and Reagents

Chemicals and reagents used in this study included chromatographic-grade methanol and acetonitrile (Merck, Darmstadt, Germany); standard chemicals of catalpol, echinacoside, and acteoside (HPLC ≥98%, Shanghai Yuan-ye Bio-Technology Co., Ltd., Shanghai, China); and DEX (Dalian Meilun Biotech Co., Ltd., Dalian, China); ALN (MSD Pharmaceutical Co., Ltd., Hangzhou, China); Ca, P, ALP, and TRAP assay kits (Nanjing Jian Cheng Bioengineering Institute, Nanjing, China); enzyme-linked immunosorbent assay (ELISA) kits for BGP, DPD, and CTX-I (Xin Yu Biological Engineering Co., Ltd., Shanghai, China); antibodies specific for OPN, CYP17A1, CYP19A1, HSD11B1, and HSD3B2 (Abcom, Cambridge, UK); antibodies specific for RUNX2, anti-rabbit IgG, anti-mouse IgG, and GAPDH (CST, Danvers, MA, USA).

4.2. Preparation of RR Extract

RR is the processed product of the dry rhizome of *Rehmannia glutinosa* Libosch. In this study, RR was purchased from Shanghai De Kang Pharmaceutical Co., Ltd. and authorized by Professor Qin Luping, Department of Pharmacognosy, School of Pharmacy of the Second Military Medical University. The voucher specimen (RR 20170328) was deposited in the herbarium of Second Military Medical University. Dried RR (350 g) was cut into small pieces and reflux-extracted with 2.8 L distilled water at 60 °C three times. The extract of RR was concentrated with a vacuum evaporator, and dissolved in an appropriate volume of distilled water, and then adjusted to a concentration of 0.1 g/mL, 0.2 g/mL, and 0.4 g/mL, equivalent to crude drugs for animal experiments, or 0.2 mg/L, 1 mg/L, and 5 mg/L, equivalent to crude drugs for in vitro experiments. The dose of the RR extract was converted according to the clinical dosage of humans.

4.3. UHPLC-MS Analysis of RR Extract

UHPLC-MS analysis was performed on an Agilent 1290 Infinity LC system coupled to an Agilent 6538 accurate-mass quadrupole time-of-flight (Q-TOF) mass spectrometer (Agilent, Palo Alto, CA, USA). Chromatographic separations were performed on an Acquity UHPLC HSS T3 column (2.1 × 100 mm, 2.5 μm, Waters, Milford, MA, USA) at 25 °C, and the injection volume was 3 μL at a flow rate of 0.4 mL/min. The mobile phase consisted of 0.1% formic acid (A) and ACN modified with 0.1% formic acid (B). The gradient program was as follows: 5% B over 0–2 min, 5–95% B over 2–13 min, and 95% B over 13–19 min. The capillary voltage was 4 kV for positive ion mode and 3.5 kV for negative ion mode. The drying gas flow rate was 11 L/min at 350 °C. The nebulizer pressure was 45 psig, the fragmentor voltage was 120 V, and the skimmer voltage was 60 V. Data were collected in a centroid mode and the mass range was m/z 100–1100 using an extended dynamic range.

4.4. Animal Treatment and Samples Collection

Female Sprague-Dawley (SD) rats aged 12 weeks and weighing 180–220 g were purchased from Slacom (Shanghai, China), and maintained at the Experimental Animal Center of the Second Military Medical University. The animals were housed at 24 ± 0.5 °C with a 12-h light and 12-h dark cycle with free access to food and water. After seven-day acclimatization, animals were randomly divided into six groups according to their body weights (n = 8 per group): Normal (saline) group, DEX (DEX 2.5 mg/kg + saline) group, DEX + ALN (DEX 2.5 mg/kg + ALN 1 mg/kg) group, DEX + RR-L (DEX 2.5 mg/kg + RR 1 g/kg) group, DEX + RR-M (DEX 2.5 mg/kg + RR 2 g/kg) group, and DEX + RR-H (DEX 2.5 mg/kg + RR 4 g/kg) group. At the first week, all rats except for those in the normal group were injected with DEX daily via the caudal vein. Then, the rats were injected with DEX via the caudal vein twice a week and orally administered with different dosages of RR daily for eight weeks.

The day before the end of the experiment, rats were housed individually in metabolic cages for 24 h without providing food to collect urine samples. Then, all rats were anesthetized with an intraperitoneal (i.p.) injection of 300 mg/kg chloral hydrate. The blood was collected from the abdomen artery, and centrifuged at 3000 rpm for 10 min to collect the sera. Serum samples were stored at −80°C for biochemical determination and metabolomics profiling. The right femur was prepared for micro-computed tomography scanning. All studies were conducted in accordance with the NIH publication and Second Military Medical University principles for laboratory animal use and care.

4.5. Micro-CT Analysis and Biochemical Marker Measurement

The measurement of trabecular micro-architecture was performed on an micro-CT system (eXplore Locus, GE Healthcare, Boston, MA, USA) with the voltage set at 80 kV, current at 80 µA, angular rotation at 360°, and angular step at 0.4°. The femur was scanned from the proximal growth plate in the distal direction (14 µm/slice). The ROI was selected at a distance of 0.16 mm from the distal end of the growth plate. BMD, BMC, TMD, TMC, Tb.Th., Tb.Sp., BVF, and BS/BV were measured.

The U-Ca, S-Ca, S-P, ALP, and TRAP levels were measured by standard colorimetric methods using commercially available assay kits. The BGP, DPD, and CTX-I levels were measured using the ELISA kits and the micro-plate reader (Thermo Fisher Scientific Inc., Pittsburgh, PA, USA).

4.6. UHPLC-Q-TOF/MS Metabolomics Analysis

Rat urine samples (100 µL) in the control, DEX, and DEX+RR-M groups were added into 300 µL methanol solutions containing 5 µg/mL 2-chloro-L-phenylalanine as the internal standard. The mixed solution was homogenized by vortex for 5 min and centrifuged at 13,000 rpm, 4 °C for 15 min. A total of 150 µL supernatant was filtered through a 0.22 µm membrane for metabolomics studies. The method of UHPLC-Q-TOF/MS metabolomics analysis was the same as that mentioned in Section 4.3. The mobile phase consisted of 0.1% formic acid (A) and ACN modified with 0.1% formic acid (B), and the gradient program was as follows: 5% B over 0–2 min, 5–15% B over 2–8 min, 15–30% B over 8–10 min, 30–95% B over 10–13 min, and 95% B over 13–15 min. The reference ions were 121.0509 and 922.0098 in positive mode, and 112.9856 and 1033.9881 in negative mode. The QC samples were used every eight urine samples to evaluate the stability during sequence analysis.

4.7. Data Processing and Multivariate Analysis

All UHPLC-MS raw data were transformed into common data format (.mzdata) files using Agilent MassHunter qualitative software. The program XCMS (http://metlin.scripps.edu/download/)

was used for peak alignment, peak extraction, and automatic integration. After mean-centering and pareto-scaling procedures, the retention time (RT)-m/z pairs, observations, and relative ion intensities of all detected ions were imported into SIMCA-P 11.0 software package (Umetrics, Umea, Sweden) for principal component analysis (PCA) and PLS-DA. HMDB (http://www.hmdb.ca/) and Metlin database (https://metlin.scripps.edu/) were selected for metabolites matching based on a combination of database queries using exact mass measurements. Additionally, the model of PLS-DA was evaluated according to the cross-validation of R^2, Q^2 value, and permutation test. An independent sample t-test was performed for statistical analysis using SPSS version 20.0 (IBM, USA) and $p < 0.05$ was considered statistically significant. A heat map of the different metabolites was processed by MEV-MultiExperiment Viewer 4.8.1. The pathway analysis of potential biomarkers was performed with MetaboAnalyst (http://www.metaboanalyst.ca/) and KEGG pathway database (http://www.genome.jp/kegg/).

4.8. Osteoblasts Culture

Female Wistar rats aged 24 h were purchased from the Experimental Animal Center of the Second Military Medical University (Shanghai, China). Primary osteoblasts were prepared from the calvarias according to literature [28], and cultured in α-MEM supplemented with 10% FBS at 37 °C in a humidified atmosphere containing 5% CO_2. All studies were conducted in accordance with the NIH publication and Second Military Medical University principles for laboratory animal use and care.

4.9. Osteoblastic MTT and ALP Activity Assay

Osteoblasts were injured with DEX (10 μM), and at the same time treated with RR (0.2, 1 and 5 mg/L) for 48 h in an MTT assay and for seven days in an ALP activity assay. In the MTT assay, 20 μL of 5 mg/mL MTT was added into plates after drugs treatment. The medium was discarded and the formazan crystals that formed in the cells were dissolved in 150 μL of DMSO. Optical density (OD) was measured at 570 nm. For the ALP activity assay, the cells were lysed after drug treatment, and the total protein concentration was measured using a BCA-protein assay kit. The ALP activity was measured according to the conversion of colorless p-nitrophenyl phosphate to colored p-nitrophenol.

4.10. Osteoblastic Bone Matrix Mineralization Assay

Osteoblasts were cultured in osteogenic differentiation medium (α-MEM with 10% FBS, 50 μg/mL ascorbic acid, and 10 mM β-glycerophosphate) for 12 days. Cells were injured with DEX (10 μM), and at the same time treated with RR (0.2, 1 and 5 mg/L) for another nine days in osteogenic differentiation medium. After washing, cells were fixed with ice-cold 4% paraformaldehyde for 10 min. Then, 0.1% Alizarin Red staining solution (pH 8.3) was added and incubated for 30 min at 37 °C. The staining of Alizarin Red was incubated with 5% (v/w) cetylpyridinium chloride for 30 min at 37 °C and OD was measured at 570 nm.

4.11. Western Blotting

Osteoblasts were injured with DEX (10 μM), and at the same time treated with RR (0.2, 1 and 5 mg/L) for 48 h. Then, cells were lysed and centrifuged at 12,000 rpm, 4 °C for 10 min. The protein concentration of the supernatants was determined using the BCA kit. Each sample (20 μg protein) was separated by SDS-PAGE (10% gel) and transferred to polyvinylidene fluoride (PVDF) membranes. The membranes were then blocked in 5% BSA, and incubated with the primary antibodies overnight at 4 °C. After washing with TBS-T, the membranes were incubated with a second antibody for 1 h at room temperature. Immunoreaction signals were detected using electrochemiluminescence (ECL) reagent (Tanon, Shanghai, China), and exposed on a Gel imaging system (Tanon-5200 Multi, Shanghai, China).

4.12. Statistical Analysis

The data were expressed as the mean ± standard deviation (SD) and group differences were determined by one way analysis of variance (ANOVA) with the Turkey test. The analyses were performed using SPSS version 20.0 and $p < 0.05$ was considered statistically significant.

Supplementary Materials: The following are available online, Figure S1: Representative total ion chromatograms (TIC) in metabolomics study; Figure S2: Fig. S2 Quality control (QC) superposed graph in metabolomics study.

Author Contributions: H.X. and L.Q. conceived and designed the research; T.X., X.D. and Y.J. performed and analyzed the data of the metabolomics study; L.L., Z.D. and Y.S. performed and analyzed the data of pharmacological experiments; T.X. and Q.Z. wrote the manuscript. All authors read and approved the manuscript.

Funding: This research was funded by National High-tech R&D Program of China (863 Program, Grant no. 2013AA093003), and National Natural Science Foundation of China (Grant no. U1505226, U1603283).

Conflicts of Interest: The authors declared no conflict of interest.

References

1. Seibel, M.J.; Cooper, M.S.; Zhou, H. Glucocorticoid-induced osteoporosis: Mechanisms, management, and future perspectives. *Lancet Diabetes Endocrinol.* **2013**, *1*, 59–70. [CrossRef]
2. Yang, Y.; Nian, H.; Tang, X.; Wang, X.; Liu, R. Effects of the combined Herba Epimedii and Fructus Ligustri Lucidi on bone turnover and TGF-β1/Smads pathway in GIOP rats. *J. Ethnopharmacol.* **2017**, *201*, 91–99. [CrossRef] [PubMed]
3. Mak, W.; Shao, X.; Dunstan, C.R.; Seibel, M.J.; Zhou, H. Biphasic Glucocorticoid-dependent regulation of Wnt expression and its inhibitors in mature osteoblastic cells. *Calcif. Tissue Int.* **2009**, *85*, 538–545. [CrossRef] [PubMed]
4. Abrahamsen, B. Adverse effects of bisphosphonates. *Calcif. Tissue Int.* **2010**, *86*, 421–435. [CrossRef] [PubMed]
5. Pozzi, S.; Marcheselli, R.; Sacchi, S.; Baldini, L.; Angrilli, F.; Pennese, E.; Quarta, G.; Stelitano, C.; Caparotti, G.; Luminari, S.; et al. Bisphosphonate-associated osteonecrosis of the jaw: A review of 35 cases and an evaluation of its frequency in multiple myeloma patients. *Leuk. Lymphoma* **2007**, *48*, 56–64. [CrossRef] [PubMed]
6. Liu, C.; Ma, R.; Wang, L.; Zhu, R.; Liu, H.; Guo, Y.; Zhao, B.; Zhao, S.; Tang, J.; Li, Y.; et al. Rehmanniae Radix in osteoporosis: A review of traditional Chinese medicinal uses, phytochemistry, pharmacokinetics and pharmacology. *J. Ethnopharmacol.* **2017**, *198*, 351–362. [CrossRef] [PubMed]
7. Oh, K.O.; Kim, S.W.; Kim, J.Y.; Ko, S.Y.; Kim, H.M.; Baek, J.H.; Ryoo, H.M.; Kim, J.K. Effect of Rehmannia glutinosa Libosch extracts on bone metabolism. *Clin. Chim. Acta* **2003**, *334*, 185–195. [CrossRef]
8. Xia, B.; Xu, B.; Sun, Y.; Xiao, L.; Pan, J.; Jin, H.; Tong, P. The effects of Liuwei Dihuang on canonical Wnt/β-catenin signaling pathway in osteoporosis. *J. Ethnopharmacol.* **2014**, *153*, 133–141. [CrossRef]
9. Ge, J.; Xie, L.; Chen, J.; Li, S.; Xu, H.; Lai, Y.; Qiu, L.; Ni, C. Liuwei Dihuang Pill treats postmenopausal osteoporosis with Shen (Kidney) yin deficiency via Janus kinase/signal transducer and activator of transcription signal pathway by up-regulating cardiotrophin-like cytokine factor 1 expression. *Chin. J. Integr. Med.* **2016**, *24*, 1–8.
10. Gao, Z. ER, PR are up-regulated by rehmannia in aging female mice. *J. Shanxi Coll. Tradit. Chin. Med.* **2000**, *1*, 1–3.
11. Chao, J.; Huo, T.I.; Cheng, H.Y.; Tsai, J.C.; Liao, J.W.; Lee, M.S.; Qin, X.M.; Hsieh, M.T.; Pao, L.H.; Peng, W.H. Gallic acid ameliorated impaired glucose and lipid homeostasis in high fat diet-induced NAFLD mice. *PLoS ONE* **2014**, *9*, e96969. [CrossRef] [PubMed]
12. Weinstein, R.S. Glucocorticoid-Induced Osteoporosis and Osteonecrosis. *Endocrinol. Metab. Clin. N. Am.* **2012**, *41*, 595–611. [CrossRef]
13. Vimalraj, S.; Arumugam, B.; Miranda, P.J.; Selvamurugan, N. Runx2: Structure, function, and phosphorylation in osteoblast differentiation. *Int. J. Biol. Macromol.* **2015**, *78*, 202–208. [CrossRef] [PubMed]
14. Fujita, T.; Azuma, Y.; Fukuyama, R.; Hattori, Y.; Yoshida, C.; Koida, M.; Ogita, K.; Komori, T. Runx2 induces osteoblast and chondrocyte differentiation and enhances their migration by coupling with PI3K-Akt signaling. *J. Cell Biol.* **2004**, *166*, 85–95. [CrossRef] [PubMed]

15. Yodthong, T.; Kedjarune-Leggat, U.; Smythe, C.; Wititsuwannakul, R.; Pitakpornpreecha, T. l-Quebrachitol Promotes the Proliferation, Differentiation, and Mineralization of MC3T3-E1 Cells: Involvement of the BMP-2/Runx2/MAPK/Wnt/β-Catenin Signaling Pathway. *Molecules* **2018**, *23*, 3086. [CrossRef] [PubMed]
16. Khosla, S.; Monroe, D.G. Regulation of Bone Metabolism by Sex Steroids. *Cold Spring Harb. Perspect. Med.* **2017**, *8*, a031211. [CrossRef]
17. Matsuzaki, Y.; Honda, A. Dehydroepiandrosterone and its derivatives: Potentially novel anti-proliferative and chemopreventive agents. *Curr. Pharm. Des.* **2006**, *12*, 3411–3421. [CrossRef] [PubMed]
18. Miller, W.L. Androgen biosynthesis from cholesterol to DHEA. *Mol. Cell Endocrinol.* **2002**, *198*, 7–14. [CrossRef]
19. Marx, C.E.; Bradford, D.W.; Hamer, R.M.; Naylor, J.C.; Allen, T.B.; Lieberman, J.A.; Strauss, J.L.; Kilts, J.D. Pregnenolone as a novel therapeutic candidate in schizophrenia: Emerging preclinical and clinical evidence. *Neuroscience* **2011**, *191*, 78–90. [CrossRef]
20. Maurya, S.W.; Dev, K.; Singh, K.B.; Rai, R.; Siddiqui, I.R.; Singh, D.; Maurya, R. Synthesis and biological evaluation of heterocyclic analogues of pregnenolone as novel anti-osteoporotic agents. *Bioorg. Med. Chem. Lett.* **2017**, *27*, 1390–1396. [CrossRef]
21. Yantsevich, A.V.; Dichenko, Y.V.; Mackenzie, F.; Mukha, D.V.; Baranovsky, A.V.; Gilep, A.A.; Usanov, S.A.; Strushkevich, N.V. Human steroid and oxysterol 7α-hydroxylase CYP7B1: Substrate specificity, azole binding and misfolding of clinically relevant mutants. *FEBS J.* **2014**, *281*, 1700–1713. [CrossRef] [PubMed]
22. Mohamad Asri, S.F.; Mohd Ramli, E.S.; Soelaiman, I.N.; Mat Noh, M.A.; Abdul Rashid, A.H.; Suhaimi, F. Piper sarmentosum Effects on 11β-Hydroxysteroid Dehydrogenase Type 1 Enzyme in Serum and Bone in Rat Model of Glucocorticoid-Induced Osteoporosis. *Molecules* **2016**, *21*, 1523. [CrossRef] [PubMed]
23. Atanasov, A.G.; Odermatt, A. Readjusting the glucocorticoid balance: An opportunity for modulators of 11beta-hydroxysteroid dehydrogenase type 1 activity? *Endocr. Metab. Immune Disord. Drug Targets* **2007**, *7*, 125–140. [CrossRef] [PubMed]
24. Eijken, M.; Hewison, M.; Cooper, M.S.; de Jong, F.H.; Chiba, H.; Stewart, P.M.; Uitterlinden, A.G.; Pols, H.A.P.; van Leeuwen, J.P.T.M. 11β-Hydroxysteroid Dehydrogenase Expression and Glucocorticoid Synthesis Are Directed by a Molecular Switch during Osteoblast Differentiation. *Mol. Endocrinol.* **2005**, *19*, 621–631. [CrossRef] [PubMed]
25. Bulun, S.E. Aromatase and estrogen receptor α deficiency. *Fertil. Steril.* **2014**, *101*, 323–329. [CrossRef] [PubMed]
26. Carson, J.A.; Manolagas, S.C. Effects of sex steroids on bones and muscles: Similarities, parallels, and putative interactions in health and disease. *Bone* **2015**, *80*, 67–78. [CrossRef] [PubMed]
27. Somner, J.; McLellan, S.; Cheung, J.; Mak, Y.T.; Frost, M.L.; Knapp, K.M.; Wierzbicki, A.S.; Wheeler, M.; Fogelman, I.; Ralston, S.H.; et al. Polymorphisms in the P450 c17 (17-Hydroxylase/17,20-Lyase) and P450 c19 (Aromatase) Genes: Association with Serum Sex Steroid Concentrations and Bone Mineral Density in Postmenopausal Women. *J. Clin. Endocrinol. Metab.* **2004**, *89*, 344–351. [CrossRef] [PubMed]
28. Gu, G.; Hentunen, T.A.; Nars, M.; Härkönen, P.L.; Väänänen, H.K. Estrogen protects primary osteocytes against glucocorticoid-induced apoptosis. *Apoptosis* **2005**, *10*, 583–595. [CrossRef] [PubMed]

Sample Availability: Samples of the compounds catalpol, echinacoside, and acteoside are available from the authors.

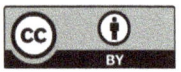

© 2019 by the authors. Licensee MDPI, Basel, Switzerland. This article is an open access article distributed under the terms and conditions of the Creative Commons Attribution (CC BY) license (http://creativecommons.org/licenses/by/4.0/).

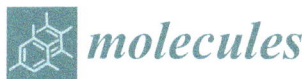

Review

Use of Cannabidiol in the Treatment of Epilepsy: Efficacy and Security in Clinical Trials

Serena Silvestro, Santa Mammana, Eugenio Cavalli, Placido Bramanti and Emanuela Mazzon *

IRCCS Centro Neurolesi "Bonino-Pulejo", Via Provinciale Palermo, Contrada Casazza, 98124 Messina, Italy; silvestro9110@gmail.com (S.S.); santa.mammana@irccsme.it (S.M.); eugenio.cavalli@irccsme.it (E.C.); placido.bramanti@irccsme.it (P.B.)

* Correspondence: emanuela.mazzon@irccsme.it; Tel.: +39-090-6012-8172

Academic Editors: Raffaele Capasso and Lorenzo Di Cesare Mannelli
Received: 20 March 2019; Accepted: 11 April 2019; Published: 12 April 2019

Abstract: Cannabidiol (CBD) is one of the cannabinoids with non-psychotropic action, extracted from *Cannabis sativa*. CBD is a terpenophenol and it has received a great scientific interest thanks to its medical applications. This compound showed efficacy as anti-seizure, antipsychotic, neuroprotective, antidepressant and anxiolytic. The neuroprotective activity appears linked to its excellent anti-inflammatory and antioxidant properties. The purpose of this paper is to evaluate the use of CBD, in addition to common anti-epileptic drugs, in the severe treatment-resistant epilepsy through an overview of recent literature and clinical trials aimed to study the effects of the CBD treatment in different forms of epilepsy. The results of scientific studies obtained so far the use of CBD in clinical applications could represent hope for patients who are resistant to all conventional anti-epileptic drugs.

Keywords: cannabidiol; treatment-resistant epilepsy; clinical trials

---

1. Introduction

Cannabis sativa L. is an ancient medicinal plant wherefrom over 100 cannabinoids are extracted [1]. Among them, the most studied are Δ^9–tetrahydrocannabinol (Δ^9–THC), a psychoactive compound, and the CBD, a non-psychotropic phytocannabinoid [2]. CBD is a cyclohexene which is substituted in position 1 by a methyl group, by a 2,6-dihydroxy-4-pentylphenyl group at position 3, and with a prop-1-en-2-yl group at position 4 (Figure 1). Most cannabinoids exert their action by interacting with cannabinoid receptors, but CBD shows a low affinity for these receptors. Nevertheless, it affects the activity of other receptors such as serotonin receptors [5-HT], opioid receptors [ORs], and non-endocannabinoid G protein-coupled receptors (GPCRs) [3] and other targets (ion channels and enzymes).

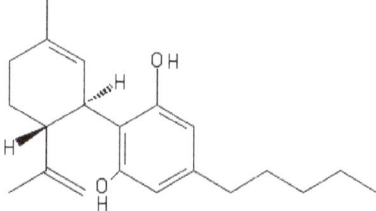

Figure 1. Structure of CBD.

In recent years, the scientific community has shown interest in this compound due to its good safety profile and neuroprotective properties [4] in several neurodegenerative diseases, including Amyotrophic Lateral Sclerosis [5], Parkinson's [6,7], Huntington's [8] and Alzheimer's diseases [9–11]. This neuroprotective action is due to its anti-inflammatory [12,13] and antioxidant [14,15] properties. CBD shows anti-inflammatory properties in several experimental studies, modulating some pro-inflammatory cytokines such as interleukin-1β (IL-1β) [16], interleukin-6 (IL-6) [17,18] and tumor necrosis factor α (TNF-α) [16,18], as well as regulation of cell cycle and immune cells' functions [19]. Furthermore, another mechanism by which CBD performs its anti-inflammatory action is mediated by interaction with the Transient Potential Vanilloid Receptor Type 1 (TRPV1). TRPV1 receptor is a nonselective cation channel that, when activated, allows the influx of Ca^{2+}. The sensitivity but also the density of TRPV1 is increased during neuro-inflammatory conditions. The binding of CBD to TRPV1 leads to a desensitization of these receptors, with a consequent reduction in inflammation [20]. The CBD also carry out a potent antioxidant activity, modulating the expression of inducible nitric oxide synthase and nitrotyrosine as well as reducing production of reactive oxygen species [21]. CBD is also generating interest due to its therapeutic properties such as antidepressant [22], antipsychotic [23], analgesic [24], and antitumor [25]. In addition, it has been shown that CBD can significantly reduce two important forms of anxiety, namely obsessive-compulsive disorder [26] and post-traumatic stress disorder [27,28].

Moreover, for a long time, the CBD has been investigated for its anticonvulsant effects [29–31]. Several studies confirmed its efficacy in the treatment of epileptic seizures, especially in pediatric age [32,33]. In 2016, the first results of phase III clinical trials showed beneficial effects of CBD (Epidiolex®; GW Pharmaceutical, Cambridge, UK) in treatment-resistant seizure disorders, including Lennox-Gastaut Syndrome (LGS) and Dravet syndromes (DS).

Epilepsy is a chronic neurological disorder. About 30% of epilepsy patients are affected by Treatment-Resistant Epilepsy (TRE) due to the failure of common anti-epileptic therapies [34]. This form of epilepsy is characterized by recurrent seizures that negatively affect the quality of life.

The purpose of this review is to provide an overview of recent clinical trials registered on ClinicalTrial.gov. These trials study the use of different CBD formulation in patients affected by severe forms of drug-resistant epilepsy. Moreover, we have described studies approved by local ethics committees published in PubMed.

2. Epilepsy

According to the World Health Organization, epilepsy affects more than 50 million people worldwide. Epilepsy is the most common neurological disorders characterized by recurrent seizures [35]. A "seizure" is a paroxysmal transient phenomenon determined by an abnormal excessive or synchronous neuronal activity in the brain [36]. Epilepsy can also cause deficit sensorimotor, cognitive, compromising quality of life and an increased risk of premature death [37]. The International League Against Epilepsy, according to the point of onset, classifies epileptic seizures into focal, generalized and unknown seizures [38]. Focal convulsions caused by an anomalous electrical activity in a circumscribed part of the brain and are classified into simple and complex. Simple focal convulsions are characterized by motor, sensory and sensory manifestations without loss of consciousness. On the contrary, complex focal convulsions involve a loss of consciousness [39]. Generalized seizures begin in one or more areas of the brain and can then spread to the entire brain. Generalized seizures are divided into crises absences, characterized by a rapid and transient loss of consciousness; tonic crises that cause muscle stiffening; atonic crisis, characterized by loss of muscular control; clonic seizures that cause rhythmic muscle movements; myoclonic seizures, characterized by muscle contraction and localized tremors. Finally, tonic-clonic seizures represent the most serious type of epileptic seizures, last about 5–10 min and are characterized by intense generalized contractions to the whole body [39,40]. The unknown seizures are called so when the beginning of a seizure is not known. These seizures can also be defined as "epileptic spasms" characterized by sudden extension or flexion of the limbs. Is defined Secondary Epilepsy when the onset is caused by several factors such as head trauma, infectious diseases (meningitis, AIDS, viral encephalitis), developmental disorders, alcohol or drug abuse, and other pathological conditions (brain tumors, stroke).

The most well-known epilepsies are DS, Sturge-Weber Syndrome (SWS), Tuberous Sclerosis Complex (TSC) and West Syndrome (WS) and LGS. DS is a rare encephalopathy, which has its onset in the first year of life [41]. DS is associated with the mutation in the gene encoding the α1 subunit of the voltage gated sodium channel (*SCN1A*) [42]. SWS is caused by a somatic mutation of the *GNAQ* gene (9q21) that encodes the G_q protein, involved in the intracellular signal of several G protein-coupled receptors that control the function of various growth factors and vasoactive peptides [43]. Patients manifest neurological abnormalities of variousdegrees, focal epileptic seizures [44]. TSC is an autosomal dominant disease, caused by a mutation of two genes: *TSC1* (localized on chromosome 9p34.3) that encodes for hamartin and *TSC2* (localized on chromosome 16p13.3) that encodes for tubulin. Often TSC patients present generalized epilepsy. WS or Infantile Spasm (IS) is the epileptic encephalopathy. This syndrome is characterized by genetic heterogeneity and the mutated gene most frequently observed in patients with this syndrome is *CDKL5* (cyclin-dependent kinase-like 5) [45]. WS is characterized by the association between axial spasm discharges and psychomotor retardation [46]. LGS is a severe epileptic encephalopathy of childhood. This syndrome is a rare condition likely associated with a genes mutation. Nevertheless, to date, it is quite unclear how the involved genes may cause this syndrome mainly characterized by recurrent seizures from early in life. An epileptic form that does not respond to therapy with at least two or three appropriately selected anti-epileptic drugs (AEDs) is defined as TRE and this is estimated to affect 30% of patients [47,48].

3. Common Antiepileptic Drugs

AEDs are the mainstay for the treatment of epilepsy and are intended to mitigate seizures. Epileptogenic discharges occur as a result of neuronal hyperexcitability caused by voltage-dependent ion channels and neurotransmitter concentrations alteration. AEDs primarily act reducing neuronal excitability blocking excitatory neurotransmitter action such as glutamic acid and enhancing inhibitory neurotransmitters such as γ-aminobutyric acid (GABA). Furthermore, the antiepileptic actions of most AEDs are due to the modulation of voltage-gated ion channels such as sodium (Na^+) and calcium (Ca^{2+}). The neuronal Na^+ and Ca^{2+} channels are responsible for the rise of the action potential and for the intrinsic excitability control of the neuronal system [49]. Some AEDs act inactivating a single voltage-dependent channel while others instead simultaneously inactivate bothchannels. Both of these mechanisms result in a reduction for neuronal hyperexcitability. Examples of drugs that perform interacting with a single channel are phenytoin that selectively blocks the Na^+ channel [50] and ethosuximide that blocks the T-type Ca^{2+} channel [51]. Instead, carbamazepine, lamotrigine, oxcarbazepine and zonisamide control seizures blocking both these voltage-dependent ion channels [52].

There are also anti-epileptics that act enhancing the GABAergic system. GABA is the main inhibitory neurotransmitter of the nervous system that acts on GABA receptors, ligand-dependent ionic receptors that increase chlorine conductance. AEDs are responsible for increasing GABA transmission reducing neuronal excitability. Drugs that exert their action through these mechanisms are benzodiazepines, phenobarbital, stiripentol, tiagabine and vigabatrin. Benzodiazepines (such as clobazam diazepam, lorazepam, clonazepam) phenobarbital and stiripentol enhance the inhibitory transmission of GABA by allosteric activation of the $GABA_A$ receptor thus increasing the frequency of chloride (Cl^-) channel openings [53,54]. Vigabatrin, instead, is an inhibitor of GABA transaminase, the enzyme responsible for the catabolism of GABA [55]. In addition to enhancing the inhibitory transmission of GABA, other drugs exert their antiepileptic action, also exploiting the blockage of the Ca^{2+} and Na^+ channels. Among the AEDs that perform their action through these effects are included, felbamate, lamotrigine and topiramate [56]. Other drugs are valproic acid and levetiracetam that perform their mechanism of action enhancing the transmission of GABA and blocking Ca^{2+} channels [57,58].

The anticonvulsant and neuroprotective efficacy of some drugs is also given by the inhibitory action of neurotransmitters, such as glutamate. Glutamate (or glutamic acid) is the most common excitatory neurotransmitter and is responsible for excitatory transmission on neurons. Felbamate and topiramate also perform their mechanism of action inhibiting glutamate thus decreasing l' hyperexcitability neuronal [59,60].

The choice of drugs is mainly linked to the identification of the type of seizure and epileptic syndrome. For patients with epilepsy, effective seizure control is the determining factor for a good quality of life. AED dosages must be individualized to maximize therapeutic effects and avoid side effects. The early childhood epilepsy syndrome such as DS, LGS and WS present no easy medical management due to the fact that subjects often show convulsion resistant to the available treatment. Therefore, of safe and effective therapies arenecessary to reduce the risk of neurological sequelae. The drugs preferentially used in particular forms of pediatric epilepsy are phenobarbital, phenytoin, benzodiazepine, topiramate, levetiracetam and valproic acid [61].

4. Cannabidiol and Molecular Targets in Epilepsy

CBD shows a low affinity for endocannabinoid receptors and it carries out its mechanisms of action by interacting with other molecular targets. One of the most important ion channel targets towards which the CBD shows a high affinity is the Transient Receptor Potential Vanilloid (TRPV).

Specifically, TRPV1 is a non-selective channel that shows a high Ca^{2+} permeability and is involved in the modulation of seizures and in epilepsy. In fact, when active, it promotes the release of glutamate and the increase in Ca^{2+}, with consequent neuronal excitability [62]. The antiepileptic action of CBD does not seem to be due to direct interaction with these molecular targets. However, it has been observed that the CBD agonist action towards TPRV1 determines one a desensitization of these channels with consequent normalization of intracellular Ca^{2+} [63]. T-Type Ca^{2+}, are another class of ion channels with which CBD interacts. These channels control Ca^{2+} peaks in neurons and they are involved in the regulation of cell excitability. The activation of these channels due to a hyperpolarization of the membranes of neurons determines an increase in the concentration of intracellular Ca^{2+}, in this way the T-Type Ca^{2+} channels increase the excitability of neurons. This mechanism is often observed in pathophysiological conditions such as epilepsy [49]. The interaction of the CBD with the T-type Ca^{2+} channels causes a blockage of these channels, this mechanism could be responsible for the antiepileptic action, even if there are no studies available that confirm this. Receptors represent other molecular targets that have been evaluated to describe their potential role in epilepsy through interaction with CBD. Serotonin receptor (5-hydroxytryptamine [5-HT]) belonging to the superfamily of the G protein-coupled receptors are divided into seven distinct classes (5-HT$_1$ to 5-HT$_7$). These receptors may depolarize or hyperpolarize neurons, modifying the conductance and/or concentration ionic within the cells. This suggests that 5-HT receptors are involved in epilepsy even though their role is still not entirely clear [64]. CBD shows a high affinity towards two subtypes of serotonin receptors: 5-HT$_{1A}$ e 5-HT$_{2A}$. These receptors can have different functions and regulatory characteristics, in fact, for example, the activation of 5HT$_1$ receptors in the hippocampus causes an increase of neurotransmission; in contrast, in raphe nuclei, activation of 5-HT$_{1A}$ receptors produces the inhibition of serotonergic neurons [65]. The dysregulation of brain neurotransmission mediated by 5-HT$_2$ might results responsible for the pathophysiology of depression and epilepsy [66]. However, although the role of serotonin receptors in epilepsy is unclear, 5-HT$_{1A}$ e 5-HT$_{2A}$ subtypes may represent a valid therapeutic target through which CBD can perform its anti-epileptic action [61,67]. Opioid receptors (OR) are G-protein-coupled receptors involved in a variety of brain disorders, including epilepsy [68,69]. The CBD at high micromolar concentrations determines the blocking of μ and δ OR, and this block would seem to generate anticonvulsant actions, even if there are still no studies to support this theory. The CBD also shows a good affinity towards the orphan G-protein-coupled receptor (GPR55), a class of receptors involved in the modulation of the synaptic transmission. The agonist action of CBD towards these receptors would seem to attenuate synaptic transmission with consequent antiepileptic effects [70].

An important enzyme target of CBD involved in epilepsy is cytochrome P450 (CYP450). CBD inhibits CYP450 [71], but this mechanism does not seem to be directly involved in the antiepileptic mechanism. It seems to be responsible for the hepatic metabolism of a variety of AEDs, as shown by the combined administration of CBD and clobazam (CLB) [72].

5. Cannabidiol: Clinical Trials for Epilepsy

In the last decades, some clinical studies were conducted in order to investigate the potential effects of the efficacy of CBD in the management of epilepsy. This review provides an overview of the studies recorded on http://clinicaltrial.gov, distributing them into complete trials (see Table 1) and ongoing trials. All trials test the use of CBD as an adjunct to common AEDs and most of them assess the efficacy and safety of CBD especially in infants, children and teenagers. Trials exploring the combination of CBD/Δ^9-THC have been excluded. In addition, we included further studies that have been approved by local ethics committees (see Table 2). In the description of these clinical trials, attention was also paid to the possible interactions of CBD with other anti-epileptic drugs.

5.1. Completed Clinical Trials

All clinical studies (phases 1, 2 and 3) reported below assess the safety and/or efficacy of CBD in addition to common AEDs. Most of these studies enrolled pediatric patients (0.5 to 17 years) with diagnoses of genetically based epilepsy, LGS, DS and WS, resistant to common antiepileptic treatments. The following trials collect data on administration short-term CBD (from 10 days to 3 months).

A phase 1/2 clinical trial NCT02324673 has evaluated efficacy and safety of the CBD oral solution at three different doses (10, 20 and 40 mg/kg/day) administered for 10 consecutive days in sixty-one children (1–17 years) with drug-resistant forms of epilepsy. It was to assess the plasma concentration of the CBD and its metabolite (7-hydroxycannabidiol, 7-OH-CBD) in blood samples collected at baseline, at day 1 and at day 10 post-treatment at different time points (1, 2, 4, 8, 12, 24, 48, 72 h). On day one, the plasma concentrations of CBD and its metabolite increase in a dose-dependent manner. These levels, instead, decrease at the 10th day. Moreover, both at the first and at the tenth day CBD concentrations are double those of its metabolite. A negative change in clinical global impression of severity score at the end of treatment has shown an improvement of illness in all dosage. An improvement, in a dose-dependent manner, has also been observed in daily seizure activity. Serious Adverse Events (SAEs) such as apnoea, skin eruption and thrombophlebitis, were observed in 5% of patients that received medium-dose CBD and in 9.5% that received high-dose. Further no-serious Adverse Events (AEs), such as anaemia, gastrointestinal disorders (diarrhoea, flatulence, constipation, gastroesophageal reflux disease, nausea), nervous system disorders (somnolence, psychomotor hyperactivity, seizure, ataxia) were respectively observed in 65% of patients treated with low-dose CBD, in 45% treated with medium dose and in 80.95% treated with high-dose. The results of this study showed that CBD can be considered safe and tolerable even at high concentrations.

A phase 2, multi-center clinical trial (NCT02551731) enrolled 9 children (6 months to 36 months) with a diagnosis of WS (Infantile Spasms) who have not responded to first-line therapies. CBD in oral solution was administered at the initial dose of 20 mg/kg/day or 40 mg/kg/day. The protocol provided the division of the study into two parts: Part A and Part B. In Part A was evaluated the efficacy, defined as complete resolution of spasms and hypsarrythmia (if present at baseline) confirmed by video-electroencephalogram (EEG) and safety at day 14 of treatment. Instead, in Part B was evaluated the efficacy and the long-term safety up to 64 weeks of treatment. In Part A, 14.3% of children showed complete resolution of spasms and hypsarrhythmia (when present at baseline) on day 14. Only in 33% showed AEs, while no SAEs were recorded. No results of Part B of the clinical trial were recorded because only one subject has completed the study. Then, these results confirm the efficacy and safety of the CBD oral solution after 14 days of treatment.

Table 1. Completed cannabidiol clinical trials in epilepsy (https://clinicaltrials.gov/). The table shows the efficacy and safety of CBD in different forms of epilepsy. In all studies, CBD is used as adjunctive therapy to conventional antiepileptic drugs.

Identifier	Study Title	Subjects	Conditions	CBD Dose	Concomitant AEDs	Efficacy	Security	Ref
NCT02987114	A Study to Evaluate the Safety, Tolerability and Efficacy of Oral Administration of PTL101 (Cannabidiol) as an Adjunctive Treatment for Pediatric Intractable Epilepsy	16 children (2 to 15 years)	Pediatric Intractable Epilepsy	25–450 mg/kg/day	-	-	-	-
NCT02324673	Cannabidiol Oral Solution in Pediatric Participants With Treatment-resistant Seizure Disorders	61 children (1 to 17 years)	Resistant Seizure Disorders	10, 20, 40 mg/kg/day	-	Improvement of illness	SAEs in 5% of patients with medium-dose and in 9.5% with high-dose	-
NCT02551731	Cannabidiol Oral Solution for Treatment of Refractory Infantile Spasms	9 infants (6 to 36 Months)	Refractory Infantile Spasms	20–40 mg/kg/day	-	Complete resolution of spasm in 14.3% of children after 14 days of treatment	No SAEs were recorded	-
NCT02318602	Cannabidiol Oral Solution as an Adjunctive Treatment for Treatment-resistant Seizure Disorder	52 children and young adults (1 to 18 years)	Treatment-resistant Seizure Disorder	10, 20, 40 mg/kg/day	-	-	SAEs in 77.78% of infants, in 38.46% of children and in 0% of adults	-
NCT02224703	GWPCARE2 A Study to Investigate the Efficacy and Safety of Cannabidiol (GWP42003-P) in Children and Young Adults With Dravet Syndrome	150 children and young adults (2 to 18 years)	Dravet Syndrome	10, 20 mg/kg/day	-	-	-	-
NCT02695537	Safety, and Tolerability of Epidiolex In Patients (Ages 1–19 Years) With Intractable Epilepsy	100 children and young adults (1 to 18 years)	Intractable Epilepsy	5–50 mg/kg/day	CLB, Valproate, Levetiracetam, Phenobarbital, Clonazepam, Phenytoin, Carbamazepine, Lamotrigine, Oxcarbazepine, Ethosuximide, Topiramate, Vigabatrin, Zonisamide, Eslicarbazepine, Ezogabine, Pregabalin, Perampanel, Rufinamide, Lacosamide	Reduction of seizures of 63.6% after 12 weeks of treatment	4 children with concomitant valproate showed elevate damage of liver function	[78]
							Improvement of AE Profile	[79]
NCT02270412	University of Alabama at Birmingham (UAB) Adult CBD Program	100 children and adults (15 to 99 years)	Epilepsy Seizures	5–50 mg/kg/day			4 children with concomitant valproate showed elevate damage of liver function	[78]
						Reduction of seizures of 63.6% after 12 weeks of treatment	Improvement of AE Profile	[79]

Table 1. Cont.

Identifier	Study Title	Subjects	Conditions	CBD Dose	Concomitant AEDs	Efficacy	Security	Ref
NCT02224560	Efficacy and Safety of GWP42003-P for Seizures Associated With Lennox-Gastaut Syndrome in Children and Adults (GWPCARE3)	225 children and adults (2 to 55 years)	Epilepsy Lennox Gastaut Syndrome	10, 20 mg/kg/day	CLB Valproate Lamotrigine Levetiracetam Rufinamide	The median percent reduction in seizures frequency from baseline was 37.2% in the 10 mg/kg/day CBD group; 41.9% in the 20 mg/kg/day CBD group	SAEs were reported in 19.40% of patients at the dose of 10 mg/kg/day of the CBD and in 15.85% at the 20 mg/kg/day	[75]
NCT02091206	A Dose-ranging Pharmacokinetics and Safety Study of GWP42003-P in Children With Dravet Syndrome (GWPCARE1)	34 children (4 to 10 years)	Dravet Syndrome	5, 10, 20 mg/kg/day	CLB Valproate Stiripentol Levetiracetam Topiramate	-	TEAEs in 5 patients; SAE in 10% of patients at the dose of 5 mg/kg/day, in 25% at the 10 mg/kg/day and in 11.11% at the 20 mg/kg/day dose. 6 patients with concomitant valproate had elevated ALT or AST	[73]
NCT02091375	Antiepileptic Efficacy Study of GWP42003-P in Children and Young Adults With Dravet Syndrome (GWPCARE1)	120 children, young adults (2 to 18 years)	Dravet Syndrome	20 mg/kg/day	CLB Valproate Stiripentol Levetiracetam Topiramate	The median frequency of seizures decreased from 12.4 to 5.9, compared to the placebo-treated group	SAEs in 16.39% of patients	[74]
NCT02224690	A Study to Investigate the Efficacy and Safety of Cannabidiol (GWP42003-P; CBD) as Adjunctive Treatment for Seizures Associated With Lennox-Gastaut Syndrome in Children and Adults (GWPCARE4)	171 children and adults (2 to 55 years)	Lennox-Gastaut Syndrome	20 mg/kg/day	CLB Valproate Lamotrigine Levetiracetam Rufinamide	The monthly frequency of seizures decreased by a median of 43.9% from baseline in the CBD group	Serious TEAEs occurred in 4 patients, SAEs in 23.26% of patients. 16 of the 36 patients on valproate had transaminase elevations	[76]
NCT02224573	GWPCARE5 - An Open Label Extension Study of Cannabidiol (GWP42003-P) in Children and Young Adults With Dravet or Lennox-Gastaut Syndromes	264 children, and adults (2 years and older)	Dravet Syndrome Lennox-Gastaut Syndrome	-	CLB Valproate Stiripentol Levetiracetam Topiramate	The monthly frequency of seizures decreased by a median ranged from 38% to 44%	SAEs in 29.2% of patients	[77]
NCT02565108	A Randomized Controlled Trial to Investigate Possible Drug-drug Interactions Between Clobazam and Cannabidiol	20 adults (18 to 65 years)	Epilepsy	20 mg/kg/day	CLB	All participants reduced the maintenance dose of CBD from 10% for the day	2 patients withdrew from the study due to SAEs (seizure cluster)	-
NCT02564952	An Open-label Extension Study to Investigate Possible Drug-drug Interactions Between Clobazam and Cannabidiol	18 adults (18 to 65 years)	Epilepsy	Initial 20 mg/kg/d titrated to maximum dose of 30 mg/kg/day	CLB	-	SAEs in 11% of patients	-

CBD: Cannabidiol; TEAEs: Treatment-emergent adverse events; SAEs: serious adverse events; AST: aspartate transferase; ALT: alanine transferase.

Table 2. Data obtained from trials authorized by local ethics committees (https://www.ncbi.nlm.nih.gov/pubmed/). The table shows the efficacy and safety of CBD in different forms of epilepsy. In all studies, CBD is used as adjunctive therapy to conventional antiepileptic drugs.

Study Design	Subjects	Conditions	CBD Dose	Concomitant AEDs	Efficacy	Safety	Ref
A prospective, open-label, expanded access study	214 children and adults (1 to 30 years)	Drug Resistant Epilepsy	Initial 2–5 mg/kg/day titrated to maximum dose of 50 mg/kg/day	CLB Valproate	The median reduction in monthly motor seizure was of 36.5%	Treatment-related SAEs were recorded in 20 patients; SAEs were reported in 30% of patients. Thrombocytopenia and elevated liver function test in patients with concomitant valproate	[83]
A prospective, open-label study	Children and adults (1 to 30 years)	Drug Resistant Epilepsy	Initial 2–5 mg/kg/day, titrated to maximum dose of 50 mg/kg/day	-	Overall quality of life significantly improved in 48 patients, The median monthly seizures frequency was 13.9	-	[86]
A prospective, multicentre, open-label study	55 children and adults (1 to 30 years)	Epilepsy Dravet Syndrome CDKL5 deficiency disorder Aicardi Doose syndromes Dup15q syndromes	Initial 5 mg/kg/day titrated to maximum dose of 50 mg/kg/day	CLB Valproic acid Levetiracetam Rufinamide Felbamate Topiramate	Median monthly convulsive seizure frequency decreased from baseline by 51.4% at week 12 and by 59.1% at week 48	A serious treatment-emergent AEs such as status epilepticus (9%) and respiratory infection (5%)	[87]
A prospective, open-label study	40 children (1 to 17 years)	Drug Resistant Epilepsy	Initial 5 mg/kg/day titrated to maximum dose of 25 mg/kg/day	-	12 patients reported substantial improvement of the condition	4 patients withdrew from the study because of AEs; SAEs were reported in 15 patients	[88]
A prospective, multiple center, open-label study	607 children (average age 13 years)	Drug Resistant Epilepsy	Initial 2–10 mg/kg/day to maximum dose of 50 mg/kg/day		A median monthly seizure frequency of 51% was recorded after 12 months of treatment and maintained at weeks 96	SAEs were reported in 33% of patients;	[89]
Expanded access program	5 infants (1 to 45 months)	Sturge–Weber Syndrome	2–25 mg/kg/day	Levetiracetam Valproic acid Felbamate CLB Rufinamide Perampanel Clorazepate Oxcarbazepine Lacosamide Topiramate	50% of seizures reductions in all patients; Improvements in quality of life in all patients	AEs were recorded during the study	[85]

Table 2. *Cont.*

Study Design	Subjects	Conditions	CBD Dose	Concomitant AEDs	Efficacy	Safety	Ref
Retrospective study	210 children (≤19 years)	Epilepsy	2.9, 5.8 mg/kg/day	CLB	50% in seizures reduction in 33% of patients in the CBD group; in 44% of CBD + CLB and in 38% of CLB group	AEs in 36% of patients in the CLB group and in 7% of patients in CBD + CLB group	[80]
Expand access investigational new drug (IND) trial	13 children and young (4 to 19 years)	Refractory Epilepsy	5–25 mg/kg/day	CLB	50% of reduction in seizures in 69.23% of patients	No serious AEs in 77% of patients	[72]
Open-label, fixed-sequence trial	78 healthy subjects	-	750 mg twice daily	CLB Stiripentol Valproate	-	Moderate AEs in 8 patients; mild AEs in most of patients	[81]
Expanded access study	18 children and adults (2 to 31 years)	Tuberous Sclerosis Complex	5–50 mg/kg/day	CLB Lacosamide Levetiracetam Lamotrigine Valproic acid Rufinamide	4 patients recorded a reduction in seizure rate greater than 80%; 1 patient became seizures-free	AEs in 66.7% of patients	[82]
Expanded access program	26 children (1 to 17 years)	Refractory epilepsy	5–25 mg/kg/day	CLB	A 50% reduction in seizures	SAEs in 23.1% of patients	[84]

CBD: Cannabidiol; TEAEs: Treatment-emergent adverse events; SAEs: serious adverse events.

The patients that concluded the clinical trials NCT02324673 and NCT02551731 have been involved in the completed phase 3 open-label clinical-trial NCT02318602. The participants were divided for an age range into three groups: infants (1 to <2 years of age), children (2 to <12 years of age) and teenagers (12 to <17 years of age). All individuals continued the treatment with CBD at the same dose of trials NCT02324673 (10, 20 and 40 mg/kg daily) and NCT02551731 (20 mg/kg daily) for 48 weeks. The first outcome of this clinical trial was to evaluate the safety of CBD as adjunctive therapy for children with treatment-resistant convulsive disorders. Patients following treatment with established AEDs were continued uninterrupted, dose adjustments were allowed if necessary based on safety concerns or changes in seizure control. SAEs such as seizures, status epilepticus and mental status changes occurred in 77.78% of infants, in 38.46% of children and 0% of teenagers. No serious AEs (anemia, diarrhoea, constipation, vomiting, infection of the upper respiratory tract, nasopharyngitis, otitis media and influenza) occurred in 88.89% of infants, in 92.31% of children and 88.24% of teenagers. In all patients, no significant changes were observed as respect to baseline in laboratory values or in vital signs. These results show that while the administration of CBD cannot be considered safe in infants, but it was generally well tolerated in adults.

The multicenter, open-label clinical trial, NCT03196934, is an extension of the NCT02318602 trial. The aim of this study is to assess the long-term safety of CBD oral solution as an adjunctive treatment for pediatric subjects with a treatment-resistant seizure. No result is available today.

Six randomized, double-blind, placebo-controlled studies were funded by GW Pharmaceuticals for evaluated the activity of the new formulation of purified CBD oral solution (GWP42003-P or Epidiolex), an epileptic medication and now Food and Drug Administration (FDA) approved for the treatment of seizures associated with DS and LGS in patients two years of age or older.

The first clinical trial GWPCARE1 was divided into two parts: Part A (NCT02091206) and Part B (NCT02091375). NCT02091206, a double-blind randomization study (phase 2), to evaluate the safety of multiple doses of the CBD oral solution (GWP42003-P) in 34 children (4 to 10 years) with DS. All patients before enrolment had to have stabilized all AEDs at least 1 month before and the therapy stability had to be maintained during the study. Participants were randomized to one of the three doses (5, 10 and 20 mg/kg/day) of active drug or placebo at a 4:1 ratio. In addition, patients had to take their usual dose of antiepileptic drugs 2 h before CBD administration. The primary outcome was to assess the incidence of Treatment-Emergent AEs (TEAEs). A pharmacokinetic evaluation was also performed by measuring the plasma concentrations of CBD and its metabolites 7-OH-CBD and 7-carboxycannabidiol (7-COOH-CBD), and of the most common antiepileptic drugs taken by patients. Serious TEAEs, such as pyrexia and convulsions, occurred in five patients: one at the dose of 5 mg/kg/day, two at the dose of 10 mg/kg/day, one at the dose of 20 mg/kg/day and one in the placebo group. No serious TEAEs (such as pyrexia, somnolence, decreased appetite, sedation, vomiting, ataxia and abnormal behaviour) reported in 80% of patients at 5 mg/kg/day of CBD, in 62.5% at the 10 mg/kg/day dose, in 77.78% at the 20 mg/kg/day dose and in 85.71% of placebo group. SAEs such as status epilepticus, convulsion, parvovirus infection, rash maculopapular, occurred in 10% of patients who received 5 mg/kg daily of CBD, in 25% at the 10 mg/kg daily, in 11.11% at the 20 mg/kg daily and in the 14.29% in placebo group. CBD was generally well-tolerated at the 5–20 mg/kg/day dose range. Elevated transaminases (ALT or AST) were only reported with concomitant use of valproate. The study showed that exposure to CBD and its metabolites increased in a dose-dependent manner, and 7-COOH-CBD was the most abundant circulating metabolite at all doses and times. In fact, at the end of treatment, 7-COOH-CBD levels were 13–17 times higher than those of CBD. The results also showed a pharmacokinetic interaction of CBD with CLB, resulting in an increment of the metabolite N-desmethylclobazam [N-CLB] in plasma exposure of the patients. An elevation in N-CLB, was absent in patients co-administered with stiripentol, possibly reflecting prior inhibition of the CYP2C19 isoenzyme [73].

All doses of CBD were well-tolerated and the 20 mg/kg/day dose was chosen by the for Part B (NCT02091375) study. NCT02091375 enrolled 120 children (2 to 10 years) with DS and drug-resistant epileptic seizures. Patients received either the CBD oral solution at a dose of 20 mg/kg/day ($n = 61$)

or placebo (*n* = 59), for 14 weeks, in addition to the standard antiepileptic treatment. During CBD-treatment, SAEs (status epilepticus, convulsion and somnolence) occurred in 16.39% of patients and in 5.8% of the placebo group. Instead, non-serious AEs (diarrhoea, vomiting, pyrexia, fatigue, upper respiratory tract infection, nasopharyngitis, decreased appetite, somnolence, lethargy, headache, convulsion, cough, irritability, gamma-glutamyltransferase increased, transaminases increased, weight decreased) occurred in 75.41% of patients who had taken CBD at the dose of 20 mg/kg/day and in 47.46% of the placebo group. The results suggested that, following the administration of CBD, the median frequency of seizures decreased from 12.4 to 5.9, compared to a decrease from 14.9 to 14.1 in the placebo-treated group. In 43% of patients treated with CBD and in 27% of patients in the placebo group occurred a reduction in seizure frequency by 50% or more and 3 patients were free of seizures [74]. Although the administration of CBD has caused high rates of AEs, CBD appears to be efficacy in the treatment of patients with DS.

Subsequently, GW launched a second Phase 3 trial, GWCARE2 (NCT02224703), to evaluate DS patients' responses to either a low (10 mg/kg/day) or a high dose (20 mg/kg/day) of GWP42003-P for 14 weeks. The study, still recruiting, plans to enroll 150 participants, both children and adults (2 to 18 years). The results are not available.

The phase 3 clinical trial NCT02224560 (GWPCARE3) included 225 patients with LGS (2 to 55 years) with two or more seizures/week. This study was to evaluate the safety and efficacy of the CBD oral solution (GWP42003-P) as an adjunctive treatment of other antiepileptic drugs. The patients were divided into 3 groups and treated with CBD at the dose of 10 mg/kg/day or 20 mg/kg/day or with placebo for 14 weeks. During the treatment, SAEs such as pneumonia, status epilepticus, elevated aspartate aminotransferase concentration, elevated alanine aminotransferase concentration and elevated γ-glutamyltransferase concentration, occurred in 19.40% of patients treated with 10 mg/kg/day of CBD, in 15.85% treated with 20 mg/kg/day and in 10.53% of the placebo group. Increases in serum aminotransferase concentrations occurred only in patients treated with placebo. While, non-serious AEs (diarrhea, vomiting, decreased appetite, pyrexia, fatigue, somnolence, upper respiratory tract infection, nasopharyngitis) have been observed in 53.73% of 10 mg/kg daily group, in 76.83% of 20 mg/kg/day group, and in 52.63% of the placebo group. A median percent reduction from baseline in drop-seizure frequency was 37.2% in the 10 mg/kg/day CBD group, 41.9% in the 20 mg/kg/day CBD group, and 17.2% in the placebo group. The results reported by the authors show that the addition of the CBD to conventional antiepileptic therapy reduces the frequency of seizures in a dose-dependent manner [75].

The phase 3 clinical trial NCT02224690 (GWPCARE4) included 171 patients (aged between 2 and 55 years) with a diagnosis of LGS. Participants had to have taken one or more antiepileptic drugs (the most used was lamotrigine, valproate and CLB) at a stable dose for at least 4 weeks prior to screening as well as interventions for epilepsy. The first endpoint was to aim the efficacy of the CBD oral solution (GWP42003-P) as adjunctive treatment in reducing the number of drop seizures when compared to the placebo. The secondary endpoint was to assess the safety of CBD by measuring AEs using standard severity measures. Individuals were divided into two groups: 85 received placebo and 86 received a CBD at a dose of 20 mg/kg/day for 14 weeks. SAEs (pneumonia, viral infection, alanine aminotransferase increased, aspartate aminotransferase increased, γ-glutamyltransferase increased) occurred in the 23.26% of CBD group and in 4.71% of patients in the placebo group. Serious TEAEs (increased levels of alanine aminotransferase, aspartate aminotransferase and γ-glutamyltransferase) occurred in four patients in the CBD group. Instead, the most common no serious-AEs (vomiting, diarrhoea, loss of appetite and drowsiness) occurred in the 61.63% of CBD group and in 50.59% of patients in the placebo group. After 14 weeks of treatment, the monthly frequency of seizures decreased by a median of 43.9% from baseline in the CBD group. A reduction in seizures frequency of 50% or more, was reported in 44% of patients in the CBD group and in 24% of patients in the placebo group. The study found that in many patients treated with antiepileptic drugs that included CLB, a higher onset of somnolence was observed. High levels of transaminases were recorded in patients treated with valproate. Nevertheless, the high rate of AEs, the results showed that the administration of long-term CBD oral solution in patients with LGS determines the reduction in seizure frequency compared to placebo [76].

Subsequently, all patients who completed the treatment period in NCT02091206, NCT02091375, NCT02224703, NCT02224560 or NCT02224690 were included in the sixth clinical trial GWPCARE5 (NCT02224573). The results of this study will help to understand the safety of CBD administered over long periods. Patients received an oral solution of CBD (100 mg/mL), titrated from 2.5 to 20 mg/kg/day over a 2-week period, in addiction with their existing treatment. The median treatment duration was 274 days. SAEs such as status epilepticus and convulsion occurred in 29.2% of patients. Commonly reported AEs (diarrhoea, pyrexia, decreased appetite and somnolence) occurred in 93.2% of patients. 17.2% of patients from GWPCARE1 that taking valproic acid, had liver transaminase elevations. In patients from GWPCARE1 Part B, the monthly frequency of seizures from baseline decreased by a median of ranged from 38% to 44% in 12-week periods up to week 48.85% of patients reported an improvement in the overall condition after 48 weeks of treatment. This trial showed that long-term CBD treatment was safe and efficacy to reduce seizure frequency in patients with treatment-resistant DS [77].

A randomized controlled trial NCT02565108 (phase 2) included twenty patients (aged 18 to 65 years) with diagnosed epilepsy treated with CLB. This study examined the possible drug-drug interactions between CLB and CBD. Participants before enrolment followed a stable therapy for at least a month with antiepileptic drugs, including CLB. Patients received CBD oral solution (GWP42003-P) at a dose of 20 mg/kg/day after taking CLB for 21 consecutive days. 75% of patients in the CBD group and 50% of patients in the placebo group showed non-serious AEs (diarrhea, nausea, vomiting, dizziness, somnolence, sedation, dermatitis). Results showed that all participants reduced the maintenance dose of CBD of 10%/day.

Eighteen participants who completed trial NCT02565108 were transferred to the open-label extension (OLE) trial NCT02564952. The OLE phase was a safety study. Initially, all participants received CBD at a dose of 20 mg/kg/day, thereafter the dose was decreased or increased to a maximum of 30 mg/kg/day. All individuals during the study continued to receive CLB. In addition to CLB, participants could not take more than two other AEDs during the study. Only seven of the 18 participants completed the study, 11.11% showed SAEs (status epilepticus, seizure, alanine aminotransferase abnormal, aspartate aminotransferase abnormal γ-glutamyltransferase abnormal). While, 94.44% of patients presented no-serious AEs such as diarrhoea, vomiting, headache, hyponatraemia, dizziness, seizure, somnolence, irritability, respiratory tract infection. The high rate of AEs in the concomitant use of the CBD and CLB for prolonged periods of time may be unsafe.

The clinical trials of phase I NCT02695537 and NCT02700412, will evaluate prospectively and longitudinally the safety and tolerability of CBD oral solution (Epidiolex) at various doses, between 5 mg/kg/day and 25 mg/kg/day with additional titration in some cases up to 50 mg/kg/day. These two trials will enroll both 100 patients with drug-resistant epilepsy. Clinical trial NCT02695537 will enroll patients aged 1 to 18 years, while the NCT02700412 patients aged 17 to 99 years. However, Gaston, et al. [78] evaluated possible CBD interactions with antiepileptic drugs typically used in 39 adults and 42 children of these trials. An analysis was carried out to check for non-uniform changes in both the CBD dose and the dose of other AEDs. In the two combined arms (pediatric and adult) the results recorded linear increases in serum levels of topiramate, rufinamide and [N-CLB] and linear decreases in CLB levels correlate with increasing CBD does. However, there were no significant changes in the levels of other AEDs analyzed (valproate, levetiracetam, phenobarbital, clonazepam, phenytoin, carbamazepine, lamotrigine, oxcarbazepine, ethosuximide, vigabatrin, ezogabine, pregabalin, perampanel and lacosamide). During the study, six adults and eight children showed sedation. The intake of concomitant CBD and valproate resulted in high levels of AST and ALT. Liver function tests showed elevated damage greater than three times the normal limit in four children who dropped out of the study, while the damages of about twice the upper normal limit in eight adults were resolved with valproate withdrawal. A major onset of somnolence following the concomitant administration of CBD and CLB and high levels of transaminases following co-administration of CBD and valproate was also recorded in another study [73] and in clinical trial NCT02224690. In conclusion, the results obtained by the researchers show that the use of CBD with other drugs can be considered safe. On the contrary concomitant use of CBD with valproate is not recommended as a significant liver dysfunction has been observed. Probably because CBD enhances the toxic action of valproate. The interaction between CBD and CLB was also highlighted. Since both of these drugs are metabolized of the cytochrome P450 pathway, this interaction can often induce high plasma levels of n-CLB. Therefore, it is important to monitor this drug-drug interaction. However, as the adverse effects occurring, in this case, are not serious, the concomitant use of CBD with CLB can be considered safe and above all effective, especially in pediatric patients with refractory epilepsy. Part of the results of NCT02695537 and NCT02700412 were described by Szaflarski, et al. [79]. The study showed the efficacy and safety of Epidiolex in 72 children and 60 adults. The results obtained show an average reduction of all types of seizures of 63.6% with difference significant between baseline and 12 weeks. The reduction in seizures seems to have remained stable, in fact, there were no significant differences between 12 and 24 weeks and between 24 and 48 weeks. The severity of the seizures assessed by the Chalfont Seizure Severity Scale (CSSS) also showed an improvement from a baseline score of 80.7 to enroll at 39.3 at 12 weeks with CSSS scores stable even between 12 and 24 weeks and between 24 and 48 weeks. The analysis of AE Profile indicates a significant improvement in the presence/severity of adverse events between the baseline and 12 weeks with stable AEDs thereafter without significant differences between 12 and 24 weeks and between 24 and 48 weeks. The results of this study show significant improvements in the profile of adverse events, in the severity of crises and in reducing the frequency of seizures as early as 12 weeks; improvements that have been maintained during the 48 weeks of treatment.

A clinical trial of phase II NCT02987114, is an open-label, single-center trial, that recruited 16 children (aged 2-15 years), with intractable epilepsy. The aim of this trial was to evaluate the safety, tolerability and efficacy of oral administration of PTL101 (formulation of seamless gelatin matrix green beads containing CBD) as adjunctive therapy for pediatric intractable epilepsy. Patients at least 4 weeks before enrolment had to have stabilized the doses of antiepileptic drugs. This clinical trial has included 4 weeks of observation of clinical parameters and 13 weeks of CBD treatment at an initial dose of 25 mg/kg daily up to the maximum dose of 450 mg/kg. Subsequently the patients were monitored for 2 weeks. The results of this study, not yet available.

The results obtained from all the completed studies show that CBD is a safe compound when combined with common AEDs. An aspect of particular interest concerns the association of CBD with valproate and CLB. In particular, some studies have shown that the association between CBD and valproate leads to a reduction in liver function related to an increase in transaminases. This alteration has been shown to be reversible and not to cause permanent liver damage. Pharmacokinetic studies have shown that CBD determines, as associated with CLB, a plasma increase in the metabolites of this benzodiazepine. All trials reporting efficacy data show that CBD is able to reduce the frequency of seizures.

5.2. Ongoing Clinical Trials

In the last 4 years, various tests have been started to evaluate the efficacy and safety of CBD as an antiepileptic. In this subsection, we have collected the trials that to date have not yet available results as they are still in the patient recruitment phase.

Two phase 2 clinical trials NCT03355300 and NCT03336242 are expecting to recruit about 30 pediatric patients (3 to 17 years), with treatment-resistant childhood absence seizure. Both studies will include three experimental treatment cohorts (20, 30 and 40 mg/kg/day). NCT03336242 will assess efficacy, safety, tolerability and pharmacokinetics of CBD oral solution after 4 weeks of treatment. This study will include a 4-week screening period and a 5 or 10 day titration period (depending on study cohort), a 4-week treatment period followed by 5-day tapering for doses >20 mg/kg/day and a 4-week follow-up period. Instead, NCT03355300 will evaluate the long-term (up to approximately 54 weeks) safety and tolerability of the CBD oral solution, monitoring the incidence of SAEs and AEs during and after treatment. For both trials, the final data collection and the results are expected by the end of the year 2019.

In the clinical trial NCT03676049, CBD will be administered as an adjunct to all current AEDs in 5–10 patients (aged between 5 and 19) with refractory epilepsy. The CBD oral solution used for treatment, with prior approval from the National Institute on Drug Abuse was prepared at the University of Mississippi, and subsequently received FDA approval for compassionate use. A dosing titration period will start with 100 mg/day, and will be titrated monthly as tolerated based on clinical response, up to 300 mg/day. During the treatment period the patients will be subjected to control visits at the baseline, at the fourth, at the eighth and at the twelfth weeks. During these visits the efficacy of the treatment will be evaluated, observing the laboratory tests, quality of life of the patient, the profile of the side effects and the crisis count. Patients who after 3 months of treatment show stability could continue the use of CBD for another 3 months.

The clinical trial NCT02461706 will assess the safety and efficacy of CBD when administered as adjunctive therapy in 50 children (2 to 16 years) who have resistant to AEDs. Patients treated with AEDs were to have stabilized doses at least 4 weeks prior to enrolling. The study established the starting dose of 25 mg/kg/day. Maximum dose titration should be achieved in most patients within 5 weeks. The patients will be clinically evaluated at baseline, once a month for three months and once every three months thereafter. In addition, to ensure the safety of the study, all patients who reached the maximum dose (more than 600 mg of daily) of the CBD will be monitored at least once a month until the steady state of the maintenance dose was reached.

A double-blind, randomized, placebo-controlled phase 3 trial (NCT02783092), is intended to evaluate the efficacy of the adjuvant use of CBD oral solution (200 mg/ml dissolved in corn oil), in patients with epilepsy. The estimated 126 patients (2 to 18 years) will be treated with CBD at the initial dose of 5 mg/kg/day, up to a maximum dose of 25 mg/kg/day. The primary outcome is to evaluate whether CBD treatment resulted in a 50% reduction in seizure frequency compared to treatment with antiepileptic drugs after 30 days. The results of this study (estimated final data collection in August 2020) will make it possible to clarify the efficacy of CBD at different doses.

The phase I clinical trial NCT02286986 is a multi-center study that to investigate the pharmacokinetics and dose-ranging tolerability, efficacy and safety of CBD (GWP42003-P), in 25 children and young adults (2 to 25 years) with epilepsy. The study was divided into two parts: Part A and Part B. Part A was used to evaluate the safety and tolerability of more ascending doses of GWP42003-P compared to placebo. The best-tolerated dose in Part A of the study was used to treat patients in Part B for 60 consecutive days. The antiepileptic efficacy of GWP42003-P compared to placebo was evaluated by monitoring the incidence in convulsions, determining the plasma concentration of GWP42003-P and its main metabolite following the escalation of multiple doses of GWP42003-P. Furthermore, was investigated the effect of GWP42003-P on the pharmacokinetics of concomitant and cognitive function, sleep quality and daytime sleepiness were also observed. The trial is still active and the results have not been published, yet.

Two phases II clinical trials NCT02607904 and NCT02607891 want to verify the possible drug-drug interactions between GWP42003-P and two antiepileptic drugs, stiripentol or valproate in patients with epilepsy. Both trials will enroll patients between 16 to 55 years. In the trials NCT02607904, patients will be treated up to a maximum dose of 30 mg/kg/day for 12 months. Instead, in NCT02607891 trials, the participants will be randomized into a 4: 1 ratio to receive GWP42003-P or corresponding placebo. The hypothesis is that levels of stiripentol or valproate may be altered as a result of using GWP42003-P. During treatment, CBD will be administered at a maximum dose of 20 mg/kg/day for 25 days. Participants had to take stiripentol or valproate and no more than two other AEDs during the blinded period of the study.

Two phases III clinical trials NCT02953548 and NCT02954887 intended to evaluate the efficacy and safety of CBD oral solution (GWP42003-P; GW Pharmaceutical) in infants with WS (Infantile Spasms). These studies weredivided into 3 phases: a pilot safety phase; a randomized central controlled phase and an open-label extension phase. The NCT02953548 will be described in the pilot phase. Two cohorts of five participants will be enrolled sequentially. GWP42003-P will be administered up to a maximum dose of 40 mg/kg/day for the 2-week treatment period. Instead, clinical trial NCT02954887 will be an extension trial that will recruit 202 infants (from 1 month to 24 months), for 1 year of treatment. The results expected from this study will allow observing if the administration of CBD will be effective in infants with WS.

Two phases III clinical trial NCT02544763 and NCT02544750 (GWPCARE6) will evaluate respectively, in a double-blinded phase and in an open-label extension phase, the efficacy of the CBD oral solution (GWP42003-P) as adjunctive therapy by monitoring the frequency of seizures in patients with TSC. NCT02544763 is expecting to recruit about 210 patients (1 to 65 years). All AEDs or interventions will be stabilized at least 1 month before the screening and the stability of the therapy will be maintained during the study. Patients will be treated with CBD at the dose of 25 or 50 mg/kg/day for 16 weeks. The efficacy of the CBD will be tested by evaluating the change in seizure frequency. Patients that will complete this blinded phase will be included in the NCT02544750 trial. The safety of CBD administration will be measured based on the incidence of AEs. All participants will be dosed up to a maximum of 50 mg/kg/day. From these two trials the results, not yet available, will help to understand if the administration of CBD can lead to a decrease in the crisis in patients with TSC.

A phase 1/2 clinical trial NCT03014440, aim to determine the safety and tolerability of CBD (Epidiolex) in addition to the anti-epileptic treatments in use, in patients aged 1 to 20 years with drug-resistant epilepsy. Antiepileptic therapy followed by patients had to be stable for at least 1 month. To date, there is no information available regarding the treatment, the doses used and the results.

The NCT02660255 is an observational, open-label, flexible dose study. The aim of this trial is to evaluate the safety and efficacy of Epidiolex, in addition to common AEDs. The study will be recruited subjects aged 1-60 years with treatment-resistant epilepsy. Patients prior to enrolment will be treated with 1–4 AEDs on stable settings from least 1 month. Epidiolex will be administered for 1 year and 9 months. To date, no superior information and results are available, yet.

The clinical trial NCT02397863 is an open-label, multi-center study including patients (1 to 18 years of age) with drug-resistant epilepsy. Patients are treated with CBD (Epidiolex), the daily dosage is up to 25 mg/kg/day with optional up-titration to a maximal daily dosage up to 50 m/kg/day until the end of treatment. Treatment was provided for a total of 52 weeks. For this study the results have not been published, yet.

Clinical trial NCT02332655 (phase 1/2) aims to assess the tolerability and optimal dose of CBD to be used as a treatment in children and young adults with SWS and drug-resistant epilepsy to define the optimal dose of Epidiolex. The study involving the recruitment of the 10 patients (aged 1 months to 45 years) already in treatment with antiepileptic drugs. Patients treated with 1–5 basic antiepileptic drugs had to have reached stable doses for a minimum of 4 weeks prior to enrolment. Treatment will start with 2 mg/kg/day. The dose will be increased by 3 mg/kg/day after seven days and then by 5 mg/kg/day every seven days up to a maximum dose of 25 mg/kg/day given for 48 weeks. From the expected results potential efficacy of CBD in refractory crises in patients with SWS will emerge.

An open-label observational study NCT02556008 will evaluate the efficacy of pure CBD for the treatment of 25 children (1 to 17 years) with severe refractory epilepsy. The pure CBD used during treatment is not approved by the FDA, therefore, investigators conducted this study through the FDA's expanded access mechanism for compassionate use. CBD will be administered as an adjunct to all current anti-epileptic therapies. Patients had to undergo therapeutic treatment with 1-3 basic antiepileptic drugs at stable doses for a minimum of 4 weeks prior to enrolment. The expected dosage of the study was 2 mg/kg/day for a first week, 3 mg/kg/day for the second week, 5 mg/kg/day for the third week up to a maximum dose of 25 mg/Kg/day. Seizure frequency will be assessed four weeks before the initiation of CBD, the next month, and at least every 3 months thereafter. The results of efficacy of CBD are not yet available. Data from these studies will be available soon, as the final data collection for many studies is expected by the end of 2019.

5.3. Clinical Trials Approved by Local Ethics Committees

In this subsection, clinical studies published in indexed journals have been described. Many of these manuscripts report the results obtained on long periods of treatment with CBD and provide important efficacy data. In addition, the common antiepileptic drugs taken by patients in association with CBD are detailed.

The study conducted by Geffrey, et al. [72], approved by Massachusetts General Hospital (MGH) Institutional Review Board (IRB) evaluated the CBD interaction with CLB. The aim of this study was to evaluate possible interactions between CBD and CLB, assessing its efficacy, safety and pharmacokinetics. For this study, 13 patients (4 to 19 years) with refractory epilepsy and treated with CLB were recruited. Patients started taking CBD at a dose of 5 mg/kg/day and treated up by 5 mg/kg/day each week to a dose of 25 mg/kg/day, for 8 weeks. CLB was administered daily at a stable dose of 0.5 mg/kg that was decreased during the study when side effects were observed. The plasma levels of CBD, CLB and [N-CLB] were measured at baseline and at weeks 4 and 8 of treatment. The results of the efficacy study showed a 50% convulsion reduction in nine out of 13 subjects, corresponding to a 70% response rate. In two patients, however, there was an increase in the frequency of seizures during the treatment period, therefore the dose of CLB was reduced. Increases in plasma levels of CBD, CLB and its metabolite were recorded. Already in the fourth week, the mean of CBL levels had been an increase of 60 ± 80%, while the mean in [N-CLB] was an increase of 500 ± 300%. The results of the safety study show that in 77% subjects AEs were reported as somnolence ($n = 6$), ataxia ($n = 2$), irritability ($n = 2$), restless sleep ($n = 1$), urinary retention ($n = 1$), tremor ($n = 1$) and loss of appetite (n = 1). After adjusting the doses of CLB all AEs were resolved. Therefore, the results reported by the authors show an interaction between CBD and CLB, and that CBD influences [N-CLB] levels much more than CLB levels.

The efficacy of the interaction between CBD and CLB was also seen in a study conducted by Porcari, et al. [80]. This study was approved by the Vanderbilt University Institutional Review Board. In this retrospective study, the aim is to define the efficacy of CBD alone or in association with CLB in 209 children ($\leq$ 19 years) with epilepsy. The duration of treatment in patients receiving CBD was 1.1 years, while patients received CBD + CLB for 1.3 years, and for 2.5 years received CLB. The reduction of antiepileptic drugs was seen in 21% of the CBD group, in 26% CBD + CLB and in 18% of CLB group. No-seizures were observed in 14% of patients in the CBD group, in 9% of patients in the CBD + CLB group and in 11% of patients in the CLB group. The results reported by the authors show a reduction of the crises > of 50% in 33% of the CBD group, in 44% of the CBD + CLB group and in 38% of the CLB group. It was also observed that LGS was the most commonly observed syndrome in all cohorts, and in these patients, the response rate was 58% with CBD, 52% with CBD and CLB and 40% with CLB alone. The sedation was the most common AEs reported in 36% of patients in the CLB group, in 7% of patients in the CBD + CLB group and in 0% of CBD group. This retrospective study suggests that CBD is useful in the treatment of refractory epilepsy with benefits that cannot be attributed to the interaction with CLB and increased levels of its active metabolite.

Morrison, et al. [81] conducted a pharmacokinetic study that evaluated the possible drug-drug interactions between CLB, stiripentol or valproate and CBD (Epidiolex). This study was approved by the Independent Ethics Committee of the Foundation Evaluation of Ethics in Biomedical Research, Assen, The Netherlands. For this open-label phase I study, were enrolled 78 healthy subjects. The primary outcome was to evaluate the interaction of multiple CBD administration as a perpetrator drug with antiepileptic drugs (victim) at steady-state plasma concentrations: CLB (and its active metabolite, *N*-desmethylclobazam); stiripentol and valproate (and its potentially hepatotoxic metabolite, 4-ene-VPA). On the contrary, was also evaluated the interaction of CBD (victim drug) and its metabolites 7-OH-CBD and 7-COOH-CBD at steady-state plasmatic concentrations, with multiple doses of CLB, stiripentol or valproate as perpetrators drugs. CBD was given at 750 mg twice daily, CLB at 10 mg/kg/day, stiripentol at 750 mg and valproate at 750 mg twice a day. The results showed a significant interaction between CBD and CLB. When CLB was used as the victim drug, significant increases in its metabolite [N-CLB] were recorded. These increases are related to an inhibition of the CPY2C19. In addition, the concentrations of the active metabolite 7-OH-CBD increased when was co-administered with CLB. Stiripentol, however, increased by 28% when it is at steady-state plasma concentrations alone, and by 50% following co-administration with CBD. The 50% increase in stiripentol concentration may be caused by an inhibition of CPY2C19 by the CBD. Instead, co-administration of stiripentol with CBD not caused an increase in CBD concentrations, but caused a 29% increase of 7-OH-CBD and 13% of 7-COOH-CBD. The interaction of the CBD and valproate did not affect the pharmacokinetics of the two drugs. Regarding the safety study, six subjects were withdrawn due to adverse events; three when CLB was added to the steady-state CBD and three when the valproate was added to the steady-state CBD. Two subjects reported SAEs when CLB was co-administered to CBD. Moderate AEs were reported in eight subjects; instead mild AEs were reported in most subjects. The results obtained by the authors can be concluded by saying that the co-administration of drugs was moderately tolerated. Furthermore, the drug-drug bidirectional interaction noted when CLB was co-administered with CBD, suggests a dose reduction for CLB when administered with CBD.

Another study to evaluate the efficacy of the CBD oral solution (GWP42003-P) as a therapy for drug-resistant epilepsy in TSC was conducted by Hess, et al. [82] (approved by Massachusetts General Hospital Institutional Review Board and U.S. Food and Drug Administration). Of the 56 patients enrolled in this study, only 18 patients (aged 2 to 31 years) were evaluated because they were affected by TSC. At the time of enrolment, patients were taking between one and seven anti-epileptic drugs, such as lacosamide ($n = 14$), CLB ($n = 10$), levetiracetam ($n = 7$), lamotrigine ($n = 5$), valproic acid ($n = 3$) and rufinamide ($n = 3$). Treatment started at a dose of 5 mg/kg/day. This dose was increased by 5 mg/kg/day every week up to the initial maximum dose of 50 mg/kg daily, for 12 months. After the third month of treatment, doses of the CBD and concomitant AEDs could be adjusted monthly in almost all patients in order to optimize seizure control. 15 patients achieved the initial maximum dose of 25 mg/kg/day of CBD, while five achieved the highest dose of 50 mg/kg/day of the CBD, and at this dose, none reported CBD-related AEs. Instead, six patients decreased the dose of CBD during the study in order to alleviate AEs and interactions with concurrent AEDs. 66.7% of patients reported AEs and among them, drowsiness, ataxia and diarrhoea. Three months after the treatment, in four patients a reduction in seizure rate greater than 80% was recorded and one patient became seizure-free and he remained free until the twelfth month. The results also show that in patients took CBD and CLB the response rate after 3 months of treatment was 58.3% against 33.3% in patients who did not take CLB. Given the results reported by the authors in this study, the CBD can be considered valid and safe in the treatment of refractory epilepsy in the TSC.

Five patients enrolled in this study were included in another multicentre analysis of CBD expanded-access conducted by Devinsky, et al. [83] (in 11 epilepsy centers in the USA). The aim of this study was to assess safe, tolerated and effective of CBD (Epidiolex) in children and young adults with severe, intractable, treatment-resistant epilepsy (the most common epilepsy syndrome treated were DS and LGS). This study was approved by the institutional review boards at each study site. CBD was used in addition to anti-epileptic treatment. For this trial, 214 patients were enrolled (1 to 30 years); of these 162 patients after the first dose of CBD were monitored for 12 weeks and were included in the safety and tolerability analysis while 137 patients (64%) were included in the efficacy analysis. Patients started the treatment with CBD at the initial dose of 2–5 mg/kg daily up to a maximum dose of 50 mg/kg daily for 12 weeks. In the safety study, SAEs were observed in 30% of patients. Treatment-related serious AEs, such as status epilepticus, diarrhoea, pneumonia and weight loss were recorded in 20 individuals. Instead, in 79% of patients showed no serious AEs, the most common were decreased appetite, fatigue, somnolence, diarrhoea, convulsions, status epilepticus, sedation, lethargy. After 12 weeks of treatment, results showed a median reduction in monthly motor seizures of 36.5%.

In the patients with DS (n = 32), the treatment led to a median reduction of monthly motor convulsions of 49%, in 16 patients a reduction of 50%. Instead, for patients with LGS (n = 30), an average reduction of 36.8% in motor crises was recorded. Findings obtained from this study showed that CBD seems to reduce the frequency of seizures and also shows an appropriate safety profile, even in patients with DS and LGS.

Another study conducted by Sands, et al. [84] assessed the long-term safety, tolerability and efficacy of CBD to children with refractory epilepsy. This study was approved by the Human Research Ethics Committee of the UCSF Benioff Children's Hospital. The CBD oral solution (Epidiolex) was administered in addition to other anti-epileptic treatments in 26 patients (aged 1 to 17 years). The doses of concomitant antiepileptic drugs had to be stable during the 4-week of baseline period and had to remain stable during the first three months of treatment. CBD was administered at the starting dose of 5 mg/kg daily and subsequently, weekly dosage was measured in increments of 5 mg/kg daily up to a maximum dose of 25 mg/kg daily. The duration of therapy ranged from 4 to 53 months. The patients underwent blood tests performed during the baseline period, after 1, 2 and 3 months and thereafter every 3 months from treatment. Furthermore, the minimum concentrations of antiepileptic drugs were evaluated. The frequency of seizures and AEs was monitored during the treatment period. The primary outcome of the study was to test the efficacy of CBD in terms of > 50% reduction in the frequency of motor seizures. Fifteen of 26 patients discontinued treatment, one due to a status epilepticus, one for severe weight loss, all others for lack of efficacy. Instead, six patients showed SAEs as status epilepticus (n = 3), catatonia (n = 2) and hypoalbuminemia (n = 1). 21 out of 26 patients reported no serious AEs among which the most frequent were: reduced appetite (n = 10), diarrhoea (n = 9), and weight loss (n = 8). In patients showing significant weight loss, the doses of CBD were reduced. Changes in the concentrations of antiepileptic drugs were observed in four patients. Three of them reported increased CLB concentrations, one reported an increment in phenobarbital contractions. In three patients was observed an increment in aspartate aminotransferase and alanine transferase levels when CBD was co-administered with valproate. The reduction in the frequency of seizures > 50%, was rediscovered in 38.4% of patients after 3 months of treatment, in 56.7% after 6 months, in 42.3% after 9 months, in 38.4% after 12 months, 42.3% after 18 months and 34.6% after 24 months. In conclusion, after 24 months of treatment, of the 26 patients enrolled, only nine continued CBD as adjunctive therapy. Of these patients, seven had a 50% reduction in the frequency of motor crises, three of which remained completely free of seizures. Only seven of the nine patients who continued treatment showed a reduction in seizure frequency > 50% after 36 months. The results reported by the authors showed that long-term CBD results in a clinically significant reduction in seizure frequency, and a low percentage of SAEs. Moreover, because treatment was stopped after a few months in most patients, the number of patients exposed to CBD for a long time is low and the rate of adverse effects over time may be underestimated.

Using the same CBD formulation (Epidiolex) and the same administration doses Kaplan, et al. [85] conducted a study that was approved by the Federal Drug Administration for the use of Epidiolex in the treatment of pediatric medically refractory epilepsy in SWS. In this study, five patients (aged 1 months to 45 years) were enrolled. The maximum dose of 25 mg/kg daily was tolerated only by two patients, while in the other three the maximum tolerated dose was 20 mg/kg per day. Three participants withdrew from the study, two due to lack of efficacy (week 38 and week 9), while one due to the temporary increase in seizures during dose titration, but later re-enrolled. Three subjects remain in the extension phase of the study continued to take CBD for more than a year. All subjects reported at least one CBD-related adverse event during the study such as temporarily increased seizures, behavioral issues, increased aspartate aminotransferase and fatigue. All transient AEs resolved spontaneously after dose changes in concomitant anticonvulsants or CBD. Seizure reduction above 50% was seen in two patients at weeks 14 and in three patients with bilateral brain involvement. Instead, subjects reported improvements in quality of life during the treatment. As suggested by the results obtained from this study, CBD appears to be well tolerated and a valid candidate as adjunctive therapy for seizures management in individuals with SWS.

Rosenberg, et al. [86] belonging to the same research group of Devinsky, et al. [83] prolonged the study for evaluating the Quality of Life of Childhood Epilepsy (QOLCE) before and after treatment with CBD (Epidolex). The study was approved by the NYU Langone Medical Center institutional ethics board. For this study were enrolled patients (aged 1–30) with intractable treatment-resistant epilepsy. In addition to the baseline antiepileptic drugs, patients were given CBD at the initial dose of 2–5 mg/Kg daily up to the maximum dose of 50 mg/Kg daily for 12 weeks. After 12 weeks of treatment with CBD, the median monthly seizures frequency was 13.9 and the median percent change from baseline was −39.4%. In addition, the results indicated an improvement of 8.2 ± 9.9 points in patient QOLCE. In fact, patients showed an improvement in behaviour, in memory, in energy/fatigue, in control/impotence, in other cognitive functions and in global quality of life.

The same research group of Devinsky, et al. [87], conducted a study for evaluating the safety and efficacy of long-term CBD administration in patients with severe childhood-onset epilepsy, and with CDKL5 deficiency disorder and Aicardi, Doose syndromes and Dup15q syndromes. This study was approved by the IRB at each institution. For this study, 55 patients aged between 1 and 30 were enrolled (with 55 in the safety group and 50 in the efficacy group). Patients were given a pharmaceutical compound of Highly purified CBD (Epidolex). Treatment included 144 weeks of Epidiolex administration in addition to anti-epileptic therapies at the starting dose of 5 mg/Kg per day. During treatment, an increase of 2–10 mg/kg per day was carried out every two weeks up to the maximum dose of 50 mg/kg per day. The efficacy study showed that the percent change in median monthly convulsive seizure frequency for all patients after treatment decreased from baseline of 51.4% to week 12 and of 59.1% to week 48 with a no significant change between weeks 12 and 48. After 12 weeks of follow-up was reported a decrease of 50% or more of seizures in 50% of patients and in 57% at 48 weeks. The safety results of the drug showed that of the 55 patients,10 patients withdrew by week 48, including 5 by weeks 12 and 48 due to lack of efficacy ($n = 4$) and AEs ($n = 1$). A total of 15 (27%) participants withdrew by week 144 of extended follow-up. There were no deaths during the study. SAEs that occurred during treatment were convulsions (9%), status epilepticus (9%) and respiratory infection (5%). While other adverse events reported more frequently were diarrhea (29%), drowsiness (22%) and fatigue (22%). These results can demonstrate the safety and tolerability of long-term treatment with CBD and the reduction in seizure frequency in these four aetiologies of epilepsy.

Chen, et al. [88] conducted an open-label study, the aim was to assess the tolerability and safety of CBD (Epidiolex) in the treatment of drug-resistant epilepsy in children. Sydney Children's Hospital Network Human Research Ethics Committee approved the protocol for this study. Children ($n = 40$; mean age 8.5 years) with drug-resistant epilepsy and uncountable daily seizures in focal/multifocal epilepsy, epileptic encephalopathy, LGD and DS, were enrolled. CBD was administrated in addition to anti-epileptic therapy at the initial dose of 5 mg/Kg daily for 12 weeks. The initial dose was increased every week by 5 mg/Kg daily up to a maximum dose of 25 mg/Kg daily. During the treatment five children withdrew from the study, two because he had an increase in the frequency of the seizures, one because has manifested significant somnolence, one for respiratory depression and one because their transaminase level was elevated. SAEs occurred in 15 out of patients, the frequent recurring to treatment were increased seizure number (in eight patients), intercurrent illness (in five patients), liver function disorder (in all patients), hyperlipidemia (in all patients), severe somnolence with anorexia and respiratory depression (in one patient). Over-therapeutic phenytoin levels are another SAEs manifested in two participants were considered related to treatment and occurred at doses of 10 mg/kg/day and 20 mg/kg/day. All participants showed AEs not all attributable to treatment. While, AEs that occurred frequently (15 individuals) and linked to the treatment was the drowsiness (AEs spontaneously resolved the 10 participants), and gastrointestinal disorders (nausea, vomiting, diarrhoea) in nine patients, somnolence (13 individuals) and increased seizures (two individuals).

Instead, 12 children showed an improvement in health in general. The results reported in this study show that Epidiolex can be considered useful as adjuvant therapy. The presence of adverse events and possible interactions with antiepileptic drugs are important aspects to be taken into consideration.

Szaflarski, et al. [89] conducted an open-label, Expanded-Access Program (EAP) in 25 epilepsy centers in the USA, and it was approved by an institutional review board at each site. The aim of this study was to evaluate the safety and efficacy of CBD oral solution (Epidiolex), in addition to common AEDs in patients with different forms of treatment-resistant epilepsies (TREs). For the study, 607 patients with a mean age of 13 were enrolled. All patients were included in the safety study, while 508 were included in the efficacy study. Treatment involved a 4-week baseline period followed by a 96-week treatment period. During treatment, patients received Epidiolex at the initial dose of 2–10 mg/Kg up to a maximum dose of 25-50 mg/Kg daily. 146 patients (mostly due to lack efficacy [15%] or AEs [5%]) from the safety study group and 136 patients (mostly due to lack efficacy [15%] or AEs [4%]) from the efficacy group were withdrawn from the study. SAEs were found in 33% of patients such as convulsion (9%), status epilepticus (7%), pneumonia (5%), and vomiting (3%). Instead, AEs manifested in 88% of patients the most common were diarrhea (29%), somnolence (22%), and convulsion (17%). Already after 12 weeks of treatment, the median monthly frequency of seizure convulsions was reduced by 51% and by 48 % the frequency of total seizures. These reductions remained stable during the 96 weeks of treatment. Between weeks 12 and 96 the average dose of CBD was 25 mg/kg daily, 55% of patients at follow-up had reduced the dose. Half of the patients taking concomitant CLB and valproate reduced the dose compared to baseline during the study. While, most of those who take simultaneously levetiracetam, had remained at their basal doses. The data obtained from this study show that CBD as an adjunct treatment to common AEDs can be used in the long-term effective treatment in patients with TRE.

A very interesting data in these studies is the pharmacokinetics and interaction of CBD with common AEDs. The interaction of these drugs is very complex and is linked to the individual metabolites produced and to the possible metabolic pathways that are involved. Specifically, the study conducted by Geffrey, et al. [72] shows a bidirectional drug-drug interaction when CBD is administered with the CLB for long period of time. Therefore, CLB determines an increase in serum levels of the CBD metabolite (7-OH-CBD) and conversely, CBD causes an increase in the metabolite of CLB (n-CLB). CBD is an inhibitor of CYP2C19, an enzyme involved in the degradation of n-CLB, these explain how the CBD associated with CLB causes elevated plasma levels of this metabolite. In contrast, CBD does not influence the pharmacokinetics of valproate and stiripentol when co-administered, moreover, stiripentol causes a slight decrease in CBD metabolites (7-OH-CBD 7-COOH-CBD) while valproate causes a slight increase of 7-OH-CBD. The mechanisms by which these interactions take place are not yet known but do not cause clinically relevant effects. However, the CBD shows good safety profiles, the interaction with these two drugs does not require the interruption of therapy. The modulation of the dose of these AEDs will be sufficient to resolve the adverse events. In conclusion, the results of these studies show that the administration of CBD as an addition to the common AEDs for long periods of time leads to clinically significant reductions in the frequency of convulsive and total seizures in different etiologies of epilepsy. Furthermore, an improvement in the quality of life of these patients was also observed.

6. Conclusions

The CBD is a compound extensively studied for its potential efficacy for the treatment of epilepsy. In this review, we reported the studies conducted in infants, children and teenagers affected by epilepsy resistant to common AEDs.

To date, available safety data show that the administration of CBD associated with other AEDs causes non-serious adverse events, which can be resolved reducing the dose of CBD and/or common AEDs. In this context, particular attention should be paid when CBD is associated with valproate and CLB. Specifically, abnormal liver function was noted in participants taking concomitant valproate, therefore, it is necessary to monitor serum levels of these compounds and their respective metabolites. Instead, when CBD is associated with CLB it induces an increase in its metabolites. Since the adverse effects are not serious, this association can be considered safe.

The available results also highlight the efficacy of CBD as adjunctive to common AEDs. The mechanism by which CBD interacts with other AEDs is not yet fully known, as many metabolic pathways involved in this interaction are still unknown. In addition, not all the molecular targets used by the CBD to exercise its antiepileptic action are yet known. However, the results obtained to date encourage the use of CBD associated with AEDs.

Author Contributions: S.S. wrote the manuscript; S.M. contributed to bibliographic research; E.C. contributed in graphical support; P.B. and E.M. revised the manuscript.

Funding: This study was supported by current research fund 2019, Ministry of Health, Italy.

Acknowledgments: This manuscript was supported by grants of the Italian Ministry of Health.

Conflicts of Interest: The authors declare no conflict of interest.

References

1. ElSohly, M.A.; Slade, D. Chemical constituents of marijuana: the complex mixture of natural cannabinoids. *Life Sci.* **2005**, *78*, 539–548. [CrossRef]
2. Burstein, S. Cannabidiol (CBD) and its analogs: a review of their effects on inflammation. *Bioorganic Med. Chem.* **2015**, *23*, 1377–1385. [CrossRef] [PubMed]
3. Bih, C.I.; Chen, T.; Nunn, A.V.; Bazelot, M.; Dallas, M.; Whalley, B.J. Molecular targets of cannabidiol in neurological disorders. *Neurotherapeutics* **2015**, *12*, 699–730.
4. Sanchez, A.; Garcia-Merino, A. Neuroprotective agents: cannabinoids. *Clin. Immunol.* **2012**, *142*, 57–67. [CrossRef] [PubMed]
5. Rajan, T.S.; Scionti, D.; Diomede, F.; Grassi, G.; Pollastro, F.; Piattelli, A.; Cocco, L.; Bramanti, P.; Mazzon, E.; Trubiani, O. Gingival stromal cells as an in vitro model: Cannabidiol modulates genes linked with amyotrophic lateral sclerosis. *J. Cell. Biochem.* **2017**, *118*, 819–828. [CrossRef] [PubMed]
6. Santos, N.A.G.; Martins, N.M.; Sisti, F.M.; Fernandes, L.S.; Ferreira, R.S.; Queiroz, R.H.C.; Santos, A.C. The neuroprotection of cannabidiol against MPP+-induced toxicity in PC12 cells involves trkA receptors, upregulation of axonal and synaptic proteins, neuritogenesis, and might be relevant to Parkinson's disease. *Toxicol. Vitr.* **2015**, *30*, 231–240. [CrossRef]
7. Chagas, M.H.N.; Zuardi, A.W.; Tumas, V.; Pena-Pereira, M.A.; Sobreira, E.T.; Bergamaschi, M.M.; dos Santos, A.C.; Teixeira, A.L.; Hallak, J.E.; Crippa, J.A.S. Effects of cannabidiol in the treatment of patients with Parkinson's disease: an exploratory double-blind trial. *J. Psychopharmacol.* **2014**, *28*, 1088–1098. [CrossRef] [PubMed]
8. Consroe, P.; Laguna, J.; Allender, J.; Snider, S.; Stern, L.; Sandyk, R.; Kennedy, K.; Schram, K. Controlled clinical trial of cannabidiol in Huntington's disease. *Pharmacol. Biochem. Behav.* **1991**, *40*, 701–708. [CrossRef]
9. Vallée, A.; Lecarpentier, Y.; Guillevin, R.; Vallée, J.-N. Effects of cannabidiol interactions with Wnt/β-catenin pathway and PPARγ on oxidative stress and neuroinflammation in Alzheimer's disease. *Acta Biochim. Et Biophys. Sin.* **2017**, *49*, 853–866. [CrossRef]
10. Watt, G.; Karl, T. In vivo evidence for therapeutic properties of cannabidiol (CBD) for Alzheimer's disease. *Front. Pharmacol.* **2017**, *8*, 20. [CrossRef]
11. Diomede, F.; Scionti, D.; Piattelli, A.; Grassi, G.; Pollastro, F.; Bramanti, P.; Mazzon, E.; Trubiani, O. Cannabidiol modulates the expression of Alzheimer's disease-related genes in mesenchymal stem cells. *Int. J. Mol. Sci.* **2016**, *18*, 26.
12. Oláh, A.; Tóth, B.I.; Borbíró, I.; Sugawara, K.; Szöllõsi, A.G.; Czifra, G.; Pál, B.; Ambrus, L.; Kloepper, J.; Camera, E. Cannabidiol exerts sebostatic and antiinflammatory effects on human sebocytes. *J. Clin. Investig.* **2014**, *124*, 3713–3724. [CrossRef]
13. Mecha, M.; Feliú, A.; Iñigo, P.; Mestre, L.; Carrillo-Salinas, F.; Guaza, C. Cannabidiol provides long-lasting protection against the deleterious effects of inflammation in a viral model of multiple sclerosis: a role for A2A receptors. *Neurobiol. Dis.* **2013**, *59*, 141–150. [CrossRef] [PubMed]

14. Chen, J.; Hou, C.; Chen, X.; Wang, D.; Yang, P.; He, X.; Zhou, J.; Li, H. Protective effect of cannabidiol on hydrogen peroxide-induced apoptosis, inflammation and oxidative stress in nucleus pulposus cells. *Mol. Med. Rep.* **2016**, *14*, 2321–2327. [CrossRef] [PubMed]
15. Borges, R.; Batista, J.; Viana, R.; Baetas, A.; Orestes, E.; Andrade, M.; Honório, K.; da Silva, A. Understanding the molecular aspects of tetrahydrocannabinol and cannabidiol as antioxidants. *Molecules* **2013**, *18*, 12663–12674. [CrossRef]
16. Soares, R.Z.; Vuolo, F.; Dall'Igna, D.M.; Michels, M.; Crippa, J.A.d.S.; Hallak, J.E.C.; Zuardi, A.W.; Dal-Pizzol, F. Evaluation of the role of the cannabidiol system in an animal model of ischemia/reperfusion kidney injury. *Rev. Bras. Ter. Intensiva* **2015**, *27*, 383–389. [CrossRef]
17. González-García, C.; Torres, I.M.; García-Hernández, R.; Campos-Ruíz, L.; Esparragoza, L.R.; Coronado, M.J.; Grande, A.G.; García-Merino, A.; López, A.J.S. Mechanisms of action of cannabidiol in adoptively transferred experimental autoimmune encephalomyelitis. *Exp. Neurol.* **2017**, *298*, 57–67. [CrossRef] [PubMed]
18. Castillo, A.; Tolón, M.; Fernández-Ruiz, J.; Romero, J.; Martinez-Orgado, J. The neuroprotective effect of cannabidiol in an in vitro model of newborn hypoxic–ischemic brain damage in mice is mediated by CB2 and adenosine receptors. *Neurobiol. Dis.* **2010**, *37*, 434–440. [CrossRef] [PubMed]
19. Jean-Gilles, L.; Gran, B.; Constantinescu, C.S. Interaction between cytokines, cannabinoids and the nervous system. *Immunobiology* **2010**, *215*, 606–610. [CrossRef] [PubMed]
20. Rajan, T.S.; Giacoppo, S.; Iori, R.; De Nicola, G.R.; Grassi, G.; Pollastro, F.; Bramanti, P.; Mazzon, E. Anti-inflammatory and antioxidant effects of a combination of cannabidiol and moringin in LPS-stimulated macrophages. *Fitoterapia* **2016**, *112*, 104–115. [CrossRef] [PubMed]
21. Esposito, G.; De Filippis, D.; Maiuri, M.C.; De Stefano, D.; Carnuccio, R.; Iuvone, T. Cannabidiol inhibits inducible nitric oxide synthase protein expression and nitric oxide production in β-amyloid stimulated PC12 neurons through p38 MAP kinase and NF-κB involvement. *Neurosci. Lett.* **2006**, *399*, 91–95. [CrossRef] [PubMed]
22. Linge, R.; Jiménez-Sánchez, L.; Campa, L.; Pilar-Cuéllar, F.; Vidal, R.; Pazos, A.; Adell, A.; Díaz, Á. Cannabidiol induces rapid-acting antidepressant-like effects and enhances cortical 5-HT/glutamate neurotransmission: role of 5-HT1A receptors. *Neuropharmacology* **2016**, *103*, 16–26. [CrossRef] [PubMed]
23. Bhattacharyya, S.; Morrison, P.D.; Fusar-Poli, P.; Martin-Santos, R.; Borgwardt, S.; Winton-Brown, T.; Nosarti, C.; O'Carroll, C.M.; Seal, M.; Allen, P. Opposite effects of Δ-9-tetrahydrocannabinol and cannabidiol on human brain function and psychopathology. *Neuropsychopharmacology* **2010**, *35*, 764. [CrossRef]
24. Maione, S.; Piscitelli, F.; Gatta, L.; Vita, D.; De Petrocellis, L.; Palazzo, E.; de Novellis, V.; Di Marzo, V. Non-psychoactive cannabinoids modulate the descending pathway of antinociception in anaesthetized rats through several mechanisms of action. *Br. J. Pharmacol.* **2011**, *162*, 584–596. [CrossRef] [PubMed]
25. Massi, P.; Solinas, M.; Cinquina, V.; Parolaro, D. Cannabidiol as potential anticancer drug. *Br. J. Clin. Pharmacol.* **2013**, *75*, 303–312. [CrossRef]
26. Deiana, S.; Watanabe, A.; Yamasaki, Y.; Amada, N.; Arthur, M.; Fleming, S.; Woodcock, H.; Dorward, P.; Pigliacampo, B.; Close, S. Plasma and brain pharmacokinetic profile of cannabidiol (CBD), cannabidivarine (CBDV), Δ^9-tetrahydrocannabivarin (THCV) and cannabigerol (CBG) in rats and mice following oral and intraperitoneal administration and CBD action on obsessive–compulsive behaviour. *Psychopharmacology* **2012**, *219*, 859–873.
27. Shannon, S.; Opila-Lehman, J. Effectiveness of cannabidiol oil for pediatric anxiety and insomnia as part of posttraumatic stress disorder: a case report. *Perm. J.* **2016**, *20*, 108. [CrossRef]
28. Elms, L.; Shannon, S.; Hughes, S.; Lewis, N. Cannabidiol in the Treatment of Post-Traumatic Stress Disorder: A Case Series. *J. Altern. Complementary Med.* **2018**. [CrossRef]
29. Carlini, E.; Leite, J.; Tannhauser, M.; Berardi, A. Cannabidiol and Cannabis sativa extract protect mice and rats against convulsive agents. *J. Pharm. Pharmacol.* **1973**, *25*, 664–665. [CrossRef]
30. Consroe, P.; Benedito, M.A.; Leite, J.R.; Carlini, E.A.; Mechoulam, R. Effects of cannabidiol on behavioral seizures caused by convulsant drugs or current in mice. *Eur. J. Pharmacol.* **1982**, *83*, 293–298. [CrossRef]
31. Jones, N.A.; Hill, A.J.; Smith, I.; Bevan, S.A.; Williams, C.M.; Whalley, B.J.; Stephens, G.J. Cannabidiol displays antiepileptiform and antiseizure properties in vitro and in vivo. *J. Pharmacol. Exp. Ther.* **2010**, *332*, 569–577. [CrossRef]
32. Mudigoudar, B.; Weatherspoon, S.; Wheless, J.W. Emerging antiepileptic drugs for severe pediatric epilepsies. In *Seminars in pediatric neurology*; Elsevier: Amsterdam, The Netherlands, 2016; pp. 167–179.

33. Hussain, S.A.; Zhou, R.; Jacobson, C.; Weng, J.; Cheng, E.; Lay, J.; Hung, P.; Lerner, J.T.; Sankar, R. Perceived efficacy of cannabidiol-enriched cannabis extracts for treatment of pediatric epilepsy: a potential role for infantile spasms and Lennox–Gastaut syndrome. *Epilepsy Behav.* **2015**, *47*, 138–141. [CrossRef]
34. Kwan, P.; Arzimanoglou, A.; Berg, A.T.; Brodie, M.J.; Allen Hauser, W.; Mathern, G.; Moshé, S.L.; Perucca, E.; Wiebe, S.; French, J. Definition of drug resistant epilepsy: consensus proposal by the ad hoc Task Force of the ILAE Commission on Therapeutic Strategies. *Epilepsia* **2010**, *51*, 1069–1077. [CrossRef]
35. Gloss, D.; Vickrey, B. Cannabinoids for epilepsy. *Cochrane Database Syst. Rev.* **2014**. [CrossRef]
36. Fisher, R.S.; Boas, W.V.E.; Blume, W.; Elger, C.; Genton, P.; Lee, P.; Engel Jr, J. Epileptic seizures and epilepsy: definitions proposed by the International League Against Epilepsy (ILAE) and the International Bureau for Epilepsy (IBE). *Epilepsia* **2005**, *46*, 470–472. [CrossRef]
37. Sabaz, M.; Lawson, J.A.; Cairns, D.R.; Duchowny, M.S.; Resnick, T.J.; Dean, P.M.; Bye, A.M. Validation of the quality of life in childhood epilepsy questionnaire in American epilepsy patients. *Epilepsy Behav.* **2003**, *4*, 680–691. [CrossRef]
38. Fisher, R.S.; Cross, J.H.; French, J.A.; Higurashi, N.; Hirsch, E.; Jansen, F.E.; Lagae, L.; Moshé, S.L.; Peltola, J.; Roulet Perez, E. Operational classification of seizure types by the International League Against Epilepsy: Position Paper of the ILAE Commission for Classification and Terminology. *Epilepsia* **2017**, *58*, 522–530. [CrossRef]
39. Johnson, E.L. Seizures and Epilepsy. *Med. Clin.* **2019**, *103*, 309–324. [CrossRef]
40. Stafstrom, C.E.; Carmant, L. Seizures and epilepsy: an overview for neuroscientists. *Cold Spring Harb. Perspect. Med.* **2015**, *5*, a022426. [CrossRef]
41. Dravet, C.; Bureau, M.; Oguni, H.; Fukuyama, Y.; Cokar, O. Severe myoclonic epilepsy in infancy (Dravet syndrome). *Epileptic Syndr. InfancyChild. Adolesc.* **2005**, *4*, 89–113.
42. Escayg, A.; MacDonald, B.T.; Meisler, M.H.; Baulac, S.; Huberfeld, G.; An-Gourfinkel, I.; Brice, A.; LeGuern, E.; Moulard, B.; Chaigne, D. Mutations of SCN1A, encoding a neuronal sodium channel, in two families with GEFS+ 2. *Nat. Genet.* **2000**, *24*, 343. [CrossRef]
43. Shirley, M.D.; Tang, H.; Gallione, C.J.; Baugher, J.D.; Frelin, L.P.; Cohen, B.; North, P.E.; Marchuk, D.A.; Comi, A.M.; Pevsner, J. Sturge–Weber syndrome and port-wine stains caused by somatic mutation in GNAQ. *New Engl. J. Med.* **2013**, *368*, 1971–1979. [CrossRef]
44. Comi, A.M. Presentation, diagnosis, pathophysiology and treatment of the neurologic features of Sturge-Weber Syndrome. *Neurol.* **2011**, *17*, 179. [CrossRef]
45. Archer, H.L.; Evans, J.; Edwards, S.; Colley, J.; Newbury-Ecob, R.; O'Callaghan, F.; Huyton, M.; O'Regan, M.; Tolmie, J.; Sampson, J. CDKL5 mutations cause infantile spasms, early onset seizures, and severe mental retardation in female patients. *J. Med. Genet.* **2006**, *43*, 729–734. [CrossRef]
46. Pellock, J.M.; Hrachovy, R.; Shinnar, S.; Baram, T.Z.; Bettis, D.; Dlugos, D.J.; Gaillard, W.D.; Gibson, P.A.; Holmes, G.L.; Nordli, D.R. Infantile spasms: a US consensus report. *Epilepsia* **2010**, *51*, 2175–2189. [CrossRef]
47. Kwan, P.; Sills, G.J.; Brodie, M.J. The mechanisms of action of commonly used antiepileptic drugs. *Pharmacol. Ther.* **2001**, *90*, 21–34. [CrossRef]
48. O'Connell, B.K.; Gloss, D.; Devinsky, O. Cannabinoids in treatment-resistant epilepsy: a review. *Epilepsy Behav.* **2017**, *70*, 341–348. [CrossRef]
49. Catterall, W.A. Forty Years of sodium channels: Structure, function, pharmacology, and epilepsy. *Neurochem. Res.* **2017**, *42*, 2495–2504. [CrossRef]
50. Lucas, P.T.; Meadows, L.S.; Nicholls, J.; Ragsdale, D.S. An epilepsy mutation in the $\beta1$ subunit of the voltage-gated sodium channel results in reduced channel sensitivity to phenytoin. *Epilepsy Res.* **2005**, *64*, 77–84. [CrossRef]
51. Kostyuk, P.; Molokanova, E.; Pronchuk, N.; Savchenko, A.; Verkhratsky, A. Different action of ethosuximide on low-and high-threshold calcium currents in rat sensory neurons. *Neuroscience* **1992**, *51*, 755–758. [CrossRef]
52. Sitges, M.; Chiu, L.M.; Reed, R.C. Effects of levetiracetam, carbamazepine, phenytoin, valproate, lamotrigine, oxcarbazepine, topiramate, vinpocetine and sertraline on presynaptic hippocampal Na+ and Ca 2+ channels permeability. *Neurochem. Res.* **2016**, *41*, 758–769. [CrossRef]
53. Holtyn, A.F.; Tiruveedhula, V.P.B.; Stephen, M.R.; Cook, J.M.; Weerts, E.M. Effects of the benzodiazepine GABAA $\alpha1$-preferring antagonist 3-isopropoxy-β-carboline hydrochloride (3-ISOPBC) on alcohol seeking and self-administration in baboons. *Drug Alcohol Depend.* **2017**, *170*, 25–31. [CrossRef]

54. Fisher, J.L. The anti-convulsant stiripentol acts directly on the GABAA receptor as a positive allosteric modulator. *Neuropharmacology* **2009**, *56*, 190–197. [CrossRef]
55. Walters, D.C.; Arning, E.; Bottiglieri, T.; Jansen, E.E.; Salomons, G.S.; Brown, M.N.; Schmidt, M.A.; Ainslie, G.R.; Roullet, J.-B.; Gibson, K.M. Metabolomic analyses of vigabatrin (VGB)-treated mice: GABA-transaminase inhibition significantly alters amino acid profiles in murine neural and non-neural tissues. *Neurochem. Int.* **2019**, *125*, 151–162. [CrossRef]
56. Curry, W.J.; Kulling, D.L. Newer antiepileptic drugs: gabapentin, lamotrigine, felbamate, topiramate and fosphenytoin. *Am. Fam. Physician* **1998**, *57*, 513–520.
57. Ghodke-Puranik, Y.; Thorn, C.F.; Lamba, J.K.; Leeder, J.S.; Song, W.; Birnbaum, A.K.; Altman, R.B.; Klein, T.E. Valproic acid pathway: pharmacokinetics and pharmacodynamics. *Pharm. Genom.* **2013**, *23*, 236. [CrossRef]
58. Madeja, M.; Margineanu, D.G.; Gorji, A.; Siep, E.; Boerrigter, P.; Klitgaard, H.; Speckmann, E.-J. Reduction of voltage-operated potassium currents by levetiracetam: a novel antiepileptic mechanism of action? *Neuropharmacology* **2003**, *45*, 661–671. [CrossRef]
59. Srinivasan, J.; Richens, A.; Davies, J.A. Effects of felbamate on veratridine-and K+-stimulated release of glutamate from mouse cortex. *Eur. J. Pharmacol.* **1996**, *315*, 285–288. [CrossRef]
60. Kanda, T.; Kurokawa, M.; Tamura, S.; Nakamura, J.; Ishii, A.; Kuwana, Y.; Serikawa, T.; Yamada, J.; Ishihara, K.; Sasa, M. Topiramate reduces abnormally high extracellular levels of glutamate and aspartate in the hippocampus of spontaneously epileptic rats (SER). *Life Sci.* **1996**, *59*, 1607–1616. [CrossRef]
61. Theodore, W.H.; Wiggs, E.A.; Martinez, A.R.; Dustin, I.H.; Khan, O.I.; Appel, S.; Reeves-Tyer, P.; Sato, S. Serotonin 1A receptors, depression, and memory in temporal lobe epilepsy. *Epilepsia* **2012**, *53*, 129–133. [CrossRef]
62. Naziroglu, M. TRPV1 Channel: A Potential Drug Target for Treating Epilepsy. *Curr. Neuropharmacol.* **2015**, *13*, 239–247. [CrossRef]
63. Vilela, L.R.; Lima, I.V.; Kunsch, E.B.; Pinto, H.P.P.; de Miranda, A.S.; Vieira, E.L.M.; de Oliveira, A.C.P.; Moraes, M.F.D.; Teixeira, A.L.; Moreira, F.A. Anticonvulsant effect of cannabidiol in the pentylenetetrazole model: Pharmacological mechanisms, electroencephalographic profile, and brain cytokine levels. *Epilepsy Behav. EB* **2017**, *75*, 29–35. [CrossRef]
64. Gharedaghi, M.H.; Seyedabadi, M.; Ghia, J.-E.; Dehpour, A.R.; Rahimian, R. The role of different serotonin receptor subtypes in seizure susceptibility. *Exp. Brain Res.* **2014**, *232*, 347–367. [CrossRef]
65. Theodore, W.H. Does serotonin play a role in epilepsy? *Epilepsy Curr.* **2003**, *3*, 173–177. [CrossRef]
66. Guiard, B.P.; Di Giovanni, G. Central serotonin-2A (5-HT2A) receptor dysfunction in depression and epilepsy: the missing link? *Front. Pharmacol.* **2015**, *6*, 46. [CrossRef]
67. Theodore, W.H.; Hasler, G.; Giovacchini, G.; Kelley, K.; Reeves-Tyer, P.; Herscovitch, P.; Drevets, W. Reduced hippocampal 5HT1A PET receptor binding and depression in temporal lobe epilepsy. *Epilepsia* **2007**, *48*, 1526–1530. [CrossRef]
68. Chung, P.C.S.; Kieffer, B.L. Delta opioid receptors in brain function and diseases. *Pharmacol. Ther.* **2013**, *140*, 112–120. [CrossRef]
69. Snead, O.C., III. Opiate-induced seizures: a study of μ and δ specific mechanisms. *Exp. Neurol.* **1986**, *93*, 348–358. [CrossRef]
70. Kaplan, J.S.; Stella, N.; Catterall, W.A.; Westenbroek, R.E. Cannabidiol attenuates seizures and social deficits in a mouse model of Dravet syndrome. *Proc. Natl. Acad. Sci.* **2017**, *114*, 11229–11234. [CrossRef]
71. Yamaori, S.; Ebisawa, J.; Okushima, Y.; Yamamoto, I.; Watanabe, K. Potent inhibition of human cytochrome P450 3A isoforms by cannabidiol: role of phenolic hydroxyl groups in the resorcinol moiety. *Life Sci.* **2011**, *88*, 730–736. [CrossRef]
72. Geffrey, A.L.; Pollack, S.F.; Bruno, P.L.; Thiele, E.A. Drug–drug interaction between clobazam and cannabidiol in children with refractory epilepsy. *Epilepsia* **2015**, *56*, 1246–1251. [CrossRef]
73. Devinsky, O.; Patel, A.D.; Thiele, E.A.; Wong, M.H.; Appleton, R.; Harden, C.L.; Greenwood, S.; Morrison, G.; Sommerville, K.; Group, G.P.A.S. Randomized, dose-ranging safety trial of cannabidiol in Dravet syndrome. *Neurology* **2018**. [CrossRef]
74. Devinsky, O.; Cross, J.H.; Laux, L.; Marsh, E.; Miller, I.; Nabbout, R.; Scheffer, I.E.; Thiele, E.A.; Wright, S. Trial of cannabidiol for drug-resistant seizures in the Dravet syndrome. *New Engl. J. Med.* **2017**, *376*, 2011–2020. [CrossRef]

75. Devinsky, O.; Patel, A.D.; Cross, J.H.; Villanueva, V.; Wirrell, E.C.; Privitera, M.; Greenwood, S.M.; Roberts, C.; Checketts, D.; VanLandingham, K.E. Effect of Cannabidiol on Drop Seizures in the Lennox–Gastaut Syndrome. *New Engl. J. Med.* **2018**, *378*, 1888–1897. [CrossRef]
76. Thiele, E.A.; Marsh, E.D.; French, J.A.; Mazurkiewicz-Beldzinska, M.; Benbadis, S.R.; Joshi, C.; Lyons, P.D.; Taylor, A.; Roberts, C.; Sommerville, K. Cannabidiol in patients with seizures associated with Lennox-Gastaut syndrome (GWPCARE4): a randomised, double-blind, placebo-controlled phase 3 trial. *Lancet* **2018**, *391*, 1085–1096. [CrossRef]
77. Devinsky, O.; Nabbout, R.; Miller, I.; Laux, L.; Zolnowska, M.; Wright, S.; Roberts, C. Long-term cannabidiol treatment in patients with Dravet syndrome: An open-label extension trial. *Epilepsia* **2019**, *60*, 294–302. [CrossRef]
78. Gaston, T.E.; Bebin, E.M.; Cutter, G.R.; Liu, Y.; Szaflarski, J.P.; Program, U.C. Interactions between cannabidiol and commonly used antiepileptic drugs. *Epilepsia* **2017**, *58*, 1586–1592. [CrossRef]
79. Szaflarski, J.P.; Bebin, E.M.; Cutter, G.; DeWolfe, J.; Dure, L.S.; Gaston, T.E.; Kankirawatana, P.; Liu, Y.; Singh, R.; Standaert, D.G. Cannabidiol improves frequency and severity of seizures and reduces adverse events in an open-label add-on prospective study. *Epilepsy Behav.* **2018**, *87*, 131–136. [CrossRef]
80. Porcari, G.S.; Fu, C.; Doll, E.D.; Carter, E.G.; Carson, R.P. Efficacy of artisanal preparations of cannabidiol for the treatment of epilepsy: Practical experiences in a tertiary medical center. *Epilepsy Behav.* **2018**, *80*, 240–246. [CrossRef]
81. Morrison, G.; Crockett, J.; Blakey, G.; Sommerville, K. A Phase 1, Open-Label, Pharmacokinetic Trial to Investigate Possible Drug-Drug Interactions Between Clobazam, Stiripentol, or Valproate and Cannabidiol in Healthy Subjects. *Clin. Pharmacol. Drug Dev.* **2019**. [CrossRef]
82. Hess, E.J.; Moody, K.A.; Geffrey, A.L.; Pollack, S.F.; Skirvin, L.A.; Bruno, P.L.; Paolini, J.L.; Thiele, E.A. Cannabidiol as a new treatment for drug-resistant epilepsy in tuberous sclerosis complex. *Epilepsia* **2016**, *57*, 1617–1624. [CrossRef]
83. Devinsky, O.; Marsh, E.; Friedman, D.; Thiele, E.; Laux, L.; Sullivan, J.; Miller, I.; Flamini, R.; Wilfong, A.; Filloux, F. Cannabidiol in patients with treatment-resistant epilepsy: an open-label interventional trial. *Lancet Neurol.* **2016**, *15*, 270–278. [CrossRef]
84. Sands, T.T.; Rahdari, S.; Oldham, M.S.; Nunes, E.C.; Tilton, N.; Cilio, M.R. Long-term safety, tolerability, and efficacy of cannabidiol in children with refractory epilepsy: results from an expanded access program in the US. *Cns Drugs* **2019**, *33*, 47–60. [CrossRef]
85. Kaplan, E.H.; Offermann, E.A.; Sievers, J.W.; Comi, A.M. Cannabidiol treatment for refractory seizures in Sturge-Weber syndrome. *Pediatric Neurol.* **2017**, *71*, 18–23.e12. [CrossRef]
86. Rosenberg, E.C.; Louik, J.; Conway, E.; Devinsky, O.; Friedman, D. Quality of Life in Childhood Epilepsy in pediatric patients enrolled in a prospective, open-label clinical study with cannabidiol. *Epilepsia* **2017**, *58*, e96–e100. [CrossRef]
87. Devinsky, O.; Verducci, C.; Thiele, E.A.; Laux, L.C.; Patel, A.D.; Filloux, F.; Szaflarski, J.P.; Wilfong, A.; Clark, G.D.; Park, Y.D. Open-label use of highly purified CBD (Epidiolex®) in patients with CDKL5 deficiency disorder and Aicardi, Dup15q, and Doose syndromes. *Epilepsy Behav.* **2018**, *86*, 131–137. [CrossRef]
88. Chen, K.A.; Farrar, M.; Cardamone, M.; Gill, D.; Smith, R.; Cowell, C.T.; Truong, L.; Lawson, J.A. Cannabidiol for treating drug-resistant epilepsy in children: the New South Wales experience. *Med. J. Aust.* **2018**, *209*, 217–221. [CrossRef]
89. Szaflarski, J.P.; Bebin, E.M.; Comi, A.M.; Patel, A.D.; Joshi, C.; Checketts, D.; Beal, J.C.; Laux, L.C.; De Boer, L.M.; Wong, M.H. Long-term safety and treatment effects of cannabidiol in children and adults with treatment-resistant epilepsies: Expanded access program results. *Epilepsia* **2018**, *59*, 1540–1548. [CrossRef]

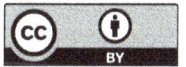

© 2019 by the authors. Licensee MDPI, Basel, Switzerland. This article is an open access article distributed under the terms and conditions of the Creative Commons Attribution (CC BY) license (http://creativecommons.org/licenses/by/4.0/).

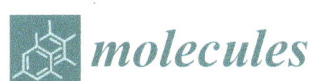

Article

Hepatotoxicity of a Cannabidiol-Rich Cannabis Extract in the Mouse Model

Laura E. Ewing [1,2], Charles M. Skinner [1,3], Charles M. Quick [4], Stefanie Kennon-McGill [1], Mitchell R. McGill [1,2,3], Larry A. Walker [5,6], Mahmoud A. ElSohly [5,6,7], Bill J. Gurley [3,8] and Igor Koturbash [1,3,*]

1. Department of Environmental and Occupational Health, University of Arkansas for Medical Sciences, Little Rock, AR 72205, USA; leewing@uams.edu (L.E.E.); cmskinner@uams.edu (C.M.S.); skennonmcgill@uams.edu (S.K.-M.); mmcgill@uams.edu (M.R.M.)
2. Department of Pharmacology and Toxicology, University of Arkansas for Medical Sciences, Little Rock, AR 72205, USA
3. Center for Dietary Supplements Research, University of Arkansas for Medical Sciences, Little Rock, AR 72205, USA; gurleybillyj@uams.edu
4. Department of Pathology, University of Arkansas for Medical Sciences, Little Rock, AR 72205, USA; quickcharlesm@uams.edu
5. National Center for Natural Products Research, University of Mississippi, University, MS 38677, USA; lwalker@olemiss.edu (L.A.W.); melsohly@olemiss.edu (M.A.E.)
6. ElSohly Laboratories, Inc. (ELI), Oxford, MS 38655, USA
7. Department of Pharmaceutics and Drug Delivery, School of Pharmacy, University of Mississippi, University, MS 38677, USA
8. Department of Pharmaceutical Sciences, University of Arkansas for Medical Sciences, Little Rock, AR 72223, USA
* Correspondence: ikoturbash@uams.edu; Tel.: +1-501-526-6638; Fax: +1-501-526-6931

Received: 11 April 2019; Accepted: 29 April 2019; Published: 30 April 2019

Abstract: The goal of this study was to investigate Cannabidiol (CBD) hepatotoxicity in 8-week-old male B6C3F$_1$ mice. Animals were gavaged with either 0, 246, 738, or 2460 mg/kg of CBD (acute toxicity, 24 h) or with daily doses of 0, 61.5, 184.5, or 615 mg/kg for 10 days (sub-acute toxicity). These doses were the allometrically scaled mouse equivalent doses (MED) of the maximum recommended human maintenance dose of CBD in EPIDIOLEX® (20 mg/kg). In the acute study, significant increases in liver-to-body weight (LBW) ratios, plasma ALT, AST, and total bilirubin were observed for the 2460 mg/kg dose. In the sub-acute study, 75% of mice gavaged with 615 mg/kg developed a moribund condition between days three and four. As in the acute phase, 615 mg/kg CBD increased LBW ratios, ALT, AST, and total bilirubin. Hepatotoxicity gene expression arrays revealed that CBD differentially regulated more than 50 genes, many of which were linked to oxidative stress responses, lipid metabolism pathways and drug metabolizing enzymes. In conclusion, CBD exhibited clear signs of hepatotoxicity, possibly of a cholestatic nature. The involvement of numerous pathways associated with lipid and xenobiotic metabolism raises serious concerns about potential drug interactions as well as the safety of CBD.

Keywords: cannabidiol; hepatotoxicity; liver injury; natural products; phytochemical

1. Introduction

Cannabidiol (CBD) is a non-psychotropic phytochemical present in *Cannabis sativa* that has gained significant popularity over the last decade. It is a major component of EPIDIOLEX®, a drug indicated for the treatment of drug-resistant epileptic seizures associated with Dravet and Lennox-Gastaut syndromes [1,2]. CBD has also been proposed as treatment for a number of other neuropsychiatric disorders for which clinical trials are currently ongoing [3].

CBD has also been marketed for a wide range of other indications, including 'anti-cancer', 'anti-inflammatory', 'sleep promotion', 'relaxation', 'normal cartilage and joint function', 'antioxidant effects', and 'pain management' just to name a few. The vast majority of those effects, however, were documented either in vitro or in clinical trials with equivocal results [4,5]. Apart from its purported salutary effects, accumulating evidence from pre-clinical in vivo studies and large-scale clinical trials, implies that CBD may elicit several potentially negative health outcomes. Specifically, numerous reports have demonstrated neurological, cardiovascular and reproductive toxicities subsequent to CBD use [6–14]. The authors of a large clinical trial that utilized CBD (dose regimen 2.5–30 mg/kg/day) to treat 278 patients with Dravet syndrome reported adverse events in 93% of subjects [15]. Another recent study inferred a strong genotoxic potential for CBD at concentrations commonly detected in human blood [16]. Furthermore, CBD may have a high drug interaction potential as it modulates numerous cytochrome P450 enzymes responsible for xenobiotic metabolism [17–21].

Of particular concern is the risk for CBD-induced hepatotoxicity [22]. Animal studies have reported increased liver weights in rhesus monkeys and elevated liver enzymes in dogs when CBD was administered at doses as low as 2 mg/kg of body weight [14,23]. In recent clinical trials, elevated liver enzymes were observed in 5–20% of patients treated with CBD, and a few patients were withdrawn due to the threat of fulminant liver failure [1,2,24].

The number of 'CBD-containing' products, available mostly online, is growing exponentially. However, the U. S. Food and Drug Administration (FDA) prohibits sales of CBD as a dietary supplement or food ingredient on the grounds that any 'article' that has been approved as a new drug or authorized for investigation as a new drug cannot be marketed as an ingredient in dietary supplements or conventional foods per the Food, Drug, & Cosmetic Act (FDCA) [21 U.S.C. §321(ff)(3)(B) and 21 U.S.C. §331(II), respectively] [25]. Furthermore, a clear regulatory oversight exists which has led to an uncontrolled CBD market that, in turn, threatens the health of a trusting general public. For instance, in a series of tests performed by the FDA on a panel of 'CBD-containing products', a large fraction either did not contain the label-claimed quantity of CBD or they were contaminated with Δ9-tetrahydrocannabidiol (THC) [26]. Furthermore, a recent independent analysis performed by CosumerLab.com, revealed that CBD doses in commercially-available products ranged from as little as 2.2 mg to as much as 22.3 mg, further amplifying concerns of potential toxicity [27].

As expansion of the CBD market seems inevitable, additional scientific studies are needed in order to support any required regulatory actions. For instance, if CBD is to be considered as a food additive, it will have to be filed as a new dietary ingredient (NDI) or a GRAS (generally recognized as safe) notice will need to be submitted to FDA. The latter will require a number of toxicity studies, the majority of which, in the case of CBD, remain to be performed. Analysis of genotoxic potential of CBD, the first toxicity test recommended by the FDA, was recently performed and the results published [16]. Therefore, we proceeded to the next set of recommended tests designed to address the short-term toxicity of a CBD-rich extract in a rodent model. Since liver injury is the primary concern for CBD, this study was designed to investigate the hepatotoxicity potential of CBD. The data collected in this study will provide important information for both industry and regulatory agencies in regards to the short-term toxicity of CBD. Furthermore, the results of these studies will aid in selecting appropriate models and doses for long-term studies (i.e., sub-chronic and chronic toxicity as well as carcinogenicity and reproductive toxicity studies) as well as the determination of a no observable effect level (NOEL) for selected endpoints.

2. Results

2.1. Acute Toxicity Study

For acute toxicity studies, a dose of 246 mg/kg was chosen as an initial dose as this is a MED analogous to those used in recent clinical trials (MED of 20 mg/kg CBD) [1,2]. Subsequently, we used doses of 738 and 2460 mg/kg CBD as 3× and 10× doses, respectively.

Mice at 738 mg/kg and 2460 mg/kg groups developed a sub-lethargic condition which presented as decreased appetite and slow response to exogenous stimuli at 4–5 h after CBD administration. This was still evident in mice receiving the 2460 mg/kg dose at the 24 h time-point. Administration of 2460 mg/kg CBD led to marginal body weight loss (9.5% from control) whereas the response in 738 mg/kg mice was mixed, with 4 mice exhibiting patterns of substantial weight loss (11%–15%) while two gained body weight (~10%) (Figure 1A). Further, 738 mg/kg caused significant increases in liver-to-body weight ratios (18%, $p < 0.005$), while 2460 mg/kg was characterized by an uneven distribution of these values (Figure 1B), even when using pre-gavage body weights to calculate organ to body weight ratios. No significant differences in kidney- and heart-to-body weight ratios were observed (Supplementary Figure S1A,B). No appreciable histomorphological differences were observed between control and experimental mice (Supplementary Figure S2). A small dose-dependent increase in total glutathione (GSH + GSSG) was observed in mice gavaged with CBD; however, increased levels of oxidized glutathione (GSSG) and GSSG/GSH ratio were also observed in mice gavaged with 2460 mg/kg CBD (Figure 1C–E).

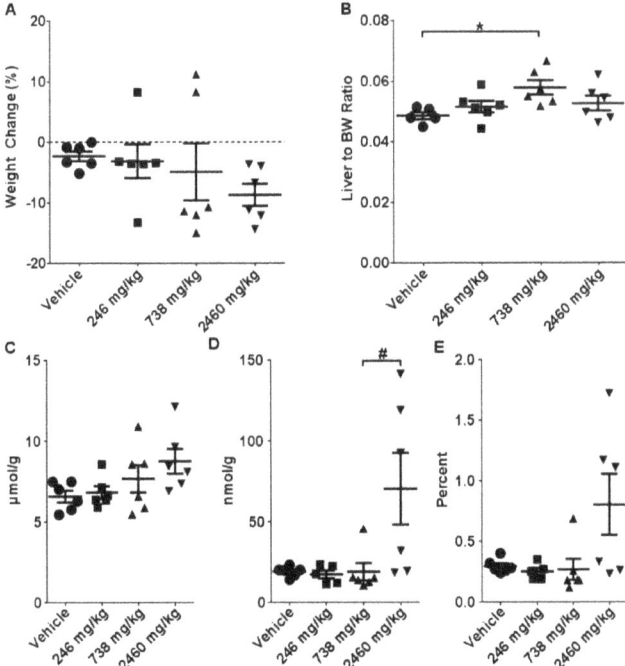

Figure 1. Effects of single gavage with CBD. Mice were gavaged with 246, 738, or 2460 mg/kg of CBD in sesame oil with tissues harvested at 24 h. (**A**) Body weight change, (**B**) liver to body weight ratios, intrahepatic concentrations of (**C**) total glutathione (GSH), (**D**) reduced glutathione (GSSG), and (**E**) GSH/GSSG ratio. Data are presented as mean ± SEM ($n = 6$). * indicates a significant difference as calculated with a One-Way ANOVA and Tukey's post-hoc test, and # indicates a significant difference as calculated with a Kruskal-Wallis test with a Dunn's post-hoc test ($p < 0.05$).

Clinical biochemistry analysis revealed moderate, but statistically significant ($p < 0.01$–0.001), dose-dependent increases in both AST and ALT serum levels (Table 1, Supplementary Figure S3A,B). Administration of 2460 mg/kg CBD led to marked elevations of total bilirubin (>20-fold, $p < 0.001$) (Table 1, Supplementary Figure S3C). No significant differences were observed in ALP or GGT (Supplementary Figure S3D–E).

Table 1. Clinical chemistry parameters 24 h after dosing with CBD oil. Cells in bold italics are significantly different from vehicle (One-Way ANOVA, indicated by *, or Kruskal-Wallis with appropriate post-hoc test). Data presented as mean ± SEM (n = 6/group).

	Vehicle	246 mg/kg	738 mg/kg	2460 mg/kg
ALT	27.5 ± 2.7	31.7 ± 2.6	*38.7 ± 4.3* *	*57.0 ± 8.0* *
AST	51.0 ± 2.0	58.7 ± 1.8	*80.3 ± 3.7* *	*120.8 ± 14.3* *
ALP	110.8 ± 2.9	106.0 ± 4.5	90.3 ± 8.8	98.8 ± 4.2
GGT	4.7 ± 0.2	4.3 ± 0.5	5.5 ± 0.3	4.2 ± 0.8
Total Bilirubin	0.1 ± 0.0	0.1 ± 0.0	0.13 ± 0.0	*2.1 ± 0.1*

Gene expression analysis of a panel of cytochromes and UDP-glucuronosyltransferases revealed significant and mostly dose-dependent increases in many isoforms (Figure 2). Of particular interest was the striking up-regulation of *Cyp2b10* (homologous to human *CYP2B6*) that exceeded 1000-fold at 2460 mg/kg CBD ($p < 0.001$). *Cyp1a2* and *Cyp2e1*, major cytochromes involved in the metabolism of ethanol and acetaminophen (APAP), were increased by 4- and 50-fold, respectively. At the same time, *Cyp2d22*, an isoform considered non-inducible, remained unaffected, lending further credence to the findings (Figure 2).

2.2. Sub-Acute Toxicity Study

Given the overt toxicity observed with 2460 mg/kg, we used a starting CBD dose of 61.5 mg/kg for this phase of experiments. This dose is an MED of 5 mg/kg CBD, which it turn is analogous to initial target doses administered in clinical trials for treatment-resistant epilepsy [28]. Subsequently, doses of 184.5mg/kg and 615 mg/kg CBD were considered as 3× and 10× doses, respectively.

Shortly after the second gavage with CBD, overt toxicity manifested as profound lethargy, loss of appetite, and body weight loss was observed in 33% of animals (2 out of 6) in the 615 mg/kg group. Two more mice developed similar symptoms after the third gavage. Thus, the remaining four animals were terminated at the end of day 3 (6 h after the third CBD dose). The remaining mice in the 61.5 mg/kg and 184.5 mg/kg cohorts were gavaged as scheduled for 10 days and exhibited no visible signs of toxicity.

Histopathological evaluation revealed pan-hepatic cytoplasmic swelling in mice gavaged with 615 mg/kg CBD (Figure 3). Foci of cytoplasmic swelling were clearly present in mice gavaged with 184.5 mg/kg, but not in the livers of mice gavaged with 61.5 mg/kg CBD.

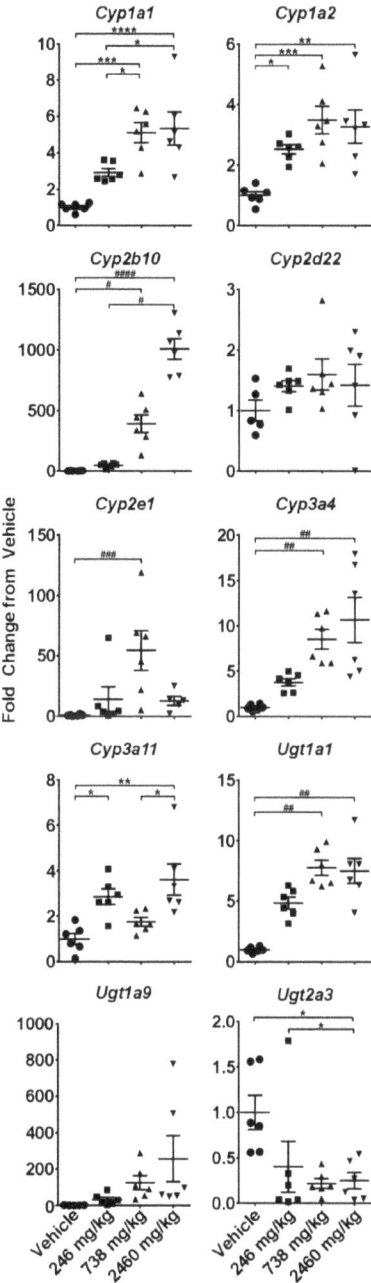

Figure 2. Effects of single gavage with CBD on intrahepatic expression of cytochrome P450s and UDP-glucuronosyltransferases. Livers were collected at 24 h and gene expression was measured using the quantitative real-time (qRT) PCR. * - indicate data analyzed by One-Way ANOVA with Tukey's post-test, and # indicate non-normal data analyzed with a Kruskal-Wallis and Dunn's post-hoc test. Data are presented as mean ± SEM fold changed from vehicle ($n = 6$), with * or # as $p < 0.05$; ** or ## as $p < 0.01$; *** or ### as $p < 0.001$; and **** or #### as $p < 0.0001$.

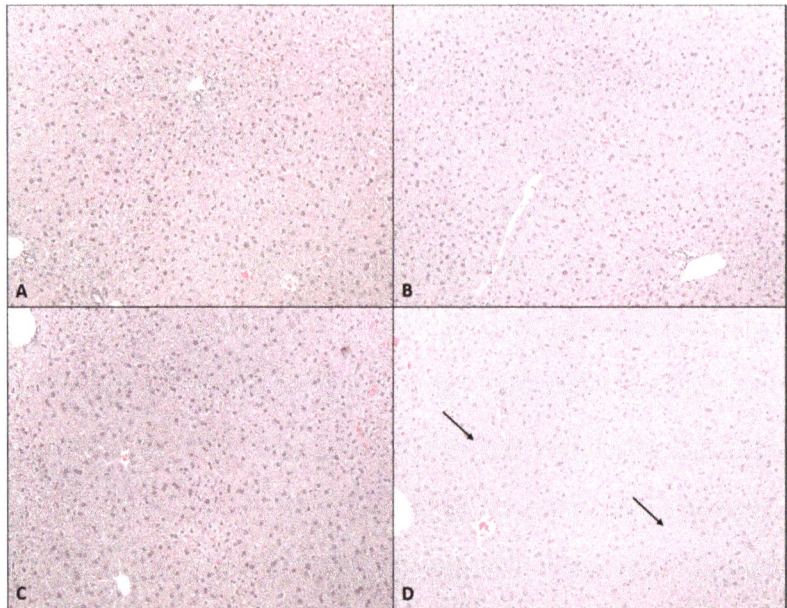

Figure 3. Effects of 2-week administration of CBD on liver histomorphology. H&E stained liver sections from (**A**) vehicle mice or those gavaged with (**B**) 61.5 mg/kg, (**C**) 184.5 mg/kg, or (**D**) 615 mg/kg CBD in sesame oil for 2 weeks. Note that 615 mg/kg group was terminated after 2–3 doses due to overt toxicity elicited by CBD.

Gavaging mice with 615 mg/kg CBD resulted in significant reductions in body weight (10%, $p < 0.05$) (Figure 4A). Furthermore, we observed a dose-dependent increase in liver-to- body weight ratios (5–30% range) (Figure 4B). Kidney-to-body weight ratios were significantly decreased in mice receiving 615 mg/kg CBD (Supplementary Figure S4). There were no significant differences in the total glutathione levels in any experimental groups and only modest changes were observed in GSSG and GSSG/GSH ratios (Figure 4C–E).

Analysis of clinical biochemistry parameters revealed that mice receiving 615 mg/kg CBD had significantly elevated total bilirubin, and moderately high levels of ALT and AST (Table 2, Supplementary Figure S3). However, no significant changes in any of these parameters were observed at lower CBD doses.

Gene expression analysis of a panel of cytochrome P450s (CYPs) and UDP-glucuronosyltransferases (UGTs) revealed similar patterns of response as that observed in the acute study phase. Up-regulation of CYP and UGT genes appeared dose-dependent, especially in the case of *Cyp2b10* and *Ugt1a9*, with significant changes occurring, in many instances, after the lowest CBD dose (61.5 mg/kg) (Figure 5).

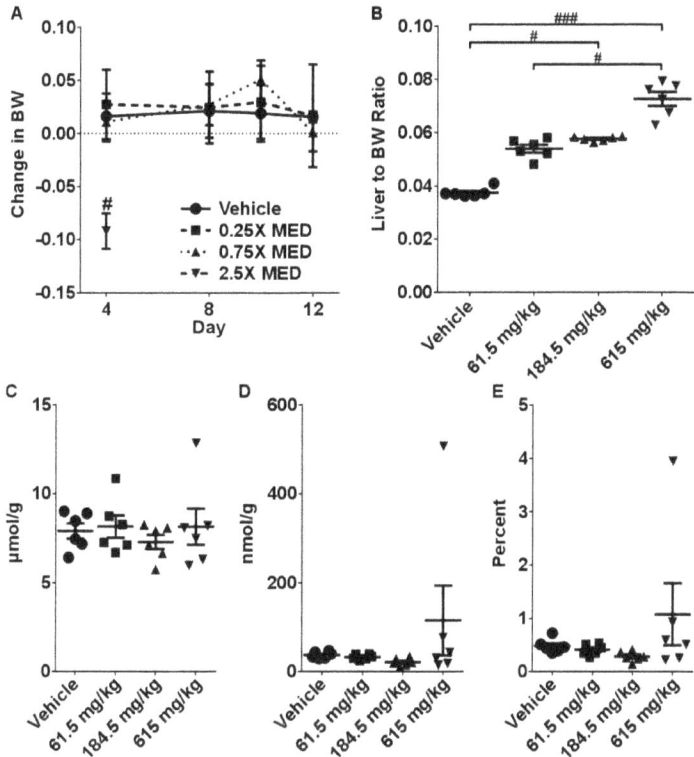

Figure 4. Effects of 2-week administration of CBD on: (**A**) Body weight dynamics, (**B**) Liver to body weight ratio. Intrahepatic concentrations of (**C**) total glutathione (GSH), (**D**) reduced glutathione (GSSG), and (**E**) GSH/GSSG ratio. Data are presented as mean ± SEM ($n = 6$). # indicates a significant difference as calculated with a Kruskal-Wallis test with a Dunn's post-hoc test with # representing $p < 0.05$; and ### $p < 0.001$.

Table 2. Clinical chemistry parameters after dosing with CBD oil for two weeks. Cells in bold italics are significantly different from vehicle (One-Way ANOVA, indicated by *, or Kruskal-Wallis with appropriate post-hoc test). Data presented as mean ± SEM ($n = 6$/group).

	Vehicle	61.5 mg/kg	184.5 mg/kg	615 mg/kg
ALT	40.0 ± 3.6	41.3 ± 14.8	32.3 ± 4.3	115.4 ± 51.2
AST	66.7 ± 6.7	74.7 ± 6.7	68.2 ± 3.9	157.0 ± 48.9
ALP	112.2 ± 3.5	112.7 ± 4.6	104.0 ± 2.0	113.2 ± 12.2
GGT	5.2 ± 0.3	4.0 ± 0.4	4.7 ± 0.2	5.0 ± 0.3
Total Bilirubin	0.1 ± 0.0	0.1 ± 0.02	0.23 ± 0.02	***1.5 ± 0.7*** *

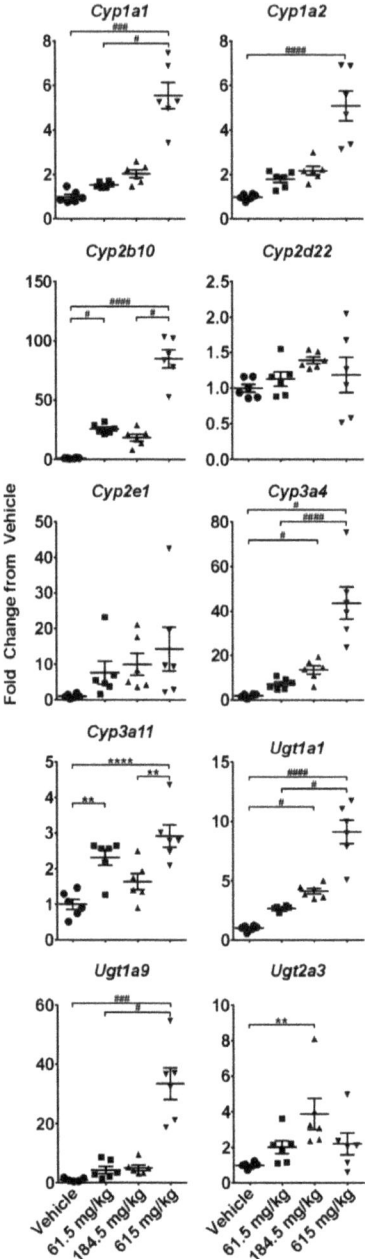

Figure 5. Effects of a two-week administration of CBD on intrahepatic expression of cytochrome P450s and UDP-glucuronosyltransferases. Livers were collected 6 h after the last gavage and gene expression was measured using the quantitative real-time (qRT) PCR. * - indicate data analyzed by One-Way ANOVA with Tukey's post-test, and # indicate non-normal data analyzed with a Kruskal-Wallis and Dunn's post-hoc test. Data are presented as mean ± SEM fold changed from vehicle ($n = 6$), with * or # as $p < 0.05$; ** or ## as $p < 0.01$; *** or ### as $p < 0.001$; and **** or #### as $p < 0.0001$.

2.3. Hepatotoxicity Gene Expression Analysis

Given that CBD-induced hepatotoxicity was observed in both study phases, we further investigated the mechanistic underpinnings of this toxicity. For this purpose, we employed a gene expression array comprised of 84 genes recognized as biomarkers of liver toxicity. These genes have been linked to pathologies such as cholestasis, steatosis, phospholipidosis, non-genotoxic hepatocarcinogenicity, necrosis, and generalized hepatotoxicity. This approach was successful in previous studies into herb-induced liver injury [29–31].

During the acute phase, 22 genes were significantly ($p < 0.05$ ANOVA) down-regulated and 26 genes were significantly up-regulated in mice livers. The vast majority of affected genes (32) were dysregulated in a dose-dependent manner (Table 3). Furthermore, several genes, including *Fmo1*, *Lgr5*, and *Lss*, exhibited a biphasic response, where the up-regulation observed at lower doses was succeeded by down-regulation at higher dose(s).

Table 3. Gene-markers of hepatotoxicity affected by CBD administration. Genes that are significantly up- or down-regulated sorted by greatest fold changed at the highest dose (2460 mg/kg or MED of 200 mg/kg). Cells in bold italics indicate those significantly different from vehicle (One-Way ANOVA, indicated by *, or Kruskal-Wallis test with appropriate post-hoc comparison). Genes that are commonly and significantly dysregulated in both the acute and sub-acute studies are highlighted in yellow. Data presented as mean ± SEM (n = 6/group) fold change from vehicle.

	Up-Regulated					
	Single Dose			2 Week Dosing		
Gene	246 mg/kg	738 mg/kg	2460 mg/kg	61.5 mg/kg	184.5 mg/kg	615 mg/kg
Krt8	32.6 ± 18.5	32.2 ± 0.4	46.9 ± 25.1	0.7 ± 0.1	0.8 ± 0.2	*8.7 ± 4.2* *
Map3k6	4.9 ± 1.9	1.6 ± 0.2	38.0 ± 17.3	1.7 ± 0.9	0.8 ± 0.1	8.6 ± 2.9
Cdkn1a	*0.3 ± 0.1*	0.5 ± 0.2	22.7 ± 6.9	*0.3 ± 0.1*	0.4 ± 0.1	9.3 ± 3.7
Hmox1	0.9 ± 0.1	2.8 ± 0.6	*19.0 ± 8.8* *	1.5 ± 0.4	1.5 ± 0.3	2.4 ± 1.2
Nqo1	3.6 ± 0.8	*4.92 ± 1.0* *	*9.7 ± 1.7* *	1.0 ± 0.1	1.1 ± 0.1	*6.2 ± 1.2* *
Ugt1a1	4.8 ± 0.5	7.8 ± 0.6	7.5 ± 1.0	2.7 ± 0.1	*4.1 ± 0.2*	*9.1 ± 0.9*
Rplp2	1.0 ± 0.1	1.5 ± 0.2	*5.7 ± 0.8* *	0.5 ± 0.1	0.5 ± 0.1	0.7 ± 0.2
Abcb1a	1.5 ± 0.4	1.0 ± 0.2	*5.6 ± 0.8*	2.1 ± 0.5	2.1 ± 0.2	*6.4 ± 1.8* *
Slc39a6	2.0 ± 0.3	1.4 ± 0.1	*5.5 ± 1.3*	1.1 ± 0.2	0.9 ± 0.1	2.9 ± 1.1
Aldoa	2.8 ± 0.9	2.1 ± 0.2	*5.4 ± 1.4*	1.3 ± 0.1	1.1 ± 0.1	*2.8 ± 0.5* *
Pla2g12a	1.6 ± 0.3	2.0 ± 0.3	*5.3 ± 0.6*	1.7 ± 0.3	1.4 ± 0.1	*3.5 ± 0.3*
Ubc	1.3 ± 0.1	1.1 ± 0.2	*4.8 ± 0.6* *	0.6 ± 0.1	1.1 ± 0.1	1.6 ± 0.3
Abcc3	2.6 ± 0.6	2.4 ± 0.4	*4.5 ± 1.2*	1.2 ± 0.2	1.1 ± 0.1	*2.2 ± 0.3* *
Abcc2	1.4 ± 0.2	1.6 ± 0.3	*3.9 ± 0.3* *	1.2 ± 0.1	0.9 ± 0.0	3.4 ± 1.3
Gsr	1.9 ± 0.5	*2.7 ± 0.3* *	*3.9 ± 0.4* *	0.8 ± 0.1	0.9 ± 0.1	*2.9 ± 0.5* *
Icam1	1.9 ± 0.4	1.2 ± 0.2	*3.8 ± 0.9*	0.8 ± 0.1	0.7 ± 0.1	1.9 ± 0.6
Cyp3a11	*2.9 ± 0.3* *	1.6 ± 0.2	*3.6 ± 0.7* *	*2.3 ± 0.2* *	1.6 ± 0.2	*2.9 ± 0.3* *
Txnrd1	1.3 ± 0.2	1.6 ± 0.3	*3.5 ± 0.4*	1.4 ± 0.3	1.0 ± 0.2	2.6 ± 1.0
Lss	*3.2 ± 0.5*	2.2 ± 0.1	0.3 ± 0.0	0.5 ± 0.2	*0.4 ± 0.2* *	0.9 ± 0.7
Pgk1	1.7 ± 0.4	1.3 ± 0.1	*3.1 ± 0.9*	0.9 ± 0.0	1.0 ± 0.1	1.6 ± 0.3
Ddx39	1.1 ± 0.1	*2.2 ± 0.6* *	*2.6 ± 0.3* *	0.9 ± 0.1	0.6 ± 0.1	3.1 ± 0.7
Psme3	1.2 ± 0.2	1.0 ± 0.1	*2.6 ± 0.5*	1.0 ± 0.1	0.8 ± 0.1	1.5 ± 0.3
Ipo4	1.1 ± 0.1	*1.9 ± 0.3* *	*2.5 ± 0.2* *	0.8 ± 0.1	0.9 ± 0.1	1.7 ± 0.4
Osmr	1.4 ± 0.2	1.0 ± 0.2	*2.4 ± 0.3* *	0.7 ± 0.1	0.4 ± 0.1	1.5 ± 0.6
Krt18	1.5 ± 0.2	*2.0 ± 0.2* *	*2.2 ± 0.4* *	0.7 ± 0.1	0.7 ± 0.1	3.2 ± 0.9
Timm10b	1.3 ± 0.1	*1.7 ± 0.2* *	*1.9 ± 0.3* *	1.0 ± 0.1	1.1 ± 0.2	1.7 ± 0.4
Tfrc	2.0 ± 0.1	3.3 ± 0.6	1.8 ± 0.1	1.3 ± 0.1	0.7 ± 0.1	*2.6 ± 0.3* *
Mrps18b	0.8 ± 0.0	0.9 ± 0.1	*1.7 ± 0.2* *	1.0 ± 0.1	0.8 ± 0.1	1.6 ± 0.3

Table 3. Cont.

	Down-Regulated					
	Single Dose			2 Week Dosing		
Gene	20 mg/kg	60 mg/kg	200 mg/kg	5 mg/kg	15 mg/kg	50 mg/kg
Igfals	1.1 ± 0.1	*0.5 ± 0.1 **	*0.02 ± 0.0 **	0.8 ± 0.1	0.9 ± 0.2	*0.2 ± 0.1 **
Lgr5	1.2 ± 0.1	*0.5 ± 0.1 **	*0.04 ± 0.0 **	*0.4 ± 0.0 **	*0.3 ± 0.1 **	*0.2 ± 0.0 **
Car3	0.8 ± 0.1	*0.2 ± 0.0 **	*0.1 ± 0.1 **	*0.5 ± 0.1 **	*0.5 ± 0.0 **	*0.1 ± 0.0 **
Atp8b1	1.4 ± 0.3	0.5 ± 0.1	*0.2 ± 0.0*	0.6 ± 0.1	0.5 ± 0.1	0.4 ± 0.1
Ppara	*0.7 ± 0.1**	*0.6 ± 0.0 **	*0.2 ± 0.0 **	*0.5 ± 0.1 **	*0.5 ± 0.1 **	*0.3 ± 0.1 **
Avpr1a	1.1 ± 0.2	0.8 ± 0.1	*0.2 ± 0.0 **	*0.5 ± 0.1 **	*0.3 ± 0.1 **	*0.3 ± 0.1 **
Abcb11	1.1 ± 0.2	*0.5 ± 0.0 **	*0.2 ± 0.0 **	0.6 ± 0.1	0.7 ± 0.1	*0.3 ± 0.1 **
Mcm10	1.9 ± 0.5	1.4 ± 0.1	0.2 ± 0.0	0.9 ± 0.2	0.6 ± 0.1	*0.2 ± 0.0 **
Fabp1	*0.6 ± 0.0 **	*0.4 ± 0.0 **	*0.2 ± 0.1 **	0.8 ± 0.1	*0.7 ± 0.0 **	*0.1 ± 0.0 **
Fads1	0.7 ± 0.1	0.6 ± 0.0	*0.2 ± 0.0*	0.9 ± 0.1	0.8 ± 0.1	0.6 ± 0.2
Cdc14b	0.9 ± 0.1	0.7 ± 0.1	*0.3 ± 0.0*	*0.6 ± 0.1 **	0.7 ± 0.1	*0.4 ± 0.1 **
Mbl2	1.3 ± 0.1	0.7 ± 0.0	*0.3 ± 0.0 **	0.9 ± 0.1	0.9 ± 0.1	*0.6 ± 0.1 **
Asah1	1.1 ± 0.1	0.9 ± 0.1	*0.4 ± 0.1 **	0.8 ± 0.1	0.7 ± 0.1	0.6 ± 0.1
Lpl	0.7 ± 0.0	0.4 ± 0.1	0.5 ± 0.1	0.4 ± 0.1	0.5 ± 0.1	*0.2 ± 0.1*
Emc9	1.3 ± 0.2	0.7 ± 0.0	*0.5 ± 0.0*	0.9 ± 0.1	0.9 ± 0.1	0.6 ± 0.1
Rhbg	0.9 ± 0.1	*0.5 ± 0.0 **	*0.5 ± 0.1 **	0.7 ± 0.1	1.0 ± 0.1	0.6 ± 0.2
L2hgdh	0.9 ± 0.1	0.8 ± 0.0	*0.5 ± 0.1 **	0.7 ± 0.1	0.7 ± 0.1	*0.4 ± 0.1 **
Cxcl12	1.2 ± 0.2	0.8 ± 0.1	0.5 ± 0.1	0.8 ± 0.0	*0.7 ± 0.0 **	*0.4 ± 0.1 **
Maob	1.0 ± 0.1	0.8 ± 0.1	*0.6 ± 0.0 **	0.8 ± 0.1	0.8 ± 0.1	*0.6 ± 0.1 **
Rdx	1.1 ± 0.1	0.8 ± 0.1	*0.6 ± 0.0 **	0.7 ± 0.1	0.8 ± 0.1	0.7 ± 0.1
B2m	1.0 ± 0.1	*0.6 ± 0.0 **	0.7 ± 0.1	0.9 ± 0.1	0.8 ± 0.1	*0.6 ± 0.1 **
Cryl1	1.0 ± 0.2	0.4 ± 0.0	*0.7 ± 0.1*	0.8 ± 0.1	0.8 ± 0.1	0.6 ± 0.1
Ipo8	1.4 ± 0.1	*0.8 ± 0.1 **	0.9 ± 0.1	0.9 ± 0.1	0.7 ± 0.1	*0.5 ± 0.2 **
Srebf1	1.2 ± 0.1	0.7 ± 0.1	0.9 ± 0.1	0.8 ± 0.1	0.7 ± 0.1	*0.7 ± 0.1 **
Scd1	0.6 ± 0.1	*0.3 ± 0.0 **	0.9 ± 0.3	0.5 ± 0.1	0.6 ± 0.0	*0.1 ± 0.0*
Dnajb11	1.3 ± 0.2	1.1 ± 0.1	1.1 ± 0.2	0.7 ± 0.1	*0.4 ± 0.1 **	0.9 ± 0.1
Tagln	1.0 ± 0.1	0.8 ± 0.2	1.2 ± 0.7	0.6 ± 0.1	*0.5 ± 0.1 **	*0.3 ± 0.1 **
Abcb4	1.1 ± 0.3	0.6 ± 0.1	1.4 ± 0.4	0.8 ± 0.1	0.6 ± 0.1	*0.4 ± 0.1 **
Fasn	2.2 ± 0.3	1.4 ± 0.1	1.5 ± 0.5	0.5 ± 0.0	*0.4 ± 0.1 **	0.5 ± 0.2

During the sub-acute phase, 21 genes were significantly down-regulated and 12 genes were significantly up-regulated. Unlike the acute phase, only 15 affected genes were dysregulated in a dose-dependent manner. Another 15 genes were affected only at the high CBD dose (i.e., 615 mg/kg CBD).

Expression of a substantial number of genes (21) was affected during both study phases. The largest subset of dysregulated genes (9) was associated with general hepatotoxicity. Of these, *Aldoa*, *Gsr*, *Krt8*, *Krt18*, *Nqo1*, and *Pla2g12a* were up-regulated, whereas *Avpr1a*, *Car3*, and *Igfals* were down-regulated.

All the gene expression data is summarized in Supplementary Table S3.

2.4. Dose-Response Analysis

Dose-response was also evaluated with linear and log regression models, with the best fit model meeting at least three of the following criteria: lowest AICc, lowest standard deviation of residuals, lowest absolute sum of squares, and/or highest R^2 value (at least 0.5) (Supplementary Table S4). In the 24 h acute study, AST, *Cyp1a1*, *Cyp1a2*, *Cyp2b10*, *Cyp3a4*, *Gsr*, *Ipo4*, *Nqo1*, *Timm10b*, and *Ugt1a1* had an increasing response with CBD dose ($R^2 > 0.5$) and *Abcb11*, *Car3*, *Cdc14b*, *Fabp1*, *Fads1*, *Igfals*, *L2hgdh*, *Lgr5*, *Maob*, *Mbl2*, and *Ppara* had a decreasing response with CBD dose ($R^2 > 0.5$). Similar responses for some of the parameters were seen in the two-week acute study: increasing responses in *Cyp2b10*,

Ugt1a1, and liver to body weight ratios; and decreasing responses with *Atp8b1*, *Avpr1a*, *Car3*, *Cdc14b*, *Cxcl12*, *Fabp1*, *L2hgdh*, *Lgr5*, *Ppara*, *Scd1*, and *Tagln*. The parameters in common between the two time points were *Cyp2b10*, *Ugt1a1*, *Car3*, *Fabp1*, *L2hgdh*, *Lgr5*, and *Ppara*, which, aside from *Cyp2b10* and *Ugt1a1*, were down-regulated.

3. Discussion

The marketing of products containing CBD, a non-psychotropic constituent of the *Cannabis sativa* plant, has grown rapidly in the last five years. It has been successfully utilized for therapy of treatment-resistant epilepsy and may have a number of other beneficial health effects. However, to our knowledge, there is a lack of comprehensive toxicological studies devoted to CBD safety that are critical for further marketing of CBD and CBD-containing products.

In this study, we demonstrated that CBD, when delivered orally to mice in the form of a concentrated CBD-enriched Cannabis extract, has the potential to cause liver injury. In the acute toxicity study, the highest CBD dose (2460 mg/kg), exhibited clear evidence of hepatotoxicity as indicated by marked increases in serum ALT, AST, and total bilirubin as well as increased intrahepatic concentrations of oxidized glutathione. Interestingly, this dose did not result in consistent increases in liver-to-body weight ratio; however, a similar response was observed in rhesus monkeys injected with sub-lethal or lethal doses of CBD [14]. Although 2460 mg/kg (MED of 200 mg/kg CBD) is not applicable to most real-life scenarios, it does provide critical information regarding the potential consequences of CBD overdose as well as for doses needed for further sub-chronic and chronic toxicity studies. Single administration of lower doses (246 mg/kg and 738 mg/kg CBD) caused only increases in liver-to-body weight ratios among the generally liver-focused toxicological responses measured.

The administration of CBD caused dose-dependent and sometimes dramatic induction of major cytochromes and UDP-glucuronosyltransferases (Supplemental Table S3). Induction of murine Cyp isoforms by CBD has been noted previously following sub-chronic dosing [19]. Of particular concern is the induction of *Cyp2e1* and *Cyp2b10*. The former isoform is a central participant in the biotransformation of ethanol and APAP, while the latter plays a role in the metabolism of a number of prescription medications including bupropion, clobazam, cyclophosphamide, ketamine, propofol, and several others. Furthermore, CYP2B6 and CYP3A4, the human homologues of *Cyp2b10* and *Cyp3a11* (another CYP induced in this study), are central in the metabolism (N-demethylation) of clobazam, an anti-seizure medication used in the treatment of epilepsy. Interestingly, recent clinical studies have noted that serum concentrations of N-desmethylclobazam, the active metabolite of clobazam, are markedly increased when co-administered with CBD (Epidiolex®) [32]. Such clinical observations appear to support the inductive effects of CBD on CYPs noted in this study. To what extent, however, the induction of murine Cyps by CBD is translatable to humans remains to be determined. Clearly, additional clinical studies investigating CBD-mediated drug interactions are needed, especially if Epidiolex® is to be prescribed for other medical conditions, but more importantly as CBD gains popularity across the U.S. following its descheduization as a result of the passage of the Agriculture Improvement Act of 2018, otherwise known as the 2018 Farm Bill [33].

The 10 day sub-acute study also revealed that CBD doses above 50 mg/kg MED, although well tolerated after single administration, were toxic when repetitively delivered. The observed general toxicity was, in part, mediated by liver injury as numerous signatures of hepatotoxicity were observed, including pan-hepatic cytoplasmic swelling, increases in liver-to-body weight ratios, and elevated ALT, AST, and total bilirubin. No measurable toxicological responses associated with liver injury were observed in mice gavaged with CBD at 184.5 mg/kg (MED of 15 mg/kg CBD) or lower, however, foci of hepatocyte cytoplasmic swelling were often detected. These findings are in line with observations from recent clinical trials in which 5–20% of patients exhibited increases in liver enzymes during chronic CBD administration at doses of 20 mg/kg [1,2,24]. Taken together, this evidence suggests that, despite some inter-species differences in CBD disposition, the mouse is a reliable model for assessing the safety of this popular cannabinoid.

Another important finding of this study was the wide palette of molecular responses elicited by CBD, particularly the dysregulation of more than 50 genes involved in hepatotoxicity. To our knowledge, the magnitude of such a response has not been observed in previous studies utilizing similar gene expression arrays aimed at examining the hepatotoxicity of bromobenzene, carbon tetrachloride, dimethyl nitrosamine, or OxyELITE-Pro, a botanical dietary supplement linked to severe liver injury in humans [29,30,34]. The involvement of numerous enzymatic pathways in response to CBD exposure suggests that liver injury associated with this cannabinoid occurs via various mechanisms. Of particular concern was the up-regulation of genes associated with oxidative stress, in particular *Hmox1*, *Nqo1*, and *Txnrd1*. These findings, coupled with increased levels of oxidized glutathione, infer a strong pro-oxidant trait to CBD, thereby bringing into question its claimed 'antioxidant' properties.

Importantly, a number of genes were differentially regulated at low and high doses of CBD, resulting in a biphasic or hormetic response. For instance, the expression of lanosterol synthase (*Lss*), a gene responsible for the biosynthesis of cholesterol, steroid hormones, and vitamin D, was up-regulated after 246 and 738 mg/kg CBD, but substantially down-regulated with a CBD dose of 2460 mg/kg. Interestingly, previous studies have also described a biphasic response to CBD, where low doses were stimulatory, while higher doses were inhibitory [35]. More strikingly, cyclin dependent kinase inhibitor 1A (*Cdkn1a*) was down-regulated after exposure to non-toxic doses of CBD, but significantly up-regulated at doses associated with either overt toxicity (2460 mg/kg CBD) or mortality (615 mg/kg CBD) in acute and sub-acute studies, respectively. Previous studies have demonstrated that down-regulation of *Cdkn1a*, also known as *p21*, stimulates liver regeneration, while overexpression inhibits this process [36–38]. Furthermore, a recent report of *Cdkn1a* up-regulation resulting from acute cholestatic injury was proposed as a biomarker for impaired liver regeneration [39]. Elevated total bilirubin in conjunction with up-regulation of *Cdkn1a* and a number of other gene-markers of cholestatic liver injury (i.e., *Abcb1a*, *Abcc2*, *Abcc3*, *Atp8b1*, and *Rdx*) and down-regulation of fatty acid metabolism-related genes (*Car3*, *Fabp1*, and *Ppara*) observed in our study, suggest that CBD-induced liver injury may be cholestatic, though ALP and GGT were not elevated. Future studies are needed to confirm this hypothesis.

In conclusion, the results of these studies demonstrate that, despite the beneficial effects of CBD in the treatment of certain therapy-resistant seizures, it poses a risk for liver injury. Furthermore, the probability of CBD-drug interactions appears quite high. Therefore, additional studies are needed to examine the toxicity of chronic low-dose CBD exposure as well as explore CBD's potential to interact with other medications. Such studies will provide important information regarding the range of CBD doses that can be deemed safe for the purpose of regulatory decision-making.

4. Materials and Methods

4.1. CBD Extract Characterization, Dosing Solution, and Dose Calculations

CBD extract was prepared following GMP procedures from the leaves and flowering tops by the extraction of CBD rich cannabis plant material (5.61% of CBD and 0.2% THC) using hexane as the extraction solvent. The extract was then evaporated to dryness followed by raising the temperature to 80 °C to effect complete decarboxylation of the extract. The final extract was analyzed using GC/MS for its cannabinoid content, solvent residue, heavy metals, bacterial and fungal counts and aflatoxin content following USP procedures. The results showed the following: cannabidiol content 57.9%; other cannabinoids: cannabichromene 2.03%, Δ^9-tetrahydrocannabinol 1.69%, cannabigerol 1.07%, Δ^8-tetrahydrocannabinol <0.01%; tetrahydrocannabivarin <0.01%. Residual solvent <0.5%; loss on drying 0.32%; heavy metals: lead, mercury, cadmium, and arsenic were not detected; aflatoxins: AFB_1, AFB_2, AGF_1, AFG_2 were not detected.

Doses of the CBD extract were calculated based on the CBD content listed above to deliver the required dose of CBD. For simplicity, the 'CBD-rich cannabis extract' will be referred to as 'CBD' throughout this manuscript. The extract was diluted in sesame oil to prepare the gavage solution. Allometric scaling for CBD mouse equivalent doses (MED) was determined per the recommendation of Wojcikowski and Gobe which, in turn, is based upon the FDA Industry Guidance for Estimating the Maximum Safe Starting Dose in Initial Clinical Trials for Therapeutics in Adult Volunteers [40]. The scaling factor of 12.3, commonly used for mice weighing between 11–34 g, was used to calculate the MED for CBD. The MED was based on the maximum recommended human maintenance dose of CBD (Epidiolex®), which is 20 mg/kg. For the 1× dose, the quantity of CBD administered was 20 mg/kg × 0.025 kg (average mouse weight in our study) × 12.3 (scaling factor for mice) = 6.15 mg total CBD delivered in 300 µL of gavage solution or 246 mg/kg. Consequently, 3× dose = 18.45 mg total CBD in 300 µL gavage solution or 738 mg/kg), and 10× dose = 61.5 mg total CBD in 300 µL gavage solution or 2460 mg/kg). In the sub-acute study, the dose of 61.5 mg/kg (MED of 5 mg/kg CBD) was considered as 1× dose. Consequently, the doses of 184.5 mg/kg (MED of 15 mg/kg CBD) and 615 mg/kg (MED of 50 mg/kg CBD) were considered as 3× and 10×, respectively. Control mice received 300 µL of sesame oil.

4.2. Animals

Male B6C3F$_1$/J mice, 8 weeks of age (standard age of mice used in safety assessment studies), were purchased from Jackson Laboratories (Bar Harbor, ME, USA) and were housed at the UAMS Division of Laboratory Animal Medicine (DLAM) facility. B6C3F$_1$/J mice are characterized by an average sensitivity to hepatotoxicants and are widely used by both the FDA and pharmaceutical industry to investigate the potential for xenobiotics to produce hepatotoxicity. Animals were given one week to acclimate before the initiation of studies. Animal experiments were conducted in two stages. In the first stage (acute toxicity), mice were gavaged with a single dose of either 246, 738, or 2460 mg/kg of CBD (MED of 20, 60, and 200 mg/kg, respectively) and 24 h later animals were euthanized and tissues/organs were harvested. During the second stage (sub-acute toxicity), mice were gavaged with CBD extract for ten days (Mon-Fri) with (MED of 61.5, 184.5, and 615 mg/kg, respectively) for reasons explained later in the Results. Mice were terminated six hours after the last gavage.

To avoid any potential fasting-exacerbated toxicity, food and water were provided *ad libitum*. Each animal was individually identified with an ear tag. Animal body weights were measured and recorded twice a week. All procedures were approved by the UAMS Institutional Animal Care and Use Committee (protocol number: AUP # 3701), and all personnel followed the appropriate safety precautions.

4.3. Blood Sampling and Clinical Biochemistry

To measure the effects of CBD extract on a panel of liver enzymes characteristic for drug-induced liver injury, blood was collected at the end of each experimental stage described above. Blood was collected from the retroorbital plexus with a heparinized micro-haematocrit capillary tube (Fisher Scientific, Pittsburg, PA, USA) and placed into a 1.1 mL Z-gel microtube (Sarstedt, Newton, NC, USA). Tubes were kept on ice and centrifuged at 10,000 rpm for 20 min; serum samples were then immediately aliquoted and delivered to the Veterinary Diagnostic Laboratory at the Arkansas Livestock and Poultry Commission (Little Rock, AR, USA) on dry ice where the samples were processed the same day.

4.4. Histopathological Assessment

Livers were excised and a 1 mm section was obtained from the left lateral lobe and another from the right medial lobe. Sections were fixed in 4% formalin for 24 h, then briefly rinsed in PBS and stored in 70% ethanol for 24 h. Livers were then processed at the UAMS Pathology Core Facility, stained with hematoxylin eosin, and evaluated by a board-certified pathologist in a blinded fashion.

For histologic assessment purposes, each liver was represented by two sections obtained from different locations within the liver. Each section was initially evaluated at magnifications of ×40 and ×100. Sections were further evaluated at ×200 and ×400 to check for the presence of mitotic figures, necrotic foci, and apoptotic bodies.

4.5. Glutathione Analysis

Glutathione was measured using a modified Tietze assay [41]. Briefly, liver tissue was homogenized in 3% sulfosalicylic acid. One aliquot was diluted in N-ethylmaleimide (NEM) to mask reduced glutathione (GSH) and facilitate measurement of oxidized glutathione (GSSG), while another was diluted in 0.1 M HCl for measurement of total (GSH + GSSG) glutathione. After removal of NEM by solid phase extraction with a C18 column, glutathione was measured in both aliquots using a colorimetric glutathione reductase cycling detection method [41].

4.6. Analysis of mRNA Levels of Major Cytochromes and Transporter Genes

Total RNA was extracted from flash frozen liver tissue using the RNeasy Mini Kit (QIAGEN, Germantown, MD, USA). Following purification, 1000 ng were reverse transcribed with the High Capacity cDNA Reverse Transcription Kit (Thermo Fisher, Waltham, MA, USA). Primers were added at a final concentration of 5 µM (Supplementary Table S1). Gene expression values were normalized to the internal control gene *Hprt* and expressed as fold change according to the ΔΔCt method.

4.7. Hepatotoxicity Gene Expression Array

Total RNA was extracted as described above. The cDNA was diluted to 5 ng/µL and 105 µL was mixed with an equal volume of 2× TaqMan® Fast Advanced Master Mix. For real-time PCR, 100 µL of the mix was applied to each of two channels on a TaqMan Low Density Hepatotoxicity Array (TLDA) (Supplementary Table S2) (Thermo Fisher, Waltham, MA, USA). Four biological samples were loaded onto each array with six replicates analyzed per group. Analysis was performed using the ExpressionSuite Software v1.1 (Thermo Fisher, Waltham, MA, USA).

4.8. Statistical Analysis

All statistical analyses were performed with Graphpad Prism 6 software (Graphpad Software, San Diego, CA, USA). Treatment groups were compared with their respective untreated group using ANOVA followed by Tukey's multiple comparison test. In cases where the data was not normally distributed as indicated by a positive Brown-Forsythe test, a Kruskal-Wallis with Dunn's multiple comparison test was used instead. Comparisons were considered significant at $p < 0.05$. To evaluate trends in dose-dependent responses, all parameters were analyzed with regression analyses within Prism using log(dose) as the independent variable. We used three different models to determine best fit: linear regression with y-intercept constrained to 0, linear regression with unconstrained y-intercept, and log(agonist) vs response (three parameters). Regression models were excluded if the model was ambiguous, interrupted, or not converged or if the 95% confidence intervals were calculated to be 'very wide'. Models for each response parameter were compared using the goodness of fit parameters R^2 (higher being better), standard deviation of residuals (lower being better; noted as Sy.x), AICc (lower being better), and the absolution sum of squares (lower being better), with the model having best goodness of fit parameters being considered the better model.

Supplementary Materials: The following are available online, Figure S1: Kidney- and Heart-to Body-Weight Ratio in Mice Gavaged with Single Dose of CBD, Figure S2: Effects of Single Dose of CBD on Liver Histomorphology, Figure S3: Kidney- and Heart-to-Body-Weight Ratio in Mice Gavaged with CBD for 10 Days, Figure S4: Kidney- (A) and heart- (B) to-body-weight ratio in mice gavaged with CBD for 10 days, Table S1: Forward and Reverse Primer Sequences for Cyp P450s and UGTs, Table S2: Custom Taqman Low Density Hepatotoxicity Array Gene Targets, Table S3: Commonly dysregulated genes sorted by function, including CYPs, Ugts, and hepatotoxicity markers, Table S4: Dose-response analysis with linear and log regression models.

Author Contributions: Conceptualization, L.A.W, M.A.E., B.J.G. and I.K.; Data curation, L.E.E. and I.K.; Formal analysis, L.E.E., C.M.S., C.M.Q., S.K.-M., M.R.M., M.A.E., B.J.G. and I.K.; Funding acquisition, M.R.M. and I.K.; Investigation, L.A.W., C.M.S., M.R.M., M.A.E., B.J.G. and I.K.; Methodology, M.A.E.; Resources, B.J.G.; Writing—original draft, M.R.M., M.A.E., B.J.G. and I.K.

Funding: This work was supported by the National Institute of General Medical Sciences [grant # P20 GM109005 to IK], the American Association for the Study of Liver Diseases (AASLD) Foundation [Pinnacle Research Award to MRM], and the Arkansas Biosciences Institute.

Acknowledgments: The authors are thankful to Robin Mulkey and Bridgette Engi for excellent animal care at the UAMS Animal Facility.

Conflicts of Interest: Quick serves as a scientific consultant for Allergen. The other authors have no conflicts of interest to disclose.

References

1. Devinsky, O.; Cross, J.H.; Wright, S. Trial of Cannabidiol for Drug-Resistant Seizures in the Dravet Syndrome. *N. Eng. J. Med.* **2017**, *377*, 699–700. [CrossRef]
2. Thiele, E.A.; Marsh, E.D.; French, J.A.; Mazurkiewicz-Beldzinska, M.; Benbadis, S.R.; Joshi, C.; Lyons, P.D.; Taylor, A.; Roberts, C.; Sommerville, K.; et al. Cannabidiol in patients with seizures associated with Lennox-Gastaut syndrome (GWPCARE4): A randomised, double-blind, placebo-controlled phase 3 trial. *Lancet* **2018**, *391*, 1085–1096. [CrossRef]
3. Crippa, J.A.; Guimaraes, F.S.; Campos, A.C.; Zuardi, A.W. Translational Investigation of the Therapeutic Potential of Cannabidiol (CBD): Toward a New Age. *Front. Immunol.* **2018**, *9*, 2009. [CrossRef] [PubMed]
4. Olah, A.; Toth, B.I.; Borbiro, I.; Sugawara, K.; Szollosi, A.G.; Czifra, G.; Pal, B.; Ambrus, L.; Kloepper, J.; Camera, E.; et al. Cannabidiol exerts sebostatic and antiinflammatory effects on human sebocytes. *J. Clin. Investig.* **2014**, *124*, 3713–3724. [CrossRef] [PubMed]
5. Hampson, A.J.; Grimaldi, M.; Axelrod, J.; Wink, D. Cannabidiol and (-)Delta9-tetrahydrocannabinol are neuroprotective antioxidants. *Proc. Natl. Acad Sci. USA* **1998**, *95*, 8268–8273. [CrossRef]
6. Carvalho, R.K.; Santos, M.L.; Souza, M.R.; Rocha, T.L.; Guimaraes, F.S.; Anselmo-Franci, J.A.; Mazaro-Costa, R. Chronic exposure to cannabidiol induces reproductive toxicity in male Swiss mice. *J. Appl. Toxicol.* **2018**, *38*, 1215–1223. [CrossRef]
7. Carvalho, R.K.; Souza, M.R.; Santos, M.L.; Guimaraes, F.S.; Pobbe, R.L.H.; Andersen, M.L.; Mazaro-Costa, R. Chronic cannabidiol exposure promotes functional impairment in sexual behavior and fertility of male mice. *Reprod Toxicol.* **2018**, *81*, 34–40. [CrossRef]
8. Carty, D.R.; Thornton, C.; Gledhill, J.H.; Willett, K.L. Developmental Effects of Cannabidiol and Delta9-Tetrahydrocannabinol in Zebrafish. *Toxicol. Sci.* **2018**, *162*, 137–145. [CrossRef] [PubMed]
9. Schonhofen, P.; de Medeiros, L.M.; Bristot, I.J.; Lopes, F.M.; De Bastiani, M.A.; Kapczinski, F.; Crippa, J.A.; Castro, M.A.; Parsons, R.B.; Klamt, F. Cannabidiol Exposure During Neuronal Differentiation Sensitizes Cells Against Redox-Active Neurotoxins. *Mol. Neurobiol.* **2015**, *52*, 26–37. [CrossRef]
10. ElBatsh, M.M.; Assareh, N.; Marsden, C.A.; Kendall, D.A. Anxiogenic-like effects of chronic cannabidiol administration in rats. *Psychopharmacology (Berl)* **2012**, *221*, 239–247. [CrossRef]
11. Mato, S.; Victoria Sanchez-Gomez, M.; Matute, C. Cannabidiol induces intracellular calcium elevation and cytotoxicity in oligodendrocytes. *Glia* **2010**, *58*, 1739–1747. [CrossRef]
12. Usami, N.; Yamamoto, I.; Watanabe, K. Generation of reactive oxygen species during mouse hepatic microsomal metabolism of cannabidiol and cannabidiol hydroxy-quinone. *Life Sci.* **2008**, *83*, 717–724. [CrossRef]
13. Jadoon, K.A.; Tan, G.D.; O'Sullivan, S.E. A single dose of cannabidiol reduces blood pressure in healthy volunteers in a randomized crossover study. *JCI Insight* **2017**, *2*. [CrossRef]
14. Rosenkrantz, H.; Fleischman, R.W.; Grant, R.J. Toxicity of short-term administration of cannabinoids to rhesus monkeys. *Toxicol. Appl. Pharmacol.* **1981**, *58*, 118–131. [CrossRef]
15. Devinsky, O.; Nabbout, R.; Miller, I.; Laux, L.; Zolnowska, M.; Wright, S.; Roberts, C. Long-term cannabidiol treatment in patients with Dravet syndrome: An open-label extension trial. *Epilepsia* **2018**. [CrossRef]
16. Russo, C.; Ferk, F.; Misik, M.; Ropek, N.; Nersesyan, A.; Mejri, D.; Holzmann, K.; Lavorgna, M.; Isidori, M.; Knasmuller, S. Low doses of widely consumed cannabinoids (cannabidiol and cannabidivarin) cause DNA damage and chromosomal aberrations in human-derived cells. *Arch. Toxicol.* **2018**. [CrossRef] [PubMed]
17. Yamaori, S.; Ebisawa, J.; Okushima, Y.; Yamamoto, I.; Watanabe, K. Potent inhibition of human cytochrome P450 3A isoforms by cannabidiol: Role of phenolic hydroxyl groups in the resorcinol moiety. *Life Sci.* **2011**, *88*, 730–736. [CrossRef]

18. Jones, G.; Pertwee, R.G. A metabolic interaction in vivo between cannabidiol and 1-tetrahydrocannabinol. *Br. J. Pharmacol.* **1972**, *45*, 375–377. [CrossRef]
19. Bornheim, L.M.; Everhart, E.T.; Li, J.; Correia, M.A. Induction and genetic regulation of mouse hepatic cytochrome P450 by cannabidiol. *Biochem. Pharmacol.* **1994**, *48*, 161–171. [CrossRef]
20. Narimatsu, S.; Watanabe, K.; Matsunaga, T.; Yamamoto, I.; Imaoka, S.; Funae, Y.; Yoshimura, H. Inhibition of hepatic microsomal cytochrome P450 by cannabidiol in adult male rats. *Chem. Pharm. Bull. (Tokyo)* **1990**, *38*, 1365–1368. [CrossRef] [PubMed]
21. Bornheim, L.M.; Correia, M.A. Selective inactivation of mouse liver cytochrome P-450IIIA by cannabidiol. *Mol. Pharmacol.* **1990**, *38*, 319–326. [PubMed]
22. Marx, T.K.; Reddeman, R.; Clewell, A.E.; Endres, J.R.; Beres, E.; Vertesi, A.; Glavits, R.; Hirka, G.; Szakonyine, I.P. An Assessment of the Genotoxicity and Subchronic Toxicity of a Supercritical Fluid Extract of the Aerial Parts of Hemp. *J. Toxicol.* **2018**, *2018*, 8143582. [CrossRef] [PubMed]
23. Gamble, L.J.; Boesch, J.M.; Frye, C.W.; Schwark, W.S.; Mann, S.; Wolfe, L.; Brown, H.; Berthelsen, E.S.; Wakshlag, J.J. Pharmacokinetics, Safety, and Clinical Efficacy of Cannabidiol Treatment in Osteoarthritic Dogs. *Front. Vet. Sci.* **2018**, *5*, 165. [CrossRef] [PubMed]
24. Devinsky, O.; Patel, A.D.; Cross, J.H.; Villanueva, V.; Wirrell, E.C.; Privitera, M.; Greenwood, S.M.; Roberts, C.; Checketts, D.; VanLandingham, K.E.; et al. Effect of Cannabidiol on Drop Seizures in the Lennox-Gastaut Syndrome. *N. Eng. J. Med.* **2018**, *378*, 1888–1897. [CrossRef] [PubMed]
25. FDA. Federal Food, Drug, and Cosmetic Act (FD&C Act). Available online: https://www.fda.gov/regulatory-information/laws-enforced-fda/federal-food-drug-and-cosmetic-act-fdc-act (accessed on 29 April 2019).
26. FDA. Warning Letters and Test Results for Cannabidiol-Related Prodcuts. Available online: https://www.fda.gov/newsevents/publichealthfocus/ucm484109.htm (accessed on 29 April 2019).
27. ConsumerLab. Product Reviews: CBD & Hemp Extract Supplements, Lotions, and Balms Review. Available online: https://www.consumerlab.com/reviews/cbd-oil-hemp-review/cbd-oil/#whatclfound (accessed on 29 April 2019).
28. Szaflarski, J.P.; Bebin, E.M.; Comi, A.M.; Patel, A.D.; Joshi, C.; Checketts, D.; Beal, J.C.; Laux, L.C.; De Boer, L.M.; Wong, M.H.; et al. Long-term safety and treatment effects of cannabidiol in children and adults with treatment-resistant epilepsies: Expanded access program results. *Epilepsia* **2018**, *59*, 1540–1548. [CrossRef] [PubMed]
29. Skinner, C.M.; Miousse, I.R.; Ewing, L.E.; Sridharan, V.; Cao, M.; Lin, H.; Williams, D.K.; Avula, B.; Haider, S.; Chittiboyina, A.G.; et al. Impact of obesity on the toxicity of a multi-ingredient dietary supplement, OxyELITE Pro (New Formula), using the novel NZO/HILtJ obese mouse model: Physiological and mechanistic assessments. *Food Chem. Toxicol.* **2018**, *122*, 21–32. [CrossRef]
30. Miousse, I.R.; Skinner, C.M.; Lin, H.; Ewing, L.E.; Kosanke, S.D.; Williams, D.K.; Avula, B.; Khan, I.A.; ElSohly, M.A.; Gurley, B.J.; et al. Safety assessment of the dietary supplement OxyELITE Pro (New Formula) in inbred and outbred mouse strains. *Food Chem. Toxicol.* **2017**, *109*, 194–209. [CrossRef]
31. Gurley, B.J.; Miousse, I.R.; Nookaew, I.; Ewing, L.E.; Skinner, C.M.; Jenjaroenpun, P.; Wongsurawat, T.; Kennon-McGill, S.; Avula, B.; Bae, J.Y.; et al. Decaffeinated Green Tea Extract Does Not Elicit Hepatotoxic Effects and Modulates the Gut Microbiome in Lean B6C3F1 Mice. *Nutrients* **2019**, *11*, 776. [CrossRef]
32. Gaston, T.E.; Szaflarski, J.P. Cannabis for the Treatment of Epilepsy: An Update. *Curr. Neurol. Neurosci. Rep.* **2018**, *18*, 73. [CrossRef]
33. Agriculture Improvement Act of 2018. In *Public Law 115–334*; National Archives: Washington, DC, USA, 2018; pp. 115–334.
34. Minami, K.; Saito, T.; Narahara, M.; Tomita, H.; Kato, H.; Sugiyama, H.; Katoh, M.; Nakajima, M.; Yokoi, T. Relationship between hepatic gene expression profiles and hepatotoxicity in five typical hepatotoxicant-administered rats. *Toxicol. Sci.* **2005**, *87*, 296–305. [CrossRef]
35. Jenny, M.; Santer, E.; Pirich, E.; Schennach, H.; Fuchs, D. Delta9-tetrahydrocannabinol and cannabidiol modulate mitogen-induced tryptophan degradation and neopterin formation in peripheral blood mononuclear cells in vitro. *J. Neuroimmunol.* **2009**, *207*, 75–82. [CrossRef]
36. Hui, T.T.; Mizuguchi, T.; Sugiyama, N.; Avital, I.; Rozga, J.; Demetriou, A.A. Immediate early genes and p21 regulation in liver of rats with acute hepatic failure. *Am. J. Surg.* **2002**, *183*, 457–463. [CrossRef]

37. Buitrago-Molina, L.E.; Marhenke, S.; Longerich, T.; Sharma, A.D.; Boukouris, A.E.; Geffers, R.; Guigas, B.; Manns, M.P.; Vogel, A. The degree of liver injury determines the role of p21 in liver regeneration and hepatocarcinogenesis in mice. *Hepatology* **2013**, *58*, 1143–1152. [CrossRef]
38. Lehmann, K.; Tschuor, C.; Rickenbacher, A.; Jang, J.H.; Oberkofler, C.E.; Tschopp, O.; Schultze, S.M.; Raptis, D.A.; Weber, A.; Graf, R.; et al. Liver failure after extended hepatectomy in mice is mediated by a p21-dependent barrier to liver regeneration. *Gastroenterology* **2012**, *143*, 1609–1619.e4. [CrossRef] [PubMed]
39. Dondorf, F.; Fahrner, R.; Ardelt, M.; Patsenker, E.; Stickel, F.; Dahmen, U.; Settmacher, U.; Rauchfuss, F. Induction of chronic cholestasis without liver cirrhosis - Creation of an animal model. *World J. Gastroenterol.* **2017**, *23*, 4191–4199. [CrossRef] [PubMed]
40. Wojcikowski, K.; Gobe, G. Animal studies on medicinal herbs: Predictability, dose conversion and potential value. *Phytother. Res.* **2014**, *28*, 22–27. [CrossRef]
41. McGill, M.R.; Jaeschke, H. A direct comparison of methods used to measure oxidized glutathione in biological samples: 2-vinylpyridine and N-ethylmaleimide. *Toxicol. Mech. Methods* **2015**, *25*, 589–595. [CrossRef] [PubMed]

Sample Availability: Tissue samples from experimental animals are available from the authors.

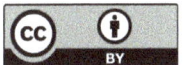

© 2019 by the authors. Licensee MDPI, Basel, Switzerland. This article is an open access article distributed under the terms and conditions of the Creative Commons Attribution (CC BY) license (http://creativecommons.org/licenses/by/4.0/).

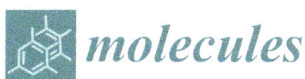

Communication

Anti-Amyloidogenic and Cyclooxygenase Inhibitory Activity of *Guettarda speciosa*

Mario A. Tan [1,2,3,4,*], Mark Wilson D. Lagamayo [2], Grecebio Jonathan D. Alejandro [2,3,4] and Seong Soo A. An [1,*]

1. Department of Bionano Technology, Bionano Research Institute, Gachon University, 1342 Sungnam-daero, Sujung-gu, Seongnam-si, Gyeonggi-do 461-701, Korea
2. Graduate School, University of Santo Tomas, Manila 1015, Philippines; mwdlagamayo@gmail.com (M.W.D.L.); gdalejandro@ust.edu.ph (G.J.D.A.)
3. Research Center for the Natural and Applied Sciences, University of Santo Tomas, Manila 1015, Philippines
4. College of Science, University of Santo Tomas, Manila 1015, Philippines
* Correspondence: matan@ust.edu.ph (M.A.T.); seong.an@gmail.com (S.S.A.A.); Tel.: +63-2-7314031 (M.A.T.); +82-31-750-8755 (S.S.A.A)

Academic Editors: Raffaele Capasso, Lorenzo Di Cesare Mannelli and Nicola Volpi
Received: 23 September 2019; Accepted: 11 November 2019; Published: 14 November 2019

Abstract: *Guettarda speciosa* is known in traditional folk medicine for treating cough, cold, sore throat, fever, wounds, epilepsy, and headaches. To discover the scientific pharmacological potential of *G. speciosa*, we explore its anti-inflammatory, cytotoxicity, and inhibition of amyloid-*beta* (Aβ) aggregation effects. Cyclooxygenase assay of the *G. speciosa* CHCl$_3$ (GSC) extract and *G. speciosa* MeOH (GSM) extract are more selective to COX-1 inhibition with a 50% inhibitory concentration (IC$_{50}$) of 3.56 µg/mL for the GSC extract and 4.98 µg/mL for the GSM extract. Neuroblastoma SH-SY5Y inhibition and thioflavin T assay amyloid-*beta* (Aβ) aggregate inhibition of the GSM and GSC extracts showed their potential therapeutic effects against Alzheimer's disease. The putative compounds from the LC-MS analysis could be responsible for the observed activities. The results suggest that *G. speciosa* possesses anti-inflammatory and anti-neurodegenerative properties and a promising lead as a source of pharmacologically active compounds.

Keywords: Alzheimer's disease; COX-1; cytotoxicity; *Guettarda speciosa*; thioflavin T

---

1. Introduction

Guettarda speciosa L. (Rubiaceae) is a perennial shrub or small tree, which grows in coastal habitats in tropical areas. This species is the only representative of the genus *Guettarda* L. in the Philippines [1]. The genus is widely distributed from East Africa to South and Southeast Asia and the South Pacific [2]. It is regarded as a medicinal plant used in traditional folk medicine for treating postpartum infection, cough, cold, sore throat, dysentery, fever, boils, wounds, epilepsy, and headache [3–6]. In African medicinal plants, the flower decoction was combined with *Ocimum americanum* L. and *O. gratissimum* L. to treat malaria, while the roots are used for diarrhea (decoction), rheumatism (rubdown on articulations), and pelvic pain (massage) [7]. These traditional folkloric claims were corroborated by pharmacological studies including the antiepileptic activity of the inner bark extract from India [5] and the anti-inflammatory activity in murine macrophages of the methanolic extract from Indonesia [8]. Phytochemical analysis has elaborated the presence of iridoids and their glucosides, phenolics, glycerol derivatives, steroids, triterpenoids [9,10], and fatty acids [11]. There is limited information on the biological activities and chemical constituents associated with *G. speciosa*.

To address this gap, and in the interest of searching for medicinal Rubiaceae plants from the Philippines with potential anti-inflammatory and anti-neurodegenerative activities [12–15], we herein describe the acute toxicity, cyclooxygenase inhibition, and anti-amyloidogenic activity of the extracts of G. speciosa.

2. Results

2.1. Acute Oral Toxicity

No death was observed among the animals over the 14-day period. Hence, assessment of the acute oral toxicity indicated that the G. speciosa MeOH (GSM) extract was safe and nontoxic up to 2000 mg/kg following the Organization for Economic Co-operation and Development (OECD) 425 guidelines. Prominent signs of toxicity and abnormalities were also not observed. Moreover, the post toxicity and gross necropsy study showed that all vital organs, such as the liver, kidneys, and stomach, were comparable to the control group as indicated in the histopathological results (Figure 1) analyzed by a licensed veterinarian.

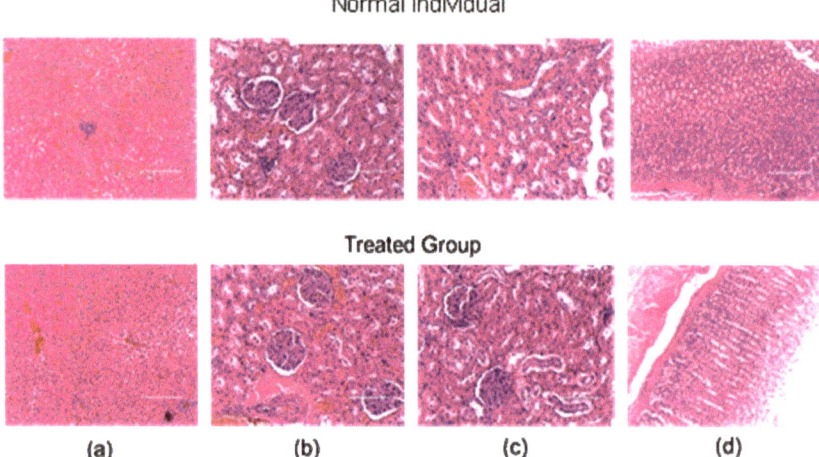

Figure 1. Histopathological examination of (**a**) liver, (**b**) left kidney, (**c**) right kidney, and (**d**) stomach in normal and G. *speciosa* extract-treated (GSM) groups. No significant changes were observed in the examined vital organs of the GSM-treated groups when compared to the normal control group.

2.2. COX-1 and COX-2 Assay

Aerial parts of G. *speciosa* were extracted with MeOH to afford the crude extract (GSM). Various extracts of G. *speciosa* with varying polarity were prepared using solvent partitioning. Nonpolar compounds are contained in the G. *speciosa* hexane (GSH) extract, semi-polar compounds in the G. *speciosa* CHCl$_3$ (GSC) extract, and polar compounds in the G. *speciosa* aqueous (GSA) extract. All the extracts were dried free of solvents prior to use in the succeeding experiments.

The cyclooxygenase screening assay results of the G. *speciosa* extracts (Figure 2) showed a greater inhibition to the COX-1 enzyme as compared to the COX-2. The extracts were initially tested at a concentration of 10 µg/mL. More than 50% inhibition for the COX-1 enzyme was observed for GSC (66.68% ± 2.77) and GSM (62.25% ± 2.39) extracts. None of the extracts gave a 50% inhibition using COX-2 enzyme with the GSC extract exhibiting the highest inhibition with 30.85% ± 5.11. Interestingly, the GSM extract exhibited a negative inhibition with COX-2 (−9.98% ± 5.62). The percentage inhibition of the extracts had a significant difference when compared to the positive control, indomethacin (4.0 mM) (85.1–86.3%), at $p < 0.05$.

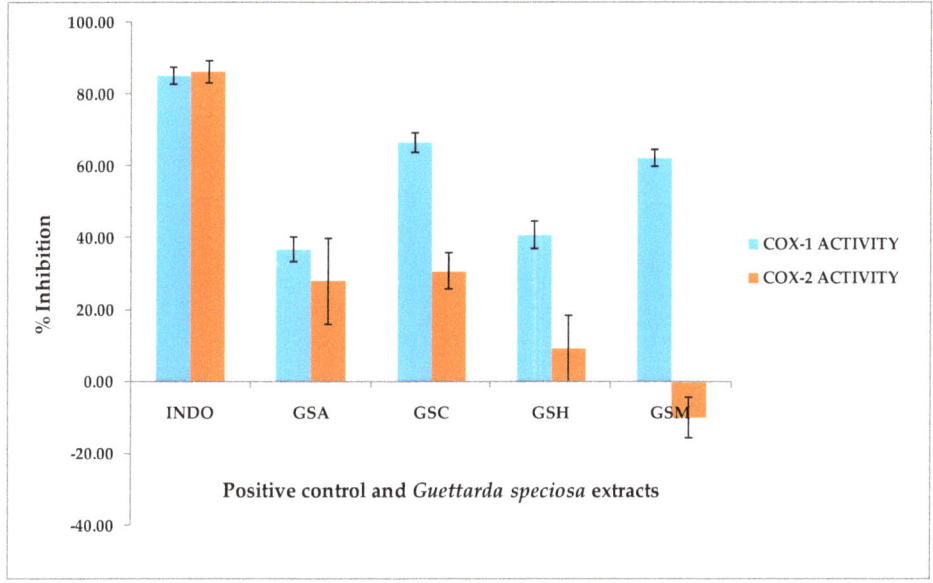

Figure 2. In vitro cyclooxygenase screening of *Guettarda speciosa* (*G. speciosa*) extracts at a concentration of 10 μg/mL. The *G. speciosa* extracts exhibited an inhibition to the COX-1 enzyme with the chloroform GSC and methanol GSM extracts showing a greater than 50% inhibition. Indomethacin (4.0 mM) (INDO) was used as the positive control. GSA—*G. speciosa* aqueous extract; GSC—*G. speciosa* $CHCl_3$ extract; GSH—*G. speciosa* hexane extract; GSM—*G. speciosa* MeOH extract.

Based on the screening results, the 50% inhibitive concentration (IC_{50}) of the GSC and GSM extracts for COX-1 were also determined using seven concentrations (0.5, 1, 5, 10, 40, 70, and 100 μg/mL). The results indicate an IC_{50} of 3.56 μg/mL for the GSC extract and 4.98 μg/mL for the GSM extract. Because of the promising results in the cyclooxygenase assay, the GSM and GSC extracts were further evaluated via cell viability and thioflavin T assays.

2.3. Cell Viability

The cytotoxicity of the GSM and GSC extracts was explored against neuroblastoma SH-SY5Y utilizing the ATP luminescence assay. The ATP serves as the cell's most important chemical energy storage for all biological processes. When cells are exposed to environmental or metabolic stressors (depleted iron and carbon sources), their ability to produce ATP is impeded. Hence, cellular ATP measurement is a good indication of a cell's metabolic health and subsequent viability. As illustrated in Figure 3, the GSM extract exhibited a 17% cell growth inhibition using the smallest concentration of 0.39 μg/mL, followed by 25% growth inhibition at 0.78 μg/mL. Surprisingly, an almost similar trend was observed, using 12.5, 6.25, 3.13, and 1.56 μg/mL concentrations with cell growth inhibitions at 35–38%. The highest concentration at 50 μg/mL showed a cell growth inhibition of 57%. Compared to the negative control, a significant difference was shown on the cell cytotoxicity of the extracts at all the given concentrations ($p < 0.05$). Cytotoxicity was also observed on the GSC extracts in a concentration-dependent manner from 0.39 to 50 μg/mL as observed in Figure 3. A 62% cell growth inhibition was noted on the 50 μg/mL, followed by the 25 μg/mL with 50% inhibition. The lowest concentration, 0.39 μg/mL, showed only a 6% cell growth inhibition with a cell viability of 94%. Statistical analyses also indicated a significant difference on the percentage cell viability of the GSC extracts when compared to the control (100% cell viability), with the exception of the lowest concentration (0.39 μg/mL).

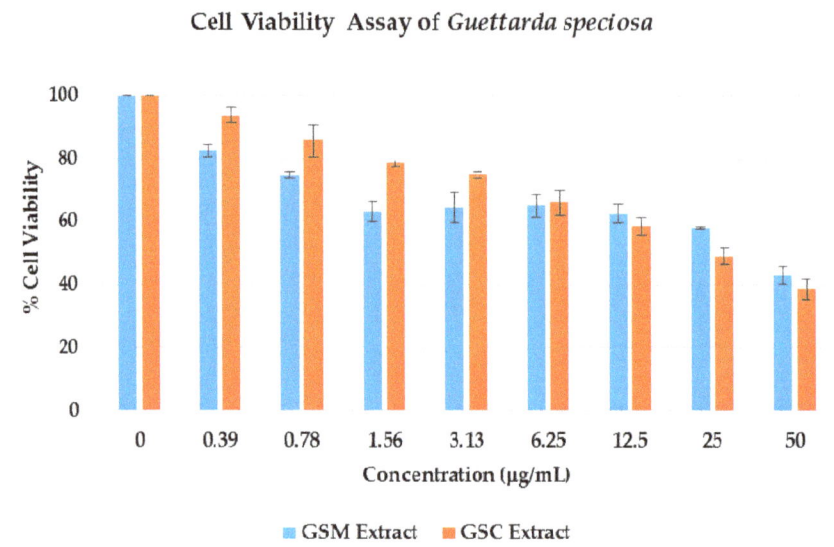

Figure 3. Effect of *Guettarda speciosa* MeOH (GSM) and CHCl$_3$ (GSC) extracts on cell viability in neuroblastoma SH-SY5Y cells. Cell viability was determined using the ATP luminescence assay. The results indicate % cell viability vs. the negative control (mean ± SD of triplicate measurement). All of the extracts exhibited a significant difference on the % cell viability on the negative control vs. the plant extracts at $p < 0.05$, except for the GSC extract at 0.39 µg/mL).

Through the cell viability ATP luminescence assay, the half maximal inhibitory concentration of the cell population death was determined. The GSM extract inhibited the growth of SH-SY5Y cells with an IC$_{50}$ value of 43.44 µg/mL. The GSC extract was found to be more active with an IC$_{50}$ of 8.049 µg/mL. SH-SY5Y cells have been used in many neurological studies, such as Parkinson's disease (PD), Alzheimer's disease (AD), and traumatic brain injury (TBI) [16]. The cell viability of the neuroblastoma SH-SY5Y cells against the GSM extracts may suggest promising leads with respect to the identification of potential bioactive secondary metabolites in neurological diseases.

2.4. Thioflavin T (ThT) Assay

The abnormal aggregation of β-amyloid (Aβ), tau protein accumulation, decreased acetylcholine, oxidative stress, and neuroinflammation of the nervous system are some of the pathological hallmarks associated with Alzheimer's disease. To address whether the GSM and GSC extracts are capable of inhibiting the aggregation of Aβ, we also utilized thioflavin T (ThT) assay using phenol red as the positive control (Table 1). The GSC extract at 50 µg/mL exhibited the highest inhibition of the Aβ fibril formation with 65.78%. This is also statistically comparable ($p < 0.05$) to the inhibition of the positive control at 69.85%. The GSM extract gave a 54.71% inhibition but is statistically different from the positive control ($p < 0.05$). The observed activity of the GSC and GSM extracts may be attributed to the presence of secondary metabolites, which could be capable of inhibiting the Aβ fibril formation.

Table 1. Thioflavin T (ThT) assay results of *Guettarda speciosa* extracts.

	Aβ$_{1-42}$ Aggregation Inhibition (%) [a]
Phenol Red (50 μM) [b]	69.85 ± 0.29
GSM Extract (50 μg/mL)	54.71 ± 2.92
GSM Extract (5 μg/mL)	17.20 ± 0.85
GSC Extract (50 μg/mL)	65.78 ± 3.12 *
GSC Extract (5 μg/mL)	24.63 ± 1.19

[a] The values are expressed as mean ± SD of three trial experiments. [b] The positive control. * No significant difference with the positive control at $p < 0.05$. GSM—*G. speciosa* MeOH extract; GSC—*G. speciosa* CHCl$_3$ extract.

2.5. Metabolite Profiling

A total of nine putatively identified compounds were determined from the GSM extract using LC-MS analysis. Optimized run method produced the LC chromatogram as shown in Figure 4, where the Y-axis represents the % signal intensity and the X-axis is the retention time in minutes. The compounds presented (Table 2 and Figure 5) are those that fall within the "good match" standards of the Traditional Chinese Medicine (TCM) library [17,18]. These putatively identified nine compounds were also previously isolated from the different *Guettarda* species based on the available literature data. Loganin (**3**) was isolated from *G. platypoda* DC. [19] and *G. pohliana* Müll. Arg. [20]; rotundic acid (**7**) from *G. angelica* Mart. ex Müll. Arg. [21] and *G. platypoda* [22]; quinovic acid (**9**) from *G. angelica* [23] and *G. platypoda* [22,24]; strictosidine (**1**), sickingine (**5**), 5-caffeoylquinic acid (**6**), and 4,5-dicaffeoylquinic acid (**8**) from *G. acreana* K. Krause [3]; sweroside (**2**) from *G. platypoda* [24] and *G. pohliana* [20]; and β-sitosterol (**4**) from *G. platypoda* [22]. Interestingly, the putatively identified compounds exhibit diverse biological activities as reported in the literature (Table 2). The putatively identified metabolites with their reported activities in the literature may explain the biological activities exhibited by the extracts in this study. Several compounds were identified to have anti-inflammatory activity (**2**, **4**, and **6**), cytotoxicity (**2** and **3**), and neuroprotective (**3**) activity.

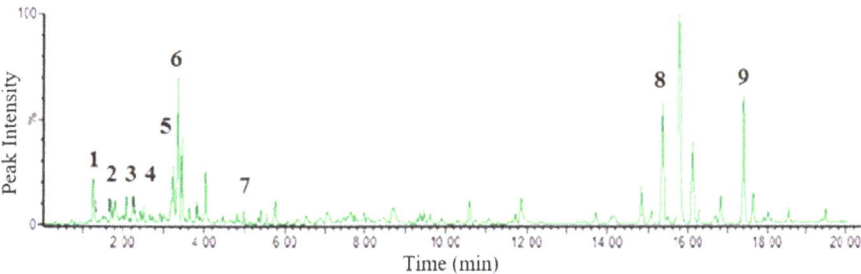

Figure 4. Chromatogram of *G. speciosa* MeOH (GSM) extract. Nine putative compounds were identified utilizing the UNIFI data analysis software and comparing the acquired MS spectra to library matching using the Traditional Chinese Medicine (TCM) library that is incorporated in the UNIFI analysis software. All of these compounds were previously isolated from other *Guettarda* species. The x-axis is the retention time in minutes, while the y-axis is the peak % signal intensity.

Table 2. LC-MS putative compounds from *G. speciosa* (GSM) extract.

RT	Exact Mass		Elemental Composition	Error (ppm)	Putative Identity	Biological Activity
	Calculated	Observed				
1.27	530.22644	530.22500	$C_{27}H_{34}N_2O_9$	−2.63	Strictosidine (1)	Antimicrobial [25]
2.26	358.12638	358.12690	$C_{16}H_{22}O_9$	1.45	Sweroside (2)	Cytotoxic [26]; Antigenotoxic [27]; Antiosteoporotic [28]; Anti-inflammatory [29]
2.35	390.15259	390.15900	$C_{17}H_{26}O_{10}$	2.35	Loganin (3)	Antigenotoxic [27]; Neuroprotective [30]; Cytotoxic [31]
2.42	414.38617	414.38650	$C_{29}H_{50}O$	0.72	β-Sitosterol (4)	Anti-inflammatory [32,33]; Antipyretic [33] Anthelminthic, Antimutagenic, Analgesic [34]
3.25	528.21100	528.21050	$C_{27}H_{32}N_2O_9$	−0.94	Sickingine (5)	
3.37	354.09509	354.09430	$C_{16}H_{18}O_9$	−2.25	5-Caffeoylquinic acid (6)	Antimicrobial [35] Anti-inflammatory [36]
4.93	488.35019	488.35210	$C_{30}H_{48}O_5$	3.88	Rotundic acid (7)	Antimicrobial [37,38]
15.37	516.45500	516.45460	$C_{25}H_{24}O_{12}$	−0.77	4,5-Dicaffeoylquinic acid (8)	Antipigmentation [39]
17.35	486.33453	486.33290	$C_{30}H_{46}O_5$	−3.28	Quinovic acid (9)	

RT—retention time in minutes.

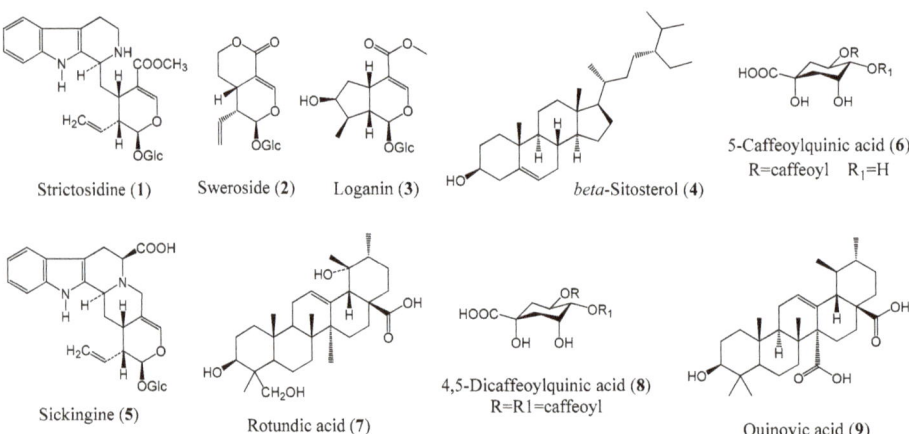

Figure 5. Structures of putatively identified compounds from *G. speciosa*.

3. Discussion.

In our continuous study using endemic Rubiaceae species indigenous to the Philippines, we described the potential therapeutic effects of *G. speciosa* extracts. The leaf extracts of *G. speciosa*, free from any trace of solvents, have been shown to inhibit *in vitro* the aggregation of $A\beta_{1-42}$, cyclooxygenase-1 enzyme, and cell growth of neuroblastoma SH-SY5Y cells. These biological activities may be ascribed to the compounds that were characterized using untargeted LC-MS. Natural products from plants continue to be the source of pharmacologically active compounds with diverse structures in the treatment or prevention of various diseases. In this experiment, these compounds were defined as indole alkaloids (1, 5), iridoids (2, 3), steroid (4), triterpenoids (7, 9), and polyhydroxy cyclic acids (6, 8). Pharmacological studies on *G. platypoda* have reported the synergistic action of quinic acid glycosides with β-sitosterol and triterpenes with anti-inflammatory activity, while the mechanism of β-sitosterol is comparable to hydrocortisone [32]. Most of the Rubiaceae species also contained iridoids and indole alkaloids [40], which are known to possess anti-inflammatory activities [41,42].

This study also described the inclination of the *G. speciosa* extracts to COX-1 inhibition as compared to the COX-2 enzyme. Both COX-1 and COX-2 perform a complex function in the mechanism of central nervous system (CNS) inflammation [43]. Most studies prefer a COX-2 inhibition, because COX-1 is involved in the cytoprotective function in the gastrointestinal system. Moreover, the suppression of COX-1 can result in side effects, including ulcers and bleeding [44]. Several studies have reconsidered the advantages of selective COX-1 inhibition. As stated, COX-1-dependent prostaglandin synthesis is implicated in pathological progressions, including atherosclerosis, cancer, endothelial dysfunction, neuroinflammation, preterm labor, and pain [43,45].

Alzheimer's disease (AD) is the most common cause of neurodegenerative dementia in elderly people, often associated with a progressive memory loss and other cognitive impairments [12]. Abnormal β-amyloid (Aβ) deposition, tau protein aggregation, a decreased level of acetylcholine, oxidative stress, and neuroinflammation of the nervous system are numerous causes associated with enhanced AD progression [46]. Although there is no cure for AD, currently, only five compounds (donezipil, tacrine, rivastigmine, galantamine, and memantine) are available and approved in the market to reduce the symptoms associated with AD [47]. The biological activity of the GSM extracts to inhibit the Aβ aggregation exhibits the potential of this medicinal plant as a new pharmacologically active material or therapeutic agent to minimize the effect of AD. To the best of our knowledge, this is the first report on the SH-SY5Y cytotoxicity, Aβ aggregation prevention, and COX-1 inhibition activities associated with *G. speciosa*.

4. Materials and Methods

4.1. Plant Materials

Fresh leaves of *G. speciosa* were collected from Bantayan Island, Cebu, Philippines (11°12′60.00″ N, 123°43′59.99″ E) in April 2017. The plant was collected and identified by Grecebio Jonathan Alejandro, a Philippine Rubiaceae specialist. A voucher specimen was kept at the University of Santo Tomas Herbarium (USTH 014369).

4.2. Extraction and Fractionation of Extracts

Air-dried, ground leaves of *G. speciosa* (1.7 kg) were placed in a percolator and extracted with MeOH. The ground leaves were allowed to soak overnight. The extract was drained, collected, and concentrated under reduced pressure using a rotary evaporator. A total of 15.0 L MeOH was used with the extraction process repeated thrice. The procedure obtained 207 g of the MeOH extract (GSM), and a portion (158 g) was suspended in distilled H_2O (300 mL) and partitioned exhaustively with hexane (2500 mL). The combined hexane layer was dried with anhydrous Na_2SO_4 and concentrated under reduced pressure to obtain the hexane extract (GSH, 23.2 g). The aqueous layer was partitioned exhaustively with $CHCl_3$ (2800 mL). The collected $CHCl_3$ layer was dried with anhydrous Na_2SO_4 and concentrated under reduced pressure to obtain the $CHCl_3$ extract (GSC, 10.7 g). The aqueous layer was freeze-dried using a lyophilizer (Thermo Fisher Scientific, Singapore) to obtain the aqueous extract (GSA, 18.7 g).

4.3. Animal Study

The experiment protocol (UST-IACUC code number RC2017-890915) was approved by the Institutional Animal Care and Use Committee (IACUC) at the Research Center for Natural and Applied Sciences (RCNAS), University of Santo Tomas (UST), and was further issued by the Philippine Bureau of Animal Industry and Animal Research Permit.

Six female Sprague-Dawley rats were used to assess the acute oral toxicity following the OECD 425 guidelines. The animals were housed in the UST-RCNAS Animal House and acclimatized to laboratory conditions for seven days before conducting the experiment. They were fed with standard rodent pellets and given access to clean drinking water. The laboratory conditions were maintained at a temperature of 25 ± 3 °C, humidity at 60 ± 4%, and a 12/12 h light/dark cycle.

4.4. Acute Oral Toxicity (OECD 425 Guidelines)

All animals were fasted for 24 h to determine their actual weight before receiving the crude extract. One rat served as a normal control group and was treated only with water as the vehicle medium. The animals were given 2000 mg/kg GSM via gastric gavage. The animals were observed periodically for 24 h for signs of toxicity; thereafter, they were observed daily for 14 days. The animals were then sacrificed by CO_2 inhalation. Gross necropsy, observation of gross pathological changes, and microscopic examination of all livers, kidneys, and stomachs of the test animals were performed by a licensed veterinarian.

4.5. COX-1 and COX-2 Assay

The cyclooxygenase assay was based on a previous protocol [15] as follows. The following were added to 150 µL of 100 mM Tris: 10 µL of 10 ppm plant extracts in DMSO, 10 µL of 1000 µM Hemin, and 10 µL of 250 U/mL COX-2 or COX-1 enzyme (Cayman Chemicals, Singapore). Indomethacin (Sigma Aldrich, St. Louis, MO, USA) was used as the positive control, and DMSO served as the negative control. The mixture was incubated at 25 °C for 15 min. After incubation, 10 µL of 200 µM amplex red was added to the mixture. Then, 10 µL of 2000 µM arachidonic acid (Sigma Aldrich, St. Louis, MO, USA) was added, and the reaction fluorescence absorbance was monitored for 2 min using Varioskan Flash (Thermo Scientific, Waltham, MA, USA) with excitation and emission wavelengths at 535 and 590 nm, respectively. The percent inhibition of the samples and the positive control were determined based on the averaged slope of each replicate using the following formula:

$$\% \text{ Inhibition} = [(\text{Slope uninhibited} - \text{Slope inhibited})/\text{Slope uninhibited}] * 100. \qquad (1)$$

"Slope uninhibited" is the slope of the line from the fluorescence intensity vs. time plot of the negative control group, and "slope inhibited" is the slope of the line from the fluorescence intensity vs. time plot of the samples/positive control. The method above was also done for the GSM and GSC extracts at different effective well concentrations (0.5, 1, 5, 10, 40, 70, and 100 µg/mL) to obtain the IC_{50} in µg/mL. Three trials consisting of three replicates per trial were done for each concentration of each sample.

4.6. Cell Viability Assay

The neuroblastoma cells (SH-SY5Y) were purchased from the American Type Culture Collection (ATCC, Manassas, VA, USA). SH-SY5Y cells were maintained in Dulbecco's modified eagle media (DMEM) supplemented with 10% fetal bovine serum (FBS), 1% kanamycin, and 1% penicillin. Cell cultures were maintained at 37 °C in 5% CO_2 and passaged once per week. The SH-SY5Y cells were subcultured into a 96-well plate at 2×10^5 cells/well and incubated for 24 h. After incubation, the cells were treated with plant extracts at different concentrations and incubated for another 72 h. The medium was removed, and the wells were washed with phosphate-buffered saline (PBS). Fresh medium (100 µL) was added and incubated for another 30 min. After incubation, CellTiter-Glo® luminescent reagent (100 µL; Promega, Madison, WI, USA) was added, and the luminescence was measured using a PerkinElmer Victor-3® multi-plate reader (PerkinElmer, Waltham, MA, USA) [48]. The 50% inhibitive concentrations of the plant extracts were calculated using a nonlinear regression curve fit (GraphPad Prism ver. 6, San Diego, CA, USA). The values representing cell viability were expressed as means ± standard deviation (SD) of three trial experiments.

4.7. Thioflavin T (ThT) Fluorescense Assay

Aβ$_{1-42}$ (Aggresure™)(10 μM, 30 μL) in PBS (pH 7.4) was incubated with (20 μL) or without the tested extracts at 37 °C for 24 h in a 384-well plate. Then, 20 μL ThT solution (50 μM) in glycine-NaOH buffer (pH 9) was added. The fluorescence signal was measured (excitation wavelength, 450 nm; emission wavelength, 510 nm) using a PerkinElmer Victor-3® multi-plate reader. The percentage of aggregation inhibition was calculated using the following equation: $[(1-I_{Fi}/I_{Fc}) * 100\%]$, where I_{Fi} and I_{Fc} are the fluorescence absorbance with and without the inhibitors, respectively, after subtracting the background fluorescence of the ThT solution [46].

4.8. Untargeted LC-MS Metabolite Profiling

Untargeted LC–MS/MS analysis of the GSM extract was performed using a Xevo G2-S Qtof (Waters Corp., Singapore). The separation was achieved using a BEH HSS T3 column (50 × 2.1 mm internal diameter). The system delivered a constant flow of 0.4 mL/min, and the mobile phase consisted of 5% CH$_3$CN and 0.1% HCOOH. The injection volume was 1 μL. For operation in MS/MS mode, a mass spectrometer with an electrospray interface (ESI) was used, and the parameters were set as follows: capillary voltage, 3.0 kV for negative mode; source temperature, 120 °C; desolvation temperature, 400 °C; cone gas flow, 100 L/h; and desolvation gas flow, 1000 L/h. Low collision energy at 6 V, high collision energy at 20–50 V, and lock mass solution at 1 ng/μL were used to calibrate mass accuracy. All LC–MS/MS data were processed by the MassLynx version 3.5 NT Quattro data acquisition software (Milford, MA, USA). For putative compound identification, accurate mass screening was carried out using the UNIFI data analysis software (San Mateo, CA, USA). The acquired MS spectra were subjected to library matching using the Traditional Chinese Medicine (TCM) library that is integrated within the UNIFI analysis software. Annotation of the candidate masses was based on the accurate mass match, isotopic ratio match, and precursor ion intensity counts. The criteria for a component ID to be considered a good match were as follows: a mass accuracy error ≤ 5 mDa or ≥ −5 mDa and a response precursor for precursor ion ≥2000.

4.9. Statistical Analysis

All values were reported as mean values with standard deviations (mean ± SD). Statistical significance of the data was analyzed by one-way ANOVA and Levene's test followed by Tukey's honestly significant difference (HSD) test (GraphPad Prism 5 software package, version 5.02, GraphPad Software Inc., San Diego, CA, USA), and $p < 0.05$ was considered statistically significant.

5. Conclusions

This study has demonstrated the first therapeutic potential of *G. speciosa* on neuroblastoma cytotoxicity, cyclooxygenase-1 inhibition, and the control of Aβ aggregation. The results of the untargeted LC-MS metabolite profiling also describe several compounds, which might be pharmacologically relevant. Hence, deeper understanding of the chemistry and pharmacological aspect of *G. speciosa* is warranted as this plant is being utilized in traditional folk medicine. It also presents its significance as a prospective biologically active material for further development of novel and safer plant-based agents and/or pharmacologically relevant natural products for anti-inflammatory or anti-neurodegenerative diseases.

Author Contributions: M.A.T. and S.S.A.A. conceptualized the research and wrote the manuscript; M.A.T. and M.W.D.L. performed the experiments; G.J.D.A. collected and authenticated the plants.

Funding: This research was funded by the National Research Foundation of Korea (NRF) Grants awarded by the Korean government (MEST, No. 2017R1A2B4012636). The Philippine DOST-NSC-SEI for the thesis grant was awarded to M.W.D.L.

Acknowledgments: The Pascual Pharma Corporation is gratefully acknowledged for the LC-MS analysis. We also thank Felicidad Christina Ramirez for the help on the statistical analyses.

Conflicts of Interest: The authors declare no conflicts of interest.

References

1. Alejandro, G.J.D. The Current Status of the Philippine Rubiaceae. *Phil. J. Syst. Biol.* **2007**, *1*, 47–60. [CrossRef]
2. Puff, C.; Chayamarit, K.; Chamchumroon, V. *Rubiaceae of Thailand: A Pictorial Guide to Indigenous and Cultivated Genera*; Forest Herbarium, National Park, Wildlife and Plant Conservation Department: Prachachon, Bangkok, 2005.
3. Capasso, A.; Balderrama, L.; Sivila, S.C.; De Tommasi, N.; Sorrentino, L.; Pizza, C. Phytochemical and pharmacological studies of *Guettarda acreana*. *Planta Med.* **1998**, *64*, 348–352. [CrossRef] [PubMed]
4. Gandhimathi, R.; Saravana, K.A.; Senthil Kumar, K.K.; Kusuma, P.K.; Uma, M.J. Pharmacological studies of anti-diarrhoeal activity of *Guettarda speciosa* (L.) in experimental animals. *J. Pharm. Sci. Res.* **2009**, *2*, 61–67.
5. Saravana Kumar, A.; Gandhimathi, R. Effect of *Guettarda speciosa* extracts on biogenic amines concentrations in rat brain after induction of seizure. *Int. J. Pharm. Pharm. Sci.* **2009**, *1*, 237–243.
6. Mohotti, S.; Rajendran, S.; Muhammad, T.; Strömstedt, A.; Adhikari, A.; Burman, R.; deSilva, E.; Göransson, U.; Hettiarachchi, C.; Gunasekera, S. Screening for bioactive metabolites in Sri Lankan medicinal plants by microfractionation and targeted isolation of antimicrobial flavonoids from *Derris scandens*. *J. Ethnopharm.* **2020**, *246*, 112158. [CrossRef]
7. Kaou, A.M.; Mahiou-Leddet, V.; Hutter, S.; Aïnouddine, S.; Hassani, S.; Yahaya, I.; Azas, N.; Ollivier, E. Antimalarial activity of crude extracts from nine African medicinal plants. *J. Ethnopharm.* **2008**, *116*, 74–83. [CrossRef]
8. Le, H.T.; Cho, Y.C.; Cho, S. Methanol extract of *Guettarda speciosa* Linn. inhibits the production of inflammatory mediators through the inactivation of Syk and JNK in macrophages. *Int. J. Mol. Med.* **2018**, *41*, 1783–1791. [CrossRef]
9. Cai, W.-H.; Matsunami, K.; Otsuka, H.; Shinzato, T.; Takeda, Y. A glycerol α-D-glucuronide and a megastigmane glycoside from the leaves of *Guettarda speciosa* L. *J. Nat. Med.* **2011**, *65*, 364–369. [CrossRef]
10. Inouye, H.; Takeda, Y.; Nishimura, H.; Kanomi, A.; Okuda, T.; Puff, C. Chemotaxonomic studies of Rubiaceous plants containing iridoid glycosides. *Phytochem.* **1988**, *27*, 2591–2598. [CrossRef]
11. Mongrand, S.; Badoc, A.; Patouille, B.; Lacomblez, C.; Chavent, M.; Bessoule, J. Chemotaxonomy of the Rubiaceae family based on leaf fatty acid composition. *Phytochem.* **2005**, *66*, 549–559. [CrossRef]
12. Bagyinszky, E.; Giau, V.V.; Shim, K.; Suk, K.; An, S.S.A.; Kim, S. Role of inflammatory molecules in the Alzheimer's disease progression and diagnosis. *J. Neurol. Sci.* **2017**, *376*, 242–254. [CrossRef] [PubMed]
13. Giau, V.V.; An, S.S.A. Epitope mapping immunoassay analysis of the interaction between β-amyloid and fibrinogen. *Int. J. Mol. Sci.* **2019**, *20*, 496. [CrossRef] [PubMed]
14. Olivar, J.E.; Sy, K.; Villanueva, C.; Alejandro, G.J.; Tan, M.A. Alkaloids as chemotaxonomic markers from the Philippine endemic *Uncaria perrottetii* and *Uncaria lanosa* f. *philippinensis*. *J. King Saud. Univ. Sci.* **2018**, *30*, 283–285. [CrossRef]
15. Tan, M.A.; Callanta, R.B.; Apurillo, C.C.; delaCruz, T.E.; Alejandro, G.J.; Ysrael, M.C. Anti-inflammatory and antimicrobial constituents from the leaves of *Villaria odorata*. *Acta. Manil.* **2014**, *62*, 47–52.
16. Wu, G.-J.; Chen, W.-F.; Hung, H.-C.; Jean, Y.-H.; Sung, C.-S.; Chakraborty, C.; Lee, H.-P.; Chen, N.-F.; Wen, Z.-H. Effects of propofol on proliferation and anti-apoptosis of neuroblastoma SH-SY5Y cell line: New insights into neuroprotection. *Brain Res.* **2011**, *1384*, 42–50. [CrossRef]
17. Chen, C.-Y. TCM database in Taiwan: The world's largest traditional Chinese medicine database for drug screening *in silico*. *Plos ONE* **2011**, *6*, 15939. [CrossRef]
18. He, M.; Grkovic, T.; Evans, J.R.; Thornburg, C.C.; Akee, R.K.; Thompson, J.R.; Whitt, J.A.; Harris, M.J.; Loyal, J.A.; Britt, J.R.; et al. The NCI library of traditional Chinese medicinal plant extracts- Preliminary assessment of the NCI-60 activity and chemical profiling of selected species. *Fitoterapia* **2019**, *137*, 104285. [CrossRef]
19. Aquino, R.; De Simone, F.; Senatore, F.; Pizza, C. Iridoids and secoiridoids from *Guettarda platypoda*. *Pharm. Res.Commun.* **1988**, *20*, 105–108. [CrossRef]

20. De Oliveira, P.R.; Testa, G.; Medina, R.P.; De Oliveira, C.M.; Kato, L.; Da Silva, C.C.; Santin, S.M. Cytotoxic activity of *Guettarda pohliana* Müll. Arg. (Rubiaceae). *Nat. Prod. Res.* **2013**, *27*, 1677–1681. [CrossRef]
21. Sousa, M.P.; Matos, M.E.; Machado, M.I.; Filho, R.B.; Vencato, I.; Mascarenhas, Y.P. Triterpenoids from *Guettarda angelica*. *Phytochem.* **1984**, *23*, 2589–2592. [CrossRef]
22. Bhattacharyya, J.; De Almeida, M. Isolation of the constituents of the root-bark of *Guettarda platypoda*. *J. Nat. Prod.* **1985**, *48*, 148–149. [CrossRef]
23. Matos, M.E.; Sousa, M.P.; Machado, M.L.; Filho, R.B. Quinovic acid glycosides from *Guettarda angelica*. *Phytochem.* **1986**, *25*, 1419–1422. [CrossRef]
24. Ferrari, F.; Messana, I.; Botta, B. Constituents of *Guettarda platypoda*. *J. Nat. Prod.* **1986**, *49*, 1150–1151. [CrossRef]
25. Luijendijk, T.J.; van der Meijden, E.; Verpoorte, R. Involvement of strictosidine as a defensive chemical in *Catharanthus roseus*. *J. Chem. Ecol.* **1996**, *22*, 1355–1366. [CrossRef] [PubMed]
26. Han, X.-L.; Li, J.-D.; Yang, C.; Li, Z.-Y. Sweroside eradicated leukemia cells and attenuated pathogenic processes in mice by inducing apoptosis. *Biomed. Pharm.* **2017**, *95*, 477–486. [CrossRef] [PubMed]
27. Deng, S.; West, B.J.; Jarakae Jensen, C. UPLC-TOF-MS characterization and identification of bioactive iridoids in *Cornus mas* fruit. *J. Anal. Methods Chem* **2013**. [CrossRef]
28. Sun, H.; Li, L.; Zhang, A.; Zhang, N.; Lu, H.; Sun, W.; Wang, X. Protective effects of sweroside on human MG-63 cells and rat osteoblast. *Fitoterapia* **2013**, *84*, 174–179. [CrossRef]
29. Wang, R.; Dong, Z.; Lan, X.; Liao, Z.; Chen, M. Sweroside alleviated LPS-induced inflammation via SIRT1 mediating NF-κB and FOXO1 signaling pathways in RAW 264.7 cells. *Molecules* **2019**, *24*, 872. [CrossRef]
30. Xu, Y.-D.; Sun, M.-F.; Zhu, Y.-L.; Chu, M.; Shi, Y.-W.; Lin, S.-L.; Yang, X.-S.; Shen, Y.-Q. Neuroprotective effects of loganin on MPTP-induced Parkinson's disease mice: Neurochemistry, Glial reaction and autophagy studies. *J. Cell Biochem.* **2017**, *118*, 3495–3510. [CrossRef]
31. Khan, M.; Garg, A.; Srivastava, S.K.; Darokar, M.P. Acytotoxic agent from *Strychnosnux-vomica* and biological evaluation of its modified analogues. *Med. Chem. Res.* **2012**, *21*, 2975–2980. [CrossRef]
32. Pina, E.M.; Araujo, F.W.; Souza, I.A.; Bastos, I.V.; Silva, T.G.; Nascimento, S.C.; Militao, G.C.; Soares, L.A.; Xavier, H.S.; Melo, S.J. Pharmacological screening and acute toxicity of bark roots of *Guettarda platypoda*. *Rev. Bras. Farm.* **2012**, *22*, 1315–1322. [CrossRef]
33. Gupta, M.B.; Nath, R.; Srivastava, N.; Shanker, K.; Kishor, K.; Bhargava, K.P. Anti-inflammatory and antipyretic activities of β-sitosterol. *Planta Med.* **1980**, *39*, 157–163. [CrossRef] [PubMed]
34. Villasenor, I.M.; Angelada, J.; Canlas, A.P.; Echegoyen, D. Bioactivity studies on β-sitosterol and its glucoside. *Phytother. Res.* **2002**, *16*, 417–421. [CrossRef] [PubMed]
35. Bajko, E.; Kalinowska, M.; Borowski, P.; Siergiejczyk, L.; Lewandowski, W. 5-O-Caffeoylquinicacid: A spectroscopic study and biological screening for antimicrobial activity. *LWT Food Sci. Technol.* **2016**, *65*, 471–479. [CrossRef]
36. Toyama, D.O.; Ferreira, M.; Romoff, P.; Favero, O.A.; Gaeta, H.H.; Toyama, M.H. Effect of chlorogenic acid (5-caffeoylquinic acid) isolated from *Baccharis oxyodonta* on the structure and pharmacological activities of secretory phospholipase A2 from *Crotalus durissus terrificus*. *Biomed. Res. Int.* **2014**, *2014*. [CrossRef] [PubMed]
37. Haraguchi, H.; Kataoka, S.; Okamoto, S.; Hanafi, M.; Shibata, K. Antimicrobial triterpenes from *Ilex integra* and the mechanism of antifungal action. *Phytother. Res.* **1999**, *13*, 151–156. [CrossRef]
38. Nguyen, H.T.; Ho, D.V.; Vo, H.Q.; Le, A.T.; Nguyen, H.M.; Kodama, T.; Ito, T.; Morita, H.; Raal, A. Antibacterial activities of chemical constituents from the aerial parts of *Hedyoti spilulifera*. *Pharm. Biol.* **2017**, *55*, 787–791. [CrossRef]
39. Tabassum, N.; Lee, J.H.; Yim, S.H.; Batkhuu, G.J.; Jung, D.W.; Williams, D.R. Isolation of 4,5-O-dicaffeoylquinic acid as a pigmentation inhibitor occurring in *Artemisi acapillaris* Thunberg and its validation *in vivo*. *Evid. Based Complement. Altern. Med.* **2016**, *2016*. [CrossRef]
40. Martins, D.; Nunez, C.V. Secondary metabolites from Rubiaceae species. *Molecules* **2015**, *20*, 13422–13495. [CrossRef]
41. Chadha, N.; Silakari, O. Indoles as therapeutics of interest in medicinal chemistry: Bird's eye view. *Eur. J. Med. Chem.* **2017**, *134*, 159–184. [CrossRef]
42. Viljoen, A.; Mncwangi, N.; Vermaak, I. Anti-inflammatory iridoids of botanical origin. *Curr. Med. Chem.* **2012**, *19*, 2104–2127. [CrossRef] [PubMed]

43. Perrone, M.G.; Scilimati, A.; Simone, L.; Vitale, P. Selective COX-1 inhibition: A therapeutic target to be reconsidered. *Curr. Med. Chem.* **2010**, *17*, 3769–3805. [CrossRef] [PubMed]
44. Bjarnason, I.; Scarpignato, C.; Holmgren, E.; Olszewski, M.; Rainsford, K.D.; Lanas, A. Mechanism of damage to the gastrointestinal tract from nonsteroidal anti-inflammatory drugs. *Gastroenterology* **2018**, *154*, 500–514. [CrossRef] [PubMed]
45. Hošek, J.; Leláková, V.; Bobál, P.; Pížová, H.; Gazdová, M.; Malaník, M.; Jakubczyk, K.; Vesely, O.; Landa, P.; Temml, V.; et al. Prenylated stilbenoids affect inflammation by inhibiting the NF-κB/AP-1 signaling pathway and cyclooxygenases and lipoxygenase. *J. Nat. Prod.* **2019**, *82*, 1839–1848. [CrossRef]
46. Xia, C.-L.; Tang, G.-H.; Guo, Y.-Q.; Xu, Y.-K.; Huang, Z.-S.; Yin, S. Mulberry Diels-Alder-type adducts from *Morus alba* as multi-targeted agents for Alzheimer's disease. *Phytochem.* **2019**, *157*, 82–91. [CrossRef]
47. Alghazwi, M.; Smid, S.; Musgrave, I.; Zhang, W. *In vitro* studies of the neuroprotective activities of astaxanthin and fucoxanthin against amyloid beta (Aβ$_{1-42}$) toxicity and aggregation. *Neurochem. Int.* **2019**, *124*, 215–224. [CrossRef]
48. Tran, A.V.; Shim, K.H.; Vo Thi, T.T.; Kook, J.K.; An, S.S.A.; Lee, S.W. Targetted and controlled drug delivery by multifunctional mesoporous silica nanoparticles with internal fluorescent conjugates and external polydopamine and graphene oxide layers. *Acta. Biomater.* **2018**, *74*, 397–413. [CrossRef]

Sample Availability: Samples of the plant extracts are available from the authors.

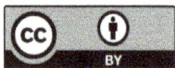

© 2019 by the authors. Licensee MDPI, Basel, Switzerland. This article is an open access article distributed under the terms and conditions of the Creative Commons Attribution (CC BY) license (http://creativecommons.org/licenses/by/4.0/).

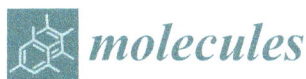

Article

Mulberry Fruit Cultivar 'Chiang Mai' Prevents Beta-Amyloid Toxicity in PC12 Neuronal Cells and in a *Drosophila* Model of Alzheimer's Disease

Uthaiwan Suttisansanee [1], Somsri Charoenkiatkul [1], Butsara Jongruaysup [2], Somying Tabtimsri [3], Dalad Siriwan [4,*,†] and Piya Temviriyanukul [1,*,†]

1. Institute of Nutrition, Mahidol University, Salaya, Phuttamonthon, Nakhon Pathom 73170, Thailand; uthaiwan.sut@mahidol.ac.th (U.S.); somsri.chr@mahidol.ac.th (S.C.)
2. Office of Sericulture Conservation and Standard Conformity Assessment, The Queen Sirikit Department of Sericulture, Ministry of Agriculture and Cooperatives, Bangkok 10900, Thailand; butsara_2000@hotmail.com
3. The Queen Sirikit Department of Sericulture Center (Kanchanaburi), Nong Ya, Mueang Kanchanaburi District, Kanchanaburi 71000, Thailand; yodyingtts@gmail.com
4. Institute of Food Research and Product Development, Kasetsart University, Chatuchak, Bangkok 10900, Thailand
* Correspondence: dalad.s@ku.th (D.S.); piya.tem@mahidol.ac.th (P.T.)
† These authors contributed equally to this work.

Received: 25 March 2020; Accepted: 14 April 2020; Published: 15 April 2020

Abstract: Alzheimer's disease (AD) is the most common form of dementia, characterized by chronic neuron loss and cognitive problems. Aggregated amyloid beta (Aβ) peptides, a product of cleaved amyloid precursor protein (APP) by beta-secretase 1 (BACE-1), have been indicated for the progressive pathogenesis of AD. Currently, screening for anti-AD compounds in foodstuffs is increasing, with promising results. Hence, the purpose of this study was to investigate the extraction conditions, phytochemical contents, and anti-AD properties, targeting Aβ peptides of *Morus* cf. *nigra* 'Chiang Mai' (MNCM) both in vitro and in vivo. Data showed that the aqueous extract of MNCM contained high amounts of cyanidin, keracyanin, and kuromanin as anthocyanidin and anthocyanins. The extract also strongly inhibited cholinesterases and BACE-1 in vitro. Moreover, MNCM extract prevented Aβ-induced neurotoxicity and promoted neurite outgrowth in neuronal cells. Interestingly, MNCM extract reduced Aβ$_{1-42}$ peptides and improved locomotory coordination of *Drosophila* co-expressing human APP and BACE-1, specifically in the brain. These findings suggest that MNCM may be useful as an AD preventive agent by targeting Aβ formation.

Keywords: *Morus* species; Alzheimer's disease; anthocyanins; anthocyanidins; amyloid peptides; beta-secretase 1; *Drosophila melanogaster*

1. Introduction

Alzheimer's disease (AD) is the most common form of dementia and a public health concern worldwide. AD is the fifth leading cause of death among people over 65 years old [1] and growth of AD prevalence is expected. In the USA, the care cost for dementia patients has been estimated at $290 billion, rendering a huge economic problem for society [2]. AD is a chronic neurodegenerative disorder that is characterized by the loss of cholinergic neurons, low levels of acetylcholine, and aggregation of neurotoxic amyloid beta plaque. Loss of cholinergic neurons located in the basal forebrain leads to reduced production of the neurotransmitter, acetylcholine, which is involved in memory and cognitive functions. Hence, inhibition of acetylcholine-degrading enzymes, cholinesterases (acetylcholinesterase (AChE) and butyrylcholinesterase (BChE)), may improve attention span and cognitive ability [3]. The accumulation of amyloid beta or beta amyloid (Aβ) peptides results from the cleavage of transmembrane amyloid precursor protein (APP) by β-site amyloid precursor protein cleaving enzyme 1 or beta-secretase 1 (BACE-1) as one of the AD hallmarks [4]. The Aβ peptides, either as $Aβ_{1-40}$ or $Aβ_{1-42}$, are secreted and aggregated as a dense senile plaque due to their hydrophobic properties. However, familial AD patients usually exhibit a higher ratio of $Aβ_{1-42}$ in the brain, indicating that $Aβ_{1-42}$ may be used as a marker for AD pathogenesis [5]. Therefore, besides cholinesterase inhibitors, BACE-1 inhibitors could be a target of interest for AD prevention.

Several epidemiological reports have documented that the consumption of fruits and vegetables may prevent or delay the onset of degenerative diseases, including AD and dementia [6,7]. Anthocyanins are flavonoids and occur in fruits and vegetables, mostly in berries. It has been shown that anthocyanins prevent streptozotocin-induced sporadic dementia of Alzheimer's type by decreasing AChE activity in both the cerebral cortex and hippocampus of rats [8]. Furthermore, anthocyanins, including cyanidin-3-glucoside, delphinidin-3-glucoside, and petunidin-3-glucoside, suppressed BACE-1 expression in the hippocampal neurons of $Aβ_{1-42}$-treated rats [9]. These data support the postulation that anthocyanin-rich foodstuffs may exert anti-AD properties and promote AD prevention and treatment.

The mulberry tree belongs to the family Moraceae. Three important mulberries are widely grown as *Morus alba*, *Morus rubra*, and *Morus nigra* [10]. Interestingly, *M. nigra* has been reported to have the highest amounts of anthocyanins compared to other species [10,11]. *M. nigra* is generally known as black mulberry. This plant is cultivated in Africa, South America, and Asian countries, including Thailand. Almost all parts of *M. nigra* are utilized for both food and pharmacological properties. Its leaves have been demonstrated to have antinociceptive, anti-inflammatory, and antidiabetic properties [12], while the fruits have historically been used as food because they are rich in nutrition elements, flavonols, and anthocyanins [11,13]. The fruits are also used in traditional medicine as they exert a wide range of health benefits, such as antimicrobial, anti-inflammatory, and antioxidative stress properties [12,14]. Evidence showed that compounds isolated from *M. alba* as artoindonesianin O and inethermulberrofuran C exhibited anti-AD properties [15,16]; however, little is known about the anthocyanin-rich *M. nigra*. Therefore, here, the anti-AD properties of *M. nigra* were investigated. A well-characterized *Morus* cf. *nigra* 'Chiang Mai' (MNCM) that is widely planted in Thailand was used in this study. The mulberry fruits of the mentioned cultivar were determined for their extraction conditions, phytochemical contents, antioxidative stress, and inhibitory activity against AChE, BChE, and BACE-1 in vitro. The extract was also determined for its anti-AD properties, targeting Aβ peptides in the adrenal phaeochromocytoma (PC12) neuronal cells and in a *Drosophila* model of AD. These flies were developed for studying potential therapeutic approaches since human APP and BACE-1 are co-expressed specifically in the central nervous system (CNS), representing the production of Aβ peptides in humans.

2. Results

2.1. Extraction Optimization of Morus cf. nigra 'Chiang Mai' (MNCM)

To optimize the extraction conditions regarding anti-AD properties of MNCM, aqueous ethanol was utilized as a solvent for anthocyanins extraction. First, the sample (30 mg/mL) was extracted with 0–100% (*v/v*) aqueous ethanol at 30°C for 30 min. The results suggested that acetylcholinesterase (AChE) inhibition was optimally achieved when extraction was performed under 0% (*v/v*) ethanol (or ultrapure water) (Table 1). Inhibition decreased with an increasing percentage of ethanol to 20% (*v/v*), and then completely diminished.

Table 1. Effects of different percentages of aqueous ethanol on MNCM extraction regarding AChE inhibition.

Independent Variable (Solvents, % (v/v) Aqueous Ethanol)	Dependent Variable % AChE Inhibition	Controlled Variables
0% (v/v) (ultrapure water)	40.29 ± 1.27 [a]	
20% (v/v)	27.07 ± 1.36 [b]	
40% (v/v)	ND *	• Extraction temperature 30 °C
60% (v/v)	ND *	• Shaking time 30 min
80% (v/v)	ND *	• Extraction concentration 30 mg/mL
100% (v/v) (absolute ethanol)	ND *	

Values expressed are mean ± standard deviation (SD) of triplicate experiments (n = 3). Lower letter case indicates significant differences in each column at $p < 0.05$ calculated by one-way analysis of variance (ANOVA) and Duncan's multiple comparison test. * ND = not detected.

The effects of shaking time on AChE inhibition were then investigated by utilizing water extraction of MNCM. The shaking time varied from 0.5 to 6 h and was applied with fixed conditions of a 30 °C extraction temperature and 30 mg/mL extraction concentration. The results suggested that AChE inhibition was continuously elevated with an increased shaking time and achieved the significantly highest inhibition at the 2-h shaking time (Table 2). However, AChE inhibition started to decline after reaching this optimal shaking time.

Table 2. Effects of different shaking times on MNCM extraction regarding AChE inhibition.

Independent Variable (Shaking Time, h)	Dependent Variable % AChE Inhibition	Controlled Variables
0.5	27.63 ± 0.42 [c]	
1	33.63 ± 0.97 [b]	• Extraction temperature 30 °C
2	43.35 ± 3.32 [a]	• Extraction solvent of water
4	30.18 ± 1.15 [c]	• Extraction concentration 30 mg/mL
6	28.41 ± 0.58 [c]	

Values expressed are mean ± standard deviation (SD) of triplicate experiments (n = 3). Lower letter case indicates significant differences in each column at $p < 0.05$ calculated by one-way analysis of variance (ANOVA) and Duncan's multiple comparison test.

The last parameter for MNCM extraction was the extraction temperature. The effect of temperature (30–90 °C) on AChE inhibition using water extraction conditions of a 2-h shaking time and 30 mg/mL extraction concentration was investigated. The results indicated that AChE inhibition increased with increasing extraction temperature and reached optimal inhibition at 50 °C (Table 3). However, when raising the extraction temperature above 50 °C, AChE inhibition declined to the lowest inhibition at 90 °C.

Table 3. Effect of different temperatures on MNCM extraction regarding AChE inhibition.

Independent Variable (Temperature, °C)	Dependent Variable % AChE Inhibition	Controlled Variables
30	27.89 ± 1.36 [b]	
50	32.20 ± 2.67 [a]	• Extraction solvent of water
70	23.66 ± 2.16 [c]	• Shaking time of 2 h
90	11.29 ± 0.18 [d]	• Extraction concentration 30 mg/mL

Values expressed are mean ± standard deviation (SD) of triplicate experiments (n = 3). Lower letter case indicates significant differences in each column at $p < 0.05$ calculated by one-way analysis of variance (ANOVA) and Duncan's multiple comparison test.

Thus, the optimized extraction conditions of MNCM to achieve the highest AChE inhibition were aqueous-based extraction (ultrapure water) using a 50 °C extraction temperature and 2-h shaking time.

2.2. Antioxidant Activities of MNCM Extract

Antioxidant activities were determined using MNCM extracted under optimized extraction conditions as mentioned above. Antioxidant activities determined by the 2,2-diphenyl-1-picrylhydrazyl (DPPH) radical scavenging assay suggested that MNCM extract exhibited scavenging activity of 0.40 ± 0.03 µmol TE/100 g DW, while the chelating ability of ferrous ion was 21.33 ± 0.35 µmol TE/g DW as investigated by the ferric ion reducing antioxidant power (FRAP) assay. The antioxidant capacity measured by the oxygen radical absorbance capacity (ORAC) assay was determined at 132.21 ± 8.88 µmol TE/g DW.

2.3. Phytochemical Analysis

It was found that MNCM extracted under optimized extraction conditions exhibited total phenolic contents (TPCs) of 6.93 ± 0.58 mg GAE/g DW. The only anthocyanin detected in MNCM extracted under acidic methanol was cyanidin, with a content of 233.77 ± 24.02 µg/g DW, while anthocyanins were detected as cyanidin-3-O-rutinoside or keracyanin (610.99 ± 9.17 µg/g DW) and cyanidin-3-O-glucoside or kuromanin (730.97 ± 3.61 µg/g DW) utilizing high performance liquid chromatography (HPLC) analysis (Figure S1).

2.4. MNCM Extract Inhibits Cholinesterase and BACE-1 Activities in Vitro

The MNCM extracted under optimized extraction conditions inhibited the key enzymes involved in AD, including AChE, BChE, and BACE-1, at different percentages. The AChE inhibitory activity of MNCM extract with 55.36 ± 4.02% inhibition was lower than BChE inhibition with 81.43 ± 4.56% inhibition at the final extract concentration of 5 mg/mL. Under the same extract concentration, BACE-1 inhibition was reported at 66.34 ± 5.32%.

2.5. MNCM Extract Prevents Aβ Peptide-Induced Toxicity and Promotes Neurite Outgrowth

To investigate the neuroprotective effect of MNCM extract on PC12 neuronal cells, the cytotoxicity of MNCM extract was studied. PC12 cells were exposed with various concentrations of MNCM extract (50–200 µg/mL) for 24, 48, and 72 h. Results from the resazurin assay (Figure 1A) displayed that all concentrations of MNCM aqueous extract were not toxic to PC12 cells even after 72 h of treatment. We then selected these four concentrations for further analysis.

As mentioned above, MNCM is rich in anthocyanins and anthocyanidins, resulting in antioxidant activities. In addition, free radicals are also involved in the pathogenesis of AD [17]. Therefore, the protective effects of MNCM extract against H_2O_2, an oxidative stress inducer, were determined. Pre-treatment of PC12 cells with MNCM extracts (50–200 µg/mL) for 24 h significantly protected cells from oxidative stress-induced cell death in a dose-dependent manner compared with non-pretreated cells, as seen in Figure 1B, confirming the antioxidant activities in vitro.

It is well established that Aβ peptide-induced neuronal toxicity occurs via oxidative stress induction [18]. As illustrated in Figure 1C, PC12 cells were pre-treated with MNCM extract for 24 h before adding Aβ_{25-35} peptides. The Aβ_{25-35} peptides are widely used in AD study. Moreover, they have short fragments but retain active domains of Aβ_{1-42}. In addition, the Aβ_{25-35} and Aβ_{1-42} peptides induce neural toxicity in a similar fashion [19]. Figure 1C shows that non-pretreated cells gave approximately 40% cell viability after exposure to Aβ_{25-35} peptides, whereas MNCM extract prevented Aβ peptide-induced toxicity in a dose-dependent manner, similar to Figure 1B. It seemed likely that the 200 µg/mL extract could diminish all adverse effects of Aβ peptides compared with the DI treatment.

Neurite outgrowth is a vital mechanism in neuronal growth and differentiation, and defects in the process might lead to neurodegenerative disorders like AD [20]. Therefore, we determined the effects of MNCM extract on neurite outgrowth. The results in Figure 1D and Figure S2 show that cells without nerve growth factor (NGF) or MNCM extract contained a lower percentage of neurite-bearing cells, whereas nerve growth factor (NGF) stimulated neurite outgrowth as previously reported. A dose-dependent manner of MNCM extract in stimulating neurite outgrowth was observed. Intriguingly, a high dose of MNCM extract at 200 µg/mL activated neurite outgrowth similar to the NGF-treated cells.

In conclusion, aqueous extract of MNCM was not toxic to PC12 cells, prevented H_2O_2 or Aβ peptide-induced cell death, and promoted neurite outgrowth.

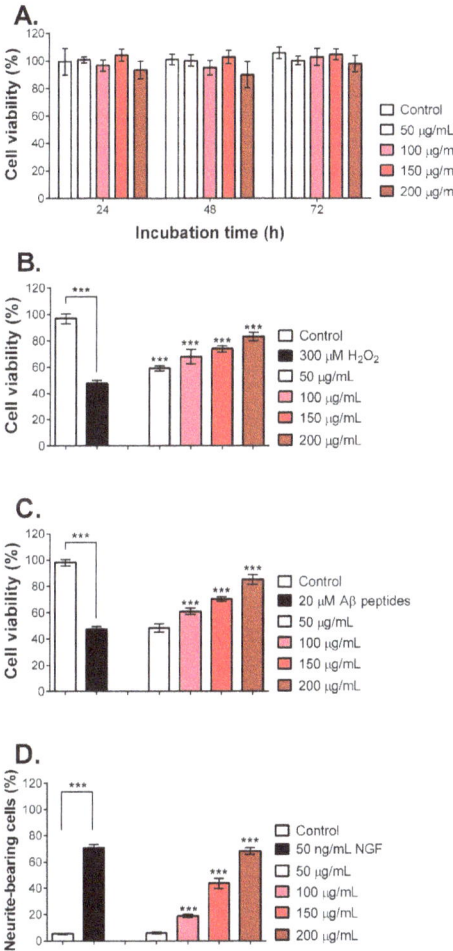

Figure 1. (**A**) Determination of safe doses of MNCM extract on the cell viability of PC12 cells after 24, 48, and 72 h of MNCM extract treatment, the percentage of cell viability is displayed. (**B**) Preventive effects of MNCM extract on H_2O_2-induced cell death, cells were pre-treated with the extract (50–200 µg/mL) for 24 h, then 300 µM of H_2O_2 was added for another 24 h. The percentage of cell viability is illustrated. (**C**) Preventive effects of MNCM aqueous extract on Aβ peptide-induced cell death, cells were pre-treated with MNCM extract (50–200 µg/mL) for 24 h, then 20 µM of Aβ peptides were added for another 24 h. The percentage of cell viability is illustrated. (**D**) Effects of MNCM extract (50–200 µg/mL) on neurite outgrowth compared with the nerve growth factor (NGF, 50 ng/mL). The data are represented as the percentage of neurite-bearing cells. The bar graphs are representative of three experiments and show mean ± standard deviation (SD). The one-way ANOVA followed by Tukey's test was used to determine the differences between groups. ***, $p < 0.001$.

2.6. MNCM Extract Reduces Aβ$_{1-42}$ by Inhibiting BACE-1 Activity in a Drosophila Model of AD

To further investigate the anti-AD properties of MNCM extract in vivo, we employed a *Drosophila* model to our advantage by co-expressing human APP and BACE-1 specifically in the CNS of fly brains, thereby representing the amyloidogenic pathway. These short memory-deficient AD flies proved to be a useful tool to delineate the preventive effects of food or phytochemicals on the Aβ pathway [21]. First, we investigated safe doses of MNCM extract in *Drosophila* larvae. Larvae were exposed to MNCM extracts (0–1 mg/mL), and then the hatched flies were scored. As seen in Figure 2A, compared to the DI treatment, MNCM extracts up to 500 μg/mL were not toxic, whereas toxicity was observed at 1 mg/mL of MNCM extract. Thus, MNCM extracts at 150, 250, and 500 μg/mL were selected and used for further analysis.

It is known that the cleavage of APP by BACE-1 results in Aβ peptides as AD hallmarks. Hence, the flies were treated with MNCM extract at the indicated concentration from one day after eclosion, and donepezil, an AD drug, was used as the control. After 28 days, heads were collected, and the levels of Aβ$_{1-42}$ peptides were quantified. The data showed that donepezil and 500 μg/mL of MNCM extract reduced Aβ$_{1-42}$ peptide formation by approximately 2 fold compared with DI-treated flies (Figure 2B). A lesser reduction was also observed at 250 μg/mL of MNCM extract, while MNCM extract at 150 μg/mL was not potent enough to reduce Aβ$_{1-42}$ formation, consistent with the cell study.

AD leads to a progressive decline in locomotory coordination. This ability can be measured by the climbing assay in *Drosophila*. Therefore, we tested whether MNCM extract ameliorated Aβ$_{1-42}$-induced motor dysfunction in the AD flies. Using the same treatment as above, at day 28, flies were recorded for their climbing index. As shown in Figure 2C, the DI-treated flies representing AD exhibited an extremely reduced ability to climb compared to the AD-free flies (elav-GAL4), suggesting severe locomotory coordination possibly from high amounts of Aβ$_{1-42}$ peptides (Figure 2B). Interestingly, the climbing index was rescued in a dose-dependent manner when flies were exposed to MNCM extracts at 250 and 500 μg/mL and donepezil.

To test whether MNCM extract acts as a BACE-1 inhibitor and leads to a reduction in Aβ$_{1-42}$ peptides, fly brain lysates at day 28 of treatment were prepared and determined for BACE-1 activity. It was found that MNCM extract at 150 μg/mL and the DI control had the same BACE-1 activity (Figure 2D). However, flies treated with donepezil, and 250 and 500 μg/mL MNCM extract showed significantly decreased BACE-1 activity in AD fly brains. Donepezil is claimed to be a cholinesterase inhibitor, and its BACE-1 inhibitory activity has been documented [22].

In summary, aqueous extract of MNCM reduced Aβ$_{1-42}$ formation and improved locomotor dysfunctions by inhibiting BACE-1 activity in the *Drosophila* model of AD.

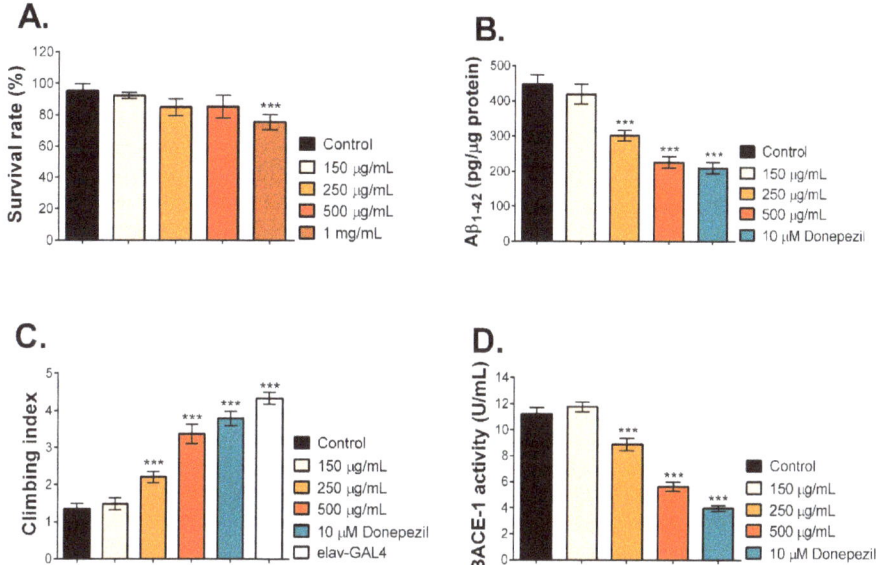

Figure 2. (**A**) Determination of safe doses of MNCM extract in fly larvae, the third-instar larvae were fed with MNCM extract (150 µg/mL–1 mg/mL). The surviving flies were counted within 5 days after the first eclosion and the percentage of the survival rate was calculated. (**B**) Effects of MNCM extract on the accumulation of Aβ_{1-42} peptides in fly brains. Flies were treated with MNCM extract (150–500 µg/mL) for 28 days, and after that fly heads were lysed and subjected for ELISA. (**C**) Effects of MNCM extract (150–500 µg/mL) on the locomotory coordination (climbing) of AD flies after 28 days of treatment. (**D**) Effects of MNCM extract on the BACE-1 activity in fly brains. Flies were treated with MNCM extract (150–500 µg/mL) for 28 days, then fly heads were lysed and subjected for BACE-1 activity determination. The data are representative of three replicates and show mean ± standard deviation (SD). The one-way ANOVA followed by Tukey's test was used to determine the differences between groups. ***, $p < 0.001$.

3. Discussion

AD is a complex and progressive neurodegenerative disorder and an effective therapy is lacking. Therefore, the identification of novel AD therapeutic agents is urgently required. It is well-documented that oxidative stress and the expression of cholinesterases and BACE-1 play a vital role in AD initiation and progression [3,4,17]; thus, an ideal AD therapeutic agent should function against different AD pathogenic mechanisms [23]. Plants and their bioactive constituents are of great interest due to their safety and efficacy. Indeed, many plant-derived compounds, including phenolic acids and flavonoids, have been reported for their anti-AD properties toward oxidative stress, AChE, BChE, and BACE-1 activities [23,24].

Mulberry has been recognized to be rich in anthocyanins as members of the flavonoids, and especially for *M. nigra*. Therefore, this project aimed to study the anti-AD properties of aqueous extracts of *M.* cf. *nigra* 'Chiang Mai' fruit (MNCM), which is widely grown in Thailand. The major findings were (i) MNCM extract was rich in anthocyanins and anthocyanidins, especially cyanidin, kuromanin, and keracyanin, which are probably involved in antioxidative stress; (ii) MNCM extract exhibited up to 50% inhibitory activity against AChE, BChE, and BACE-1; (iii) MNCM extract protected neuronal cells from H_2O_2 or Aβ peptide-induced toxicity and promoted neurite outgrowth; and (iv) MNCM extract reduced Aβ_{1-42} peptides by inhibiting BACE-1 activity in a *Drosophila* model of AD.

Previous reports suggested that mulberry exhibited different degrees of phenolics and antioxidant activities depending on both internal factors (such as cultivars and stages of maturity) and external factors (such as detection methods and extraction conditions) [25,26]. Comparing water-extracted MNCM with the TPCs of 6.39 mg GAE/g DW, five cultivars of Korean mulberries (*M. alba*) extracted under 70% (*v/v*) aqueous ethanol exhibited lower TPCs, ranging from 2.2 to 2.6 mg GAE/g DW [25]. Besides, water-extracted MNCM also exhibited higher TPCs than methanolic-extracted *M. alba* collected in North Serbia, with the TPCs ranging from 1.05 to 2.16 mg GAE/g DW [27]. As for antioxidant activities, these values seemed to be greatly affected by both internal and external factors. In comparison to MNCM with ORAC activity of 132.21 ± 8.88 µmol TE/g DW, it was previously suggested that juices from different maturity stages of thornless blackberry exhibited ORAC activities ranging from 86.8–204.1 µmol TE/g DW, while those from red raspberry ranged of 40.8–114.9 µmol TE/g DW [28]. In the same study, juices from various cultivars of ripe strawberry exhibited ORAC activities of 120.8–172.3 µmol TE/g DW. The FRAP activity of MNCM (21.33 ± 0.35 µmol TE/g DW) was comparable to raspberry (28.11 µmol TE/g DW) and cranberry (22.41 µmol TE/g DW) extracted under a mixture of 70% (*v/v*) aqueous methanol (MeOH) and 70% (*v/v*) aqueous acetone (1:1, *v/v*) [29]. Interestingly, the FRAP activity of MNCM was higher than blackcurrant and blueberry (17.81 and 17.27 µmol TE/g DW, respectively) but lower than those of blackberry and black chokeberry (11.63 and 33.16 µmol TE/g DW, respectively) [29]. However, the DPPH radical scavenging activity (0.40 ± 0.03 µmol TE/100 g DW or approximately 0.44 µmol TE/100 g fresh weight with 90% moisture content) of MNCM was lower than blackberries, black mulberries (*M. nigra*), bilberries, and blackthorns ranging from 1.6–8.4 µmol TE/100 g frozen fruit extracted under acidified MeOH (0.1% HCl) [30].

Interestingly, keracyanin (60%) and kuromanin (38%) were the two main anthocyanins detected in mulberry [31,32]. Keracyanin (610.90 µg/g DW) and kuromanin (730.97 µg/g DW) detected in MNCM extract were in the range of those detected in Korean mulberries (30.6–486.7 µg keracyanin/g DW and 93.2–1364.9 µg kuromanin/g DW) [25]. The aqueous extract of MNCM provided good inhibitory activities against AChE, BChE, and BACE-1. It was previously reported that 18 commercially available mulberries (*M. alba*) in Poland, extracted under 80% (*v/v*) aqueous methanol, exhibited AChE inhibitory activity in the range of 2.6–37.9% [33]. However, this paper failed to indicate the extract concentration in the enzyme assay, and this cannot be used for comparison with MNCM extract. Considering the predominant anthocyanins and anthocyanidin detected in mulberry, cyanidin was able to inhibit AChE, with IC_{50} of 14.43 µM, while its BChE inhibitory activity was slightly higher [34]. Compared to cyanidin, its anthocyanin glycosides, including keracyanin and kuromanin, with insignificantly different cholinesterase inhibition, exhibited lower inhibitory activity against AChE and BChE [34]. However, an in vitro report on the BACE-1 inhibitory activity of these anthocyanidins and anthocyanidins remains unwritten.

After studying the anti-AD properties in vitro regarding AChE, BChE, and BACE-1, we also examined the anti-AD effects of MNCM extract on PC12 neuronal cells. As shown in Figure 1B,C, pre-treatment with MNCM extract evidently protected cells from H_2O_2 or Aβ peptide-induced toxicity. It may be possible that MNCM extract exerted its effective antioxidative properties based on the high amounts of anthocyanins and anthocyanidins as previously mentioned. Furthermore, it has been found that $Aβ_{25-35}$ peptides cause PC12 apoptosis by triggering oxidative stress, lipid peroxidation, and intracellular calcium ($[Ca^{2+}]_i$), similar to that of H_2O_2 [35,36], indicating that $Aβ_{25-35}$ peptides lead to mitochondrial dysfunction. Mitochondria is an organelle function in ATP synthesis and Ca^{2+} homeostasis, thus its impairment will provoke $[Ca^{2+}]_i$ release and the apoptotic protease-activating factor 1 (Apaf1)-mediated intrinsic apoptotic pathway. Indeed, $Aβ_{25-35}$ peptides induced Apaf1-mediated cell death, while pre-treatment with ethanolic extract of Chinese *M. nigra* for 24 h followed by $Aβ_{25-35}$ exposure downregulated Apaf1 [37]. Previous studies showed that cyanidin and kuromanin attenuate Aβ-induced PC12 neurotoxicity by maintaining mitochondrial stability [38]. Interestingly, MNCM extract was high in cyanidin, kuromanin, and keracyanin, indicating that MNCM extract may play a role in maintaining mitochondrial stability, which eventually leads to reduced

Aβ$_{25-35}$-mediated cell death. Additionally, kuromanin has been reported to reverse ethanol-induced inhibition of neurite outgrowth [39]. Neurite outgrowth is in neuron growth, and poor neurite outgrowth is observed in AD [20]. MNCM extract activated the neurite outgrowth of PC12 cells (Figure 1D). A high dose of MNCM extract at 200 µg/mL activated neurite outgrowth better than that of NGF-exposed cells. This could be because MNCM may enhance the expression of NGF as demonstrated in *M. fructus* [40].

To elucidate the anti-AD properties of MNCM extract in depth, a *Drosophila* co-expressing human APP and BACE-1 was employed. The fruit fly has emerged as a promising alternative model for AD drug screening since transgenic flies carrying AD-related genes demonstrated AD characteristics as in humans [41]. Flies also possess a unique approach for AD study because the elav-GAL4 driver can drive the expression of AD proteins in the brain at an early stage. This was in accordance with one of the present strategies for anti-AD agents to target at the earlier stages [42]. As illustrated in Figure 2B,C,D, MNCM extract inhibited BACE-1 activity, resulting in decreased Aβ$_{1-42}$ peptides and improved locomotor functions in AD flies, in a dose-dependent fashion. The data raise the hypothesis that MNCM extract may penetrate the blood–brain barrier (BBB) and restrain BACE-1 function. It is important to consider that several neurotherapeutic agents worked well in the cell study but not in animal models since they failed to cross the BBB. BACE-1 is a rate-limiting enzyme responsible for amyloid peptide production, thereby making it ideal for AD therapy [43]. Anthocyanins and anthocyanidins are able to cross the BBB, especially kuromanin, and are located in the brain regions contributing to cognitive functions [44,45]. Thus, the present data support that MNCM could be further developed as a potential natural product for AD prevention by targeting BACE-1. Furthermore, in this study, MNCM was extracted by water, making it useful for further application as a functional food for neuroprotection.

4. Materials and Methods

4.1. Mulberry Collection and Preparation

Morus cf. *nigra* 'Chiang Mai' (MNCM) was sourced from the Queen Sirikit Department of Sericulture. The sample was identified based on the morphology and nuclear ribosomal internal transcribed spacer (nITS) (GenBank: MK946679.1) and deposited at the Bangkok Herbarium (BK), Bangkok, Thailand. The Herbarium voucher specimen is B. Jongruaysup et al. 12-1 (BK). Fruits of uniform color and ripening stage were selected and cleaned before being freeze-dried. Samples were then ground to a fine powder and extracted using ultrapure water (Smart2Pure 3 UV™ Water Purification System, Thermo Fisher Scientific, Waltham, MA, USA) at 50 °C for 2 h.

4.2. In Vitro Antioxidant Activity

The in vitro antioxidant activity of the mulberry extract was performed from a well-established protocol for 2,2-diphenyl-1-picrylhydrazyl (DPPH) scavenging activity, oxygen radical absorbance capacity (ORAC), and ferric ion reducing antioxidant power (FRAP) assays [46–49].

4.3. Total Phenolic Contents, Anthocyanin, and Anthocyanidin Determination

Total phenolic contents (TPCs) were determined using Folin-Ciocalteu reagent as described by Thuphairo et al. 2019 [24]. Gallic acid was used as a reference matter, and the TPCs were reported as mg gallic acid equivalent (GAE)/g dried matter (DW) [24]. To determine anthocyanins and anthocyanidins, the mulberry powder was extracted under acidic conditions. The extracts were collected by filtering through a 0.45-µm polytetrafluoroethylene (PTFE) syringe filter. The HPLC analysis (an UtiMate HPLC with an HPG-3400SD pump and a photodiode array detector from DIONEX, Sunnyvale, CA, USA) was performed using Thermo Scientific Chromeleon Chromatography Data System (CDS) software (DIONEX, Sunnyvale, CA, USA) and a Reprosil-Pur ODS-3 column (250 mm × 4.6 mm, 5 µm from Dr. Maisch GmbH, Ammerbuch, Germany). For anthocyanidin analysis, a constant flow rate of 1 mL/min at ambient temperature was employed with an isocratic solvent of 82% Milli-Q water containing 0.4% (*v/v*) trifluoroacetic acid (TFA) (Solvent A) and 18% acetonitrile containing 0.4% (*v/v*) TFA (Solvent B) over 60 min. For anthocyanin analysis, a constant flow rate of 1 mL/min at ambient temperature was employed. The solvent system is shown in Table 4.

Table 4. Solvent system of anthocyanin analysis using HPLC.

Time (min)	Solvent A	Solvent B
0	88	12
6	88	12
8	85	15
25	85	15
25	88	12
30	88	12

Solvent A = Milli-Q water containing 0.4% (*v/v*) TFA; solvent B = acetonitrile containing 0.4% (*v/v*) TFA.

Samples were kept in the autosampler at 4 °C until injection (20 μL). The presence of anthocyanins and anthocyanidins was visualized at 525 and 530 nm, respectively. Anthocyanins (cyanidin-3-O-glucoside (kuromanin), cyanidin-3-O-rutinoside (keracyanin), cyanidin-3,5-O-diglucoside (cyanin), cyanidin-3-O-galactoside (idaein), pelargonidin-3,5-O-diglucoside (pelargonin), malvidin-3-O-galactoside (primulin), and petunidin-3-O-glucoside) and anthocyanidins (cyanidin, delphinidin, pelargonidin, peonidin, petunidin, and malvidin) were used as standards to identify anthocyanins and anthocyanidins in the sample by comparing their retention times (R_t) and UV-vis spectral fingerprints. All chemicals were received from Sigma-Aldrich (St. Louis, MO, USA).

4.4. Determination of Cholinesterases and Beta-Secretase 1 (BACE-1) Inhibitory Activities

Inhibitory activity of MNCM extract against AChE was carried out as previously reported [24,50,51]. In brief, a mixture containing 20 ng of *Electrophorus electricus* AChE (1000 units/mg, 100 μL), 16 mM 5,5-dithio-bis-(2-nitrobenzoic acid) (DTNB, 10 μL), 0.8 mM acetylthiocholine (40 μL), and the extract (50 μL) were well-mixed. The initial velocity was measured at 412 nm using a microplate reader (Synergy™ HT 96-well UV-visible spectrophotometer using Gen5 data analysis software from BioTek Instruments, Inc., Winooski, VT, USA). Percentage of inhibition was then calculated as follows:

$$\% \text{ inhibition} = \left(1 - \frac{B-b}{A-a}\right) \times 100, \qquad (1)$$

where A is the initial velocity of the reaction with enzyme, a is the initial velocity of the reaction without enzyme, B is the initial velocity of the enzyme reaction with extract, and b is the initial velocity of the reaction with extract but without enzyme.

Inhibitory activity of MNCM extract against BChE was determined similarly to AChE, except that 100 ng of equine serum BChE (≥10 units/mg protein, 100 μL) and 0.1 mM butyrylthiocholine (BTCh) were used as the reaction enzyme and substrate, respectively [24,50]. All chemicals and reagents for cholinesterase inhibitory activities were purchased from Sigma-Aldrich (St. Louis, MO, USA).

The BACE-1 activity was determined using a BACE-1 activity detection kit (Sigma-Aldrich, St. Louis, MO, USA) following the manufacturer's instructions and expressed as the percentage of BACE-1 inhibition.

4.5. Cell Culture and Cytotoxicity Analysis by Resazurin Assay

The PC12 neuronal cells were obtained from the American Type Culture Collection (ATCC, Manassas, VA, USA) and cultured in Roswell Park Memorial Institute 1640 (RPMI1640), 10% (*v/v*) fetal bovine serum (FBS) (Thermo Fisher Scientific, Waltham, MA, USA) and 1% (*v/v*) penicillin-streptomycin (Sigma-Aldrich, St. Louis, MO, USA) at 37 °C in a humidified atmosphere containing 5% CO_2.

For cytotoxicity analysis, each well of a 96-well plate of 1×10^4 exponentially growing PC12 cells was seeded and cultured overnight. Then, the cells were exposed to 50, 100, 150 and 200 µg/mL of MNCM extracts for 24, 48, and 72 h. At the indicated time, 20 µL of resazurin dye (CellTiter-Blue®, Promega, Madison, WI, USA) was added. One hour later, the fluorescence (emission = 585 nm, excitation = 570 nm) was measured. Cells treated with deionized water (DI) were used as a negative control.

4.6. Prevention of Hydrogen Peroxide (H_2O_2) and Aβ Peptide-Induced Toxicity

Each well of a poly-D-lysine (PDL)-coated 96-well plate of PC12 cells was plated and cultured overnight at a density of 2×10^4 cells/mL. Then, the cells were treated with MNCM extracts for 24 h (50, 100, 150, and 200 µg/mL). After that, 300 µM of H_2O_2 (Merck, Darmstadt, Germany) or 20 µM of amyloid peptide (Aβ$_{25-35}$) (Bachem, Bubendorf, Switzerland) were added. Forty-eight hours later, cell survival was measured by the resazurin assay, as mentioned above.

4.7. Determination of Neurite Outgrowth

Each well of a poly-D-lysine (PDL)-coated 6-well plate of PC12 cells was seeded and cultured overnight at a density of 1×10^4 cells/mL. Cells were then treated with MNCM extracts at 50, 100, 150, and 200 µg/mL in RPMI1640 with 0.5% FBS for one week, and the medium was changed every two days. The nerve growth factor (NGF) (Sigma-Aldrich, St. Louis, MO, USA) at 50 ng/mL was used as a positive control. Before analysis under a phase-contrast microscope, the neurite-bearing cells were fixed with 4% paraformaldehyde. The percentage of neurite-bearing cells was expressed. At least three independent experiments were carried out.

4.8. Drosophila Stocks and Culture

Fly stocks (elav-GAL4 (8760) and UAS-APP-BACE-1) (33798)) were obtained from the Bloomington Stock Center at Indiana University. After eclosion, F1 progeny flies obtained from the mating between elav-GAL4 and UAS-APP-BACE-1 were cultured on Formula 4-24 blue® medium (Carolina, Burlington, NC, USA) containing MNCM extract or DI (control) at 28 °C for 28 days. Flies were transferred to fresh media every 2–3 days. The *Drosophila* study was approved by Mahidol University-Institute Animal Care and Use Committee (MU-IACUC) (COA.No.MU-IACUC 2018/022).

4.9. Climbing Assay

The assay was determined following the published method [52]. At day 28 after treatment, 20 to 30 flies were placed in a transparent tube. After tapping, their rate of climb to the top of the tube was recorded and analyzed. At least three independent experiments were performed.

4.10. Quantification of Aβ Peptide by Enzyme-Linked Immunosorbent Assay (ELISA)

Quantification of Aβ peptide was performed as reported with slight modification [53]. The heads of F1 progeny flies at day 28 were collected and homogenized in 5 M guanidine-HCl containing 2X Halt protease inhibitor cocktail (Thermo Fisher Scientific, Waltham, MA, USA). Then, the protein concentration was measured using the BCA protein assay kit (Thermo Fisher Scientific, Waltham, MA, USA). Before sample loading, a serial dilution of supernatants was made with ELISA diluent buffer containing protease inhibitor cocktail. After following the manufacturer's instructions (human Aβ$_{42}$ ELISA kit (Thermo Fisher Scientific, Waltham, MA, USA)) the samples were measured at 450 nm. The concentration of Aβ$_{1-42}$ peptides was calculated and compared with standard recombinant human Aβ$_{1-42}$.

4.11. Determination of BACE-1 Activity in Fly Brain Lysate

The heads of F1 progeny flies at day 28 were collected and homogenized in T-PER tissue protein extraction reagent (Thermo Fisher Scientific, Waltham, MA, USA). Then, the protein concentration and BACE-1 activity were measured as mentioned above within the same day.

Supplementary Materials: The following are available online at http://www.mdpi.com/1420-3049/25/8/1837/s1, Figure S1: High-performance liquid chromatography (HPLC) chromatograms of (A.) cyanidin chloride standard (B.) kuromanin and keracyanin standard (C.) anthocyanidin analysis of MNCM extract and (D.) anthocyanin analysis of MNCM extract. The retention times (R_t) of cyanidin chloride, kuromanin and keracyanin in MNCM extract was also indicated; Figure S2: Representative images from the neurite outgrowth study showing neurite-bearing cells of (A.) control, (B.) MNCM extract-treated cells at 50 µg/mL, (C.) MNCM extract-treated cells at 100 µg/mL, (D.) MNCM extract-treated cells at 150 µg/mL, (E.) MNCM extract-treated cells at 200 µg/mL, and (F.) NGF-treated cells at 50 ng/mL.

Author Contributions: B.J. and S.T. initial technical support and provided samples. U.S. performed experiments, interpreted the results and generated the figures and tables, wrote the manuscript. D.S. and P.T. supervised, interpreted the results and designed the research, wrote the manuscript, reviewed the manuscript. S.C. suggested and reviewed the manuscript. All authors have read and agree to the published version of the manuscript.

Funding: This study was supported by Biodiversity-Based Economy Development Office (BEDO) (grant No. 22/2561), and partially supported by Grants-in-Aid from JSPS Core to-Core Program B. Asia-Africa Science Platforms.

Acknowledgments: We thank Kanchana Pruesapan, Plant Varieties Protection Division, Department of Agriculture, Bangkok for identification of the sample. We also thank Woorawee Inthachat for artwork editing and personal assistant.

Conflicts of Interest: All authors declare that there are no conflicts of interest.

References

1. Wang, H.; Naghavi, M.; Allen, C.; Barber, R.M.; A Bhutta, Z.; Carter, A.; Casey, D.C.; Charlson, F.; Chen, A.Z.; Coates, M.M.; et al. Global, regional, and national life expectancy, all-cause mortality, and cause-specific mortality for 249 causes of death, 1980–2015: A systematic analysis for the Global Burden of Disease Study 2015. *Lancet* **2016**, *388*, 1459–1544. [CrossRef]
2. Alzheimer's association. Alzheimer's disease facts and figures. *Alzheimer's Dement* **2015**, *11*, 321–387.
3. Ferreira-Vieira, T.H.; Guimaraes, I.M.; Silva, F.R.; Ribeiro, F. Alzheimer's Disease: Targeting the Cholinergic System. *Curr. Neuropharmacol.* **2016**, *14*, 101–115. [CrossRef] [PubMed]
4. Hardy, J.; Selkoe, D.J. The amyloid hypothesis of Alzheimer's disease: Progress and problems on the road to therapeutics. *Science* **2002**, *297*, 353–356. [CrossRef] [PubMed]
5. Citron, M.; Diehl, T.S.; Gordon, G.; Biere, A.L.; Seubert, P.; Selkoe, D.J. Evidence that the 42- and 40-amino acid forms of amyloid β protein are generated from the β-amyloid precursor protein by different protease activities. *Proc. Natl. Acad. Sci. USA* **1996**, *93*, 13170–13175. [CrossRef]
6. Dai, Q.; Borenstein, A.R.; Wu, Y.; Jackson, J.C.; Larson, E.B. Fruit and Vegetable Juices and Alzheimer's Disease: The Kame Project. *Am. J. Med.* **2006**, *119*. [CrossRef]
7. Loef, M.; Walach, H. Fruit, vegetables and prevention of cognitive decline or dementia: A systematic review of cohort studies. *J. Nutr. Health Aging* **2012**, *16*, 626–630. [CrossRef]
8. Pacheco, S.M.; Soares, M.S.P.; Gutierres, J.M.; Gerzson, M.F.B.; Carvalho, F.B.; Azambuja, J.H.; Schetinger, M.R.C.; Stefanello, F.M.; Spanevello, R.M. Anthocyanins as a potential pharmacological agent to manage memory deficit, oxidative stress and alterations in ion pump activity induced by experimental sporadic dementia of Alzheimer's type. *J. Nutr. Biochem.* **2018**, *56*, 193–204. [CrossRef]
9. Badshah, H.; Kim, T.H.; Kim, M.O. Protective effects of Anthocyanins against Amyloid beta-induced neurotoxicity in vivo and in vitro. *Neurochem. Int.* **2015**, *80*, 51–59. [CrossRef]
10. Özgen, M.; Serce, S.; Kaya, C. Phytochemical and antioxidant properties of anthocyanin-rich *Morus nigra* and *Morus rubra* fruits. *Sci. Hortic.* **2009**, *119*, 275–279. [CrossRef]
11. Chen, H.; Yu, W.; Chen, G.; Meng, S.; Xiang, Z.; He, N. Antinociceptive and Antibacterial Properties of Anthocyanins and Flavonols from Fruits of Black and Non-Black Mulberries. *Molecules* **2017**, *23*, 4. [CrossRef] [PubMed]

12. Lim, S.H.; Choi, C.-I. Pharmacological Properties of *Morus nigra* L. (Black Mulberry) as A Promising Nutraceutical Resource. *Nutrients* **2019**, *11*, 437. [CrossRef] [PubMed]
13. Koyuncu, F.; Cetinbas, M.; Ibrahim, E. Nutritional constituents of wild–grown black mulberry (*Morus nigra* L.). *J. Appl. Bot. Food Qual.* **2014**, *87*, 93–96.
14. Imran, M.; Khan, H.; Shah, M.; Khan, R.; Khan, F. Chemical composition and antioxidant activity of certain *Morus* species. *J. Zhejiang Univ. Sci. B* **2010**, *11*, 973–980. [CrossRef]
15. Qiao, A.; Wang, Y.; Zhang, W.; He, X. Neuroprotection of Brain-Targeted Bioactive Dietary Artoindonesianin O (AIO) from Mulberry on Rat Neurons as a Novel Intervention for Alzheimer's Disease. *J. Agric. Food Chem.* **2015**, *63*, 3687–3693. [CrossRef] [PubMed]
16. Xia, C.-L.; Tang, G.; Guo, Y.-Q.; Xu, Y.-K.; Huang, Z.-S.; Yin, S. Mulberry Diels-Alder-type adducts from *Morus alba* as multi-targeted agents for Alzheimer's disease. *Phytochemistry* **2019**, *157*, 82–91. [CrossRef]
17. Chen, Z.; Zhong, C. Oxidative stress in Alzheimer's disease. *Neurosci. Bull.* **2014**, *30*, 271–281. [CrossRef]
18. Butterfield, D.A.; Boyd-Kimball, D. Oxidative Stress, Amyloid-β Peptide, and Altered Key Molecular Pathways in the Pathogenesis and Progression of Alzheimer's Disease. *J. Alzheimer's Dis.* **2018**, *62*, 1345–1367. [CrossRef]
19. Frozza, R.L.; Horn, A.P.; Hoppe, J.B.; Simao, F.; Gerhardt, D.; Comiran, R.A.; Salbego, C.G. A comparative study of beta-amyloid peptides Abeta1–42 and Abeta25–35 toxicity in organotypic hippocampal slice cultures. *Neurochem. Res.* **2009**, *34*, 295–303. [CrossRef]
20. Dowjat, W.K.; Wisniewski, T.; Efthimiopoulos, S.; Wisniewski, H.M. Inhibition of neurite outgrowth by familial Alzheimer's disease-linked presenilin-1 mutations. *Neurosci. Lett.* **1999**, *267*. [CrossRef]
21. Wang, X.; Kim, J.-R.; Lee, S.-B.; Kim, Y.-J.; Jung, M.Y.; Kwon, H.W.; Ahn, Y.-J. Effects of curcuminoids identified in rhizomes of *Curcuma longa* on BACE-1 inhibitory and behavioral activity and lifespan of Alzheimer's disease Drosophila models. *BMC Complement. Altern. Med.* **2014**, *14*. [CrossRef] [PubMed]
22. Liu, R.; Liu, Y.C.; Meng, J.; Zhu, H.; Zhang, X. A microfluidics-based mobility shift assay to identify new inhibitors of beta-secretase for Alzheimer's disease. *Anal. Bioanal. Chem.* **2017**, *409*, 6635–6642. [CrossRef]
23. Mancini, F.; De Simone, A.; Andrisano, V. Beta-secretase as a target for Alzheimer's disease drug discovery: An overview of in vitro methods for characterization of inhibitors. *Anal. Bioanal. Chem.* **2011**, *400*, 1979–1996. [CrossRef]
24. Thuphairo, K.; Sornchan, P.; Suttisansanee, U. Bioactive Compounds, Antioxidant Activity and Inhibition of Key Enzymes Relevant to Alzheimer's Disease from Sweet Pepper (*Capsicum annuum*) Extracts. *Prev. Nutr. Food Sci.* **2019**, *24*, 327–337. [CrossRef]
25. Bae, S.-H.; Suh, H. Antioxidant activities of five different mulberry cultivars in Korea. *LWT* **2007**, *40*, 955–962. [CrossRef]
26. Oki, T.; Kobayashi, M.; Nakamura, T.; Okuyama, A.; Masuda, M.; Shiratsuchi, H.; Suda, I. Changes in Radical-scavenging Activity and Components of Mulberry Fruit During Maturation. *J. Food Sci.* **2006**, *71*, 18–22. [CrossRef]
27. Natić, M.; Dabić, D.Č; Papetti, A.; Akšić, M.F.; Ognjanov, V.; Ljubojević, M.; Tešić, Ž. Analysis and characterisation of phytochemicals in mulberry (*Morus alba* L.) fruits grown in Vojvodina, North Serbia. *Food Chem.* **2015**, *171*, 128–136. [CrossRef]
28. Wang, S.Y.; Lin, H.-S. Antioxidant activity in fruits and leaves of blackberry, raspberry, and strawberry varies with cultivar and developmental stage. *J. Agric. Food Chem.* **2000**, *48*, 140–146. [CrossRef] [PubMed]
29. Kim, J.-S. Antioxidant Activities of Selected Berries and Their Free, Esterified, and Insoluble-Bound Phenolic Acid Contents. *Prev. Nutr. Food Sci.* **2018**, *23*, 35–45. [CrossRef]
30. Ştefănuţ, M.N.; Căta, A.; Pop, R.; Mosoarca, C.; Zamfir, A.D. Anthocyanins HPLC-DAD and MS Characterization, Total Phenolics, and Antioxidant Activity of Some Berries Extracts. *Anal. Lett.* **2011**, *44*, 2843–2855. [CrossRef]
31. Pawlowska, A.M.; Oleszek, W.; Braca, A. Quali-quantitative Analyses of Flavonoids of *Morus nigra* L. and *Morus alba* L. (Moraceae) Fruits. *J. Agric. Food Chem.* **2008**, *56*, 3377–3380. [CrossRef] [PubMed]
32. Qin, C.; Li, Y.; Niu, W.; Ding, Y.; Zhang, R.; Shang, X. Analysis and characterisation of anthocyanins in mulberry fruit. *Czech. J. Food Sci.* **2010**, *28*, 117–126. [CrossRef]
33. Polumackanycz, M.; Sledzinski, T.; Goyke, E.; Wesolowski, M.; Viapiana, A. A Comparative Study on the Phenolic Composition and Biological Activities of *Morus alba* L. Commercial Samples. *Molecules* **2019**, *24*, 3082. [CrossRef] [PubMed]

34. Szwajgier, D. Anticholinesterase Activities of Selected Polyphenols—A Short Report. *Pol. J. Food Nutr. Sci.* **2014**, *64*, 59–64. [CrossRef]
35. Ye, J.; Meng, X.; Yan, C.; Wang, C. Effect of Purple Sweet Potato Anthocyanins on β-Amyloid-Mediated PC-12 Cells Death by Inhibition of Oxidative Stress. *Neurochem. Res.* **2009**, *35*, 357–365. [CrossRef]
36. Hong, H.; Liu, G.-Q. Protection against hydrogen peroxide-induced cytotoxicity in PC12 cells by scutellarin. *Life Sci.* **2004**, *74*, 2959–2973. [CrossRef]
37. Song, N.; Yang, H.; Pang, W.; Qie, Z.; Lu, H.; Tan, L.; Li, H.; Sun, S.; Lian, F.; Qin, C.; et al. Mulberry extracts alleviate abeta 25-35-induced injury and change the gene expression profile in PC12 cells. *Evid Based Complement. Alternat Med.* **2014**, 1–9. [CrossRef]
38. Zheng, Z.-C.; Cho, N.C.; Wang, Y.; Fu, X.-T.; Li, D.-W.; Wang, K.; Wang, X.-Z.; Li, Y.; Sun, B.-L.; Yang, X.-Y. Cyanidin suppresses amyloid beta-induced neurotoxicity by inhibiting reactive oxygen species-mediated DNA damage and apoptosis in PC12 cells. *Neural Regen. Res.* **2016**, *11*, 795–800. [CrossRef]
39. Chen, G.; Bower, K.A.; Xu, M.; Ding, M.; Shi, X.; Ke, Z.; Luo, J. Cyanidin-3-Glucoside Reverses Ethanol-Induced Inhibition of Neurite Outgrowth: Role of Glycogen Synthase Kinase 3 Beta. *Neurotox. Res.* **2009**, 15. [CrossRef] [PubMed]
40. Kim, H.G.; Oh, M.S. Memory-enhancing effect of Mori Fructus via induction of nerve growth factor. *Br. J. Nutr.* **2012**, *110*, 86–94. [CrossRef]
41. Pandey, U.B.; Nichols, C.D. Human disease models in Drosophila melanogaster and the role of the fly in therapeutic drug discovery. *Pharmacol. Rev.* **2011**, 63. [CrossRef]
42. Chintamaneni, M.; Bhaskar, M. Biomarkers in Alzheimer's disease: A review. *ISRN Pharmacol.* **2012**. [CrossRef] [PubMed]
43. Ghosh, A.K.; Gemma, S.; Tang, J. beta-Secretase as a therapeutic target for Alzheimer's disease. *Neurotherapeutics* **2008**, *5*, 399–408. [CrossRef] [PubMed]
44. Fornasaro, S.; Ziberna, L.; Gasperotti, M.; Tramer, F.; Vrhovšek, U.; Mattivi, F.; Passamonti, S. Determination of cyanidin 3-glucoside in rat brain, liver and kidneys by UPLC/MS-MS and its application to a short-term pharmacokinetic study. *Sci. Rep.* **2016**, *6*, 22815. [CrossRef] [PubMed]
45. Afzal, M.; Redha, A.; AlHasan, R. Anthocyanins Potentially Contribute to Defense against Alzheimer's Disease. *Molecules* **2019**, *24*, 4255. [CrossRef] [PubMed]
46. Benzie, I.; Strain, J. The Ferric Reducing Ability of Plasma (FRAP) as a Measure of "Antioxidant Power": The FRAP Assay. *Anal. Biochem.* **1996**, *239*, 70–76. [CrossRef]
47. Fukumoto, L.R.; Mazza, G. Assessing Antioxidant and Prooxidant Activities of Phenolic Compounds. *J. Agric. Food Chem.* **2000**, *48*, 3597–3604. [CrossRef]
48. Ou, B.; Hampsch-Woodill, M.; Prior, R.L. Development and validation of an improved oxygen radical absorbance capacity assay using fluorescein as the fluorescent probe. *J. Agric. Food Chem.* **2001**, *49*, 4619–4626. [CrossRef]
49. Sripum, C.; Kukreja, R.K.; Charoenkiatkul, S.; Kriengsinyos, W.; Suttisansanee, U. The effect of extraction conditions on antioxidant activities and total phenolic contents of different processed Thai Jasmine rice. *Int. Food Res. J.* **2017**, *24*, 1644–1650.
50. Jung, H.A.; Min, B.S.; Yokozawa, T.; Lee, J.-H.; Kim, Y.S.; Choi, J.S. Anti-Alzheimer and antioxidant activities of *Coptidis Rhizoma* alkaloids. *Biol. Pharm. Bull.* **2009**, *32*, 1433–1438. [CrossRef]
51. Nantakornsuttanan, N.; Thuphairo, K.; Kukreja, R.K.; Charoenkiatkul, S.; Suttisansanee, U. Anti-cholinesterase inhibitory activities of different varieties of chili peppers extracts. *Int. Food Res. J.* **2016**, *23*, 1953–1959.
52. Jantrapirom, S.; Piccolo, L.L.; Yoshida, H.; Yamaguchi, M. A new Drosophila model of Ubiquilin knockdown shows the effect of impaired proteostasis on locomotive and learning abilities. *Exp. Cell Res.* **2018**, *362*, 461–471. [CrossRef] [PubMed]
53. Sofola-Adesakin, O.; Khericha, M.; Snoeren, I.; Tsuda, L.; Partridge, L. pGluAbeta increases accumulation of Abeta in vivo and exacerbates its toxicity. *Acta Neuropathol. Commun.* **2016**, *4*, 109. [CrossRef] [PubMed]

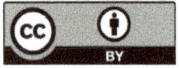

© 2020 by the authors. Licensee MDPI, Basel, Switzerland. This article is an open access article distributed under the terms and conditions of the Creative Commons Attribution (CC BY) license (http://creativecommons.org/licenses/by/4.0/).

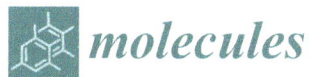

Article

Study on the Antinociceptive Activity and Mechanism of Action of Isolated Saponins from *Siolmatra brasiliensis* (Cogn.) Baill

Thais Biondino Sardella Giorno [1,2], Carlos Henrique Corrêa dos Santos [3], Mario Geraldo de Carvalho [3], Virgínia Cláudia da Silva [4], Paulo Teixeira de Sousa Jr. [4], Patricia Dias Fernandes [1,2,*] and Fabio Boylan [5]

1. Federal University of Rio de Janeiro, Institute of Biomedical Sciences, Laboratory of Pharmacology of Pain and Inflammation, Rio de Janeiro 21941-902, Brazil; thais.sardella.farma@hotmail.com
2. Federal University of Rio de Janeiro, Institute of Biomedical Sciences, Graduate Program in Pharmacology and Medicinal Chemistry, Rio de Janeiro 21941-902, Brazil
3. Federal Rural University of Rio de Janeiro, Department of Chemistry, Seropédica 23890-000, Brazil; caio.chcs@msn.com (C.H.C.d.S.); mgeraldo@ufrrj.br (M.G.d.C.)
4. Federal University of Mato Grosso, Department of Chemistry, Cuiabá 78935-901, Brazil; vcsvirginia@yahoo.com.br (V.C.d.S.); pauloteixeiradesousa@gmail.com (P.T.d.S.J.)
5. Trinity College Dublin, Trinity Biomedical Sciences Institute, School of Pharmacy and Pharmaceutical Sciences, Dublin 2, Ireland; fabio.boylan@tcd.ie
* Correspondence: patricia.dias@icb.ufrj.br; Tel.: +5521-3938-6442

Academic Editors: Raffaele Capasso and Lorenzo Di Cesare Mannelli
Received: 4 November 2019; Accepted: 9 December 2019; Published: 14 December 2019

Abstract: Infusions of roots of *Siolmatra brasiliensis* (Cogn.) Baill, ("taiuiá", "cipó-tauá") are used for toothache pain and ulcers. We aimed to study the antinociceptive effects and identify the possible mechanism of action of this plant and its isolated substances (cayaponoside A1, cayaponoside B4, cayaponoside D, and siolmatroside I). Hydroethanol extract (HE), ethyl acetate fraction (EtOAc), and isolated saponins were evaluated in chemical and thermal models of pain in mice. Animals were orally pretreated and evaluated in the capsaicin- or glutamate-induced licking and in the hot plate tests. The antinociceptive mechanism of action was evaluated using the hot plate test with the following pretreatments: Atropine (cholinergic antagonist), naloxone (opioid antagonist), or L-NAME (nitric oxide synthase inhibitor). All extracts and isolated saponins increased the area under the curve in the hot plate test. Tested substances induced a higher effect than the morphine-treated group. Our data suggest that stems of *S. brasiliensis* and their isolated substances present antinociceptive effects. Cholinergic and opioidergic pathways seem to be involved in their mechanism of action. Taken together our data corroborate the traditional use of the plant and expands the information regarding its use.

Keywords: *Siolmatra brasiliensis*; antinociceptive activity; cayaponoside A1; cayaponoside B4; cayaponoside D; siolmatroside I; pain; analgesia

1. Introduction

Siolmatra brasiliensis (Cogn.) Baill is a climbing plant belonging to the Cucurbitaceae family that occurs in the central region of Brazil, especially in Cerrado and Pantanal where it is popularly known as "taiuiá" or "cipó-tauá" [1]. Its roots are considered a purifying and antisyphilis agent [2]. Infusions prepared with roots are widely used in traditional medicine as an analgesic for treatment of toothache [2] and for the treatment of ulcers [3]. Due to the presence of cucurbitacins, compounds responsible for the bitter tang and high toxicity, Lima et al. [1] showed some toxicological effects of

S. brasiliensis only at very high doses (i.e., 2 g/kg). In a recent study, Dos Santos et al. [3] performed a regional ethnopharmacological use of the infusion of *S. brasiliensis* stems in Mato Grosso (Brazil) and demonstrated that the crude hydroethanol extract reduced the hyperglycemia and glycosuria in diabetic mice. On the other hand, our continuous search for evidences for the traditional use of Brazilian species led us to hear about the popular use of *S. brasiliensis* to treating pain as a result of toothache. On that basis, the aim of the present work was to investigate the antinociceptive effect of *S. brasiliensis* extract and its previously isolated saponins: Cayaponoside A1, cayaponoside B4, cayaponoside D, and siolmatroside I, and suggest the mechanism of their antinociceptive activity. In this regard we used atropine (cholinergic antagonist), naloxone (opioid antagonist), or L-NAME (nitric oxide synthase inhibitor) to evaluate the participation of these pathways in the antinociceptive effect of *S. brasiliensis*. It is important to mention that siolmatroside I (a dammarane type saponin) was described by our research group for the first time in the plant kingdom.

2. Results

2.1. Assessment of Side Effects and Toxicity

A single oral administration of HE, EtOAc, or the isolated saponins (SI, D, B4, and A1) were evaluated against a possible toxic effect when administered orally. Doses of 150 mg/kg of extracts or 10 mg/kg of each isolated saponins were used. After periods of 1, 3, 6, and every 24 h until five days post-oral administration animals were evaluated regarding behaviour alterations. We also evaluated food and water intake every 24 h until the fifth day. Results obtained indicated that none of the extract or isolated saponins induced compartmental alterations, did not change the amount of food and water intake, and did not induce any mucosal lesion five days after their administration, presenting visual conditions similar to those for the vehicle (supplementary material, Tables S1–S4).

2.2. Antinociceptive Effect of HE, EtOAc, SI, D, B4, and A1 in the Hot Plate Test

The hot plate model was used to evaluate the supraspinal antinociceptive effect of the tested substances. As it can be observed in Figure 1A and B, all three doses of HE and EtOAc significantly increased the time necessary for mice to respond to the stimulus. Maximal effects were observed at 150- or 120-min post-administration, respectively, and they returned to basal levels after this period. When data obtained in time course assays were converted to a graph of area under the curve (AUC) it could be noted that all doses increased these values. Furthermore, higher doses (30 and 100 mg/kg) of EtOAc were significantly even when compared to the morphine-treated group (Figure 1C and D). Although a lower dose (30 mg/kg) of HE presented higher area under the curve values than higher dose (100 mg/kg) (7001 ± 1260 versus 4697 ± 1483) a statistical significance between both groups was not observed (Figure 1A and B).

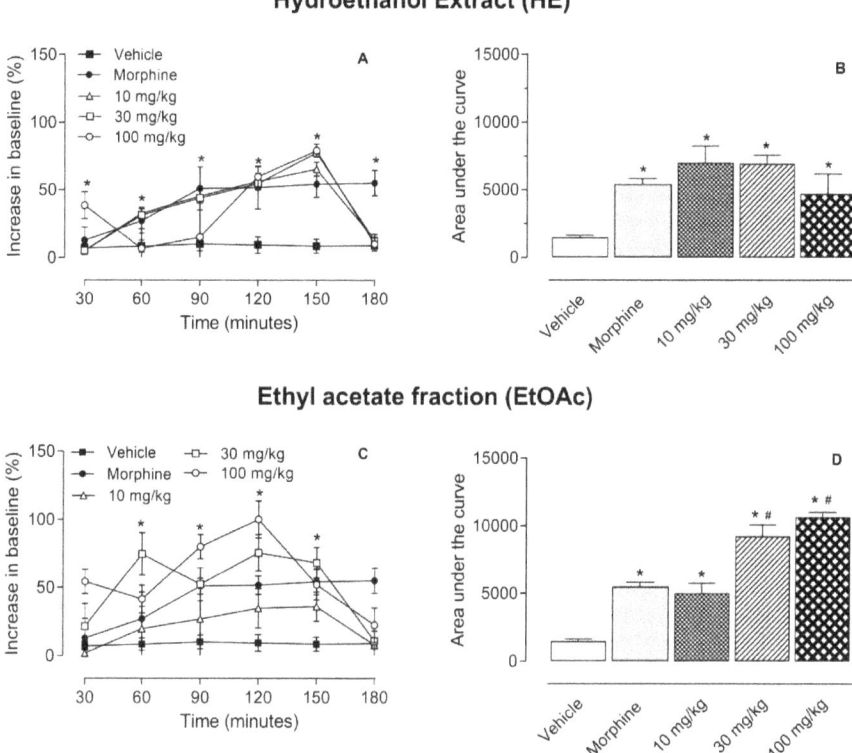

Figure 1. Effects of hydroethanol extract (HE, graphs **A** and **B**) or ethyl acetate fraction (EtOAc, graphs **C** and **D**) of *S. brasiliensis* in the hot plate model. Animals were orally pretreated with different doses of HE, EtOAc, morphine (2.5 mg/kg) or vehicle. The results are presented as mean ± SD. (n = 6 per group) of increase in baseline (graphs **A** and **C**) or area under the curve (graphs **B** and **D**) calculated by Prism Software 5.0. Statistical significance was calculated by ANOVA followed by Dunnett's test. * $p < 0.05$ when comparing to vehicle-treated group; # $p < 0.05$ when comparing treated mice with the morphine-treated group.

The next step was the evaluation of the saponins isolated from ethyl acetate fraction using this same model. The doses were chosen based on the yield of each saponin after isolation from the ethyl acetate fraction. Data shown in Figure 2 demonstrated that doses of 1 and 3 mg/kg of all saponins presented a significant antinociceptive effect increasing the AUC. It is interesting to note that SI (at the doses of 1 and 3 mg/kg) presented an effect higher than that observed for the positive control group (morphine-treated mice).

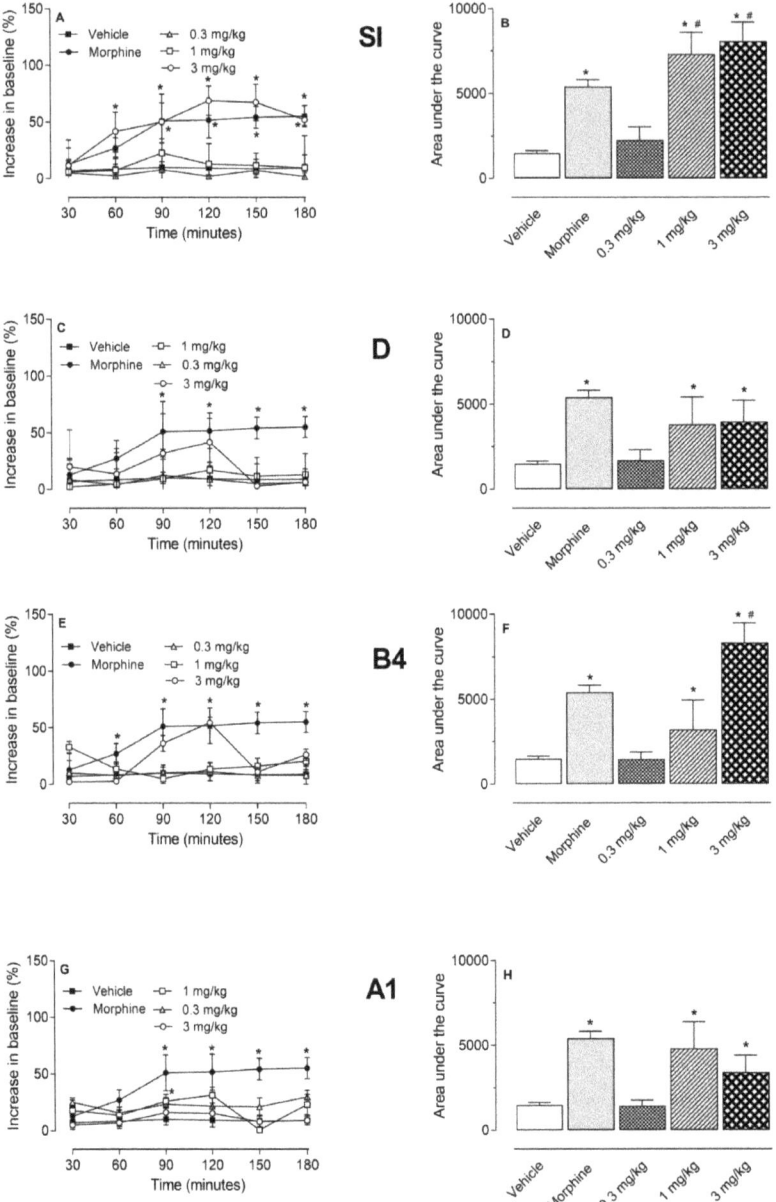

Figure 2. Effects of Saponins isolated from the ethyl acetate fraction of the stems of *S. brasiliensis*: siolmatroside I (SI), cayaponoside D (D), cayaponoside B4 (B4), and cayaponoside A1 (A1) in the hot plate model. Animals were orally pretreated with different doses of A1, B4, D, I, morphine (2.5 mg/kg), or vehicle. The results are presented as mean ± SD. (n = 6 per group) of increase in baseline (graphs **A**, **C**, **E**, and **G**) or area under the curve (graphs **B**, **D**, **F**, and **H**) calculated by Prism Software 5.0. Statistical significance was calculated by ANOVA followed by Dunnett´s test. * $p < 0.05$ when comparing to vehicle-treated group; # $p < 0.05$ when comparing treated mice with the morphine-treated group.

2.3. Investigation of the Mechanism of Action of EtOAc, SI, D, B4, and A1 in the Hot Plate Model

As the ethanol extract, ethyl acetate fraction and its isolated saponins (SI, D, B4, and A1) showed that the significant antinociceptive effect was decided to further investigate the role of different nociceptive pathways involved in the transmission of nociceptive stimulus or the activation of pathways involved in the control of nociception. None of the receptor antagonists (atropine and naloxone) or enzyme inhibitor (L-NAME) demonstrated any antinociceptive effect per se in the hot plate model (Data not shown). As the intention was to observe an inhibitory effect, we decided to use the higher dose of the extract, fraction (100 mg/kg), or isolated saponins (3 mg/kg). The pretreatment with atropine (muscarinic receptor antagonist, 1 mg/kg, i.p.) or naloxone (opioid receptor antagonist, 1 mg/kg, i.p.) reversed the antinociceptive effect of HE and EtOAc (Figure 3A), SI, D, B4, and A1 (Figure 3B). The inhibitor of nitric oxide synthase enzyme (L-NAME, 3 mg/kg, i.p.) reversed the antinociceptive effect EtOAc (Figure 3A), SI, B4, and A1 (Figure 3B).

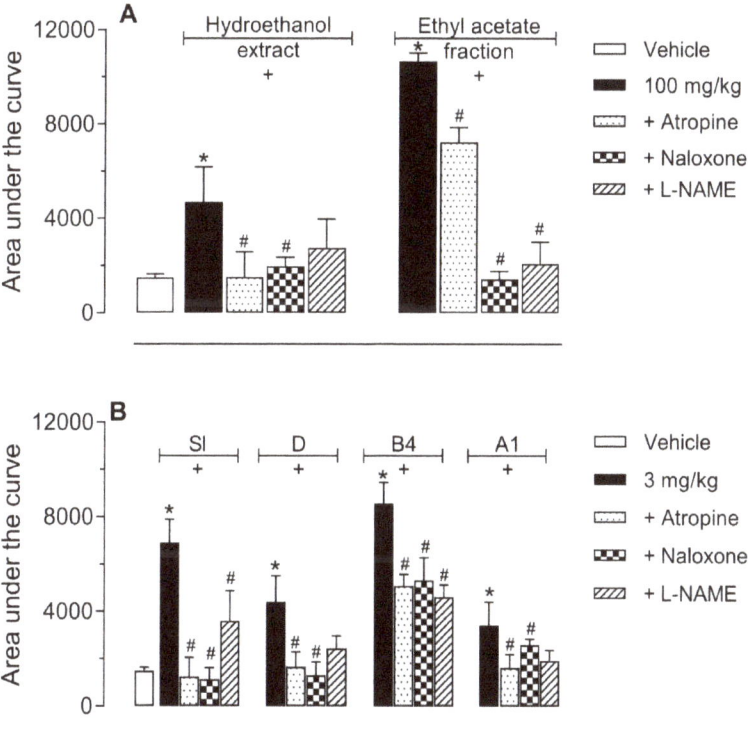

Figure 3. Effects of different antagonists on the antinociceptive activity of HE, EtOAc (graph **A**), siolmatroside I (SI), cayaponoside D (D), cayaponoside B4 (B4), and cayaponoside A1 (A1) (graph **B**) in the hot plate model. Animals were pretreated with atropine (1 mg/kg, i.p.), naloxone (1 mg/kg, i.p.) or L-NAME (3 mg/kg, i.p.), 15 min prior to oral administration of HE, EtOAc (100 mg/kg), SI, D, B4, and A1 (3 mg/kg). The results are present as mean ± SD. (n = 6 per group) of the area under the curve calculated by Prism Software 5.0. Statistical significance was calculated by ANOVA followed by Dunnett´s test. * $p < 0.05$ when comparing HE, EtOAc, SI, D, B4, and A1-treated mice to the vehicle-treated group; # $p < 0.05$ when comparing antagonist or inhibitor pretreated mice with the HE, EtOAc, SI, D, B4, or A1-treated group.

2.4. Antinociceptive Effect of HE, EtOAc, SI, D, B4, and A1 in the Capsaicin- or Glutamate-Induced Nociception

The results depicted in Figure 4A show that HE and EtOAc produced a significantly and dose-dependent reduction in the capsaicin-induced neurogenic pain. Pretreatment of animals with HE (at 10, 30, or 100 mg/kg doses) significantly reduced the paw licking induced by capsaicin by 22.2%, 50.4%, and 65.3% (52.1 ± 4.1; 33.5 ± 3.1, and 23.4 ± 1.7 s, respectively). Same doses of EtOAc demonstrated 40.7%; 54.2% and 67.8% reduction (40 ± 1.5; 30.9 ± 1.5; 21.7 ± 1.2 s, respectively) when compared to vehicle-treated animals (67.5 ± 1.9 s). Oral treatment of mice with A1 or SI significantly inhibited the capsaicin-induced licking pain at the doses of 0.3, 1, and 3 mg/kg, with the following results: 43.1 ± 1.4 (36.1%), 34.9 ± 1.1 (48.3%), 26.4 ± 1.2 (60.9%), and 49.0 ± 1.2 (27.4%), 38.8 ± 1.1 (42.5%), 32.8 ± 2.0 s (51.4%), respectively, when comparing with vehicle-treated mice (67.5 ± 1.9 s). Only the dose of 3 mg/kg of B4 and D demonstrated a significant effect (Figure 4C).

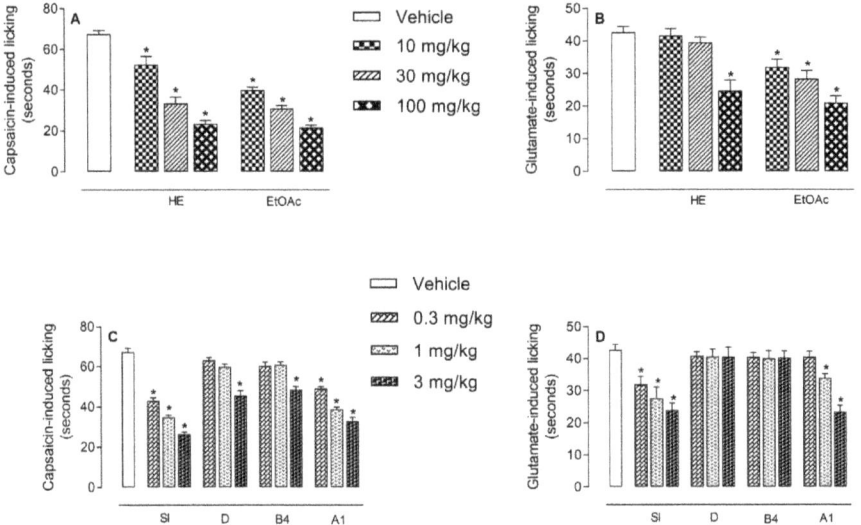

Figure 4. Antinociceptive effect of HE, EtOAc (graphs **A** and **B**), siolmatroside I (SI), cayaponoside D (D), cayaponoside B4 (B4), and cayaponoside A1 (A1) (graphs **C** and **D**) on the licking response induced by capsaicin or glutamate in mice, respectively. Animals were pretreated with different doses of HE, EtOAc, SI, D, B4, and A1 or vehicle 60 min before the injection of capsaicin (1.6 ng/paw) or glutamate (3.7 ng/paw). The results are presented as mean ± SD. (n = 6 per group) of the time that the animal spent licking the capsaicin-injected paw. Statistical significance was calculated by ANOVA followed by Dunnett´s test. * $p < 0.05$ when compared to vehicle-treated mice.

We also observed that HE (at 100 mg/kg, p.o.) produced a significant reduction (41.9%) of glutamate-induced licking response (24.8 ± 3.2 s) when compared to vehicle-treated mice (42.7 ± 1.8 s). While EtOAc, at all doses, significantly and dose-dependently inhibited the glutamate-induced pain behavior (31.9 ± 2.5, 28.4 ± 2.9, and 21 ± 2.1 s, to 10, 30, and 100 mg/kg, respectively) when comparing with the vehicle-treated group, leading to an inhibition of 25.3%, 33.5%, and 50.8%, respectively (Figure 4B). Among the isolated saponins, only SI (0.3, 1, and 3 mg/kg p.o.) was effective in reducing (31.9 ± 2.6, 27.6 ± 3.6, and 23.8 ± 5 s) the glutamate-induced nociceptive response corresponding to an inhibition of 5.3%, 34.6%, and 44.3%, respectively. The cayaponoside A1 reduced the paw licking at the doses of 1 and 3 mg/kg (34.0 ± 1.5 and 23.3 ± 2.1 s) producing a reduction of 20.4% and 45.4%, respectively (Figure 4D).

3. Discussion

This study investigated the antinociceptive activity of *S. brasiliensis* confirming its popular use and contributing to the pharmacological knowledge of this plant.

To the best of our knowledge this is the first study showing that hydroethanol extract (HE) of *S. brasiliensis* stems, one of its fraction (EtOAc) and two saponins isolated from this fraction (A1 and SI) have antinociceptive activity when administered orally in different models of thermal and chemical nociception in mice.

When a chemical, mechanical, or thermal stimulus occurs in mice paw, there is activation of nociceptors that transmit nociceptive information to the somatosensory cortex, for example, present in the central nervous system (CNS) producing an organized response, resulting in an elevation of motor response and/or licking of the paw [4]. The administration of HE, EtOAc, SI, D, B4, and A1, produced a rapid effect and time course of action similar to morphine.

Several saponins have already been related to the antinociceptive/anti-inflammatory activity. Examples to cite are saponins from *Ipomoea involucrate* [5], *Pterodone marnatus* [6], and Xeromphisnilotica [7]. Saponins isolated from *S. brasiliensis* in this study belong to the cucurbitane (A1, B4, D) and dammarane (SI) types. Cucurbitanes have been shown to possess a good antinociceptive and anti-inflammatory action as demonstrated recently in a *Momordica charantia* review paper [8].

Knowing that several endogenous systems are involved in pain control, the mechanism of antinociceptive action of HE, EtOAc, SI, D, B4, and A1 was also investigated. Atropine, a non-selective muscarinic receptor antagonist, was used to assess the involvement of the cholinergic system. Some studies show that activation of the muscarinic receptor (subtype M2) may reduce the response of peripheral nociceptors in front of noxious stimuli. The stimulation of the M2 and M4 muscarinic receptors in the dorsal horn of the spinal cord contributes to the analgesic effect through the release of inhibitory interneurons, reducing nociceptive transmission [9]. Our results showed the reversal of the antinociceptive effect of HE, EtOAc, SI, D, B4, and A1 when atropine was used suggesting that the effects of extract, fraction, or isolated saponins may involve, at least in part, activation of muscarinic receptors and consequently cholinergic pathway.

Our data also indicated that the opioid system could be involved in the antinociception caused by HE, EtOAc, SI, D, and B4. Opioid receptors (μ, δ, and κ) can be found in peripheral, spinal, and supraspinal regions. The downward pain modulation also involves the participation of opioid receptors, which promotes reduction in synaptic release of γ-aminobutyric acid (GABA) to the spinal cord rostral medial projections and periaqueductal gray; subsequently leading to spinal disinhibited projections of adrenergic neurons in the locus coeruleus [10]. In this context, the extract and isolated substances tested in this work may exert their antinociceptive effects through the opioid system at the peripheral level, spinal, and/or supraspinal. Literature reviews have already demonstrated that saponins may present an antinociceptive activity. The investigation of the mechanism of action of a *Polygonum verticillatum* methanol extract rich in saponins showed the involvement of the opioid pathway [11], similarly to what was observed in our study for the ethanol extract of *S. brasiliensis*, its EtOAc fraction, two curcubitane, and one dammarane type of saponin.

The knowledge of the dual role of nitric oxide (NO) in nociceptive transmission and its contribution to antinociception by opioid pain killers and anti-inflammatory drugs motivated us to assess whether the antinociception of HE, EtOAc, SI, D, B4, and A1 involve nitrergic pathway. NO present in the dorsal horn of the spinal cord can stimulate the release of neurokinin A, substance P, CGRP, and glutamate by primary afferent fibers facilitating nociceptive transmission. Activation of NMDA type receptors by NO is involved in central sensitization mechanism [10]. In this context, our results showed that the antinociceptive effect of EtOAc, SI, B4, and A1 was reversed by pretreatment with L-NAME suggesting that the antinociceptive effect of EtOAc and the three substances involves the inhibition of NOS activity and/or indirect reduction in NO levels.

Hydroethanol extract, ethyl acetate fraction, and the isolated substances SI and A1 also presented an inhibitory effect against the neurogenic nociception induced by intraplantar injection of capsaicin.

It is an amine extracted from red pepper that stimulates nerve endings causing intense thermal and nociceptive pain [9,11,12]. Studies have shown that capsaicin acts through vanilloid receptor type-1 (TRPV-1) expressed on nociceptive fibers [13] and in the dorsal root ganglion of the spinal cord, trigeminal ganglia, and CNS [14]. The stimulation of TRPV-1 receptors is mediated by the release of several neurotransmitters, including glutamate and substance P, from the peripheral and central terminals of primary sensory neurons thus contributing to nociceptive processing [15,16]. Our data suggest that extracts and isolated saponins reduce licking behavior induced by capsaicin. We have no means to attest that the observed effect is mediated through a direct action on peripherals and/or central vanilloid receptors, but we can suggest that part of the effect is mediated by capsaicin pathway.

We also suggest that at least part of the inhibitory effect observed can also occur due to an effect against the glutamate pathway since it was observed that EtOAc reduced glutamate-induced licking response. It is most probably that the effect of *S. brasiliensis* extract, fraction, and SI occurs due to a direct combination of effects in the capsaicin and glutamate systems. It is also suggested that isolated saponins D and B4 do not present an effect against both neurogenic substances.

Taken together our data suggest *S. brasiliensis* and the isolated substances siolmatroside I (SI), cayaponoside D (D), cayaponoside B4 (B4), and cayaponoside A1 (A1) present significant antinociceptive effects. Cholinergic and opioidergic pathways seem to be involved in their mechanism of action. We also demonstrated that the siolmatroside I was the most active saponin identified in the plant. Taken together our data corroborate the traditional use of the plant and expands the information regarding its use.

4. Methods

4.1. Plant Material

Stems of *S. brasiliensis* were collected in Jangada/Mato Grosso State, Brazil and identified by Dr. Vali Joana Pott (Department of Biology, UFMT, Cuiabá, Brazil). A voucher specimen was deposited at the herbarium of the UFMT under the number CGMS: 31643.

4.2. Extraction and Isolation

Air dried stems of *S. brasiliensis* (2.07 kg) were powdered and subjected to extraction with a mixture of EtOH:H$_2$O (7:3) (3 × 6 L) (named hydroethanol, HE extract). The HE extract was concentrated under reduced pressure and circulation oven (45 °C). HE (149 g) was suspended in a mixture of MeOH:H$_2$O (1:1) (1 L) and subjected to a liquid–liquid partition between chloroform, ethyl acetate, and n-butanol. Cayaponoside A1 [17] (A1), cayaponoside B4 [18] (B4), cayaponoside D [17] (D), and siolmatroside I (SI) were isolated by us from the ethyl acetate fraction, as described previously [3] (Figure 5).

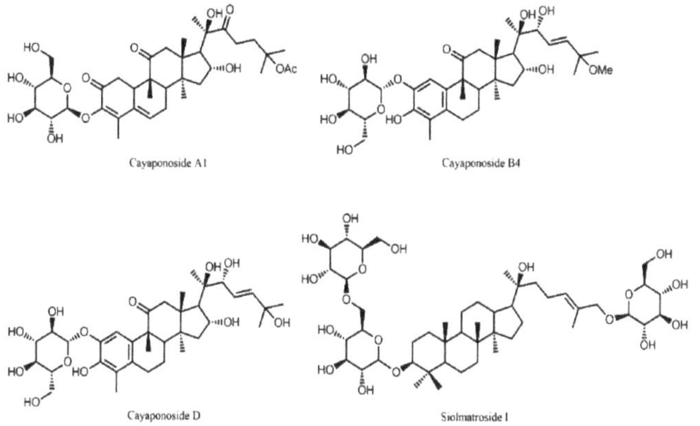

Figure 5. Saponins isolated from the ethyl acetate fraction of the stems of *S. brasiliensis*: Cayaponoside A1, cayaponoside B4, cayaponoside D, and siolmatroside I.

4.3. Animals

Animals used in this study (Swiss Webster mice (25–30g)) were donated by Instituto Vital Brazil (Niterói, Rio de Janeiro, Brazil) and maintained in a room with light-dark cycle of 12 h, 22 ± 2 °C, 60% to 80% humidity and food and water provided ad libitum. Before each test, the animals were acclimatized to the laboratory for at least 1 h. Twelve hours before each experiment the animals received only water in order to avoid food interference with substances absorption. Animals were daily monitored to assess their physical conditions and that with any signs of suffering were euthanized. None of the animals used became severely ill or died at any time prior to the experimental endpoint. At the end of each assay, animals were euthanized following AVMA guidelines. The experimental protocols used in this work have been carried out in accordance with the Guide for the Care and Use of Laboratory Animals as adopted and promulgated by the US National Institutes of Health, and were approved by the rules advocated by Law 11,794, of 8 October 2008 by the National Council of Animal Experimentation Control (CONCEA) and were approved by the Ethics Committee of Animal Use (CEUA)/UFRJ and received the number 31/19 and 34/19.

4.4. Extracts, Isolated Substances, and Control Drugs' Administration

Hydroethanol extract, fractions, and the isolated substances were dissolved in dimethylsulfoxide (DMSO, Sigma-Aldrich, St. Louis, MO, USA) in order to prepare a stock solution at 200 mg/mL. The hydroethanol extract (HE) and the ethyl acetate fraction (EtOAc) were tested at doses of 10, 30, or 100 mg/kg. Siolmatroside I (SI), cayaponoside D (D), cayaponoside B4 (B4), and cayaponoside A1 (A1) were tested at doses of 0.3, 1, or 3 mg/kg. All of them were administered by oral gavage in a final volume of 0.1 mL per animal randomly divided into groups of 6 to 8 mice. The final amount of DMSO used in higher dose (100 mg/kg) had no effect per se. Morphine (2.5 mg/kg) was used as a reference drug and was administered by oral gavage at the intervals indicated in each protocol. Control group was the given vehicle (ultrapure water with the same amount of DMSO used in higher dose).

4.5. Drugs and Reagents

Morphine sulfate and naloxone hydrochloride (both dissolved in phosphate buffer saline, PBS) were kindly provided by Cristália (São Paulo, Brazil). Atropine sulfate monohydrate (in PBS), capsaicin (in DMSO), L-glutamic acid hydrochloride (glutamate, in PBS), L-nitroarginine methyl ester (L-NAME, in PBS) were purchased from Sigma-Aldrich (St. Louis, MO, USA). All drugs were diluted just before their use.

4.6. Acute Toxicity

Acute toxicity parameters were determined following the method described by Lorke [19]. Oral dose of the HE, EtOAc (150 mg/kg), or isolated saponins (SI, D, B4, A1, 10 mg/kg) were administered to groups of ten mice (five males and five females). Parameters such as convulsion, sedation, reflex, hyperactivity, increased or decreased respiration, and food and water intake were observed at 1, 3, 6, 12, and every 24 h over a period of five days to analyze the behaviour of the animals. After that, mice's stomachs were removed in order to search for ulcers (single or multiple erosion, ulcer or perforation) and instances of hyperemia were counted.

4.7. Hot Plate Test

Mice were orally treated with substances, vehicle, or morphine and immediately placed on a hot plate apparatus (Insight Equipment, Brazil) set at 55 ± 1 °C. The time necessary for mice that licked their fore- and/or hind-paws (named reaction time) was measured at intervals of 30 min post-oral administration. Baseline was calculated with the use of measurements obtained at 60 and 30 min before the administration of the compounds, vehicle, or morphine and considered as a normal reaction of the animal to the temperature. The calculation of area under the curve (AUC) of responses from 30 min after drug administration until the end of the experiment was used to indicate the antinociception. The following formula based on the trapezoid rule was used to calculate the AUC: AUC = 30 × IB ((min 30) + (min 60) + ... + (min 180)/2), where IB is the increase from baseline (in %) [20,21].

4.8. Analysis of the Mechanisms of Action of Hydroethanol Extract (HE), Ethyl Acetate Fraction (EtOAc), and its Isolated Saponins

To investigate the involvement of the cholinergic, opioid, or nitrergic system in the mechanism of action of substances, some specific receptor antagonists and/or enzyme inhibitors were used. After 15 min of intraperitoneal administration of atropine (muscarinic receptor antagonist, 1 mg/kg), naloxone (opioid receptor antagonist, 1 mg/kg), or L-nitro arginine methyl ester (L-NAME, inhibitor of nitric oxide synthase enzyme, 3 mg/kg) mice received oral administration of HE or EtOAc (100 mg/kg each), SI, D, B4, or A1 (3 mg/kg each). Based on data from literature [22,23] and previous data from our own laboratory [24], dose response curves with agonists and respective antagonist were previously constructed and the dose of antagonist that reduced in 50% the agonist effect was chosen for these assays. The antinociceptive effect was evaluated in the hot plate test as described above.

4.9. Capsaicin- and Glutamate-Induced Nociception

The animals were pretreated 60 min before the intraplantar injection of capsaicin or glutamate with substances or vehicle by oral gavage. After treatment, mice received an intraplantar injection of capsaicin (20 µL, 1.6 µg/paw) or glutamate (20 µL, 3.7 ng/paw). Immediately animals were individually placed in a transparent box and the time that the animal kept licking the capsaicin- or glutamate-injected paw was recorded during a period of 5 min [25] and 15 min [26], respectively. The time mice spent licking the injected paw was recorded and this was considered as the nociceptive reaction.

4.10. Statistical Analysis

Experimental groups were composed of 6–8 mice and the results were presented as mean ± S.D. Statistical significance between groups was determined using the application of analyses of variance (ANOVA) followed by Dunnett´s post-test. Differences were considered significant (*) when $p < 0.05$. The area under the curve (AUC) was calculated using Prism Software 5.0 (Graph Pad Software, La Jolla, CA, USA).

5. Conclusion

Our work validated for the first time the antinociceptive activity in peripheral and central models of analgesia of *S. brasiliensis* ethanol extract, its ethyl acetate fraction, and its isolated saponins cayaponoside A1, cayaponoside B4, cayaponoside D, and siolmatroside I. The actions are mediated by opioid, nitrergic, and cholinergic systems and, in part by vanilloid receptors. Our study confirms that this species may be used for treating pain processes corroborating with its traditional use and contributing to the pharmacological knowledge of this Brazilian species.

Supplementary Materials: The following are available online. Table S1: Toxic effects of hydroethanol extract (HE), ethyl acetate fraction (EtOAc), siolmatroside I (SI), cayaponoside D (D), cayaponoside B4 (B4) and cayaponoside A1 (A1) observed at 1, 3, 6 or 12 hours post-oral administration. Table S2: Toxic effects of hydroethanol extract (HE), ethyl acetate fraction (EtOAc), siolmatroside I (SI), cayaponoside D (D), cayaponoside B4 (B4) and cayaponoside A1 (A1) observed at 1, 2, 3, 4 or 5 days post-oral administration; Table S3: Effects of hydroethanol extract (HE), ethyl acetate fraction (EtOAc), siolmatroside I (SI), cayaponoside D (D), cayaponoside B4 (B4) and cayaponoside A1 (A1) in water and food intake observed at 1, 2, 3, 4 or 5 days post-oral administration; table S4: Effects of hydroethanol extract (HE), ethyl acetate fraction (EtOAc), siolmatroside I (SI), cayaponoside D (D), cayaponoside B4 (B4) and cayaponoside A1 (A1) in the presence of ulcers or hyperemia 5 days post-oral administration.

Author Contributions: Conceptualization, T.B.S.G., M.G.d.C., P.T.d.S., F.B., and P.D.F.; Data curation, T.B.S.G., C.H.C.d.S., and P.D.F.; Formal analysis, T.B.S.G., C.H.C.d.S., M.G.d.C., V.C.d.S., F.B., and P.D.F.; Funding acquisition, M.G.d.C. and P.D.F.; Investigation, T.B.S.G., C.H.C.d.S., and P.T.d.S.; Methodology, T.B.S.G., C.H.C.d.S., and V.C.d.S.; Project administration, P.D.F.; Resources, V.C.d.S., P.T.d.S., and P.D.F.; Supervision, M.G.d.C. and P.D.F.; Writing—original draft, T.B.S.G.; Writing—review and editing, M.G.d.C., F.B., and P.D.F.

Funding: This research was funded by Conselho Nacional de Desenvolvimento Científico e Tecnológico (CNPq, Grant support and fellowship to PDF), Fundação Carlos Chagas Filho de Apoio à Pesquisa do Estado do Rio de Janeiro (FAPERJ, Grant support and fellowship to PDF and TBSG), Conselho de Administração de Pessoal de Ensino Superior (CAPES, fellowship to TBSG). FB also wishes to acknowledge the High Education Authority's Programme for Research in Third-Level Institutions Cycle 5's funding support for TBSI and to reinforce the importance of SFI programme ISCA-Brazil (Grant no. SFI/13/ISCA/2843).

Acknowledgments: Alan Minho for technical assistance and Instituto Vital Brazil (Niterói City, Brazil) for mice donation.

Conflicts of Interest: The authors declare no conflict of interest.

References

1. Lima, A.P.; Barbosa, C.E.S.; Pereira, F.C.; Vilanova-Costa, C.A.S.T.; Ribeiro, A.S.B.B.; Silva, H.D.; Azavedo, N.R.; Gomes-Klein, V.R.; Silveira-Lacerda, E.P. *Siolmatra brasiliensis* (Cogn.) Baill., Cucurbitaceae, acute toxicity in mice. *Rev. Bras. Farm.* **2010**, *20*, 917–921. [CrossRef]
2. Pott, A.; Pott, V.J. *Plantas do Pantanal*; Embrapa: Brasília, Brazil, 1994.
3. Santos, C.H.C.; Borges, I.P.; Silva, V.C.; Sousa, P.T.; Kawashita, N.H.; Baviera, A.M.; Carvalho, M.G. A new dammarane saponin and other triterpenoids from *Siolmatra brasiliensis* and evaluation of the antidiabetic activity of its extract. *Pharm. Biol.* **2016**, *54*, 1–9.
4. Mogil, J.S.; Adhikari, S.M. Hot and cold nociception are genetically correlated. *J. Neurosci.* **1999**, *19*, RC25. [CrossRef]
5. Ijeoma, U.F.; Aderonke, S.O.; Ogbonna, O.; Augustina, M.A.; Ifeyinwa, C.N. Antinociceptive and anti-inflammatory activities of crude extracts of Ipomoea involucrata leaves in mice and rats. *Asian Pac. J. Trop. Med.* **2011**, *4*, 121–124. [CrossRef]
6. Negri, G.; Mattei, R.; Mendes, F.R. Antinociceptive activity of the HPLC- and MS-standardized hydroethanolic extract of *Pterodon emarginatus* vogel leaves. *Phytomedicine* **2014**, *21*, 1062–1069. [CrossRef]
7. Adzu, B.; Amizan, M.B.; Okhale, S.E. Evaluation of antinociceptive and anti-inflammatory activities of standardised root bark extract of *Xeromphis nilotica*. *J. Ethnopharmacol.* **2014**, *158*, 271–275. [CrossRef]
8. Dandawate, P.R.; Subramaniam, D.; Padhye, S.B.; Anant, S. Bitter melon: A panacea for inflammation and cancer. *Chin. J. Nat. Med.* **2016**, *14*, 81–100. [CrossRef]
9. Wess, J.; Duttaroy, A.; Gomeza, J.; Zhang, W.; Yamada, M.; Felder, C.C.; Bernardini, N.; Reeh, P.W. Muscarinic receptor subtypes mediating central and peripheral antinociception studied with muscarinic receptor knockout mice: A review. *Life Sci.* **2003**, *72*, 2047–2954. [CrossRef]

10. Cury, Y.; Picolo, G.; Gutierrez, V.P.; Ferreira, S.H. Pain and analgesia: The dual effect of nitric in the nociceptive system. *Nitric Oxide* **2011**, *25*, 243–254. [CrossRef]
11. Khana, H.; Saeeda, M.; Gilanib, A.; Khanc, M.A.; Dard, A.; Khana, I. The antinociceptive activity of *Polygonatum verticillatum* rhizomes in pain models. *J. Ethnopharmacol.* **2010**, *127*, 521–527. [CrossRef]
12. Binotti, R.S.; Melo, A.M.T.; Oliveira, C.H.; De Nucci, G. Pimenta-vermelha (*Capsicum fructescens*—SOLANACEAE). *J. Bras. Fitomed.* **2003**, *1*, 6–11.
13. Jancso, G. Selective degeneration of chemo sensitive primary sensory neurons induced by capsaicin: Glial changes. *Cell Tissue Res.* **1978**, *195*, 145–152. [CrossRef]
14. Palazzo, E.; De Novellis, V.; Marabese, I.; Cuomo, D.; Rossi, F.; Berrino, L.; Rossi, F.; Maione, S. Interaction between vanilloid and glutamate receptors in the central modulation of nociception. *Eur. J. Pharm.* **2002**, *439*, 69–75. [CrossRef]
15. Afrah, A.W.; Stiller, C.O.; Olgart, L.; Brodin, E.; Gustafsson, H. Involvement of spinal N-methyl-D-aspartate receptors in capsaicin-induced in vivo release of substance P in the rat dorsal horn. *Neurosci. Lett.* **2001**, *316*, 83–86. [CrossRef]
16. Medvedeva, Y.V.; Kim, M.S.; Usachev, Y.M. Mechanisms of prolonged presynaptic Ca2þ signaling and glutamate release induced by TRPV1 activation in rat sensory neurons. *J. Neurosci.* **2008**, *28*, 5295–5311. [CrossRef]
17. Himeno, E.; Nagao, T.; Honda, J.; Okabe, H.; Irino, N.; Nakasumi, T. Structures of new non-aromatized *nor*-cucurbitacin glucosides in the roots of *Cayaponia tayuya*. *Chem. Pharm. Bull.* **1993**, *41*, 986–988. [CrossRef]
18. Himeno, E.; Nagao, T.; Honda, J.; Okabe, H.; Irino, N.; Nakasumi, T. Studies on the constituents of *Cayaponia tayuya* (Vell.) Cogn. I. Structures of Cayaponosides, new 29-nor-1,2,3,4,5,10-hexadehydrocucurbitacins glucosides. *Chem. Pharm. Bull.* **1994**, *42*, 2295–2300. [CrossRef]
19. Lorke, D. A new approach to practical acute toxicity testing. *Arch. Toxicol.* **1983**, *54*, 275–287. [CrossRef]
20. Sahley, T.L.; Berntson, G.G. Antinociceptive effects of central and systemic administration of nicotine in the rat. *Psychopharmacology* **1979**, *65*, 279–283. [CrossRef]
21. Matheus, M.E.; Berrondo, L.F.; Vieitas, E.C.; Menezes, F.S.; Fernandes, P.D. Evaluation of the antinociceptive properties from *Brillantaisia palisotii* Lindau stems extracts. *J. Ethnopharmacol.* **2005**, *102*, 377–381. [CrossRef]
22. Otuki, M.F.; Ferreira, J.; Lima, F.V.; Meyre-Silva, C.; Malheiros, A.; Muller, L.A.; Cani, G.S.; Santos, A.R.; Yunes, R.A.; Calixto, J.B. Antinociceptive properties of mixture of alpha-amyrin and beta-amyrintriterpenes: Evidence for participation of protein kinase C and protein kinase A pathways. *J. Pharm. Exp.* **2005**, *313*, 310–318. [CrossRef] [PubMed]
23. Tabarelli, Z.; Berlese, D.B.; Sauzem, P.D.; Rubin, M.A.; Missio, T.P.; Teixeira, M.V.; Sinhorin, A.P.; Martins, M.A.P.; Zanatta, N.; Bonacorso, H.G.; et al. Antinociceptive effect to novel pyrazolines in mice. *Braz. J. Med. Biol. Res.* **2004**, *37*, 1531–1540. [CrossRef] [PubMed]
24. Pinheiro, M.M.G.; Bessa, S.O.; Fingolo, C.E.; Kuster, R.M.; Matheus, M.E.; Menezes, F.S.; Fernandes, P.D. Antinociceptive activity of fractions from *Couroupita guianensis* Aubl. leaves. *J. Ethnopharmacol.* **2010**, *127*, 407–413. [CrossRef] [PubMed]
25. Sakurada, T.; Katsumata, K.; Tanno, K.; Sakurada, S.; Kisara, K. The Capsaicin test in mice for evaluating tachykinin antagonists in the spinal cord. *Neuropharmacology* **1992**, *31*, 1279–1285. [CrossRef]
26. Beirith, A.; Santos, A.R.S.; Calixto, J.B. Mechanisms underlying the nociception and paw oedema caused by injection of glutamate into the mouse paw. *Brain Res.* **2002**, *924*, 219–228. [CrossRef]

Sample Availability: Samples of the compounds hydroethanol extract (HE), ethyl acetate fraction (EtOAc), siolmatroside I (SI), cayaponoside D (D), cayaponoside B4 (B4) and cayaponoside A1 (A1) are available from the authors.

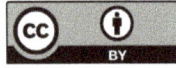

© 2019 by the authors. Licensee MDPI, Basel, Switzerland. This article is an open access article distributed under the terms and conditions of the Creative Commons Attribution (CC BY) license (http://creativecommons.org/licenses/by/4.0/).

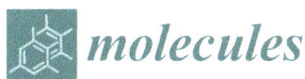

Article

Comprehensive Chemical Profiling and Multidirectional Biological Investigation of Two Wild *Anthemis* Species (*Anthemis tinctoria* var. *Pallida* and *A. cretica* subsp. *tenuiloba*): Focus on Neuroprotective Effects

Giustino Orlando [1,†], Gokhan Zengin [2,†], Claudio Ferrante [1,*], Maurizio Ronci [3], Lucia Recinella [1], Ismail Senkardes [4], Reneta Gevrenova [5], Dimitrina Zheleva-Dimitrova [5], Annalisa Chiavaroli [1], Sheila Leone [1], Simonetta Di Simone [1], Luigi Brunetti [1], Carene Marie Nancy Picot-Allain [6], Mohamad Fawzi Mahomoodally [6], Kouadio Ibrahime Sinan [2] and Luigi Menghini [1]

1. Department of Pharmacy, University "G. d'Annunzio" of Chieti-Pescara, 66100 Chieti, Italy
2. Department of Biology, Faculty of Science, Selcuk University, Konya 42130, Turkey
3. Department of Medical, Oral and Biotechnological Sciences, University "G. d'Annunzio" of Chieti-Pescara, 66100 Chieti, Italy
4. Department of Pharmaceutical Botany, Faculty of Pharmacy, Marmara University, Istanbul 34668, Turkey
5. Department of Pharmacognosy, Faculty of Pharmacy, Medical University of Sofia, 1431 Sofia, Bulgaria
6. Department of Health Sciences, Faculty of Science, University of Mauritius, Réduit 80837, Mauritius
* Correspondence: claudio.ferrante@unich.it; Tel.: +39-0871-355-4755
† These authors contributed equally to this work.

Academic Editors: Raffaele Capasso and Lorenzo Di Cesare Mannelli
Received: 1 July 2019; Accepted: 14 July 2019; Published: 16 July 2019

Abstract: Ethyl acetate (EA), methanol (MeOH), and aqueous extracts of aerial parts of *Anthemis tinctoria* var. *pallida* (ATP) and *A. cretica* subsp. *tenuiloba* (ACT) were investigated for their phenol and flavonoid content, antioxidant, and key enzyme inhibitory potentials. All extracts displayed antiradical effects, with MeOH and aqueous extracts being a superior source of antioxidants. On the other hand, EA and MeOH extracts were potent against AChE and BChE. Enzyme inhibitory effects against tyrosinase and α-glucosidase were observed, as well. We also studied *Anthemis* extracts in an ex vivo experimental neurotoxicity paradigm. We assayed extract influence on oxidative stress and neurotransmission biomarkers, including lactate dehydrogenase (LDH) and serotonin (5-HT), in isolated rat cortex challenged with K^+ 60 mM Krebs-Ringer buffer (excitotoxicity stimulus). An untargeted proteomic analysis was finally performed in order to explore the putative mechanism in the brain. The pharmacological study highlighted the capability of ACT water extract to blunt K^+ 60 mM increase in LDH level and 5-HT turnover, and restore physiological activity of specific proteins involved in neuron morphology and neurotransmission, including NEFMs, VAMP-2, and PKCγ, thus further supporting the neuroprotective role of ACT water extract.

Keywords: *Anthemis*; oxidative stress; neurotransmission; proteomic; phytomedicine

1. Introduction

Anthemis L is the second largest genus in Asteraceae family including more than 210 species, which are distributed in western Eurasia, Mediterranean and a small part of eastern Africa. According to the Flora of Turkey, the Anthemideae are divided into three subgenera (*Anthemis*, *Maruta* and *Cota*) and the subgenus *Anthemis* includes four sections; *Hiorthia*, *Anthemis*, *Maruta*, and *Chia* [1–3]. In Turkey, the genus is represented by 81 taxa belonging to 51 species, 29 (54%) of which are endemic. Species belonging to *Anthemis* genus are commonly referred to as "Papatya", in Turkey [1,4,5].

The species belonging to *Anthemis* genus are known to possess various biological properties and have found broad use in pharmaceutics, cosmetics, and food chemistry. The flowers of *Anthemis* species are well-documented for their use as antiseptic and healing herbs, with flavonoids, and essential oils being the main active components [2,6]. Extracts, tinctures, salves, and tisanes are extensively used as antispasmodic, anti-inflammatory, antibacterial and sedative agents, in Europe [5]. Extracts are also used to clean wounds and ulcers, and as therapy for irradiated skin injuries, cystitis and dental afflictions [2]. The antimicrobial activity of essential oils of several *Anthemis* species have been previously reported [7–10]. Moreover, *Anthemis* species are widely used to treat intestinal disorders, kidney stones, and hemorrhoids in traditional medicine. The plant is also used as antispasmodic medications and to stimulate menstrual flow. It is documented that the seed oil has been used in the treatment of earaches and deafness [11–13].

Anthemis genus is mainly characterized by the presence of sesquiterpene lactones, flavonoids and essential oils. Sesquiterpene lactones belonging to germacranolides, eudesmanolides, and guaianolides have been gained attention because of their chemo-ecological functions, biological activities and taxonomic significance. They are the major classes of secondary metabolites in *Anthemis* genus [2,3,14]. The essential oil compositions of several *Anthemis* species has also been investigated [2,12,15,16].

A. tinctoria var. *pallida* (ATP) is a rounded perennial plant measuring between 20 to 45 cm. The flowers are white or cream [17]. ATP, commonly known as yellow chamomile, produces a yellow dye used in food industry for production of diary and butchery products. Decoction of ATP flower is traditionally taken to treat shortness of breath, bronchitis, stomachache, anxiety, and to strengthen hair [18]. Aerial part of *Anthemis* species has been reported to exhibit antimicrobial property [17]. However, there is no record of the use of *A. cretica* subsp. *tenuiloba* (ACT) by folk populations, in Turkey.

To the best of our knowledge, there are no reports in literature investigating chemical profile and biological activities of ATP and ACT. Thus, we aimed to determine the chemical characterization and biological effects of these two *Anthemis* species. Phytochemical profiles of ethyl acetate (EA), methanol (MeOH) and aqueous extracts were performed by ultra-high-performance liquid chromatography coupled with electrospray ionization high resolution mass spectrometry (UHPLC-ESI/HRMS). The samples were assayed for evaluating antioxidant and enzyme inhibitory potential, as well.

Finally, considering both the traditional antianxiety effect of *A. tinctoria*, the relationships between anxiety and brain oxidative/inflammatory stress [19], alongside with the well-established multi-target protective effects exerted by flavonoid fraction, in the brain [20], we studied the putative protective role of *Anthemis* extracts in isolated rat cortex challenged with a neurotoxicity stimulus (K^+ 60 mM). The influence of extract supplementation on the levels of specific biomarkers of oxidative stress and neurotransmission, including lactate dehydrogenase (LDH) and serotonin (5-HT), was investigated using validated analytical methods. An untargeted proteomic profile was also performed on rat cortex homogenate, in order to explore the putative mechanism of action of *Anthemis* extracts. It is expected that results presented in this study will support the protective effects of the studied *Anthemis* extracts as potential pharmacological agents.

2. Results and Discussion

2.1. Total Phenolic and Flavonoid Contents

Phenolic compounds are of increasing interest mainly due to their diverse chemical structure and wide biological activity valuable in the prevention of some chronic or degenerative diseases. To this end, the evaluation of the phytochemical profile of plant extracts is important. In the present study, the total phenol and flavonoid contents of EA, MeOH, and aqueous extracts of ATP and ACT were illustrated in Table 1. The phenolic content of ATP and ACT ranged from 26.46 to 100.09 mg GAE/g and 21.31 to 47.61 mg GAE/g, respectively. Highest phenolic content was observed in the MeOH extract of

ATP, followed by its aqueous extract. Whilst for ACT, MeOH extract contained the highest amount of phenols, followed by EA extract. Regarding the total flavonoid content, the results showed that EA (ATP: 45.82 an ACT: 46.26 mg RE/g) and MeOH (ATP: 48.54 and ACT: 45.08 mg RE/g) extracts of both species were rich in flavonoids.

Table 1. Total phenol and flavonoid content of *Anthemis* extracts *.

Plant Names	Solvents	Total Phenol Content (mg GAE/g)	Total Flavonoid Content (mg RE/g)
A. tinctoria var. *pallida*	EA	26.46 ± 1.11 [d]	45.82 ± 0.40 [b]
	MeOH	100.09 ± 2.83 [a]	48.54 ± 0.57 [a]
	Aqueous	86.74 ± 1.80 [b]	23.10 ± 0.13 [d]
A. cretica subsp. *tenuiloba*	EA	21.31 ± 1.58 [e]	46.26 ± 0.25 [b]
	MeOH	46.73 ± 0.80 [c]	45.08 ± 0.26 [c]
	Aqueous	47.61 ± 1.89 [c]	21.17 ± 0.24 [e]

* Values expressed are means ± S.D. of three parallel measurements. GAE: Gallic acid equivalent; RE: Rutin equivalent. Different letters indicate significant differences in the extracts ($p < 0.05$).

2.2. LC-MS Results

In the present study, 70 compounds were tentatively identified by UHPLC-ESI/MS in both ACT and ATP extracts. The negative ion mode was used for analysis of acylquinic acids and flavonoids, while positive ion mode was used for sesquiterpenes determination (Table 2).

2.2.1. Acylquinic Acids

Twenty nine acylquinic acids were identified in tested *Anthemis* extracts (Table 2). The acylquinic acids elucidation was based on the hierarchical key developed by Clifford and colleagues [21,22]. Peaks **4**, **5**, **6**, and **7** were identified as 3-*O*-, 1-*O*-, 5-*O*- and 4-*O*-caffeoylquinic acids ($[M - H]^-$ at m/z 353.088), respectively, according to the relative abundance of the characteristic fragment ions at m/z 191.055 [quinic acid − H]$^-$, 179.034 [caffeic acid − H]$^-$, 173.045 [quinic acid − H − H_2O]$^-$, and 135.044 [caffeic acid − H − CO_2]$^-$ [21,22]. Compounds **4** and **6** were identified by comparison with neochlorogenic and chlorogenic acid, respectively. In the same manner, peaks **1**, **2**, and **3** were assigned as 3-*O*-, 5-*O*-, and 1-*O*-*p*-coumaroylquinic acids ($[M - H]^-$ at m/z 337.093), while peaks **8**, **9**, **10**, and **11** ($[M - H]^-$ at m/z 367.103) were assigned as 3-*O*-, 1-*O*- 5-*O*-, and 4-*O*-feruloylquinic acid (Table 4). With respect to the diacylquinic acids, peaks **12–15** were related to 3,4-*O*-, 1,5-*O*, 3,5-*O*, and 4,5-*O*-dicaffeoylquinic acids ($[M - H]^-$ at m/z 515.120); **12** and **13** were identified by comparison with standards. The presence of **14** was evidenced by the relative abundance of the ions at m/z 191.055, 179.034, and 135.043 [21–23], while the ion at 173.044 was prominent for **15**. Compounds **16–24**, $[M - H]^-$ at m/z 529.136 were tentatively identified as caffeoylferuloylquinic acids [21,22]. Among the tricaffeoylquinic acids, peaks **25–29** were related to ($[M - H]^-$ at m/z 677.152). Compounds **26**, **28**, and **29** yielded indicative fragment ions at 173.045 deduced 4-substituted CQA [22]. According to the presence of weak signal at m/z 203.034, the relative intensity of the fragment ion at m/z 335.078, and lipophilicity, peaks **26**, **28**, and **29** were tentatively assigned as 1,3,4-*O*-, 1,4,5-*O*-, and 3,4,5-*O*-tricaffeoylquinic acid, while **25** and **27** were related to 3,4,5-*O*-tricaffeoylquinic acid and its isomer.

2.2.2. Flavonoids

Based on literature and comparison with standards, 15 flavonoid aglycones **30–44** (most of them methoxylated), twelve glycosides, and one caffeoyl-*O*-flavonoid were identified in the studied extracts (Table 4). Regarding **41–43** ($[M - H]^-$ at m/z 345.061), the fragment ion at m/z 287.020, due to consecutive loss of 2CH_3^- and CO is more intense in the product-ion spectra of **43** than **41** and **42**. Probably methoxylation of **43** in both A- and C-rings provides very stable fragments due to concurrent methyl loss [24]. Fragment ion at m/z 121.028 (^{1,2}B) (for **41** and **42**) were attributed to the Retro-Diels Alder

(RDA) cleavages of the flavonoid skeleton specific for 3′,4′-dihydroxy flavonols [25]. Thus, according to literature, **41–43** were tentatively identified as eupatolitin, spinatoside, and spinacetin, respectively.

The fragmentation fingerprints of **52** and **56** were associated with isorhamnetin derivatives, witnessed by the abundant fragment ion at m/z 315.051 supported by the ions at m/z 300.027 and 133.028 [24]. Fragmentation patterns and monoisotopic profiles of **52** was in good agreement with those of caffeoyl-O-isorhamnetin. The fragmentation of [M − H]$^-$ at m/z 609.1472 (**56**) yielded abundant ion at m/z 315.0517 ([M − H − 294.095]$^-$ indicating the loss of hexose and pentose moieties.

2.2.3. Sesquiterpenes

Thirteen sesquiterpene lactones including one eudesmanolide, three germacranolides, and nine guaianolides, were tentatively identified in both ACT and ATP extracts. Concerning compound **58** ([M + H]$^+$ at m/z 229.122), its fragmentation pattern involved losses of 18 Da (H$_2$O), 28 Da (CO) and 46 Da (CO$_2$H) suggesting chamazulene carboxylic acid, a degradation product of proazulenic sesquiterpene lactones, e.g., matricarin [25]. Similar fragmentation patterns were observed in spectra of **59** and **60**. In addition, a loss of 44 Da (CO$_2$) and fragment ions at m/z 185.095 ([M + H − 16 − 44]$^+$ and 95.049 (C$_6$H$_7$O) due to the overall fracture of lactone ring, suggested dehydroleucodin or isodehydroleucodin [26]. Accordingly, **61** was assigned as leucodin ([M + H]$^+$ at m/z 247.132), where C-13 was saturated in a methyl group. **68** and **69** were tentatively identified as matricarin and its isomer, due to the concomitant loss of (CO$_2$ + H$_2$O) at m/z 245.117 from the additional acetyl group [3]. Three isobaric sesquiterpene lactones **63–65** shared the same [M + H]$^+$ at m/z 263.127 (exact mass). Peaks **63–65** demonstrated difference of 15.995 Da, in comparison to **61**, suggesting the presence of an additional hydroxyl group. Thus **63–65** were tentatively assigned to hydroxyleucodin and its isomers [27]. In the same manner, peaks **62**, isobaric pair **66/67**, and **70** were ascribed as parthenolide, stizolin, and ludalbine, respectively, previously identified in *Anthemis* species [3].

2.3. Antioxidant Activity

Oxidative stress-related diseases often arise as a result of the imbalance between the production of free radicals and reactive oxygen/nitrogen species, and antioxidant defences. These diseases can be managed/prevented using natural antioxidants that represent promising therapeutic candidates [29]. Different antioxidant assays are needed to obtain certain information regarding antioxidant profile of herbal extracts. From this point, the antioxidant capacity of different extracts of ATP and ACT were evaluated using multiple assays based on different mechanisms and the results were presented in Table 3.

Table 2. Peak assessment of compounds in *Anthemis* extracts.

Peak №	Accurate Mass [M − H]$^-$ m/z	Molecular Formula	MS/MS Data m/z	t_R min	Exact Mass [M − H]$^-$ m/z	Delta ppm	Tentative Structure	Ref.
			Acylquinnic acids					
			Monoacylquinic acids					
1	337.0946	$C_{16}H_{17}O_8$	337.0946 (3.1), 191.0557 (7.7), 173.0453 (2.5), 163.0390 (100), 119.0488 (22.8)	3.05	337.0929	5.071	3-*p*-coumaroyl-quinic acid [1,2,6]	[19]
2	337.0932	$C_{16}H_{17}O_8$	337.0932 (7.2), 191.0554 (100), 173.0445 (6.7), 163.0390 (5.8), 119.0489 (5.5), 93.0329 (17.6)	4.07	337.0929	0.829	5-*p*-coumaroyl-quinic acid [1,2,3,5,6]	[19]
3	337.0930	$C_{16}H_{17}O_8$	337.0930 (5.9), 191.0554 (100), 173.0446 (1.9), 163.0391 (2.4), 127.0391 (1.5), 119.0487 (1.4), 111.0439 (1.3), 93.0331 (5.3), 85.0280 (7.1)	4.74	337.0929	0.473	1-*p*-coumaroyl-quinic acid [1,2,5,6]	[19]
4	353.0879	$C_{16}H_{17}O_9$	353.0879 (32.4), 191.0553 (100), 179.0341 (60.7), 173.0443 (4.1), 161.0233 (3.9), 135.0439 (50.7), 111.0438 (0.9), 93.0333 (4.5), 85.0279 (8.7)	2.47	353.0867	0.325	neochlorogenic (3-caffeoylquinic) acid [1,2,3,4,6]	*
5	353.0879	$C_{16}H_{17}O_9$	353.0879 (29.9), 191.0554 (47.7), 179.0341 (70.1), 173.0447 (100), 135.0439 (57.7), 111.0436 (3.3), 93.331 (22.6), 85.0280 (8.6)	2.48	353.0867	0.240	1-caffeoylquinic acid [1,2,3,4,6]	[19]
6	353.0880	$C_{16}H_{17}O_9$	353.0880 (3.8), 191.0554 (100), 179.0338 (1.4), 173.0446 (0.9), 161.0234 (2.1), 135.0441 (1.1), 111.0435 (1.2), 93.0331 (2.7), 85.0279 (0.4)	3.30	353.0867	0.495	chlorogenic (5-caffeoylquinic) acid [1,2,3,4,5,6]	*
7	353.0880	$C_{16}H_{17}O_9$	353.0880 (28.1), 203.6057 (0.1), 191.0554 (100), 179.0341 (58.3), 173.0446 (4.6), 161.0233 (3.9), 135.0438 (51.8), 111.0437 (2.2), 93.0330 (4.82), 85.0279 (10.2)	5.92	353.0867	0.665	4-caffeoylquinic acid [1,2,3,4,6]	[19]
8	367.1043	$C_{17}H_{19}O_9$	367.1043 (12.5), 193.0500 (100), 173.0453 (3.9), 149.0598 (2.9), 134.0361 (65.7), 127.0395 (1.0), 111.0439 (1.4), 93.0331 (2.9)	3.54	367.1034	2.410	3-feruloylquinic acid [1,2,5,6]	[19]
9	367.1039	$C_{17}H_{19}O_9$	367.1039 (49.3), 161.0234 (100), 127.0390 (1.7), 85.0281 (13.4)	3.97	367.1034	1.238	1-feruloylquinic acid [1,2,5,6]	[19]
10	367.1035	$C_{17}H_{19}O_9$	367.1035 (14.1), 193.0499 (6.7), 191.0555 (100), 173.0447 (18.2), 134.0447 (10.9), 111.0437 (3.9), 93.0331 (26.2), 85.0280 (5.3)	4.52	367.1034	−0.015	5-feruloylquinic acid [1,2,3,4,5,6]	[19]
11	367.1030	$C_{17}H_{19}O_9$	367.1030 (11.8), 193.0499 (17.1), 173.0446 (100), 111.0435 (3.1), 93.0331 (24.0)	4.78	367.1034	−1.322	4-feruloylquinic acid [1,2,5,6]	[19]

Table 2. Cont.

Peak №	Accurate Mass [M − H]− m/z	Molecular Formula	MS/MS Data m/z	t_R min	Exact Mass [M − H]− m/z	Delta ppm	Tentative Structure	Ref.
			Diacylquinic acids					
12	515.1196	$C_{25}H_{23}O_{12}$	515.1196 (100), 353.0880 (18.5), 335.0788 (6.4), 203.0331 (1.3), 191.0554 (29.5), 179.0341 (58.1), 173.0446 (65.7), 161.0235 (19.8), 135.0439 (57.5), 127.0389 (3.6), 111.0436 (4.7), 93.0330 (18.7), 85.0277 (4.3)	5.79	515.1184	0.137	3,4-dicaffeoylquinic acid [1,2,3,4,5,6]	*
13	515.1199	$C_{25}H_{23}O_{12}$	515.1199 (21.8), 353.0881 (83.1), 335.0782 (2.6), 191.0554 (100), 179.0341 (48.6), 173.0445 (10.6), 161.0233 (12.4), 135.0439 (57.5), 127.0387 (2.8), 93.0332 (6.4), 85.0280 (9.0)	5.96	515.1184		1,5-dicaffeoylquinic acid [1,2,3,4,5,6]	*
14	515.1204	$C_{25}H_{23}O_{12}$	515.1204 (22.6), 353.0880 (87.4), 191.0555 (100), 179.0342 (52.0), 173.0455 (9.8), 161.0235 (8.9), 135.0438 (51.7), 93.0333 (2.8), 85.0281 (8.6),	6.14	515.1184	1.787	3,5-dicaffeoylquinic acid [3,4]	[28]
15	515.1199	$C_{25}H_{23}O_{12}$	515.1199 (75.6), 353.0880 (60.6), 203.0343 (3.1), 191.0555 (34.7), 179.0342 (72.3), 173.0447 (100), 135.0440 (48.1), 127.0384 (1.2), 111.0439 (3.7), 93.0330 (17.2), 85.0280 (4.2)	6.34	515.1184	0.720	4,5-dicaffeoylquinic acid [1,2,3,4,5,6]	[28]
16	529.1356	$C_{26}H_{25}O_{12}$	529.1356 (100), 367.1037 (8.3), 353.0889 (7.4), 349.0935 (5.2), 335.0774 (11.8), 193.0499 (60.5), 191.0555 (9.2), 179.0342 (42.1), 173.0446 (48.1), 161.0235 (24.6), 149.0596 (1.1), 134.0361 (56.0), 111.0437 (8.9), 93.0331 (14.7), 85.0276 (2.7)	6.00	529.1351	0.889	3-feruloyl-5-caffeoylquinic acid [1,2,4,5,6]	[28]
17	529.1357	$C_{26}H_{25}O_{12}$	529.1357 (55.4), 367.1038 (25.6), 193.0499 (2.6), 179.0342 (3.0), 173.0449 (1.9), 161.0234 (100), 135.0441 (12.7), 134.0367 (4.3), 127.0380 (0.5), 93.0331 (1.1), 85.0279 (3.2)	6.92	529.1351	1.003	1-feruloyl-5-caffeoylquinic acid [1,2,3,5]	[28]
18	529.1354	$C_{26}H_{25}O_{12}$	529.1354 (38.3), 367.1040 (39.6), 353.0883 (44.99), 193.0506 (15.6), 191.0555 (100), 179.0343 (41.61), 173.0454 (14.8), 161.0239 (13.0), 135.0440 (52.3), 134.0363 (21.5), 93.0332 (14.2), 85.0281 (7.4)	7.00	529.1351	0.436	3-caffeoyl-5-feruloylquinic acid [1,2,3,4]	[28]
19	529.1352	$C_{26}H_{25}O_{12}$	529.1352 (66.9), 367.1044 (100), 193.0504 (12.1), 179.0333 (57.2), 173.0447 (76.9), 161.0236 (15.6), 135.0439 (73.7), 134.0365 (49.6), 93.0331 (76.7)	7.12	529.1351	0.077	4-feruloyl-5-caffeoylquinic acid [4,5,6]	[28]
20	529.1361	$C_{26}H_{25}O_{12}$	529.1361 (14.2), 367.1036 (60.3), 193.0499 (14.5), 173.0447 (100), 161.0239 (1.1), 134.0362 (17.5), 127.0392 (1.0), 111.0436 (3.4), 93.0330 (24.9),	7.23	529.1351	1.816	3-caffeoyl-4-feruloylquinic acid [1,2,3,6]	[28]

Table 2. *Cont.*

Peak №	Accurate Mass [M − H]⁻ m/z	Molecular Formula	MS/MS Data m/z	t_R min	Exact Mass [M − H]⁻ m/z	Delta ppm	Tentative Structure	Ref.
21	529.1388	$C_{26}H_{25}O_{12}$	529.1388 (83.7), 353.0898 (56.5), 191.0550 (75.9), 179.0346 (79.9), 173.0448 (100), 161.0237 (11.9), 135.0439 (69.8), 93.0330 (38.2)	7.28	529.1351	6.880	4-caffeoyl-5-feruloylquinic acid [4,5,6]	[28]
22	529.1356	$C_{26}H_{25}O_{12}$	529.1356 (74.2), 367.1031 (21.5), 349.0925 (2.1), 191.0554 (1.2), 179.0341 (30.5), 173.0446 (4.94), 161.0234 (100), 135.0439 (49.6), 93.0331 (1.9)	7.34	529.1351	0.776	1-feruloyl-3-caffeoylquinic acid [1,2,3,5]	[28]
23	529.1348	$C_{26}H_{25}O_{12}$	529.1348 (100), 367.1052 (45.3), 179.0348 (10.3), 173.0449 (60.2), 161.0237 (24.0), 135.0441 (16.4), 111.0439 (13.0), 93.0331 (77.1)	7.44	529.1351	−0.717	4-feruloyl-?-caffeoylquinic acid [4,6]	**
24	529.1353	$C_{26}H_{25}O_{12}$	529.1353 (74.9), 367.1037(19.5), 349.0932 (4.4), 179.0341 (73.22), 161.0234 (62.3), 135.0439 (100), 134.0364 (12.4), 93.0331 (0.6), 85.0276 (0.5)	7.71	529.1351	0.304	1-feruloyl-3-caffeoylquinic acid-isomer [1,2,5,6]	**
			Triacylquinic acids					
25	677.1523	$C_{34}H_{29}O_{15}$	677.1523 (2.9), 515.1105 (44.5), 353.0903 (3.7), 341.0888 (4.4), 191.0552 (9.6), 179.0341 (100), 173.0446 (6.0), 161.0230 (4.6), 135.0439 (79.8), 111.0443 (1.0), 93.0331 (1.6)	4.85	677.1512	1.634	1,3,5-tricaffeoylquinic acid [1,2,4,5,6]	[28]
26	677.1524	$C_{34}H_{29}O_{15}$	677.1524 (89.2), 515.1190 (17.3), 353.0879 (25.83), 341.0876 (8.0), 335.0772 (23.0), 323.0791 (5.1), 203.1523 (0.9), 191.0552 (30.6), 179.0341 (71.0), 173.0446 (54.7), 161.0233 (46.0), 135.0439 (100), 127.0388 (4.3), 111.0437 (7.8), 93.0330 (19.3), 85.0280 (1.9)	5.26	677.1512	1.812	1,3,4-tricaffeoylquinic acid [1,2,3,5,6]	[28]
27	677.1529	$C_{34}H_{29}O_{15}$	677.1529 (52.3), 515.1200 (55.7), 353.0878 (26.0), 341.0900 (15.6), 191.0553 (57.3), 179.0338 (75.3), 173.0449 (31.1), 161.0236 (34.66), 135.0439(100), 93.0328 (7.5)	5.37	677.1512	2.447	1,3,5-tricaffeoylquinic acid [2,5,6] isomer	**
28	677.1524	$C_{34}H_{29}O_{15}$	677.1524 (87.1), 515.1281 (24.3), 353.0878 (26.2), 341.0880 (31.5), 335.0787 (2.3), 323.0779 (10.6), 191.0555 (34.4), 179.0342 (94.0), 173.0447 (78.7), 161.0235 (21.9), 135.0439 (100), 111.0439 (2.2), 93.0331 (24.8), 85.0279 (4.8)	5.66	677.1512	1.812	1,4,5-tricaffeoylquinic acid [1,2,5,6]	[28]
29	677.1519	$C_{34}H_{29}O_{15}$	677.1519 (88.4), 515.1203 (30.3), 353.0881 (55.6), 335.0779 (19.1), 203.0344 (1.3), 191.0554 (57.4), 179.0341 (79.9), 173.0447 (100), 161.0234 (33.1), 135.0439 (95.5), 111.0437 (1.1), 93.0331 (28.3), 85.0278 (6.3)	7.85	677.1512	0.985	3,4,5-tricaffeoylquinic acid [1,2,3,4,5]	[28]

245

Table 2. Cont.

Peak №	Accurate Mass [M − H]− m/z	Molecular Formula	MS/MS Data m/z	t_R min	Exact Mass [M − H]− m/z	Delta ppm	Tentative Structure	Ref.
			Flavonoids					
30	269.0457	$C_{15}H_9O_5$	269.0457 (100), 151.0027 (6.39), 149.0233 (5.74), 117.0332 (22.24), 107.0124 (5.35)	8.73	269.0444	0.644	apigenin [1,2,3,4,5,6]	*
31	285.0406	$C_{15}H_9O_6$	285.0406 (100), 151.0028 (5.92), 133.0282 (25.08), 107.0126 (3.32)	7.82	285.0393	0.452	luteolin [1,2,3,4,5,6]	*
32	287.0566	$C_{15}H_{11}O_6$	287.0566 (14.91), 151.0025 (100), 135.0435 (89.99), 125.0231 (5.03), 107.0124 (13.58)	7.53	287.0550	1.842	eriodictyol [1,2,3,4,5,6]	[24]
33	299.0561	$C_{16}H_{11}O_6$	299.0561 (58.00), 284.0328 (100), 256.0382 (0.86), 227.0350 (3.45), 211.0393 (2.22)	8.91	299.0550	0.029	diosmetin [1,2,3,4,5,6]	*
34	299.0562	$C_{16}H_{11}O_6$	299.0562 (95.99), 284.9335 (100), 227.047 (2.78), 151.0033 (3.67), 107.0123 (2.84)	9.09	299.0550	0.430	3,4',7-trihydroxy-3'-methoxyflavone [1,2,3,4,5,6]	[23]
35	301.0352	$C_{15}H_9O_7$	301.0352 (100), 300.0273 (24.24), 178.9976 (21.40), 151.0025 (49.72), 121.0282 (16.11), 107.0124 (14.15)	7.83	301.0342	−0.717	quercetin [1,2,3,4,5,6]	*
36	315.0512	$C_{16}H_{11}O_7$	315.0512 (61.55), 300.0279 (100), 271.0252 (28.24), 255.030 (11.23), 227.0349 (2.28), 136.9872 (2.51),	8.34	315.0499	0.584	nepetin [4,5,6]	Mass bank
37	315.0513	$C_{16}H_{11}O_7$	315.0513 (86.15), 301.0315 (11.76), 300.0276 (100), 243.0303 (0.70), 165.9890 (1.63), 136.9868 (9.78)	7.90	315.0499	0.965	rhamnetin [1,2,3,4,5,6]	*
38	315.0514	$C_{16}H_{11}O_7$	315.0514 (100), 301.0316 (3.73), 300.0273 (41.59), 243.0298 (1.08), 151.0025 (7.85), 107.0126 (6.32)	9.26	315.0499	1.156	isorhamnetin [1,2,3,4,5,6]	*
39	329.0670	$C_{17}H_{13}O_7$	329.0607 (14.45), 314.0436 (100), 299.0198 (25.08), 271.0250 (47.23), 133.0282 (5.34), 107.2971 (0.52)	9.25	329.0655	0.954	jaceosidin [1,3,4,6]	Mass bank
40	331.0463	$C_{16}H_{11}O_8$	331.0463 (100), 316.0226 (56.40), 287.0199 (15.97), 271.0246 (5.47), 270.0176 (4.09), 165.9897 (19.03)	7.80	331.0448	1.086	patuletin [1,3,4,6]	[23]
41	345.0618	$C_{17}H_{13}O_8$	345.0618 (91.18), 330.0384 (100), 315.0150 (50.33), 287.0201 (15.30), 121.0280 (1.86)	8.36	345.0604	0.694	eupatuletin [4,5,6]	**
42	345.0618	$C_{17}H_{13}O_8$	345.0618 (100), 330.0385 (95.66), 315.0150 (46.41), 287.0198 (14.78), 121.0284 (7.72)	8.40	345.0604	0.694	spinatoside [1,2,3]	[23]
43	345.0619	$C_{17}H_{13}O_8$	345.0619 (100), 330.0385 (42.35), 315.0145 (4.01), 301.0388 (6.46), 287.0199 (40.72)	9.38	345.0604	0.694	spinacetin [1,2,3]	[23]
44	359.0775	$C_{18}H_{15}O_8$	359.0775 (100), 344.0539 (49.89), 329.0304 (52.64), 301.0359 (6.67), 287.0139 (4.46)	9.95	359.0761	0.750	jaceidin [1,2,3,4,5,6]	[23]

Table 2. Cont.

Peak №	Accurate Mass [M − H]⁻ m/z	Molecular Formula	MS/MS Data m/z	t_R min	Exact Mass [M − H]⁻ m/z	Delta ppm	Tentative Structure	Ref.
45	431.0981	$C_{21}H_{19}O_{10}$	431.0981 (100), 269.0440 (27.72), 268.0378 (57.01)	6.17	431.0972	−0.673	apigenin-7-O-glucoside 1,2,3,4,5,6	*
46	447.0934	$C_{21}H_{19}O_{11}$	447.0934 (100), 327.0507 (0.95), 285.0405 (99.96), 151.0030 (7.20), 133.0280 (5.74), 107.0123 (4.57)	5.45	447.0921	0.348	luteolin-7-O-glucoside 1,2,3,4,5,6	*
47	461.0725	$C_{21}H_{17}O_{12}$	461.0725 (42.84), 285.0406 (100), 151.0025 (3.72), 133.0280 (10.72), 107.0121 (1.50)	5.46	461.0714	−0.150	luteolin-7-O-glucuronide 1,2,3	*
48	461.1094	$C_{22}H_{21}O_{11}$	461.1094 (100), 446.0858 (28.76), 299.0554 (12.48), 284.0313 (9.73), 283.0250 (21.41), 269.0467 (2.08), 255.0300 (73.76), 227.0345 (0.67), 151.0028 (0.86)	6.37	461.1078	2.220	diosmetin-O-glucoside 1,2,3	**
49	463.0887	$C_{21}H_{19}O_{12}$	463.0887 (100), 372.1873 (4.84), 301.0360 (93.71), 300.0282 (27.20)	4.77	463.0871	1.038	isoquercitrin 1,2,3,4,5,6	*
50	463.0903	$C_{21}H_{19}O_{12}$	463.0903 (100), 301.0349 (47.50), 300.0276 (66.34)	5.29	463.0871	4.601	hyperoside 1,2,3,4,5,6	*
51	477.1041	$C_{22}H_{21}O_{12}$	477.1041 (100), 315.0496 (14.04), 314.0434 (53.04), 300.0274 (5.68), 285.0411 (6.84), 243.0297 (22.73), 271.0249 (27.98), 151.0032 (3.66)	6.10	477.1027	0.442	isorhamnetin-7-O-glucoside 1,2,3,4,5,6	*
52	493.0777	$C_{25}H_{17}O_{11}$	493.0777 (11.58), 315.0512 (99.41), 314.0435 (100), 300.0277 (14.30), 285.0411 (13.30), 243.0293 (34.06), 227.0341 (4.04), 177.0182 (16.10), 151.0030 (4.86), 133.0283 (12.50)	9.12	493.0765	0.194	caffeoyl-O-isorhamnetin 1,3	**
53	493.0974	$C_{22}H_{21}O_{13}$	493.0974 (100), 331.0463 (96.71), 316.0224 (22.61), 287.0196 (26.93), 271.0253 (9.58), 165.9891 (8.24)	5.63	493.0976	−0.257	patuletin-O-hexoside 4,5,6	**
54	593.1504	$C_{27}H_{29}O_{15}$	593.1504 (97.39), 318.6214 (6.24), 285.0405 (100), 284.0327 (60.74), 227.0352 (29.58)	5.71	593.1500	−1.354	luteolin-7-O-rutinoside 1,2,3,4,5,6	*
55	609.1467	$C_{27}H_{29}O_{16}$	609.1467 (72.52), 343.0477 (1.65), 301.0354 (100), 300.0278 (38.67), 178.9970 (1.59), 151.0027 (13.46),121.0279 (1.84), 107.0123 (4.76)	5.17	609.1450	0.923	rutin 1,2,3,4,5,6	*
56	609.1472	$C_{27}H_{29}O_{16}$	609.1472 (96.84), 411.8945 (5.23), 315.0517 (100), 300.0275 (48.87), 133.0284 (7.86)	5.43	609.1450	2.149	isorhamnetin-O-pentosyl-hexoside 4,5,6	**
57	623.1613	$C_{28}H_{31}O_{16}$	623.1613 (5.57), 315.0514 (100), 301.0306 (1.22), 300.0279 (16.19), 151.0025 (7.85), 107.0125 (3.48)	6.08	623.1606	−0.703	isorhamnetin-3-O-rutinoside 1,2,3,4,5,6	*

Table 2. *Cont.*

Peak №	Accurate Mass [M − H]⁻ *m/z*	Molecular Formula	MS/MS Data *m/z*	t_R min	Exact Mass [M − H]⁻ *m/z*	Delta ppm	Tentative Structure	Ref.
			Sesquiterpenes					
58	229.1220	$C_{15}H_{17}O_2$	229.1220 (100), 211.1116 (12.69), 201.1272 (19.57), 183.1167 (40.99), 91.0548 (6.40),	6.10	229.1223	−3.643	chamazulene carboxylic acid [1,2,3]	[25]
59	245.1170	$C_{15}H_{17}O_3$	245.1170 (100), 227.1067 (44.35), 217.1222 (20.20), 201.0910 (20.68), 199.1116 (75.08), 185.0959 (28.15), 95.0497 (66.93)	10.48	245.1172	−0.942	dehydroleucodin/ isodehydroleucodin [1,2,3]	[26]
60	245.1171	$C_{15}H_{17}O_3$	245.1171 (84.77), 227.1065 (44.23), 217.1225 (17.55), 201.0910 (17.75), 199.1116 (63.86), 185.0960 (18.51), 95.0497 (100)	10.48	245.1172	−0.942	dehydroleucodin/ isodehydroleucodin [1,2,3]	[26]
61	247.1325	$C_{15}H_{19}O_3$	247.1325 (100), 229.1220 (90.72), 211.1113 (8.83), 201.1271 (37.99), 187.0752 (37.99), 183.1167 (22.85), 91.0548 (9.16)	9.79	247.1328	−1.663	desacetoxymatricarin [1,2,3,4,5,6]	**
62	249.1481	$C_{15}H_{21}O_3$	249.1481 (100), 231.1378 (30.41), 213.1277 (9.04), 203.1431 (10.25), 193.0856 (5.87), 189.1272 (11.79), 159.1167 (22.04), 119.0857 (16.94), 105.0702 (18.62), 95.0860 (10.61)	10.42	249.1485	−0.451	parthenolide [1,2,3,4,5,6]	**
63	263.1275	$C_{15}H_{19}O_4$	263.1275 (100), 245.1170 (55.39), 227.1061 (9.88), 219.1021 (15.59), 217.1223 (47.56), 203.1065 (10.39), 199.1115 (21.45), 191.0704 (28.72), 95.0497 (96.99)	10.52	263.1277	−0.316	hydroxyleucodin [1,2,3]	**
64	263.1274	$C_{15}H_{19}O_4$	263.1274 (100), 245.1171 (33.08), 227.1063 (4.95), 219.1012 (14.30), 217.1224 (16.65), 203.1065 (10.12), 199.1117 (15.19), 191.0702 (79.26), 95.0497 (20.99)	11.22	263.1277	−0.406	hydroxyleucodin isomer [1,2,3]	**
65	263.1275	$C_{15}H_{19}O_4$	263.1275(100), 245.1170 (51.98), 227.1063 (11.55), 219.1014 (34.60), 217.1223 (47.24), 203.1067 (12.57), 199.1117 (22.59), 191.0702 (32.46), 95.0497 (81.14)	11.22	263.1277	−0.406	hydroxyleucodin isomer [1,2,3]	**
66	265.1432	$C_{15}H_{21}O_4$	265.1432 (8.16), 247.1326 (34.45), 229.1221 (100), 211.1115 (3.94), 201.1273 (20.45), 187.0752 (14.30), 183.1168 (7.67), 91.0548 (5.66)	6.04	265.1434	−0.813	stizolin [1,3]	**
67	265.1429	$C_{15}H_{21}O_4$	265.1429 (24.21), 247.1325 (100), 229.1222 (71.63), 219.1372 (36.25), 201.1272 (55.14), 187.1111 (17.50), 183.1174 (17.90), 91.0548 (13.40)	9.78	265.1434	−1.982	stizolin isomer [1,3]	**

Table 2. Cont.

Peak №	Accurate Mass [M − H]⁻ m/z	Molecular Formula	MS/MS Data m/z	t_R min	Exact Mass [M − H]⁻ m/z	Delta ppm	Tentative Structure	Ref.
68	305.1360	$C_{17}H_{21}O_5$	305.1360 (44.97), 287.1268 (3.27), 269.1206 (1.63), 263.1274 (42.58), 245.1170 (100), 227.1065 (63.42), 217.1220 (60.59), 109.1116 (23.36), 201.0903 (12.29), 185.0958 (19.24), 181.1010 (44.17), 171.1166 (56.51), 105.0703 (50.85), 95.0496 (25.16)	7.05	305.1383	−7.538	matricarin [3]	**
69	305.1363	$C_{17}H_{21}O_5$	305.1363 (23.50), 263.1279 (20.85), 245.1170 (100), 227.1063 (29.92), 217.1216 (19.51), 201.0911 (2.62), 185.0961 (16.47), 181.1009 (28.17), 171.1167 (31.70), 131.0857 (46.50), 95.0496 (3.40)	5.42	305.1383	−6.654	matricarin isomer [3]	**
70	307.1544	$C_{17}H_{21}O_5$	307.1544 (2.15), 289.1433 (0.75), 267.2721 (0.18), 247.1325 (2.63), 229.1219 (100), 211.1115 (0.95), 183.1168 (2.88)	9.67	307.1540	1.366	ludalbin [1,2,3]	**

[1] -A. cretica MeOH extract. [2] -A. cretica aqueous extract, [3] -A. cretica EA extract, [4] -A. palida MeOH extract, [5] -A. palida aqueous extract, [6] -A. palida EA extract. *-comparison with standard substance **-tentatively identification.

Table 3. Antioxidant properties of Anthemis extracts *.

Plant Names	Solvents	Phosphomolybdenum (mmol TE/g)	DPPH (mg TE/g)	ABTS (mg TE/g)	CUPRAC (mgTE/g)	FRAP (mgTE/g)	Metal Chelating Abilitiy (mg EDTAE/g)
A. tinctoria var. pallida	Ethyl acetate	2.59 ± 0.19 [b]	40.30 ± 0.78 [e]	45.52 ± 5.53 [f]	113.31 ± 2.26 [d]	47.63 ± 3.77 [f]	39.01 ± 4.42 [a]
	Methanol	2.99 ± 0.14 [a]	407.07 ± 8.88 [a]	320.11 ± 5.67 [a]	691.17 ± 12.07 [a]	362.12 ± 2.63 [a]	28.28 ± 1.81 [c]
	Aqueous	2.65 ± 0.02 [b]	298.40 ± 6.74 [b]	303.16 ± 8.57 [b]	584.01 ± 8.71 [b]	316.34 ± 4.15 [b]	33.59 ± .16 [b]
A. cretica subsp. tenuiloba	Ethyl acetate	1.69 ± 0.08 [cd]	45.47 ± 2.16 [e]	57.13 ± 3.89 [e]	112.87 ± 4.41 [d]	55.74 ± 2.27 [e]	21.90 ± 0.81 [d]
	Methanol	1.77 ± 0.08 [c]	97.22 ± 0.22 [c]	112.41 ± 2.35 [d]	223.09 ± 6.17 [c]	143.21 ± 1.77 [d]	20.93 ± 1.70 [d]
	Aqueous	1.56 ± 0.05 [d]	86.74 ± 2.46 [d]	127.68 ± 0.45 [c]	214.45 ± 1.39 [c]	130.86 ± 1.81 [c]	39.64 ± 1.34 [a]

* Values expressed are means ± S.D. of three parallel measurements. TE: Trolox equivalent; EDTAE: EDTA equivalent. Different letters indicate significant differences in the extracts ($p < 0.05$).

Based on the experimental results (Table 3), it can be noticed that for both species, MeOH extract exhibited the highest total antioxidant activity. According to data presented in Table 3, ATP MeOH extract (DPPH: 407.07 ± 8.88 and ABTS: 320.11 ± 5.67 mg TE/g), followed by the aqueous extract (DPPH: 298.40 ± 6.74 and ABTS: 303.16 ± 8.57 mg TE/g) showed higher radical scavenging activity in both assays. Likewise, ACT MeOH (DPPH: 97.22 ± 0.22 and ABTS: 112.41 ± 2.35 mg TE/g) and aqueous extracts (DPPH: 86.74 ± 2.46 and ABTS: 127.68 ± 0.45 mg TE/g) showed potent radical scavenging activity.

CUPRAC and FRAP assays were employed to assess the reducing capacity of different extracts. CUPRAC method evaluates the conversion of Cu (II) into Cu (I) while FRAP assay measures the reducing potential of an antioxidant reacting with the colourless TPTZ/Fe^{3+} complex to form a blue TPTZ/Fe^{2+} complex at low pH [30]. Remarkable reducing potencies were displayed by MeOH (CUPRAC: 691.17 ± 12.07 and FRAP: 362.12 ± 2.63) and aqueous (CUPRAC: 584.01 ± 8.71 and FRAP: 316.34 ± 4.15 mg TE/g) extracts of APT. EA extract displayed the lowest reducing capacity. This trend was also observed as regards ACT extracts (Table 3).

Chelation of pro-oxidant metals is recognized as one of the most important mechanisms of action of antioxidants. Particularly, iron is the most powerful and abundant pro-oxidant and transition metal which causes oxidative changes of cellular components, such as, lipids and proteins [31]. Evaluation of iron chelating activity showed that ATP and ACT extracts possessed notable chelation potential, with the highest activity displayed by ATP EA extract (39.01 ± 4.42 mg EDTAE/g) and ACT aqueous extract (39.64 ± 1.34 mg EDTAE/g).

2.4. Enzyme Inhibitory Activity

The enzyme inhibitory effect of ATP and ACT extracts was determined against cholinesterases, α-amylase, α-glucosidase, and tyrosinase and the results were presented in Table 4. EA and MeOH extracts of ATP and ACT exhibited potent inhibitory activity against AChE, with the highest activity observed for ATP MeOH extract (3.28 ± 0.43 mg GALAE/g) and ACT EA extract (4.68 ± 0.21 mg GALAE/g). On the other hand, ATP EA extract (3.48 ± 0.21 mg GALAE/g), ACT EA extract (2.51 ± 0.34 mg GALAE/g), and ACT MeOH extract (1.15 ± 0.05 mg GALAE/g) showed inhibitory effect against BChE. Both AChE and BChE hydrolyze acetylcholine and terminate the synaptic transmission [31]. While enhanced AChE activity is associated with early stages of AD, BChE activity is found to increase with the progression of the disease. Therefore, both enzymes are considered as legitimate therapeutic targets for managing AD [32,33].

Table 4. Enzyme inhibitory activity of *Anthemis* extracts *.

Plant Names	Solvents	AChE Inhibition (mg GALAE/g)	BChE Inhibition (mg GALAE/g)	Tyrosinase Inhibition (mg KAE/g)	Amylase Inhibition (mmol ACAE/g)	Glucosidase Inhibition (mmol ACAE/g)
A. tinctoria var. pallida	Ethyl acetate	1.33 ± 0.03 [c]	3.48 ± 0.21 [a]	124.60 ± 0.15 [b]	0.78 ± 0.05 [a]	21.94 ± 1.91 [b]
	Methanol	3.28 ± 0.43 [b]	na	124.48 ± 1.23 [b]	0.54 ± 0.02 [c]	9.15 ± 2.26 [c]
	Aqueous	na	na	72.10 ± 1.64 [d]	0.11 ± 0.01 [d]	4.95 ± 0.25 [d]
A. cretica subsp. tenuiloba	Ethyl acetate	4.68 ± 0.21 [a]	2.51 ± 0.34 [b]	128.73 ± 0.71 [a]	0.65 ± 0.01 [b]	24.16 ± 0.12 [a]
	Methanol	3.45 ± 0.26 [b]	1.15 ± 0.05 [c]	128.85 ± 1.41 [a]	0.52 ± 0.06 [c]	4.49 ± 0.93 [d]
	Aqueous	na	na	88.95 ± 0.49 [c]	0.09 ± 0.01 [d]	2.49 ± 0.17 [e]

* Values expressed are means ± S.D. of three parallel measurements. GALAE: Galatamine equivalent; KAE: Kojic acid equivalent; ACAE: Acarbose equivalent; na: not active. Different letters indicate significant differences in the extracts ($p < 0.05$).

Based on the results (Table 4), it can be observed that the extracts of both species showed remarkable inhibitory activity against tyrosinase with values ranging from 124.60 ± 0.15 to 72.10 ± 1.64 mg KAE/g and from 128.85 ± 1.41 to 88.95 ± 0.49 mg KAE/g for ATP and ACT, respectively. The lowest inhibitory activity against tyrosinase was detected for the aqueous extracts of both species. Tyrosinase is a key enzyme in melanin biosynthesis which is responsible for skin pigmentation. However, excessive melanin production could lead to various skin disorders such as melasma, lentigines, age spots, and post-inflammatory hyperpigmentation. Thus, tyrosinase inhibitors, used as hypopigmenting agents, became increasingly important for medicinal and cosmetic products [34].

Type II diabetes is a growing pandemic and poses an enormous public health challenge for almost every country worldwide. α-Amylase and α-glucosidase are considered as key therapeutic targets for the management of type II diabetes. α-Amylase and α-glucosidase are carbohydrate hydrolysing enzymes, responsible for the breakdown of carbohydrates into glucose [35,36]. The present study showed that all ATP and ACT extracts displayed weak α-amylase inhibitory effects, despite being active α-glucosidase inhibitors. The highest inhibitory effect against α-amylase (0.78 and 0.65 ACAEs/g extract, for ATP and ACT, respectively) and α-glucosidase (21.94 and 24.16 ACAEs/g extract, for ATP and ACT, respectively) was displayed by EA extracts.

2.5. Multivariate Analysis

In an attempt to compare the difference between extract activity, multivariate statistic (sPLS-DA) was carried out by using principal component analysis (PCA) and partial least squares projection to latent structures. PCA is very useful in reducing the dimension of data with minimum loss of information. Figure 1 showed the score plots of projected extracts on principal components PC1 vs. PC2 and PC1 vs. PC3. PCA allowed analysis of biological activities disparity between the extracts. The first three components defining most of variance were found to be the best to clearly classify the extracts (Figure 1C). Nevertheless, the result obtained did not facilitate us for a better discrimination and classification of extracts. Thus, it was considered necessary to apply sPLS-DA, a supervised multivariate analysis known to offer many advantages over PCA, notably by erecting more parsimonious and easily interpretable models compared to PCA.

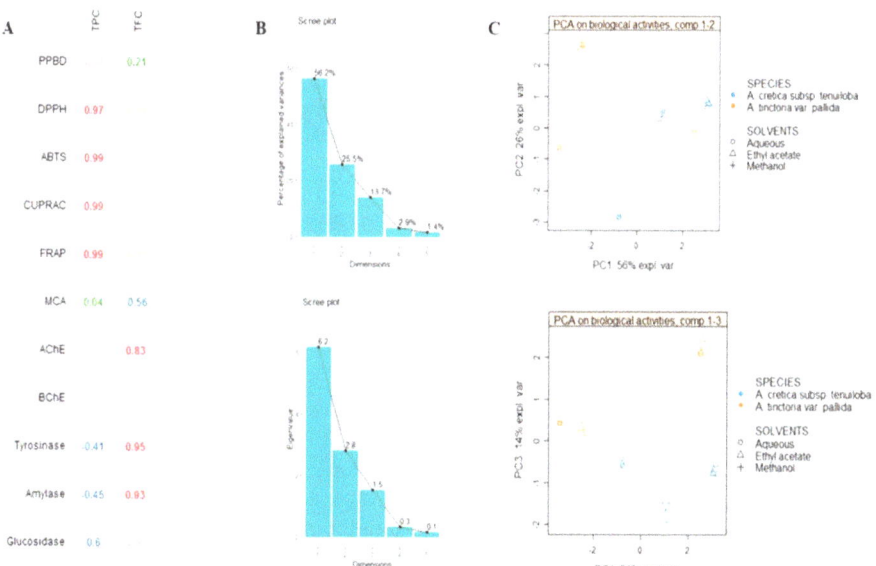

Figure 1. (**A**): Relationship between total phenol content (TPC), total flavonoid content (TFC) and biological activities. (**B,C**): results of preliminary multivariate analysis with PCA (**B**: Percentage of explained variance and Eigen value per component, **C**: PCA sample plot on PC1 vs. PC2 and PC1 vs. PC3 respectively).

Firstly, analysed species were used as class membership criteria to assess whether they were characterized by distinctive biological activities. sPLS-DA samples plot was reported in Figure 2; as shown, a clear separation between *A. cretica* subsp. *tenuiloba* and *A. tinctoria* var. *pallida* was achieved, thus suggesting distinctive biological activities. Afterwards, with the aim to identify the most discriminant biological activities providing the differences overviewed in the sPLS-DA samples plot, VIP (variable importance in projection) plot was generated (Figure 2). Five biological activities including PPBD, DPPH, ABTS, CUPRAC and FRAP possessed a VIP score upper 1, which suggested them as discriminants for the two species.

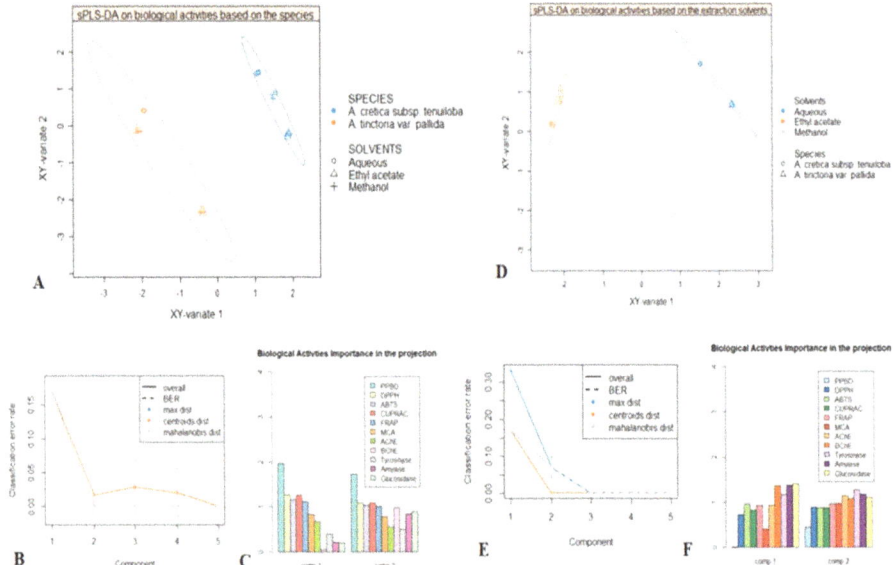

Figure 2. Supervised analysis with sPLS-DA. **A**: sPLS-DA samples plot with confidence ellipse plots considering the species as class membership criteria. **B**: Performance of the model (BER) for three prediction distances using 10 × 5-fold cross-validation. **C**: VIP score plot displaying the biological activities having highly contributed to the discrimination of both studied species. **D**: Factorial plan 1-2 of the sPLS-DA with confidence ellipse plots according to the extraction conditions as class membership criteria. **E**: The model performance per component for the three prediction distances using 5-fold cross-validation repeated 10 times. **F**: VIP score plot showing the biological activities outlining the difference between the three extraction conditions.

Secondly, sPLS-DA was performed considering three different extraction conditions, in order to evaluate the effect of extraction solvents on biological activities. As shown in samples plot (Figure 2) the subspace formed by the first two components showed that methanol, water and ethyl acetate extracts were well separated. Next, the prediction performance and the number of components necessary for the final model were evaluated according to BER (Balanced Error Rate). The performance of our model reached its best for two components, which suggested ncomp = 2 for a final sPLS-DA model (Figure 2). Subsequently, the biological activities having highly contributed to the separation of used solvents were identified. As it could be seen in Figure 2, AChE, BChE, tyrosinase, α-amylase and α-glucosidase were the most contributing biological activities (Figure 2).

2.6. Multidirectional Biological Evaluation

The biological activity of *Anthemis* extracts was formerly evaluated through allelopathy assay, a validated pharmacognostic test for discriminating herbal extract phytotoxicity. Particularly, we investigated the effects of scalar extract concentrations (100 µg/mL–10 mg/mL) on seedling germination of three commercial lettuce varieties, namely Canasta (C), Romana verde (RV), and Romana bionda (RB). After challenging the seeds with *Anthemis* water and EA extracts, we observed that germination process was unaffected in the tested concentration range (Figure 3A–E). Conversely, ATP MeOH extract displayed concentration-dependent inhibition of seedling germination, in the range 1–10 mg/mL (Figure 3F). The root elongation rate test revealed evident inhibitory effect, in the range 1–10 mg/mL. On the other hand, extracts resulted biocompatible at the lowest tested concentration (100 µg/mL), with percentage elongation rate ≥70% compared to vehicle untreated group. The results of elongation rate test suggest a further toxicological investigation, with independent methods in order to confirm the biocompatibility limit, as described below.

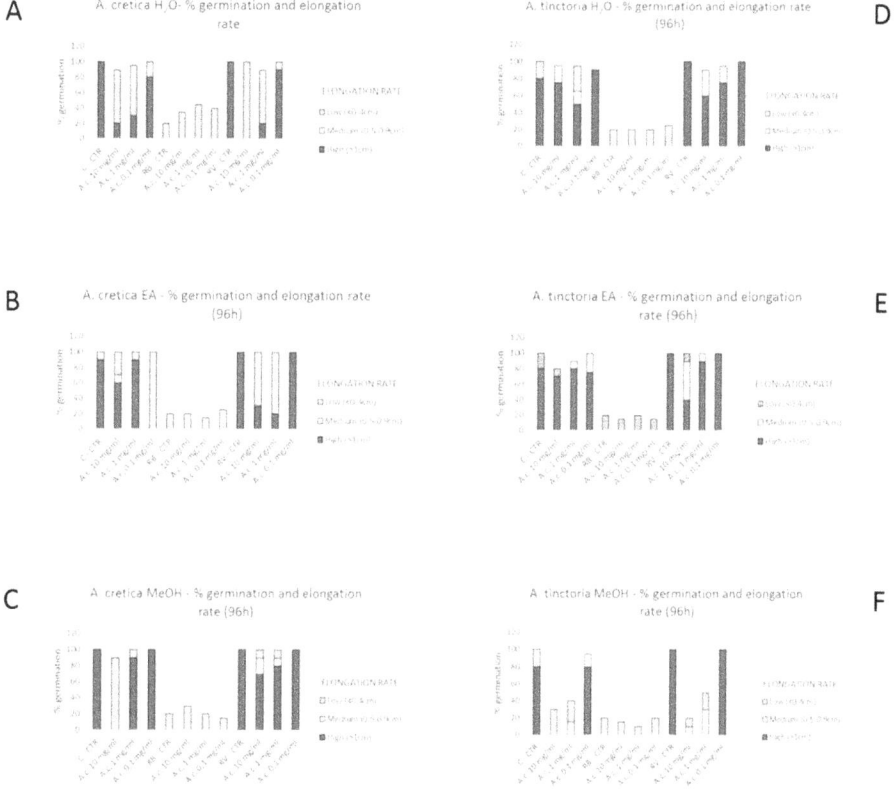

Figure 3. Seedling germination and growth of Canasta (C), Romana verde (RV) and Romana bionda (RB) seeds challenged with *A. tinctoria and A. Cretica* extracts. Results are expressed as root and hypocotyl (seedling) length ± SD at different concentrations and mean of GP after the fourth day since the sowing. (**A**): Effect of *A. cretica* water extract on seedling germination. (**B**): Effect of *A. cretica* ethyl acetate (EA) extract on seedling germination. (**C**): Effect of *A. cretica* water methanol (MeOH) on seedling germination. (**D**): Effect of *A. tinctoria* water extract on seedling germination. (**E**): Effect of *A. tinctoria* ethyl acetate (EA) extract on seedling germination. (**F**): Effect of *A. tinctoria* water methanol (MeOH) on seedling germination.

The potential toxicity of water, MeOH and EA extracts of *Anthemis* species (0.1–20 mg/mL) was also investigated through brine shrimp (*Artemia salina* Leach) lethality assay. Evaluation of lethality induced on brine shrimp, *Artemia salina* Leach, is considered predictive of cytotoxicity [37]. The results of this test revealed LC$_{50}$ values < 10 mg/mL, for all tested extracts.

Additionally, we evaluated the activity of *Anthemis* extracts on HypoE22 cell line viability. According to brine shrimp and allelopathy assays, we tested the extracts at 100 µg/mL. MTT test revealed that *Anthemis* extracts were well tolerated by HypoE22 cells, with a resulting cell viability ≥70% (Figure 4). This concentration was used for subsequent ex vivo investigations aimed to elucidate extract neuroprotective effects, as following reported.

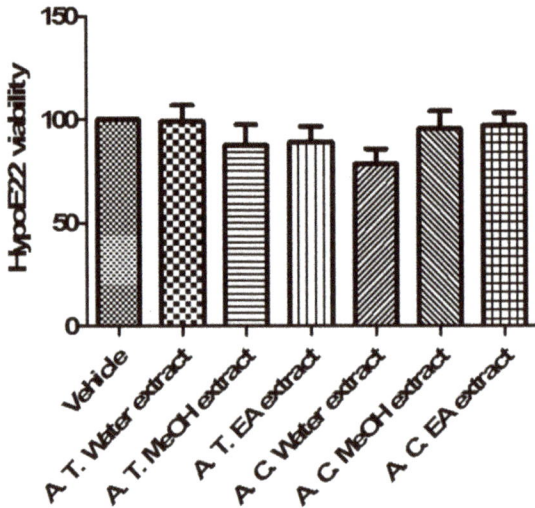

Figure 4. Effect of *A. tinctoria* (A. T.) and *A. cretica* (A. C.) extracts (100 µg/mL) on HypoE22 cell line viability (MTT test). Data are means ± SD of three experiments performed in triplicate.

Cortical spreading depression (CSD) is a pathophysiological and mass depolarization of neurons and glial cells which is characterized by a change in ion and water distribution across neuron membrane associated with cytotoxic effects, including neuron death [38]. In physiological conditions, neurotransmitter release is elicited by depolarizing-stimuli (K$^+$ 9–15 mM) which, through the increased passage of Ca^{2+} ions across nerve terminals via voltage-sensitive calcium channels (VSCCs), stimulates classical neurotransmitter exocytosis. On the other hand, in CSD, the neurotransmitter release increases possibly through additional mechanisms, including membrane transporter reversal [39]. Particularly, excitotoxicity depolarizing-stimuli (K$^+$ ≥ 50 mM) were reported to increase significantly 5-HT overflow [40] which could stimulate neurotransmitter turnover, thus explaining the cortical 5-HT depletion induced by CSD, in vivo [41]. CSD has been recently described as a potential triggering mechanism in migraine with *aura*, via the activation of trigeminal nociceptive system, both peripherally and centrally [42]. While low 5-HT state could play a pivotal role in migraine attack, through multiple effects, including the reduction of pain perception threshold, the increased tendency of having headache and the interference with the control of cerebrovascular nociception [41]. A chronic reduction of 5-HT is also seen in migraineurs and in depressed patients, while amitriptyline and venlafaxine are first-choice drugs for treating patients suffering from migraine with comorbid depression [43]. Considering the role played by 5-HT in anxiety and migraine [41,43], and the traditional use of *Anthemis* species in anxiety [18], we tested ATP and ACT extracts (100 µg/mL) in isolated cortex specimens challenged with an excitotoxicity stimulus constituted by K$^+$ (60 mM) Krebs-Ringer buffer. The results indicated that ATP and ACT EA extracts and ACT water extracts were able to completely blunt K+ (60 mM)-induced 5HIIA/5-HT ratio (Figure 5), which has long been considered as a valuable index of 5-HT degradation, in the brain [44,45]. On the other hand, MeOH extracts were ineffective in modifying K$^+$ (60 mM)-induced

5-HT degradation (Figure 5). Conversely, MeOH extracts revealed a more selective enzyme inhibition on AChE (Table 4). Recently, pilocarpine, a muscarinic receptor agonist, was able to antagonize CSD effects, after sub-convulsing dose administration [46], thus suggesting a role played by acetylcholine signaling stimulation, in CSD. Actually, extract capacity to improve 5-HT and acetylcholine pathways could be related to their antiradical activity (Table 3) [47]. Previously, antioxidant herbal extracts were shown to blunt oxidative stress-induced reduction of neurotransmitter level, in the brain [48,49]. Specifically, water *Harpagophytum procumbens* extract was able to prevent cortex 5-HT depletion induced by amyloid β-peptide [48], possibly through concomitant antioxidant mechanisms, that have been, at least partially, displayed by *Anthemis* extracts, as well. Whereas multiple studies also pointed out the efficacy of isolated secondary metabolites, including polyphenols and tocopherols, in blunting oxidative stress-induced monoamine depletion, thus further suggesting a putative role in managing clinical symptoms related to neurodegenerative diseases [50,51].

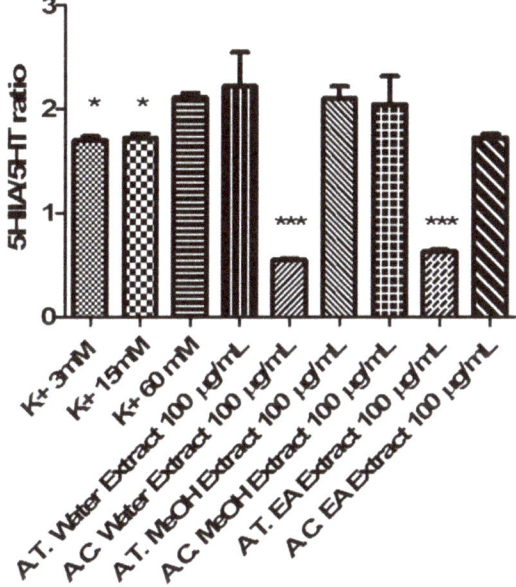

Figure 5. Effect of *A. tinctoria* (A. T.) and *A. cretica* (A. C.) extracts (100 μg/mL) on serotonin (5-HT) turnover, expressed as 5HIIA/5-HT ratio. Turnover was evaluated on isolated rat cortex challenged with basal (K^+ 3mM) and depolarizing stimuli (K^+ 15 mM; K^+ 60 mM). Data are means ± SD of three experiments performed in triplicate. ANOVA, $p < 0.0001$; post-hoc, * $p < 0.05$, *** $p < 0.001$ vs. K^+ 60 mM control group.

On the other hand, after evaluating the effects of *Anthemis* extracts (100 μg/mL) on LDH, a well-recognized marker of tissue damage [52], we observed that ACT EA and MeOH extracts, alongside with ATP water and EA extracts, revealed effective in blunting K^+ (60 mM)-induced LDH level (Figure 6). Considering the results of qualitative fingerprint analysis, we could hypothesize that the observed effects might be related to the presence of flavonoids and terpenes such as apigenin, patuletin, jaceosidin, quercetin, luteolin, and parthenolide.

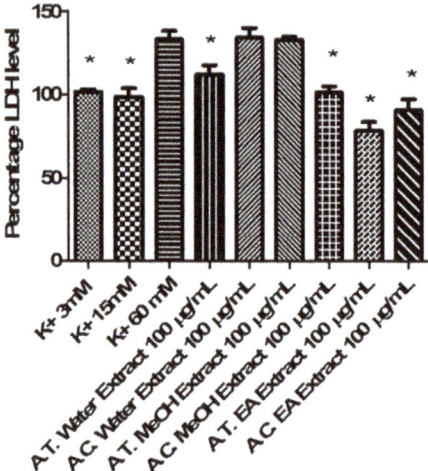

Figure 6. Effect of *A. tinctoria* (A. T.) and *A. cretica* (A. C.) extracts (100 µg/mL) on lactate dehydrogenase (LDH) level, measured on isolated rat cortex challenged with basal (K^+ 3mM) and depolarizing stimuli (K^+ 15 mM; K^+ 60 mM). Data are means ± SD of three experiments performed in triplicate. ANOVA, $p < 0.0001$; post-hoc, * $p < 0.05$ vs. K^+ 60 mM control group.

In agreement with the antiradical activity (Table 2) and blunting effect on 5-HT turnover (Figure 5), ACT water extract samples has been subjected to a further proteomic study, in order to deepen our knowledge about the putative mechanism of action related to neuroprotective effects. The deepening about ACT water extract was performed in comparison with the corresponding ATP extract that, despite showing a null effect on 5-HT turnover (Figure 5), displayed a significant inhibitory effect on K^+ (60 mM)-induced LDH level (Figure 6).

Particularly, untargeted proteomic analysis showed that K^+ 60 mM was able to significantly downregulate neurofilament (NFEM) proteins (Figure 7A/Supplementary Data 1), expressed along the axons and involved in axonal diameter regulation. Reduced NFEM levels have long been related to neurodegeneration [53]. The treatment of isolated rat cortex with ACT water extract was able to prevent NFEM downregulation, restoring the activity of NEFM proteins during K^+ 15 mM physiologic depolarizing stimulus. While ATP water extract did not exert any relevant effect on NFEM level, in isolated rat cortex challenged with K^+ 60 mM (Figure 7B/Supplementary Data 2). Conversely, K^+ 60 mM stimulus led to significant upregulation of protein C kinase γ (PKCγ) and vesicle-associated membrane protein-2 (VAMP-2) (Figure 7A/Supplementary Data 2), compared to physiologic depolarizing stimulus (K^+ 15 mM). VAMP-2 is placed on the membranes of neuronal endings'synaptic vesicles, playing a key role in synaptic vesicle fusion to the presynaptic neuronal ending membrane [54]. Multiple studies suggested upregulation of VAMP-2 level during hypoxia [55,56], which is strictly related to high K^+ concentration-induced CNS injury [39]. PKCγ plays multiple roles in neuronal cells and eye tissues, such as regulation of the neuronal receptors GRIA4/GLUR4 and GRIN1/NMDAR1, modulation of receptors and neuronal functions related to sensitivity to opiates, pain and alcohol, mediation of synaptic function and cell survival after ischemia, and inhibition of gap junction activity after oxidative stress. Its level is positively related to migraine pathogenesis [57]. Additionally, PKCγ gene expression was observed in histidine triad nucleotide-binding protein 1 (Hint1) KO mice, that also showed increased anxiety-related behavior, compared to wild type control mice [58]. Also in this case, treatment of isolated rat cortex with ACT water extract was able to restore the activity of both VAMP-2 and PKCγ during K^+ 15 mM-depolarizing stimulus (Figure 7A/Supplementary Data 2), further supporting the neuroprotective effects of this extract against the burden of oxidative stress and inflammation occurring in CSD.

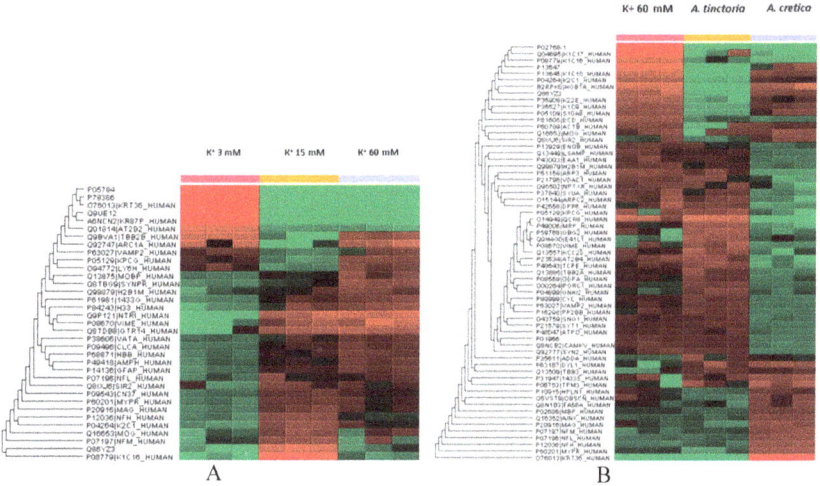

Figure 7. Panel **A**: Untargeted proteomic analysis performed on rat cortex challenged with basal (K^+ 3mM) and depolarizing stimuli (K^+ 15 mM; K^+ 60 mM). The activity of the detected proteins was calculated in comparison with the calibrator of the experiment (K^+ 60 mM). Panel **B**: Untargeted proteomic analysis showing the effects of *A. tinctoria* and *A. cretica* water extracts (100 µg/mL) on rat cortex challenged with excitotoxicity depolarizing stimulus (K^+ 60 mM). T The activity of the detected proteins was calculated in comparison with the calibrator of the experiment (K^+ 60 mM). In subfigure **A**, it is showed that K^+ 60 mM depolarizing stimulus downregulated NEFMs and upregulated VAMP-2 and PKCγ levels. On the other hand, as depicted in subfigure **B**, *A. cretica* water extract (100 µg/mL) was able to restore the activity of specific proteins involved in neuron morphology and neurotransmission, including NEFMs, VAMP-2, and PKCγ. After treating rat cortex with that *A. cretica* water extract, the activity of these proteins was similar to that measured after challenging the brain tissue with physiologic depolarizing stimulus (K^+ 15 mM).

3. Materials and Methods

3.1. Plant Material and Preparation of Extracts

Sampling of the plant species (*Anthemis tinctoria* L. var. *pallida* DC. and *A. cretica* L. subsp. *tenuiloba* (DC.) Grierson) was done in Kastamonu (Hanonu) of Turkey in 2018. The collected plant identity was confirmed by the botanist Dr. Ismail Senkardes (Marmara University, Faculty of Pharmacy, Istambul, Turkey). Aerial parts were collected from wild full blooming plants and dried in ventilated oven (in the dark, temperature 40 °C) until constant weight. Afterwards, dried materials were powdered.

Methanol and ethyl acetate extracts were prepared through maceration method (5 g plant material in 100 mL solvents for 24 h). After that, extracts were filtered and then concentrated by using one rotary evaporator under *vacuo*. Regarding water extracts, infusion method was selected (5 g plant was kept in 100 mL boiling water in 20 min). The infusions were filtered and then lyophilized. All extracts were stored at +4 °C, avoiding light exposure.

3.2. Assays for Total Phenolic and Flavonoids

With reference to our earlier report [59], total bioactive components namely total phenols (TPC) and flavonoids (TFC) were measured by spectrophotometric assays. Gallic acid was the standard for phenols, while rutin was selected for flavonoids.

3.3. Antioxidant and Enzyme Inhibition Assays

Antioxidant properties of *Anthemis* extracts were determined by different in vitro assays namely FRAP, CUPRAC, DPPH, ABTS, chelating and phospomolybdenum assays. Regarding enzyme inhibitory properties, some enzymes including tyrosinase, cholinesterase, α-amylase and α-glucosidase were selected. All experimental procedures were given in our earlier report [59].

3.4. UHPLC-ESI/HRMS Analysis

Neochlorogenic acid (3-CQA) (4), chlorogenic acid (5-CQA) (6), apigenin (30), luteolin (31), quercetin (35), isoquercitrin (49), hyperoside (50), luteolin-7-*O*-rutinoside (54), and rutin (55) were obtained from Extrasynthese (Genay, France). 3,4-*O*-diCQA (12), 3,4-*O*-diCQA (13), diosmetin (33), rhamnetin (37), isorhamnetin (38), luteolin-7-*O*-glucuronide (47), isorhamnetin-7-*O*-glucoside (51), and isorhamnetin-3-*O*-rutinoside (57) were purchased from PhytoLab (Vestenbergsgreuth, Germany).

The UHPLC-ESI/HRMS analyses were carried out on a Q Exactive Plus heated electrospray ionization (HESI-II) – high resolution mass spectrometer (HRMS) (ThermoFisher Scientific, Inc., Bremen, Germany) equipped with an ultra-high-performance liquid chromatography (UHPLC) system Dionex Ultimate 3000RSLC (ThermoFisher Scientific, Inc.) [60].

3.5. Statistical Analysis for Antioxidant and Enzyme Inhibitory Assays

To interpret data gathered, R version 3.5.1 software (The R Foundation, St. Louis, MO, USA) with corrplot and mixOmics packages was used to perform univariate and multivariate statistical analyses. One way analysis of variance (ANOVA) and Tukey's post hoc test were employed to compare bioactive compounds and biological activities between the samples. Also, relationships between bioactive compounds and biological activities were evaluated by the estimation of Pearson's correlation. For multivariate analysis, biological activities of samples were firstly analyses by PCA to pinpoint similarities or differences between samples. Then sPLS-DA was applied by using the species and different extraction condition as class memberships respectively. This allowed better comparison between the two studied species and gauged the effect of the different extraction solvents on biological activities.

3.6. Pharmacological Assays

3.6.1. Allelopathy Bioassay

Allelopathy bioassay was carried on the seeds of three commercial lettuces [Canasta (C), Romana verde (RV) and Romana bionda (RB)], because of their fast germination rate and high sensitivity. The detailed procedure has been extensively reported in our recent paper [61]. Seeds were treated with scalar *Anthemis* extract concentrations (0.1–10 mg/mL) and considered germinated for observed root length ≥ 1 mm, after the third day of treatment.

3.6.2. *Artemia salina* Lethality Bioassay

Artemia salina lethality bioassay was performed as previously reported [61]. Brielfy, brine shrimp larvae were bred at 25–28 °C for 24 h in presence of *Anthemis* extracts (0.1–20 mg/mL) dissolved in incubation medium (artificial sea water). After incubation period (24 h) with extracts, the number of surviving shrimps was evaluated and their vitality was compared to untreated control group. Experiments were carried out in triplicate, and percentage mortality was calculated with the following equation: $((T - S)/T) \times 100$, where T and S are the total number of incubated larvae and survival napulii, respectively.

3.6.3. In Vitro Studies

Rat hypothalamic Hypo-E22 cells were cultured in DMEM (Euroclone), as previously reported [48]. The effects of *Anthemis* extracts (100 µg/mL) on Hypo-E22 cell line viability was evaluated through 3-(4,5-dimethylthiazol-2-yl)-2,5-diphenyltetrazolium bromide (MTT) test.

3.6.4. Ex Vivo Cortical Spreading Depression Paradigm

Male adult Sprague-Dawley rats (200–250 g) were sacrificed by CO_2 inhalation (100% CO_2 at a flow rate of 20% of the chamber volume per min) and cortex specimens were immediately collected and maintained in thermostatic shaking bath at 37 °C for 1 h (incubation period), in Krebs-Ringer buffer at different K^+ concentrations, as described below:

K^+ 3 mM: corresponding to basal condition;
K^+ 15 mM: corresponding to physiologic depolarizing-stimulus;
K^+ 60 mM: corresponding to excitotoxicity depolarizing-stimulus.

The present experimental paradigm reproduced the neural pathophysiological condition named cortical spreading depression (CSD), and was designed according to previous ex vivo and in vivo studies, describing the use of elevated K^+ concentrations (up to 50–60 mM) to induce central nervous system (CNS) injury [38–40]. During incubation, cortex specimens were challenged with water, MeOH and EA *A. tinctoria* and *A. cretica* extracts (100 µg/mL). Afterwards, individual cortex slices were homogenized in perchloric acid solution (0.05 M) in order to extract and quantify serotonin (5-HT) and its main metabolite (5-hydroxyindoleacetic acid, 5HIIA) via HPLC coupled to electrochemical detection, as previously reported [61,62]. The results were expressed as ng/mg wet tissue. Additionally, we carried out colorimetric evaluation of LDH level [52]. Finally, an untargeted proteomic profile was performed on rat cortex homogenate, as described below, in order to further elucidate the putative mechanism of action of *Anthemis* extracts.

3.7. Protein Extraction and Filter-aided Sample Preparation

After protein quantification, a volume corresponding to 50 ug of proteins was loaded onto a Nanosep 10-kDa-cutoff filter (Pall Corporation, Michigan city, MI, USA) and digested according to the protocol we routinely use in our laboratory. Briefly, the sample was washed twice with 200 µL urea buffer (8 M urea, 100 mM Tris pH 8.5 in milliQ water) to remove the detergents present in the lysis buffer. The proteins on the filter where subsequently reduced and alkylated by adding 100 µL of DTT solution (8 mM dithiothreitol in urea buffer) and 100 µL of IAA solution (50 mM iodoacetamide in Urea buffer). For protein digestion, the buffer was exchanged with 50 mM ammonium bicarbonate, before adding trypsin to a ratio of 1:50 (enzyme:substrate). The reaction was incubated for 16 h at 37 °C, and the mixture of peptides was collected by centrifugation, acidified with 10% trifluoroacetic acid and stored at −20 °C until analysis. The detailed description of mass spectrometric analysis is reported as "Supplementary Proteomic Analysis".

3.8. Statistical Analysis for Pharmacological Assays

Statistical analysis was performed using GraphPad Prism version 5.01 for Windows (GraphPad Software, San Diego, CA, USA). Means ± S.E.M. were determined for each experimental group and analyzed by one-way analysis of variance (ANOVA), followed by Newman-Keuls comparison multiple test. Statistical significance was set at $p < 0.05$. As regards the animals randomized for each experimental group, the number was calculated on the basis of the "Resource Equation" $N = (E + T)/T$ ($10 \leq E \leq 20$; https://www.nc3rs.org.uk/experimental-designstatistics).

4. Conclusions

Results collected in the present study indicated the promising biological effects of ATP and ACT extracts. As summarized in Figure 8, tested extracts showed significant antioxidant activity and potent inhibitory effects against key enzymes, involved in Alzheimer's disease, type II diabetes, and hyperpigmentation conditions. Particularly, EA and methanol extracts of both species showed higher enzyme inhibitory activity (at least 1.5 fold: Table 4) compared to water extracts. Conversely, ACT water extract revealed more significant protective effects, as evidenced by reduced (−74%) cortex 5-HT turnover and restored activity of key proteins (i.e., NFEMs and PKCγ) involved in neuron morphology and neurotransmission, in the selected model of neurotoxicity. In this context *A. cretica* water extract appears to be a good candidate for future investigations aimed to confirm and characterize the observed pharmacological effects, possibly through the use of independent experimental methods.

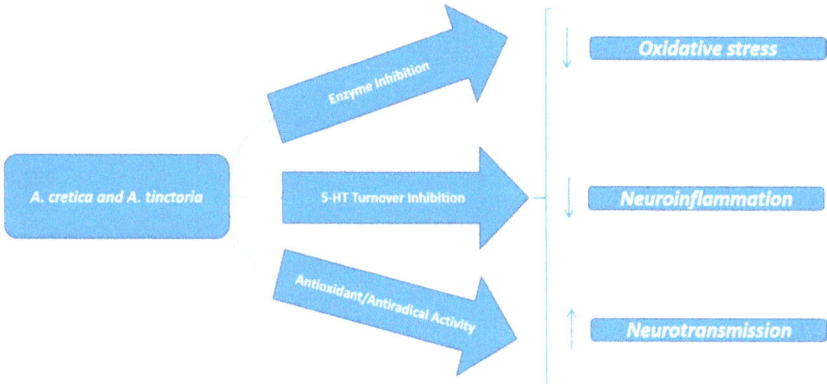

Figure 8. Protective effects induced by *A. cretica* and *A. tinctoria* extracts, as evidenced by the present pharmacological investigation.

Supplementary Materials: The following are available online. Supplementary Data 1; Supplementary Data 2; Supplementary Proteomic Analysis.

Author Contributions: Conceptualization, G.Z., L.M., G.O. and C.F.; methodology, M.R., D.Z.-D., R.G.; software, L.M.; validation, C.F., M.R., R.G. and D.Z.-D.; formal analysis, C.F., L.R.; investigation, A.C., S.L., A.M., G.M., M.P.D., S.D.S, I.S., C.M.N.P.-A., K.I.S.; resources, G.O., L.M., C.F.; data curation, C.F., G.Z.; writing—original draft preparation, C.F., G.Z.; writing—review and editing, L.M., M.F.M., G.O.; visualization, L.B.; supervision, L.B.; project administration, L.R., G.O., C.F.; funding acquisition, G.O., C.F.

Funding: This research was supported by Italian Ministry of University Grant (FAR 2017 granted to Claudio Ferrante; FAR 2017 granted to Giustino Orlando).

Conflicts of Interest: The authors declare no conflict of interest

References

1. Davis, P. *Flora of Turkey and the Aegean Islands*; Edinburgh University Press: Edinburgh, UK, 1975; Volume 5.
2. Doğan, G.; Demirpolat, A.; Bağcı, E. Composition of the Volatile Oils of Anthemis coelopoda var. coelopoda from Turkey. *Hacettepe J. Biol. Chem.* **2015**, *4*, 259–265. [CrossRef]
3. Staneva, J.D.; Todorova, M.N.; Evstatieva, L.N. Sesquiterpene lactones as chemotaxonomic markers in genus Anthemis. *Phytochemistry* **2008**, *69*, 607–618. [CrossRef] [PubMed]
4. Gonenc, T.; Argyropoulou, C.; Erdogan, T.; Gousiadou, C.; Juergenliemk, G.; Kıvçak, B.; Skaltsa, H. Chemical constituents from Anthemis wiedemanniana Fisch. & Mey. *Biochem. Syst. Ecol.* **2011**, *39*, 51–55.
5. Kilic, O.; Kocak, A.; Bagci, E. Composition of the volatile oils of two Anthemis L. taxa from Turkey. *Z. Für Nat. C* **2011**, *66*, 535–540. [CrossRef]

6. Vaverkova, S.; Habán, M.; Eerna, K. Qualitative Properties of Anthemis Tinctoria and Anthemis nobilis, (Chamaemelum nobile) under Different Environmental Conditions. Ecophysiology of Plant Production Processes in Stress Conditions. In Proceedings of the Fourth International Conference, Rackova Dolina, Slovakia, 12–14 September 2001; pp. 1–2.
7. Aboee-Mehrizi, F.; Rustaiyan, A.; Zandi, H.; Ashkezari, M.D.; Zare, M. Chemical Composition and Antimicrobial Activity of the Essential Oil of Anthemis gayana Growing in Iran. *J. Essent. Oil Bear. Plants* **2016**, *19*, 1557–1560. [CrossRef]
8. Bardaweel, S.K.; Tawaha, K.A.; Hudaib, M.M. Antioxidant, antimicrobial and antiproliferative activities of Anthemis palestina essential oil. *Bmc Complementary Altern. Med.* **2014**, *14*, 297. [CrossRef] [PubMed]
9. Kurtulmus, A.; Fafal, T.; Mert, T.; Saglam, H.; Kivcak, B.; Ozturk, T.; Demirci, B.; Baser, K. Chemical composition and antimicrobial activity of the essential oils of three Anthemis species from Turkey. *Chem. Nat. Compd.* **2009**, *45*, 900–904. [CrossRef]
10. Samadi, N.; Manayi, A.; Vazirian, M.; Samadi, M.; Zeinalzadeh, Z.; Saghari, Z.; Abadian, N.; Mozaffarian, V.-O.-A.; Khanavi, M. Chemical composition and antimicrobial activity of the essential oil of Anthemis altissima L. var. altissima. *Nat. Prod. Res.* **2012**, *26*, 1931–1934. [CrossRef] [PubMed]
11. Eser, F.; Sahin Yaglioglu, A.; Dolarslan, M.; Aktas, E.; Onal, A. Dyeing, fastness, and cytotoxic properties, and phenolic constituents of Anthemis tinctoria var. tinctoria (Asteraceae). *J. Text. Inst.* **2017**, *108*, 1489–1495. [CrossRef]
12. Kizil, S.; Kayabaşi, N.; Arslan, N. Determination of some agronomical and dyeing properties of dyer's chamomile (Anthemis Tinctoria L.). *J. Cent. Eur. Agric.* **2006**, *6*, 403–408.
13. Kültür, Ş. Medicinal plants used in Kırklareli province (Turkey). *J. Ethnopharmacol.* **2007**, *111*, 341–364. [CrossRef] [PubMed]
14. Zhang, S.; Won, Y.-K.; Ong, C.-N.; Shen, H.-M. Anti-cancer potential of sesquiterpene lactones: bioactivity and molecular mechanisms. *Curr. Med. Chem. -Anti-Cancer Agents* **2005**, *5*, 239–249. [CrossRef] [PubMed]
15. Gonenc, T.M.; Erdogan, T.F.; Demirci, B.; Baser, K.; Kivcak, B. Chemical composition of the essential oils of Anthemis coelopoda var. bourgaei and A. aciphylla var. aciphylla. *Chem. Nat. Compd.* **2012**, *48*, 332–334. [CrossRef]
16. Pavlović, M.; Kovačević, N.; Tzakou, O.; Couladis, M. Essential oil composition of Anthemis triumfetti (L.) DC. *Flavour Fragr. J.* **2006**, *21*, 297–299.
17. Uysal, I.; Celik, S.; Oldacay, M. Antimicrobial activity of Anthemis coelopoda Var. bourgaei Boiss. and Anthemis tinctoria Var. pallida DC. species having ethnobotanical features. *J. Appl. Sci.* **2005**, *5*, 639–642.
18. Özüdoğru, B.; Akaydın, G.; Erik, S.; Yesilada, E. Inferences from an ethnobotanical field expedition in the selected locations of Sivas and Yozgat provinces (Turkey). *J. Ethnopharmacol.* **2011**, *137*, 85–98. [CrossRef] [PubMed]
19. Banagozar Mohammadi, A.; Torbati, M.; Farajdokht, F.; Sadigh-Eteghad, S.; Fazljou, S.M.B.; Vatandoust, S.M.; Golzari, S.E.J.; Mahmoudi, J. Sericin alleviates restraint stress induced depressive- and anxiety-like behaviors via modulation of oxidative stress, neuroinflammation and apoptosis in the prefrontal cortex and hippocampus. *Brain Res.* **2019**, *1715*, 47–56. [CrossRef]
20. Prasanth, M.I.; Sivamaruthi, B.S.; Chaiyasut, C.; Tencomnao, T. A Review of the Role of Green Tea (Camellia sinensis) in Antiphotoaging, Stress Resistance, Neuroprotection, and Autophagy. *Nutrients* **2019**, *11*, 474. [CrossRef]
21. Clifford, M.N.; Johnston, K.L.; Knight, S.; Kuhnert, N. Hierarchical scheme for LC-MS n identification of chlorogenic acids. *J. Agric. Food Chem.* **2003**, *51*, 2900–2911. [CrossRef]
22. Clifford, M.N.; Knight, S.; Kuhnert, N. Discriminating between the six isomers of dicaffeoylquinic acid by LC-MS n. *J. Agric. Food Chem.* **2005**, *53*, 3821–3832. [CrossRef]
23. Zheleva-Dimitrova, D.; Gevrenova, R.; Zaharieva, M.M.; Najdenski, H.; Ruseva, S.; Lozanov, V.; Balabanova, V.; Yagi, S.; Momekov, G.; Mitev, V. HPLC-UV and LC–MS analyses of acylquinic acids in Geigeria alata (DC) Oliv. & Hiern. and their contribution to antioxidant and antimicrobial capacity. *Phytochem. Anal.* **2017**, *28*, 176–184. [PubMed]
24. Justesen, U. Collision-induced fragmentation of deprotonated methoxylated flavonoids, obtained by electrospray ionization mass spectrometry. *J. Mass Spectrom.* **2001**, *36*, 169–178. [CrossRef] [PubMed]
25. Smelcerovic, A.; Lamshoeft, M.; Radulovic, N.; Ilic, D.; Palic, R. LC–MS Analysis of the Essential Oils of Achillea millefolium and Achillea crithmifolia. *Chromatographia* **2010**, *71*, 113–116. [CrossRef]
26. Priestap, H.A.; Abboud, K.A.; Velandia, A.E.; Lopez, L.A.; Barbieri, M.A. Dehydroleucodin: a guaiane-type sesquiterpene lactone. *Acta Crystallogr. Sect. E Struct. Rep. Online* **2011**, *67*, o3470. [CrossRef] [PubMed]

27. Michalska, K.; Żylewski, M.; Kisiel, W. Structure elucidation and complete NMR spectral assignments of two new sesquiterpene lactone xylosides from Lactuca triangulata. *Magn. Reson. Chem.* **2008**, *46*, 1185–1187. [CrossRef] [PubMed]
28. Clifford, M.N.; Wu, W.; Kirkpatrick, J.; Kuhnert, N. Profiling the chlorogenic acids and other caffeic acid derivatives of herbal Chrysanthemum by LC– MS n. *J. Agric. Food Chem.* **2007**, *55*, 929–936. [CrossRef] [PubMed]
29. Lobo, V.; Patil, A.; Phatak, A.; Chandra, N. Free radicals, antioxidants and functional foods: Impact on human health. *Pharmacogn. Rev.* **2010**, *4*, 118. [CrossRef]
30. Zengin, G.; Lobine, D.; Mollica, A.; Locatelli, M.; Carradori, S.; Mahomoodally, M.F. Multiple pharmacological approaches on Fibigia eriocarpa extracts by in vitro and computational assays. *Fundam. Clin. Pharmacol.* **2018**. [CrossRef]
31. Ma, Y.-L.; Zhu, D.-Y.; Thakur, K.; Wang, C.-H.; Wang, H.; Ren, Y.-F.; Zhang, J.-G.; Wei, Z.-J. Antioxidant and antibacterial evaluation of polysaccharides sequentially extracted from onion (Allium cepa L.). *Int. J. Biol. Macromol.* **2018**, *111*, 92–101. [CrossRef]
32. Lionetto, M.G.; Caricato, R.; Calisi, A.; Giordano, M.E.; Schettino, T. Acetylcholinesterase as a biomarker in environmental and occupational medicine: new insights and future perspectives. *Biomed Res. Int.* **2013**, *2013*. [CrossRef]
33. Greig, N.H.; Lahiri, D.K.; Sambamurti, K. Butyrylcholinesterase: an important new target in Alzheimer's disease therapy. *Int. Psychogeriatr.* **2002**, *14*, 77–91. [CrossRef] [PubMed]
34. Pintus, F.; Sabatucci, A.; Maccarrone, M.; Dainese, E.; Medda, R. Amine oxidase from Euphorbia characias: Kinetic and structural characterization. *Biotechnol. Appl. Biochem.* **2018**, *65*, 81–88. [CrossRef] [PubMed]
35. Ali, H.; Houghton, P.; Soumyanath, A. α-Amylase inhibitory activity of some Malaysian plants used to treat diabetes; with particular reference to Phyllanthus amarus. *J. Ethnopharmacol.* **2006**, *107*, 449–455. [CrossRef] [PubMed]
36. Ouassou, H.; Zahidi, T.; Bouknana, S.; Bouhrim, M.; Mekhfi, H.; Ziyyat, A.; Aziz, M.; Bnouham, M. Inhibition of α-Glucosidase, Intestinal Glucose Absorption, and Antidiabetic Properties by Caralluma europaea. *Evid.-Based Complementary Altern. Med.* **2018**, *2018*. [CrossRef] [PubMed]
37. Ohikhena, F.U.; Wintola, O.A.; Afolayan, A.J. Toxicity Assessment of Different Solvent Extracts of the Medicinal Plant, Phragmanthera capitata (Sprengel) Balle on Brine Shrimp (Artemia salina). *Int. J. Pharmacol.* **2016**, *12*, 701–710.
38. Richter, F.; Eitner, A.; Leuchtweis, J.; Bauer, R.; Ebersberger, A.; Lehmenkühler, A.; Schaible, H.-G. The potential of substance P to initiate and perpetuate cortical spreading depression (CSD) in rat in vivo. *Sci. Rep.* **2018**, *8*, 17656. [CrossRef] [PubMed]
39. Raiteri, L.; Stigliani, S.; Zedda, L.; Raiteri, M.; Bonanno, G. Multiple mechanisms of transmitter release evoked by 'pathologically'elevated extracellular [K+]: involvement of transporter reversal and mitochondrial calcium. *J. Neurochem.* **2002**, *80*, 706–714. [CrossRef] [PubMed]
40. Sbrenna, S.; Marti, M.; Morari, M.; Calo, G.; Guerrini, R.; Beani, L.; Bianchi, C. Modulation of 5-hydroxytryptamine efflux from rat cortical synaptosomes by opioids and nociceptin. *Br. J. Pharmacol.* **2000**, *130*, 425–433. [CrossRef]
41. Supornsilpchai, W.; Sanguanrangsirikul, S.; Maneesri, S.; Srikiatkhachorn, A. Serotonin depletion, cortical spreading depression, and trigeminal nociception. *Headache J. Head Face Pain* **2006**, *46*, 34–39. [CrossRef]
42. Close, L.N.; Eftekhari, S.; Wang, M.; Charles, A.C.; Russo, A.F. Cortical spreading depression as a site of origin for migraine: Role of CGRP. *Cephalalgia* **2018**, 0333102418774299. [CrossRef]
43. Zarcone, D.; Corbetta, S. Shared mechanisms of epilepsy, migraine and affective disorders. *Neurol. Sci.* **2018**, *38*, 73–76. [CrossRef] [PubMed]
44. Lee, J.; Chang, C.; Liu, I.; Chi, T.; Yu, H.; Cheng, J. Changes in endogenous monoamines in aged rats. *Clin. Exp. Pharmacol. Physiol.* **2001**, *28*, 285–289. [CrossRef] [PubMed]
45. Brunetti, L.; Orlando, G.; Ferrante, C.; Recinella, L.; Leone, S.; Chiavaroli, A.; Di Nisio, C.; Shohreh, R.; Manippa, F.; Ricciuti, A. Peripheral chemerin administration modulates hypothalamic control of feeding. *Peptides* **2014**, *51*, 115–121. [CrossRef] [PubMed]
46. Francisco, E.D.S.; Guedes, R.C. Sub-convulsing dose administration of pilocarpine reduces glycemia, increases anxiety-like behavior and decelerates cortical spreading depression in rats suckled on various litter sizes. *Front. Neurosci.* **2018**, *12*, 897. [CrossRef] [PubMed]

47. Mollica, A.; Stefanucci, A.; Zengin, G.; Locatelli, M.; Macedonio, G.; Orlando, G.; Ferrante, C.; Menghini, L.; Recinella, L.; Leone, S. Polyphenolic composition, enzyme inhibitory effects ex-vivo and in-vivo studies on two Brassicaceae of north-central Italy. *Biomed. Pharmacother.* **2018**, *107*, 129–138. [CrossRef] [PubMed]
48. Ferrante, C.; Recinella, L.; Locatelli, M.; Guglielmi, P.; Secci, D.; Leporini, L.; Chiavaroli, A.; Leone, S.; Martinotti, S.; Brunetti, L. Protective effects induced by microwave-assisted aqueous Harpagophytum extract on rat cortex synaptosomes challenged with amyloid β-peptide. *Phytother. Res.* **2017**, *31*, 1257–1264. [CrossRef] [PubMed]
49. Romano, A.; Pace, L.; Tempesta, B.; Lavecchia, A.M.; Macheda, T.; Bedse, G.; Petrella, A.; Cifani, C.; Serviddio, G.; Vendemiale, G. Depressive-like behavior is paired to monoaminergic alteration in a murine model of Alzheimer's disease. *Int. J. Neuropsychopharmacol.* **2015**, *18*. [CrossRef]
50. Ramis, M.R.; Sarubbo, F.; Terrasa, J.L.; Moranta, D.; Aparicio, S.; Miralles, A.; Esteban, S. Chronic α-Tocopherol Increases Central Monoamines Synthesis and Improves Cognitive and Motor Abilities in Old Rats. *Rejuvenation Res.* **2016**, *19*, 159–171. [CrossRef] [PubMed]
51. Chen, M.; Wang, T.; Yue, F.; Li, X.; Wang, P.; Li, Y.; Chan, P.; Yu, S. Tea polyphenols alleviate motor impairments, dopaminergic neuronal injury, and cerebral α-synuclein aggregation in MPTP-intoxicated parkinsonian monkeys. *Neuroscience* **2015**, *286*, 383–392. [CrossRef] [PubMed]
52. Menghini, L.; Leporini, L.; Vecchiotti, G.; Locatelli, M.; Carradori, S.; Ferrante, C.; Zengin, G.; Recinella, L.; Chiavaroli, A.; Leone, S. Crocus sativus L. stigmas and byproducts: qualitative fingerprint, antioxidant potentials and enzyme inhibitory activities. *Food Res. Int.* **2018**, *109*, 91–98. [CrossRef]
53. Valdiglesias, V.; Fernández-Tajes, J.; Pásaro, E.; Méndez, J.; Laffon, B. Identification of differentially expressed genes in SHSY5Y cells exposed to okadaic acid by suppression subtractive hybridization. *Bmc Genom.* **2012**, *13*, 46. [CrossRef] [PubMed]
54. Jahn, R.; Südhof, T.C. Membrane fusion and exocytosis. *Annu. Rev. Biochem.* **1999**, *68*, 863–911. [CrossRef] [PubMed]
55. Manzur, A.; Sosa, M.; Seltzer, A.M. Transient increase in rab 3A and synaptobrevin immunoreactivity after mild hypoxia in neonatal rats. *Cell. Mol. Neurobiol.* **2001**, *21*, 39–52. [CrossRef] [PubMed]
56. Valdez, S.R.; Patterson, S.I.; Ezquer, M.E.; Torrecilla, M.; Lama, M.C.; Seltzer, A.M. Acute sublethal global hypoxia induces transient increase of GAP-43 immunoreactivity in the striatum of neonatal rats. *Synapse* **2007**, *61*, 124–137. [CrossRef] [PubMed]
57. Wu, B.; Wang, S.; Qin, G.; Xie, J.; Tan, G.; Zhou, J.; Chen, L. Protein kinase C γ contributes to central sensitization in a rat model of chronic migraine. *J. Mol. Neurosci.* **2017**, *63*, 131–141. [CrossRef] [PubMed]
58. Varadarajulu, J.; Lebar, M.; Krishnamoorthy, G.; Habelt, S.; Lu, J.; Bernard Weinstein, I.; Li, H.; Holsboer, F.; Turck, C.W.; Touma, C. Increased anxiety-related behaviour in Hint1 knockout mice. *Behav Brain Res.* **2011**, *220*, 305–311. [CrossRef] [PubMed]
59. Uysal, S.; Zengin, G.; Locatelli, M.; Bahadori, M.B.; Mocan, A.; Bellagamba, G.; De Luca, E.; Mollica, A.; Aktumsek, A. Cytotoxic and enzyme inhibitory potential of two Potentilla species (P. speciosa L. and P. reptans Willd.) and their chemical composition. *Front. Pharmacol.* **2017**, *8*, 290. [CrossRef]
60. Zengin, G.; Aktumsek, A.; Ceylan, R.; Uysal, S.; Mocan, A.; Guler, G.O.; Mahomoodally, M.F.; Glamoclija, J.; Ciric, A.; Sokovic, M. Shedding light on the biological and chemical fingerprints of three Achillea species (A. biebersteinii, A. millefolium and A. teretifolia). *Food Funct.* **2017**, *8*, 1152–1165. [CrossRef]
61. Ferrante, C.; Recinella, L.; Ronci, M.; Menghini, L.; Brunetti, L.; Chiavaroli, A.; Leone, S.; Di Iorio, L.; Carradori, S.; Tirillini, B. Multiple pharmacognostic characterization on hemp commercial cultivars: Focus on inflorescence water extract activity. *Food Chem. Toxicol.* **2019**, *125*, 452–461. [CrossRef]
62. Ferrante, C.; Orlando, G.; Recinella, L.; Leone, S.; Chiavaroli, A.; Di Nisio, C.; Shohreh, R.; Manippa, F.; Ricciuti, A.; Vacca, M. Central inhibitory effects on feeding induced by the adipo-myokine irisin. *Eur. J. Pharmacol.* **2016**, *791*, 389–394. [CrossRef]

Sample Availability: Samples of the extracts are available from the authors.

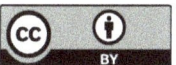

© 2019 by the authors. Licensee MDPI, Basel, Switzerland. This article is an open access article distributed under the terms and conditions of the Creative Commons Attribution (CC BY) license (http://creativecommons.org/licenses/by/4.0/).

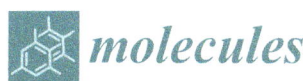

Article

Anticancer Activity of *Smallanthus sonchifolius* Methanol Extract against Human Hepatocellular Carcinoma Cells

Phyu Phyu Myint [1],[†], Thien T. P. Dao [2],[†] and Yeong Shik Kim [2],*

[1] Department of Chemistry, Loikaw University, Loikaw 09013, Myanmar
[2] College of Pharmacy and Natural Products Research Institute, Seoul National University, Seoul 08826, Korea
* Correspondence: kims@snu.ac.kr; Tel.: +82-2-880-2479
[†] These authors contributed equally to this work.

Academic Editors: Raffaele Capasso and Lorenzo Di Cesare Mannelli
Received: 22 July 2019; Accepted: 21 August 2019; Published: 22 August 2019

Abstract: Background: This research aimed to investigate the cytotoxicity of methanol extract of *Smallanthus sonchifolius* leaf (YLE) against a human hepatocellular carcinoma cell line (HepG2). This plant is currently used as a traditional herbal remedy in the treatment of liver diseases in some rural parts of Myanmar. **Methods**: The cytotoxic activity of the plant extract against the cancerous cell line was assessed using an MTT assay. YLE demonstrated a significant effect (IC50 = 58.2 ± 1.9 µg/mL) on anti-cancer activity, which was further investigated using various assays including an in vitro cell migration assay, a colony formation assay, cell cycle analysis, western blot analysis, and a ROS assay. The significance of the phytochemical constituents of YLE could be identified using LC/Q-TOF-MS techniques. **Results**: We putatively identified the active components in YLE, which were possibly melampolide-type sesquiterpenoids. YLE showed an inhibitory effect on HepG2 cell proliferation and cell migration. YLE also induced cell cycle arrest and necrosis in a dose-dependent manner. Additionally, YLE significantly suppressed ROS formation in HepG2 cells. **Conclusions**: These findings suggest that YLE is sufficient for application as a promising anti-liver drug in herbal medicine.

Keywords: *S. sonchifolius* leaf; HepG2 cells; MTT assay; cell cycle arrest; anti-liver cancer drug; antioxidant

1. Introduction

In 2018, liver cancer was the sixth most common cancer and the fourth leading cause of cancer deaths worldwide [1]. The highest incidence of this cancer can be seen in East Asia, Southeast Asia, and North and Southern Africa [2]. Based on the database of the International Agency for Research on Cancer (IARC), there were more than 69,000 new cancer cases in Myanmar in 2018 and liver cancers were in the top 5 in terms of incidence, mortality, and prevalence by cancer site [1]. Currently, the Ministry of Health and Sports from Myanmar supports the implementation of the National Cancer Control Plan, focusing on priority activities and maximizing efforts in line with the respective mandates, priorities, and areas of expertise of the partner and to achieve better results for cancer prevention, care, and control.

Testing, annual screenings, and early intervention for cancers are currently inadequate on many accounts, which include the rise in population, an inadequate supply of drugs, the cost of treatments, the side effects of several synthetic medicines, and increasing resistance to the drugs used. In most rural areas, herbal medicine has been used for decades by traditional practitioners to treat cancer problems. Medicinal plants have long been used in the treatment of liver diseases or the maintenance of a healthy liver. Yacon, or *Smallanthus sonchifolius* ((Poepp. & Endl.) H. Rob.), is a plant belonging to the Asteraceae family, native to the Andean regions of South America [3]. The plant contents include phenolic acids, flavonoids, and sesquiterpene lactones [4,5]. Yacon has been used as a functional food with multiple beneficial effects on the body, including as an antimicrobial, as an antioxidant, hypolipidemic effects, and probiotic substances [3,6]. The plant was cultivated in Myanmar in the 2000s. It has become increasingly popular as medicated green tea for diabetes patients and its use is wide-spread.

In recent years, Yacon has emerged as a potential anti-cancer agent. Previous in vitro studies indicated that the crude extract of Yacon and the phytochemicals derived from the plants exerted the cytotoxicity against breast cancer [7], colon cancer [7,8], and cervical cancer [9,10]. The anticancer property was attributed to sesquiterpene lactones in Yacon [9–11]. In addition, Yacon has been well-known to have antioxidant effects because of an abundant amount of polyphenols, which are found at high quantities in leaves or stems of the plant [6]. Recent studies have indicated that antioxidants might possess anti-tumor and hepatoprotective effects, although the mechanism needs further investigation [12].

This research aimed to evaluate the effects of Yacon leaf extract (YLE) on liver cancer in vitro using hepatocellular carcinoma HepG2 cell line, which is the most commonly used in drug metabolism and hepatotoxicity studies. HepG2 cells are nontumorigenic with high proliferation rates and an epithelial-like morphology that performs many differentiated hepatic functions [13]. The medicinal plant is of high pharmacological importance, but it is still not reported for its chemotherapeutic potential as an alternative medicine for liver cancer disease. Our results may provide scientific evidence for the therapeutic potential of this plant, as a functional food, on liver cancer.

2. Results

2.1. Cytotoxicity of YLE by MTT Assay

The sample was evaluated for cytotoxic activity on human hepatoma carcinoma cell lines (HepG2), as presented in Figure 1. The results of the MTT assay showed a dose-dependent reduction in cell viability of HepG2 cells while YLE did not affect those of non-tumor HEK 239 cells after 24 h treatment. The calculated IC_{50} of YLE on HepG2 was 58.2 ± 1.9 µg/mL.

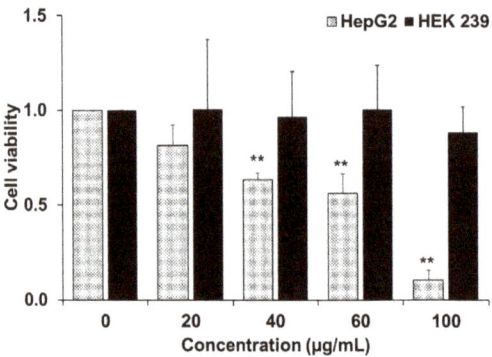

Figure 1. Cell viability of HepG2 and HEK 239 cells after being treated with different concentration of YLE. Data are presented as means ± standard deviation (S.D) ($n = 3$); ** $p < 0.01$ vs. control group.

2.2. YLE Reduces Colony Formation of HepG2 Cells

To determine the effect of YLE on the replicative potential and the longer-term viability of liver cancer cells under colony-forming culture conditions, we treated HepG2 cells with various concentrations of the extracts for 24 h or 48 h, then conducted a crystal violet-based clonogenic assay. Data showed that YLE significantly inhibited colony formation of HepG2 after 14 days. We found that cell proliferation rates gradually decreased as the concentration of the extract was increased. These findings suggest that YLE exerts its strong inhibitory effect on longer-term viability liver cancer cells in a dose-dependent manner. The full inhibitory effect of YLE on the HepG2 clonogenicity could be observed within 24 h at 100 µg/mL dose and 48 h at 80 and 100 µg/mL (Figure 2).

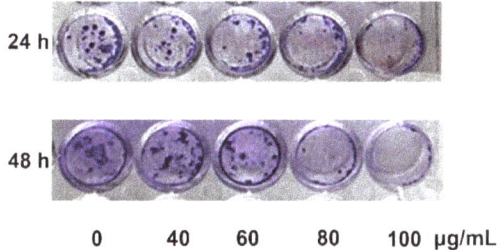

Figure 2. HepG2 cells after 24 h and 48 h treatment with YLE were allowed to grow into visible colonies for an additional 2 weeks. The figure presents one of three independent experiments.

2.3. Effect of YLE on Wound Healing in HepG2 Cells

Migration of cells plays a vital role in cancer cells survival; thus, we conducted a wound-healing assay to examine the effect of YLE on the healing process in HepG2 cells. In this study, at the start of in vitro scratch test, there were little or no cells inside the scratch region. After 24 h exposure to YLE, it was observed that the cell migrated towards the induced gap (Figure 3). The control sample migration (0 µg/mL) was noted to be the highest in all the cell lines tested. YLE significantly decreased the migration in HepG2 cells.

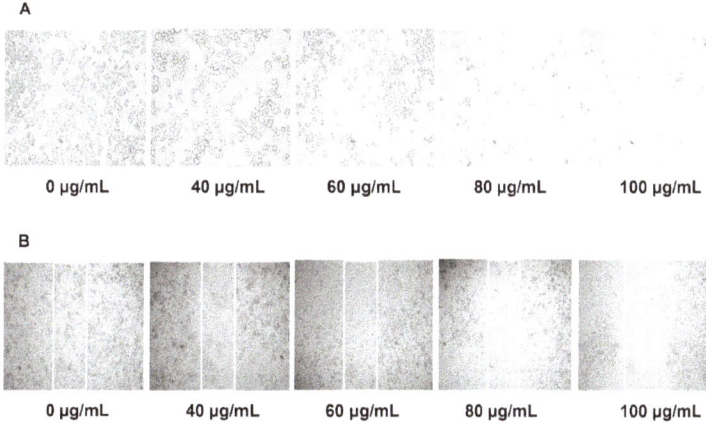

Figure 3. Effect of YLE on (**A**) cell morphology and (**B**) migration ability of HepG2 cells. The figures show one of three independent experiments.

2.4. Effect of YLE on ROS Production

To evaluate the influence of YLE on mediating ROS generation in HepG2 cells, we incubated cells with different concentrations of YLE in indicated times (3 h, 6 h, 9 h). The intracellular ROS was measured via 2′,7′-dichlorofluorescein diacetate (DCF-DA) fluorescence. As displayed in Figure 4, intracellular ROS levels were significantly decreased in a concentration-dependent manner (Figure 4A), while the cell viability of HepG2 was not affected in short-time treatment (Figure 4B). These data proved that a reduction of ROS production in HepG2 cells was not due to decreasing numbers of living cells.

The ROS-inhibitory effect of YLE showed similar patterns after 3 h and 6 h of treatment. The specific changes could be observed only at high concentrations, such as 80 and 60 µg/mL, respectively. However, after 9 h of treatment, the ROS production was inhibited notably (>50%) even at the lowest concentration (40 µg/mL) used in the experiments. These results suggest that the antioxidant effect of YLE possibly led to induced cytostasis in HepG2 cells after 24 h treatment.

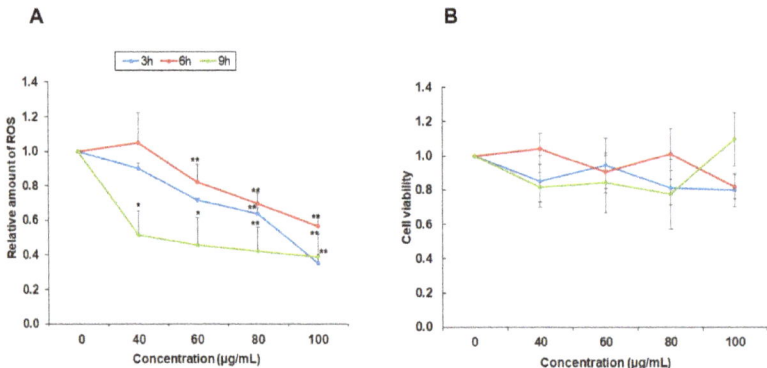

Figure 4. Effect of YLE on ROS formation of HepG2 cells. (**A**) Antioxidant effect of YLE on HepG2 cells after 3 h, 6 h, and 9 h. Data are expressed as averages ± S.D ($n = 3$); * $p < 0.05$, ** $p < 0.01$ vs. control group. (**B**) Effect of YLE on cell viability. Data indicated no specific change between treatment groups and the control group after indicated times (3 h, 6 h, 9 h).

2.5. YLE Induces Cell Cycle Arrest in HepG2 Cells

Next, we examined the effect of YLE on the cell cycle of a HepG2 liver cancer cell line after 24 h treatment using flow cytometry. Figure 5 shows the relative percentages of HepG2 cells in each phase of the cell cycle following treatment. There was a dose-dependent increase in the percentage of cells in the G0/G1 phase. The data in this study suggested that YLE could inhibit cell proliferation of HepG2 cells by inducing the cell cycle at the G0/G1 phase.

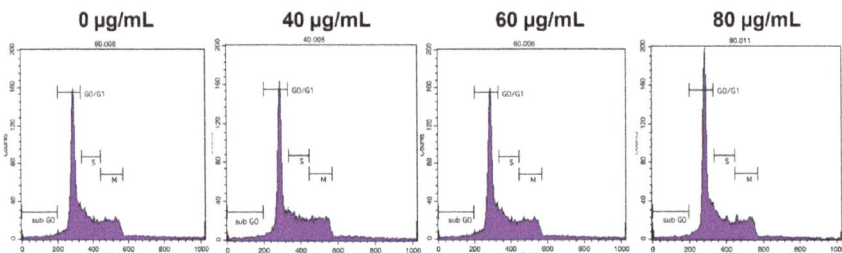

Figure 5. Effect of YLE on the cell cycle of HepG2 cells. The figure represents triplicate experiments.

2.6. YLE Induces Necrosis in HepG2 Cells

To clarify the mechanism of YLE on inducing cell death in HepG2 cells, we stained the YLE-treated cells with Annexin V/PI after 24 h exposure and measured the fluorescence by flow cytometry. The percentage of each subpopulation of cells is described in Figure 6. We found that YLE induced the loss of cell membrane integrity, which was indicated by the increase in numbers of PI-positive cells. The proportion of only the PI-positive cell population treated with 100 µg/mL YLE was approximately 20-fold higher than the one in the control group. Additionally, YLE did not trigger caspase activation or cleavage of caspase proteins, such as caspase 3 and caspase 8. These data suggest a necrotic mode of cell death induced by YLE.

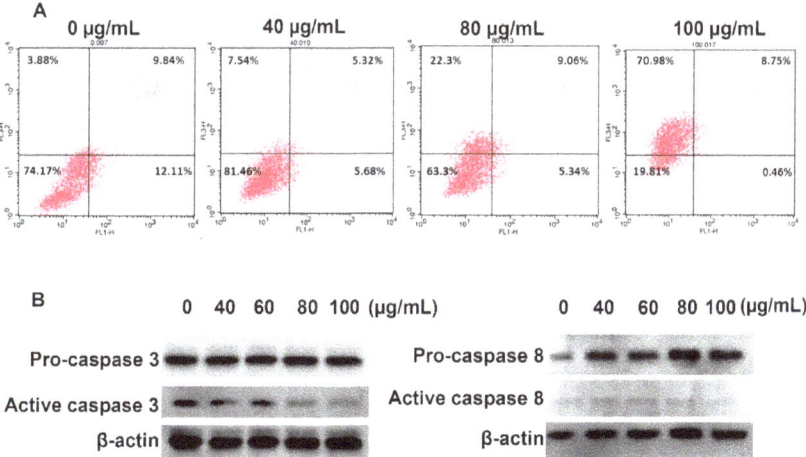

Figure 6. Effect of YLE on (**A**) the cell death mechanism and (**B**) the expression levels of proteins in HepG2 cells. The figure shows one of three independent experiments.

2.7. Metabolites Identification of Methanol Extract of YLE

In this study, we confirmed the presence of several metabolites in YLE based on the characteristic fragments in the MS spectra previously described in the literature [5]. We focused on raw formulas of several melampolide sesquiterpene lactones, which were previously described as main components in Yacon, as follows: $C_{23}H_{28}O_8$, $C_{23}H_{28}O_9$, and $C_{23}H_{28}O_{10}$ [5]. Figure 7 displays the total ion current chromatogram (TIC) of the extract (Figure 7A) and the obtained extracted-ion chromatograms (EIC) showing the series of peaks with *m/z* values corresponding to the three selected molecular formulas (Figure 7B–D). Compound 1 (retention time (rt) 11.94), compound 2 (rt. 12.81 min), and compound 3 (rt.15.13) exhibited a protonated molecular ion [M + H]$^+$ at *m/z* 465.1657 [$C_{23}H_{28}O_{10}$ + H]$^+$, *m/z* 449.1812 [$C_{23}H_{28}O_9$ + H]$^+$, and *m/z* 433.1788 [$C_{23}H_{28}O_8$ + H]$^+$, respectively. These formulas shared the common product-ions that were characterized for uvedalin moiety with *m/z* 213.0901; 241.0815; 273.1809, putatively identified as an isoform to enhydrin ($C_{23}H_{28}O_{10}$), uvedalin ($C_{23}H_{28}O_9$), and polymatin B ($C_{23}H_{28}O_8$) [5] (Figure 7E–G).

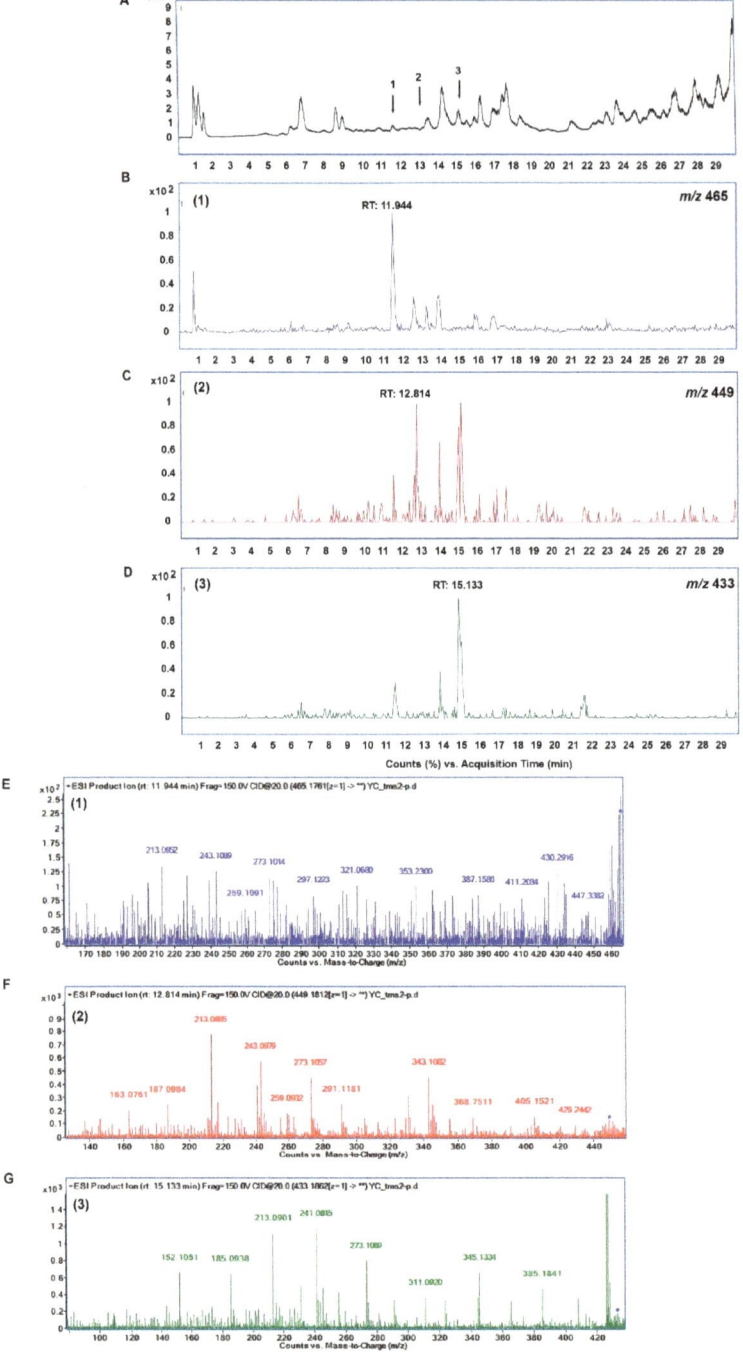

Figure 7. TIC in the positive mode of YLE (**A**). EIC of m/z 465.1761 (±10.0 ppm) [$C_{23}H_{28}O_{10}$ + H]$^+$ (**B**); EIC of m/z 449.1812 (±10.0 ppm) [$C_{23}H_{28}O_9$ + H]$^+$ (**C**); EIC of m/z 433.1862 (±10.0 ppm) [$C_{23}H_{28}O_8$ +H]$^+$ (**D**). Product-ion chromatograms of compound 1 (**E**), compound 2 (**F**), and compound 3 (**G**).

3. Discussion

Yacon (*S. sonchifolius*), a common edible plant grown throughout the world, is well known for its anti-diabetic properties [14]. It is also demonstrated to have several other pharmacological properties, including anti-inflammatory, anti-oxidant, anti-allergic, and anti-cancer effects [15]. The cytotoxicity potential of hexane, methanol, and dichloromethane extracts of Yacon leaves was assessed against MCF-7 and HT-29 cell lines by using the AlamarBlue® assay [7]. Sesquiterpene lactones from Yacon leaves, such as enhydrin, uvedalin, and their derivatives, also exhibited cytotoxic activity against MGC80-3 [16], HeLa, HL-60, and B16-F10 cell lines [9]. However, there has been no report yet to evaluate the anti-liver cancer activity of *S. sonchifolius* on liver cancer cells. Therefore, this study aimed to investigate the anti-cancer effect of YLE on HepG2 cells in terms of inhibiting cell proliferation and migration. In addition, we also examined the YLE effect on cell cycle and ROS generation in this cell line.

In the current study, YLE was found to show a potent inhibitory effect on HepG2 cell survival. Firstly, we examined the toxicity of YLE on liver cancer HepG2 cells. The calculated IC_{50} (58.2 ± 1.9 µg/mL) implied the promising inhibitory effect against these cancer cells. Indeed, the colony formation of HepG2 cells was significantly suppressed with increasing concentration of YLE up to more than 90% at 100 µg/mL, in comparison with the control, after 24 h or 48 h treatment. Taken together, these results suggested that YLE demonstrates a long-term suppressive effect on cell proliferation of HepG2 in a concentration-dependent manner.

It is known that metastasis is one of the leading causes of death from cancer and it is complicated to examine [17]. During tumor metastasis, malignant cells migrate into neighboring healthy tissues, contributing to tumor development. In this study, YLE could effectively prevent the migration of HepG2 in a dose-dependent manner. Therefore, YLE could contribute to hinder metastasis progression in hepatocellular carcinoma.

To control cancer growth, inhibition of the progression of the cell cycle is one of the essential strategies [18]. In this study, flow cytometry analysis demonstrated that the extract dose-dependently increased the percentage of cells of the G0/G1 phase of the HepG2 cell cycle. This observation reveals that YLE induces cell cycle arrest at the G0/G1 phase of the cell cycle.

In term of inducing cancer cell death, we found that YLS induced necrosis in HepG2 cells. The number of cells in the necrosis subpopulation significantly increased from 3.88% (control group) to 70.98% (100 µg/mL YLE-treatment group), whereas YLE did not activate caspase 3 or caspase 8, which regulate apoptosis in cells.

High levels of ROS in cancer cells have been found in almost all cancer cells due to high metabolomic activity and they have specific functions in cancer cell development [19]. ROS have been reported to be involved in cell proliferation, cell survival, cell cycle progression, and angiogenesis. Therefore, suppressing ROS may be a useful strategy in cancer treatment [20]. Since YLE has been reported to contain a large number of polyphenols [4], we sought to evaluate the antioxidant effect of YLE on HepG2 cells. YLE could notably reduce ROS in HepG2 in both dose and time-dependent manners. These observations may support the inhibitory effect of YLE on HepG2 cell proliferation.

The presence of sesquiterpene lactones, such as polymatin B, enhydrin, and uvedalin, was also confirmed by HPLC coupled with high-resolution mass tandem analysis [5]. These compounds have been demonstrated to have cytotoxicity as well as to induce apoptosis or necrosis in several cancer cell lines [11]. In the current study, we partly confirmed the presence of these sesquiterpenoids sharing the common fragment characteristic of the uvedalin moiety. These compounds may be significant as chemical defenses for human hepatocellular carcinoma HepG2 cells. Although the effect of individual constituents of this plant extract on HepG2 cells needs to be further investigated, the findings in the current study suggest that *S. sonchifolius* leaf could be recommended as a potential source of a chemopreventative agent against liver cancer.

4. Materials and Methods

4.1. Preparation of the Samples

The Yacon (*Smallanthus sonchifolius* ((Poepp. & Endl.) H. Rob.) leaves were collected from Pindaya Township, Shan State, in the eastern part of Myanmar. The sample was identified at the Department of Botany, University of Yangon. The leaves were cleaned, carefully dried in shadow, and powdered. About 2 g of ground powder was soaked in 20 mL methanol and shaken for 8 h at 180 rpm and 37 °C. The soaked substance was filtered throughout 110 mm filter paper (Hyundai, Seoul, South Korea). The solvent was eliminated with a rotary evaporator (SB-1200, EYELA, Shanghai, China) at 60 °C. The residue was placed in a freeze drier (Operon, Korea) to dry. The crude extract was kept in a refrigerator at 4 °C and protected from light. The experiment was performed in triplicate. Four-hundred mg of the sample extract was dissolved in 1 mL of dimethyl sulfoxide (DMSO) and then serially diluted to 100, 60, 40, and 20 µg/mL for further biological experiments. All other chemical reagents were from Sigma-Aldrich Chemical Company (St. Louis, MO, USA) unless otherwise noted.

4.2. Cell Line and Culture Medium

HepG2 and HEK 239 cell lines were obtained from the American Type Culture Collection (ATCC). Cells were cultured in Dulbecco's Modified Eagle Medium (DMEM) media supplemented with 10% (*v/v*) fetal bovine serum and 1% (*v/v*), 100 U/mL penicillin and 100 µg/mL streptomycin. Cells were cultured in an incubator at 37 °C and 5% CO_2 humidified atmosphere. Media were changed every 2 to 3 days. Reagents and media for cell culture were purchased from GenDePOT (Katy, TX, USA).

4.3. Cytotoxicity Assay (MTT Assay)

The cellular toxicity of the YLE on cultured cells was measured using 3-(4,5-dimethylthiazol-2-yl)-2, 5-diphenyl tetrazolium bromide (MTT). Cells were grown in a 96-well plate at a density of 1×10^4 cells per well. The cells are allowed to grow overnight in a cell culture incubator. Then, we treated cells with different concentrations of samples (0, 20, 40, 60, and 100 µg/mL) for 24 h. Later, cells were washed twice with phosphate buffer saline (PBS). MTT solution was added to each well (final concentration of MTT was 0.5 mg/mL) and the plate was incubated for 3 h. Finally, the medium was replaced by DMSO to solubilize the formazan crystals. The optical density was measured by absorbance at 595 nm with a microplate spectrophotometer (SpectraMax 190, Molecular Devices, San Jose, CA, USA). We identified the IC_{50} value using the ED50 Plus v1.0 online software (National Institute of Respiratory Diseases (INER), Mexico) as described elsewhere [21].

4.4. Cell Colony Formation Assay

Cells were seeded at a density of 1×10^3 cells/well in 6-well plates and allowed to attach overnight. Then, the cells were treated with YLE (0, 40, 60, 80, and 100 µg/mL) for 24 h or 48 h. After treatment, cells were continuously grown for another 2 weeks. The media were changed every 3 days. After 14 days, cells were washed with PBS and fixed with 3.7% formaldehyde solution for 30 min before being stained with 0.5% crystal violet for another 30 min at room temperature (RT). Cells were washed with water to remove the dye and then photographed.

4.5. Cell Migration Assay (Wound–Healing Assay)

We seeded cells in a 24-well plate (5×10^4 cells/well) and cultured at 37 °C, 5% CO_2 for 24 h. The 80–90% cell confluence was observed before the scratch assay was performed. We stimulated a wound using a sterile 200 µL pipette tip. After washing with PBS to remove loosened debris, cells were treated with YLE (0, 40, 60, 80, and 100 µg/mL) for 24 h at 37 °C, 5% CO_2. After treatment, cells were washed twice with PBS. The images of cells were captured under a CKX41 microscope

(Olympus, Japan) at 400× magnification. Images were processed with ProgRes Capture Pro software v.2.8.8 (JENOPTIK Optical Systems, Jena, Germany).

4.6. Reactive Oxygen Species (ROS) Production Assay

The level of intracellular ROS was determined by the change in fluorescence resulting from the oxidation of the fluorescent probe dichlorofluorescein diacetate (DCF-DA). We seeded cells at a density of 1×10^6 cells/well in 6 wells plate and then treated them with 0, 40, 60, 80, and 100 ug/mL of YLE for 3, 6, and 9 h. After indicated periods, cells were washed twice with DPBS and stained with dichlorofluorescein diacetate (DCF-DA, 10 μM) at 37 °C for 30 min in the dark. After washing twice with PBS, the fluorescence generation was measured in a microplate reader, (excitation wavelength (ext.): 485 nm; emission wavelength (emi.): 535 nm). Data were expressed as the percentage of ROS relative to untreated control groups.

4.7. Cell Cycle Analysis

HepG2 cells at a concentration of 1×10^6/well cells were cultured in 6-well plates and treated with different concentrations of YLE for 24h. After treatment, the cells were washed with PBS and harvested using a centrifuge at 1300 rpm for 3 min. Then, cells were re-suspended and fixed with 70% ethanol at −20 °C for 1 week. After fixing, we harvested cells by washing with PBS and centrifuging at 2000 rpm for 3 min. Cells were incubated with RNase (200 μg/mL) at 37 °C for 30 min to remove cellular RNA, then stained with propidium iodide (PI, 100 μg/mL) for another 10 min at RT in the dark. Finally, the cells were analyzed by flow cytometry (BD FACSCalibur, BD Biosciences, USA) according to detected signals in the FL2 channel (ext: 488 nm, emi: 564–606 nm) while data were analyzed with Cell Quest Pro software (BD Biosciences, San Jose, CA, USA).

4.8. Annexin V/PI Assay

HepG2 cells were seeded in the 6-well plates (1×10^6 cells/well). After overnight incubation, we treated cells with indicated concentrations of YLE for 24 h. Cells were washed with PBS and harvested using a centrifuge at 2000 rpm for 3 min for the following analysis. To distinguish apoptotic and necrotic cell death in HepG2 cells, we used the BD Annexin V: FITC Apoptosis Detection Kit I (BD Biosciences, San Diego, CA, USA), according to the manufacture's direction. The cells were analyzed by flow cytometry (BD FACSCalibur, San Jose, CA). Signals were detected in the FL1 channel (for Annexin V) and FL3 channel (for PI), while data were analyzed with Cell Quest Pro software.

4.9. Western Blotting

The HepG2 cells were seeded in a 6-well plate at 1×10^6 cells/well and treated with various concentrations of YLE for 24 h. The whole cells lysates were prepared by homogenizing cells in a prepared lysis buffer (20 mM HEPES (pH 7.6), 350 mM NaCl, 20% glycerol, 0.5 mM EDTA, 0.1 mM EGTA, 1% NP-40, 50 mM NaF, 0.1 mM DTT, 0.1 mM PMSF, and a protease inhibitor cocktail) on ice for 30 min, followed by collecting the supernatant using a centrifuge at 15,000 rpm for 10 min. The concentration of protein was identified using a Bradford assay. The equal amounts of proteins were separated by electrophoresis on 10% SDS gels and transferred to nitrocellulose membranes. Blots were blocked with 5% BSA for 1 h prior to incubating with the following primary antibodies: β-actin conjugated with HRP (Santa Cruz, 47778) as1:3000, pro-caspase 3 (rabbit, Santa Cruz H-277: sc-7148) as 1:1000, cleaved caspase 3 (rabbit, Abcam ab2302) as 1:1000, pro-caspase 8 (rabbit, Santa Cruz, sc-6134) as 1:1000, and cleaved caspase 8 (rabbit, Cell Signaling Technology, 9496) as 1:1000, at 4 °C overnight. After washing the membrane and incubating with goat anti-rabbit IgG (H + L) secondary antibody conjugated with HRP (GeneTex, GTX213110, 1:3000) for 1 h at RT, the bands of interest were detected using an EZWestern ECL kit (Daeillab Service, Seoul, South Korea) and then photographed on the LAS-4000 imaging system (GE Healthcare, Chicago, IL, USA).

4.10. LC-Q-TOF-MS Analysis of YLE

Since the cytotoxicity of YLE was attributed to its active ingredients, which were known to be sesquiterpenoids, we confirmed the presence of these compounds using liquid chromatography analysis in an HPLC system (Agilent Technologies, Santa Clara, CA, USA) linked to a G6530A ESI-Q-TOF MS spectrometer (Agilent Technologies). Chromatographic separations were conducted using a C18 column (2.1 × 150 mm, 3.5 µm, Agilent Technologies). The mobile phases were water with 0.1% formic acid (A) and acetonitrile with 0.1% formic acid (B). The gradient program consisted of the following: 0–15 min, 5–50% B; 15–20 min, 50% B; 20–30 min, 50–95% B; followed by 95% B for 10 min washing. The flow rate was 0.3 mL/min and the temperature was kept at 40 °C. The injection volume was 3 µL. The instrument was operated with an ESI source in positive ion mode. The mass determination was performed using the following MS conditions: Ion spray voltage of 400 kV; desolvation temperature, 350 °C; desolvation gas flow rate, 10 L/min. The fragmentor was set at 150 V. The full-scan mass spectra were acquired within an *m/z* range of 100 to 1200 *m/z* in the MS mode followed by the target MS/MS mode. Data acquisition and proceeding were performed using Mass Hunter Qualitative Analysis software (Agilent Technologies). The compounds were putatively identified based on their mass tandems in comparison with published data.

4.11. Statistical Analysis

In this study, we performed all experiments in triplicate and analyzed results using one-way ANOVA followed by a Dunnett's test (SPSS version 25.0; Chicago, IL, USA). Probabilities of $p < 0.05$ were considered significant.

5. Conclusions

In this study, we partially identified the active ingredients present in the YLE, which are possibly melampolide sesquiterpene lactones with uvedalin moiety. The results in this study indicate that YLE appears to be capable of killing malignant liver cancer cells by inhibiting the growth and migration in addition to inducing necrosis and cell cycle arrest. Furthermore, we also confirmed the antioxidant effect of YLE on liver cancer cells. To conclude, these findings suggest *S. sonchifolius* (Yacon) is a promising potential anti-liver cancer agent in the area of herbal medicine. Further research regarding the role of each active compound in YLE towards anti-liver cancer activity would be worthwhile.

Author Contributions: Conceptualization, Y.S.K. and P.P.M.; Methodology, T.T.P.D. and P.P.M.; Software, T.T.P.D.; Validation, T.T.P.D., P.P.M. and Y.S.K.; Formal Analysis, T.T.P.D. and P.P.M.; Investigation, T.T.P.D. and P.P.M.; Resources, Y.S.K. and P.P.M.; Data Curation, T.T.P.D.; Writing—Original Draft Preparation, P.P.M.; Writing—Review & Editing, T.T.P.D.; Visualization, Y.S.K. and P.P.M.; Supervision, Y.S.K.; Project Administration, Y.S.K.; Funding Acquisition, Y.S.K. and P.P.M.

Funding: This research was funded by a grant (NRF-2017R1A2B4009301) from the National Research Foundation of Korea. P.P.M was supported by the Korea Foundation for Advanced Studies (KFAS). T.T.P.D. was awarded a fellowship from the BK21 PLUS supported from the Ministry of Education.

Acknowledgments: We appreciated the technical support of Ji Yoon Lee in College of Pharmacy, SNU.

Conflicts of Interest: The authors declare no conflict of interest.

References

1. Ferlay, J.; Ervik, M.; Lam, F.; Colombet, M.; Mery, L.; Piñeros, M.; Znaor, A.; Soerjomataram, I.; Bray, F. *Global Cancer Observatory: Cancer Today*; International Agency for Research on Cancer: Lyon, France, 2018; Available online: https://gco.iarc.fr/today (accessed on 5 May 2019).
2. Siegel, R.; Ma, J.; Zou, Z.; Jemal, A. Cancer statistics, 2014. *CA Cancer J. Clin.* **2014**, *64*, 9–29. [CrossRef] [PubMed]
3. Caetano, B.F.; de Moura, N.A.; Almeida, A.P.; Dias, M.C.; Sivieri, K.; Barbisan, L.F. Yacon (*Smallanthus sonchifolius*) as a Food Supplement: Health-Promoting Benefits of Fructooligosaccharides. *Nutrients* **2016**, *8*, 436. [CrossRef] [PubMed]

4. Simonovska, B.; Vovk, I.; Andrensek, S.; Valentova, K.; Ulrichova, J. Investigation of phenolic acids in yacon (*Smallanthus sonchifolius*) leaves and tubers. *J. Chromatogr. A* **2003**, *1016*, 89–98. [CrossRef]
5. Ziarovska, J.; Padilla-Gonzalez, G.F.; Viehmannova, I.; Fernandez, E. Genetic and chemical diversity among yacon [*Smallanthus sonchifolius* (Poepp. et Endl.) H. Robinson] accessions based on iPBS markers and metabolomic fingerprinting. *Plant Physiol. Biochem.* **2019**, *141*, 183–192. [CrossRef] [PubMed]
6. De Almeida Paula, H.A.; Abranches, M.V.; de Luces Fortes Ferreira, C.L. Yacon (*Smallanthus sonchifolius*): A food with multiple functions. *Crit. Rev. Food Sci. Nutr.* **2015**, *55*, 32–40. [CrossRef] [PubMed]
7. Mendoza, R.P.; Vidar, W.S.; Oyong, G.G. In vitro cytotoxic potential of Yacon (*Smallanthus sonchifolius*) against HT-29, MCF-7 and HDFn cell lines. *J. Med. Plants Res.* **2017**, *11*, 207–217.
8. De Moura, N.A.; Caetano, B.F.; Sivieri, K.; Urbano, L.H.; Cabello, C.; Rodrigues, M.A.; Barbisan, L.F. Protective effects of yacon (*Smallanthus sonchifolius*) intake on experimental colon carcinogenesis. *Food Chem. Toxicol.* **2012**, *50*, 2902–2910. [CrossRef] [PubMed]
9. Kitai, Y.; Hayashi, K.; Otsuka, M.; Nishiwaki, H.; Senoo, T.; Ishii, T.; Sakane, G.; Sugiura, M.; Tamura, H. New Sesquiterpene Lactone Dimer, Uvedafolin, Extracted from Eight Yacon Leaf Varieties (*Smallanthus sonchifolius*): Cytotoxicity in HeLa, HL-60, and Murine B16-F10 Melanoma Cell Lines. *J. Agric. Food Chem.* **2015**, *63*, 10856–10861. [CrossRef] [PubMed]
10. Siriwan, D.; Naruse, T.; Tamura, H. Effect of epoxides and alpha-methylene-gamma-lactone skeleton of sesquiterpenes from yacon (*Smallanthus sonchifolius*) leaves on caspase-dependent apoptosis and NF-kappaB inhibition in human cercival cancer cells. *Fitoterapia* **2011**, *82*, 1093–1101. [CrossRef] [PubMed]
11. De Ford, C.; Ulloa, J.L.; Catalan, C.A.N.; Grau, A.; Martino, V.S.; Muschietti, L.V.; Merfort, I. The sesquiterpene lactone polymatin B from *Smallanthus sonchifolius* induces different cell death mechanisms in three cancer cell lines. *Phytochemistry* **2015**, *117*, 332–339. [CrossRef] [PubMed]
12. Li, S.; Tan, H.Y.; Wang, N.; Zhang, Z.J.; Lao, L.; Wong, C.W.; Feng, Y. The Role of Oxidative Stress and Antioxidants in Liver Diseases. *Int. J. Mol. Sci.* **2015**, *16*, 26087–26124. [CrossRef] [PubMed]
13. Donato, M.T.; Tolosa, L.; Gomez-Lechon, M.J. Culture and Functional Characterization of Human Hepatoma HepG2 Cells. *Methods Mol. Biol.* **2015**, *1250*, 77–93. [CrossRef] [PubMed]
14. Xiang, Z.; He, F.; Kang, T.G.; Dou, D.Q.; Gai, K.; Shi, Y.Y.; Kim, Y.H.; Dong, F. Anti-diabetes constituents in leaves of *Smallanthus sonchifolius*. *Nat. Prod. Commun.* **2010**, *5*, 95–98. [PubMed]
15. Lee, K.P.; Choi, N.H.; Kim, J.T.; Park, I.S. The effect of yacon (*Samallanthus sonchifolius*) ethanol extract on cell proliferation and migration of C6 glioma cells stimulated with fetal bovine serum. *Nutr. Res. Pract.* **2015**, *9*, 256–261. [CrossRef] [PubMed]
16. Suo, T.J.; Wang, X.T.; Li, D.W.; Aung, K.W.; Ran, X.K.; Dou, D.Q.; Dong, F. Extraction of Yacon Leaves Enhances Enhydrin Degradation. *J. Chem. Soc. Pak.* **2016**, *38*, 379–383.
17. Seyfried, T.N.; Huysentruyt, L.C. On the origin of cancer metastasis. *Crit. Rev. Oncog.* **2013**, *18*, 43–73. [CrossRef] [PubMed]
18. Vermeulen, K.; Van Bockstaele, D.R.; Berneman, Z.N. The cell cycle: A review of regulation, deregulation and therapeutic targets in cancer. *Cell Prolif.* **2003**, *36*, 131–149. [CrossRef] [PubMed]
19. Liou, G.Y.; Storz, P. Reactive oxygen species in cancer. *Free Radic. Res.* **2010**, *44*, 479–496. [CrossRef] [PubMed]
20. Kumari, S.; Badana, A.K.; Malla, R. Reactive Oxygen Species: A Key Constituent in Cancer Survival. *Biomark. Insights* **2018**, *13*, 1177271918755391. [CrossRef] [PubMed]
21. Lockwood, W.W.; Zejnullahu, K.; Bradner, J.E.; Varmus, H. Sensitivity of human lung adenocarcinoma cell lines to targeted inhibition of BET epigenetic signaling proteins. *Proc. Natl. Acad. Sci. USA* **2012**, *109*, 19408–19413. [CrossRef] [PubMed]

Sample Availability: Not available.

© 2019 by the authors. Licensee MDPI, Basel, Switzerland. This article is an open access article distributed under the terms and conditions of the Creative Commons Attribution (CC BY) license (http://creativecommons.org/licenses/by/4.0/).

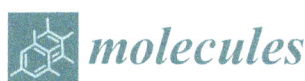

Article

Chemical Composition, Antimicrobial, Antioxidant, and Antiproliferative Properties of Grapefruit Essential Oil Prepared by Molecular Distillation

Weihui Deng, Ke Liu, Shan Cao, Jingyu Sun, Balian Zhong and Jiong Chun *

National Navel Orange Engineering Research Center, College of Life Sciences, Gannan Normal University, Ganzhou 341000, China; dwh110by@163.com (W.D.); liuke121602026@126.com (K.L.); scoral29116@163.com (S.C.); SJYnj_1997@163.com (J.S.); bal.zh@163.com (B.Z.)
* Correspondence: qczx99@163.com; Tel.: +86-797-839-3068

Academic Editor: Raffaele Capasso
Received: 3 December 2019; Accepted: 3 January 2020; Published: 5 January 2020

Abstract: Grapefruit essential oil has been proven to have wide range of bioactivities. However, bioactivity of its molecular distillate has not been well studied. In this study, a light phase oil was obtained by molecular distillation from cold-pressed grapefruit essential oil and GC-MS was used to identify its chemical composition. The antimicrobial activity of the light phase oil was tested by filter paper diffusion method, and the anticancer activity was determined by the Cell Counting Kit-8 (CCK-8) assay. Twenty-four components were detected with a total relative content of 99.74%, including 97.48% of terpenes and 1.66% of oxygenated terpenes. The light phase oil had the best antimicrobial effect on *Bacillus subtilis*, followed by *Escherichia coli*, *Staphylococcus aureus* and *Salmonellaty phimurium*. DPPH and ABTS assays demonstrated that the light phase oil had good antioxidant activity. The CCK-8 assay of cell proliferation showed that the light phase oil had a good inhibitory effect on the proliferation of HepG2 liver cancer cells and HCT116 colon cancer cells.

Keywords: grapefruit essential oil; molecular distillation; GC-MS; antimicrobial; antioxidant; anticancer activity

1. Introduction

With the frequent occurrence of food safety issues and the toxicity of synthetic chemicals, the demand for safe and natural alternatives is growing. Plant extracts have been used since ancient times, and now the focus is on their role in health promotion and their treatment and prevention properties for various diseases. In the past few decades, plant essential oils (EOs) have attracted a lot of interest due to their safety and pharmacological properties including bacteriostatic, free radical scavenging, anti-inflammatory, and inhibitory effects on malignant tumor cell proliferation [1–4]. Citrus Eos are the main aromatic by-products of the juice extraction industry and are widely used in food, cosmetics and pharmaceutical industry [5–7]. The annual global production of citrus EO is approximately 16,000 tons, and the cost is about $14,000/ton on the international market. Thus, citrus EO is of great demand and is one of the more promising market prospects [8]. Grapefruit (*Citrus paradisi* Macf.), one of the world's largest production citrus families [9], is famous for its taste and nutritional value. Grapefruit EO is extracted from grapefruit peel and has been used for a long time as a valuable ingredient for its characteristic aroma in flavor and fragrance [10,11]. Similar to most citrus EOs, its major components are terpenes and terpene oxides. Terpene oxides include alcohols, ethers, aldehydes, ketones, and esters [12–14], which are the main source of the aroma, whereas terpenes contribute less to the aroma. In spite of extensive studies on the aroma features of grapefruit EO, in recent years, more and more researchers have become interested in exploring their biological and pharmacological activities. Grapefruit EO has been reported to have a wide range of bioactivities. It was shown to inhibit the growth of food-borne spoilage bacteria and pathogenic strains [15–17]. Okunowo et al. (2013) found that grapefruit EO obtained from the peel by hydrodistillation exerted inhibitory effects against bacteria and fungi, andmay be further developed for the treatment of certain diseases [18]. Grapefruit EO has shown antioxidant activity, which was important for food preservation and disease prevention [19,20]. Ahmed et al. (2019) reported that grapefruit EO extracted by hydrodistillation had antioxidant activity by using DPPH and FRAP assays [21]. Grapefruit peel extracts have been shown to decrease the HL-60 cell viability in a concentration-dependent manner [22]. In fact, grapefruit extracts (a mixture of EO and other nonvolatile phytochemicals) could also inhibit the growth and proliferation of cancer cells such as neuroblastomas, leukemias, and prostate and lung cancer lines [23–25]. Cuthrell et al. (2006) reviewed the anticancer activities of phytochemicals found in grapefruit [26].

Most grapefruit EO samples used for bioactivity studies were made by cold-pressing, steam distillation, or hydrodistillation methods. Cold-pressing is the predominant method to extract most citrus peel EOs, including grapefruit EOs. In commercial practice, grapefruitis processed to obtain juice and other by-products. EO is one of the primary grapefruit by-products. Large-scale grapefruit EO is mainly prepared by a cold-pressing method based on John Bean FoodTech (JBT) juice extractors and its technology, which is used by 75% of the world's citrus juice production [27]. The juice and EO are extracted separately and simultaneously. The EO was extracted by mechanical rupturing of the oil sacs in the flavedo, expressing the oil as an aqueous emulsion from which it is separated by centrifuging. The EO recovery is a physical separation process and no heat is applied throughout the whole extraction procedure. The operation temperature is much lower than in the distillation procedure. Thus, the EOs will have characteristics that are closer to those of the essence present in the grapefruit matrix. Large scale production, low cost and the aroma characteristic remaining are the big advantages of the cold-pressing method. However, cold-pressed grapefruit oil contains waxes, pesticide residues, coumarins, carotenoids and other nonvolatile components [28–30], some of them also have good bioactivities that may cause bias in bioactivity research of EO. César et al. (2009) found that furanocoumarins isolated from grapefruit peel oil showed potent in vitro inhibitory activity against intestinal cytochrome P450 3A4, an enzyme involved in "grapefruit/drug" interactions in humans [28]. Steam distillation or hydrodistillation was carried out at relatively high temperature which may cause degradation of some thermal sensitive molecules [18,31]. To avoid such problems, and find a new way to use the commercial available cold-pressed grapefruit EO in biochemistry and pharmachutical fields, we used a molecular distillation method to prepare grapefruit oil samples for our bioactivity tests.

Molecular distillation is a special liquid–liquid separation technology under high vacuum, which is employed as a separation process in the food industry [32,33]. Molecular distillation can divide the EO mixture into two different phases according to the free path of different molecules at low temperature. Molecular distillation is prominent with the advantages of low temperature treatment and high vacuum application, which is very suitable for thermolabile compounds and is used for concentrating and refining EOs [34,35]. At present, there are seldom reports on the antibacterial and anticancer activity of Eos obtained by molecular distillation. In this study, the cold-pressed grapefruit EO was processed by molecular distillation technology and the light phase essential oil (LPEO) was collected. Its constituents were identified by GC-MS. The activities of LEPO were tested on microorganisms and malignant proliferating cells (HCT116 colon cancer cells and HepG2 liver cancer cells) were tested. We expect that this work can stimulate the development of new agents for food preservation and chemo-preventive anti-cancer treatments.

2. Results and Discussion

2.1. Chemical Composition of the Light Phase Grapefruit Essential Oil

The chemical composition of the grapefruit light phase essential oil (LPEO) was analyzed by GC-MS. The total ion chromatogram (TIC) of LPEO is shown in Figure 1. The relative content of each component was calculated by the peak area normalization method. The components were identified according to retention index and the NIST mass spectral library.

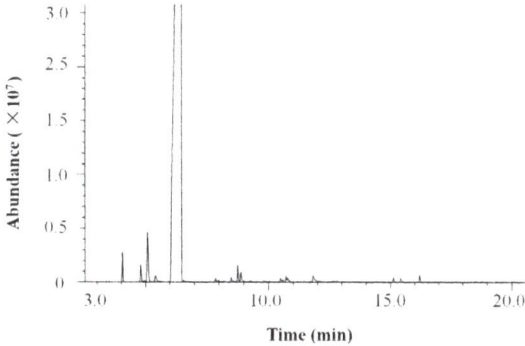

Figure 1. Total ion chromatogram of grapefruit light phase essential oil (LPEO).

As shown in Table 1, twenty-four compounds, accounting for 99.74% of the total oil were identified. Monoterpenes were the major components, accounting for 96.93% of the total oil. Limonene (93.33%) was the predominant component of monoterpenes, followed by β-myrcene (2.16%), α-pinene (0.76%), and sabinene (0.60%). Monoterpene oxide (1.62%) included carvone (0.41%), cis-limonene oxide (0.43%), and trans-limonene oxide (0.33%). The sesquiterpene (0.55%) included caryophyllene (0.20%), β-cubebene (0.14%), α-copaene (0.13%), etc. Caryophyllene oxide (0.04%) was the only sesquiterpene oxide detected. In addition, three linear aldehydes: Octanal (0.36%), decanal (0.19%), and nonanal (0.05%) were found in LPEO. Pino et al. (1999) reported the chemical composition of grapefruit EO prepared by steam distillation from solids and effluents produced during commercial oil extraction [31]. The limonene content (70.9%) in steam-distilled oil was much less than LPEO (93.33%); however, the content of myrcene (13.6%) and α-pinene (3.8%) was much higher than LPEO (myrcene 2.16% and α-pinene 0.76%). Also, Okunowo et al. (2013) reported the components of grapefruit EO obtained by hydrodistillation [18]. The content of limonene (75.07%) was closed to that of steam-distilled oil. Cold-pressed grapefruit oil was shown to have a limonene content of 93.47%, however, the corrected limonene content became 85.60% when nonvolatiles were excluded [36]. The composition of distilled samples of grapefruit EO still vary from each other according to genetic differences, soil type, maturity stages, weather types and culturing conditions etc [37].

Table 1. Chemical composition of grapefruit light phase essential oil (LPEO) by GC-MS.

No.	RI[a]	Compounds	Composition (%)
1	938	α-Pinene	0.76
2	956	Camphene	0.01
3	977	Sabinene	0.60
4	985	β-Pinene	0.05
5	992	β-Myrcene	2.16
6	1007	Octanal	0.36
7	1049	Limonene	93.33

Table 1. Cont.

No.	RI[a]	Compounds	Composition (%)
8	1053	β-Ocimene	0.02
9	1103	Linalool	0.12
10	1108	Nonanal	0.05
11	1127	trans-p-Mentha-2,8-dien-1-ol	0.16
12	1137	cis-Limonene oxide	0.43
13	1141	trans-Limonene oxide	0.33
14	1155	Citronellal	0.04
15	1199	α-Terpineol	0.13
16	1208	Decanal	0.19
17	1251	Carvone	0.41
18	1377	α-Copaene	0.13
19	1388	β-Cubebene	0.14
20	1421	Caryophyllene	0.20
21	1457	Humulene	0.03
22	1482	Germacrene D	0.01
23	1519	δ-cadinene	0.04
24	1566	Caryophyllene oxide	0.04
Total			99.74
		Monoterpene hydrocarbons	96.93
		Oxygenated monoterpenoids	1.62
		Sesquiterpene hydrocarbons	0.55
		Oxygenated sesquiterpenes	0.04
		others	0.60

RI[a], retention indices determined on HP-5 column, using the homologous series of n-alkanes (C8–C20).

2.2. Antimicrobial Activity

Grapefruit EOs prepared by cold-pressing or hydrodistillation using a Clevenger-type apparatus have shown a wide spectrum of antimicrobial activity in vitro [18,37]. However, antimicrobial activity of grapefruit EO prepared by molecular distillation has not been well studied. We tested LPEO on five microorganisms and the results obtained are shown in Table 2. The filter paper diffusion method was used to test the antibacterial activity of LPEO against different bacteria, and the activity of LPEO was evaluated according to the diameter of the inhibition zone and the minimum inhibitory concentration (MIC) values. LPEO exhibited strong antibacterial effects on the four bacteria tested. From the scale of the inhibition zone, LPEO had the strongest inhibitory effect on *B. subtilis* with a maximum diameter of 35.59 mm, followed by *E. coli*, *S. aureus*, and *S. typhimurium*. LPEO had no inhibitory activity against *P. aeruginosa* with an inhibition zone of 8.57 mm. *P. aeruginosa* belongs with *E. coli* and *S. typhimurium* to the group of Gram-negative bacteria but exhibits quite a different response to LPEO. This phenomenon may be partly due to its relatively low outer membrane permeability. LPEO molecules enter the periplasm by diffusion through the channels of nonspecific porins in the outer membrane, and this pathway in *P. aeruginosa* is 10- to 100-fold less efficient than that in *E. coli* [38]. Regarding MIC values, LPEO showed the best antimicrobial activity against *Bacillus subtilis* with a MIC value of 0.78 μL/mL. Based on the inhibition zone and MIC values, the order of sensitivity of the different bacteria was: *B. subtilis* > *E. coli* > *S. aureus* > *S. typhimurium* > *P. aeruginosa*. Since cold-pressed grapefruit oil (*Citrus paradisi* Macf.) has been evaluated as "generally recognized as safe" (GRAS) by the Expert Panel of the Flavor and Extract Manufacturers Association (FEMA) [39], and LPEO, a distillate from cold-pressed EO, showed strong sensitivity to most tested microorganisms, it appeared to be suitable to food applications. These results demonstrate that molecular distillation technology can provide a grapefruit EO fraction with good antimicrobial activity.

Table 2. The antimicrobial activity of grapefruit light phase essential oil (LPEO).

Bacterial Strain	Diameter of Inhibition Zone (mm)	MIC (µL/mL)
Bacillus subtilis (G+)	35.59 ± 1.06 [a]	0.78
Staphylococcus aureus (G+)	24.34 ± 0.52 [c]	6.25
Escherichia coli (G-)	26.86 ± 0.17 [b]	6.25
Salmonella typhimurium (G-)	21.70 ± 0.21 [d]	12.50
Pseudomonas aeruginosa (G-)	8.57 ± 0.13 [e]	25.00

Disk diameter is 6.0 mm. Zone of growth inhibition values are presented as mean± standard deviation for at least three experiments. Different superscript letters represent the significant differences at $P < 0.05$ according to Tukey's multiple range test. The scale of zone of inhibition measurement was the following (disk diameter included): ≥20 mm is strongly inhibitory; <20–16 mm is moderately/mildly inhibitory; <15–10 mm is weak inhibitory; <9–7 mm is not inhibitory.

Uysal et al. (2011) evaluated the antibacterial activities of grapefruit Eos from solvent-free microwave extraction (SFME) and hydrodistillation (HD) by the disc-diffusion method [17]. The Eos obtained from SFME and HD showed the highest activity against *S. aureus* with inhibition zones of 53 and 41 mm, respectively, higher than LPEO (24.34 mm). The activity against *E. coli* (30 mm and 28 mm) was close to our result (26.86 mm). Both of their samples and LPEO showed no obvious activity against *P. aeruginosa*. LPEO showed better activity against *S. typhimurium* (21.70 mm) than their samples (15 mm and 13 mm). Although a lot of plant EOs have shown antimicrobial activity, the reason of this capacity is not well known. It could be provoked by the major components of the EOs or due to a synergistic effect among the major components and the minor ones. Different preparation methods yield EO samples with differences in chemical composition and relative content, and cause differences in antimicrobial activity.

2.3. Antioxidant Activity

A lot of EOs have been reported to scavenge the free radicals that cause damage to the body and reduce the risk of many diseases originating from oxidative stress. In order to measure the effect of LPEO and determine its potential application in food, cosmetic or pharmaceutical industries, we evaluated its antioxidant activity using two different assays: The 2,2-diphenyl-1-picrylhydrazyl (DPPH)and 2,2′-azino-bis(3-ethylbenzthiazoline-6-sulfonic acid) radical (ABTS) assays. Butylated hydroxytoluene (BHT) was used as positive control. The IC_{50} values of BHT in DPPH and ABTS were 0.03 mg/mL and 0.01 mg/mL, which was consistent with the literature [40]. The DPPH and ABTS activities of LPEO were obtained with IC_{50} values of 22.06 ± 0.92 mg/mL and 15.72 ± 0.32 mg/mL, respectively. LPEO had better antioxidant activity than cold-pressed grapefruit EO in the DPPH assay ($EC_{50} > 40$ mg/mL) and hydrodistilled grapefruit EO in the ABTS assay ($EC_{50} = 27.5$ mg/mL) [35]. Compared with cold-pressed orange oil, LPEO had much lower antioxidant activity in the DPPH assay ($IC_{50} = 3.01 ± 0.20$ mg/mL) and better activity in the ABTS assay ($IC_{50} = 23.25 ± 0.84$ mg/mL) [41].

2.4. Antiproliferative Activity of LPEO in HepG2 and HCT116 Cancer Cells

The effects of different concentrations of LPEO on the proliferation of HepG2 liver cancer and HCT116 colon cancer cells were tested by the Cell Counting Kit-8 (CCK-8) method [42,43]. The results are shown in Figure 2. The viability rate of both cell types decreased with increasing LPEO concentration. When the concentration of LPEO was less than 0.1 µL/mL, no obvious change of viability of HepG2 cells was observed. However, when the concentration of LPEO was higher than 0.1 µL/mL, the viability of HepG2 cells significantly decreased; at the LPEO concentration of 0.3 µL/mL, the viability was 7.4%only. LPEO also had a good inhibitory effect on the growth of HCT116 colon cancer cells. At the concentration of0.05 µL/mL or higher, the viability of HCT116 cells significantly decreased. It was as low as 7.43% when the concentration of LPEO was 0.5 µL/mL. GraphPad Prism™ (Version 5.00) software (GraphPad Software, San Diego, CA, USA) was used to calculate IC_{50} values. IC_{50} value of HepG2 and HCT116 was 0.24 and 0.20 µL/mL, respectively. These results indicate that LPEO has a significant inhibitory effect on the proliferation of HepG2 hepatoma cells and HCT116 colon cancer cells in vitro.

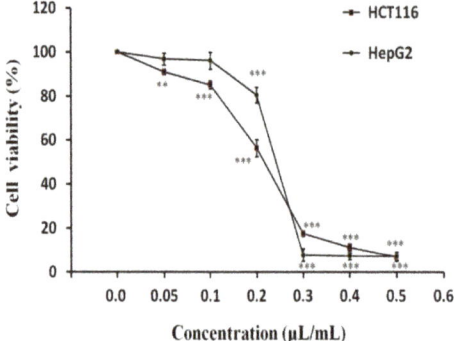

Figure 2. Effects on the viability of cancer cellsHepG2 and HCT116 as a function of LPEO concentration. Significant decreases in cell viability of cancer cells are seen at increasing LPEO concentrations compared to untreated controls (control group was set to 100%). **—Very significant at $p < 0.01$, ***—Highly significant at $p < 0.001$.

Sun et al. (2002) studied antiproliferative activity of grapefruit fruit extract on the growth of HepG2 human liver cancer cells in vitro [22]. The extract showed antiproliferative activity in a dose-dependent manner with the median effective dose (EC_{50}) value of 130.09 mg/mL. However, they did not identify the specific phytochemicals which were responsible for antiproliferative activity. Manassero et al. (2013) studied the antiproliferative activity of cold-pressed EO from mandarin peel and its principal component limonene [44]. Mandarin EO and limonene exhibited IC_{50} of 0.063 µL/mL and 0.150 µL/mL against HepG2 cells, respectively. The much higher activity of mandarin EO than LPEO (0.24 µL/mL) may attributed to other high potent phytochemicals in cold-pressed EO. We have reported antiproliferative activity of the 'Gannanzao' orange EO (GOEO) prepared by hydrodistillation, which exhibited IC_{50} of 0.29 µL/mL and 0.35 µL/mL against HepG2 cells and HCT116 colon cancer cells, respectively [43]. LPEO showed a slightly higher activity than GOEO, which may be attributed to its higher limonene content (LPEO 93.33%, GOEO 88.07%).

The discussion about anticancer activity of some EO components has been made by Mukhtar et al. [45]. Our study preliminarily tested the inhibitory effect of LPEO on the proliferation of HepG2 liver cancer cells and HCT116 colon cancer cells. The anticancer activity of LPEO and its components on cancer cells and their mode of action deserve further study.

3. Materials and Methods

3.1. Materials

Cold-pressed Marsh white grapefruit (*Citrus paradisi* Macf., Lakeland, FL, USA) EO was purchased from Ungerer Limited. 2,2-diphenyl-1-picrylhydrazyl (DPPH) was purchased from Tokyo Chemical Industry Co., Ltd. (Tokyo, Japan), 2,2′-azino-bis(3-ethylbenzthiazoline-6-sulfonic acid) (ABTS), *n*-alkanes(C8–C20)were purchased from Sigma-Aldrich (St. Louis, MO, USA). Butylated hydroxytoluene (BHT) was purchased from Macklin, Shanghai, China. The following microorganisms were purchased from Beijing, China General Microbiological Culture Collection Center (CGMCC): *Escherichia coli* (ATCC25922), *Staphylococcus aureus* (ATCC25923), *Bacillus subtilis* (ATCC6633), *Salmonella typhimurium* (ATCC14028), and *Pseudomonas aeruginosa* (ATCC9207).

3.2. Preparation of Grapefruit Light Phase EO Sample

Grapefruit light phase EO(LPEO) was obtained by molecular distillation from cold-pressed grapefruit EO (*Citrus paradisi* Macf., Lakeland, FL, USA) using a wiped-film molecular distillation apparatus (Pope Two Inch Laboratory Scale Wiped-Film Molecular Still & Evaporator, Pope Scientific Inc., Saukville, WI, USA). The evaporation temperature and operation pressure were 55 °C and 6.0 Torr, respectively. Cold-pressed grapefruit EO was fed at room temperature and the feeding rate was 3.0 mL/min. The rotational speed of the roller wiper (Pope Scientific Inc., Saukville, WI, USA) was 325 rpm, and the condenser temperature was 0 °C. The final grapefruit EO sample (LPEO) was obtained from the light phase outlet with the yield of 86%.

3.3. GC-MS Analyses

The constituents of LPEO were analyzed using an Agilent 7890B gas chromatograph coupled with an Agilent mass spectrometer detector (Agilent Technologies, Santa Clara, CA, USA). The GC was equipped with a HP-5 column (30.00 m × 0.25 mm × 0.25 μm). Mass spectra were obtained by electron ionization (EI) at 70 eV. The injector and detector were operated at 250 °C and 300 °C, respectively. The temperature program was 80 °C for 4 min, and then increased at 5 °C/min to 250 °C and held constant for 10 min. The constituents were identified by comparing their mass spectra with the National Institute of Standards and Technology (NIST, version 2010, U.S. Department of Commerce, Gaithersburg, MD, USA) data reference. The retention indices (RI) of the constituents were determined by adding a C8–C20 *n*-alkanes mixture to the essential oil before injecting in the GC-MS equipment and analyzing it under the same conditions described above.

3.4. Antimicrobial Activity Assays

3.4.1. Microbial Growth Conditions

The microbial strains were maintained in nutrient agar media at 37 °C. Subsequently, one colony from each culture was inoculated in liquid medium for 18–24 h with shaking (200 rpm) to obtain freshly cultured microbial suspensions (>10^8 CFU mL^{-1}) for test.

3.4.2. Determination of Diameter of the Inhibition Zone

LPEO was tested on five microbial strains, using filter paper diffusion method [46]. Briefly, a suspension of the tested microorganism (10^6 CFUmL^{-1}) was spread on the solid media plates. The paper discs (Whatman No. 1 filter paper, 6 mm diameter) were impregnated with 20 μL LPEO and placed on the inoculated agar. The plates inoculated with bacterial strains were incubated for 24 h at 37 °C. After incubation, diameter of the inhibition zone was measured in millimeters. Each test was performed in triplicates on at least three separate experiments.

3.4.3. Determination of Minimum Inhibitory Concentration (MIC)

MIC values of LPEO against microorganisms were determined by disc-diffusion method [46,47] Sterile filter paper discs were placed on the surface of Petri dishes and impregnated with 20 μL of EO at different concentrations (100.00, 50.00, 25.00, 12.50, 6.25, 3.125, 1.56, 0.78, 0.39, and 0.195 mg/mL) in dimethyl sulfoxide (DMSO). DMSO alone was used as negative control. After staying at 4 °C for 2 h, all Petri dishes were incubated at 37 °C for 24 h. All determinations were performed in triplicates. The minimum inhibitory concentration (MIC) values were determined as the lowest concentration of EOs that inhibited visible growth of the tested microorganism.

3.5. Free Radical-Scavenging Capacity

3.5.1. DPPH Radical-Scavenging Assay

The free radical-scavenging activity of LPEO was measured using the stable radical 2,2-diphenyl-1-picrylhydrazyl (DPPH) assay [48]. DPPH was dissolved in ethanol at concentration of 0.1 mmol L^{-1}. The absorbance of 2.7 mL DPPH solution and 0.3 mL ethanol was measured as the negative control. A different concentration of the sample solution in ethanol (0.3 mL) was pipetted into a cuvette with 2.7 mL DPPH solution. The resultant solution was incubated for 30 min at room temperature in the dark, and then monitored at 517 nm. The DPPH scavenging activity was expressed according to the following equation:

$$\text{DPPH scavenging activity (\%)} = (A_C - A_S)/A_C \times 100 \quad (1)$$

where A_C is the absorbance of the negative control, and A_S is the absorbance containing 0.3 mL sample and 2.7 mL DPPH solution. All samples were analyzed in triplicates, and the results are expressed as the mean ± standard deviation. The scavenging activity was expressed as the 50% inhibitory concentration (IC_{50}), which was defined as the sample concentration necessary to inhibit DPPH radical activity by 50% after incubation.

3.5.2. ABTS Radical-Scavenging Assay

This method was performed as described by Teles et al. [49], based on the capacity of LPEO to inhibit the 2,2'-azinobis (3-ethylbenzthiazoline-6-sulfonic acid) radical (ABTS). Twenty-five mL of ABTS (7 mM) were added to 440 µL of potassium persulfate ($K_2S_2O_8$, 140 mM), and the solution was kept in darkness for 12 h at room temperature in order to form the radical. An accurate volume of the solution was diluted in ethanol until an absorbance of 0.70 at 734 nm. Once the radical was formed, 2 mL of ABTS solution were mixed with 100µL of LPEO and the absorbance measured at 734 nm. ABTS scavenging effect was calculated using the following equation:

$$\text{ABTS scavenging activity (\%)} = (A_C - A_S)/A_C \times 100 \quad (2)$$

where A_S is the absorbance of the solution when the sample has been added and A_C is the absorbance of the ABTS solution as control. The IC_{50} was calculated from the graph of scavenging percentage against LPEO concentration. The results are expressed as the mean ± standard deviation.

3.6. Cancer Cell Culture

HCT116 colon cancer cells and HepG2 liver cancer cells were purchased from Library of Typical Culture of Chinese Academy of Sciences (Shanghai, China). HCT116 cells were cultured in Dulbecco's modified Eagle's medium (DMEM; Hyclone, UT, USA), supplemented with 10% fetal bovine serum (FBS) and 1% penicillin/streptomycin (Hyclone, UT, USA). HepG2 cells were cultured in MEM containing 10% FBS and 1% penicillin/streptomycin (Hyclone, UT, USA). The above-mentioned cells were maintained in 25 cm^2 cell culture flasks in a humidified atmosphere containing 5% CO_2 at 37 °C. Cells were fed until 90% confluence and the confluent cells were washed twice with phosphate buffered saline (PBS), treated with 0.25% trypsin (Invitrogen, MA, USA) for about 1 min, and incubated at 37 °C. When the cells were contracted and rounded under the microscope, FBS (Hyclone, UT, USA) containing medium was added, centrifuged at 200× g for 3 min, and subcultured at a split ratio of 1:3.

3.7. Antiproliferative Activity Test of LPEO

The cell proliferation inhibition rate of LPEO was evaluated by CCK-8 assay [42,43]. LPEO (50 µL) was added to the medium and mixed well. The mixture was diluted in DMSO to prepare solutions at a concentration of 0.5, 0.4, 0.3, 0.2, 0.1, 0.05, and 0.0 µL/mL, respectively. The cells were placed into 96-well plates (3 × 10³ cells/well). After 24 h, 100 µL of LPEO at different concentrations was added and continued to incubate for 48 h at 37 °C in a CO_2 incubator, after which the medium in the 96-well plate was disposed. A 100 µL of CCK-8 test solution (DojinDo, Tokyo, Japan) was added and incubated for 2 h at 37 °C. The optical density (OD) for each well was measured at 450 nm using a microplate reader (BioTek, Winooski, VT, USA). The cell viability rate at different concentrations of LPEO treatment was calculated according to the formula:

$$\text{Viability rate (\%)} = (OD_{sample} - OD_{blank})/(OD_{control} - OD_{blank}) \times 100\% \tag{3}$$

3.8. Statistical Analysis

The mean and standard deviation of three experiments were determined. Statistical analyses of the differences between mean values obtained for experimental groups were calculated using IBM SPSS Statistics 23.0. (IBM Corp. Released 2015. IBM SPSS Statistics for Windows, Version 23.0. Armonk, NY, USA). p values < 0.05 were regarded as significant, p values < 0.01 as very significant and p values < 0.001 as highly significant.

4. Conclusions

Essential oils are valuable plant extracts used in food, medicine and complementary treatment strategies [41]. The beneficial role of grapefruit EO has been widely reported. However, the bioactivities of grapefruit EO prepared by molecular distillation has not been well studied. Molecular distillation is a very useful technique to separate thermally-sensitive EOs. In our study, molecular distillation was used to remove undesired components from the cold-pressed grapefruit EO to provide light phase EO (LPEO). The chemical composition and antimicrobial activity of LPEO were studied. LPEO showed a wide spectrum of antimicrobial activity against some Gram-positive and Gram-negative microorganisms, with MIC values ranging from 0.78 to 12.50 µL/mL. LPEO might be used as a novel antimicrobial agent in the food industry. The antioxidant activity of LPEO by DPPH and ABTS was obtained with IC_{50} values of 22.06 ± 0.92 mg/mL and 15.72 ± 0.32 mg/mL, respectively. An in vitro test showed a dose-dependent antiproliferative activity of LPEO on HepG2 and HCT116 cancer cells. Thus, LPEO may potentially be used as a new complementary anticancer agent. However, this still needs further studies.

Author Contributions: J.C. and B.Z. contributed to the conception and design of the study and data analysis; W.D., K.L., J.S., and J.C. collected the plant material and performed distillation and GC-MS analysis; K.L. and S.C. carried out bioactivity test; W.D. and J.C. wrote the manuscript. All authors have read and agreed to the published version of the manuscript.

Funding: This work was supported by Foundation of Jiangxi Province Educational Committee (KJLD14079), Natural Science Foundation of Jiangxi Province (20141BBG70002), and Innovation Team Plan of Jiangxi Province (20142BCB24007).

Conflicts of Interest: The authors declare no conflict of interest.

References

1. Shaaban, H.A.H.; El-Ghorab, A.H.; Takayuki, S. Bioactivity of essential oils and their volatile aroma components: Review. *J. Essent. Oil Res.* **2012**, *24*, 203–212. [CrossRef]
2. Edris, A.E. Pharmaceutical and therapeutic potentials of essential oils and their individual volatile constituents: A review. *Phytother. Res.* **2007**, *21*, 308–323. [CrossRef] [PubMed]
3. Burt, S. Essential oils: Their antibacterial properties and potential applications in foods-A review. *Int. J. Food Microbiol.* **2004**, *94*, 223–253. [CrossRef] [PubMed]
4. Sahay, S. A review on pharmacological uses of essential oil. *Int. J. Curr. Pharm. Rev. Res.* **2015**, *6*, 71–79.
5. Hardin, A.; Crandall, P.G.; Stankus, T. Essential Oils and Antioxidants Derived From Citrus By-Products in Food Protection and Medicine: An Introduction and Review of Recent Literature. *J. Agric. Food Inf.* **2010**, *11*, 99–122. [CrossRef]

6. Fisher, K.; Phillips, C. The mechanism of action of a citrus oil blend against Enterococcus faecium and Enterococcus faecalis. *J. Appl. Microbiol.* **2009**, *106*, 1343–1349. [CrossRef]
7. Kaur, J.; Kaur, G. An insight into the role of citrus bioactives in modulation of colon cancer. *J. Funct. Foods* **2015**, *13*, 239–261. [CrossRef]
8. Shan, Y. *Comprehensive Utilization of Citrus By-Products*; Academic Press: Cambridge, MA, USA, 2016.
9. U.S. Department of Agriculture (USDA). Citrus: World Markets and Trade. Available online: http://apps.fas.usda.gov/psdonline/circulars/citrus.pdf. (accessed on 25 November 2019).
10. Nelson, E.K.; Mottern, H.H. Florida grapefruit oil. *J. Ind. Eng. Chem.* **1934**, *26*, 634–637. [CrossRef]
11. Flamini, G.; Cioni, P.L. Odour Gradients and Patterns in Volatile Emission of Different Plant Parts and Developing Fruits of Grapefruit (*Citrus paradisi* L.). *Food Chem.* **2010**, *120*, 984–992. [CrossRef]
12. Njoroge, M.S.; Koaze, H.; Karanja, P.N.; Sawamura, M. Volatile Constituents of Redblush Grapefruit (*Citrus paradisi*) and Pummelo (*Citrus grandis*) Peel Essential Oils from Kenya. *J. Agric. Food Chem.* **2005**, *53*, 9790–9794. [CrossRef]
13. Esmaeili, A.; Abednazari, S.; Abdollahzade, Y.M.; Abdollahzadeh, N.M.; Mahjoubian, R.; Tabatabaei-Anaraki, M. Peel Volatile Compounds of Apple (*Malus domestica*) and Grapefruit (*Citrus Paradisi*). *J. Essent. Oil Bear. Plants* **2012**, *15*, 794–799. [CrossRef]
14. Viuda-Martos, M.; Ruiz-Navajas, Y.; Fernández-López, J.; Pérez-Álvarez, J. Antifungal activity of lemon (*Citrus lemon* L.), mandarin (*Citrus reticulate* L.), grapefruit (*Citrus paradise* L.) and orange (*Citrus sinesis* L.) essential oils. *Food Control.* **2008**, *19*, 1130–1138. [CrossRef]
15. Negi, P.S.; Jayaprakasha, G.K. Antibacterial activity of grapefruit (*Citrus paradisi*) peel extracts. *Eur. Food Res. Technol.* **2001**, *213*, 484–487.
16. Viuda-Martos, M.; Ruiz-Navajas, Y.; Fernández-López, J.; Perez-Álvarez, J. Antibacterial activity of lemon (*Citrus limon* L.), mandarin (*Citrus reticulata* L.), grapefruit (*Citrus paradisi* L.) and orange (*Citrus sinensis* L.) essential oils. *J. Food Saf.* **2008**, *28*, 567–576. [CrossRef]
17. Uysal, B.; Sozmen, F.; Aktas, O.; Oksal, B.S.; Kose, E.O. Essential oil composition and antibacterial activity of the grapefruit (*citrus paradisi. L*) peel essential oils obtained by solvent-free microwave extraction: Comparison with hydrodistillation. *Int. J. Food Sci. Technol.* **2011**, *46*, 1455–1461. [CrossRef]
18. Okunowo, W.O.; Oyedeji, O.; Afolabi, L.O.; Matanmi, E. Essential oil of grape fruit (*Citrus paradisi*) peels and its antimicrobial activities. *Am. J. Plant. Sci.* **2013**, *4*, 1–9. [CrossRef]
19. Yang, S.A.; Jeon, S.K.; Lee, E.J.; Shim, C.H.; Lee, I.S. Comparative study of the chemical composition and antioxidant activity of six essential oils and their components. *Nat. Prod. Lett.* **2010**, *24*, 140–151. [CrossRef]
20. Teixeira, B.; Marques, A.; Ramos, C.; Neng, N.R.; Nogueira, J.M.F.; Saraiva, J.A.; Nunesa, M.L. Chemical composition and antibacterial and antioxidant properties of commercial essential oils. *Ind. Crops Prod.* **2013**, *43*, 587–595. [CrossRef]
21. Ahmed, S.; Rattanpal, H.S.; Gul, K.; Dar, R.A.; Sharma, A. Chemical composition, antioxidant activity and GC-MS analysis of juice and peel oil of grapefruit varieties cultivated in India. *J. Integr. Agric.* **2019**, *18*, 1634–1642. [CrossRef]
22. Sun, J.; Chu, Y.F.; Wu, X.; Liu, R. Antioxidant and Antiproliferative Activities of Common Fruits. *J. Agric. Food Chem.* **2002**, *50*, 7449–7454. [CrossRef]
23. Diab, K.A. In Vitro Studies on Phytochemical Content, Antioxidant, Anticancer, Immunomodulatory, and Antigenotoxic Activities of Lemon, Grapefruit, and Mandarin Citrus Peels. *Asian Pac. J. Cancer Prev.* **2016**, *17*, 3559–3567. [PubMed]
24. Cristóbal-Luna, J.M.; Álvarez-González, I.; Madrigal-Bujaidar, E.; Cevallos, G.C. Grapefruit and its biomedical, antigenotoxic and chemopreventive properties. *Food Chem. Toxicol.* **2018**, *112*, 224–234. [CrossRef] [PubMed]
25. Lin, J.; Rouseff, R.L. Characterization of aroma-impact compounds in cold-pressed grapefruit oil using time-intensity GC-olfactometry and GC-MS. *Flavour Fragr. J.* **2001**, *16*, 457–463. [CrossRef]
26. Cuthrell, K.; Marchand, L.L. Grapefruit and Cancer—A Review. In *Potential Health Benefits of Citrus*; Patil, B.S., Brodbelt, J.S., Miller, E.G., Turner, N.D., Eds.; ACS Symposium Series: Washington, DC, USA, 2006; Volume 936, pp. 235–252.
27. Berk, Z. *Citrus Fruit Processing*; Elsevier: Amsterdam, The Netherlands, 2016.
28. César, T.B.; Manthey, J.A.; Myung, K. Minor Furanocoumarins and Coumarins in Grapefruit Peel Oil as Inhibitors of Human Cytochrome P450 3A4. *J. Nat. Prod.* **2009**, *72*, 1702–1704. [CrossRef]

29. Uckoo, R.M.; Jayaprakasha, G.K.; Balasubramaniam, V.M.; Patil, B.S. Grapefruit (*Citrus paradisi* Macfad) phytochemicals composition is modulated by household processing techniques. *J. Food Sci.* **2012**, *77*, C921–C926. [CrossRef]
30. Ko, J.H.; Arfuso, F.; Sethi, G.; Ahn, K.S. Pharmacological Utilization of Bergamottin, Derived from Grapefruits, in Cancer Prevention and Therapy. *Int. J. Mol. Sci.* **2018**, *19*, 4048. [CrossRef]
31. Pino, J.; Acevedo, A.; Rabelo, J.; González, C.; Escandón, J. Chemical Composition of Distilled Grapefruit Oil. *J. Essent. Oil Res.* **1999**, *11*, 75–76. [CrossRef]
32. Busing, A.; Drotleff, A.M.; Ternes, W. Identification of α-tocotrienolquinone epoxides and development of an efficient molecular distillation procedure for quantitation of α-tocotrienol oxidation products in food matrices by high-performance liquid chromatography with diode array and fluorescence detection. *J. Agric. Food Chem.* **2012**, *60*, 8302–8313.
33. Ketenoglu, O.; Ozkan, K.S.; Yorulmaz, A.; Tekin, A. Molecular distillation of olive pomace oil - Multiobjective optimization for tocopherol and squalene. *LWT Food Sci. Technol.* **2018**, *91*, 198–202. [CrossRef]
34. Mezza, G.N.; Borgarello, A.V.; Daguero, J.D.; Pramparo, M.C. Obtention of Rosemary Essential Oil Concentrates by Molecular Distillation and Free Radical Scavenging Capacity Analysis. *Int. J. Food. Eng.* **2013**, *9*, 147–153. [CrossRef]
35. Martins, P.F.; Medeiros, H.H.R.; Sbaite, P.; Maciel, M.R.W. Enrichment of oxyterpenes from orange oil by short path evaporation. *Sep. Purif. Technol.* **2013**, *116*, 385–390. [CrossRef]
36. Wilson, C.W.; Shaw, P.E. Quantitative Composition of Cold-Pressed Grapefruit Oil. *J. Agric. Food Chem.* **1978**, *26*, 1432–1434. [CrossRef]
37. Ou, M.C.; Liu, Y.H.; Sun, Y.W.; Chan, C.F. The composition, antioxidant and antibacterial activities of cold-pressed and distilled essential oils of *Citrus paradise* and *Citrus grandis* (L.) Osbeck. *Evid. Based Complement. Altern. Med.* **2015**, *2015*, 804091. [CrossRef] [PubMed]
38. Ochs, M.M.; McCusker, M.P.; Bains, M.; Hancock, R.E. Negative regulation of the Pseudomonas aeruginosa outer membrane porin OprD selective for imipenem and basic amino acids. *Antimicrob. Agents. Chemother.* **1999**, *43*, 1085–1090. [CrossRef]
39. Cohena, S.M.; Eisenbrandb, G.; Fukushimac, S.; Gooderhamd, N.J.; Guengeriche, F.P.; Hechtf, S.S.; Rietjensg, I.M.C.M.; Bastakih, M.; Davidsenh, J.M.; Harmanh, C.L.; et al. FEMA GRAS assessment of natural flavor complexes: Citrus-derived flavoring ingredients. *Food Chem. Toxicol.* **2019**, *124*, 192–218. [CrossRef]
40. Hashim, N.A.; Ahmad, F.; Jani, N.A.; Susanti, D. In vitro Antioxidant, Antityrosinase, Antibacterial and Cytotoxicity Activities of the Leaf and Stem Essential Oil from *Piper magnibaccum* C. DC. *J. Essent. Oil Bear. Plants* **2017**, *20*, 223–232. [CrossRef]
41. Torresalvarez, C.; González, A.N.; Rodríguez, J.; Castillo, S.; Leosrivas, C.; Báezgonzález, J.G. Chemical composition, antimicrobial, and antioxidant activities of orange essential oil and its concentrated oils. *CyTA J. Food* **2017**, *15*, 129–135.
42. Tominaga, H.; Ishiyama, M.; Ohseto, F.; Sasamoto, K.; Hamamoto, T.; Suzuki, K.; Watanabe, M. A water-soluble tetrazolium salt useful for colorimetric cell viability assay. *Anal. Comm.* **1999**, *36*, 47–50. [CrossRef]
43. Liu, K.; Deng, W.; Hu, W.; Cao, S.; Zhong, B.; Chun, J. Extraction of 'Gannanzao' Orange Peel Essential Oil by Response Surface Methodology and its Effect on Cancer Cell Proliferation and Migration. *Molecules* **2019**, *24*, 499. [CrossRef]
44. Manassero, C.A.; Girotti, J.R.; Mijailovsky, S.; García de Bravo, M.; Polo, M. In vitro comparative analysis of antiproliferative activity of essential oil from mandarin peel and its principal component limonene. *Nat. Prod. Res.* **2013**, *27*, 1475–1478. [CrossRef]
45. Mukhtar, Y.M.; Adu-Frimpong, M.; Xu, X.; Yu, J. Biochemical significance of limonene and its metabolites: Future prospects for designing and developing highly potent anticancer drugs. *Biosci. Rep.* **2018**, *38*, 1–12. [CrossRef] [PubMed]
46. Borugă, O.; Jianu, C.; Mişcă, C.; Goleţ, I.; Gruia, A.T.; Horhat, F.G. Thymus vulgaris essential oil: Chemical composition and antimicrobial activity. *J. Med. Life* **2014**, *7*, 56–60. [PubMed]
47. Rota, C.; Carraminana, J.J.; Burillo, J.; Herrera, A. In vitro antimicrobial activity of essential oils from aromatic plants against selected foodborne pathogens. *J. Food Prot.* **2004**, *67*, 1252–1256. [CrossRef] [PubMed]

48. Chen, Z.; Mei, X.; Jin, Y.; Kim, E.H.; Yang, Z.; Tua, Y. Optimisation of supercritical carbon dioxide extraction of essential oil of flowers of tea (*Camellia sinensis L.*) plants and its antioxidative activity. *J. Sci. Food. Agric.* **2014**, *94*, 316–321. [CrossRef]
49. Telesa, S.; Pereirab, J.A.; Oliveirad, L.M.; Malheirob, R.; Machadoc, S.S.; Lucchesec, A.M.; Silvaa, F. Organic and mineral fertilization influence on biomass and essential oil production, composition and antioxidant activity of Lippiaoriganoides H.B.K. *Ind. Crops Prod.* **2014**, *59*, 169–176. [CrossRef]

Sample Availability: Sample of the compound LPEO is available from the authors.

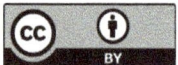

© 2020 by the authors. Licensee MDPI, Basel, Switzerland. This article is an open access article distributed under the terms and conditions of the Creative Commons Attribution (CC BY) license (http://creativecommons.org/licenses/by/4.0/).

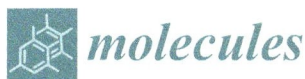

Article

Antimicrobial Activity and Chemical Constitution of the Crude, Phenolic-Rich Extracts of *Hibiscus sabdariffa*, *Brassica oleracea* and *Beta vulgaris*

Seham Abdel-Shafi [1,*], Abdul-Raouf Al-Mohammadi [2], Mahmoud Sitohy [3], Basma Mosa [1], Ahmed Ismaiel [1], Gamal Enan [1] and Ali Osman [3]

1. Botany and Microbiology Department, Faculty of Science, Zagazig University, Zagazig 44519, Egypt; shefaalab1984@gmail.com (B.M.); ahmedismaiel80@gmail.com (A.I.); gamalenan@ymail.com (G.E.)
2. Department of Science, King Khalid Military Academy, Riyadh 11495, P.O. Box 22140, Saudi Arabia; almohammadi26@hotmail.com
3. Biochemistry Department, Faculty of Agriculture, Zagazig University, Zagazig 44511, Egypt; mzsitohy@hotmail.com (M.S.); ali_khalil2006@yahoo.com (A.O.)
* Correspondence: hegazyseham@yahoo.com or sahegazy@zu.edu.eg; Tel.: +20-1289600036

Academic Editors: Raffaele Capasso and Lorenzo Di Cesare Mannelli
Received: 12 November 2019; Accepted: 22 November 2019; Published: 24 November 2019

Abstract: Crude, phenolic-rich extracts (CPREs) were isolated from different sources, such as *Hibiscus sabdariffa* (*H. sabdariffa*), *Brassica oleracea* var. capitata f. rubra (*B. oleracea*) and *Beta vulgaris* (*B. vulgaris*) and characterized. These CPREs showed potential antibacterial and antifungal activities. *H. sabdariffa* CPRE (HCPRE) is the most potent, as it inhibited all tested bacteria and fungi. Total anthocyanins content (TAC), total phenolic content (TPC) and total flavonoid content (TFC) were estimated in all three CPREs. *H. sabdariffa* contained 4.2 mg/100 g TAC, 2000 mg/100 g of TPC and 430 mg/100 g of TFC in a dry weight sample. GC–MS analysis of HCPRE showed 10 different active compounds that have antimicrobial effects against pathogenic bacteria and fungi, especially alcoholic compounds, triazine derivatives and esters. Scanning and transmission electron microscopy images of *Staphylococcus aureus* DSM 1104 and *Klebsiella pneumonia* ATCC 43816 treated with HCPRE (50 µg/mL) exhibited signs of asymmetric, wrinkled exterior surfaces, cell deformations and loss of cell shapes; and adherence of lysed cell content led to cell clumping, malformations, blisters, cell depressions and diminished cell numbers. This indicates death of bacterial cells and loss of cell contents. *Aspergillus ochraceus* EMCC516 (*A. ochraceus*, when treated with 100 µg/mL of HCPRE showed irregular cell organelles and cell vacuolation.

Keywords: *Hibiscus sabdariffa*; *Brassica oleracea*; Beta vulgaris; crude phenolic rich extract; anthocyanins; GC–MS analysis; antimicrobial

1. Introduction

The demand for effective natural antimicrobial compounds free of toxicity and environmental hazards has enormously increased as a result of the mounting increased drug resistant bacteria, nullifying drugs' effectiveness and causing widespread infections [1]. To avoid the increasingly growing antibiotic resistance, many natural products such as native or modified proteins have been investigated for their antibacterial actions as possible substitutes for the antibiotics [2–13]. Pathogenic bacteria and fungi affect agriculture, food industry, consumers and the national economy. The safe, plant-derived compounds with antimicrobial activity against pathogens are vital. For instance, carvacrol and cinnamaldehyde reduced *Campylobacter jejuni* and *Salmonella enterica* to undetectable levels at 0.2% concentration. The native cowpea seed proteins 7S and 11S were reported to strongly inhibit the in vitro growth of *Pseudomonas aeruginosa* ATCC 26853 and *Salmonella typhimurium* ATCC 14028 [14]. Additionally, soybean's glycinin basic subunit was able to inhibit methicillin-vancomycin intermediate *Staphylococcus aureus* (MRSA-VISA) while soy glycinin was competent to impede *Bacillus* spore germination [15,16].

Anthocyanins are the most important group of water-soluble pigments in nature. The word "Anthocyanin" is derived from two Greek words 'anthos' meaning flower and 'kyanos' meaning dark blue, referring to its important role as a natural colorant [17,18]. Anthocyanins are the polyphenolics that are responsible for red to purple color in plants. They are members of flavonoid group of phytochemicals [19,20]. Primary constituents that are present in flavonoid group are anthocyanins, flavanols, flavones, flavanones, etc. Anthocyanins are the hydroxyl and methoxyl derivatives of phenyl-2-benzopyrylium salts, regarded as flavonoid compounds [21].

The previous study reported two major anthocyanins, delphinidine-3-sambubioside and cyanidine-3-sambubioside, and two minor compounds, i.e., delphinidine-3-glu-coside and cyanidine-3-glucoside, present in the calyces of *Hibiscus sabdariffa* (roselle) [22]. Approximately 85% of anthocyanins were delphinidine-3-sambubioside which is the principal source of the antioxidant capacity of roselle extract [23].

The phenolic structure of anthocyanin stands behind their antioxidant activity; i.e., their capability to scavenge reactive oxygen species (ROS); i.e., superoxide (O_2^-), singlet oxygen (O_2), peroxide (ROO), hydrogen peroxide (H_2O_2), and hydroxyl radicals (OH) [24]. The herbs' antioxidant activities may be attributed to the plant pigments constituting the major components of the herbal extract. Antioxidant assays in foods and biological systems can be classified in two groups, those based on the evaluation of lipid peroxidation, and those based on the measurement of free radical scavenging power [25,26].

Roselle is widely used for treating diseases. The aqueous methanolic extract of roselle was analyzed for its phytochemical constituents, antimicrobial activity and cytotoxicity, revealing the following components, cardiac glycosides, flavonoids, saponins and alkaloids. It exhibited in vitro antibacterial activities against *Staphylococcus aureus, Bacillus stearothermophilus, Micrococcus luteus, Serratia mascences, Clostridium sporogenes, Escherichia coli, Klebsiella pneumoniae, Bacillus cereus* and *Pseudomonas fluorescence* [27].

The in vitro antimicrobial action of roselle extract was ascribed to the flavonoids, which can establish complexes with the bacterial cell walls, enhancing their permeation to the extract. The mechanism of action may include some metabolic steps, e.g., inhibition of electron transport protein translocation, phosphorylation steps, and some other enzyme dependent reactions ending with raised membrane permeability coupled with the leakage of the bacterial cell constituents [28].

Red cabbage (*Brassica oleracea* L.) has been extensively studied, due to its distinct color and potential physiological functions, arising probably from the presence of anthocyanin [29], the major pigment of this plant [30], which is composed of cyanidin-3-diglucoside-5-glucoside "cores," that are non-acetylated, mono-acetylated or di-acetylated with p-coumaric, caffeic, ferulic and sinapic acids. Anthocyanin was previously extracted from red cabbage using high pressure CO_2 [31]. Red cabbage is one of the most important vegetables belonging to the family *Cruciferae*. It is an herbaceous plant characterized by a short stem crowned up with a mass of red leaves (head). It is mainly used as salad, but can be cooked or pickled. Red cabbage is known for its medicinal properties; e.g., anticancer activity, due to the presence of indole-3-carbinol. It is an excellent source of vitamin C, vitamin B complex, potassium and calcium. The purple/red color leaves are due to a pigment belonging to anthocyanins (flavins). This color varies according to the soil pH, being more reddish in acidic soils, purple in neutral soils and greenish yellow in alkaline soil. Red cabbage is a rich source of natural antioxidants such as ascorbic acid, α-tocopherol, β-carotene and lutein [32]; oligosaccharides; and a some bioactive substances; e.g., flavonols and glucosinolates [33]. Its wide spread use in traditional medicine were ascribed to its antioxidant, anti-inflammatory and antibacterial properties. It is used for treating symptoms associated with gastrointestinal disorders; e.g., peptic and duodenal ulcers, gastritis or irritable bowel syndrome [34].

Natural colorants may be promising active biological agents. For example, phycocyanins were found to have many biological activities [35–37]. Likewise, red beet (*Beta vulgaris* L.) grows red or purple tuberous root vegetables, known as beetroot or garden beets, which are a firm, clean, globe-shaped vegetable with no mucilaginous or watery tissues, and its tubers contain freshly emerged young leaves. The biological importance of red beet is based on its high red pigment content, (betalain), which displays excellent values, meeting some applications in food and pharmaceutical products. Among many plants accumulating betalains, only red beet and prickly pear (*Opuntia ficus-indica*) are approved for food and pharmaceutical applications [38]. For example, the use of beet extract as a food colorant is approved by the US Food and Drug Administration (FDA). As a powerful antioxidant pigment, betanin may provide protection and reduce risk of cardiovascular disease and cancer [39].

Based on the potentially high content of anthocyanins and other bioactive compounds, three plants growing in Egypt were selected for this study; *Hibiscus sabdariffa* (*H. sabdariffa*), *Brassica oleracea* (*B. oleracea*) and *Beta vulgaris* (*B. vulgaris*), as the sources for isolating the crude phenolic rich extract (CPRE). These extracts (CPRE) were analyzed for total phenolics content and total flavonoids and evaluated for their antibacterial and antifungal activity by different methods.

2. Results

2.1. Chemical Characterization of Isolated CPRE

2.1.1. Total Anthocyanin, Total Phenolic and Total Flavonoid Contents

Total phenolic contents (TPC) of all samples were assayed by Folin–Ciocalteu's method, and found to be varied (Table 1). The highest amount of TPC was observed in *H. sabdariffa* CPRE (HCPRE) (2000 mg GAE/100 g dry pigment). *B. oleracea* showed the lowest amount of TPC (150 mg GAE/100 g dry pigment). The highest amounts of anthocyanin and flavonoid contents were observed with HCPRE.

Table 1. Chemical characterization of isolated pigments.

Samples	Total Anthocyanin Content (mg/100 g Dry Pigment)	Total Phenolic Content (mg GAE/100 g Dry Pigment)	Total Flavonoid Content (mg QE/100 g Dry Pigment)
H. sabdariffa	4.2	2000	430
B. oleracea	2.7	150	50
B. vulgaris	3.8	400	120

GAE: gallic acid equivalent. QE: quercetin equivalent.

2.1.2. Gas Chromatography-Mass Spectrometry (GC–MS) Analysis of HCPRE

The chemical compounds extracted from HCPRE (2000 µg/mL) were obtained by GC–MS analysis (Table 2; Figure 1). HCPRE contains ten active compounds, most of which have antimicrobial effects against pathogenic bacteria and fungi, especially alcoholic compounds, triazine derivatives, mercepto compounds and esters.

Table 2. The chemical compounds in the *Hibiscus sabdariffa* pigment (crude, phenolic-rich extracts—HCPRE) extracted, analyzed by GC–MS.

No	Classification	M. Formula	M. W.	Compound Name and Structure
1	Hydrocarbons (Alkan)-saturated compounds	$C_{22}H_{66}$	450	$CH_3(CH_2)_3OCH_3$—Dotriacontan
2	Alcoholic componds	$C_{17}H_{36}O$	256	2-Methylhexadecan-1-OL
3	Triazine derivatives	$C_5H_8ClN_5$	173	4-Amino-6-chloro-2-N-ethylamine 1,3,5-Triqazine
4	Unsat. alcoholic compound	$C_{19}H_{38}O$	280	14-Methyl-2,15-octadecadien-1-OL
5	Unsaturated ester	$C_{17}H_{22}O_2$	268	7-Methyl-2-tetradecan-1-OL acetate
6	Mercepto compound	$C_{16}H_{34}S$	258	1,1-Dimethyl tetradecyl hydrosulfide or tert-headecanethiol (com.)
7	Alkenes	$C_{19}H_{38}$	266	1-Nonadecene or Monadeca-1-ene
8	Primary alcohols	$C_{37}H_{76}O$	536	1-Heptalriaontanol or Heptatricotanol
9	Unsaturated ester	$C_{17}H_{30}O_2$	266	7-Methyl hexadeca-3,8-dienoate
10	Natural product (Cholesterol)	$C_{28}H_{48}O$	400	2-Methylene cholestan-3-oL

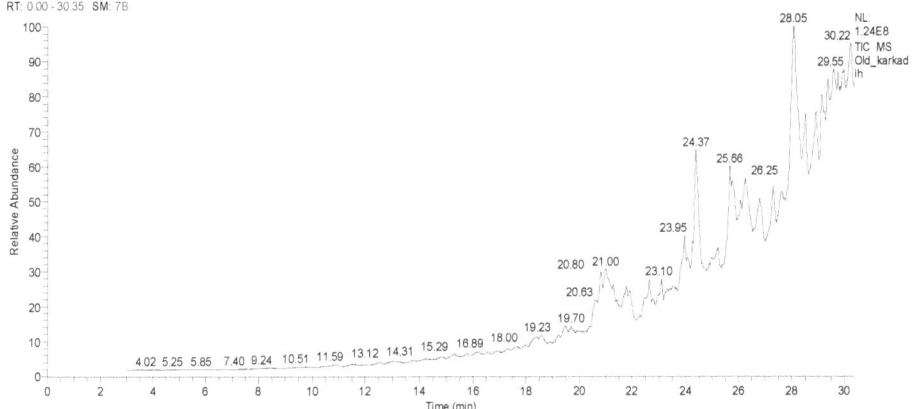

Figure 1. The TIC chromatogram of *H. sabdariffa* using GC–MS. RT—retention Time; SM—signal in method; NL—noise level.

2.2. Antimicrobial Activity of Crude Phenolic Rich Extract (CPRE) (2000 µg/mL) against Pathogenic Bacteria

The CPREs from H. sabdariffa, Brassica oleracea var. capitata f. rubra and B. vulgaris (2000 µg/mL) were tested for their antibacterial actions against S. aureus, Streptococcus pyogenes, Listeria monocytogenes, E. coli, K. pneumonia and Pseudomonas aeruginosa (Table 3). HCPRE exhibited the highest inhibition zones against the all bacteria, but B. vulgaris pigment had lower inhibition zones.

Table 3. Antibacterial activity of crude phenolic rich extracts (CPREs) (2000 µg/mL) from three plants against pathogenic bacteria using agar well diffusion assays.

Microorganisms	Inhibition Zone (mm)		
	H. sabdariffa	B. oleracea	B. vulgaris
Gram positive bacteria			
S. aureus	48 ± 8.0	38 ± 3.0 [a]	24 ± 4.0 [a]
St. pyogenes	40 ± 5.0 [b]	32 ± 2.0 [b]	10 ± 2.0 [b]
L. monocytogenes	32 ± 4.0 [c]	37 ± 3.0 [a]	13 ± 3.0 [b]
Gram negative bacteria			
E. coli	46 ± 6.0 [a]	28 ± 0.50 [c]	7 ± 0.50 [c]
K. pneumonia	48 ± 6.5 [a]	30 ± 2.0 [b]	18 ± 2.0 [a]
P. aeruginosa	32 ± 3.0 [c]	29 ± 0.50 [c]	7 ± 0.50 [c]

Means in the same column having different letters are significantly different ($p \leq 0.05$).

2.3. Minimum Inhibitory Concentrations (MICs) Values of HCPRE and B. oleracea Pigments against Bacteria

Different concentrations of extracted HCPRE were prepared (0, 25, 50, 100, 200 and 250 µg/mL) and tested for their antibacterial action (Table 4, Figure S1). The results indicated that the MIC of the pigment against Gram positive S. aureus, S. pyogenes and L. monocytogenes was 50 µg/mL; the MIC against Gram negative E. coli and P. aeruginosa was 25 µg/mL; and it was 50 µg/mL for K. pneumoniae. S. aureus and K. penuomonia are the most sensitive bacteria to HCPRE. Different concentrations of extracted B. oleracea pigment (BOP) were prepared (0, 25, 50, 100, 200 and 250 µg/mL) and tested for their antibacterial action against pathogenic bacteria (Table 4). The results showed that the MICs of the BOP against S. aureus, S. pyogenes and L. monocytogens were 25,100 and 50 µg/mL; and against E. coli, K. pneumonia and P. aeruginosa were 100, 200 and 100 µg/mL respectively. S. aureus and P. aeruginosa are the most sensitive bacteria to BOP.

Table 4. Minimum Inhibitory Concentrations (MIC) values of HCPRE and *Brassica oleracea* pigments against pathogenic bacteria using agar well diffusion assays.

Microorganisms	Inhibition Zone (mm)					
	0	25	50	100	200	250
		H. sabdariffa pigment				
Gram positive bacteria						
S. aureus	−ve	−ve	15 ± 3.0 [c]	20 ± 2.0 [b]	23 ± 3.0 [b]	28 ± 4.0 [a]
St. pyogenes	-ve	−ve	9 ± 0.5 [c]	15 ± 1.0 [b]	20 ± 2.0 [a]	22 ± 2.0 [a]
L. monocytogenes	−ve	−ve	11 ± 1.5 [c]	22 ± 3.0 [b]	23 ± 3.0 [b]	26 ± 3.0 [a]
Gram negative bacteria						
E. coli	−ve	11 ± 1.5 [c]	14 ± 2.0 [c]	20 ± 2.0 [b]	24 ± 4.0 [b]	30 ± 5.0 [a]
K. pneumonia	−ve	−ve	15 ± 3.0 [c]	20 ± 2.0 [b]	25 ± 5.0 [a]	26 ± 3.0 [a]
P. aeruginosa	−ve	10 ± 1.0	14 ± 2.0	23 ± 3.0	29 ± 6.0	30 ± 4.0
		B. oleracea pigment				
Gram positive bacteria						
S. aureus	−ve	9 ± 1.0 [c]	12 ± 2.0 [c]	16 ± 2.0 [b]	21±2.0 [a]	25±3.0 [a]
St. pyogenes	−ve	−ve	−ve	9 ± 0.5 [b]	10±1.0 [a]	11±1.0 [a]
L. monocytogenes	−ve	−ve	9 ± 1.0 [c]	12 ± 1.5 [c]	23±3.0 [b]	26±4.0 [a]
Gram negative bacteria						
E. coli	−ve	−ve	−ve	10 ± 1.0 [b]	16 ± 2.0 [a]	17 ± 2.0 [a]
K. pneumonia	−ve	−ve	−ve	−ve	11 ± 1.0 [b]	13 ± 1.5 [a]
P. aeruginosa	−ve	−ve	−ve	11 ± 1.2 [c]	15 ± 2.0 [b]	19 ± 2.5 [a]

Means in the same row having different letters are significantly different ($p \leq 0.05$).

2.4. Antifungal Activity of HCPRE against Pathogenic Fungi and MIC Values

HCPRE (2000 µg/mL) strongly inhibited all tested fungi (Table 5). Different concentrations of HCPRE extract were prepared (0, 100, 200, 300, 400 and 500 µg/mL) and tested for their antifungal actions against pathogenic fungi. The results showed that the MICs of the pigment against the fungi (*A. ochraceus, F. oxysporum, P. expansum* and *P. citrinum*) were 100 µg/mL, and according to the diameter of inhibition zones it showed that *A. ochraceus* was the most sensitive fungus to HCPRE (Table 6; Figure S2). Moreover, different concentrations of extracted *B. oleracea* pigment were prepared (0, 100, 200, 300, 400 and 500 µg/mL) and tested for their antifungal actions against pathogenic fungi.

Table 5. Antifungal activities of some plant pigments (2000 µg/mL) against pathogenic fungi using well diffusion assays.

Microorganismis	Inhibition Zone (mm)		
	H. sabdariffa	*B. oleracea*	*B. vulgaris*
A. ochraceus	45 ± 5.0 [a]	20 ± 2.0 [b]	−ve
F. oxysporum	40 ± 4.0 [b]	22 ± 3.0 [a]	−ve
P. expansum	35 ± 3.0 [c]	−ve	−ve
P. citrinum	36 ± 3.2 [c]	−ve	−ve

Means in the same column having different letters are significantly different ($p \leq 0.05$). −ve: No inhibition zone.

The results showed that the MICs of BOP against *A. ochraceus* and *F. oxysporum* were 400 and 300 µg/mL, respectively. BOP do not inhibit the growth of *P. expansum* and *P. citrinum* (Table 6, Figure S2).

Table 6. MICs of *H. sabdariffa* and *B. oleracea* pigments against pathogenic fungi using well diffusion assay.

Microorganisms	Inhibition Zone (mm)					
	0	100	200	300	400	500
			H. sabdariffa pigment			
A. ochraceus	−ve	23 ± 2.0 [c]	30 ± 3.0 [bc]	34 ± 3.0 [b]	35 ± 3.0 [b]	40 ± 5.0 [a]
F. oxysporum	−ve	12 ± 1.0 [d]	15 ± 1.5 [c]	20 ± 2.0 [b]	25 ± 2.0 [a]	26 ± 2.0 [a]
P. expansum	−ve	9 ± 0.5 [c]	20 ± 2 [b]	21 ± 2.0 [b]	28 ± 2.5 [a]	32 ± 3.0 [a]
P. citrinum	−ve	13 ± 1.5 [d]	25 ± 3.0 [c]	32 ± 3.0 [b]	33 ± 3.0 [b]	38 ± 4.0 [a]
			B. oleracea pigment			
A. ochraceus	−ve	−ve	−ve	−ve	13 ± 2.0 [b]	15 ± 1.0 [a]
F. oxysporum	−ve	−ve	−ve	9 ± 1.0 [c]	11 ± 1.0 [b]	18 ± 2.0 [a]
P. expansum	−ve	−ve	−ve	−ve	−ve	−ve
P. citrinum	−ve	−ve	−ve	−ve	−ve	−ve

−ve: No inhibition zone. Mean in the same row having different letters are significantly different ($p \leq 0.05$).

2.5. Quantitative Inhibition of Pathogenic Bacteria by Plant Pigments (Bacterial Growth Curve)

Plant pigments (*H. sabdariffa* and *B. oleraceae*) were added at their MIC values to test tubes containing 10 mL NB and inoculated with 10 µl aliquots of bacterial suspensions. Samples and untreated test tubes (controls) were incubated at 37 °C for 30 h. At appropriate time intervals, 1 mL aliquots of bacterial suspensions were withdrawn and were analyzed for their turbidity at OD600. Results are given in (Figure 2).

In the case of treating with *H. sabdariffa* pigment, almost no growth was shown in bacterial test tubes treated with pigment. However, bacteria grew rapidly in control tubes (without pigment) and turbidity went from 0.1 to almost 1.2 at OD600. Distinctive inhibition was observed at OD600, which increased only ≥0.0 in all of them. Moderate inhibition was observed for growth recorded at OD600 within 30 h in contradicting situations. In case of BOP bacteria grew rapidly in control tubes and bacterial growth inhibited in treated tubes.

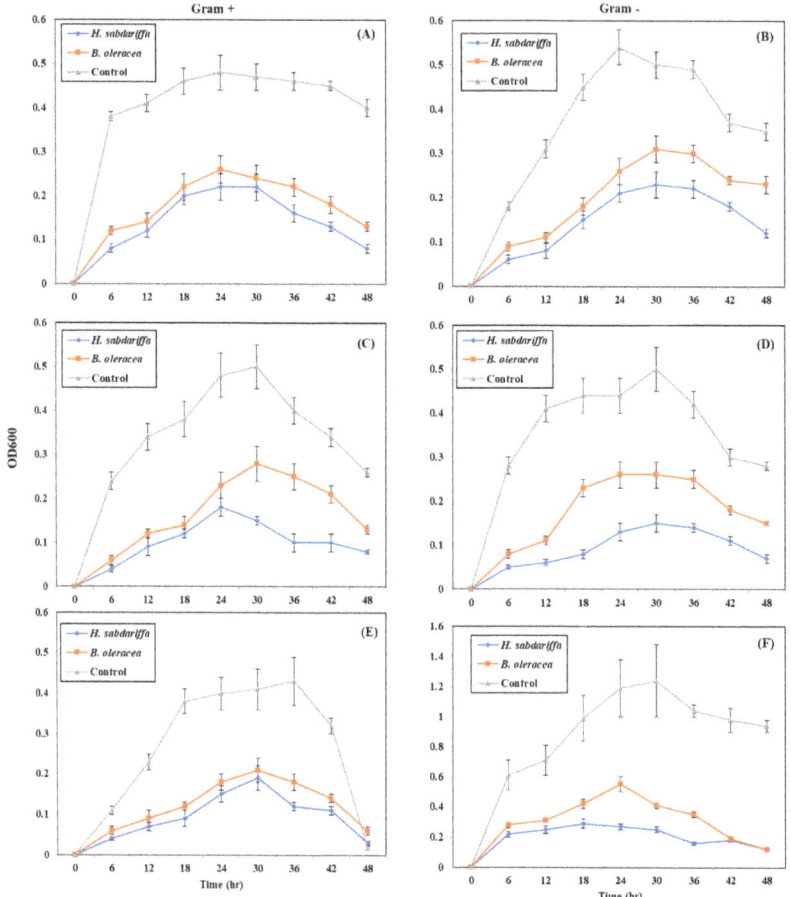

Figure 2. Quantitative inhibition of Gram-positive and Gram-negative bacteria by MIC of *H. sabdariffa* crude phenolic rich extract. (**A**) *S. aureus*; (**B**) *E. coli*; (**C**) *St. pyogenes*; (**D**) *K. pneumonia*; (**E**) *L. monocytogenes*; (**F**) *P. aeruginosa*.

2.6. SEM and TEM Microscopy Analysis

SEM images showed that the presence of HCPRE (50 µg/mL) on NB media containing *S. aureus* affected the bacterial cells and caused cell deformations, wrinkles and loss of cell shapes. The adherence of lysed cell content led to cell clumping, and this was seen after 18 h of incubation at 37 °C. HCPRE (50 µg/mL) on nutrient broth (NB) media containing *K. pneumonia* showed malformations (increases in length and decrease in width), cell depressions, diminished cell number and observed rectangular cells as loss of regular cell shapes were detected. That indicates the death of cells and loss of cellular contents. SEM images of *A. ochraceus* treated with HCPRE (100 µg/mL) showed destruction of conidia, failing in conidia formation, thinning and condensation of mycelia; then, malformation and loss of cell contents.

TEM images showed that *S. aureus* and *K. pneumonia* affected by HCPRE (50 µg/mL) on NB media showed malformed shapes, cell depress, cell vacuolation, blisters and wrinkles.

A. ochraceus, when treated with (100 µg/mL) of HCPRE showed irregular cell organelles and cell vacuolation (Figure 3A–F).

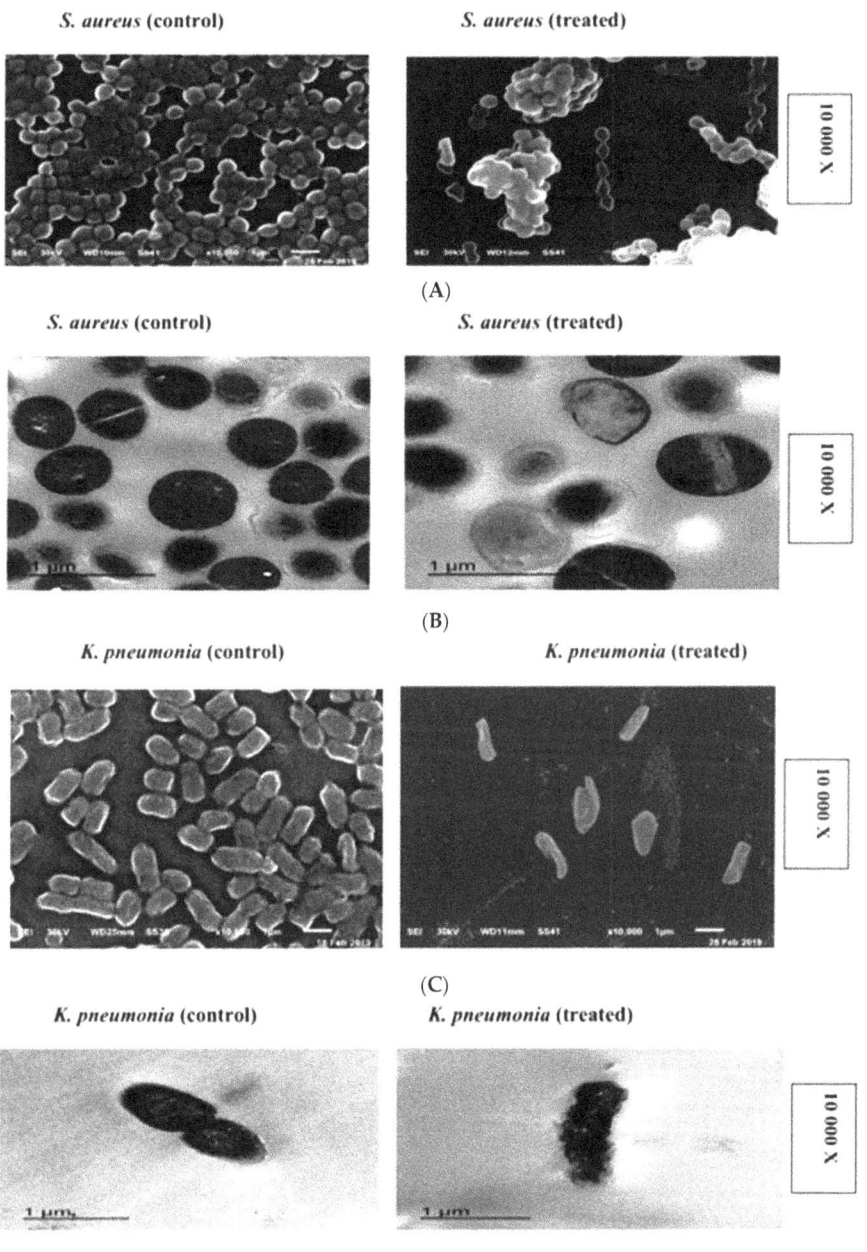

Figure 3. Cont.

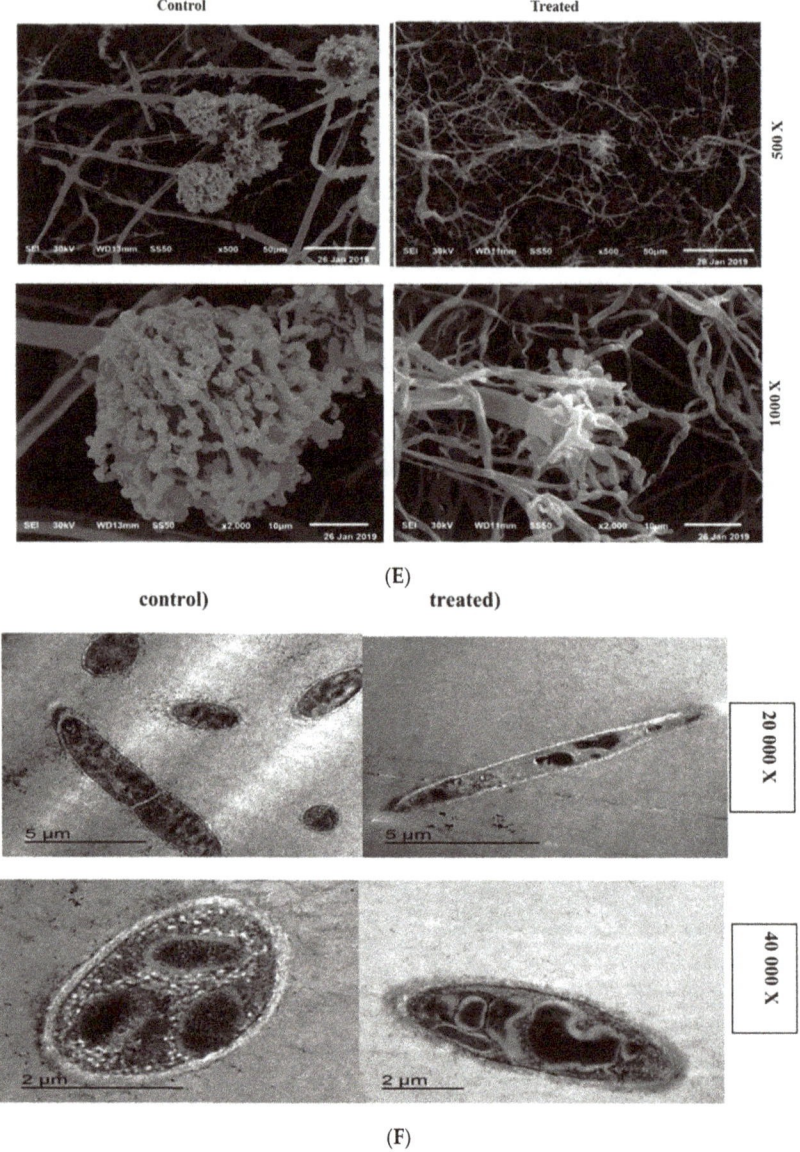

Figure 3. (**A**) SEM of *Staphylococcus aureus* affected by 50 µg/mL of HCPRE. (**B**) TEM of *S. aureus* affected by 50 µg/mL of HCPRE. (**C**) SEM of *K. pneumonia* affected by 50 µg/mL of HCPRE. (**D**) TEM of *K. pneumonia* affected by 50 µg/mL of HCPRE. (**E**) SEM of *A. ochraceus* affected by 100 µg/mL of HCPRE. (**F**) TEM of *A. ochraceus* affected by 100 µg/mL of HCPRE.

3. Discussion

Natural colorants obtained from vegetables are more available and healthy than synthetic colors [40]. The natural pigments are used in medicine and food [41]. Many bacterial organisms have developed increasing resistance against the frequently used antibiotics [42].

In this study, the pigments extracted from *H. sabdariffa* inhibited all tested bacteria and fungi. The previous studies showed that *H. sabdariffa* inhibited *S. aureus*, *B. cereus*, *E. coli*, *Clostridium sp.*, *Klebsiella pneumonia* and *Pseudomonas fluorescens* [42]. Herbal drug formulations composed of medicinal plants have been inherited from ancient times to treat many diseases, since their antimicrobial properties suggest them as potentially rich sources of various potent drugs [43]. Natural antimicrobials have enormous therapeutic potential, since they can probably conduct the required functions without any posing health hazards often associated with synthetic agents [44]. *H. sabdariffa*'s aqueous extract has strong activity against *C. albicans* [27]. Roselle can be utilized either as a distinct functional food or as an active ingredient in other functional food potentially applicable in the treatment of various degenerative diseases [45].

Based on the results, the antibacterial action of anthocyanin was concentration-dependent. HCPRE contains total anthocyanin content of 4.2 (mg/100 g) in dry pigment. Anthocyanin had relatively higher antibacterial activity than antifungal activity against the microorganisms investigated. Anthocyanins were reported to have anticarcinogenic activity against multiple cancer cell lines in vitro and in vivo tumor types [46]. *H. sabdariffa* showed antimicrobial activities against some food pathogenic microbial isolates, e.g., *E. coli* O157:H7, *Salmonella enterica* and *L. monocytogenes*, as well as veterinary, and clinical isolates. This indicated that HCPRE extract is broadly effective against different microorganisms, suggesting its application as a potential food-grade antimicrobial [28]. The antibacterial effects of roselle calyx aqueous and ethanol extracts and protocatechuic acid against food spoilage bacteria *Salmonella typhimurium* DT104, *E. coli* O157:H7, *L. monocytogenes*, *S. aureus* and *B. cereus* were examined by [47]. The inhibitory activities in a dose-dependent manner against bacteria in ground beef and apple juice were studied, and it was suggested that they might be potent agents as food additives to prevent contamination from these bacteria.

The anthocyanins and polyphenols from the *H. sabdariffa* (roselle) were extracted by an aqueous or organic solvent. The dried roselle contained total anthocyanins as cyanidine 3-glucoside 622.91 mg/100 g and 37.42 mg/100 g total phenolic content in dry weight samples [48]. A recent study identified delphinedine-3-O-sambubioside, delphinidine-3-O-glucoside and cyani-dine-3-O-sambubioside at the concentrations of 7.03 mg/g, 1.54 mg/g and 4.40 mg/g in the roselle extract. GC–MS analysis showed 10 compounds in HCPRE. All of them have previously been shown to have antimicrobial activity. It is quite known that many *Hibiscus* species contain different classes of secondary metabolites, including flavonoids, anthocyanins, terpenoids, steroids, polysaccharides, alkaloids, sesquiterpene, quinones and naphthalene groups. Some of these components have antibacterial, anti-inflammatory, antihypertensive, antifertility, hypoglycemic, antifungal and antioxidative activities [49]. The antioxidant capacity of anthocyanins is dependent on its basic structural orientation; i.e., the ring orientation will determine the readiness of a hydrogen atom from a hydroxyl group to be donated to a free radical and the capability of the anthocyanin to support an unpaired electron [25]. *H. sabdariffa* is a safe medicinal plant, having medical compounds with nutritional and medicinal properties [50].

In this study, *S. aureus* and *K. pneumonia* were affected by HCPRE (50 µg/mL), showing malformed shapes, cell depressions, cell vacuolation, blisters and wrinkles. *A. ochraceus*, when treated with (100 µg/mL) of HCPRE, showed irregular cell organelles. The anthocyanin-rich blueberry extract was capable of inhibiting the growth, adhesion and/or biofilm formation of all of the following: *P. aeruginosa*, *E. coli*, *P. mirabilis*, *A. baumannii* and *S. aureus* [51]. Roselle contains proanthocyanidins which combine or transform the structural entity of P-fimbriae of bacterial cells; thus, inhibiting their adhesion to the ur-epithelium and formation of biofilms in vitro [45]. The antimicrobial properties of eight food dyes against 10 bacteria and five fungal organisms were previously investigated, showing that the red dyes were associated with the best antibacterial activities, while the yellow ones were more linked to better antifungal activity. Besides the antimicrobial analysis, antioxidant activity, measured by three different methods, was also investigated. In all the methods, red dye was found to have greater antioxidant activity. It suggests that the addition of these dyes in food not only enhances the value addition by making the food more presentable but also shall address the issue of food supplementation with substances that are good antibiotics and antioxidants, subsequently proving to be health benefactors [52].

4. Materials and Methods

4.1. Crude Phenolic Rich Extract (CPRE) Preparation

All chemicals used in this work were supplied from Al-Gomhorya Company for chemicals and public procurement Zagazig city, Egypt. The calyx of *H. sabdariffa*; the leaves of *Brassica oleracea* var. capitata f. rubra (*B. oleracea*) and *B. vulgaris* tuberous root vegetables were obtained from local market in Egypt). The plants we used were botanically classified by Samer Teleb, Taxonomy and Flora, Botany and Microbiology Department, Faculty of Science, Zagazig University, Egypt. Milled sample (0.5 g) was soaked in 50 mL of ethanol for 24 h and the extract obtained was pre-filtered with Whatman No.4 filter (Whatman®Prepleated Qualitative Filter Paper, Grade 4V, Sigma-Aldrich, USA) before evaporation using a vacuum rotary evaporator (BüCHI-water bath-B-480, Czech Republic) at 30 °C.

4.2. Crude Phenolic Rich Extract Characterization

4.2.1. Determination of Anthocyanins

Total anthocyanin content was colorimetrically determined according to the procedure described by [53] where a known volume of the filtered extract was diluted to 100 mL with the extracting solvent and the resulting color was measured at 520 nm for water and citric acid solution extracts and at 535 nm for acidified ethanol using Spectrophotometer (JENWAY-6405 UV/VIS, Chelmsford, England). The total anthocyanin content defined as cyanidin-3-glucoside was calculated using the following Equation (1):

$$\text{Total anthocyanins} \left(\frac{\text{mg}}{100 \text{ g}}\right) = \frac{\text{Absorbance} \times \text{dilution factor}}{\text{Sample weight} \times 55.9} \times 100. \quad (1)$$

4.2.2. Determination of Total Phenolic Compounds (TPCs)

The TPCs were estimated by Foline–Ciocalteu reagent as described by [54]. One milliliter of sample (1000 µg in 1 mL) was added to 5 mL of Folin–Ciocalteu reagent (diluted with water 1:10, v/v) and 4 mL sodium carbonate (75 g/L). The tubes were vortex mixed for 15 s and left stand 30 min at 40 °C, before measuring the absorbance of the developed color at 765 nm. Gallic acid was used to establish the standard curve (20–200 µg/mL). The extent of reducing of the Folin–Ciocalteu reagent by the sample was expressed as mg of gallic acid equivalents (GAE) per g of extract. The calibration equation for gallic acid was $y = 0.001x + 0.0563$ ($R^2 = 0.9792$), where y and x are the absorbance and concentration of gallic acid in µg/mL, respectively.

4.2.3. Total Flavonoids (TFs) Determination

Total flavonoids (TFs) were estimated according to the protocol of [55] by blending 2 mL aliquot of 20 g/L $AlCl_3$ ethanol reagent with 1 mL of the extract (1000 µg in 1 mL solvent) and measuring the developed color absorbance at 420 nm after 60 min. Quercetin was used to establish the standard curve (20–200 µg/mL) and total flavonoid content was expressed as quercetin equivalent (QE), based on the standard curve. The calibration equation for quercetin was $y = 0.0012x + 0.008$ ($R^2 = 0.944$), where y is absorbance and x is concentration of quercetin in µg/mL.

4.2.4. Gas Chromatography–Mass Spectrometry (GC–MS) Analysis

The chemical composition analysis of the samples was carried out using Trace GC1310-ISQ mass spectrometer (Thermo Scientific, Austin, TX, USA) with a direct capillary column TGram negative5MS (30 mm× 0.25 mm × 0.25 µm film thickness, Thermo Scientific, Austin, TX, USA). The column oven temperature was initially held at 50 °C; then increased by 7 °C/min increments to 200 °C hold for 2 min; and the final temperature at 290 °C was reached by 15 °C/min increments and held for 2 min. The injector and MS transfer line temperatures were kept at 270 and 250 °C, respectively. Helium, the carrier gas, was pumped at a constant flow rate of 1 mL/min. The solvent delay was 3 min, and 1 µL aliquots of the diluted samples were injected automatically using an Autosampler AS1300 coupled (Thermo Scientific, Austin, TX, USA) with GC. The ion source temperature was set at 200 °C. EI mass spectra were collected at 70 eV ionization voltages over a range of m/z 45–400 within full scan mode. The chemical composition of the obtained components was concluded by comparing their retention times and mass spectra with those of WILEY 09 and NIST 11 mass spectral database.

4.3. Collection of Pathogenic Bacteria and Fungi

S. aureus DSM 1104, *St. pyogenes* ATCC 19615, *L. monocytogenes* LMG10470, *E. coli* LMG 8223, *K. pneumonia* ATCC 43816 and *P. aeruginosa* LMG 8029 were used. Also, pathogenic fungi such as *A. ochraceus* EMCC516 were obtained from Egyptian Microbial Culture Collection (Microbiological Resources Center MIRCEN, Cairo, Egypt); other fungi were *F. oxysporum*, *p. citrinium* and *P. expansum*. All bacteria and fungi used in this study were kindly offered by Botany and Microbiology Department (Laboratory of Bacteriology and Laboratory of fungi), Faculty of Science, Zagazig University, Zagazig, Egypt. Stock bacterial cultures were routinely kept at −20 °C in glass beads and were sub-cultured and propagated in brain heart infusion broth (BHIB) (Oxoid). Slope cultures were prepared fresh on nutrient agar for every experiment [11] and stored at 4 °C throughout the experimental work.

4.4. Antibacterial and Antifungal Activities of the CPREs

The antibacterial and antifungal activities of CPREs (2000 µg/mL) were tested against the experimental pathogenic bacteria and fungi by agar well-diffusion assays [56].

4.5. MIC Values of H. Sabdariffa CPRE

Pure cultures of bacterial strains were sub-cultured on BHIB at 37 °C. Each strain was spread uniformly onto an individual plate with a sterile cotton swab. Uniform wells (6 mm diameters) were made on nutrient agar (NA) plates using a gel puncturing tool. Aliquots (50 µL) of pigment solutions (0, 25, 50, 100, 200 and 250 µg/mL) were placed into each well. Sterilized distilled water was considered the negative control. After 24 h incubation at 37 °C, the diameters of the inhibition zones (mm) were measured using a transparent millimeter ruler. The pure cultures of fungal strains were sub-cultured on yeast extract agar (YES) at 30 °C. Each strain was spread uniformly onto the individual plates using sterile cotton swabs. Wells of 6 mm diameter were similarly made on YES plates. Aliquots (50 µL) of HCPRE and *B. oleracea* pigment solutions (0, 100, 200, 300, 400 and 500 µg/mL) were placed in each well. After 4 days' incubation at 30 °C, the diameters of inhibition zones (mm) were similarly measured.

4.6. Quantitative Inhibition of Pathogenic Bacteria by CPRE (Bacterial Growth Curve)

A series of test tubes each containing 10 mL of nutrient broth (NB) were inoculated with 100 µL of log phase bacterial suspension and were then treated with 50 µg/mL HCPRE for all bacteria; and 200 µg/mL *B. oleracea* pigment for *E. coli* and 100 µg/mL for other bacteria. Control test tubes contained NB with bacteria only. Samples and controls were incubated at 37 °C. Growth was determined at time 0 and after 6, 12, 18, 24, 30, 36, 42 and 48 h of incubation by the turbidity method (OD600) using a spectrophotometer (JENWAY-6405 UV/VIS, Chelmsford, England).

4.7. Scanning and Transmission Electron Microscopy (SEM-TEM)

S. aureus (Gram positive bacteria) and *K. pneumonia* (Gram negative bacteria) were selected for scanning electron microscopy (SEM) and transmission electron microscopy (TEM). Bacteria were grown on NB media and incubated at 37 °C to reach maximum level of 10^6 CFU/mL. The MIC values of about 50 μg/mL of HCPRE were added to *S. aureus* and *K. pneumonia* plates except for controls and incubated at 37 °C for 18 h. Also *A. ochraceus* was grown on YSA and incubated at 30 °C for 3 days to reach the maximum level of growth and MIC value of about 100 μg/mL of *H. sabdariffa* pigment.

4.7.1. Scanning Electron Microscopy (SEM)

SEM (JEOL-scanning electron microscope JSM-6510 L.V SEM-JAPAN) at electron microscope (EM) Unit, Mansoura University, Egypt was used to evaluate the morphological changes of tested microorganisms as described in [2,16].

4.7.2. Transmission Electron Microscopy (TEM)

TEM (JEOL JEM -2100, JAPAN) at EM Unit, Mansoura University, Egypt was used to evaluate ultrastructural changes of tested microorganisms as described in [14,57].

4.8. Statistical Analysis

The collected data were tabulated and analyzed using IBM SPSS software (version 26, IBM corporation, Chicago, IL, USA). The results were expressed as a means ± standard errors (SEs) in either tables or figures.

5. Conclusions

According to the obtained results, it can be concluded that *H. sabdariffa* pigment could be used as an antibacterial and antifungal agent. It can be efficiently and successfully used as safe, natural products. It can be prepared with low costs.

Supplementary Materials: The following are available online.

Author Contributions: M.S., G.E., A.-R.A.-M., A.I., and S.A.-S suggested the work protocol, interpreted the results and revised the manuscript. S.A.-S., A.I., A.O. and B.M. performed the laboratory experiments regarding microbiological and chemical investigations and prepared the manuscript. A.-R.A.-M. financed the publication fees.

Funding: Zagazig University, Zagazig, Egypt, supported the experimental work. A.-R.A.-M. from the Department of Science, King Khalid Military Academy, Riyadh 11495, P.O. Box 22140, Saudi Arabia, was responsible for paying the publication fees.

Acknowledgments: The authors are indebted to Zagazig University, Egypt for facilities throughout the experimental work, and thank Samer Teleb, Taxonomy and Flora, Botany and Microbiology Department, Faculty of Science, Zagazig University, Egypt for the botanical classification of the plants. Also, thanks A. H. Moustafa for his help in GC–MS analysis.

Conflicts of Interest: The authors declare no conflict of interest.

References

1. Laxminarayan, R.; Duse, A.; Wattal, C.; Zaidi, A.K.; Wertheim, H.F.; Sumpradit, N.; Vlieghe, E.; Hara, G.L.; Gould, I.M.; Goossens, H. Antibiotic resistance—The need for global solutions. *Lancet Infect. Dis.* **2013**, *13*, 1057–1098. [CrossRef]
2. Sitohy, M.Z.; Mahgoub, S.A.; Osman, A.O. In vitro and in situ antimicrobial action and mechanism of glycinin and its basic subunit. *Int. J. Food Microbiol.* **2012**, *154*, 19–29. [CrossRef] [PubMed]
3. Osman, A.; Goda, H.A.; Abdel-Hamid, M.; Badran, S.M.; Otte, J. Antibacterial peptides generated by Alcalase hydrolysis of goat whey. *LWT-Food Sci. Technol.* **2016**, *65*, 480–486. [CrossRef]
4. Sitohy, M.; Osman, A. Antimicrobial activity of native and esterified legume proteins against Gram-negative and Gram-positive bacteria. *Food Chem.* **2010**, *120*, 66–73. [CrossRef]
5. Abdel-Hamid, M.; Goda, H.A.; De Gobba, C.; Jenssen, H.; Osman, A. Antibacterial activity of papain hydrolysed camel whey and its fractions. *Int. Dairy J.* **2016**, *61*, 91–98. [CrossRef]
6. Osman, A.O.; Mahgoub, S.A.; Sitohy, M.Z. Preservative action of 11S (glycinin) and 7S (β-conglycinin) soy globulin on bovine raw milk stored either at 4 or 25 °C. *J. Dairy Res.* **2013**, *80*, 174–183. [CrossRef] [PubMed]

7. Mahgoub, S.; Osman, A.; Sitohy, M. Inhibition of growth of pathogenic bacteria in raw milk by legume protein esters. *J. Food Prot.* **2011**, *74*, 1475–1481. [CrossRef]
8. Sitohy, M.; Mahgoub, S.; Osman, A.; El-Masry, R.; Al-Gaby, A. Extent and mode of action of cationic legume proteins against Listeria monocytogenes and Salmonella Enteritidis. *Probiotics Antimicrob. Proteins* **2013**, *5*, 195–205. [CrossRef]
9. Sitohy, M.; Mahgoub, S.; Osman, A. Controlling psychrotrophic bacteria in raw buffalo milk preserved at 4 C with esterified legume proteins. *LWT-Food Sci. Technol.* **2011**, *44*, 1697–1702. [CrossRef]
10. Mahgoub, S.A.; Sitohy, M.Z.; Osman, A.O. Counteracting recontamination of pasteurized milk by methylated soybean protein. *Food Bioprocess Technol.* **2013**, *6*, 101–109. [CrossRef]
11. Abdel-Shafi, S.; Osman, A.; Enan, G.; El-Nemer, M.; Sitohy, M. Antibacterial activity of methylated egg white proteins against pathogenic Gram positive and Gram negative bacteria matching antibiotics. *SpringerPlus* **2016**, *5*, 983. [CrossRef] [PubMed]
12. Sitohy, M.Z.; Osman, A.O. Enhancing milk preservation with esterified legume proteins. *Probiotics Antimicrob. Proteins* **2011**, *3*, 48–56. [CrossRef] [PubMed]
13. Osman, A.; El-Araby, G.M.; Taha, H. Potential use as a bio-preservative from lupin protein hydrolysate generated by alcalase in food system. *J. Appl. Biol. Biotechnol.* **2016**, *4*, 76–81.
14. Abdel-Shafi, S.; Al-Mohammadi, A.-R.; Osman, A.; Enan, G.; Abdel-Hameid, S.; Sitohy, M. Characterization and Antibacterial Activity of 7S and 11S Globulins Isolated from Cowpea Seed Protein. *Molecules* **2019**, *24*, 1082. [CrossRef] [PubMed]
15. Mahgoub, S.A.; Osman, A.O.; Sitohy, M.Z. Impeding Bacillus spore germination in vitro and in milk by soy glycinin during long cold storage. *J. Gen. Appl. Microbiol.* **2016**, *62*, 52–59. [CrossRef]
16. Osman, A.; Daidamony, G.; Sitohy, M.; Khalifa, M.; Enan, G. Soybean glycinin basic subunit inhibits methicillin resistant-vancomycin intermediate *Staphylococcus aureus* (MRSA-VISA) *in vitro*. *Int. J. Appl. Res. Nat. Prod.* **2016**, *9*, 17–26.
17. Delgado-Vargas, F.; Paredes-Lopez, O. *Natural Colorants for Food and Nutraceutical Uses*; CRC Press: Boca Raton, FL, USA; London, UK; New York, NY, USA; Washington, DC, USA, 2002.
18. Delgado-Vargas, F.; Jiménez, A.; Paredes-López, O. Natural pigments: carotenoids, anthocyanins, and betalains—characteristics, biosynthesis, processing, and stability. *Critical Rev. Food Sci. Nutr.* **2000**, *40*, 173–289. [CrossRef]
19. Lila, M.A. Anthocyanins and human health: an in vitro investigative approach. *BioMed. Res. Int.* **2004**, *2004*, 306–313. [CrossRef]
20. Kumar, A.; Premoli, M.; Aria, F.; Bonini, S.A.; Maccarinelli, G.; Gianoncelli, A.; Memo, M.; Mastinu, A. Cannabimimetic plants: are they new cannabinoidergic modulators? *Planta* **2019**, *249*, 1681–1694. [CrossRef]
21. Eder, R. Pigments. In *Food Analysis by HPLC*; Nollet, L.M., Ed.; Marcel Dekker: Monticello, NY, USA, 2000; pp. 825–880.
22. Cissé, M.; Vaillant, F.; Pallet, D.; Dornier, M. Selecting ultrafiltration and nanofiltration membranes to concentrate anthocyanins from roselle extract (Hibiscus sabdariffa L.). *Food Res. Int.* **2011**, *44*, 2607–2614. [CrossRef]
23. Diessana, A.; Parkouda, C.; Cissé, M.; Diawara, B.; Dicko, M.H. Optimization of aqueous extraction of anthocyanins from Hibiscus sabdariffa L. calyces for food application. *Food Sci. Qual. Manage.* **2015**, *45*, 23–31.
24. Saed-Moucheshi, A.; Shekoofa, A.; Pessarakli, M. Reactive oxygen species (ROS) generation and detoxifying in plants. *J. Plant Nutr.* **2014**, *37*, 1573–1585. [CrossRef]
25. Miguel, M.G. Anthocyanins: Antioxidant and/or anti-inflammatory activities. *J. Appl. Pharm. Sci.* **2011**, *1*, 7–15.
26. Mastinu, A.; Kumar, A.; Maccarinelli, G.; Bonini, S.A.; Premoli, M.; Aria, F.; Gianoncelli, A.; Memo, M. Zeolite clinoptilolite: Therapeutic virtues of an ancient mineral. *Molecules* **2019**, *24*, 1517. [CrossRef] [PubMed]
27. Elmanama, A.A.; Alyazji, A.A.; Abu-Gheneima, N. Antibacterial, antifungal and synergistic effect of *Lawsonia inermis, Punica granatum* and *Hibiscus sabdariffa*. *Ann. Alquds Med.* **2011**, *7*, 33–41.
28. Fullerton, M.; Khatiwada, J.; Johnson, J.U.; Davis, S.; Williams, L.L. Determination of antimicrobial activity of sorrel (*Hibiscus sabdariffa*) on *Escherichia coli* O157, H7 isolated from food, veterinary, and clinical samples. *J. Med. Food* **2011**, *14*, 950–956. [CrossRef] [PubMed]

29. Cartea, M.E.; Francisco, M.; Soengas, P.; Velasco, P. Phenolic compounds in *Brassica* vegetables. *Molecules* **2011**, *16*, 251–280. [CrossRef]
30. Ahmadiani, N.; Robbins, R.J.; Collins, T.M.; Giusti, M.M. Anthocyanins contents, profiles, and color characteristics of red cabbage extracts from different cultivars and maturity stages. *J. Agric. Food Chem.* **2014**, *62*, 7524–7531. [CrossRef]
31. Xu, Z.; Wu, J.; Zhang, Y.; Hu, X.; Liao, X.; Wang, Z. Extraction of anthocyanins from red cabbage using high pressure CO_2. *Bioresour. Technol.* **2010**, *101*, 7151–7157. [CrossRef]
32. Isabelle, M.; Lee, B.L.; Lim, M.T.; Koh, W.-P.; Huang, D.; Ong, C.N. Antioxidant activity and profiles of common vegetables in Singapore. *Food Chem.* **2010**, *120*, 993–1003. [CrossRef]
33. Wiczkowski, W.; Szawara-Nowak, D.; Topolska, J. Red cabbage anthocyanins: Profile, isolation, identification, and antioxidant activity. *Food Res. Int.* **2013**, *51*, 303–309. [CrossRef]
34. Kapusta-Duch, J.; Kopec, A.; Piatkowska, E.; Borczak, B.; Leszczynska, T. The beneficial effects of *Brassica* vegetables on human health. *Rocz. Panstw. Zakl. Hig.* **2012**, *63*, 389–395. [PubMed]
35. Osman, A.; Abd-Elaziz, S.; Salama, A.; Eita, A.A.; Sitohy, M. Health Protective Actions of Phycocyanin Obtained from an Egyptian Isolate of Spirulina platensis on Albino Rats. *Eur. Asian J. BioSci.* **2019**, *13*, 105–112.
36. Sitohy, M.; Osman, A.; Ghany, A.; Salama, A. Antibacterial phycocyanin from Anabaena oryzae SOS13. *Int J. Appl. Res. Nat. Prod.* **2015**, *8*, 27–36.
37. Salama, A.; Ghany, A.A.; Osman, A.; Sitohy, M. Maximising phycocyanin extraction from a newly identified Egyptian cyanobacteria strain: Anabaena oryzae SOS13. *International Food Res. J.* **2015**, *22*, 517.
38. Khan, M.I. Plant betalains: Safety, antioxidant activity, clinical efficacy, and bioavailability. *Compr. Rev Food Sci. Food Saf.* **2016**, *15*, 316–330. [CrossRef]
39. Wu, L.-C.; Hsu, H.-W.; Chen, Y.-C.; Chiu, C.-C.; Lin, Y.-I.; Ho, J.-A. Antioxidant and antiproliferative activities of red pitaya. *Food Chem.* **2006**, *95*, 319–327. [CrossRef]
40. Adam Burrows, J.D. Palette of our palates: A brief history of food coloring and its regulation. *Compr. Rev. Food Sci. Food Saf.* **2009**, *8*, 394–408. [CrossRef]
41. Chaitanya Lakshmi, G. Food coloring: The natural way. *Res. J. Chem. Sci.* **2014**, *2231*, 606X.
42. Ouyang-Latimer, J.; Jafri, S.; VanTassel, A.; Jiang, Z.-D.; Gurleen, K.; Rodriguez, S.; Nandy, R.K.; Ramamurthy, T.; Chatterjee, S.; McKenzie, R. In vitro antimicrobial susceptibility of bacterial enteropathogens isolated from international travelers to Mexico, Guatemala, and India from 2006 to 2008. *Antimicrob. Agents Chemother.* **2011**, *55*, 874–878. [CrossRef]
43. Iwu, M.W.; Duncan, A.R.; Okunji, C.O. New antimicrobials of plant origin. In *Perspectives on New Crops and New Uses*; ASHS Press: Alexandria, VA, USA, 1999; pp. 457–462.
44. Giuliani, A.; Rinaldi, A.C. Beyond natural antimicrobial peptides: multimeric peptides and other peptidomimetic approaches. *Cell. Mol. Life Sci.* **2011**, *68*, 2255–2266. [CrossRef] [PubMed]
45. Riaz, G.; Chopra, R. A review on phytochemistry and therapeutic uses of *Hibiscus sabdariffa* L. *Biomed. Pharm.* **2018**, *102*, 575–586. [CrossRef] [PubMed]
46. Wang, L.-S.; Stoner, G.D. Anthocyanins and their role in cancer prevention. *Cancer Lett.* **2008**, *269*, 281–290. [CrossRef] [PubMed]
47. Chao, C.-Y.; Yin, M.-C. Antibacterial effects of roselle calyx extracts and protocatechuic acid in ground beef and apple juice. *Foodborne Pathog. Dis.* **2009**, *6*, 201–206. [CrossRef] [PubMed]
48. Abou-Arab, A.A.; Abu-Salem, F.M.; Abou-Arab, E.A. Physico-chemical properties of natural pigments (anthocyanin) extracted from Roselle calyces (*Hibiscus subdariffa*). *J. Am. Sci.* **2011**, *7*, 445–456.
49. Vasudeva, N.; Sharma, S. Biologically Active Compounds from the Genus *Hibiscus*. *Pharm. Biol.* **2008**, *46*, 145–153. [CrossRef]
50. Singh, P.; Khan, M.; Hailemariam, H. Nutritional and health importance of *Hibiscus sabdariffa*: a review and indication for research needs. *J. Nutr. Health Food Eng.* **2017**, *6*, 00212.
51. Silva, S.; Costa, E.M.; Mendes, M.; Morais, R.; Calhau, C.; Pintado, M. Antimicrobial, antiadhesive and antibiofilm activity of an ethanolic, anthocyanin-rich blueberry extract purified by solid phase extraction. *J. Appl. Microbiol.* **2016**, *121*, 693–703. [CrossRef]
52. Siva, R.; Palackan, M.G.; Maimoon, L.; Geetha, T.; Bhakta, D.; Balamurugan, P.; Rajanarayanan, S. Evaluation of antibacterial, antifungal, and antioxidant properties of some food dyes. *Food Sci. Biotechnol.* **2011**, *20*, 7–13. [CrossRef]

53. Paśko, P.; Bartoń, H.; Zagrodzki, P.; Gorinstein, S.; Fołta, M.; Zachwieja, Z. Anthocyanins, total polyphenols and antioxidant activity in amaranth and quinoa seeds and sprouts during their growth. *Food Chem.* **2009**, *115*, 994–998. [CrossRef]
54. Waterhouse, A.L. Determination of total phenolics. *Curr. protoc. Food Anal. Chem.* **2002**, *6*, I1.1.1–I1.1.8.
55. Adebiyi, O.E.; Olayemi, F.O.; Ning-Hua, T.; Guang-Zhi, Z. In vitro antioxidant activity, total phenolic and flavonoid contents of ethanol extract of stem and leaf of Grewia carpinifolia. *Beni-Suef Univer. J. Basic Appl. Sci.* **2017**, *6*, 10–14. [CrossRef]
56. Nanda, A.; Saravanan, M. Biosynthesis of silver nanoparticles from *Staphylococcus aureus* and its antimicrobial activity against MRSA and MRSE. *Nanomed. Nanotechnol. Biol. Med.* **2009**, *5*, 452–456. [CrossRef] [PubMed]
57. Abdel-Shafi, S.; Osman, A.; Al-Mohammadi, A.-R.; Enan, G.; Kamal, N.; Sitohy, M. Biochemical, biological characteristics and antibacterial activity of glycoprotein extracted from the epidermal mucus of African catfish (Clarias gariepinus). *Int. J. Biol. Macromol.* **2019**, *138*, 773–780. [CrossRef] [PubMed]

Sample Availability: Samples of the compounds are not available from the authors.

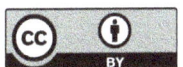

© 2019 by the authors. Licensee MDPI, Basel, Switzerland. This article is an open access article distributed under the terms and conditions of the Creative Commons Attribution (CC BY) license (http://creativecommons.org/licenses/by/4.0/).

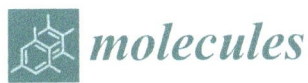

Article

Bioadhesive Polymeric Films Based on Red Onion Skins Extract for Wound Treatment: An Innovative and Eco-Friendly Formulation

Cinzia Pagano [1,†], Maura Marinozzi [1,†], Claudio Baiocchi [2], Tommaso Beccari [1], Paola Calarco [1], Maria Rachele Ceccarini [1], Michela Chielli [1], Ciriana Orabona [3], Elena Orecchini [3], Roberta Ortenzi [4], Maurizio Ricci [1], Stefania Scuota [4], Maria Cristina Tiralti [1] and Luana Perioli [1,*]

1. Department of Pharmaceutical Sciences, University of Perugia, via del Liceo 1, 06123 Perugia, Italy; cinzia.pagano@unipg.it (C.P.); maura.marinozzi@unipg.it (M.M.); tommaso.beccari@unipg.it (T.B.); paola.calarco@unipg.it (P.C.); chele@hotmail.it (M.R.C.); michela.chielli@virgilio.it (M.C.); maurizio.ricci@unipg.it (M.R.); maria.tiralti@unipg.it (M.C.T.)
2. Department of Molecular Biotechnology and Health Sciences, Sect. Analytical Chemistry, Via Pietro Giuria 5, 10125 Torino, Italy; claudio.baiocchi@unito.it
3. Department of Experimental Medicine, Sect. Pharmacology, University of Perugia, P.le L. Severi 1, Bld C/4th floor, 06132 Perugia, Italy; ciriana.orabona@unipg.it (C.O.); elena.orecchini@gmail.com (E.O.)
4. Istituto Zooprofilattico dell'Umbria e delle Marche, via G. Salvemini, 1, 06126 Perugia, Italy; r.ortenzi@izsum.it (R.O.); s.scuota@izsum.it (S.S.)
* Correspondence: luana.perioli@unipg.it; Tel.: +39-075-585-5133 or +39-075-585-5123
† These authors contributed equally to this work.

Academic Editors: Raffaele Capasso and Lorenzo Di Cesare Mannelli
Received: 29 November 2019; Accepted: 10 January 2020; Published: 13 January 2020

Abstract: The onion non-edible outside layers represent a widely available waste material deriving from its processing and consumption. As onion is a vegetable showing many beneficial properties for human health, a study aiming to evaluate the use of extract deriving from the non-edible outside layers was planned. An eco-friendly extraction method was optimized using a hydroalcoholic solution as solvent. The obtained extract was deeply characterized by in vitro methods and then formulated in autoadhesive, biocompatible and pain-free hydrogel polymeric films. The extract, very soluble in water, showed antioxidant, radical scavenging, antibacterial and anti-inflammatory activities, suggesting a potential dermal application for wounds treatment. In vitro studies showed a sustained release of the extract from the hydrogel polymeric film suitable to reach concentrations necessary for both antibacterial and anti-inflammatory activities. Test performed on human keratinocytes showed that the formulation is safe suggesting that the projected formulation could be a valuable tool for wound treatment.

Keywords: onion skins extract; hydrogel; polymeric films; anti-inflammatory; antibacterial

1. Introduction

The common onion (*Allium cepa* L.) is a worldwide cultivated vegetable used both as food and also in the health field for the presence of bioactive molecules mainly endowed with antioxidant activity [1–3]. Many scientific studies on the lipid- and glucose-lowering [4–8], anti-inflammatory [9–11], antioxidant [12–16] and antibacterial [13] properties of onion extracts have been published. Our previous work in this area reported the pungency determination [17] and the antioxidant and immune modulatory activities of purple-skin Rojo Duro onion extracts [18].

The non-edible outside layers (hereinafter referred as OL) are the main waste material obtained from onion processing and consumption. Besides rich in flavonoids [19], they are odorless and can be stored for a long time after the harvesting. The utilization of a biomass endowed with these positive peculiarities fulfills the principles of circular economy and meets the need of environmentally aware consumers [20].

The above considerations, along with the availability of onions endowed with short and traceable production-chain, pushed us to develop an innovative study based on OL use as source of active ingredients [21–25] for the preparation of dermatological products for wound treatment. The presented approach is advantageous as it proposes a new formulation by using waste materials reducing the disposal costs and the consequent environmental impact.

The work was structured as follows: (i) optimization of the extraction method according to green chemistry principles, (ii) evaluation of the extract activity in terms of antioxidant, radical scavenging, antibacterial, anti-inflammatory activities and cytotoxicity and (iii) formulation of the extract as an hydrogel film followed by its activity and safety evaluation.

2. Results

2.1. Optimization of the Extraction Procedure

The first step of the study was the set-up of the best extraction conditions in terms of recovery material, total phenol content (TPC) and antioxidant activity. On the road of biocompatibility, ultrapure water and EtOH were chosen as unique extraction solvents and the procedure was tested both at RT and 60 °C. The obtained results (Table 1) showed that increasing the temperature the recovery yield increased using both abs and 70% EtOH (Table 1); the presence of water in the extraction medium gave a higher extract recovery.

Table 1. Recovery extract yield.

Extraction Conditions: Solvent, Temperature	Recovery Yield (%) [a]
abs EtOH, RT [b]	6.4
70% EtOH, RT [b]	8.7
abs EtOH, 60 °C	7.9
70% EtOH, 60 °C	9.7

[a] mean of two experiments performed in duplicate. [b] RT room temperature.

TPC of the extracts obtained by the four different procedures was measured by the Folin–Ciocalteu method using a calibration curve of gallic acid standard solutions [18]. The calibration curve was fully validated for intra-day and inter-day precision and accuracy before the use (r = 0.9972). A statistically significant difference in TPC was observed among the samples resulting from the different extraction conditions: the use of abs EtOH increased the TPC of the corresponding extracts at both temperatures (Figure 1A). Although abs EtOH resulted a less efficient extraction solvent in terms of yield, it gave extracts with higher TPC than those obtained using 70% EtOH. Among the several protocols reported for assessing the free radical-trapping capability of phytochemicals [26], the ferric ion reducing antioxidant power (FRAP) and 2,2-diphenyl-1-picrylhydrazyl (DPPH) radical assays were chosen [27]. According to FRAP test results (Figure 1B) the highest total reducing capacity (TRC) was found in the extract obtained at 60 °C using abs EtOH. The data ranking of the four extracts was perfectly in accordance with TPC results, hypothesizing that TRC is attributable to the polyphenolic component. Again, the extract obtained in abs EtOH at 60 °C was endowed with the best performance also in DPPH assay (Figure 1C) [18]. The three assays therefore confirmed that the antioxidant component was more soluble in abs EtOH than in hydroalcoholic medium (EtOH 70%) and stable up to 60 °C. Due to the coherence of the obtained data, the extract obtained by using abs EtOH at 60 °C (hereinafter referred as OLE, outside layers extract) was selected for the further studies.

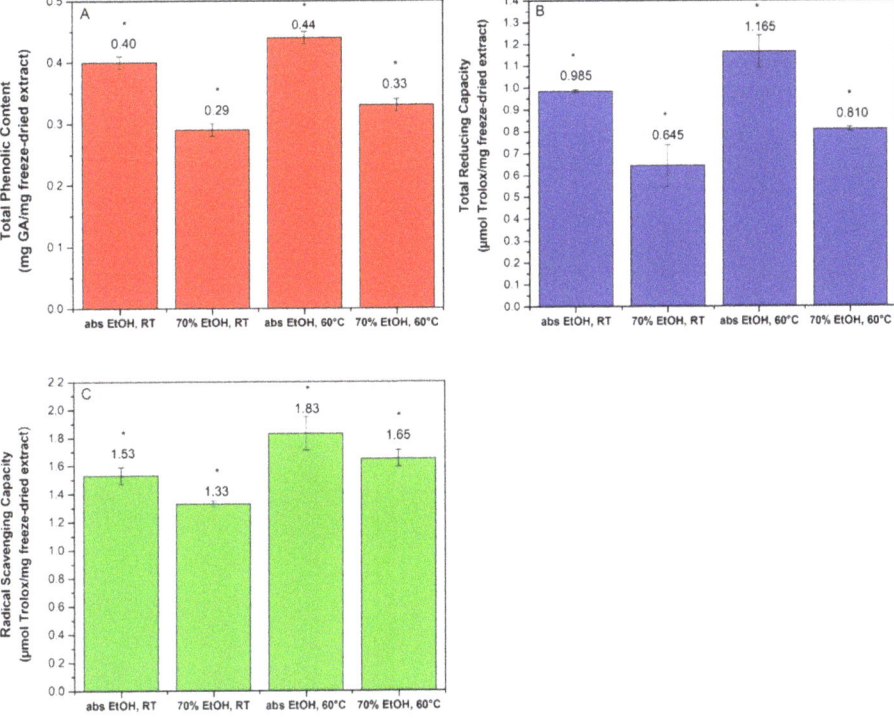

Figure 1. (**A**) Total phenol content (TPC) of the extracts obtained by the four different extraction conditions. Data are expressed as mg of GA/mg of freeze-dried extract and represent the mean of six samples, each measured in triplicate; * $p \leq 0.05$ (one-way ANOVA test). (**B**) Total reducing capacity (TRC) of the extracts obtained by the four different extraction conditions. Data are expressed as mg of GA/mg of freeze-dried extract and represent the mean of six samples, each measured in triplicate. * $p \leq 0.05$. (**C**) Radical scavenging capacity (RSC) of the extracts obtained by the four different extraction conditions. Data are expressed as mg of GA/mg of freeze-dried extract and represent the mean of six samples, each measured in triplicate; * $p \leq 0.05$ (one-way ANOVA test).

2.2. Extract Characterization

2.2.1. Fingerprint Analysis of OLE Constituents

The main OLE components were identified. The species more present were the anthocyanidine cyanidin-3-O-(6′-malonyl-glycoside) (protonated precursor ion $m/z = 535.1082$) and the flavonol quercetin (protonated precursor ion $m/z = 303.0504$). Two other anthocyanidines were present (responsible together with the previously cited one of the red color of the onion) positional isomers of cyanidin malonyl glycoside ($m/z = 535.1082$) and a cyanidin glycoside ($m/z = 449.1081$). Quercetin is only present in glycosylated form ($m/z = 465.1028$) and in much less amount in diglycosilated form ($m/z = 627.1881$). In Figure 2A a chromatogram of OLE monitored in full mass is reported showing the main components identified. The UV spectra (not reported) were highly helpful in substances identification because their shape were informative about the chemical class the various molecules belonged to. Figure 2B shows the separation of much more polar substances performed in isocratic conditions and monitored in ion negative mode. It can be detected that they show very short retention times. Epigallocatechin has anti-oxidative properties whereas the other three acidic substances possess anti-bacterial properties. A quantitative analysis for both cyanidin derivatives and quercetin was performed using quercetin and cyanidin pure standards. The obtained results were: quercetin 9.5

ppm, cyanidin-3-O(-6'-malonyl-glycoside) 5.2 ppm, cyanidin malonyl glycoside isomer 1.7 ppm and cyanidin glycoside 2.1 ppm.

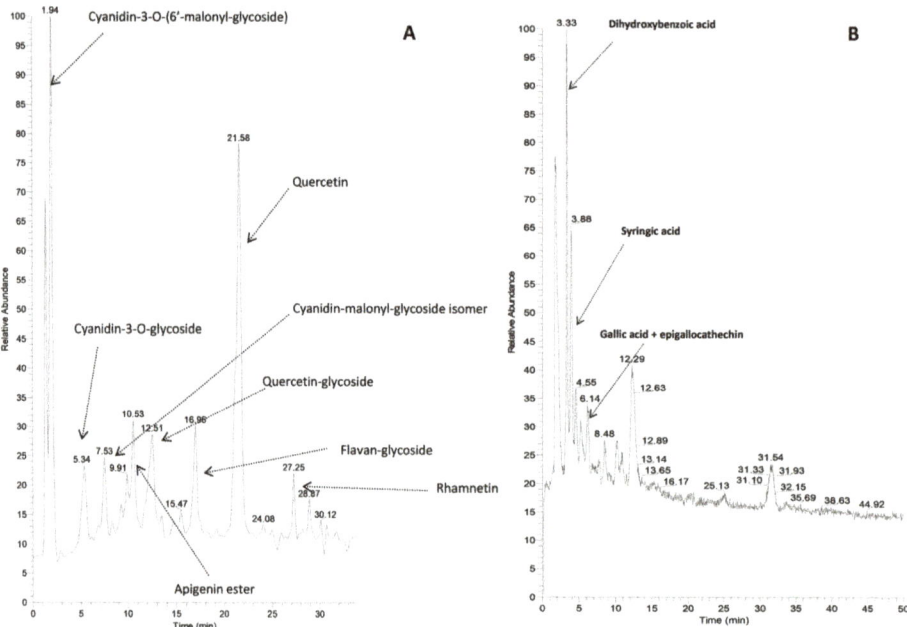

Figure 2. (**A**) Chromatographic separation of OLE constituents monitored in full mass ion positive mode and (**B**) chromatographic separation of OLE constituents monitored in full mass ion negative mode.

All these substances and the other flavonoids present in smaller amounts exhibit anti-oxidative activities combined with the anti-bacterial properties of benzoic acid derivatives.

2.2.2. Antibacterial Activity Assay

Preliminary experiments demonstrated that *Staphylococcus epidermidis*, *Staphylococcus aureus*, *Listeria innocua* and *Enterococcus faecalis* are sensitive to OLE, for this reason Minimum inhibitory (MIC) and minimum bactericidal (MBC) values were measured. The obtained results show the lowest MIC and MBC values for both *S. epidermidis* and *S. aureus* therefore the most sensitive to OLE among the investigated strains (Table 2). The values measured for *S. epidermidis* are the closest to the positive control ampicillin suggesting its greater susceptibility to OLE in comparison to the other ones.

Table 2. Minimum inhibitory (MIC) and minimum bactericidal (MBC) values of OLE and the reference antibiotic ampicillin expressed as mg/mL ± SD (n = 3).

	S. epidermidis	*S. aureus*	*L. innocua*	*E. faecalis*
OLE MIC	0.47 ± 0.00	0.94 ± 0.00	3.75 ± 0.00	3.75 ± 0.00
OLE MBC	0.94 ± 0.00	1.88 ± 0.00	7.50 ± 0.00	7.50 ± 0.00
Ampicillin MIC	0.13 ± 0.00	0.13 ± 0.00	0.50 ± 0.00	0.50 ± 0.00
Ampicillin MBC	0.50 ± 0.00	0.25 ± 0.00	1.00 ± 0.00	4.00 ± 0.00

2.2.3. Cytotoxicity Studies on RAW 264.7 and HaCaT Cell Lines

As macrophages play a key role in all phases of wound healing (inflammation, proliferation and remodeling) [28], RAW 264.7 cell model was used to evaluate OLE anti-inflammatory activity. Firstly, in order to exclude false positives, OLE cytotoxicity on the macrophage cell line RAW 264.7 stimulated with lipopolysaccharide (LPS, 50 ng/mL for 24 h) was investigated. By using eight two-fold dilutions of OLE in the 0.015–2.0 mg/mL concentration range, after 24 h of incubation, it was observed that the cell viability decreased below 75% at the concentration of 0.5 mg/mL. However, it was maintained higher than 65% up to 1 mg/mL and dropped around 50%, with an increased fraction of dead/apoptotic cells, at the concentration of 2.0 mg/mL (Figure 3A,B). For this reason, the concentration 2 mg/mL was excluded from the study focusing the attention on the concentrations range of 0.015–1.0 mg/mL for testing a potential OLE anti-inflammatory effect in LPS-treated RAW 264.7 cells.

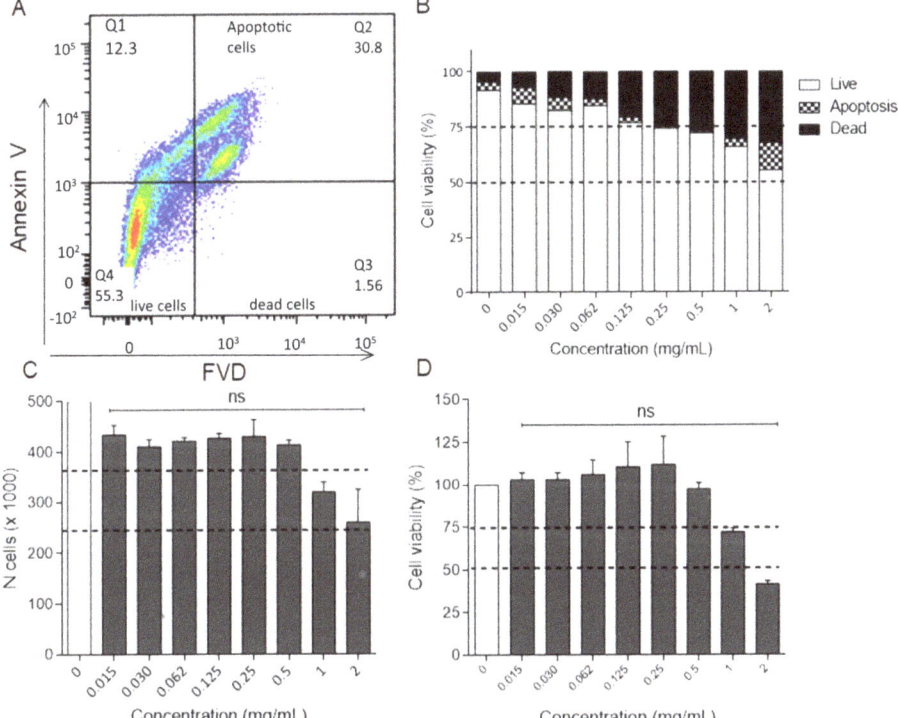

Figure 3. (**A**) LPS-activated cells were treated for 24 h with OLE at the indicated concentrations. Cells were stained using the PerCP-Annexin V and FVD 780 and analyzed by flow cytometry. Annexin V/FVD—double negative cells (lower left quadrant) represented live cells, annexin V/FVD—double positive cells (upper right quadrant) represented apoptotic cells and annexin V-negative/FVD-positive cells (lower right quadrant) indicated dead cells. A representative dot plot is shown. The percentage of viable, apoptotic and dead cells was reported in (**B**) for each OLE concentration. Data are the mean percentage of two different experiments. Evaluation of OLE cytotoxicity and safety on HaCaT cell line by (**C**) Trypan Blue exclusion and (**D**) MTT assays. Dotted lines indicate the 50% and 75% of cell viability. ns, not significant OLE-treated versus untreated group (one-way ANOVA test).

Simultaneously, Trypan Blue exclusion assay and MTT test were carried out on human immortalized keratinocyte cell line (HaCaT), in vitro model of stratum corneum, to evaluate OLE safety in the same concentration range used for RAW 264.7 cells (0.015–2.0 mg/mL). The dose-response curve obtained from Trypan Blue exclusion assay revealed that the number of cells was comparable to the negative control until 0.5 mg/mL and slightly decreased at 1 mg/mL, reaching the 50% of viability at 2.0 mg/mL (Figure 3C). Similar results were obtained by MTT assay. By using the same OLE concentration range (0.015–2.0 mg/mL), after 24 h of incubation HaCaT cells viability was around 75% up to 1 mg/mL, decreasing below 50% at 2.0 mg/mL (Figure 3D). Overall, the cytotoxicity analyses revealed that OLE is safe for both cell lines in the concentration range 0.015–0.5 mg/mL.

2.2.4. Anti-Inflammatory Activity

RAW 264.7 stimulation by LPS for 24 h induces NO synthase (iNOS) activation and thus NO release in the culture supernatant [29], detectable by using Griess reaction. The incubation of LPS stimulated RAW 264.7 with OLE for 24 h induces a significant decrease of NO release in the concentration range 0.125–1.0 mg/mL (Figure 4A). The obtained concentration curve provided an $IC_{50} = 0.230 \pm 0.022$ mg/mL for the down-regulation of NO release by OLE (Figure 4B). The release of pro-inflammatory cytokines, IL-6 and IL-1β in the same cell system was analyzed as reported in the literature [30,31]. It was observed a similar inhibitory effect exerted by OLE on the production of both cytokines in LPS-treated RAW 264.7 macrophages. Specifically, both IL-6 and IL-1β were significantly inhibited by OLE starting from the concentration of 0.030 mg/mL (Figure 4C,D). The inhibitory effect on IL-6 production was concentration-dependent, with an $IC_{50} = 0.090 \pm 0.008$ mg/mL (Figure 4E). Differently, the inhibitory effect on IL-1β production showed a concentration-dependence in the range 0.030–0.25 mg/mL, with an $IC_{50} = 0.054 \pm 0.002$ mg/mL (Figure 4F). For higher concentrations (0.5–1.0 mg/mL) a decreased inhibitory effect on IL-1β production was observed, probably due to the activation of the inflammasome in increased apoptotic RAW 264.7 cells [32,33].

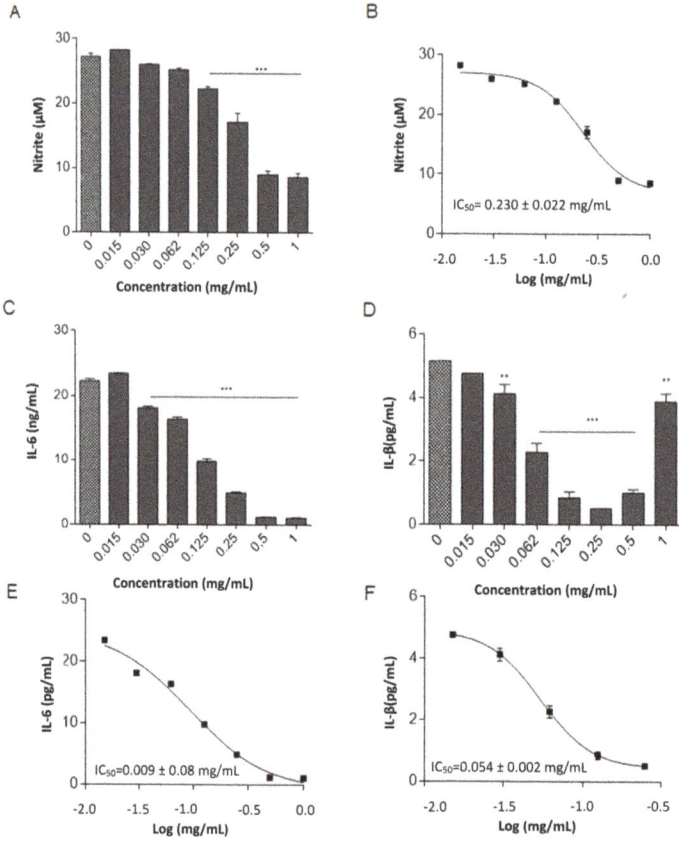

Figure 4. (**A**) LPS-activated RAW 264.7 cells were in vitro stimulated using different OLE concentrations

for 24 h. NO release in the supernatant culture was quantified by using Griess reagent. Results are reported as mean ± SD of three independent experiments, each conducted in triplicate. (**B**) *** $p < 0.0001$, OLE–treated versus LPS-treated group (one-way ANOVA test). Concentration-response curve was obtained for the determination of the IC_{50}. Results are reported as mean of two independent experiments, each conducted in triplicate. LPS-activated RAW 264.7 cells were in vitro stimulated with different concentrations of OLE for 24 h. Supernatants were collected and the concentrations of IL-6 and IL-1β were determined by ELISA test (**C,D**). ** $p < 0.001$, *** $p < 0.0001$, OLE-treated versus LPS-treated group (one-way ANOVA test). Concentration-response curves were obtained for the determination of the IC_{50}. For each curve results are reported as mean of two independent experiments, each conducted in triplicate (**E,F**).

Overall, OLE inhibited the production of inflammatory mediators in LPS-treated RAW264.7 cell line with IC_{50} lower than the highest cytotoxic concentration (i.e., 0.5 mg/mL).

2.3. Hydrogel Film Preparation

After these preliminary studies on pure OLE, a suitable dosage form was developed and characterized. The antioxidant, anti-inflammatory and antibacterial activities observed for pure OLE suggested that it could be a suitable active ingredient for wounds treatment. The wound healing process is a natural post-trauma repairing course rather complex and sensitive; its interruption can lead to the formation of non-healing chronic wounds. A chronic wound, in fact, can be defined as a lesion in which the normal healing process has been interrupted at one or more points during the phases of hemostasis, inflammation, proliferation and remodeling of the wound [34]. Diabetes, venous or arterial disease, infections, metabolic deficiencies, oxidative phenomena and inflammation are the main factors contributing to non-healing chronic wounds [35].

In order to exploit all the OLE biological activities a formulation suitable to be applied on severely injured skin was developed. This formulation should (i) auto-adhere to skin (without the aid of glue), (ii) protect the wound from mechanical solicitations, (iii) avoid occlusion and pain and (iv) be easily removable and able to promote a sustained OLE release.

In order to reach this objective, OLE was formulated in a hydrogel film for potential dermal applications. The formulation was projected and developed based on the following requirements: (i) biocompatibility, (ii) autoadhesivity to skin/wound, (iii) easy and pain-free removal (atraumatic removal) and (iv) an easy and scalable manufacturing method. The hydrogel films were prepared starting from hydrogels whose composition was optimized referring to a previous study [36] by using NaCMC (2%) and PVP K90 (0.1%) as bioadhesive polymers [37,38]. Many modifications in the composition were tested in order to find the most suitable for the hydrogel film preparation (Table S1). Differently from the previously developed films [36], bentonite nanoclay was introduced in the composition as filler [39] to improve the hydrogel film mechanical properties. A preliminary selection was made based on the following criteria: (i) hydrogel aspect (homogeneity and consistency) and physical stability, (ii) easy casting (difficult for very viscous gels) and (iii) final film appearance (detection of visible imperfection under visual inspection). Hydrogel 1 showed low consistency and instability due to bentonite particles sedimentation after 24 h from the preparation.

This phenomenon was ascribed to the low hydrogel viscosity and for this reason three new hydrogels (2, 3 and 4) were prepared with an increased amount of bentonite (Table S1) well known as rheological modifier agent [40]. The idea was that the increase of bentonite content could improve the hydrogel viscosity and thus its stability. Since, the sedimentation phenomenon was still observed, the amount of bentonite was fixed at 4.0% and NaCMC content increased until 3.0% (hydrogel 5, Table S1). These modifications allowed us to obtain a stable hydrogel, but very viscous and thick making difficult the successive casting procedure. To solve this problem hydrogel 6 was then prepared, having the same composition of hydrogel 1, with an increased NaCMC content (3.0%). The obtained hydrogel showed stability and suitable consistency to allow an easy casting.

2.4. Hydrogel Film Characterization

2.4.1. Hydrogel Film Antibacterial Activity

Starting from hydrogel 6 composition (Table S1), three different hydrogel films were prepared loaded with 1.0, 3.0 or 5.0% w/w of OLE (Table S2). The corresponding hydrogel films were submitted to antibacterial activity studies in order to evaluate their ability to reach OLE concentrations necessary active against bacteria. Thus, the hydrogel films were evaluated against the same bacterial strains resulted sensitive to the unformulated OLE: *S. epidermidis*, *S. aureus*, *L. innocua* and *E. faecalis*. Inhibition halos of different sizes were generated by the three different films on the analyzed bacterial strains as reported in Table 3. Specifically, the hydrogel film B1 produced inhibition zone just for *S. epidermidis* and *S. aureus*, while B2 and B3 hydrogel films, containing OLE in higher amount, produced similar inhibition halos for all the tested bacterial strains (Table 3). Analogously to the results obtained for the unformulated OLE, *S. epidermidis* resulted in the most sensitive strain to the loaded hydrogel film. Overall, these data suggested that the hydrogel film B2, containing 10.92 mg/cm^2 of OLE, could be the most suitable formulation for wounds application. For this reason further characterized in the next studies.

Table 3. Inhibition halos measured for the hydrogel films B1–B3. Results are expressed as mm ± SD (n = 3, n.i. = no inhibition).

Hydrogel Film (OLE mg)	S. epidermidis	S. aureus	L. innocua	E. faecalis
B1 (3.64)	23.00 ± 0.00	16.33 ± 0.58	n.i.	n.i.
B2 (10.92)	28.67 ± 0.58	20.33 ± 0.58	21.67 ± 0.58	21.00 ± 0.00
B3 (18.21)	25.67 ± 0.58	21.00 ± 0.00	21.67 ± 0.58	21.33 ± 0.58

n.i. no inhibition.

The preliminary thermal characterization of the hydrogel film B2 showed a water content of 13.6% (Figure S1) after drying and a high glass transition temperature (>200 °C; Figure S2).

2.4.2. Hydrogel Film Thickness, Swelling Behavior and Matrix Erosion Capacity

The hydrogel film B2 (circle 3.14 cm^2) in dry conditions showed a thickness of 0.43 mm (±0.05), resulting very thin. In general, the low thickness of a film for skin use represents a suitable property for ensuring imperceptibility after the application. After hydration the film thickness increased to 2.5 mm (±0.04), suggesting that its swelling after the contact with SWF should not cause an excessive increase of the dimensions that could compromise patient's acceptability during the use. The swelling ability of the hydrogel film B2 was an important parameter to be evaluated as this property is responsible for the ability to absorb exudate from the wound. Moreover, it influences the bioadhesion capacity and OLE release rate from the formulation.

The hydrogel film B2 exhibited a high capacity to absorb fluids, testified by the swelling % measured. It swelled reaching two fold its original weight after 15 min and nine fold after 8 h (Figure S3). This behavior can be attributed to the hydrophilic properties of the hydrogel film with a marked water affinity. During the experiment the hydrogel film showed also weight loss, expressed as erosion matrix % (Figure S3) and due to the gradual dissolution in the medium. The erosion % was 40% after 15 min, then reached 60% after 60 min, maintaining this extent until the 8th h. Both swelling and erosion % cannot be measured after 8 h as after this time the polymeric network resulted completely relaxed due to the very high amount of the absorbed SWF. Thus, the complete hydrogel film dissolution in SWF was observed. Based on these results, it is reasonable to think that the hydrogel film can be easily removed by washing ensuring an atraumatic and pain free removal.

2.4.3. Ex Vivo Adhesion Studies

The adhesion capability of the hydrogel film B2 was evaluated ex vivo by using pig skin samples in which a wound was simulated as reported in Figure 5. The obtained results showed a detachment force of 0.4 N ± 0.06 and detachment time of 13.00 sec ± 0.57. The measured adhesion capacity of the hydrogel film B2 can be ascribed to the combination of both hydrophobic and hydrophilic interactions. The hydrophobic interactions predominate in the case of the binding between hydrogel film and stratum corneum of the peri-wound area. The hydrophilic interactions become more important in the binding of the damaged area characterized by the presence of exudate.

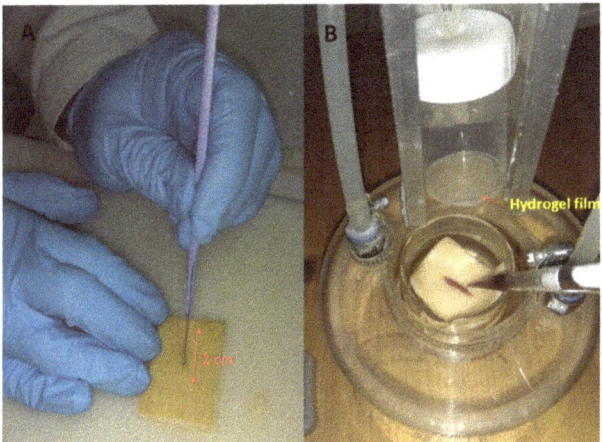

Figure 5. Skin used for the assay (**A**) and simulation of an open wound (**B**).

The obtained results suggested that the developed hydrogel film B2 possesses the suitable balance of hydrophobic and hydrophilic groups to bind wounded skin. In fact, the high swelling capacity measured (Section 3.5.2) evidenced that it is able to interact with the exudate and to swell. This event allowed the distension of NaCMC and PVP K90 polymeric chains exposing the hydrophilic groups (-OH and carboxyl groups for NaCMC and carbonyl for PVP K90) to establish interactions (mainly hydrogen bonds) with the subcutaneous tissues surrounding the wound.

The binding to the peri-wound area could mainly be attributed to hydrophobic groups (-CH_3 for NaCMC and alkyl group for PVP K90) exposed to the outer side of the film and thus available to interact with skin. This aspect is very important as the hydrogel film composition is suitable to adhere to the skin surface avoiding the use of adhesives, not recommended in the open wounds management because they are painful and discomfortable.

2.4.4. OLE In Vitro Release and Correlation with the Anti-Inflammatory Activity

The release capability of hydrogel film B2 loaded with OLE was evaluated in vitro by the Franz diffusion cell. The obtained profile (Figure 6A) shows that OLE is released just after application reaching a concentration of 0.060 mg/mL in 15 min and 0.62 mg/mL within 24 h. This suggests that the hydrogel film B2 is able to release an amount of OLE necessary to obtain the anti-inflammatory activity (Section 2.2.4) from the first minutes. At the same time OLE level remained below 1.0 mg/mL, a viable concentration for both RAW 264.7 and HaCaT cell lines (Figure 3).

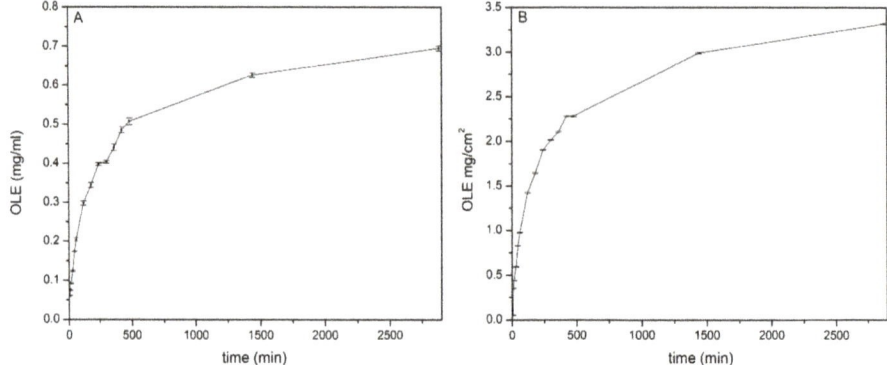

Figure 6. (A) OLE In vitro release profile of from the hydrogel film B2 represented as mg/mL vs. time and (B) mg/cm^2 vs. time.

Despite the hydrogel film B2 has been projected for one daily application, OLE release monitoring was performed until 48th h in order to evaluate if the produced concentrations remain in the safety range. As reported in Figure 6A the amount of OLE released within 48 h increased slightly (0.69 mg/mL) compared to 24th h. The concentration remained below the cytotoxic value (1.0 mg/mL) suggesting that a prolonged application time did not impair skin cells viability.

It is interesting to evaluate the amount of OLE released per unit area (mg/cm^2) as reported in Figure 6B. The hydrogel film B2 was able to produce effective concentrations per cm^2 for the antibacterial and anti-inflammatory activities. Thus, wounds of different sizes could be treated modulating the hydrogel film and is a suitable delivery system for OLE dermal applications for wounds treatment.

2.4.5. In Vitro Safety Studies of Hydrogel Film on HaCaT Cell Line

As the hydrogel film was projected for one daily application the safety studies on HaCaT cells was evaluated within 24 h. A circular film (3.14 cm^2) was incubated for 24 h at 37 °C in DMEM complete medium. Subsequently, the medium was used to treat HaCaT cells for 24 h. From the in vitro release studies it was possible to know the exact OLE amount released from the hydrogel film B2. Different concentrations comparable to OLE values (0.25, 0.5, 1, 1.5 and 2.0 mg/mL) were assayed. The obtained results from MTT assay showed very similar results compared to unformulated OLE (Figure 7) suggesting that both OLE alone and formulated in the hydrogel film B2 is cytotoxic at the concentration of 2.0 mg/mL (above the maximum concentration obtained from the hydrogel film). Thus, it is possible to conclude that both OLE and hydrogel film B2 are safe on an in vitro skin model.

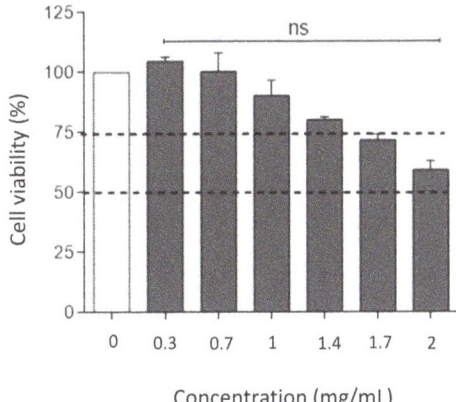

Figure 7. Evaluation of hydrogel film B2 cytotoxicity and safety on HaCaT cell line by an MTT assay. Dotted lines indicate the 50% and 75% of cell viability. ns, not significant OLE-treated versus untreated group (one-way ANOVA test).

3. Materials and Methods

3.1. Materials

Rojo Duro onion samples were provided by the farm "Azienda Agraria Turrioni Fiorella" (Cannara-Perugia, Italy). The extract from OL was prepared about five months after the onion harvesting.

Folin–Ciocalteu reagent, 2,4,6-tris(2-pyridyl)-s-triazine (TPTZ), 6-hydroxy-2,5,7,8-tetramethyl-2-carboxylic acid (Trolox), 2,2-diphenyl-1-picrylhydrazyl (DPPH), hydrochloric acid (HCl), ferric chloride ($FeCl_3$), sodium acetate (NaOAc), sodium carbonate (Na_2CO_3), acetic acid (AcOH), gallic acid (GA) and ethanol (EtOH) and bentonite nanoclay were purchased from Sigma-Aldrich (Milano, Italy). Polyvinylpyrrolidone K90 (PVP K90) was furnished by ISP (Baar, Switzerland). Sodium carboxymethylcellulose (NaCMC) was purchased from Caelo (Hilden, Germany). Ultrapure water was obtained from a reverse osmosis based Milli Q System (Millipore, Milano, Italy). Other reagent grade chemicals and solvents were used without further purification. Ultrapure water was sterilized in a steam autoclave (121 °C, 2118 millibar absolute pressure and relative pressure 1360 millibar).

The simulated wound fluid (SWF) pH 6.5 was prepared by dissolving 8.30 g of NaCl and 0.28 g of $CaCl_2$ in 1000 mL of ultrapure water [36].

3.2. Extraction Procedure

OL, usually produced during the manipulation and braiding of fresh onions, were collected, then quickly washed with ultrapure water and finally dried by a cotton towel. OL (4 g) were suspended in 160 mL of absolute (abs) or 70% EtOH and the obtained suspension kept under magnetic stirring for 90 min at room temperature (RT) or at 60 °C. The supernatant was recovered by decantation (or by the use of a Pasteur pipette) and the residue resuspended in the same starting solvent (100 mL), kept under magnetic stirring for 90 min at the same previously used temperature. In this case, the supernatant was also recovered and the second extraction step repeated once again. The collected supernatants were combined and the solvent removed by a rotary evaporator (water bath temperature 37.0 ± 0.1 °C, Buchi Italia s.r.l., Cornaredo, Italy). The obtained solid was suspended in ultrapure water (28 mL) and the resulting suspension centrifuged at 4000 rpm, 20 °C for 20 min. The supernatant solution was recovered and the pellet twice submitted to the centrifugation step using 10 mL and 6 mL of ultrapure water for suspending the second and the third pellet, respectively. The combined supernatants were freeze-dried and the obtained dry material stored at −20 °C. The procedures were performed in duplicate for each extraction method.

Folin–Ciocalteu assay [18] was performed using the sample (extract) dissolved in ultrapure water, whereas in the case of FRAP (ferric ion reducing antioxidant power) and DPPH (2,2-diphenyl-1-picrylhydrazyl) assays [18], the sample was dissolved in EtOH 75%. In any case, the solution was prepared dissolving 20 mg of freeze-dried extract in 50 mL of solvent (0.4 mg/mL).

3.3. Extract Characterization

3.3.1. Fingerprint Analysis of OLE Constituents

A qualitative evaluation of OLE constituents was performed by LC-UV-high resolution mass spectrometry. Freeze-dried OLE (100.0 mg) was solubilized in 10.0 mL of an EtOH/water (70:30) solution. The obtained solution was centrifuged and 20.0 μL of the clear supernatant were injected in a LC-UV-Vis-HRMS (High resolution mass spectrometry) system. The LC module was an Ultimate 3000 (Thermo Scientific, Rodano, Milan, Italy), the UV-Diode Array module was a Surveyor PDA Plus Detector (Thermo Scientific, Rodano, Milan, Italy), and High Resolution Mass Spectrometer was a linear ion trap linked to an Orbitrap System (LTQ XL, Thermo Scientific, Rodano, Milan, Italy).

OLE molecular species were separated by using a Luna Phenomenex RP-18 column (150 mm × 2.1 i.d., 3 μm particles). Mobile phase was a binary mixture of 0.01% formic acid aqueous solution (solvent **A**) and acetonitrile (solvent **B**) pumped through the column at a flow rate of 0.200 mL/min. Two different chromatographic conditions were used aimed to suitably separate components with very different polarity properties and mass spectrometric response. More polar compounds were separated in isocratic conditions (**A/B** = 72/28) whereas the medium polarity constituents were separated by a gradient elution program consisting of a linear gradient from **A/B** = 95/5 to **A/B** = 50/50. UV-Vis detector was programmed in the wavelength range 220–650 nm.

High resolution and LC-tandem mass spectra were acquired either in negative and in positive ion mode using a linear ion trap-Orbitrap detector equipped with an ESI source with the following parameter settings: spray voltage 4.5 kV; sheath gas flow rate 35 (arbitrary units); drying gas flow rate 25 (arbitrary units) and capillary temperature of 250 °C.

Full scan mass spectra were recorded in the range m/z 220–1200. MS/MS spectra were acquired in the range between ion trap cut-off and precursor ion m/z values. High resolution mass accuracy of recorded ions (vs. calculated) was ±5 millimass units (without internal calibration). High-resolution spectra were acquired with the resolution R = 30,000 (FWHM).

3.3.2. Antibacterial Activity Assay

OLE antibacterial activity was evaluated for four bacterial species *S. epidermidis* WDCM (world data centre for microorganisms) 00036, *S. aureus* WDCM 00034, *E. L. innocua* WDCM 00017 and *faecalis* WDCM 00087. MIC and MBC concentrations were measured using a standard microdilution technique according to Clinical Laboratory Standards Institute Guidelines, adapting the protocol as suggested by J.M. Silván et al. [41]. The bacterial suspension used for the assay was prepared using bacteria to approximately 1×10^5 CFU/mL in Muller Hilton Broth (MHB; Biolife Italiana s.r.l, Cod. 4017412). The stored strains were revitalized on Brain Heart Infusion Broth (BHI, Biolife Italiana s.r.l, Cod. 4012302) and incubated according to their own growth conditions (Table S3). At the time of use, OLE was dissolved in sterile ultrapure water to obtain the concentration required by the protocol for the evaluation of the antibacterial effect. The assayed concentrations were: 30, 15, 7.50, 3.75, 1.88, 0.94 and 0.47 mg/mL. Moreover, for each bacterial strain three controls were set up. These included antibiotic control (ampicillin), organism control (MHB and the bacterial suspension), negative control (MHB and the solution of the extract at the same concentration tested). For each bacterial species the test was performed in triplicate. The microplates were incubated according to the growth conditions of each bacterial strain tested (Table S3). After incubation, serial decimal dilutions of each well were prepared in sterile saline solution (0.9% *w/v* NaCl) and plated onto agar with 5% sheep blood (Biolife Italiana s.r.l, Cod. 4011552). Results are expressed as log CFU/mL.

3.3.3. Cell Lines and Cytotoxicity Studies

The mouse macrophage cell line RAW 264.7, obtained from the American Type Culture Collection (ATCC, Manassas, VA, USA), was used to investigate OLE anti-inflammatory activity. RAW 264.7 cells were cultured according to standard procedures in Roswell Park Memorial Institute 1640 medium (RPMI-1640), whereas HaCaT cells were cultured according to standard procedures in Dulbecco's modified Eagle's medium (DMEM). Both medium were supplemented with 10% heat-inactivated Fetal Bovine Serum (FBS), 2 mM of L-glutamine and antibiotics (100 U/mL penicillin, 100 µg/mL streptomycin; Gibco, Invitrogen, Carlsbad, CA, USA). Both cell lines were cultured at 37.0 °C in a 5% CO_2 atmosphere and the medium replaced every 3 days. RAW 264.7 and (HaCaT) were tested for mycoplasma contamination before use. RAW 264.7 cells were activated with lipopolysaccharides (LPS), serotype 055:B5 (Sigma-Aldrich, Saint Louis, MO, USA) at 50 ng/mL for 24 h. LPS-activated RAW 264.7 cells were cultured at the concentration of 1×10^6 cells/700 µL in a 24-well plate and co-treated with serial two-fold dilutions of OLE for 24 h. The percentage of live, apoptotic and dead cells, was determined by using Annexin V Apoptosis Detection Kit PerCP-eFluor™ 710 and FVD (Fixable Viability Dye eFluor™ 780; eBioscience, San Diego, CA, USA), according to the manufacturer's instructions. Specifically, each cell sample was washed and suspended in 100 µL of phosphate-buffered saline before the staining. A dilution 1:1000 of FVD was then added to the sample and incubated at 4 °C for 30 min in the dark. Annexin V-PerCP, diluted 1:20, was added and incubated for 15 min at RT in the dark. Flow cytometry analysis was performed within 4 h.

HaCaT cells were purchased from I.Z.S.L.E.R. (Istituto Zooprofilattico Sperimentale della Lombardia e dell'Emilia Romagna, Brescia, Italy) and used as model for assessing the epidermal homeostasis during wound treatment. Cells viability was assessed after treatment for 24 h with OLE both by Trypan Blue exclusion and MTT assays [42]. Cells were seeded at the density of 2×10^5 cells/well into 6-well culture plates in a final volume of 2 mL and 5×10^3 cells/well into 96-well flat bottom culture plates in a final volume of 200 µL, for Trypan Blue exclusion and MTT assay respectively. Cell viability was measured and expressed as a percentage relative to that of the control cells as previously described [43].

3.3.4. Anti-Inflammatory Activity

For the quantification of nitric oxide (NO) release, LPS-activated RAW 264.7 cells were cultured at the concentration of 0.15×10^6 cells/200 µL in a 96-well plate and co-treated with serial two-fold dilutions of OLE for 24 h. The total production of NO was detected by incubating at RT for 7 min each culture supernatant (50 µL) with 100 µL of Griess reagent (1% naphthylethylenediamine dihydrochloride in distilled water and 1% sulfanilamide in 5% concentrate H_3PO_4, mixed 1:1). Nitrite concentration was quantified by comparison with a sodium nitrite standard curve. The absorbance of samples was read at $\lambda = 530.0$ nm, by using a spectrophotometer (TECAN). The assay was conducted in triplicate.

For the quantification of IL-6 and IL-1β, LPS-activated RAW 264.7 cells were cultured at the concentration of 0.5×10^6 cells/500 µL in a 48-well plate and co-treated with serial two-fold dilutions of OLE for 24 h. IL-6 and IL-1β were determined in the culture supernatants by Mouse IL-6 Uncoated ELISA kit (Invitrogen, Carlsbad, CA, USA) and Mouse IL-1 β ELISA Ready-SET-Go!™ kit (eBioscience, San Diego, CA, USA), respectively, as described by the manufacturer's instructions. The experiments were conducted in triplicate and repeated two times.

3.4. Hydrogel Film Preparation

The hydrogel films were prepared by the solvent casting method [36] starting from a hydrogel. An OLE solution (1.0%, 3.0% or 5.0% *w/w*) was initially prepared in ultrapure water then, bentonite (1%) was dispersed in this solution. Finally, glycerol (10%), NaCMC (3.0%) and PVP K90 (0.1%) were added. The mixing was performed at 600 rpm, for 20 min, at RT using a mechanical stirrer equipped with a three blade helical impellers (DLS VELP® Scientifica, Usmate MB, Italy). In order to remove the air incorporated during the mixing, each hydrogel was degassed in a conditioning planetary mixer (Thinky mixer ARE-250) at 2000 rpm for 10 min. Afterwards, 3.5 g of the prepared mixture was casted into silicon molds (ø = 3.5 cm) and left to dry in ventilated oven at 37.0 °C ± 0.1 for 24 h. After drying, the hydrogel films were stored at RT and 40% relative humidity (RH) until use.

3.5. Hydrogel Film Characterization

3.5.1. Hydrogel Film Antibacterial Activity

The test medium and bacterial suspension used for the assay were prepared as previously reported (Section 3.3.2). The experiment was carried out on *S. epidermidis* WDCM 00036, *S. aureus* WDCM 00034, *E. faecalis* WDCM 00087 and *L. innocua* WDCM 00017. Different inoculated media were used for each bacterial strains. Sterile Petri dishes (diameter 90 mm) were filled with 20 mL of the prepared and seeded media. After medium solidification, a small square (1 cm × 1 cm) of the hydrogel film was placed in each series of plates and incubated according to their own growth conditions (Table S3). The test was conducted in triplicate for each bacterial strain. Negative control was set up using a hydrogel film OLE free. At the end of the incubation time the presence and the diameter of the inhibition halo was evaluated by a gauge.

3.5.2. Hydrogel Film Thickness, Swelling Behavior and Matrix Erosion

Hydrogel film thickness was measured in both dry and wet state by a manual micrometer (Borletti, Cremona, Italy). The thickness of the hydrogel film after hydration was measured after incubation in 10 mL of SWF thermostated at 32.0 ± 0.5 °C for 8 h. After this period, the excess of SWF was removed by filter paper and the thickness measured. The hydrogel film swelling capacity and erosion [44] were calculated using Equations (1) and (2) respectively:

$$\text{swelling \%} = \frac{W2 - W1}{W1} \times 100. \quad (1)$$

$$\text{erosion \%} = \frac{W1 - W3}{W1} \times 100. \quad (2)$$

Each hydrogel film (circles of 3.14 cm^2) was weighted (W1), immersed in 10 mL of SWF into a Petri plate (ø = 5 cm) and thermostated at 32.0 ± 0.1°C for established times (15, 30, 60, 90, 120, 180, 300 and 1440 min). After immersion, the hydrogel films were wiped off from the excess of SWF using filter paper and weighted (W2).

The erosion % was measured as follows. The swollen films were dried at 60 °C for 24 h and kept in desiccator over CaCl$_2$ (40% RH) for 48 h and after drying the weighting was repeated (W3). The obtained results represent the average of three measurements (n = 3).

3.5.3. Thermal Properties Measurement

Thermogravimetric (TGA) analysis was performed by a Netzsch STA 449C apparatus (Mettler Toledo, Milano, Italy), in air flow and heating rate of 10 °C/min, to determine the weight loss as a function of increasing temperature. Differential scanning calorimetry (DSC) analysis was performed using an automatic thermal analyzer (DSC821e, Mettler Toledo, Milano, Italy) and indium standard for temperature calibrations. Holed aluminum pans were employed in the experiments for all samples and an empty pan, prepared in the same way, was used as a reference. Samples of 3–6 mg were weighted directly into aluminum pans and thermal analyses of the samples were conducted, at a heating rate of 5 °C/min from 25 to 300 °C.

3.5.4. Ex Vivo Adhesion Studies

The hydrogel film adhesion force and time were assessed using pig skin samples (from shoulder region), obtained from large white pigs weighing 165–175 kg, furnished by the Veterinary Service of ASL N.1 Città di Castello (Perugia, Italy) and used within 12 h from pig death [36]. The ex vivo adhesion force was measured by a dynamometer (Didatronic, Terni, Italy). By means of cyanoacrylate glue the film was attached to the bottom of a cylindrical support and the porcine skin tissue (2 cm × 2 cm) on the surface of a glass support thermostated at 32.0 ± 0.5 °C. An incision of 2 cm was made by a scalpel on the skin sample in order to simulate a wound. The latter was filled with 500 µL of SWF and the hydrogel film was put in contact with the simulated wound by applying a light force (0.5 N) for 60 sec. After this time, the force was removed and the hydrogel film kept in contact with the skin for further 60 sec and then put in traction. The force necessary for film detachment to skin was measured and expressed as average of three measurements ($n = 3$).

3.5.5. In Vitro Release of Extract from The Hydrogel Film

OLE In vitro release from the hydrogel film was evaluated by vertical Franz diffusion cell (USP <1724>; PermeGear, Inc., Bethlehem, PA, USA, diameter 20 mm). A cellulose membrane (Whatman 41, Whatman GmbH, Dassel, Germany) was placed between the two chambers. The receptor chamber was filled with SWF as receptor medium (15 mL), thermostated at 32.0 °C ± 0.5 and magnetically stirred (600 rpm). The hydrogel film (circle of 3.14 cm^2) was placed on top of the cellulose membrane. The donor phase was represented by 2 mL of a 0.025-N K$_2$CO$_3$ solution (simulating air CO$_2$) [43]. All openings including donor top and receptor arm were occluded with parafilm® to prevent solvent evaporation. At regular time intervals (5, 10, 15, 30, 45, 60, 120, 240, 300, 360, 420, 480, 1440 and 2880 min) samples of the receiving phase were withdrawn and OLE content was measured by a UV-vis spectrophotometer (UV-Visible Agilent model 8453, Agilent Technologies, Cernusco sul Naviglio MI, Italy) accomplished using a standard curve in SWF (λ_{max} = 280.0 nm, r = 0.9998). All experiments were performed in triplicate, each result represents an average of three measurements and the error was expressed as standard deviation (±SD).

4. Conclusions

The manuscript described the use of the non-edible outside layers of the onion cultivar Rojo Duro for the preparation of a hydrogel film for dermal application. This study proved that medical devices could be developed by recycling a waste material from agricultural and food processing industries. The use of the non-edible outside layers as a source of active ingredients is an efficient and smart approach for avoiding the expensive disposal procedures while producing a high-value added product.

The extract (OLE) deriving from the non-edible outside layers was obtained by using eco-friendly solvents thus without the production of further waste. OLE showed interesting antioxidant, radical scavenging, anti-inflammatory and antibacterial activities. As these properties were suitable for wounds treatment, OLE was formulated as autoadhesive biocompatible hydrogel film for application on injured skin with the aim to promote the healing process through synergic mechanisms. This could represent an effective alternative to conventional antibacterial therapies, limiting the use of antibiotics and thus the resistance problem.

OLE (10.92 mg/cm^2) was released from the hydrogel film by a sustained release reaching effective concentrations to (i) exert the antibacterial activity against *S. epidermidis*, *S. aureus* and *E. faecalis* (common strains responsible for wounds infections); (ii) obtain the anti-inflammatory activity and at the same time and iii) maintain cells viability.

The hydrogel film is biocompatible, its composition is simple (PVP K90, NaCMC, bentonite), allows a rapid adhesion to skin, without the use of adhesives, a mechanical protection of the wound and an easy/pain-free removal by washing. Moreover, the hydrogel film is self-applicable. The last property, together to that described above, fulfills the compliance of the patient. The hydrogel film is green, scalable and cheap, thus resulting advantageous for the industry.

The obtained results suggest that the developed formulation represents an innovative and effective strategy useful for wounds treatment.

Supplementary Materials: The following are available online at http://www.mdpi.com/1420-3049/25/2/318/s1, Figure S1: The TGA curve shows three steps: the first one until 200 °C corresponding to the vaporization of residual water (13.6%), the second step until 500 °C due to the decomposition of the organic components, the third one above 500 °C characterized by a mineral residue (22.78%) due to bentonite content. Figure S2. PVP K90 shows a broad endothermic peak between 45 and 120 °C due to the evaporation of bound water or moisture. For bentonite it is detectable a broad band between 60 and 100 °C attributable to adsorbed water loss. NaCMC shows a glass transition temperature (Tg) at 75 °C, corresponding and an exothermic peak at 284 °C due to the melting and the crystallization transition. Pre OLE thermogram shows that thermal process occurs at 80 °C probably related to the loss of volatile constituent of the sample (ethanol). No thermal decomposition was observed in the temperature range investigated. For the hydrogel film B2 a glass transition temperature (Tg) at 228 °C was observed. The spectra are shown in arbitrary units (a.u.) and shifted for clarity. Figure S3. Swelling % and erosion % of the hydrogel film B2 in SWF thermostated at 32 °C for 480 min. Table S1. Hydrogels compositions. Table S2. Compositions of hydrogels loaded with different OLE percentages. Table S3. Bacterial strains and growth conditions.

Author Contributions: Conceptualization, M.M. and L.P.; Data curation, C.B., M.M., M.R.C., C.O., R.O. and L.P.; Formal analysis, C.P., P.C., C.B., M.R.C., M.C., E.O., R.O. and M.R.; Funding acquisition, M.M., S.S., M.C.T. and L.P.; Investigation, C.P., M.M., T.B., C.O., C.B., S.S. and L.P.; Methodology, C.P., M.M., C.B., T.B., C.O. and L.P.; Resources, M.M., T.B., C.O., S.S., C.B. and L.P.; Supervision, C.P., M.M., M.R., M.C.T. and L.P.; Validation, P.C., C.B., M.R.C., M.C., E.O. and R.O.; Visualization, C.P., M.M., T.B., C.O., S.S. and L.P.; Writing—original draft, C.P., M.M., T.B., C.O., M.R., S.S. and L.P.; Writing—review and editing, C.P., M.M., M.R.C., C.O., R.O., M.C.T. and L.P. All authors have read and agreed to the published version of the manuscript.

Funding: This research was financed by MIUR-Fondo d'Ateneo per la Ricerca di Base 2015.

Acknowledgments: Authors sincerely acknowledge Marco Marani (Department of Pharmaceutical Sciences) for technical assistance, Fiorello Turrioni and "Azienda Agraria Turrioni Fiorella" (Cannara, Perugia, Italy) for providing Rojo Duro onion skins, Simonetta De Angelis from ASL N. 1 (Città di Castello, Perugia, Italy), for providing pig skin samples.

Conflicts of Interest: The authors declare no conflict of interest.

References

1. Ninfali, P.; Mea, G.; Giorgini, S.; Rocchi, M.; Bacchiocca, M. Antioxidant capacity of vegetables, spices and dressings relevant to nutrition. *Br. J. Nutr.* **2005**, *93*, 257–266. [CrossRef] [PubMed]
2. Wong, S.; Leong, L.; Williamkoh, J. Antioxidant activities of aqueous extracts of selected plants. *Food Chem.* **2006**, *99*, 775–783. [CrossRef]
3. Slimestad, R.; Fossen, T.; Vågen, I.M. Onions: A Source of Unique Dietary Flavonoids. *J. Agric. Food Chem.* **2007**, *55*, 10067–10080. [CrossRef] [PubMed]
4. Kim, J.; Cha, Y.-J.; Lee, K.-H.; Park, E. Effect of onion peel extract supplementation on the lipid profile and antioxidative status of healthy young women: A randomized, placebo-controlled, double-blind, crossover trial. *Nutr. Res. Pract.* **2013**, *7*, 373–379. [CrossRef]
5. Lee, J.-S.; Cha, Y.-J.; Lee, K.-H.; Yim, J.-E. Onion peel extract reduces the percentage of body fat in overweight and obese subjects: A 12-week, randomized, double-blind, placebo-controlled study. *Nutr. Res. Pract.* **2016**, *10*, 175–181. [CrossRef]
6. Kim, K.-A.; Yim, J.-E. Antioxidative Activity of Onion Peel Extract in Obese Women: A Randomized, Double-blind, Placebo Controlled Study. *J. Cancer Prev.* **2015**, *20*, 202–207. [CrossRef]
7. Jung, J.Y.; Lim, Y.; Moon, M.S.; Kim, J.Y.; Kwon, O. Onion peel extracts ameliorate hyperglycemia and insulin resistance in high fat diet/streptozotocin-induced diabetic rats. *Nutr. Metab.* **2011**, *8*, 18. [CrossRef]
8. Kim, S.-H.; Jo, S.-H.; Kwon, Y.-I.; Hwang, J.-K. Effects of Onion (*Allium cepa* L.) Extract Administration on Intestinal α-Glucosidases Activities and Spikes in Postprandial Blood Glucose Levels in SD Rats Model. *Int. J. Mol. Sci.* **2011**, *12*, 3757–3769. [CrossRef]
9. Albishi, T.; John, J.A.; Al-Khalifa, A.S.; Shahidi, F. Antioxidant, anti-inflammatory and DNA scission inhibitory activities of phenolic compounds in selected onion and potato varieties. *J. Funct. Foods* **2013**, *5*, 930–939. [CrossRef]

10. Kim, O.Y.; Lee, S.-M.; Do, H.; Moon, J.; Lee, K.-H.; Cha, Y.-J.; Shin, M.-J. Influence of Quercetin-rich Onion Peel Extracts on Adipokine Expression in the Visceral Adipose Tissue of Rats. *Phyther. Res.* **2011**, *26*, 432–437. [CrossRef]
11. Kim, K.-A.; Yim, J.-E. The Effect of Onion Peel Extract on Inflammatory Mediators in Korean Overweight and Obese Women. *Clin. Nutr. Res.* **2016**, *5*, 261–269. [CrossRef] [PubMed]
12. De Dicastillo, C.; Navarro, R.; Guarda, A.; Galotto, M. Development of Biocomposites with Antioxidant Activity Based on Red Onion Extract and Acetate Cellulose. *Antioxidants* **2015**, *4*, 533–547. [CrossRef] [PubMed]
13. Ye, C.L.; Dai, D.H.; Hu, W.L. Antimicrobial and antioxidant activities of the essential oil from onion (*Allium cepa* L.). *Food Control* **2013**, *30*, 48–53. [CrossRef]
14. Shon, M.Y.; Choi, S.D.; Kahng, G.G.; Nam, S.H.; Sung, N.J. Antimutagenic, antioxidant and free radical scavenging activity of ethyl acetate extracts from white, yellow and red onions. *Food Chem. Toxicol.* **2004**, *42*, 659–666. [CrossRef]
15. Petropoulos, S.A.; Fernandes, Â.; Barros, L.; Ferreira, I.C.F.R.; Ntatsi, G. Morphological, nutritional and chemical description of "Vatikiotiko", an onion local landrace from Greece. *Food Chem.* **2015**, *182*, 156–163. [CrossRef]
16. Benkeblia, N. Free-radical scavenging capacity and antioxidant properties of some selected onions (*Allium cepa* L.) and garlic (*Allium sativum* L.) extracts. *Braz. Arch. Biol. Technol.* **2005**, *48*, 753–759. [CrossRef]
17. Ianni, F.; Marinozzi, M.; Scorzoni, S.; Sardella, R.; Natalini, B. Quantitative Evaluation of the Pyruvic Acid Content in Onion Samples with a Fully Validated High-Performance Liquid Chromatography Method. *Int. J. Food Prop.* **2016**, *19*, 752–759. [CrossRef]
18. Lisanti, A.; Formica, V.; Ianni, F.; Albertini, B.; Marinozzi, M.; Sardella, R.; Natalini, B. Antioxidant activity of phenolic extracts from different cultivars of Italian onion (*Allium cepa*) and relative human immune cell proliferative induction. *Pharm. Biol.* **2016**, *54*, 799–806. [CrossRef]
19. Rodrigues, A.S.; Almeida, D.P.F.; Simal-Gándara, J.; Pérez-Gregorio, M.R. Onions: A Source of Flavonoids. In *Flavonoids—From Biosynthesis to Human Health*; InTech: London, UK, 2017.
20. Zuin, V.G.; Ramin, L.Z. Green and Sustainable Separation of Natural Products from Agro-Industrial Waste: Challenges, Potentialities, and Perspectives on Emerging Approaches. *Top. Curr. Chem.* **2018**, *376*, 3. [CrossRef]
21. Ko, M.-J.; Cheigh, C.-I.; Cho, S.-W.; Chung, M.-S. Subcritical water extraction of flavonol quercetin from onion skin. *J. Food Eng.* **2011**, *102*, 327–333. [CrossRef]
22. Brüll, V.; Burak, C.; Stoffel-Wagner, B.; Wolffram, S.; Nickenig, G.; Müller, C.; Langguth, P.; Alteheld, B.; Fimmers, R.; Naaf, S.; et al. Effects of a quercetin-rich onion skin extract on 24 h ambulatory blood pressure and endothelial function in overweight-to-obese patients with (pre-)hypertension: A randomised double-blinded placebo-controlled cross-over trial. *Br. J. Nutr.* **2015**, *114*, 1263–1277. [CrossRef]
23. Ramos, F.A.; Takaishi, Y.; Shirotori, M.; Kawaguchi, Y.; Tsuchiya, K.; Shibata, H.; Higuti, T.; Tadokoro, T.; Takeuchi, M. Antibacterial and Antioxidant Activities of Quercetin Oxidation Products from Yellow Onion (*Allium cepa*) Skin. *J. Agric. Food Chem.* **2006**, *54*, 3551–3557. [CrossRef]
24. Suh, H.; Lee, J.; Cho, J.; Kim, Y.; Chung, S. Radical scavenging compounds in onion skin. *Food Res. Int.* **1999**, *32*, 659–664. [CrossRef]
25. Lee, K.A.; Kim, K.-T.; Kim, H.J.; Chung, M.-S.; Chang, P.-S.; Park, H.; Pai, H.-D. Antioxidant activities of onion (*Allium cepa* L.) peel extracts produced by ethanol, hot water, and subcritical water extraction. *Food Sci. Biotechnol.* **2014**, *23*, 615–621. [CrossRef]
26. Frankel, E.N.; Meyer, A.S. The problems of using one-dimensional methods to evaluate multifunctional food and biological antioxidants. *J. Sci. Food Agric.* **2000**, *80*, 1925–1941. [CrossRef]
27. Marinozzi, M.; Sardella, R.; Scorzoni, S.; Ianni, F.; Lisanti, A.; Natalini, B. Validated Pungency Assessment of Three Italian Onion (*Allium cepa* L.) Cultivars. *Agric. Food* **2014**, *2*, 532–541.
28. Krzyszczyk, P.; Schloss, R.; Palmer, A.; Berthiaume, F. The role of macrophages in acute and chronic wound healing and interventions to promote pro-wound healing phenotypes. *Front. Physiol.* **2018**, *9*, 419. [CrossRef]
29. Kwon, H.K.; Song, M.J.; Lee, H.J.; Park, T.S.; Kim, M.; Park, H.J. Pediococcus pentosaceus-Fermented Cordyceps militaris Inhibits Inflammatory Reactions and Alleviates Contact Dermatitis. *Int. J. Mol. Sci.* **2018**, *19*, 3504. [CrossRef]

30. Chen, B.-C.; Liao, C.-C.; Hsu, M.-J.; Liao, Y.-T.; Lin, C.-C.; Sheu, J.-R.; Lin, C.-H. Peptidoglycan-Induced IL-6 Production in RAW 264.7 Macrophages Is Mediated by Cyclooxygenase-2, PGE 2/PGE 4 Receptors, Protein Kinase A, IκB Kinase, and NF-κB. *J. Immunol.* **2006**, *177*, 681–693. [CrossRef]
31. Jeong, D.; Dong, G.Z.; Lee, H.J.; Ryu, J.H. Anti-Inflammatory Compounds from *Atractylodes macrocephala*. *Molecules* **2019**, *24*, 1859. [CrossRef]
32. An, Z.; Su, J. Acinetobacter baumannii outer membrane protein 34 elicits NLRP3 inflammasome activation via mitochondria-derived reactive oxygen species in RAW264.7 macrophages. *Microbes Infect.* **2018**, *3*, 143–153. [CrossRef]
33. Escandell, J.; Recio, M.; Giner, R.; Máñez, S.; Ríos, J. Bcl-2 is a negative regulator of interleukin-1β secretion in murine macrophages in pharmacological-induced apoptosis. *Br. J. Pharmacol.* **2010**, *160*, 1844–1856. [CrossRef]
34. Han, G.; Ceilley, R. Chronic Wound Healing: A Review of Current Management and Treatments. *Adv. Ther.* **2017**, *34*, 599–610. [CrossRef]
35. Latifa, K.; Sondess, S.; Hajer, G.; Manel, B.-H.-M.; Souhir, K.; Nadia, B.; Abir, J.; Salima, F.; Abdelhedi, M. Evaluation of physiological risk factors, oxidant-antioxidant imbalance, proteolytic and genetic variations of matrix metalloproteinase-9 in patients with pressure ulcer. *Sci. Rep.* **2016**, *6*, 29371. [CrossRef]
36. Pagano, C.; Ceccarini, M.R.; Calarco, P.; Scuota, S.; Conte, C.; Primavilla, S.; Ricci, M.; Perioli, L. Bioadhesive polymeric films based on usnic acid for burn wound treatment: Antibacterial and cytotoxicity studies. *Colloids Surf. B Biointerfaces* **2019**, *178*, 488–499. [CrossRef]
37. Djekic, L.; Martinović, M.; Dobričić, V.; Ćalija, B.; Medarević, Đ.; Primorac, M. Comparison of the Effect of Bioadhesive Polymers on Stability and Drug Release Kinetics of Biocompatible Hydrogels for Topical Application of Ibuprofen. *J. Pharm. Sci.* **2019**, *108*, 1326–1333. [CrossRef]
38. Poonguzhali, R.; Basha, S.K.; Kumari, V.S. Nanostarch Reinforced with Chitosan/Poly (vinyl pyrrolidone) Blend for In Vitro Wound Healing Application. *Polym. Plast. Technol. Eng.* **2018**, *57*, 1400–1410. [CrossRef]
39. Jose, T.; George, S.C.; Maya, M.G.; Maria, H.J.; Wilson, R.; Thomas, S. Effect of Bentonite Clay on the Mechanical, Thermal, and Pervaporation Performance of the Poly (vinyl alcohol) Nanocomposite Membranes. *Ind. Eng. Chem. Res.* **2014**, *53*, 16820–16831. [CrossRef]
40. Abu-Jdayil, B. Rheology of sodium and calcium bentonite–water dispersions: Effect of electrolytes and aging time. *Int. J. Miner. Process.* **2011**, *98*, 208–213. [CrossRef]
41. Silván, J.M.; Mingo, E.; Hidalgo, M.; de Pascual-Teresa, S.; Carrascosa, A.V.; Martinez-Rodriguez, A.J. Antibacterial activity of a grape seed extract and its fractions against Campylobacter spp. *Food Control* **2013**, *29*, 25–31. [CrossRef]
42. Ceccarini, M.R.; Vannini, S.; Cataldi, S.; Moretti, M.; Villarini, M.; Fioretti, B.; Albi, E.; Beccari, T.; Codini, M. In Vitro Protective Effects of Lycium barbarum Berries Cultivated in Umbria (Italy) on Human Hepatocellular Carcinoma Cells. *BioMed Res. Int.* **2016**, *2016*, 7529521. [CrossRef]
43. Pagano, C.; Perioli, L.; Latterini, L.; Nocchetti, M.; Ceccarini, M.R.; Marani, M.; Ramella, D.; Ricci, M. Folic acid-layered double hydroxides hybrids in skin formulations: Technological, photochemical and in vitro cytotoxicity on human keratinocytes and fibroblasts. *Appl. Clay Sci.* **2019**, *168*, 382–395. [CrossRef]
44. Perioli, L.; Ambrogi, V.; Angelici, F.; Ricci, M.; Giovagnoli, S.; Capuccella, M.; Rossi, C. Development of mucoadhesive patches for buccal administration of ibuprofen. *J. Control Release* **2004**, *99*, 73–82. [CrossRef]

Sample Availability: Samples of OLE and films are available from the authors.

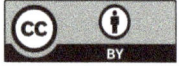

© 2020 by the authors. Licensee MDPI, Basel, Switzerland. This article is an open access article distributed under the terms and conditions of the Creative Commons Attribution (CC BY) license (http://creativecommons.org/licenses/by/4.0/).

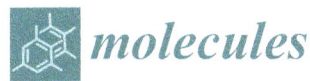

Review

Bee Products in Dermatology and Skin Care

Anna Kurek-Górecka [1,*], Michał Górecki [2], Anna Rzepecka-Stojko [2], Radosław Balwierz [1] and Jerzy Stojko [3]

1. Silesian Academy of Medical Sciences in Katowice, Mickiewicza 29, 40-085 Katowice, Poland; radoslaw.balwierz@gmail.com
2. Department of Drug Technology, Faculty of Pharmaceutical Sciences in Sosnowiec, Medical University of Silesia, Jedności 8, 41-200 Sosnowiec, Poland; mgorecki@sum.edu.pl (M.G.); annastojko@sum.edu.pl (A.R.-S.)
3. Department of Toxycology and Bioanalysis, Faculty of Pharmaceutical Sciences in Sosnowiec, Medical University of Silesia, Ostrogórska 30, 41-200 Sosnowiec, Poland; jstojko@sum.edu.pl
* Correspondence: akurekgorecka@interia.pl

Academic Editors: Raffaele Capasso and Lorenzo Di Cesare Mannelli
Received: 27 December 2019; Accepted: 26 January 2020; Published: 28 January 2020

Abstract: Honey, propolis, bee pollen, bee bread, royal jelly, beeswax and bee venom are natural products which have been used in medicine since ancient times. Nowadays, studies indicate that natural bee products can be used for skin treatment and care. Biological properties of these products are related to flavonoids they contain like: chrysin, apigenin, kaempferol, quercetin, galangin, pinocembrin or naringenin. Several pharmacological activities of phenolic acids and flavonoids, and also 10-hydroxy-*trans*-2-decenoic acid, which is present in royal jelly, have been reported. Royal jelly has multitude of pharmacological activities: antibiotic, antiinflammatory, antiallergenic, tonic and antiaging. Honey, propolis and pollen are used to heal burn wounds, and they possess numerous functional properties such as: antibacterial, anti-inflammatory, antioxidant, disinfectant, antifungal and antiviral. Beeswax is used for production of cosmetics and ointments in pharmacy. Due to a large number of biological activities, bee products could be considered as important ingredients in medicines and cosmetics applied to skin.

Keywords: bee products; flavonoids, phenolic acids; skin care; therapeutic properties

1. Introduction

Nowadays, alternative medicine, which employs natural biologically active substances obtained from bee products, is getting more and more attention. Bee products have been used not only in treatment, but also for skin care as ingredients of cosmetics. The effect of bee products on the skin has also been proved by numerous studies, and the use of honey, propolis, bee pollen and bee venom in wound healing highlights their curative value [1–4]. Each bee product possesses specific active substances which determine its use for various skin problems. Honey, propolis, bee pollen, bee bread, beeswax and bee venom are the bee products which are used for medicinal purposes and cosmetic production.

Honey is a natural product which is made by bees from nectar and honeydew. Honey is a supersaturated solution of carbohydrates with numerous properties and wide use. Propolis, also called bee glue, is a resinous substance collected by bees from buds of trees, shrubs, and green plants. Both, propolis and honey were used in antiquity for embalming bodies, whereas folk medicine used honey for wound healing and pain relief [5]. Bee pollen is collected from plants and transported to the hive in form of pollen loads. The formation of loads involves moisturizing pollen with nectar or honey. Pollen for winter supplies, which is deposited in the honeycomb cells, undergoes lactic fermentation and produces bee bread. Bee bread and bee pollen are bactericidal and bacteriostatic agents [6,7]. Beeswax is a substance produced by glands located in the bee abdomen. Wax obtained from honeycombs constitutes a valuable ingredient used in cosmetology and pharmacy. Bee venom also called apitoxin produced by honeybee. It consists a complex mixture of different peptides and mast cell degranulating peptide, which therapeutic and cosmetic properties are used in many areas [8].

2. Selected Compounds of Bee Products

The chemical composition of bee products is quite diversified, and depends on the botanical composition, geographical origin, time of collection and environmental conditions [9–11]. However, each product made by bees has a specified composition and content of biologically active substances, which give specific properties to each bee product. The chemical composition determines the curative and properties of these products.

Honey contains at least 181 ingredients [12]. Honey is a supersaturated carbohydrates solution containing mainly glucose and fructose [13]. Moreover, honey can have in its composition of sucrose, rhamnose, trehalose, nigerobiose, isomaltose, maltose, maltotetraose, maltotriose, maltulose, melezitose, melibiose, nigerose, palatinose, raffinose, and erlose [14,15]. It also contains enzymes, namely, glucose oxidase, amylase, catalase, peroxidase, invertase, and lysozyme. Glucose oxidase produces hydrogen peroxide which is one of responsible substances for the bactericidal activity of honey [16]. Honey contains also organic acids: gluconic acid, citric acid, malic acid, lactic acid, succinic acid, oxalic acid, tartaric acid, formic acid, acetic acid, benzoic acid, and pyromucic acid. The acids originate from bee bodies and enzymatic conversions which occur during honey production. The content of these acids is higher in mature honeys. Phenolic acids and flavonoids, which are responsible for many biological properties and have antioxidative activity, are also important ingredients of honey. The group of phenolic acids includes derivatives of hydroxycinnamic acid and hydroxybenzoic acid. The derivatives of hydroxycinnamic acid are *p*-coumaric acid, caffeic acid, ferulic acid, and sinapic acid. Whereas, the derivatives of hydroxybenzoic acid include *p*-hydroxybenzoic, vanillic, syringic, salicylic and gallic acids and ellagic acid as a dimer of gallic acid [15]. In honey, flavonoids are represented by naringenin, hesperetin, pinocembrin, chrysin, galangin, quercetin and kaempferol. However, a significant decrease in the concentration of galangin, kaempherol, and myricetin is observed after honey has been heated, while pasteurization causes a substantial decrease in myricetin concentration [17]. Honey contains also essential oils, whose composition includes terpenes (thymol, bisabolol, farnesol, and cineol). Other components of honey comprise water, amino acids and proteins. Proline (50–80%) dominates among amino acids, and its increased presence indicates honey maturity [14]. Vitamins constitute a small group of compounds present in honey, and they are mainly: thiamine, riboflavin, pyridoxine, *p*-aminobenzoic acid, folic acid, pantothenic acid, and vitamins A, C, E. Honey contains also minerals: phosphorus, potassium, calcium, magnesium, sulfur, iron, copper, manganese, and zinc. Although there is only a small amount of trace-elements in honey, they are highly bioavailable. It was reported that copper, calcium, zinc, iron, manganese and magnesium from honey are characterized a bioavailability of 80–90% [18].

In terms of chemical composition, propolis is a very diverse product. At present, at least 300 active compounds have been identified in it [19]. Phenolic acids (caffeic, ferulic, chlorogenic, *p*-coumaric), benzoic acid, cinnamic acid and flavonoids are the most important biologically active compounds. Among flavonoids, we can enumerate chrysin, luteolin, apigenin, galangin, kaempherol, quercetin, pinostrobin, pinocembrin, and terpene compounds, whose content is 0.5% (bisabolol), and alcohols (cetyl, myricyl, mannitol and inositol) [20–22]. Propolis contains also minerals (calcium, magnesium, manganese, zinc, copper, iron, cobalt and selenium), vitamins (B1, B2, B6, C and E) and enzymes (succinate dehydrogenase, glucose-6-phosphatase, adenosine triphosphatase, acid phosphatase) [22,23].

Bee pollen comprises at least 200 biologically active substances. Proteins constitute about 22.7% of bee pollen composition, including 10.4% essential amino acids: methionine, lysine, threonine, histidine, leucine, isoleucine, valine, phenylalanine, tryptophan. Digestible carbohydrates constitute 30.8%, while the percentage of reducing sugars is 25.7%. Among the fatty acids present in bee pollen, we can list acids such as gamma-linolenic acid, arachidonic acid, and linoleic acid (0.4%). Additionally, nucleic acids and nucleosides are valuable components of bee pollen [2,24]. It contains also vitamins (B1, B2, B3, B5, B6, C, H, E) and minerals (potassium, calcium, phosphorus, iron, zinc, copper, manganese) [9].

Protein content in bee bread is 12% lower than its content in bee pollen. The content of reducing sugars increases by 40–50%, whereas the content of lactic acid rises to 3.1%. Bee bread contains vitamin K and enzymes which cannot be found in bee pollen [25,26]. Bee bread is also a good source of phenolic components. Among bee bread from different parts of the Baltic Region the *p*-coumaric acid, ferulic acid, caffeic acid, kaempherol, isorhamnetin, naringenin and quercetin were identified [27].

Royal jelly contains peptides: jelleines I, II, III, IV, proteins, carbohydrates, lipids, vitamins and minerals [28]. Among proteins we can list royalisin and enzymes: amylase, invertase, catalase, acid phosphatase, and lysozyme. Proteins of royal jelly are rich in exogenous amino acids. The carbohydrates in royal jelly are mainly monosaccharides: fructose, glucose and oligosaccharides. Lipids play an important role in royal jelly composition [29]. 10-hydroxy-*trans*-2-decenoic acid, 3-hydroxydodecanoic acid, and 11-oxododecanoic acid can be included into the most valuable ones [28]. 10-hydroxy-*trans*-2-decenoic acid (10H2DA) is the main and specific lipid component of this product. 10H2DA is used as a marker to validate the quality of royal jelly [28,30]. Royal jelly contains also volatile compounds such as phenol, guaiacol and methyl salicylate. In royal jelly, there are also present trace amounts of such bio-elements as potassium, sodium, magnesium, phosphorus, sulfur, calcium, zinc, iron, and copper. Royal jelly contains mainly vitamins from group B: thiamine, riboflavin, pyridoxine, pantothenic acid, nicotinic acid and biotin and it is also contains phenolic compounds: ferulic acid, quercetin, kaempherol, galangin and fisetin, pinocembrin, naringin and hesperidin, apigenin, acacetin, and chrysin [31,32].

Esters of acids and fatty alcohols are main constituents of beeswax and subsequent components, in respect of amount, are free fatty acids [33]. Among the latter, 10-hydroxy-*trans*-2-decenoic acid (10H2DA) exhibits antibacterial effect, which is important. Beeswax is composed of hydrocarbons and free fatty alcohols [34,35]. Free fatty alcohols such as triacontanol, octacosanol, hexacosanol, and tetracosanol are antioxidative and anti-inflammatory. Other substances are triterpenes, β-carotene, volatile compounds and phenolic compounds. Among flavonoids, the main role is played by chrysin, which relieves inflammation, has antimicrobial and regenerative effects. Sterols have a regenerative effect, whereas an antiseptic effect is provided by three components: 10-hydroxy-*trans*-2-decenoic acid, chrysin, and squalene [34,36].

Bee venom contains different peptides including melittin, apamine, adolapin, sekapin, prokamin and mast cell degranulating peptide [37]. Peptides are main components of bee venom. Among peptides especially melittin plays important role in inducing reactions associated with bee stings. Melittin induces membrane permeabilization and lyses cells. It possesses also biologically active amines like histamine, epinephrine, dopamine, norepinephrine and enzymes like phospholipase A2, hyaluronidase, acid phosphomonoesterase, lysophospholipase. Bee venom has another components than peptides including lipids, carbohydrates and free amino acids [8,38,39].

3. Bee Products as Raw Material for Medicines and Cosmetics Production

Honey in cosmetics is named "Honey" or "Mel" according to the International Nomenclature of Cosmetic Ingredient (INCI), it is an emollient or humectant, and exhibits moisturizing properties. Some cosmetics contain derivatives of honey, defined in the INCI as "Mel Extract" with moisturizing properties, "Hydrogenated Honey" which is humectant, and antistatic "Hydroxypropyltrimonium Honey". Hydroxypropyltrimonium honey is used in shampoos and hair conditioners. More often the concentration of honey in cosmetics is up to 10%. Higher concentrations (up to 70%) are obtained by dispersing in oils, gels or polymer entrapment [40].

Most frequently, propolis has a form of aqueous or ethanol extracts. According to the INCI nomenclature, in cosmetics we can find it under the following names: propolis and propolis extract. Ethanol extracts of propolis are most frequently used. To obtain them, propolis is extracted with 70%

ethanol, and then the extract is concentrated in reduced pressure conditions [41]. An aqueous extract of propolis is used in antifungal cosmetics, while propolis dissolved in fats is used to produce lipsticks.

Royal jelly can most frequently be found in cosmetics in a lyophilized form, and the higher percentage content of lyophilized royal jelly is, the less viscous cream becomes. However, royal jelly content does not affect emulsion stability. Preparations with a higher content of royal jelly are well absorbed, and do not leave greasy film. Creams with royal jelly have moisturizing properties especially in concentration of 0.5% and 1% [42].

In cosmetic manufacturing, bee pollen is used in a form of aqueous, lyophilized and lipid extracts. Active substances can be extracted with water, propylene glycols, glycerin and oils. Bee pollen extacts are used in cosmetic in concentrations 0.5–5% [43]. In natural cosmetics, dried grains of bee pollen—micronized and added to cosmetics—are also used.

Beeswax is used in cosmetics after honey has been removed from honeycombs, wax has been melted, and impurities have been separated. To do this, various types of wax extractors are used: solar, electric or steam ones. Yellow wax (*Cera flava*) or white wax (*Cera alba*) is used to produce cosmetics [34].

According to INCI, bee venom or apitoxin are defined as bee venom powder. It is yellow light powder obtained by collecting a large amount of bee venom by electric stunning with using a bee venom collector without harming the honey bee. Then bee venom has to be purified under strict laboratory conditions. In next step purified bee venom is diluted in water, centrifuged, lyophilized and refrigerated for use as cosmetic ingredient [44]. It is used as a cosmetic ingredients which possesses antiaging, anti-inflammatory and antibacterial, antifungal and antiviral effects. Bee venom is used to produce antiphotoaging and anti-acne products [8,44]. Bee venom is used in treatment psoriasis, atopic dermatitis and alopecia [39].

4. The Effect of Bee Products on the Skin

4.1. Honey

Honey is used in medicine including due to its antimicrobial effect, which results from the following factors: hydrogen peroxide, high osmotic pressure, high acidity, the presence of phenolic acids, flavonoids and lysozyme [45]. Honey inhibits the growth of bacteria and fungi by reducing their development on the skin surface. Honey is particularly suitable as a dressing for wounds and burns, and has also been included in treatments against pityriasis, tinea, seborrhea, dandruff, diaper dermatitis, psoriasis, hemorrhoids, and anal fissure [40]. Pinocembrin and lysozyme are responsible for antifungal properties. Lysozyme inhibits growth of yeast-like fungi [46]. The effect of honey on healing postsurgical wounds was documented [1]. Among 52 patients incisions on skin were covered with honey dressing. The aesthetic outcome after third and six months was rated. The width of the scars was smaller in compare to conventional dressing. After 5-day application of honey dressing, an analgesic effect was obtained and wound healing was accelerated in women after plastic surgeries. Honey induced extracellular Ca^{2+} entry results in wound healing. It is similar to role plays by Ca^{2+} signaling in tissue regeneration [47]. Moreover honey regulates the process of epithelial mesenchymal transition (EMT) and it has a positive impact on wound healing. The effect on EMT depends on the floral and origin of the honey [48]. Honey is the apitherapeutic agent in topical wounds treatment due to killing bacteria, ability to bacterial biofilm penetration, lowering wounds pH, Reducing pain and inflammation, promoting fibroblast migration and keratinocyte closure, promoting collagen deposition so honey has a potential role in the area of tissue engineering and regeneration. Honey should be considered to incorporate it to the biomaterial tissue templates for tissue regeneration. Honey was used in electrospun templates, cryogels or hydrogels [49]. The main problem of use honey in tissue engineering are: cytotoxicity of high concentrations of honey, the lack of prolonged release rates of the honey over time. So future research should focus on these aspects. Among different types of honey, a strong antibacterial effect was observed in manuka honey which contains larger amount of methylglyoxal than European honeys [50]. The antibiotic activity of manuka honey is estimated by

Unique Manuka Factor (UMF) and methylglyoxal (MGO) markers [46]. Due to an increased content of glucose oxidase, a higher level of hydrogen peroxide than in European honeys can be observed [51]. Hydrogen peroxide is responsible for produce free radicals, which cause oxidative damage to bacterial cell walls. The antimicrobial effect of honey from New Zealand is also evident in undiluted honeys and it is not abolished by catalases, which differentiates manuka honey from other types of honey. This type of honey is used in the treatment of various wounds, including burns. The inhibition value against *Staphylococcus aureus* FDA 209P of manuka honey in dilutions from 1:2 to 1:128 is determined in the range of 2.0–4.5 [50]. Manuka honey is used in medicine to heal burns, ulcers and wounds difficult to heal, and brings satisfactory results. Manuka honey also soothes gum inflammation, and inhibits the formation of dental plaque, fights thrush, and prevents periodontitis [52]. Another variety of honey with antibacterial activity is Revamil from The Netherlands. The antibiotic factor in Revamil is the peptide defensin-1 [46]. Bee defensin-1 permeabilizes bacteria and inhibits their RNA, DNA and protein synthesis [49]. However in other varieties of honey also the phenolic compounds are responsible for antibacterial effect.

Honey is a bee product with a high nutritional value and regenerative properties that is why it is used in skin care products. A high content of carbohydrates, the presence of fruit acids and trace elements are responsible for its nutritional and regenerative effects. Thanks to osmosis, microcirculation in the dermal tissue is stimulated, which results in its better nutrition and oxygenation. In this way, metabolic processes are also stimulated, which leads to eliminating harmful metabolites, and increasing regenerative processes. Additionally, honey has hygroscopic properties, absorbing metabolites, and causing detoxification of the dermal tissue. This results in an increase in the skin tension, improvement of its elasticity, revitalizing its color, and smoothing out wrinkles [52]. Fruit acids, as honey components, provide an exfoliating effect for dead skin cells. Honey can be used as peeling agent in a sugared form [53]. As a result, many valuable nutritional components, including vitamins, can diffuse through the skin more easily. Xerosis is relieved by fatty acids and mineral salts in honey. Honey soothes skin irritations, it is a good cosmetic for chapped lips, rough, cracked hands, and frost bites. Honey is used in balms and bath products because of its toning, relaxing, conditioning effects related to the high content of simple sugars, the presence of essential oils, and bioelements [53]. Due to the presence of flavonoids, honey can also play an important role in sun protection by preventing skin irritation [40].

4.2. Propolis

Propolis is widely used in medicine. Thanks to its antiseptic properties it is used in dermatology to treat staphylococcal, streptococcal and fungal infections. Purulent skin infections, hidradenitis, intertrigo, cheilosis, and thrush, among other things, are treated with propolis. As reported the Propol T, which is a propolis preparation, is highly effective in treatment of skin burns [54]. There are comparable therapeutic effects when propolis and sulfathiazole are used, however, bee glue is safer, and has fewer adverse effects. Propolis is not only antimicrobial and anti-inflammatory but also it increases cicatrization and reduces pain. Chrysin, which is a flavonoid, provides an analgesic effect. Propolis used to treat burn wounds in pigs increased fibrolast proliferation, activation and growth capacity. Propolis stimulates glycosaminoglycan accumulation what is needed for granulation, tissue growth and wound closure. Propolis as apitherapeutic agent is more effectively than silver sulfadiazine. Accumulation of collagen type I in matrix of an injury stimulates the repair process because collagen type I is indispensable for the keratinocyte migration and reepithelization. Moreover, propolis increased accumulation of collagen type III what accelerates healthy process. The usage of propolis ointment to treat burns as a topical apitherapeutic product could contribute to reepithelization [3]. Topically applied propolis decreased persistent inflammatory in diabetic wounds by normalizing neutrophil and neutrophil elastase. Caffeic acid is responsible for anti-inflammatory effect of propolis [55]. Genistein from propolis accelerated wound healing and stimulated wound angiogenesis in mice with diabetes type-1 [56]. Furthermore propolis may be effective in healing in different animal models including animals with burns and diabetic wounds [3,55,56]. Moreover propolis is highly effective in the treatment of *Acne vulgaris*. Researchers confirmed the limitation of occurrence of *Cutibacterium acnes*, i.e., a bacterium which plays a key role in acne vulgaris pathogenesis, after ethanol extract of propolis was applied to the skin [57]. The ethanol extract of propolis inhibits also *Staphylococcus epidermidis*. Propolis is used to manufacture cosmetics for the skin with acne, and to produce drugs against bacterial and fungal infections [58]. Propolis in the concentration of 5–20% has regenerative, repair effects and protects against external factors. It can be used to produce anti-bedsores preparations, since it firms the dermal tissue and protects it against pathogenic microbes [59]. Propolis protects also from ultraviolet radiation, since it can absorb UV light due to the presence of caffeic acid, coumaric acid, and ferulic acid. Propolis is a good additive to sun blockers (creams, lotions, sticks, and lipsticks) due to its properties of a natural filter, as well as antioxidative, anti-inflammatory and regenerative effects [60]. Other researchers showed that Romanian propolis had photoprotective effects against UVB after topical application to 30 Swiss mice [61]. Propolis is also used to produce protective lipsticks. It is regenerative and antiviral in cold sores caused by herpex simplex virus. Flavones and flavonols from propolis, especially galangin, kaempferol, quercetin, have a high antiviral activity against herpes simplex virus type 1 in vitro [62]. Nolkemper et al. observed that both, aqueous and ethanol extracts of propolis were strongly antiviral against herpes simplex type 2 (HSV-2) [63]. Skin care with products based on propolis is helpful against fungal problems of the skin due to the presence of flavonoids (pinocembrin and pinobanksin), phenolic acids (caffeic acid) and terpenes [59]. Pinocembrin isolated from propolis inhibits the mycelial growth of *Penicillium italicum* by interfering energy homeostasis and cell membrane damage of the pathogen [64]. Shampoos with bee glue can be a natural alternative in treatment of dandruff and prevention of its recurrence due to its antifungal and anti-seborrheic properties. Propolis has also been used for manufacturing toothpastes. Bee glue inhibits the formation of dental plaque and is antimicrobial, thereby it reduces dental caries development. Propolis ethanol extracts inhibit the growth of cariogenic bacteria, which include mainly *Staphylococcus mutant* and *Staphylococcus sobrinus*. Glucosyltransferase makes bacteria produce glucan they feed on, which is insoluble in water. Propolis eliminates cariogenic bacteria, inhibits the activity of glucosyltransferase, and reduces adherent abilities of bacteria [65]. The conducted studies showed that the use of toothpaste with propolis reduced dental plaque by 34.3% annually, whereas normal paste reduced the plaque by 31.9%. After two-year use of the paste with propolis a further reduction of plaque by 12.4% was observed, while normal paste managed to reduce it only by 5%. Rinsing the mouth with water with 0.5% propolis content complements the oral cavity care. After 21 days, this solution was able to reduce dental plaque by 18.1% [66]. Propolis smoothes out wrinkles and has antiaging properties. A huge role is played here by antioxidants such as phenolic compounds and flavonoids which neutralize an unfavorable effect of free radicals on the skin. Bee glue lightens and smoothens the skin, reduces signs of fatigue and moisturizes it [59].

4.3. Royal Jelly

Royal jelly has a broad spectrum of biological activities which determine the effect of royal jelly on the skin, namely, antibacterial, anti-inflammatory, immunomodulatory, anti-allergic, antioxidant, toning, moisturizing, and antiaging [67]. Royal jelly is a bee product with strong antimicrobial activity within skin tissue, which is already evident in 20% concentration. Due to its anti-inflammatory activity, royal jelly relieves periodontal diseases, inflammation of the oral cavity, tongue and throat. Anti-inflammatory activity and wound healing results from its ability to inhibit the production of pro-inflammatory cytokines (TNF-α, IL-6, IL-1). Royal jelly has a protective effect on blood vessels and relieves hemorrhoids, and varicose veins of the lower extremities. It is used to treat lichen, ulcers, burns, bed sores, shingles, in all cases where the regeneration of epidermis is expected, wound epithelialization, nutritional effect, healing and antimicrobial activity. The effect of 5% royal jelly on ulcers on the diabetic foot has been studied. The treatment lasted 3 months and involved dressing the wound with 5% sterile royal jelly 3 times a week. Among eight treated ulcers, seven were cured, and in one case an improvement was observed [68]. Royal jelly promotes wound reepithelization. The keratinocytes are responsible for the elevated production of MMP-9 (matrix metalloproteinase-9) after incubation with a water extract of royal jelly. After applying water extract of royal jelly increased keratinocyte migration and wound closure rates. The component of royal jelly responsible for stimulating MMP-9 production is defensin-1. Moreover defensin-1 promotes reepithelization and wound closure. Similarly as in honey, defensin-1 is responsible for cutaneous wound closure by enhancing keratinocyte and MMP-9 secretion [69]. Royal jelly is effective in the treatment of wounds, and is successfully used in cosmetics for problem skin care. Royal jelly is an ingredient of preparations normalizing sebum secretion, for seborrheic skin, acne-prone skin where frequently skin lesions and small wounds occur [31]. Due to stimulating metabolism in tissues, royal jelly improves regenerative processes of tissues. Regenerative, nutritional and healing properties are used in balms, creams, and lotions. Immunomodulatory and antiallergenic activities of royal jelly are related to the properties of fatty acids, isolated from it. Both, 10HDA and 3-10-dihydroxydecanoic acid modulate immune response and lower the concentration of IL-2 and IL-10. Anti-inflammatory and immunomodulatory activities of royal jelly were used to treat atopic dermatitis, hypertrophy, hyperkeratosis and epidermis and dermis inflammation, possibly through a blend of TNF-specific low adjustment of IFN-gamma specific production and high adjustment of nitric-oxide synthase (NOS) expression [70]. 10-hydroxy-*trans*-2-decenoic acid, which is present in royal jelly, stimulates fibroblast production of collagen by inducting the production of transforming growth factor. As a result, royal jelly affects the production of collagen, which is an important factor that supports the skin [28]. Royal jelly is highly moisturizing, and affects hydration of the stratum corneum by retaining water in it. In consequence, the skin become more elastic and better moisturized [42].

4.4. Bee Pollen

Bee pollen, another bee product, can also affect the skin. Bee pollen is a potent antifungal, antimicrobial, antiviral, anti-inflammatory, immunostimulating agent, and it also facilitates the granulation process of burn healing [71]. Pollen ethanol extract is antimicrobial against *Staphylococcus aureus, Escherichia coli, Klebsiella pneumoniae, Pseudomonas aeruginosa,* and has an antifungal activity against *Candida albicans.* Flavonoids and phenolic acids provide antifungal and antibacterial properties of bee pollen. Anti-inflammatory activity of bee pollen is due to inhibiting the activity of enzymes participating in the development of inflammation, i.e., cyclooxygenase II and lipoxygenase. Phenolic acids, fatty acids and phytosterols are responsible for anti-inflammatory characteristics. Additionally, kaempferol inhibits hyaluronidase and elastase, which suppresses inflammatory response. Besides, topical application of ointment with pollen extract to treat burns has been studied, since bee pollen can regenerate damaged tissues [2].

Bee pollen is an active ingredient in cosmetics, usually in the concentration of 0.5–5% [43]. Its significant effect on the skin tissue is due to a high content of flavonoids. Their presence allows bee pollen to strengthen and seal capillaries, which is also increased by high vitamin C content, and that is why bee pollen is used in creams for couperose skin. Bee pollen affects cell metabolism, boosts regeneration and stimulates mitotic division. Bee pollen is used to produce shampoos and conditioners. Its sebo-balancing activity, which involves reducing sebum secretion, is used in preparations for oily hair. Bee pollen normalizes the activity of sebaceous glands due to presence of zinc, methionine and phospholipids. Moreover, sulphur containing amino acids, mainly cysteine, present in bee pollen strengthen hair shaft. Bee pollen is also added to anti-dandruff shampoos, since it limits fungal growth and stops itching of the scalp, but it still has moisturizing, conditioning and regenerating properties. Other researchers inform that a good solution would be to mix ethyl esters of essential unsaturated fatty acids from flaxseeds with bee pollen. Essential fatty acids (EFA) would play the role of lipid fraction solvent. Preparations with omega-3 and omega-6 acids enriched with diverse properties of bee pollen could help in the care of atopic skin, sensitive skin, and the skin more vulnerable to scarring [43].

4.5. Beeswax

When compared to other bee products, beeswax has the smallest range of biological activities. Kędzia [34] wrote that beeswax was added to ointments, liniments and creams used in treatment of various dermatoses, e.g., boils, wounds, atopic dermatitis, psoriasis, diaper dermatitis caused by *Candida albicans*. Beeswax is mainly used as an emulsifying agent. In cosmetics, beeswax is used as a stiffener, a substance providing elasticity, plasticity and increasing skin adhesiveness. Beeswax is the base for lipsticks, sticks and creams [72]. Beeswax has lubricating, softening activities and reduces transepidermal water loss from skin. Sterols, which are also components of intercellular space, provide these characteristics of beeswax. Squalene, 10-hydroxy-*trans*-2-decenoic acid and flavonoids (chrysin) provide antiseptic properties to this product, and protect the skin against pathogenic microorganisms. Beeswax constitutes a protective barrier against many external factors by forming a film on the skin surface. β-carotene present in beeswax is a valuable source of vitamin A, into which it is converted. Vitamin A delays collagen degradation, stimulates mitotic division in the epidermis, thus leads to sooner regeneration of the skin after damage [34,36].

The main effects of flavonoids and phenolic acids present in above bee products on the skin are presented in Table 1.

Table 1. Main effects of selected flavonoids and phenolic acids on skin.

Group	Representative	Structure	Effect
Flavones	Chrysin		anti-inflammatory [73], antibacterial & antiviral [74], antioxidant [22]
	Apigenin		antiviral & antifungal [74], anti-allergic [75], antioxidant [22]
Flavonols	Galangin		antiviral [62], antifungal [76], antioxidant [22]
	Kaempferol		anti-inflammatory [77], antifungal & antiviral [74], antioxidant [22], UV photoprotective [78]
	Quercetin		anti-allergic [2], antiviral & antifungal [74], antibacterial [12], antioxidant [79], UV photoprotective [78], anti-inflammatory [77]

Table 1. Cont.

Group	Representative	Structure	Effect
Flavanones	Pinocembrin		antifungal [76], antioxidant [22]
	Naringenin		UV photoprotective [80], antioxidant [79], anti-inflammatory [77], antiviral [74]
Phenolic acids	p-Coumaric		antiviral [20], antibacterial [46]
	Caffeic		anti-inflammatory [55], antiviral [20], antibacterial [46], antifungal [59]
	Ferulic		antibacterial [46], photoprotective [60]

4.6. Bee Venom

Bee venom has been used in medicine in treatment but also as a cosmetic ingredient. Bee venom has a wide spectrum of biological activity. It exhibit antibacterial and anti-inflammatory effects so it can be used as a ingredient of anti-acne products. Bee venom shows inhibitory effects on *Cutibacterium acnes*. *Cutibacterium acnes* is the main factor inducing the inflammation in acne. An et al. [81] showed that topical application bee venom on mice skin, which previous obtained intradermally injected *Cutibacterium acnes* into ears, limited number of inflammatory cells and also reduced level of tumor necrosis factor (TNF)-α and interleukin IL-1β. Moreover, bee venom inhibited Toll like receptor (TLR2) and CD14 expression in tissue which has been injected *C. acnes*. These results indicate that bee venom can be used as anti-acne agent. Another researchers [82] also showed positive effects of cosmetics containing bee venom on acne vulgaris. Purified bee venom reduced number of *C. acnes* at concentration of 0.5 mg. Bee venom possesses bactericidal and bacteriostatic effects thanks to melittin [38]. It has a significant antibacterial effect against *Staphylococcus aureus*, *Staphylococcus epidermidis* and *Staphylococcus pyrogenes* [39,83]. Melittin is a toxic peptide that causes destruction of the bacterial cell wall [38]. Bee venom can be used in fungi and viral skin infections. The antifungal effect of bee venom against *Trichophyton mentagrophytes*, *Trichophyton rubrum*, *Candida albicans* and *Malassezia furfur* was proved [84–86]. Antiviral effect of bee venom on herpes simplex virus has been studied. Bee venom suppressed the replication this virus [87]. Moreover bee venom is a potential inhibitor of 5 α-reductase, which is responsible for converse testosterone into dihydrotestosterone and plays important role as hair growth promoter, what was confirmed in study on alopecia. Bee venom in different concentrations 0.001%, 0.005% and 0.01% was applied in compare 2% minoxidil. Researchers showed that bee venom promoted hair growth and inhibited transition from the anagen to catagen phase. Additionally bee venom inhibited the expression of SRD5A2 which encodes a 5-α-reductase [88]. Bee venom can play role as a new therapy in localized plaque psoriasis. Intradermal bee venom and intradermal bee venom combined with oral propolis constitute effective treatment of localized plaque psoriasis. Bee venom reduces level of IL-1β, TNF-α, and IL-6. Bee venom contains melittin, which blocks the expression of inflammatory genes. Additionally bee venom inhibits the COX-2 expression, so decrease production of prostaglandins which take part in inflammatory process [89]. Bee venom compounds possess various, sometime opposing immune-related effects. Some components of bee venom like apamin, histamine, mast cell degranulating (MCD) peptide and phospholipase A2 (PLA2) increase inflammatory response, while polypeptide adolapin inhibits prostaglandins synthesis and inhibit the activity of bee venom PLA2 and human lipoxygenase [90]. Anti-inflammatory effect of bee venom is used also in treatment atopic dermatitis. Patients who applied emollient with bee venom had lower eczema area, severity index and visual analogue scale value than patients who applied emollient without bee venom [84]. The biological activities of bee venom have been used in wounds healing. The mechanism of wound healing is associated with expressions of TGF-β1, fibronectin, vascular endothelial growth factor (VEGF) and collagen-I. The research, which was conducted in mice showed decreasing of wound size and increasing epithelial proliferation. Topical use of bee venom is effective especially in reducing size of wounds in animal model [83]. The bee venom is using in wound dressing combined with polyvinyl alcohol and chitosan. 4% bee venom in wound dressing in diabetic rats accelerated healing and limited inflammatory process [91]. Another study showed that 6% bee venom with chitosan supported wound healing [92]. Researchers indicated that bee venom stimulated human epidermal keratinocyte proliferation and migration. Bee venom joined with hydrogel increased collagen formation. Bee venom supports wound healing due to its anti-inflammatory, anti-microbial and also antioxidant activity. Effective action of bee venom is very important in human melanoma A2058 cells. Tu et al. exhibited that bee venom leads to apoptosis cell death by induction hydroxyl radicals [93]. Recently bee venom also has been used as antiwrinkle agent. As a cosmetic ingredient bee venom serum at a concentration of 0.006% was applied at amount 4 mL twice a day for 12 weeks among twenty-two women from South Korea. It caused decreasing total wrinkle area, total wrinkle count and wrinkle depth. Moreover bee venom possesses antimelanogenic activity by inhibiting tyrosinase-related proteins [94]. The study conducted by Han et al. [44] reported that bee venom exhibits photoprotective activity by reducing of the protein levels of matrix metalloproteinases. Bee venom effectively inhibits photoaging processes so it can be used for photodamaged skin. Gel containing 0.06% bee venom did not lead to photosensitive dermatitis what has been confirmed on animal model [8,44].

5. Allergic Adverse Effects of Bee Products

The use of bee products for cosmetic as well as medicine production can involve the occurrence of allergic reactions. An allergy to honey is seldom, and the most frequent allergen from honey that causes hypersensitivity reactions is bee pollen. Additionally, bee protein in honey can cause an allergy. Honey used to treat dermatoses undergoes thorough filtration to eliminate particles of bee pollen, which are the main cause of honey allergic reactions. Honey allergy is very rare but sometimes causes IgE-mediated hypersensitivity reaction [95]. In 2010 Basista conducted studies on beekeepers. None of them was hypersensitive to honey [96]. More than 26 allergenic substances were determined in propolis composition. Most frequently, an allergic reaction is caused by esters of caffeic acid and cinnamic acid derived from poplar buds. In hypersensitive people, they cause a contact allergic reaction. Due to the presence of these esters in other materials, cross allergic reaction can occur. The most potent alergens are: LB-1, i.e., the compound consisting of 3-methyl-2-butyl-caffeate (54.2%), 3-methyl-3-butyl-caffeate (28.3%), 2-methyl-2-butylcaffeate (4.3%), caffeic acid (1.3%), benzyl caffeate (1.0%), caffeic acid phenethyl ester (CAPE, 7.9%) and benzyl salicylate. An allergy to propolis is rare, and an allergic response was more frequently reported after topical application than an oral one. In the years 1989–2006, the World Health Organization registered only 26 notifications about side effects after the contact with bee glue, of which just six were considered certain, and the remaining ones were not fully credible. In healthy individuals, an allergy to propolis is rarely observed (0.64–1.3%), however, it occurs more frequently in people treated for allergies (1.2–6.7%). This hypersensitivity is manifested by atopic eczema after the application of ethanol extract of propolis [97]. Moreover, topical application of royal jelly in the form of ointments can cause skin rashes and eczemas [67]. Allergic and irritation reaction of bee venom have been associated with presence components likes: phospholipase A2, melittin, hyaluronidase. Phospholipase A2 is a major allergen which is responsible for inducing immuno-globulin E (IgE) [98]. Melittin causes cell lysis and fusion in addition to activation of phospholipase A2. Hyaluronidase is a next allergen in venom, which is responsible for changes in cell membranes. It caused spread of venom toxin through the gaps between cells. However, bee venom can be toxic when large amount of venom is inoculated into body [98]. However, Han et al. indicates that long term topically treatment with bee venom is safe what confimed their study [94].

6. Conclusions

Bee products constitute an important component of medicines and cosmetics. Honey is regenerative and antimicrobial due to its high osmolarity, the presence of hydrogen peroxide and lysozyme. Manuka honey thanks to the presence of methylglyoxal is a potent antiseptic agent. Propolis is a bee product rich in phenolic compounds, which determine antimicrobial, UV protective, analgesic, antioxidative and regenerative activities. Royal jelly is characterized by the presence of royalisin and jelleines peptides. It also contains 10-hydroxy-*trans*-2-decenoic acid which improves the production of collagen and is antiseptic. Bee pollen is rich in unsaturated fatty acids, vitamins, flavonoids and hydroxy acids. Beeswax plays the most important role as emulsifier of the cosmetic forms. Moreover, bee venom is an attractive and effective natural toxin rich in peptides. It plays an important role in treatment and care skin especially in photodamage, acne, atopic dermatitis, alopecia or psoriasis. Bee venom exhibits anti-inflammatory, antimicrobial, antifungal and antiviral action. Each of the bee products is characterized by the content of certain active substances, which differentiates one bee product from another, and causes that each of them is worth using for a different skin problem. The effect of bee products on the skin has been proved by numerous studies, whose results are satisfactory, and the use of these product in wound healing highlights their curative value. The advantage of medicines and cosmetics based on bee products is their effectiveness with minimal side effects. Table 2 summarizes skin diseases where the therapeutic application of bee products has been studied.

Table 2. The summary of the skin diseases where the therapeutic application of bee products has been studied.

Bee Product	Components	Effect	Disease	Reference
Honey	pinocembrin, lysozyme	antifungal	tinea	[13,46,64]
	methylglyoxal, defensin-1 peptide, lysozyme, glucose oxidase, phenolic acids	antibacterial	wounds, burns, ulcers	[13,16,45,46,50]
	fruits acids, sugars	exfoliating	wrinkles	[13]
	quercetin, naryngenin, kaempferol, chrysin	anti-inflammatory	wounds, gum inflammation	[49,52]
	carbohydrates, fruit acids, trace elements	regenerative	wounds	[40,49,52,53]
Propolis	chrysin	analgesic	wounds	[3]
	caffeic acid, quercetin	anti-inflammatory	wounds	[19,55]
	pinocembrin, galangin, caffeic acid	antibacterial	acne, wounds	[19,57,65,66]
	pinocembrin, pinobanksin, quercetin, kaempherol, caffeic acid, *p*-coumaric acid, terpenes,	antifungal	tinea, fungal infections	[19,59]
	galangin, kaempferol, quercetin	antiviral	infection of *Herpes simplex* virus	[62,63]
	caffeic acid, *p*-coumaric acid, ferulic acid, quercetin, kaempferol	photoprotective	photoaging	[60]
	phenolic acids, flavonoids	antiaging	wrinkles	[59]
	genistein	stimulates angiogenesis	diabetic wound	[56]

Table 2. *Cont.*

Bee Product	Components	Effect	Disease	Reference
Royal jelly	defensin-1 peptide, ferulic acid	antibacterial	wounds, diabetic foot ulcers, acne	[32,67,68]
	10-hydroxydecanoic acid, 3-10-dihydroxydecanoic acid, amino, gamma globulin	antiinflammatory	atopic dermatitis, wounds, hypertrophy, hyperkeratosis	[67]
	10-hydroxy-*trans*-2-decenoic acid, 10-hydroxydecanoic acid	antiaging	wrinkles	[67]
	10-hydroxydecanoic acid, 3-10-dihydroxydecanoic acid	immunomodulatory and antiallergenic	autoimmune and inflammatory diseases	[70]
Bee pollen	pinocembrin, apigenin, quercetin, kaempferol, ferulic acid, *p*-coumaric acid	antifungal	tinea	[2,24,43]
	kaempferol, phenolic acids	antimicrobial	burns	[2,6,24,43]
	phenolic acids, fatty acids, phytosterols, kaempferol, quercetin	antiinflammatory	atopic dermatitis, burns	[2,43]
	methionine, zinc, phospholipids	sebo-balancing	acne	[43]
Beeswax	squalene, 10-hydroxy-*trans*-2-decenoic acid, chrysin	antibacterial	wounds, atopic dermatitis, psoriasis	[34,36]
	sterols	reduce transepidermal water loss	atopic dermatitis	[34]
Bee venom	melittin	antimicrobial	wounds, acne	[39,81–83,92]
	melittin, apamin	antifungal	tinea	[84–86]
	melittin	antiviral	herpes simplex infections	[84–87]
	not reported	photoprotective, antimelanogenic	hiperpigmentation	[44,94]
	melittin, adolapin	antiinflammatory	plaque psoriasis, wounds, atopic dermatitis	[83,84,89,91,92]
	phospholipase A2	pigmentation effect	vitiligo	[39]
	not reported	promote hair growth	alopecia	[88]
	not reported	antiwrinkle	wrinkles	[44,94]

Author Contributions: A.K.-G. designed the review; coordinated and participated in the writing of all sections and wrote Abstract, Sections 1–3, Sections 4.1, 4.6 and 6 and collaborated in the creation of Table 1; M.G. wrote Section 4.3 and created Tables 1 and 2 and collaborated in the writing of Section 4.2; A.R.-S. wrote Section 4.2 and collaborated in the writing of Section 5; R.B. wrote Sections 4.4 and 4.5; J.S. wrote the Section 5. All authors were involved in the editing process. All authors have read and agreed to the published version of the manuscript.

Funding: This work was funded by medical University of Silesia, Katowice, Poland grant number KNW-1-163/N/9/O.

Acknowledgments: The authors thanks to medical University of Silesia, Katowice, Poland and Silesian Academy of Medical Sciences in Katowice for their financial support.

Conflicts of Interest: The authors declare no conflict of interest.

References

1. Goharshenasan, P.; Amini, S.; Atria, A.; Abtahi, H.; Khorasani, G. Topical application of honey on surgical wounds: A randomized clinical trial. *Compl. Med. Res.* **2016**, *23*, 12–15. [CrossRef] [PubMed]
2. Komosińska-Vassev, K.; Olczyk, P.; Kaźmierczak, J.; Mencner, L.; Olczyk, K. Bee pollen: Chemical composition and therapeutic application. *Evid. Based Compl. Altern. Med.* **2015**, *2015*. [CrossRef] [PubMed]
3. Olczyk, P.; Wisowski, G.; Komosińska-Vassev, K.; Stojko, J.; Klimek, K.; Olczyk, M.; Koźma, E.M. Propolis modifies collagen types I and III accumulation in the matrix of burnt tissue. *Evid. Based Compl. Altern. Med.* **2013**, *2013*. [CrossRef] [PubMed]

4. Hozzein, W.; Badr, G.; Al-Ghamdi, A.; Sayed, A.; Al-Waili, N.; Garraud, O. Topical application of propolis enhances cutaneous wound healing by promoting TGF-beta/smad-mediated collagen production in a streptozotocin-induced type I diabetic mouse model. *Cell. Physiol. Biochem.* **2015**, *37*, 940–954. [CrossRef] [PubMed]
5. El-Soud, A.; Helmy, N. Honey between traditional uses and recent medicine. *Macedon. J. Med. Sci.* **2012**, *5*, 205–214. [CrossRef]
6. Abouda, Z.; Zerdani, I.; Kalalou, I.; Faid, M.; Ahami, M.T. The antibacterial activity of Moroccan bee bread and bee pollen (fresh and dried) against pathogenic bacteria. *Res. J. Microbiol.* **2011**, *6*, 376–384. [CrossRef]
7. Cornara, L.; Biagi, M.; Xiao, J.; Burlando, B. Therapeutic properties of bioactive compounds from different honeybee products. *Frontiers Pharmacol.* **2017**, *8*, 412. [CrossRef]
8. Han, S.M.; Lee, G.G.; Park, K.K. Skin sensitization study of bee venom (*Apis mellifera* L.) in guinea pigs. *Toxicol. Res.* **2012**, *28*, 1–4. [CrossRef]
9. Campos, M.G.; Bogdanov, S.; de Almeida-Muradian, L.B.; Szczesna, T.; Mancebo, Y.; Frigerio, C.; Ferreira, F. Pollen composition and standardisation of analytical methods. *J. Apic. Res.* **2008**, *47*, 156–161. [CrossRef]
10. Ciucure, C.T.; Geană, E.I. Phenolic compounds profile and biochemical properties of honeys in relationship to the honey floral sources. *Phytochem. Anal.* **2019**, *30*, 481–492. [CrossRef]
11. Ciulu, M.; Spano, N.; Pilo, M.I.; Sanna, G. Recent advances in the analysis of phenolic compounds in unifloral honeys. *Molecules* **2016**, *21*, 451. [CrossRef] [PubMed]
12. Viuda-Martos, M.; Ruiz-Navajas, Y.; Fernández-López, J.; Pérez-Álvarez, J.A. Functional properties of honey, propolis, and royal jelly. *J. Food Sci.* **2008**, *73*, 117–124. [CrossRef] [PubMed]
13. Ball, D.W. The chemical composition of honey. *J. Chem. Educ.* **2007**, *84*, 1643. [CrossRef]
14. Borawska, M.; Arciuch, L.; Puścion-Jakubik, A.; Lewoc, D. Content of sugars (fructose, glucose, sucrose) and proline in different varieties of natural bee honey. *Probl. Hig. Epidemiol.* **2015**, *96*, 816–820.
15. Da Silva, P.M.; Gauche, C.; Gonzaga, L.V.; Costa, A.C.O.; Fett, R. Honey: Chemical composition, stability and authenticity. *Food Chem.* **2016**, *196*, 309–323. [CrossRef] [PubMed]
16. Sak-Bosnar, M.; Sakač, N. Direct potentiometric determination of diastase activity in honey. *Food Chem.* **2012**, *135*, 827–831. [CrossRef]
17. Truchado, P.; Ferreres, F.; Bortolotti, L.; Sabatini, A.G.; Tomás-Barberán, F.A. Nectar flavonol rhamnosides are floral markers of acacia (*Robinia pseudacacia*) honey. *J. Agric. Food Chem.* **2008**, *56*, 8815–8824. [CrossRef]
18. Stecka, H.; Gręda, K.; Pohl, P. Total content and the bioavailable fraction of calcium, cooper, iron, magnesium, manganese and zinc in polish commercial bee honeys. *Bromatol. Chem. Toksykol.* **2012**, *45*, 111–116.
19. De Castro, S.L. Propolis: Biological and pharmacological activities. Therapeutic uses of this bee-product. *ARBS Ann. Rev. Biomed. Sci.* **2001**, *3*, 49–83. [CrossRef]
20. Schnitzler, P.; Neuner, A.; Nolkemper, S.; Zundel, C.; Nowack, H.; Sensch, K.H.; Reichling, J. Antiviral activity and mode of action of propolis extracts and selected compounds. *Phytother. Res.* **2010**, *24*, 20–28. [CrossRef]
21. Kurek-Górecka, A.; Rzepecka-Stojko, A.; Górecki, M.; Stojko, J.; Sosada, M.; Świerczek-Zięba, G. Structure and antioxidant activity of polyphenols derived from propolis. *Molecules* **2013**, *19*, 78–101. [CrossRef] [PubMed]
22. Olczyk, P.; Komosińska-Vassev, K.; Ramos, P.; Mencner, L.; Olczyk, K.; Pilawa, B. Free radical scavenging activity of drops and spray containing propolis—An EPR examination. *Molecules* **2017**, *22*, 128. [CrossRef] [PubMed]
23. Mărghitaş, L.A.; Dezmirean, D.S.; Bobiş, O. Important developments in Romanian propolis research. *Evid. Based Compl. Altern. Med.* **2013**. [CrossRef] [PubMed]
24. Feás, X.; Vázquez-Tato, M.P.; Estevinho, L.; Seijas, J.A.; Iglesias, A. Organic bee pollen: Botanical origin, nutritional value, bioactive compounds, antioxidant activity and microbiological quality. *Molecules* **2012**, *17*, 8359–8377. [CrossRef]
25. DeGrandi-Hoffman, G.; Eckholm, B.J.; Huang, M. A comparison of bee bread made by Africanized and European honey bees (*Apis mellifera*) and its effects on hemolymph protein titers. *Apidologie* **2013**, *44*, 52–63. [CrossRef]
26. Urcan, A.C.; Criste, A.D.; Dezmirean, D.S.; Mărgăoan, R.; Caeiro, A.; Campos, M.G. Similarity of data from bee bread with the same taxa collected in India and Romania. *Molecules* **2018**, *23*, 2491. [CrossRef]
27. Isidorov, V.A.; Isidorova, A.G.; Sczczepaniak, L.; Czyżewska, U. Gas chromatographic–mass spectrometric investigation of the chemical composition of beebread. *Food Chem.* **2009**, *115*, 1056–1063. [CrossRef]

28. Sugiyama, T.; Takahashi, K.; Mori, H. Royal jelly acid, 10-hydroxy-*trans*-2-decenoic acid, as a modulator of the innate immune responses. *Endocr. Metabol. Immun. Disord.-Drug Targets* **2012**, *12*, 368–376. [CrossRef]
29. Koya-Miyata, S.; Okamoto, I.; Ushio, S.; Iwaki, K.; Ikeda, M.; Kurimoto, M. Identification of a collagen production-promoting factor from an extract of royal jelly and its possible mechanism. *Biosci. Biotech. Biochem.* **2004**, *68*, 767–773. [CrossRef]
30. Antinelli, J.F.; Zeggane, S.; Davico, R.; Rognone, C.; Faucon, J.P.; Lizzani, L. Evaluation of (E)-10-hydroxydec-2-enoic acid as a freshness parameter for royal jelly. *Food Chem.* **2003**, *80*, 85–89. [CrossRef]
31. Bartosiuk, E.; Borawska, M.H. Royall jelly—Application in cosmetics. *Pol. J. Cosmetol.* **2013**, *16*, 80–84.
32. Ramadan, M.F.; Al-Ghamdi, A. Bioactive compounds and health-promoting properties of royal jelly: A review. *J. Funct. Foods.* **2012**, *4*, 39–52. [CrossRef]
33. Fratini, F.; Cilia, G.; Turchi, B.; Felicioli, A. Beeswax: A minireview of its antimicrobial activity and its application in medicine. *Asian Pacif. J. Tropic. Med.* **2016**, *9*, 839–843. [CrossRef] [PubMed]
34. Kędzia, B.; Hołderna-Kędzia, E. The use of beeswax in medicine. *Pasieka* **2014**, *3*. Available online: https://pasieka24.pl/index.php/pl-pl/pasieka-czasopismo-dla-pszczelarzy/108-pasieka-3-2014/1319-wykorzystanie-wosku-pszczelego-w-lecznictwie (accessed on 12 July 2019).
35. Waś, E.; Szczęsna, T.; Rybak-Chmielewska, H. Hydrocarbon composition of beeswax (*Apis mellifera*) collected from light and dark coloured combs. *J. Apic. Sci.* **2014**, *2*, 99–106. [CrossRef]
36. Buchwald, R.; Breed, M.D.; Bjostad, L.; Hibbard, B.E.; Greenberg, A.R. The role of fatty acids in the mechanical properties of beeswax. *Apidologie* **2009**, *4*, 585–594. [CrossRef]
37. Son, D.J.; Lee, J.W.; Lee, Y.H.; Song, H.S.; Lee, C.K.; Hong, J.T. Therapeutic application of anti-arthritis, pain-releasing, and anti-cancer effects of bee venom and its constituent compounds. *Pharmacol. Ther.* **2007**, *115*, 246–270. [CrossRef]
38. Pałgan, K.; Bartuzi, Z. Biological properties of bee venom. *Alerg. Astma Immun.* **2009**, *14*, 17–19.
39. Kim, H.; Park, S.-Y.; Lee, G. Potential therapeutic applications of bee venom on skin disease and its mechanisms: A literature review. *Toxins* **2019**, *11*, 374. [CrossRef]
40. Burlando, B.; Cornara, L. Honey in dermatology and skin care: A review. *J. Cosm. Dermatol.* **2013**, *12*, 306–313. [CrossRef]
41. Kurek-Górecka, A.M.; Sobczak, A.; Rzepecka-Stojko, A.; Górecki, M.T.; Wardas, M.; Pawłowska-Góral, K. Antioxidant activity of ethanolic fractions of Polish propolis. *Z. Naturforsch. C* **2012**, *67*, 545–550. [CrossRef] [PubMed]
42. Bocho-Janiszewska, A.; Sikora, A.; Rajewski, J.; Łobodzin, P. Application of royall jelly in moisturizing creams. *Pol. J. Cosmetol.* **2013**, *16*, 314–320.
43. Basista, K.; Sodzawiczny, K. Bee pollen—A new natural material, possibilities of use in medicine and cosmetology. *Gazeta Farmaceutyczna* **2011**, *12*, 30–32.
44. Han, S.M.; Hong, I.P.; Woo, S.O.; Kim, S.G.; Jang, H.R.; Park, K.K. Evaluation of the skin phototoxicity and photosensitivity of honeybee venom. *J. Cosmet. Dermatol.* **2017**, *16*, 68–75. [CrossRef] [PubMed]
45. Bogdanov, S. Nature and origin of the antibacterial substances in honey. *LWT-Food Sci. Technol.* **1997**, *30*, 748–753. [CrossRef]
46. Kędzia, B.; Hołderna-Kędzia, E. Contemporary opinions on the mechanism of antimicrobial action of honey. *Postep. Fitoter.* **2017**, *4*, 290–297. [CrossRef]
47. Martinotti, S.; Laforenza, U.; Patrone, M.; Moccia, F.; Ranzato, E. Honey-Mediated Wound Healing: H_2O_2 Entry through AQP3 Determines Extracellular Ca^{2+} Influx. *Int. J. Mol. Sci.* **2019**, *20*, 764. [CrossRef]
48. Nordin, A.; Sainik, N.Q.A.V.; Zulfarina, M.S.; Naina-Mohamed, I.; Saim, A.; Idrus, R.B.H. Honey epithelial to mesenchymal transition in wound healing: An evidence-based review. *Wound Med.* **2017**, *18*, 8–20. [CrossRef]
49. Minden-Birkenmaier, B.A.; Bowlin, G.L. Honey-based templates in wound healing and tissue engineering. *Bioengineering* **2018**, *5*, 46. [CrossRef]
50. Hołderna-Kędzia, E.; Ostrowski-Maissner, H.; Kędzia, B. Estimation of anibiotic activity of New Zeland manuka honey by the method of serial dilutions in liquid medium. *Postep. Fitoter.* **2008**, *2*, 70–75.
51. Allen, K.L.; Molan, P.C.; Reid, G.M. A survey of the antibacterial activity of some New Zealand honeys. *J. Pharm. Pharmacol.* **1991**, *43*, 817–822. [CrossRef] [PubMed]

52. Marwicka, J.; Gałuszka, R.; Gałuszka, G.; Podolska, A.; Żurawski, Ł.; Niemyska, K. Analysis of bee honey properties and its use in dietetics and cosmetology. *Kosmetologia Estetyczna* **2014**, *2*, 107–110.
53. Majewska, K.; Zaprutko, L. Honey—Natural product with many properties. *Kosmet. Kosmetol.* **2010**, *5–6*, 8–12.
54. Olczyk, P.; Komosińska-Vassev, K.; Winsz-Szczotka, K.; Stojko, J.; Klimek, K.; Gajewski, K.; Olczyk, K. The evaluation of chosen extracellular matrix enzymes activity during regeneration of experimental thermal injuries. *Leczenie Ran* **2014**, *11*, 97–101. [CrossRef]
55. Al-Waili, N.; Hozzein, W.N.; Badr, G.; Al-Ghamdi, H.; Al-Waili, H.; Salom, K.; Al-Waili, T. Propolis and bee venom in diabetic wounds; a potential approach that warrants clinical investigation. *Afr. J. Tradit. Complement. Altern. Med.* **2015**, *12*, 1–11. [CrossRef]
56. Tie, L.; An, Y.; Han, J.; Xiao, Y.; Xiaokaiti, Y.; Fan, S.; Liu, S.; Chen, A.F.; Li, X. Genistein accelerates refractory wound healing by suppressing superoxide and FoxO1/iNOS pathway in type 1 diabetes. *J. Nutr. Biochem.* **2013**, *24*, 88–96. [CrossRef]
57. Ali, B.M.M.; Ghoname, N.F.; Hodeib, A.A.; Elbadawy, M.A. Significance of topical propolis in the treatment of facial acne vulgaris. *Egypt J. Dermatol. Venerol.* **2015**, *35*, 29–36. [CrossRef]
58. Bankova, V. Recent trends and important developments in propolis research. *Evid. Based Complement. Altern. Med.* **2005**, *2*, 29–32. [CrossRef]
59. Sawicka, D.; Borawska, M.H. The use of propolis in skin diseases. *Derm. Estet.* **2013**, *1*, 13–17.
60. Nisakorn, S. Natural products as photoprotection. *J. Cosmet. Dermatol.* **2015**, *14*, 47–63. [CrossRef]
61. Bolfa, P.; Vidrighinescu, R.; Petruta, A.; Dezmirean, D.; Stan, L.; Vlase, L.; Damian, G.; Catoi, C.; Filip, A.; Clichici, S. Photoprotective effects of Romanian propolis on skin of mice exposed to UVB irradiation. *Food Chem. Toxicol.* **2013**, *62*, 329–342. [CrossRef] [PubMed]
62. Amoros, M.; Simõs, C.M.O.; Girre, L.; Sauvager, F.; Cormier, M. Synergistic effect of flavones and flavonols against herpes simplex virus type 1 in cell culture. Comparison with the antiviral activity of propolis. *J. Nat. Prod.* **1992**, *55*, 1732–1740. [CrossRef] [PubMed]
63. Nolkemper, S.; Reichling, J.; Sensch, K.H.; Schnitzler, P. Mechanism of herpes simplex virus type 2 suppression by propolis extracts. *Phytomedicine* **2010**, *17*, 132–138. [CrossRef] [PubMed]
64. Peng, L.; Yang, S.; Cheng, Y.J.; Chen, F.; Pan, S.; Fan, G. Antifungal activity and action mode of pinocembrin frompropolis against *Penicillium italicum*. *Food Sci. Biotechnol.* **2012**, *21*, 1533–1539. [CrossRef]
65. Koo, H.; Rosalen, P.L.; Cury, J.A.; Park, Y.K.; Bowen, W.H. Effects of compounds found in propolis on Streptococcus mutans growth and on glucosyltransferase activity. *Antimicrob. Agents Chemother.* **2002**, *46*, 1302–1309. [CrossRef]
66. Kędzia, B. Propolis in the treatment of dental caries. *Postęp. Fitoter.* **2011**, *2*, 113–121.
67. Pavel, C.I.; Mărghitaş, L.A.; Bobiş, O.; Dezmirean, D.S.; Şapcaliu, A.; Radoi, I.; Mădaş, M.N. Biological activities of royal jelly—Review. *Sci. Pap. Anim. Sci. Biotechnol.* **2011**, *44*, 108–118.
68. Siavash, M.; Shokri, S.; Haghighi, S.; Mohammadi, M.; Shahtalebi, M.A.; Farajzadehgan, Z. The efficacy of topical royal jelly on diabetic foot ulcers healing: A case series. *J. Res. Med. Sci.* **2011**, *16*, 904–909.
69. Bucekova, M.; Sojka, M.; Valachova, I.; Martinotti, S.; Ranzato, E.; Szep, Z.; Majtan, V.; Klaudiny, J.; Majtan, J. Bee-derived antibacterial peptide, defensin 1, promotes wound re-epithelialisation in vitro and in vivo. *Sci. Rep.* **2017**, *7*, 7340. [CrossRef]
70. Taniguchi, Y.; Kohno, K.; Inoue, S.I.; Koya-Miyata, S.; Okamoto, I.; Arai, N.; Iwaki, K.; Ikeda, M.; Kurimoto, M. Oral administration of royal jelly inhibits the development of atopic dermatitis-like skin lesions in NC/Nga mice. *Intern. Immunopharmacol.* **2003**, *3*, 1313–1324. [CrossRef]
71. Kroyer, G.; Hegedus, N. Evaluation of bioactive properties of pollen extracts as functional dietary food supplement. *Innov. Food Sci. Emerg. Technol.* **2001**, *2*, 171–174. [CrossRef]
72. Kasparaviciene, G.; Savickas, A.; Kalveniene, Z.; Velziene, S.; Kubiliene, L.; Bernatoniene, J. Evaluation of beeswax influence on physical properties of lipstick using instrumental and sensory methods. *Evid. Based Compl. Altern. Med.* **2016**. [CrossRef] [PubMed]
73. Ahad, A.; Ganai, A.A.; Mujeeb, M.; Siddiqui, W.A. Chrysin, an anti-inflammatory molecule, abrogates renal dysfunction in type 2 diabetic rats. *Toxicol. Appl. Pharmacol.* **2014**, *279*, 1–7. [CrossRef] [PubMed]
74. Narayana, K.R.; Reddy, M.S.; Chaluvadi, M.R.; Krishna, D.R. Bioflavonoids classification, pharmacological, biochemical effects and therapeutic potential. *Indian J. Pharmacol.* **2001**, *33*, 2–16.
75. Majewska, M.; Czeczot, H. Flavonoids in prevention and therapy. *Farmakol. Pol.* **2009**, *65*, 369–377.

76. Agüero, M.B.; Gonzalez, M.; Lima, B.; Svetaz, L.; Sánchez, M.; Zacchino, S.; Feresin, G.E.; Schmeda-Hirschmann, G.; Palermo, J.; Wunderlin, D.; et al. Argentinean propolis from *Zuccagnia punctata* Cav.(Caesalpinieae) exudates: Phytochemical characterization and antifungal activity. *J. Agric. Food Chem.* **2009**, *58*, 194–201. [CrossRef]
77. Hämäläinen, M.; Nieminen, R.; Vuorela, P.; Heinonen, M.; Moilanen, E. Anti-inflammatory effects of flavonoids: Genistein, kaempferol, quercetin, and daidzein inhibit STAT-1 and NF-κB activations, whereas flavone, isorhamnetin, naringenin, and pelargonidin inhibit only NF-κB activation along with their inhibitory effect on iNOS expression and NO production in activated macrophages. *Mediat. Inflamm.* **2007**, *2007*, 2007. [CrossRef]
78. Saric, S.; Sivamani, R.K. Polyphenols and sunburn. *Int. J. Mol. Sci.* **2016**, *17*, 1521. [CrossRef]
79. Burda, S.; Oleszek, W. Antioxidant and antiradical activities of flavonoids. *J. Agric. Food Chem.* **2001**, *49*, 2774–2779. [CrossRef]
80. Fernández-García, E. Photoprotection of human dermal fibroblasts against ultraviolet light by antioxidant combinations present in tomato. *Food Funct.* **2014**, *5*, 285–290. [CrossRef]
81. An, H.J.; Lee, W.R.; Kim, K.H.; Lee, S.J.; Han, S.M.; Lee, K.G.; Lee, C.K.; Park, K.K. Inhibitory effects of bee venom on Cutibacterium acnes-induced inflammatory skin disease in an animal model. *Int. J. Mol. Med.* **2014**, *34*, 1341–1348. [CrossRef] [PubMed]
82. Han, S.M.; Lee, K.G.; Pak, S.C. Effects of cosmetics conatining purified honeybee (*Apis mellifera* L.) venom on acne vulgaris. *J. Integr. Med.* **2013**, *11*, 320–326. [CrossRef] [PubMed]
83. Han, S.M.; Lee, K.; Yeo, J.; Baek, H.; Park, K. Antibacterial and anti-inflammatory effects of honeybee (*Apis mellifera*) venom against acne-inducing bacteria. *J. Med. Plants Res.* **2010**, *4*, 459–464.
84. You, C.E.; Moon, S.H.; Lee, K.H.; Kim, K.H.; Park, C.W.; Seo, S.J.; Cho, S.H. Effects of emollient containing bee venom on atopic dermatitis: A double-blinded, randomized, base-controlled, multicenter study of 136 patients. *Ann. Dermatol.* **2016**, *28*, 593–599. [CrossRef] [PubMed]
85. Park, C.; Lee, D.G. Melittin induces apoptotic features in candida albicans. *Biochem. Biophys. Res. Commun.* **2010**, *394*, 170–172. [CrossRef]
86. Prakash, S.; Bhargava, H. Apis cerana bee venom: It's antidiabetic and anti-dandru activity against malassezia furfur. *World Appl. Sci. J.* **2014**, *32*, 343–348.
87. Uddin, M.B.; Lee, B.H.; Nikapitiya, C.; Kim, J.H.; Kim, T.H.; Lee, H.C.; Kim, C.G.; Lee, J.S.; Kim, C.J. Inhibitory effects of bee venom and its components against viruses in vitro and in vivo. *J. Microbiol.* **2016**, *54*, 853–866. [CrossRef]
88. Park, S.; Erdogan, S.; Hwang, D.; Hwang, S.; Han, E.H.; Lim, Y.H. Bee venom promotes hair growth in association with inhibiting 5α-reductase expression. *Biol. Pharm. Bull.* **2016**, *39*, 1060–1068. [CrossRef]
89. Hegazi, A.G.; Abd Raboh, F.A.; Ramzy, N.E.; Shaaban, D.M.; Khader, D.Y. Bee venom and propolis as new treatment modality in patients with localized plaque psoriases. *Int. Res. J. Med. Med. Sci.* **2013**, *1*, 27–33.
90. Tusiimire, J.; Wallace, J.; Woods, N.; Dufton, M.J.; Parkinson, J.A.; Abbott, G.; Clements, C.J.; Young, L.; Park, J.K.; Jeon, J.W.; et al. Effect of Bee Venom and Its Fractions on the Release of Pro-Inflammatory Cytokines in PMA-Differentiated U937 Cells Co-Stimulated with LPS. *Vaccines* **2016**, *4*, 11. [CrossRef]
91. Amin, M.A.; Abdel-Raheem, I. Accelerated wound healing and anti-inflammatory effects of physically cross linked polyvinyl alcohol-chitosan hydrogel containing honey bee venom in diabetic rats. *Arch. Pharmcol. Res.* **2014**, *37*, 1016–1031. [CrossRef] [PubMed]
92. Amin, M.; Abdel-Raheem, I.; Madkor, H. Wound healing and anti-inflammatory activities of bee venom-chitosan blend films. *J. Drug. Delivery. Sci. Technol.* **2008**, *18*, 424–430. [CrossRef]
93. Tu, W.-C.; Wu, C.-C.; Hsieh, H.-L.; Chen, C.-Y.; Hsu, S.-L. Honeybee venom induces calcium -dependent but caspase-independent apoptotic cell death in human melanoma A 2058 cells. *Toxicon* **2008**, *52*, 318–329. [CrossRef] [PubMed]
94. Han, S.M.; Hong, I.P.; Woo, S.O.; Chun, S.N.; Park, K.K.; Nicholls, Y.M.; Pak, S.C. The beneficial effects of honeybee-venom serum on facial wrinkles in humans. *Clin. Interv. Aging* **2015**, *10*, 1587–1592. [CrossRef]
95. Kędzia, B.; Hołderna-Kędzia, E. Allergic effects of honey on the human body. *Pasieka* **2011**, *6*. Available online: https://pasieka24.pl/index.php/pl-pl/pasieka-czasopismo-dla-pszczelarzy/53-pasieka-6-2011/543-alergenne-oddzialywanie-miodu-na-organizm-czlowieka (accessed on 7 July 2019).
96. Basista, K. Honey—Biological and pro-health activity and its allergic potential. *Alerg. Immunol.* **2012**, *9*, 97–100.

97. Basista-Sołtys, K.; Filipek, B. Allergic potential of propolis—A literature review. *Alerg. Astma Immunol.* **2013**, *18*, 32–38.
98. Elieh Ali Komi, D.; Shafaghat, F.; Zwiener, R.D. Immunology of Bee Venom. *Clin. Rev. Allergy Immunol.* **2018**, *54*, 386–396. [CrossRef]

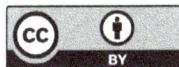

© 2020 by the authors. Licensee MDPI, Basel, Switzerland. This article is an open access article distributed under the terms and conditions of the Creative Commons Attribution (CC BY) license (http://creativecommons.org/licenses/by/4.0/).

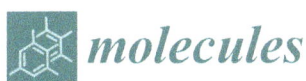

Article

Ulva intestinalis Protein Extracts Promote In Vitro Collagen and Hyaluronic Acid Production by Human Dermal Fibroblasts

Justine Bodin [1,2], Amandine Adrien [2], Pierre-Edouard Bodet [1], Delphine Dufour [2], Stanislas Baudouin [2], Thierry Maugard [1] and Nicolas Bridiau [1,*]

[1] Equipe BCBS (Biotechnologies et Chimie des Bioressources pour la Santé), La Rochelle Université, UMR CNRS 7266 LIENSs, Avenue Michel Crépeau, 17042 La Rochelle, France; justine.bodin1@univ-lr.fr (J.B.); pierreedouard.bodet@univ-lr.fr (P.-E.B.); thierry.maugard@univ-lr.fr (T.M.)

[2] SEPROSYS, Séparations, Procédés, Systèmes, 12 Rue Marie-Aline Dusseau, 17000 La Rochelle, France; amandine.adrien@seprosys.com (A.A.); delphine.dufour@seprosys.com (D.D.); stanislas.baudouin@seprosys.com (S.B.)

* Correspondence: nicolas.bridiau@univ-lr.fr; Tel.: +33-5-46-45-87-91; Fax: +33-5-46-45-82-65

Academic Editors: Raffaele Capasso and Lorenzo Di Cesare Mannelli
Received: 1 April 2020; Accepted: 21 April 2020; Published: 30 April 2020

Abstract: With the increase in life expectancy, reducing the visible signs of skin aging has become a major issue. A reduction in collagen and hyaluronic acid synthesis by fibroblasts is a feature of skin aging. The green seaweed, *Ulva intestinalis*, is an abundant and rich source of nutrients, especially proteins and peptides. The aim of this study was to assess the potential cosmetic properties of a protein fraction from *Ulva intestinalis* (PROT-1) containing 51% of proteins and 22% of polysaccharides, and its enzymatic peptide hydrolysates on human dermal fibroblasts. PROT-1 was extracted using a patented acid- and solvent-free process (FR2998894 (B1)). The biochemical characterization and chromatographic analysis showed a main set of proteins (25 kDa). To demonstrate the anti-aging potential of PROT-1, fibroblast proliferation and collagen and hyaluronic acid production were assessed on fibroblast cell lines from donors aged 20 years (CCD-1059Sk) and 46 years (CCD-1090Sk). PROT-1 induced a significant increase in collagen and hyaluronic acid production per cell, and a reduction in cell proliferation without increasing cell mortality. These effects were reversed after protein hydrolysis of PROT-1, showing the central role of proteins in this promising anti-aging property.

Keywords: *Ulva intestinalis*; seaweed proteins; human dermal fibroblast; collagen; hyaluronic acid; anti-aging

1. Introduction

In recent years, people have started to pay more attention to skin health and beauty. The cosmetic industry is growing and many studies have focused on skin aging inhibition and delay. Wrinkles, laxity and dryness are features of aging [1]. Skin aging is a complex biological process that can be divided into two basic processes, intrinsic and extrinsic aging. Intrinsic aging is genetically inherited (genetic, hormonal and metabolic processes, cellular metabolism); extrinsic aging is due to external factors such as air pollution, toxins, nicotine consumption, lifestyle influence, chemicals and chronic light exposures, which contribute to accelerate its consequences [2]. One of the major consequences of skin aging is a reduction and alteration of extracellular matrix (ECM) components such as elastin, collagen and hyaluronic acid (HA) [3]. For this reason, maintaining collagen and HA levels in the dermis is essential to maintain a healthy skin.

HA is an ECM anionic glycosaminoglycan composed of D-glucuronic acid and *N*-acetyl-D-glucosamine, synthesized by fibroblasts and keratinocytes [4]. It plays an important role in normal dermis, of water retention and activation of tissue/fibroblast proliferation. A decrease in HA level results in impaired hydration and elastic properties of the skin [5].

Collagen is the main structural protein in the extracellular space. There are several types of collagen: in the dermis, type 1 collagen represents most of the total collagen and is involved in skin tension, elasticity and flexibility. The type 1 collagen subunit is a fibril-forming heterotrimeric protein composed of two alpha-1 chains and one alpha-2 chain which fold into a stable and highly ordered triple helix [6]. Collagen degradation is related to the expression of fibroblast-secreted matrix metalloproteinases (MMP). Indeed, during the aging process, the MMP expression increases, causing collagen degradation and reducing skin firmness [7,8].

The cosmetic industry is constantly looking for novelty, especially atypical molecules. From this point of view, the marine environment is likely to open up many new possibilities [9]. Marine macroalgae are abundant and sustainable sources of compounds for nutraceutical and cosmetic applications [10]. Among these interesting biomolecules, seaweed proteins have a high potential. The protein content of seaweeds depends on and differs according to the species, season and environmental growth conditions. Some seaweeds such as *Rhodophyta* or *Chlorophyta* contain high protein levels and are a potential renewable source to isolate biomolecules with a nutritional interest [11,12]. Green seaweeds of the *Ulva* genus can contain up to 44% of proteins [13]. *Ulva* species also contain a high level of carbohydrates and are rich sources of vitamins and minerals [14]. Green seaweeds have various biological activities, including anticoagulant, anti-aging, antimicrobial and antifungal, antioxidant, mitogenic, immunomodulatory, anti-cholesterol and many other potential activities [15–17]. Among the *Ulva* genus, the edible macroalga *Ulva intestinalis* contains 19.5% of proteins during summer [18]. In addition, it has been shown that a protein hydrolysate derived from *Ulva lactuca* exhibited an anti-aging activity. This protein hydrolysate, which was composed of numerous amino acids, including lysine, histidine, arginine, aspartic acid, proline, glycine, serine, glutamic acid, alanine, threonine, tyrosine, isoleucine, leucine, and phenylalanine, optimized cellular respiration, stimulated collagen production in the skin and inhibited elastase activity [19].

In this study, we used a previously developed acid-free and solvent-free procedure to extract and purify proteins from *Ulva intestinalis* (Scheme 1) [20]. Then, we developed a hydrolysis procedure of the obtained protein fraction (PROT-1) to produce a protein fraction of reduced molecular weight (MW), H-PROT-1, in order to assess the influence of MW on collagen and hyaluronic acid production by normal human dermal fibroblast (NHDF) cell lines from donors aged 20 and 46 years.

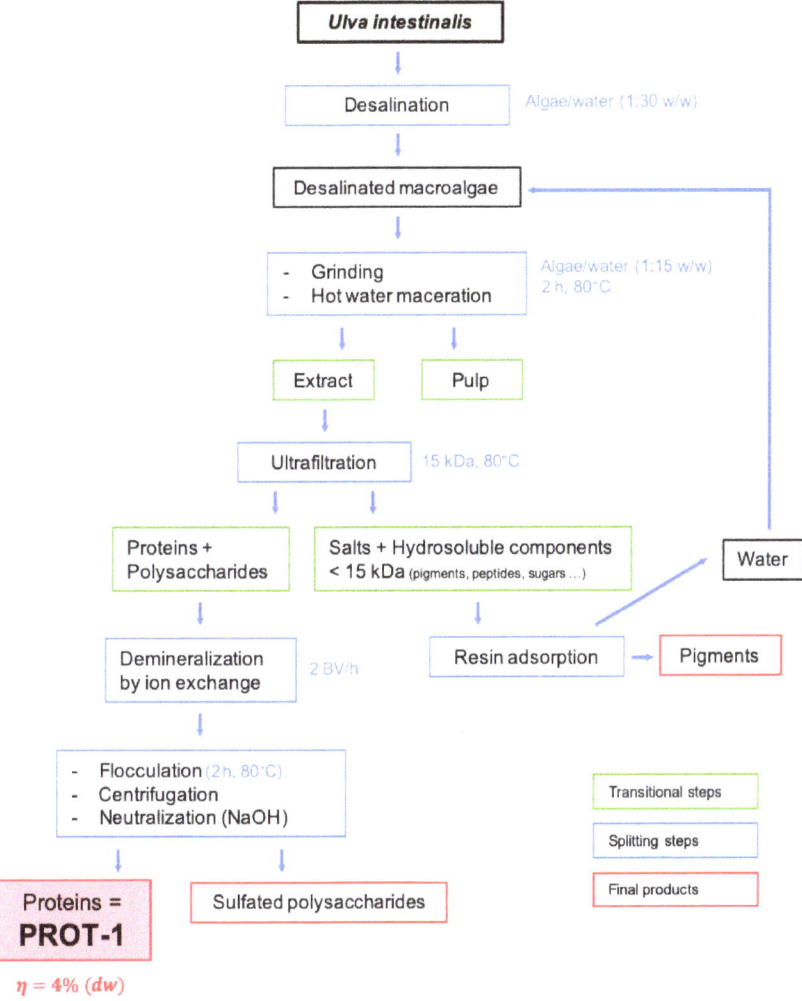

Scheme 1. Different steps and yield (η) of the extraction procedure developed by SEPROSYS [20].

2. Results and Discussion

2.1. Production and Characterization of Protein Fraction (PROT-1) and Protein Hydrolysates (H-PROT-1)

Ulva intestinalis material was shown to contain 26 ± 2.8% ($w/w_{dry\ material}$) of proteins, as determined by the Kjeldahl method, which was within the high values reported for green seaweeds of the *Ulva* genus (7–33% ($w/w_{dry\ material}$)) [21].

The protein fraction PROT-1 was extracted by following the patented Seprosys process illustrated on Scheme 1 [20]. The extracted protein fraction represented 4% ($w/w_{dry\ material}$) (21 g) of the desalinated dry macroalgae (on 500 g of algae). The efficiency of the aqueous and solvent-free protein extraction differs depending on the starting sample and protein accessibility. Indeed, some components such as polysaccharides may interfere with algae protein extract. The yield obtained here was in the average of the yields of protein aqueous extraction found in the literature [22].

The total amino acid composition of PROT-1 was determined after acid hydrolysis under strong acidic conditions at 100 °C for 2 h, using UHPLC-HRMS analysis of the amino acid mixture obtained after neutralization. Figure 1 shows that the fraction was mainly composed of leucine (27.2%), isoleucine (23.3%) and valine (28.4%). According to Lewis et al., major amino acids composing *Ulva intestinalis* seaweeds are proline, methionine and aspartic acid [23], which is different from what we found. However, amino acid composition of the alga can drastically vary with respect to the season, period or geographic place of harvest, but also to its growth stage [24], which could explain these differences.

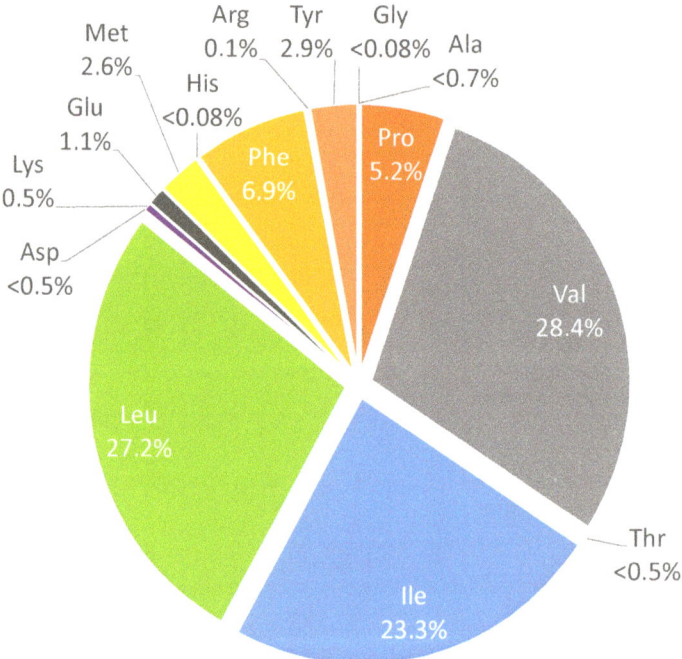

Figure 1. Total amino acids composition of the PROT-1 fraction determined after acid hydrolysis and UHPLC-HRMS analysis.

The PROT-1 fraction was also enzymatically-hydrolyzed by using the protease preparation Flavourzyme®, in order to obtain a fraction containing low MW peptides, thereafter referred as PROT-1 hydrolysates (H-PROT-1 (t2h), (t4h), (t6h), (t24h)). The enzymatic hydrolysis procedure was optimized to determine the optimal conditions (data not shown). In order to follow the time-course of hydrolysis, a monitoring method involving a separation by high-performance liquid size exclusion chromatography (HPL-SEC) was developed, and the MW of protein and peptide sets was estimated using standards of known MW. Figure 2 shows the enzymatic hydrolysis time-course of the PROT-1 fraction. The analyses showed that this fraction contained a major set of proteins with a MW of about 25 kDa, eluted at 12 min, and a set of proteins with a MW higher than 400 kDa, eluted at 7 min. During the hydrolysis, a shifting of the main peak towards higher retention times was observed, which reflected a decrease in molecular weight. For example, at t1h, two major peaks at 13.4 and 13.9 min corresponding to sets of proteins of 7.2 and 5.1 kDa, respectively, were observed. Furthermore, the profile observed after 6 h of depolymerization was probably the consequence of a profound enzymatic hydrolysis of peptides, causing the liberation of amino acids that were not or not much detected on the chromatograms, due to their very low molar extinction coefficient compared to polypeptides.

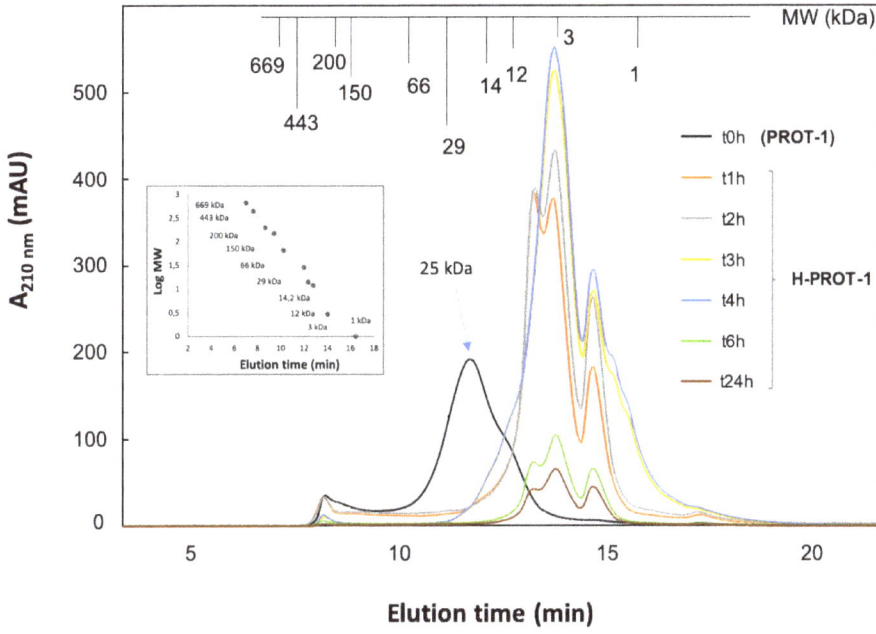

Figure 2. Standard curve and time-course HPLC-SEC profiles of PROT-1 enzymatic hydrolysis catalyzed by the protease preparation Flavourzyme®.

The PROT-1 fraction contained 51% of proteins and 22% of polysaccharides (Table 1). The presence of polysaccharides may be explained by two reasons: the presence of a cell wall mucilage containing polysaccharides [25] and the well-known presence of glycoproteins in algae of the *Ulva* genus [26]. The protein purity of the fraction could be improved by controlling the presence and composition of anionic and neutral polysaccharides composing the mucilage. To characterize PROT-1 and its hydrolysates obtained after enzymatic hydrolysis, all samples were analyzed using SDS-PAGE (Figure 3). Lane 1 contains the size markers and lane 2 contains PROT-1. The visible trail in lane 2 indicates a polydisperse set of proteins, very likely due to the partial hydrolysis of proteins that could occur during the extraction step under harsh conditions, especially during flocculation. This protein trail disappeared in accordance with the time-course of the enzymatic hydrolysis, showing its efficiency. The presence of a band at 25 kDa at t2h is in line with the results reported by Rouxel et al. on the existence of a water-soluble protein with a MW of 25 kDa in *Ulva intestinalis* [27]. The intensity of this band at 25 kDa and others corresponding to low MW (around 10 kDa) decreased throughout hydrolysis, which is consistent with the HPLC-SEC analyses.

Table 1. Biochemical composition of the PROT-1 fraction.

Fraction	Ashes	Proteins	Neutral Sugars	Uronic Acids	Lipids	Polyphenols
			% ($w/w_{dry\ extract}$)			
PROT-1	20	51	22	6	<1	<1

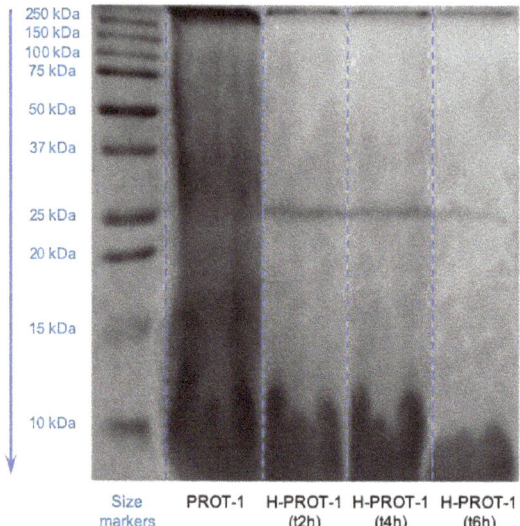

Figure 3. SDS-PAGE analysis of the PROT-1 fraction followed during enzymatic hydrolysis catalyzed by the protease preparation Flavourzyme®.

Table 2 lists the peptides that were identified in the H-PROT-1 (t1h) fraction using UHPLC-HRMS. 88 peptides were identified, more precisely 14 dipeptides, 4 tripeptides, 17 tetrapeptides, 14 pentapeptides, and 39 peptides of 6 to 15 amino acids. The amino acid composition of these 88 peptides was then determined according to their sequences and showed that these peptides were mostly composed of leucine or isoleucine (17.1%), alanine (9.7%), and glycine, glutamic acid, aspartic acid, tyrosine, threonine and serine in similar proportions, between 7.1% and 7.9% (Figure 4).

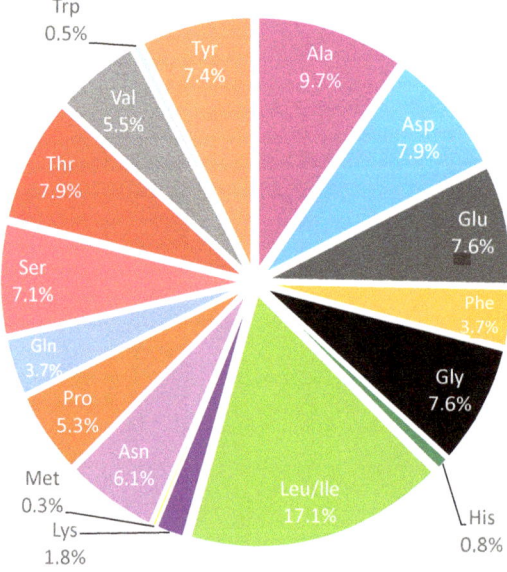

Figure 4. Amino acid composition of the 88 peptides identified in the H-PROT-1 (t1h) fraction by UHPLC-HRMS.

Table 2. Peptide sequences identified by UHPLC-HRMS in the H-PROT-1 (t1h) fraction.

Entry	Retention Time (min)	Ion	Experimental Monoisotopic Mass (Da)	Mass Accuracy (ppm)	Peptide or Amino Acid
1	2.58	[M + H]⁺	233.1130	0.86	VD
2	3.20	[M + H]⁺	508.1899	2.56	EGESS
3	3.81	[M + H]⁺	247.1284	2.02	VE
4	4.16	[M + H]⁺	246.1456	2.84	I/LN
5	5.65	[M + H]⁺	247.1289	2.02	I/LD
6	5.65	[M + H]⁺	247.1294	2.02	EV
7	6.67	[M + H]⁺	294.1545	2.72	I/L-hexose
8	8.21	[M + H]⁺	261.1452	0.77	I/LE
9	8.81	[M + H]⁺	261.1452	0.77	I/LE
10	9.57	[M + H]⁺	590.2798	2.88	ETVNQ
11	9.80	[M + H]⁺	404.2132	1.98	I/LSAN
12	10.40	[M + H]⁺	419.2135	0.00	TVAE
13	10.70	[M + H]⁺	449.2243	1.56	TEVT
14	10.93	[M + H]⁺	328.1394	0.61	F-hexose
15	11.32	[M + H]⁺	418.2293	0.96	I/LSAQ
16	11.52	[M + H]⁺	555.2410	0.18	TGYTN
17	11.52	[M + H]⁺	203.14	4.43	AI/L
18	11.83	[M + H]⁺	546.2520	0.18	DAI/LNN
19	12.46	[M + H]⁺	502.2625	1.00	AI/LNGQ
20	12.66	[M + H]⁺	295.1294	1.69	FE
21	12.87	[M + H]⁺	475.2515	0.84	AI/LSNA
22	13.41	[M + H]⁺	367.1506	0.27	W-hexose
23	14.27	[M + H]⁺	350.1740	1.43	I/LMS
24	14.48	[M + H]⁺	526.2163	4.18	SAYDA
25	14.48	[M + H]⁺	526.2163	4.18	* DADA
26	15.29	[M + H]⁺	440.1667	0.68	EEY
27	16.18	[M + H]⁺	403.2188	0.07	DVVA
28	16.65	[M + H]⁺	237.1241	3.08	AF
29	17.22	[M + H]⁺	205.0982	2.44	W
30	17.60	[M + H]⁺	229.1552	2.18	I/LP
31	18.01	[M + H]⁺	492.2662	0.61	SI/LTTA
32	19.09	[M + H]⁺	458.2607	0.59	I/LPQT
33	19.09	[M + H]⁺	458.2607	0.59	QPI/LT
34	19.98	[M + H]⁺	295.1659	2.03	I/LY
35	21.39	[M + H]⁺	302.2077	0.66	I/LI/LG
36	21.76	[M + H]⁺	416.2517	1.20	* GSI/LA
37	21.76	[M + H]⁺	416.2517	1.20	NVI/LA
38	22.01	[M + H]⁺	409.2078	1.00	VGAY
39	22.01	[M + H]⁺	409.2078	1.00	I/LNY
40	22.25	[M + H]⁺	552.2316	1.81	EAEFG
41	22.64	[M + H]⁺	411.7227	6.07	YTI/LDPP *
42	22.64	[M + H]⁺	295.1654	0.34	YI/L
43	23.03	[M + 2H]²⁺	720.3186	0.99	QAAEAAESGDFKSE
44	23.25	[M + 2H]²⁺	841.8622	-	* QSDWSEAEAAHS
45	23.45	[M + H]⁺	777.3397	0.40	NQAAEAAESGDESKF
46	23.65	[M + H]⁺	459.2179	3.64	EEYTFTK
47	23.65	[M + H]⁺	459.2179	3.64	KFTTYEE
48	23.65	[M + H]⁺	459.2179	3.64	KFYTTEE
49	23.85	[M + H]⁺	550.2878	1.13	(I/L)GTYP
50	24.12	[M + H]⁺	790.4323	2.21	TI/LATI/LSNA
51	24.32	[M + H]⁺	329.1500	1.28	YF
52	24.53	[M + H]⁺	373.2276	3.22	KDTVI/LI/LG
53	24.53	[M + 2H]²⁺	766.8573	-	* KDI/LI/LI/L *
54	25.18	[M + H]⁺	401.2756	0.72	VVAI/L
55	25.18	[M + H]⁺	600.3360	1.33	SPGGI/LGI/L
56	25.18	[M + H]⁺	600.3360	1.33	SNI/LPGI/L
57	25.58	[M + H]⁺	873.3639	1.57	(YG)YGDI/LDA
58	25.58	[M + H]⁺	873.3639	1.57	(YG)GI/LDYDA
59	25.58	[M + H]⁺	873.3639	1.57	(YG)DI/LGYDA
60	25.58	[M + H]⁺	873.3639	1.57	(YG)DYGI/LDA
61	25.58	[M + H]⁺	873.3639	1.57	(DI/L)GYGYDA
62	25.86	[M + H]⁺	687.2986	0.17	DI/LGYGY

Table 2. Cont.

Entry	Retention Time (min)	Ion	Experimental Monoisotopic Mass (Da)	Mass Accuracy (ppm)	Peptide or Amino Acid
63	26.07	[M + H]$^+$	579.3143	0.98	NVI/LAY
64	26.07	[M + 2H]$^{2+}$	590.7799	3.71	QEYENI/LI/LGSQ
65	26.07	[M + H]$^+$	555.2821	1.31	YI/LYP
66	26.73	[M + H]$^+$	431.2497	0.86	DI/LAI/L
67	27.04	[M + H]$^+$	401.2756	0.72	I/LVGI/L
68	24.69	[M + 2H]$^{2+}$	604.7886	7.87	DSTWI/LTTAI/LSN
69	28.26	[M + 2H]$^{2+}$	566.2830	5.14	SG(Q/AG)QEI/LI/LDI/LE
70	28.26	[M + 2H]$^{2+}$	566.2830	5.14	QSGQEI/LI/LDI/LE
71	28.26	[M + 2H]$^{2+}$	566.2830	5.14	TNGQEI/LI/LDI/LE
72	28.46	[M + H]$^+$	726.4041	1.13	EI/LSPPI/LA
73	28.46	[M + H]$^+$	726.4041	1.13	ESI/LPPI/LA
74	28.46	[M + H]$^+$	726.4041	1.13	DTI/LPAI/LP
75	30.26	[M + H]$^+$	577.3329	2.72	AFI/LI/LN
76	30.47	[M + H]$^+$	645.4180	4.34	TI/LI/LVI/LS
77	30.47	[M + H]$^+$	645.4180	4.34	I/LI/LTVI/LS
78	30.47	[M + H]$^+$	645.4180	4.34	VI/LTI/LI/LS
79	30.88	[M + H]$^+$	938.4491	2.66	EI/LTDTVNF
80	30.88	[M + H]$^+$	938.4491	2.66	ETI/LDTVNF
81	31.35	[M + 2H]$^{2+}$	640.3069	4.08	EGESSI/LTTAI/LSNA
82	31.35	[M + 2H]$^{2+}$	640.3069	4.08	E(SG/DG/TG)ESI/LTTAI/LSNA
83	31.89	[M + 2H]$^{2+}$	616.3179	6.44	(AP)EI/LI/LTVDYNP
84	31.89	[M + 2H]$^{2+}$	616.3179	6.44	PVVDI/LTVDYNP
85	32.13	[M + H]$^+$	558.3867	0.95	I/LTVI/LI/L
86	32.50	[M + H]$^+$	746.4453	0.74	PI/LI/LGI/LYA
87	32.70	[M + H]$^+$	890.4997	-	* I/LTI/LP
88	32.70	[M + H]$^+$	890.4997	-	* YEI/LP
89	32.70	[M + H]$^+$	675.4078	0.25	I/LPGI/LI/LY
90	32.70	[M + H]$^+$	675.4078	0.25	I/LPI/LGI/LY
91	33.17	[M + 2H]$^{2+}$	634.3411	4.10	SI/LDI/LPHI/LPTQF
92	33.37	[M + 2H]$^{2+}$	691.8536	3.45	SI/LDI/LDPHI/LPTQF

* undetermined amino acids; () undetermined sequence.

2.2. Assessment of PROT-1 and H-PROT-1 Cytotoxicity on NHDF

The aim of this part was to assess the cytotoxicity of the PROT-1 and H-PROT-1 fractions (t2h, t4h, t6h and t24h) on NHDF at 10, 100 and 500 µg/mL. Two fibroblast cell lines were used: one from a 20-year old woman (line 1059) and one from a 46-year old woman (line 1090). These two cell lines were used to determine whether the effects could vary according to the age of the donor skin.

Figure 5 shows the effect of PROT-1 and H-PROT-1 on fibroblast viability. PROT-1 decreased fibroblast proliferation, reducing by 18%, 28% and 42% the proliferation of the 1059-cell line at 10, 100 and 500 µg/mL, respectively. The effect was less marked for the 1090-cell line as there was no effect on cell proliferation at 10 and 100 µg/mL but a decrease of 53% was observed at 500 µg/mL. Thus, a slight difference was observed between both cell lines. The 1059-cell line was rapidly affected by the extract, at a lower concentration than the 1090 cell line. The effect of the low MW peptide fractions H-PROT-1 (t2h, t4h, t6h and t24h) on fibroblast proliferation was lower compared to that of PROT-1 on both cell lines. Indeed, in the wells treated with H-PROT-1 (t24h), the cell viability reached 79% for the 1059-cell line and 78% for the 1090-cell line. These results showed that decreasing the MW of PROT-1 proteins led to a reduced effect on cell proliferation for both cell lines.

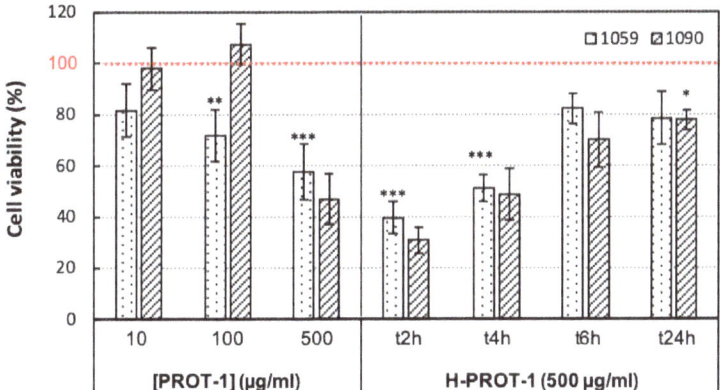

Figure 5. Effect of PROT-1 and H-PROT-1 on fibroblast proliferation in vitro (MTT assay). Results are expressed as the mean relative percentage of viable fibroblasts compared to the negative control (100%). Significant differences between values obtained with samples and negative control ($n = 20$) are indicated by * ($p < 0.05$), ** ($p < 0.01$) and *** ($p < 0.001$).

Figure 6 shows the effect of the PROT-1 fraction and H-PROT-1 hydrolysates on the cell mortality by necrosis, compared to the negative control. PROT-1 had no effect on cell mortality while a slight decrease in cell mortality was observed with H-PROT-1 at t2h, t4h and t6h: −8% (cell line 1059) and −7% (cell line 1090) for example at t4h. Except for the highest concentration of PROT-1, 500 µg/mL, which led to a very slight increase in cell mortality (+7% for the 1059-cell line and +9.5% for the 1090-cell line), no deleterious effect was observed on fibroblasts.

Overall, PROT-1 decreased cell proliferation without increasing cell mortality by necrosis. Besides, we did not observe any alteration of the fibroblast morphology when checking the cells with optical microscopy. PROT-1 thus appeared to have a cytostatic effect on both cell lines in a similar way, but this effect was reduced after enzymatic protein hydrolysis. This would therefore indicate that the molecular weight or the distinctive structure of some PROT-1 proteins is related to this cytostatic effect.

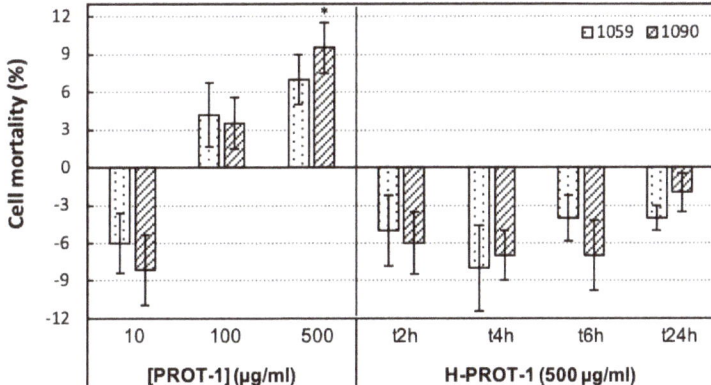

Figure 6. Effect of PROT-1 and H-PROT-1 on fibroblast mortality in vitro (LDH assay). Results are expressed as the mean relative percentage of living fibroblasts compared to the negative control (0%). Significant differences between values obtained with samples and negative control ($n = 8$) are indicated by * ($p < 0.05$).

2.3. Effect of PROT-1 and H-PROT-1 on Collagen Production

In this part of the study, the effect of the PROT-1 and H-PROT-1 fractions on collagen production was assessed. Hyaluronic acid (HA) was used as a positive control. Indeed, HA is recognized by CD44 receptors on the cell surface, which activates signaling pathways involved in the stimulation of fibroblast proliferation and collagen production [28,29].

The protein fractions showed a higher activity than the positive control (Figures 7 and 8). More specifically, at a HA concentration of 1000 µg/mL, the collagen production per well was increased by 30.5% for the 1059 cell line (Figure 7) and by 28.5% for the 1090 cell line (Figure 8), while PROT-1 induced a significant dose-dependent rise in collagen production per well by 51.9% and 151.8% at 100 and 500 µg/mL, respectively, for the 1059 cell line, and by 52.5% and 79.5% at 100 and 500 µg/mL, respectively, for the 1090 cell line. However, the reduction of PROT-1 proteins MW led to a strong decrease in collagen production. Indeed, after 24 h of hydrolysis, the collagen production per well did not significantly differ from the control conditions.

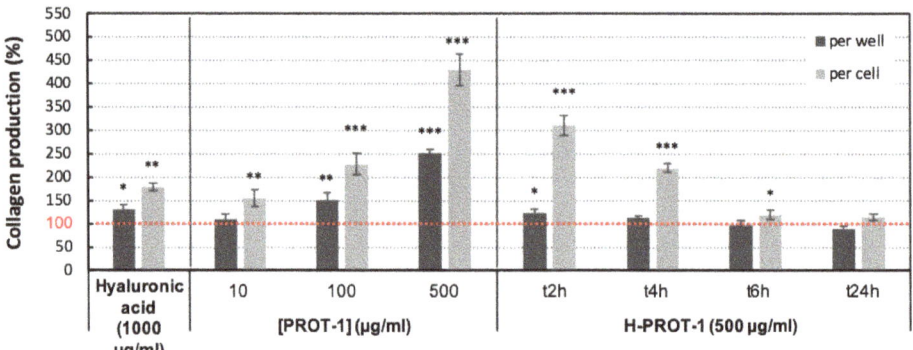

Figure 7. Collagen production per well and per cell by the human dermal fibroblast cell line 1059. Results are expressed as the mean relative percentage of production, compared to the negative control (100%). Significant differences between values obtained with samples and negative control ($n = 9$) are indicated by * ($p < 0.05$), ** ($p < 0.01$) and *** ($p < 0.001$).

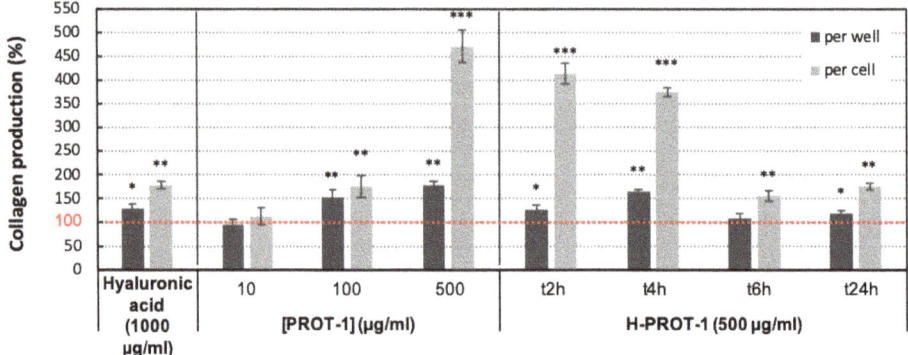

Figure 8. Collagen production per well and per cell by the human dermal fibroblast cell line 1090. Results are expressed as the mean relative percentage of production, compared to the negative control (100%). Significant differences between values obtained with samples and negative control ($n = 9$) are indicated by * ($p < 0.05$), ** ($p < 0.01$) and *** ($p < 0.001$).

We also studied the collagen production per cell. In the presence of HA at a concentration of 1000 µg/mL, the collagen production per cell increased in a similar way with both cell lines, by about

80%. The results obtained with the PROT-1 fraction were very interesting as they showed a very high dose-dependent increase in collagen production per cell, compared to the negative control: +55%, +128% and +331% for the 1059 cell line (Figure 7) and +13%, +76% and +371% for the 1090 cell line (Figure 8), at 10, 100 and 500 µg/mL, respectively. It is noteworthy, however, that this pro-collagen activity was lost when hydrolyzing proteins in the fraction PROT-1, particularly for the 1059 cell line. Indeed, the production of collagen per cell did not significantly increase in presence of H-PROT-1 at t24h. This effect seemed even closely related to the degradation of proteins in the H-PROT-1 fraction as the pro-collagen activity of the PROT-1 fraction decreased in accordance with the time-course of the enzymatic hydrolysis reaction. These results suggest that the native structure of the proteins that are responsible for the pro-collagen activity of the PROT-1 fraction is essential. The results obtained with the 1090 cell line were very similar, except that this cell line remained slightly more stimulated by the H-PROT-1 fractions.

These results are of particular interest as the pro-collagen activity of the PROT-1 and even H-PROT-1 fractions appeared to be superior to that of hyaluronic acid, which is a pro-collagen active compound usually used in anti-aging skin care cosmetic formulations [30,31]. Furthermore, this activity could be explained by the induction of a cell metabolic redirection, which would also be in accordance with the cytostatic effect of the fractions that we previously observed. It means that fibroblast moved towards collagen biosynthesis pathway(s) rather than cell growth. Indeed, fibroblasts underwent a rapid decrease in cell viability but no significant change in cell mortality and morphology. Kmail et al. showed a very similar behavior of hepatic macrophages in contact with extracts from *Asparagus aphyllus, Crataegus aronia,* and *Ephedra alata,* which induced a significant cytostatic effect on macrophage cultures, highlighted by MTT and LDH tests. These authors observed a decrease in cell viability but no cytotoxicity of these antidiabetic extracts [32].

The very significant decrease in the pro-collagen activity that was observed with the hydrolyzed protein fractions confirmed that the proteins were the molecules responsible for the collagen synthesis stimulation in PROT-1. This result was consistent with what Ko et al. highlighted when assessing the effect of a protein extract from *Ulva pertusa* on the proliferation and type I collagen synthesis of replicative senescent fibroblasts [33], as well as the pro-collagen activity of a protein extract from *Ulva lactuca*, AOSAINE®, developed by BiotechMarine. It was also consistent with the work of Montanari and Guglielmo, who reported a tripeptide of sequence Lys-Val-Lys, which was shown to promote collagen synthesis by human fibroblasts by 75% when associated to an *Ulva lactuca* aqueous extract [34]. On the contrary, our results differed from what the same authors found when they extracted water-soluble proteins from *Ulva lactuca* and produced a polypeptide containing the sequence Arg-Gly-Asp, after depolymerization of these proteins. This polypeptide was shown to promote collagen I production by stimulating the proliferation of fibroblasts and not collagen biosynthesis. Similarly, Honma et al. demonstrated that peptide sequences Leu-Glu-His-Ala, Leu-Asp-His-Ala or Leu-Glu-His-Ala-Phe, could promote extra-cellular collagen production by NHDF [35]. Nevertheless, the mechanisms of actions involved in the activities of these peptides or proteins remain unclear. The protein extract from *Ulva pertusa* was proved to directly inhibit MMP-1, which could explain its activity by preventing type I collagen degradation. Joe et al. reported that an extract from *Ecklonia stolonifera,* containing phlorotannins, could inhibit NF-kB or Ap-1 reporter gene expression and therefore suppress the expression of MMP-1 in NHDP, which led to the increase in collagen production [36]. A very similar activity was also shown with a peptide from *Chlorella vulgaris* [37]. At last, a pentadecapeptide from *Pyropia yezoensis* (Asp-Pro-Lys-Gly-Lys-Gln-Gln-Ala-Ile-His-Val-Ala-Pro-Ser-Phe), was shown to be able to activate the TGF-β/Smad signaling pathway, leading to increased type 1 collagen expression and upregulated transcription factor specificity protein 1 (Sp1) expression, which is reportedly involved in type 1 collagen expression [38].

None of these peptide sequences was found in the 88 peptide sequences identified in the H-PROT-1 (t1h) fraction, obtained after 1 h of PROT-1 hydrolysis by the enzyme preparation Flavourzyme®. Nevertheless, one tripeptide sequence Thr-Val-Asn, including a central valine and two external polar amino acids, was found in the peptides eluted at 9.57 and 30.88 min (entries 10, 79 and 80 in Table 2). This sequence is similar to that of the tripeptide Lys-Val-Lys, which was proved to exhibit a pro-collagen activity by Montanari and Guglielmo [34]. Besides, two tripeptide sequences very close to tripeptide sequences included in the pentadecapeptide from *Pyropia yezoensis* (... -Asp-Pro-Lys- ... and ... -Gln-Ala-Ile- ...) were found in the peptides eluted at 23.03, 23.45 and 33.37 min (entries 43, 45 and 92 in Table 2): Asp-Pro-His and Gln-Ala-Ala, respectively. Indeed, the only variation in the sequences is located on the third amino acid, which is very similar in terms of property: another basic amino acid for the first one and another hydrophobic amino acid for the second one. However, despite these similarities, this does not mean that polypeptides or proteins exhibiting these sequences in the PROT-1 fraction are responsible for its pro-collagen activity, as biological functions of tripeptide sequences occurring in large peptide structures would not be necessarily the same as those of smaller peptides. Further studies involving the assessment of these particular peptides or proteins after purification are needed to understand their structure–function relationship.

The MMP-1 inhibition potential of the PROT-1 fraction was also evaluated but showed no significant inhibition (data not shown). In conclusion, the increase in collagen production induced by this fraction was probably not due to a decrease in the extracellular fibrillar collagen degradation directly associated with MMP-1 inhibition, contrary to what was shown by Ko et al. in their study of an *Ulva pertusa* protein extract [33]. The increase in collagen production might therefore be linked to the effect of the PROT-1 fraction on an intra-cellular mechanism, e.g., a biosynthesis pathway such as NF-kB or TGF-β/Smad signaling pathways, chaperone synthesis pathway (maintenance of conformation) or inhibition of MMP synthesis.

2.4. Effects of PROT-1 and H-PROT-1 on Hyaluronic Acid Production

Moisturization is the first step to fight against skin aging, by improving elastic properties of the skin [5]. A major component of the skin ECM, hyaluronic acid, plays a key role in skin moisturization by retaining water in the dermis, and thus lubricating the skin [39].

In this part of the study, the effects of PROT-1 and H-PROT-1 on the HA production by both the 1059 and 1090 fibroblast cell lines were investigated by an ELISA-like assay. TGF-β is known to stimulate HA production by dermal fibroblasts [40] and was then used as a positive control. Figures 9 and 10 show that the HA production of both cell lines treated with the PROT-1 fraction was very significantly increased, compared to the negative control, and even to the positive control, TGF-β. More precisely, a TGF-β concentration of 10 µg/mL increased HA production per well and per cell of both cell lines, by about 45%, as PROT-1 induced a dose-dependent increase in hyaluronan production per well, especially with the 1059 cell line, reaching +46% and +87.3% at 100 and 500 µg/mL, respectively. However, unlike TGF-β, the PROT-1 fraction strongly and dose-dependently stimulated the HA production per cell, again mainly with the 1059 cell line; strong increases of 115%, 206% and 323% were indeed observed at 10, 100 and 500 µg/mL, respectively (Figure 9). The enzymatic hydrolysis of the PROT-1 fraction led to a loss of its pro-hyaluronic acid activity, which was very similar to what was previously observed for its pro-collagen activity. Indeed, the H-PROT-1 hydrolysates obtained after 2, 6 and 24 h induced a significant drop of HA production per cell of both cell lines at 500 µg/mL, more specifically a maximal reduction close to 245% after 24 h. This effect was particularly substantial for the 1059 cell line, which showed a strong and quick decrease in HA production. Indeed, the activity was 30% lower than that of the negative control after 6 h of hydrolysis. This loss of activity was slightly less significant with the 1090 cell line, as the HA production per cell was stimulated by the H-PROT-1 (t6h) fraction by about 42%. However, no stimulation could be observed at t24h. These results indicate that the native structure of the active proteins, which seems to be essential for their pro-collagen activity, is necessary for their pro-hyaluronic acid activity as well. They also confirm that fibroblast cell lines 1059 and 1090 are not equally stimulated by PROT-1 or H-PROT-1 fractions, pointing out that the physiological state of dermal fibroblasts might affect their stimulatory capacity.

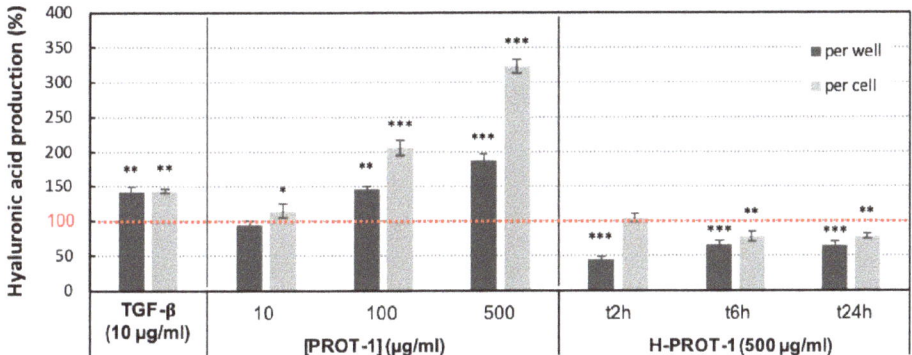

Figure 9. Hyaluronic acid production per well and per cell by the human dermal fibroblast cell line 1059. Results are expressed as the mean relative percentage of production, compared to the negative control (100%). Significant differences between values obtained with samples and negative control ($n = 9$) by * ($p < 0.05$), ** ($p < 0.01$) and *** ($p < 0.001$).

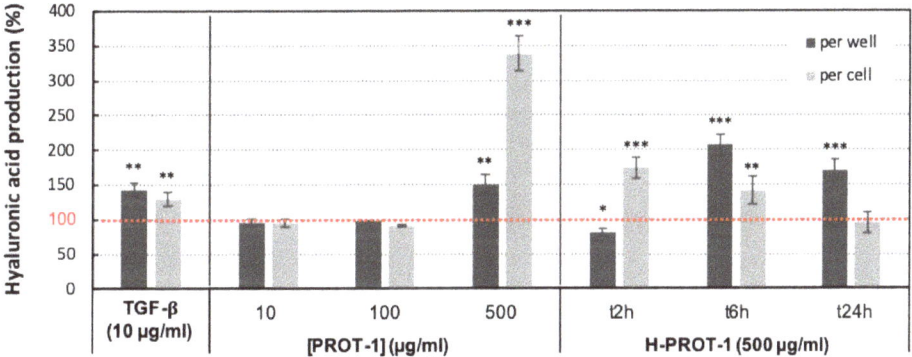

Figure 10. Hyaluronic acid production per well and per cell by the human dermal fibroblast cell line 1090. Results are expressed as the mean relative percentage of production, compared to the negative control (100%). Significant differences between values obtained with samples and negative control ($n = 9$) by * ($p < 0.05$), ** ($p < 0.01$) and *** ($p < 0.001$).

Finally, TGF-β seemed to mainly enhance HA production by stimulating cell growth while the activity of PROT-1 fractions completely differed. The fact that these fractions highly promoted HA production per cell, compared to their effect on HA production per well, suggests that they would be able to directly induce HA biosynthesis by the fibroblasts rather than their growth. Fayat et al. showed that a brown seaweed aqueous extract from *Padina pavonica* inhibited the hyaluronidase [41]. This could be a way to further explore to better understand the mechanism of action involved in the pro-hyaluronic acid activity of the PROT-1 fraction.

3. Material and Methods

3.1. Material

All chemicals and reagents were purchased from Merck (Darmstadt, Germany). Fetal bovine serum, penicillin–streptomycin, trypsin–EDTA, and Eagle's Minimum Essential Medium (EMEM) were purchased from Eurobio Ingen (Les Ulis, France). ELISA-like hyaluronic acid assay microplates were purchased from R&D systems (Wiesbaden, Germany). Human dermal fibroblasts (CCD-1059Sk, lot number 62062292, and CCD-1090Sk, lot number 204756) were obtained from ATCC Cell (Manassas,

VA, USA). They were derived from the skin of a 20- and 46-year old woman, according to the provider's information.

The green macroalga *Ulva intestinalis*, was cultivated and purchased from the aquaculture farm Algorythme on the Island of Ré (Ars-en-Ré, France). They were collected in summer 2017.

3.2. Methods

3.2.1. Protein Extraction & SEPROSYS Extraction Procedure

First, 500 g of dehydrated *Ulva intestinalis* material was washed in 15 L of deionized water (1/30 (w/w)) for 10 min at room temperature (RT) and wrung with a fabric cone to remove as much water as possible (Scheme 1). The washed algae were then ground in 5 L of deionized water at 80 °C until obtaining 2-mm particles. The 5 L suspension of minced algae in water was transferred in a thermostated tank at 80 °C containing 2.5 L of deionized water. Extraction was processed under constant agitation with a bladed stirrer at a rotation speed of 10 spins/min for 2 h. The pulps were then removed from the tank and filtered with the fabric cone to collect the aqueous extract. Then, 13 L of extract was recovered and filtered with an ultrafiltration unit equipped with a 15 kDa Kerasep KBW membrane (Novasep Process, Pompey, France). Filtration was carried out at 80 °C at a pressure of 5 bars and a circulation flow of 450 L/h (circulation speed of 5 m/s) until obtaining a retentate around 4°B. Then, 1.5 L of retentate was demineralized by passage on a column containing 100 mL of Amberlite FPA 98, a strong anionic resin in the OH^- form, in series with a column containing 200 mL of Amberlite IR 120, a strong cationic resin in the H^+ form. Circulation was processed with a peristaltic pump at a flow rate of 2 BV/h for the cationic resin. The deionized product was finally decanted in a water bath at 80 °C for 2 h (flocculation step). After centrifugation at 5000× g for 15 min at RT, the fraction, referred to as PROT-1, was neutralized to pH 7 with 1 M NaOH and lyophilized [22].

3.2.2. Enzymatic Hydrolysis of PROT-1 Proteins

Five hundred milliliters of a 10 mg/mL solution of PROT-1 fraction was prepared in deionized water and heated at 50 °C, under magnetic agitation at 500 rpm. The protease preparation Flavourzyme® was added at a ratio of 4% (v/v) and 10-mL aliquots were collected every hour for 24 h, and immediately heated at 90 °C for 20 min to inactivate the proteolytic enzymes. A control was also prepared without adding the protease preparation and similarly treated. Hydrolyzed samples, referred to as H-PROT-1 (t1h), (t2h), (t3h), (t4h), (t6h) and (t24h), were subsequently freeze-dried.

3.2.3. Biochemical Composition

The neutral sugar content was determined according to the phenol-sulfuric method [42], using rhamnose as a standard; rhamnose was chosen as it is the main moiety of the parietal water-soluble polysaccharides of seaweeds from the genus *Ulva*, the so-called ulvans, which are the major polysaccharides extracted by water maceration of these seaweeds. The protein content of the dehydrated seaweed starting material was determined by the Kjeldahl method (N× 6.25) [43] while the protein content of the PROT-1 fraction was determined by the Lowry assay [44], using bovine serum albumin as a standard. The quantification method of polyphenols was adapted from the original one [45] using gallic acid as a standard; briefly, 50 µL of Folin–Ciocalteu reagent and 200 µL of 20% sodium carbonate were successively added to 100 µL of sample and the mixture was incubated in the dark for 45 min at RT, prior to absorbance reading at 730 nm. The ash content was determined by measuring the mass loss of samples heated for 15 h at 550 °C. The lipid content was measured by the method of Chabrol and Charonnat [46] using vegetal oil as a standard.

3.2.4. High-Performance Liquid Size Exclusion Chromatography

The structural analysis and the molecular mass distribution of the proteins and peptides were assessed by high-performance liquid size exclusion chromatography (HPL-SEC), using a 1200 series

HPLC system (Agilent Technologies), equipped with two size-exclusion chromatography columns in series: TSK gel 3000 SW and TSK gel 2500 PW (TOSOH Biosciences). The temperature of analysis was stabilized at 30 °C and 30 µL of extract or standard at 1 mg/mL was injected. The products were eluted with 20 mM phosphate buffer with 0.1% NaCl (pH 7) at a flow rate of 0.8 mL/min and detected at 210 nm. The standard curve was prepared using protein and peptide standards ranging between 1000 and 669,000 Da (thyroglobulin, 669 kDa; apoferritin, 443 kDa; β-amylase, 200 kDa; alcohol dehydrogenase, 150 kDa; albumin, 66 kDa; carbonic anhydrase, 29 kDa; α-lactalbumin, 14.2 kDa; cytochrome c, 12 kDa; insulin, 3 kDa; α-casomorphin 1-4, 1 kDa).

3.2.5. Ultra-High-Performance Liquid Chromatography Coupled to High Resolution Mass Spectrometry Analysis (UHPLC-HRMS)

The total amino acid composition of the PROT-1 fraction was determined using an UHPLC system, "Acquity UPLC H-class", (Waters, Milford, MA, USA) coupled to a HRMS system, "XEVO G2 S Q-TOF", equipped with an electrospray ionization source (Waters, Manchester, England). The UHPLC system was formed by a quaternary pump (Quaternary Solvent Manager, Waters) and an automatic injector (Sample Manager-FTN, Waters) equipped with a 10 µL injection loop. Analyses were performed according to the UHPLC and MS parameters given in Table 3. The standard curve for each of the 20 essential amino acids was prepared using a standard solution at a concentration within the range 1–25 mg/L. The detection and quantification of total amino acids was performed after total acid hydrolysis of the sample. Briefly, 10 mg of the sample was solubilized in 1 mL of 1 M HCl and heated at 100 °C for two hours. After cooling at room temperature, the solution was neutralized by adding 1 M NaOH and filtered through a 0.22 µm filter prior to analysis, starting from a 2.5 mg/mL sample solution solubilized in water/methanol/formic acid 95:5:0.5 ($v/v/v$).

Table 3. Ultra-high-pressure liquid chromatography (UHPLC) and mass spectrometry (MS) parameters used to determine the total amino acid composition of the PROT-1 fraction and to elucidate the peptide sequences obtained in the H-PROT-1 (t1h) fraction.

	Total amino Acid Composition Determination	Elucidation of Peptide Sequences
UHPLC Parameters		
Column	Acquity UPLC HSST3 (150 mm × 2.1 mm × 1.7 µm) maintained at 25 °C	
Flow rate (µL·min^{-1})		0.3 mL·min^{-1}
Gradient used for the total amino acid composition determination: water/methanol 95:5 (v/v) (**A**)/water/methanol 50:50 (v/v) (**B**) + 0.5% (v/v) formic acid	0 min: 100% A; 2 min: 100% A; 7 min: 30% A; 8 min: 100% A; 13 min: 100% A.	
Gradient used for the elucidation of peptide sequences: water (**A**)/acetonitrile (**B**) + 0.1% (v/v) formic acid		0 min: 100% A; 2 min: 100% A; 2.5 min: 99% A; 3 min: 99% A; 3.5 min: 98% A; 4 min: 97% A; 5.5 min: 97% A; 8.5 min: 95% A; 10 min: 95% A; 15 min: 90% A; 18 min: 90% A; 22 min: 80% A; 27 min: 80% A; 30 min: 70% A; 34 min: 70% A; 36 min: 0% A; 38 min: 0% A; 40 min: 100% A; 45 min: 100% A.
Injection		5 µL (4 °C)
MS Parameters		
Mode	ESI$^+$ MS^E, centroid: - Function 1, low energy, 5 eV - Function 2, high energy, ramping from 10 to 30 eV	ESI$^+$ MS/MS DDA, centroid: - Transition from MS to MS/MS and MS/MS to MS when ion intensity becomes higher than 500,000/s and lower than 10,000/s (or after 10 s), respectively - Collision energy ramping from 15 to 35 eV
Source temperature		120 °C
Desolvation temperature		500 °C
Gas flow rate of the cone		50 L/h
Desolvation gas flow rate		300 L/h
Capillary voltage		3 kV
Sampling cone voltage		35 V
Source offset		80 V
Acquisition mass range	50–1200 m/z (0.5 scans/s)	50–2500 m/z (0.5 scans/s)
Lock-mass	Leucine Enkephaline (MW = 555.62 Da,1 ng/µL) with a flow-rate of 5 µL/min	

The sequence elucidation of peptides obtained in the H-PROT-1 (t1h) fraction was carried out after filtration of a 10 mg/mL sample aqueous solution on a 50 kDa membrane (Amicon Ultra 0.5 mL centrifugal filters, Merck) and analyzed using the same UHPLC-HRMS system. Analyses were performed according to the UHPLC and MS parameters given in Table 3.

The acquisitions and data processing were carried out using the Waters "Mass Lynx 4.1 version" software. The peptide sequences were checked using "Fragment ion calculator" software online (Institute for Systems Biology, Seatle, WA, USA), after the MS/MS fragmentation analysis.

3.2.6. SDS-PAGE

SDS-PAGE was carried out using a Protean II xi cell electrophoresis unit from BIORAD (Hercules, CA, USA) with a stacking gel of 5% (w/v) and a separating gel of 17% (w/v) acrylamide in Tris-HCl 25 mM, pH 8.3, glycine 0.18 M and SDS 0.1% (w/v). The separation was performed at 75 mA for 2 h. The protein bands were stained by Coomasie brilliant blue. The size markers (10–250 kDa) were purchased from Precision Plus Protein™ Standard, BIORAD (Hercules, CA, USA).

3.2.7. Cell Culture

Cells were cultured in EMEM supplemented with 10% (v/v) fetal bovine serum and 1% (v/v) antibiotic solution (10,000 U/mL penicillin, 10 mg/mL streptomycin), used as the complete culture medium. Cell lines 1059 and 1090 were cultured in a temperature-controlled humidified incubator with 5% CO_2 at 37 °C. The cells were grown in 75 cm^2 ventilated Falcon culture flasks (BD Biosciences, Franklin Lakes, NJ, USA) and subcultured by trypsinization (0.05% (w/v) trypsin, PAN Biotech, Aidenbach, Germany). The culture medium was changed every two or three days. Cells were used between the third and ninth passages for the experiments.

3.2.8. Cell Viability

The MTT assay was used according to the method described by Mosmann [47]. This is a colorimetric assay allowing assessing cell viability, based on the reduction of a yellow tetrazolium salt, 3-(4,5-dimethylthiazol-2-yl)-2,5-diphenyltetrazolium bromide (MTT), by viable cells. In the presence of mitochondrial succinate dehydrogenase found in active living cells, the tetrazolium ring of MTT is reduced and forms a violet product, formazan. The yellow solution becomes purple and the intensity of the purple coloration is proportional to the number of viable cells. The MTT test is used to determine cell growth and cell viability.

Briefly, cells were seeded in 96-well Falcon microplates (BD Biosciences, Franklin Lakes, NJ, USA) at 5×10^4 cells/mL in 100 µL of complete culture medium and incubated for 24 h. The medium was then removed and 100 µL of PROT-1 or H-PROT-1 (at 10, 100 or 500 µg/mL) prepared in complete culture medium was added in the wells. After 48 h, 25 µL of MTT (5% (w/v) in PBS) was added in each well and the microplates were incubated for 4 h at 37 °C. The medium was then removed and 200 µL of dimethyl sulfoxide was added in each well. The microplates were then incubated for 10 min prior to absorbance reading at 550 nm using a Fluostar Omega microplate reader (BMG LABTECH, Ortenberg, Germany).

3.2.9. LDH Assay

This method is based on the fact that, during cell death, the loss of the cell membrane integrity leads to the release of cytoplasmic enzymes, such as lactate dehydrogenase (LDH), into the extra-cellular medium. It measures the activity of LDH released by damaged cells in the cell supernatant, good marker of cell death [48].

LDH release was measured with a commercially available LDH assay kit (Cytotoxicity Detection Kit, Roche, France), following the supplier's instructions. Briefly, LDH that is released in the cell environment reduces NAD^+ into NADH and H^+ through the oxidation of lactate into pyruvate. Thereafter, a catalyst (diaphorase) transfers H/H^+ from NADH and H^+ to a tetrazolium salt (iodonitrotetrazolium, INT), to form a red colored formazan salt. The absorbance of the red colored formazan salt produced was measured at 492 nm using a Fluostar Omega microplate reader (BMG LABTECH, Ortenberg, Germany).

3.2.10. Collagen Quantification

NHDF were seeded at a density of 5×10^4 cells/well in 24-well culture microplates in complete culture medium. After 24 h, the medium was removed and 500 µL of PROT-1 or H-PROT-1 (at 10, 100 or 500 µg/mL) or a negative or positive control in EMEM containing 1% (v/v) antibiotic solution was added in each well. The microplates were incubated for 48 h at 37 °C and the collagen production was then measured using the Sirius Red staining procedure [49]. Briefly, the medium was removed and the cells were washed twice with PBS and then fixed for 1 h with 1 mL of Bouin's solution at RT. Following fixation, the Bouin's solution was removed and cells were washed twice with deionized water. The cells were then stained with 1 mL of Sirius Red solution (0.5 g of Sirius Red 80 in 500 mL of saturated aqueous solution of picric acid) for 1 h under stirring at RT. Samples were then washed successively with deionized water and 0.01 M HCl to remove unbound dye. The bound dye was finally solubilized in 500 µL of 0.1 M NaOH for 1 h under stirring and absorbance was read at 550 nm using a Fluostar Omega microplate reader (BMG LABTECH, Ortenberg, Germany).

Results were then expressed as the mean relative percentage of collagen production, compared to the negative control, using the following equations:

$$collagen\ production\ per\ well\ (\%) = \frac{[collagen]_{sample}}{[collagen]_{negative\ control}} \times 100 \qquad (1)$$

$$collagen\ production\ per\ cell\ (\%) = \frac{collagen\ production\ per\ well\ (\%)}{cell\ viability\ (\%)} \times 100 \qquad (2)$$

3.2.11. Hyaluronic Acid Quantification

Hyaluronic acid produced and secreted by fibroblasts in the extra-cellular medium was quantified using an ELISA-like hyaluronic acid assay plate (R&D Systems, Minneapolis, MN, USA). Briefly, cells were seeded at 5×10^4 cells/mL in 100 µL of complete culture medium in 96-well Falcon microplates (BD Biosciences, Franklin Lakes, NJ, USA) and cultured for 24 h. The medium was then removed and 150 µL of positive (10 µg/mL of TGF-β) or negative control prepared in incomplete culture medium, was added in the wells. After 48 h, the hyaluronic acid concentration in the supernatants was measured according to the manufacturer's instructions.

Results were then expressed as the mean relative percentage of hyaluronic acid production, compared to the negative control, using the following equations:

$$hyaluronic\ acid\ production\ per\ well\ (\%) = \frac{[hyaluronic\ acid]_{sample}}{[hyaluronic\ acid]_{negative\ control}} \times 100 \qquad (3)$$

$$hyaluronic\ acid\ production\ per\ cell\ (\%) = \frac{hyaluronic\ acid\ production\ per\ well\ (\%)}{cell\ viability\ (\%)} \times 100 \qquad (4)$$

3.2.12. Statistical Analysis

All data are presented as means ± standard deviations of at least triplicates. The student's t-test (independent, two-sided) was used to determine significant differences between experimental and control samples, using Sigma Plot 12.5 (Systat Software Inc., San Jose, CA, USA).

4. Conclusions

In this study, a protein-rich fraction extracted from *Ulva intestinalis* (PROT-1) was produced using an acid- and solvent-free procedure. PROT-1 contained various sets of proteins. The major one exhibited a MW close to 25 kDa. We showed that the PROT-1 fraction significantly increased in vitro collagen and hyaluronic acid production by normal human dermal fibroblasts and that these increased productions were not due to an increase in cell number but rather to an activation of cell metabolism related to collagen and hyaluronic acid biosynthesis. We also concluded that the molecular weight significantly influenced this bioactivity. Indeed, H-PROT-1 fractions, which were the enzymatic hydrolysates of the PROT-1 fraction, had no effect on fibroblast proliferation and did not stimulate collagen and hyaluronic acid biosynthesis, compared to PROT-1. Moreover, the collagen and hyaluronic acid productions were decreased in presence of some H-PROT-1 fractions, proving the protein or polypeptide origin of the pro-collagen and pro-hyaluronic acid activities of the PROT-1 fraction.

This fraction could thus be of significant interest for skin care prevention or treatment as it significantly promotes in vitro collagen and hyaluronic acid biosynthesis by dermal fibroblasts without activating cell proliferation. In vitro assessment of these pro-collagen and pro-hyaluronic acid activities, as well as cytotoxicity, are a fundamental and essential step to develop ingredients with anti-aging potential. However, according to European Cosmetic guidelines, the evaluation of cosmetics should mix instrumental measurements from both in vitro and ex vivo/in vivo model systems [50]. To further envisage the commercial human application of the PROT-1 fraction, it would consequently have to undergo ex vivo and in vivo experiments. Firstly, noninvasive ex vivo assays on reconstructed human skin models could be performed, to measure percutaneous absorption, cell renewal and/or synthesis and degradation of the MEC and its constituents, collagens and hyaluronic acid in particular. Secondly, in vivo tests might be carried out on a panel of representative volunteers, starting from a neutral and stable formulation, to determine its tolerability in terms of cutaneous (patch test) or ocular irritation, the sensation felt after applying, and its effectiveness (measurement of mechanical properties of the skin such as density, firmness, elasticity and moisture; assessment of depth and volume of wrinkles; analysis of the epidermis microrelief).

Author Contributions: Conceptualization, J.B., A.A., D.D., S.B., T.M. and N.B.; Methodology, J.B., A.A., P.-E.B. and N.B.; Software, J.B., A.A., P.-E.B. and N.B.; Validation, A.A., D.D., S.B., T.M. and N.B.; Formal Analysis, A.A., T.M. and N.B.; Investigation, J.B., A.A. and P.-E.B.; Resources, J.B., A.A., D.D., S.B., T.M. and N.B.; Data Curation, J.B., A.A., P.-E.B. and N.B.; Writing—Original Draft Preparation, J.B., A.A., T.M. and N.B.; Writing—Review & Editing, A.A. and N.B.; Visualization, J.B., A.A., D.D., S.B., T.M. and N.B.; Supervision, A.A., D.D., S.B., T.M. and N.B.; Project Administration, D.D., S.B., T.M. and N.B.; Funding Acquisition, D.D., S.B., T.M. and N.B. All authors have read and agreed to the published version of the manuscript.

Funding: This research was supported by the "Association nationale de la recherche et de la technologie", by providing a part of a PhD funding (Grant number 2016/1032).

Acknowledgments: We are very grateful to the "Association nationale de la recherche et de la technologie", for contributing to this work by providing a part of a PhD funding.

Conflicts of Interest: The authors declare no conflict of interest.

Abbreviations

RT	room temperature
ECM	extracellular matric
HA	hyaluronic acid
MMP	matrix metalloproteinase
TIMP	tissue inhibitor of metalloproteinase
SM	size markers
HPL-SEC	high-performance liquid size-exclusion chromatography
MTT	3-(4,5-dimethylthiazol-2-yl)-2,5-diphenyltetrazolium bromide
LDH	lactate dehydrogenase
TGF-β	transforming growth factor beta
AP-1	activator protein 1
NF-κB	nuclear factor-kappa B
EDTA	ethylenediaminetetraacetic acid

References

1. Kammeyer, A.; Luiten, R.M. Oxidation events and skin aging. *Ageing Res. Rev.* **2015**, *21*, 16–29. [CrossRef] [PubMed]
2. Farage, M.A.; Miller, K.W.; Elsner, P.; Maibach, H.I. Intrinsic and extrinsic factors in skin ageing: A review. *Int. J. Cosmet. Sci.* **2008**, *30*, 87–95. [CrossRef] [PubMed]
3. Naylor, E.C.; Watson, R.E.B.; Sherratt, M.J. Molecular aspects of skin ageing. *Maturitas* **2011**, *69*, 249–256. [CrossRef] [PubMed]
4. Necas, J.; Bartosikova, L.; Brauner, P.; Kolar, J. Hyaluronic acid (hyaluronan): A review. *Vet. Med. (Praha)* **2008**, *53*, 397–411. [CrossRef]
5. Manuskiatti, W.; Maibach, H.I. Hyaluronic acid and skin: Wound healing and aging. *Int. J. Dermatol.* **1996**, *35*, 539–544. [CrossRef]
6. Shoulders, M.D.; Raines, R.T. Collagen structure and stability. *Annu. Rev. Biochem.* **2009**, *78*, 929–958. [CrossRef]
7. Boisnic, S.; Branchet, M.-C. Vieillissement cutané chronologique. *EMC Dermatol. Cosmétol.* **2005**, *2*, 232–241. [CrossRef]
8. Rittié, L.; Fisher, G.J. UV-light-induced signal cascades and skin aging. *Ageing Res. Rev.* **2002**, *1*, 705–720. [CrossRef]
9. Balboa, E.M.; Conde, E.; Soto, M.L.; Pérez-Armada, L.; Domínguez, H. Cosmetics from Marine Sources. In *Springer Handbook of Marine Biotechnology*; Kim, S.-K., Ed.; Springer Handbooks; Springer: Berlin/Heidelberg, Germany, 2015; pp. 1015–1042, ISBN 978-3-642-53971-8.
10. Couteau, C.; Coiffard, L. Chapter 14—Seaweed application in cosmetics. In *Seaweed in Health and Disease Prevention*; Fleurence, J., Levine, I., Eds.; Academic Press: San Diego, CA, USA, 2016; pp. 423–441, ISBN 978-0-12-802772-1.
11. Fleurence, J. Seaweed proteins: Biochemical, nutritional aspects and potential uses. *Trends Food Sci. Technol.* **1999**, *10*, 25–28. [CrossRef]
12. van den Burg, S.; Stuiver, M.; Veenstra, F.; Bikker, P.; López-Contreras, A.; Palstra, A.; Broeze, J.; Jansen, H.; Jak, R.; Gerritsen, A.; et al. *A Triple P Review of the Feasibility of Sustainable Offshore Seaweed Production in the North Sea*; Wageningen University & Research Centre: Wageningen, The Netherlands, 2013; ISBN 978-90-8615-652-8.
13. Holdt, S.L.; Kraan, S. Bioactive compounds in seaweed: Functional food applications and legislation. *J. Appl. Phycol.* **2011**, *23*, 543–597. [CrossRef]
14. Chandini, S.K.; Ganesan, P.; Suresh, P.V.; Bhaskar, N. Seaweeds as a source of nutritionally beneficial compounds—A review. *J. Food Sci. Technol.* **2008**, *45*, 1–13.
15. Silva, M.; Vieira, L.; Almeida, A.P.; Kijjoa, A. The marine macroalgae of the genus *Ulva*: Chemistry, biological activities and potential applications. *J. Oceanogr. Mar. Res.* **2013**, *1*, 1–6. [CrossRef]
16. Adrien, A.; Bonnet, A.; Dufour, D.; Baudouin, S.; Maugard, T.; Bridiau, N. Pilot production of ulvans from *Ulva* sp. and their effects on hyaluronan and collagen production in cultured dermal fibroblasts. *Carbohydr. Polym.* **2017**, *157*, 1306–1314. [CrossRef]
17. Adrien, A.; Dufour, D.; Baudouin, S.; Maugard, T.; Bridiau, N. Evaluation of the anticoagulant potential of polysaccharide-rich fractions extracted from macroalgae. *Nat. Prod. Res.* **2017**, *31*, 2126–2136. [CrossRef]
18. Benjama, O.; Masniyom, P. Nutritional composition and physicochemical properties of two green seaweeds (*Ulva pertusa* and *U. intestinalis*) from the Pattani Bay in Southern Thailand. *Songklanakarin J. Sci. Technol.* **2011**, *33*, 575–583.
19. Majmudar, G. Compositions of Marine Botanicals to Provide Nutrition to Aging and Environmentally Damaged Skin. U.S. Patent No. 7303753B2, 4 December 2007.
20. Baudouin, S.; Dufour, D.; Yao, J. Treating Algae by Diffusing Algae in Water, Filtering Pulp, Ultrafiltration of Pressing Juice, Demineralizing Ultrafiltration Retentate and Decanting Demineralized Retentate, and Recovering Vegetable Protein and Sulfated Polysaccharide. F.R. Patent No. 2998894B1, 31 July 2015.
21. Shuuluka, D.; Bolton, J.J.; Anderson, R.J. Protein content, amino acid composition and nitrogen-to-protein conversion factors of *Ulva rigida* and *Ulva capensis* from natural populations and *Ulva lactuca* from an aquaculture system, in South Africa. *J. Appl. Phycol.* **2013**, *25*, 677–685. [CrossRef]
22. Wijesekara, I.; Lang, M.; Marty, C.; Gemin, M.-P.; Boulho, R.; Douzenel, P.; Wickramasinghe, I.; Bedoux, G.; Bourgougnon, N. Different extraction procedures and analysis of protein from *Ulva* sp. in Brittany, France. *J. Appl. Phycol.* **2017**, *29*, 2503–2511. [CrossRef]

23. Lewis, E.J.; Gonzalves, E.A. Amino acid contents of some marine algae from Bombay. *New Phytol.* **1960**, *59*, 109–115. [CrossRef]
24. Lewis, E.J.; Gonzalves, E.A. Periodic studies of the proteins, peptides, and free amino-acids in *Enteromorpha prolifera f. capillaris* and *Ulva lactuca* var. *rigida. Ann. Bot.* **1962**, *26*, 318–327. [CrossRef]
25. Wang, L.; Wang, X.; Wu, H.; Liu, R. Overview on biological activities and molecular characteristics of sulfated polysaccharides from marine green algae in recent years. *Mar. Drugs* **2014**, *12*, 4984–5020. [CrossRef]
26. Abdel-fattah, A.F.; Sary, H.H. Glycoproteins from *Ulva lactuca. Phytochemistry* **1987**, *26*, 1447–1448. [CrossRef]
27. Rouxel, C.; Bonnabeze, E.; Daniel, A.; Jérôme, M.; Etienne, M.; Fleurence, J. Identification by SDS PAGE of green seaweeds (*Ulva* and *Enteromorpha*) used in the food industry. *J. Appl. Phycol.* **2001**, *13*, 215–218. [CrossRef]
28. Girardeau-Hubert, S.; Teluob, S.; Pageon, H.; Asselineau, D. The reconstructed skin model as a new tool for investigating *in vitro* dermal fillers: Increased fibroblast activity by hyaluronic acid. *Eur. J. Dermatol.* **2015**, *25*, 312–322. [CrossRef]
29. Mast, B.A.; Diegelmann, R.F.; Krummel, T.M.; Cohen, I.K. Hyaluronic acid modulates proliferation, collagen and protein synthesis of cultured fetal fibroblasts. *Matrix* **1993**, *13*, 441–446. [CrossRef]
30. Schwach-Abdellaoui, K.; Malle, B.M. Compositions with Several Hyaluronic Acid Fractions for Cosmetic Use. W.O. Patent No. 2008003321A3, 13 March 2008.
31. Turley, E. Topically Administered, Skin-Penetrating Glycosaminoglycan Formulations Suitable for Use in Cosmetic and Pharmaceutical Applications. W.O. Patent No. 2011140630A1, 17 November 2011.
32. Kmail, A.; Lyoussi, B.; Zaid, H.; Saad, B. *In vitro* assessments of cytotoxic and cytostatic effects of *Asparagus aphyllus*, *Crataegus aronia*, and *Ephedra alata* in monocultures and co-cultures of Hepg2 and THP-1-derived macrophages. *Pharmacogn. Commun.* **2015**, *5*, 165–172. [CrossRef]
33. Ko, H.J.; Kim, G.B.; Lee, D.H.; Lee, G.S.; Pyo, H.B. The effect of hydrolyzed Jeju *Ulva pertusa* on the proliferation and type I collagen synthesis in replicative senescent fibroblasts. *J. Soc. Cosmet. Sci. Korea* **2013**, *39*, 177–186. [CrossRef]
34. Montanari, D.; Guglielmo, M. Cosmetic Composition with a Lifting Effect for Sustaining Relaxed Skin tissues. W.O. Patent No. 2008146116A2, 4 December 2008.
35. Honma, Y.; Kikuchi, K.; Uemura, H.; Inaoka, S.; Tsunetsugu, S. Peptides that Increase Collagen or Hyaluronic acid Production. U.S. Patent No. 7989590B2, 2 August 2011.
36. Joe, M.-J.; Kim, S.-N.; Choi, H.-Y.; Shin, W.-S.; Park, G.-M.; Kang, D.-W.; Kim, Y.K. The inhibitory effects of eckol and dieckol from *Ecklonia stolonifera* on the expression of matrix metalloproteinase-1 in human dermal fibroblasts. *Biol. Pharm. Bull.* **2006**, *29*, 1735–1739. [CrossRef]
37. Chen, C.-L.; Liou, S.-F.; Chen, S.-J.; Shih, M.-F. Protective effects of Chlorella-derived peptide on UVB-induced production of MMP-1 and degradation of procollagen genes in human skin fibroblasts. *Regul. Toxicol. Pharmacol.* **2011**, *60*, 112–119. [CrossRef]
38. Kim, C.-R.; Kim, Y.-M.; Lee, M.-K.; Kim, I.-H.; Choi, Y.-H.; Nam, T.-J. *Pyropia yezoensis* peptide promotes collagen synthesis by activating the TGF-β/Smad signaling pathway in the human dermal fibroblast cell line Hs27. *Int. J. Mol. Med.* **2017**, *39*, 31–38. [CrossRef] [PubMed]
39. Price, R.D.; Berry, M.G.; Navsaria, H.A. Hyaluronic acid: The scientific and clinical evidence. *J. Plast. Reconstr. Aesthet. Surg.* **2007**, *60*, 1110–1119. [CrossRef] [PubMed]
40. Tanimoto, K.; Suzuki, A.; Ohno, S.; Honda, K.; Tanaka, N.; Doi, T.; Yoneno, K.; Ohno-Nakahara, M.; Nakatani, Y.; Ueki, M.; et al. Effects of TGF-β on hyaluronan anabolism in fibroblasts derived from the synovial membrane of the rabbit temporomandibular joint. *J. Dent. Res.* **2004**, *83*, 40–44. [CrossRef] [PubMed]
41. Fayad, S.; Nehmé, R.; Tannoury, M.; Lesellier, E.; Pichon, C.; Morin, P. Macroalga *Padina pavonica* water extracts obtained by pressurized liquid extraction and microwave-assisted extraction inhibit hyaluronidase activity as shown by capillary electrophoresis. *J. Chromatogr. A* **2017**, *1497*, 19–27. [CrossRef]
42. Dubois, M.; Gilles, K.; Hamilton, J.K.; Rebers, P.A.; Smith, F. A colorimetric method for the determination of sugars. *Nature* **1951**, *168*, 167. [CrossRef]
43. Bremner, J.M. Determination of nitrogen in soil by the Kjeldahl method. *J. Agric. Sci.* **1960**, *55*, 11–33. [CrossRef]
44. Lowry, O.H.; Rosebrough, N.J.; Farr, A.L.; Randall, R.J. Protein measurement with the Folin phenol reagent. *J. Biol. Chem.* **1951**, *193*, 265–275.

45. Singleton, V.L.; Rossi, J.A. Colorimetry of total phenolics with phosphomolybdic-phosphotungstic acid reagents. *Am. J. Enol. Vitic.* **1965**, *16*, 144.
46. Chabrol, E.; Charonnat, R. Une nouvelle réaction pour l'étude des lipides: L'oléidemie. *Presse Méd.* **1937**, *45*, 1713–1714.
47. Mosmann, T. Rapid colorimetric assay for cellular growth and survival: Application to proliferation and cytotoxicity assays. *J. Immunol. Methods* **1983**, *65*, 55–63. [CrossRef]
48. Legrand, C.; Bour, J.M.; Jacob, C.; Capiaumont, J.; Martial, A.; Marc, A.; Wudtke, M.; Kretzmer, G.; Demangel, C.; Duval, D.; et al. Lactate dehydrogenase (LDH) activity of the number of dead cells in the medium of cultured eukaryotic cells as marker. *J. Biotechnol.* **1992**, *25*, 231–243. [CrossRef]
49. Tullberg-Reinert, H.; Jundt, G. In situ measurement of collagen synthesis by human bone cells with a Sirius Red-based colorimetric microassay: Effects of transforming growth factor β2 and ascorbic acid 2-phosphate. *Histochem. Cell Biol.* **1999**, *112*, 271–276. [CrossRef]
50. Dreno, B.; Araviiskaia, E.; Berardesca, E.; Bieber, T.; Hawk, J.; Sanchez-Viera, M.; Wolkenstein, P. The science of dermocosmetics and its role in dermatology. *J. Eur. Acad. Dermatol. Venereol. JEADV* **2014**, *28*, 1409–1417. [CrossRef] [PubMed]

Sample Availability: Samples of the PROT-1 and H-PROT-1 fractions are available from the authors.

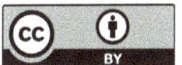

© 2020 by the authors. Licensee MDPI, Basel, Switzerland. This article is an open access article distributed under the terms and conditions of the Creative Commons Attribution (CC BY) license (http://creativecommons.org/licenses/by/4.0/).

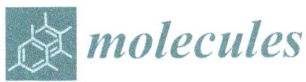

Article

Potential Photoprotective Effect of Dietary Corn Silk Extract on Ultraviolet B-Induced Skin Damage

Yeon-hee Kim [1,†], Amy Cho [1,†], Sang-Ah Kwon [1], Minju Kim [1], Mina Song [1], Hye won Han [1], Eun-Ji Shin [2], Eunju Park [2] and Seung-Min Lee [1,*]

1. Department of Food and Nutrition, BK21 PLUS Project, College of Human Ecology, Yonsei University, Seoul 03722, Korea
2. Department of Food and Nutritional Science, Kyungnam University, Changwon 51767, Korea
* Correspondence: leeseungmin@yonsei.ac.kr; Tel.: +82-2-2123-3118
† These authors contributed equally to this work.

Received: 27 May 2019; Accepted: 15 July 2019; Published: 16 July 2019

Abstract: Ultraviolet B (UVB) irradiation causes adverse effects on the skin. Corn silk contains flavonoids and other bioactive compounds and antioxidants, which may prevent skin photoaging through antioxidant and anti-inflammatory effects. We aimed to investigate the potential photoprotective effects of dietary corn silk on UVB-induced skin damage in mice and the mechanisms behind these effects on human skin cells. Oral administration of corn silk water extract (CS) (2 or 4 g/kg/day) for 19 weeks decreased epidermal thickness, wrinkle formation, and positive staining for PCNA, Ki67, and 8-OHdG, and increased collagen staining in UVB-irradiated SKH-1 hairless mice compared with controls. The pro-inflammatory NF-κB target genes (IL-1β, iNOS, and COX-2) and MMP-9 expressions were lower in the CS groups, and TGF-β/Smad signaling increased. Low skin lipid peroxidation and blood DNA oxidation levels and high blood glutathione were detected. Antioxidant transcription factor Nrf2-related catalase and SOD1 proteins and glutaredoxin mRNA levels increased. The results of CS extract treatment and UVB irradiation in HaCaT cells showed the same results in Nrf2 and NF-κB target genes. An LC-MS/MS analysis showed that the CS extract contained potential antioxidants, which might have contributed to its anti-photoaging effects in tissues and cells. CS extract may reduce UVB-induced skin damage through antioxidant and anti-inflammatory mechanisms.

Keywords: corn silk extract; photoaging; ultraviolet B; NF-κB; antioxidant; inflammation

---

1. Introduction

Skin, the largest organ in the human body, acts as a barrier against external pollutants [1]. Skin tissue is constantly exposed to solar ultraviolet (UV) radiation [2]. When the antioxidant defense system is damaged due to ultraviolet B (UVB) exposure of the skin, excessive reactive oxygen species (ROS) are generated at the irradiated sites [3], which results in various changes, including the oxidation of cellular components, DNA mutation, inflammation, and the activation of specific enzymes that degrade the extracellular matrix [4]. These changes can lead to unrestrained cell proliferation [5] and carcinogenesis [3]. Chronic exposure to UV leads to photoaging and even skin cancer [2]. Skin UVB-induced photoaging is associated with distinct clinical features, such as wrinkling and thickening of the epidermis, which is a protective layer of the skin [5,6]. There are also related histological characteristics such as disorganization of collagen in the dermis, which lies below the epidermis, fragmentation, and dispersion [7].

The antioxidant system is thought to protect against cellular damage from UV-induced oxidative stress through the scavenging of ROS or their byproducts [5]. Carotenoids, polyphenols, and vitamins E and C have been shown to act as photo-protective barriers by quenching ROS [8]. The oral administration of natural product extracts, such as French maritime pine (*Pinus pinaster*) bark, Ginkgo biloba [6], green tea (*Camellia sinensis*), and grape seed extracts [8], has been shown to prevent UV-induced skin damage. Thus, the consumption of herbal substances that are rich in antioxidant components, such as polyphenols, might offer protective effects against UVB damage [1].

Corn silk (CS, *Zea mays* L.) has been consumed as a herbal medicine in Korea [9], China, United States, and France for millennia [10]. In folk medicine, it is used for the treatment of cystitis, edema, diabetes mellitus, and prostatitis [10]. CS contains an abundance of phenolic compounds, such as flavonoids (maysin, apigmaysin, luteolin) [11,12], anthocyanins (cyanidin, peonidin) [13], chlorogenic acid, and other biologically active substances, such saponins and allantoin [11,14]. The antioxidant capacity of CS was first reported by Zoran et al., who showed a positive correlation between the polyphenol content and antioxidant activity in aqueous acetone CS extract in vitro [15]. Radical scavenging activity and iron chelating activity of CS extracts were proven in test tube experiments [16,17]. The antioxidant capacities of the CS extract have been implicated in human breast cancer cells [18], human neuroblastoma cells [19], clonal rat pancreatic β-cells [20], and CSP2, a polysaccharide isolated from the CS extract [21]. In animal experiments, ad libitum drinking of CS extract for 28 days in healthy albino mice elevated antioxidant enzyme activities and increased the content of reduced glutathione in the kidney [22]. In another animal study, dietary CS extract rescued a high salt diet-induced reduction in glutathione peroxidase [23] and alleviated radiation-induced oxidative stress in mice [24]. In addition, oral ingestion of CS-extracted flavonoids showed antioxidant effects against oxidative stress under exhaustive exercise [14] and under streptozotocin-induced diabetes [25] in mice.

The effects of CS extracts on UVB-induced damage have not been extensively studied. There were only several cell line experiments using CS constituents [26,27]. Trans-zeatin, purified from corn silk, inhibited UVB-induced MMP-1 expression in skin fibroblasts [26]. Luteolin, another flavonoid found in CS, exerted anticancer effects on UVB-irradiated mouse epidermal cells by suppressing cyclooxygenase (COX) expression and NF-κB activity [27]. The role of dietary CS extract on UVB-damaged skin and its antioxidant mechanism are still not clear. In our study, we aimed to demonstrate the effect of CS extract on preventing UVB-induced skin damage in mice and further confirm the molecular mechanisms underlying this effect in human skin cells. We hypothesized that the CS extract might contribute to its photoprotective effect through antioxidant and anti-inflammatory pathways. We investigated the effects of the oral administration or treatment of CS extract on UVB-induced damage in SKH-1 hairless mice and human skin HaCaT cells.

2. Results

2.1. DPPH and ABTS Antioxidant Capacities of CS Extract

DPPH (2,2-diphenyl-1-picryl-hydrazyl-hydrate) radical scavenging activities of CS extract varied from 18.99 to 83.92% (Figure 1A). ABTS (2,2′-azino-bis(3-ethylbenzothiazoline-6-sulphonic acid)) assay values ranged from 4.74 to 42.75% (Figure 1B). The half maximal inhibitory concentration (IC_{50}) of CS extract and the standard compound, L-ascorbic acid, in relation to DPPH and ABTS radical scavenging activities (Table 1).

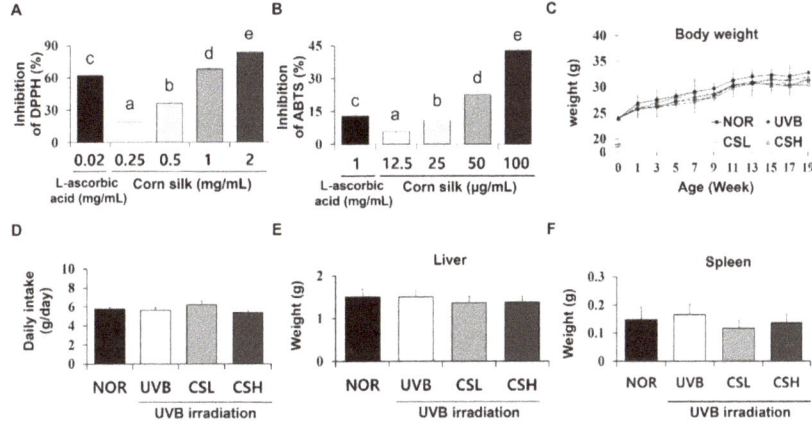

Figure 1. DPPH and ABTS antioxidative assay of corn silk (CS) extracts and the general details of SKH-1 mice during the experiment. Antioxidative effects of CS extracts were determined by DPPH (**A**) and ABTS radical scavenging activity (**B**). For the assays, CS extracts at concentrations of 1.25, 2.5, 5, 10 mg/mL and DPPH or ABTS solution were mixed at a ratio of 1:4 and 1:99. Body weight (**C**), food intake (**D**), liver weight (**E**), and spleen weight (**F**) of the mice were not significantly different across all groups (n = 8~10 per group) including normal control group (NOR), UVB-irradiated group (UVB), UVB-irradiated and low CS- (2 g/kg/day) treated group (CSL), and UVB-irradiated and high CS- (4 g/kg/day) treated group (CSH). Values are mean ± SD. The results were analyzed by one-way analysis of variance (ANOVA) followed by Duncan's post-hoc test. Different lowercase letters over bars (a, b, c, d, e) represent significant statistical differences ($p < 0.05$).

Table 1. IC_{50} values of DPPH and ABTS radical scavenging activities of corn silk (CS) extract and ascorbic acid.

Sample	IC_{50} (mg/mL)	
	DPPH	ABTS
Corn silk extract	3.60 ± 0.1	11.61 ± 0.2
L-ascorbic acid	0.08 ± 0.0	0.38 ± 0.1

Values are represented as mean ± SD of three replicates. Lower values represent higher radical scavenging activity of the corresponding sample.

2.2. Food Intake, Body Weight, and Organ Weights of Animals

Body weights of the mice were not significantly different between groups during the study period (Figure 1C). Mean daily food intake was also similar between groups (Figure 1D). Mouse liver and spleen weights were not significantly different between the groups at sacrifice (Figure 1E,F).

2.3. Effects of CS Extract on Skinfold, Epidermal Thickness, and Wrinkle Formation in UVB-Irradiated Mice

The ANTERA 3D® images of skin replicas of animal groups are presented in Figure 2A. UVB irradiation increased the epidermal thickness of the dorsal skin and the thickness of the skinfold compared with the NOR group (Figure 2B–D). However, administration of the CS extract significantly reduced the epidermal and skinfold thickness in the CSL and CSH groups compared with the UVB group (Figure 2B–D). UVB irradiation increased the values of all parameters related to wrinkle formation, including the volume of depression, the affected area of depression, the maximum valley depth, and the average wrinkle length in comparison to the NOR (Figure 2E–H). These values were significantly decreased in the CSL and CSH groups in comparison to the UVB group (Figure 2E–H).

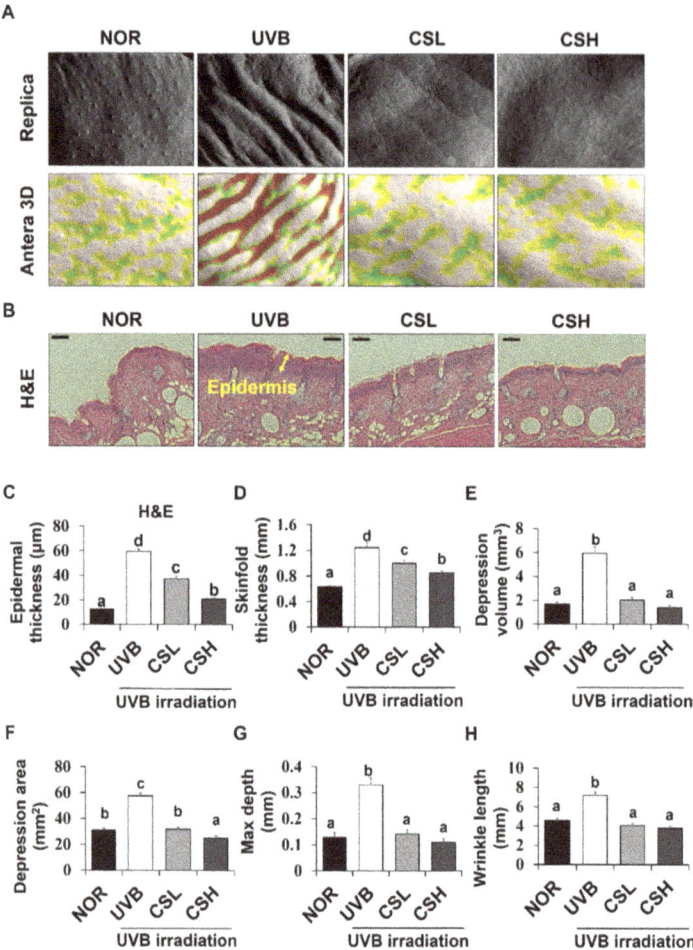

Figure 2. Effects of corn silk (CS) extract on UVB-induced wrinkle formation in the dorsal skin of SKH-1 mice at the end of the study (week 19). Photographs of the replica, replica analysis, and the backs of the mice (**A**), Hematoxylin and eosin-stained sections (original magnification 100×) (**B**), epidermal thickness (**C**), skinfold thickness (**D**), mean of skin wrinkle depression volume (**E**), mean depression area (**F**), maximum depth (**G**), and wrinkle length (**H**) are presented for normal group (NOR), UVB-irradiated group (UVB), UVB-irradiated and low CS- (2 g/kg/day) treated group (CSL), UVB-irradiated and high (4 g/kg/day) CS-treated group (CSH). Values are mean ± SD. The results were analyzed by one-way analysis of variance (ANOVA) followed by Duncan's post-hoc test. Means with different lowercase letters (a, b, c, d) represent statistically significant differences ($p < 0.05$). Bars with the same letters are not significantly different.

2.4. Effect of CS Extract on Epidermal Expression Levels of PCNA and Ki67 in UVB-Irradiated Mice

The cell proliferation levels in the dorsal skin sections of the animal groups were examined by the expression levels of proliferation marker genes PCNA (proliferating cell nuclear antigen) and Ki67 (Figure 3A–D). PCNA- and Ki67-positive cells were localized to the stratum basale (basal layer) between the epidermis and the dermis in the NOR whereas positive staining for PCNA and Ki67 were detected throughout several layers of the epidermis in the UVB group (Figure 3A,B). The positive staining levels of PCNA and Ki67 were significantly decreased in CSL and CSH groups compared with the UVB group (Figure 3C,D). Greatest reductions in the staining levels were detected in the CSH group (Figure 3C,D). The CS extract significantly rescued the UVB-induced increase in PCNA protein levels in mouse dorsal skin tissue (Figure 3E). These data indicated that the CS lessened the UVB-mediated epidermal cell proliferation.

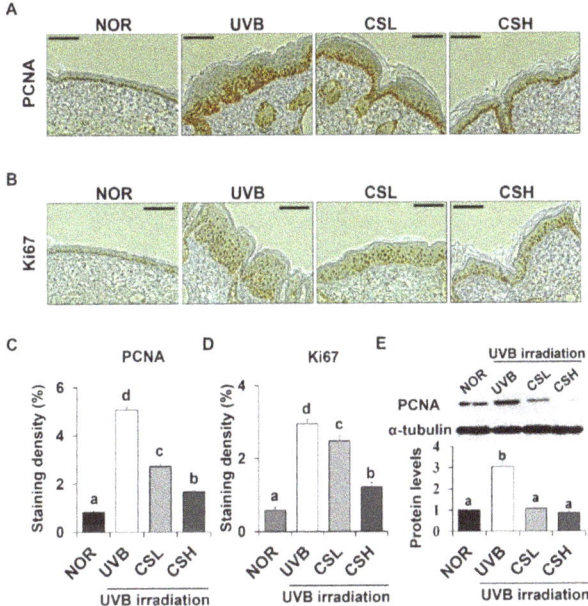

Figure 3. Effect of corn silk (CS) extract on the expression of PCNA and Ki67 in UVB-irradiated hairless mice skin. Representative images of immunohistochemical staining of PCNA (**A**) and Ki-67 (**B**) are shown. Immunostaining of each gene is depicted as brown areas at the original magnification of ×200. PCNA (**C**) and Ki-67 (**D**) were quantified using ImageJ software. Representative Western blot image and protein levels of PCNA (**E**) in mouse skin tissue are shown (repeated five times). Values are mean ± SE of the percentages of positive nuclear staining in the skin tissue or protein levels. The results were analyzed by one-way ANOVA with Duncan's post-hoc test. Bars accompanying different lowercase letters (a, b, c, d) represent statistically significant differences ($p < 0.05$), whereas the same letters represent no significant difference. Group abbreviations: Normal group (NOR), UVB-irradiated group (UVB), UVB-irradiated and low CS- (2 g/kg/day) treated group (CSL), UVB-irradiated and high CS- (4 g/kg/day) treated group (CSH).

2.5. Effect of CS Extract on Skin Collagen Fiber Content in UVB-Irradiated Mice

Skin connective tissue levels were assessed by MT and VVG staining, which detect collagen fibers (Figure 4A,B). Compared with the NOR group, the UVB group showed lower staining levels in both MT and VVG (Figure 4C,D). The CSL and CSH groups partly reverted the UVB-induced loss of the staining density and the CSH showed the strongest staining compared to other groups in both MT and VVG (Figure 4C,D). Next, protein expression levels of matrix metalloproteinase-9 (MMP-9) and Tissue inhibitors of metalloproteinases (TIMP) which regulate extracellular matrix, were examined (Figure 4E,F). Protein levels of MMP-9 and TIMP-1 in the skin were increased by UVB irradiation compared with the NOR group, but CS treatment decreased MMP-9 at both low and high doses and reduced TIMP-1 levels at the high dose (Figure 4E,F). Activation of TGF-β and Smad2/3 signaling pathway was investigated in terms of collagen production [7]. The protein levels of TGF-β were not different between the UVB and the NOR groups, but there were modest elevations of TGF-β only in the CSL and CSH groups compared with the UVB group (Figure 4G). The UVB irradiation lowered phosphorylation levels of Smad2/3 compared with the NOR group, but this reduction was significantly reverted in the CSH while not in the CSL group (Figure 4H). Procollagen type 1 levels significantly increased in the CSH than in the UVB group (Figure 4I). These results suggested that UVB-diminished TGF-β and Smad2/3 signaling pathway were re-activated in the CSH, and possibly in the CSL.

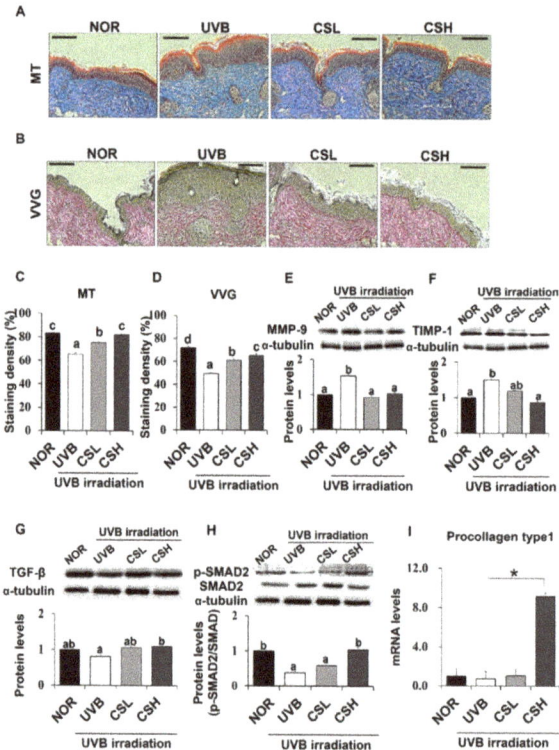

Figure 4. Effect of corn silk (CS) extract on collagen fiber content in UVB-photoaged mouse skin. Collagen fibers were stained with Masson's trichrome (MT) (**A**) and Verhoeffe Van Gieson (VVG) (**B**). Representative histological images of collagen in mouse skin tissue are presented at an original magnification of ×200. Collagen staining by MT and VVG appears blue and red, respectively. Staining density of MT (**C**) and VVG (**D**) are shown, respectively. Western blotting detected MMP-9 (**E**), TIMP-1 (**F**), TGF-β (**G**), p-SMAD2/SMAD2 (**H**), and α-tubulin expression levels in the UVB-irradiated dorsal skin protein extract of hairless mouse by using specific antibodies for each protein. Blot image is a representation of three individual experiments. The blots were quantified using ImageJ software and the signal intensities were normalized to the value of α-tubulin, except for p-SMAD2, which was normalized to the expression of SMAD2. The mRNA expression of procollagen type 1 was assessed by q-PCR analysis and was normalized to the intensity value of GAPDH, quantified using ImageJ (**I**). Values are mean ± SE. Mean values not assigned with the same letter (a, b, c, d) are significantly different, analyzed by ANOVA ($p < 0.05$). Group abbreviations: Normal group (NOR), UVB-irradiated group (UVB), UVB-irradiated and low (2 g/kg/day) CS-treated group (CSL), UVB-irradiated and high (4 g/kg/day) CS-treated group (CSH).

2.6. Effect of CS Extract on Oxidative Stress and Skin Antioxidation Genes

To investigate the effects of CS on UVB-induced oxidative stress, skin and blood oxidative stress-related markers were examined. The UVB group showed significant positive staining of 8-OHdG, an oxidative DNA damage marker, in the skin epidermis compared to the NOR group (Figure 5A,B). However, CS treatment reduced 8-OHdG levels, with a greater reduction in the CSH group (Figure 5A,B). In addition, lipid peroxidation products measured by Thiobarbituric acid reactive substances (TBARS) in the skin were significantly decreased in the CSH group (Figure 5C). UVB also increased the percentage of tail DNA and tail length of PBMC cells, indicating more DNA damage compared with NOR (Figure 5D,E). However, the tail DNA and tail length of PBMC cells were reduced in the CSL and CSH groups (Figure 5D,E). Plasma GSH, an antioxidant molecule, was slightly decreased in the UVB group compared with that in the NOR group ($p = 0.041$), but significantly increased in CSL (Figure 5F). These results indicated that the CS extract decreased UVB-induced skin and blood oxidative damage.

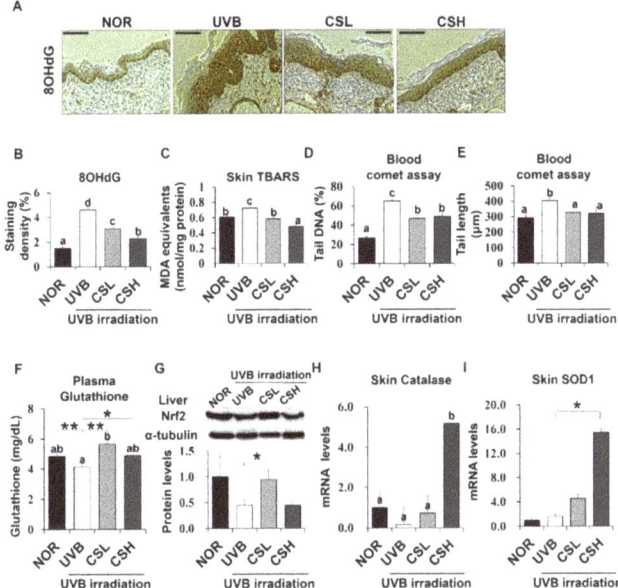

Figure 5. Effect of Corn Silk (CS) extract on antioxidant gene expressions in response to UVB-induced oxidative stress in mouse skin and liver. The UVB-induced formation of DNA/RNA damage marker, 8OHdG, was detected by immunohistochemistry. Representative images (**A**) and quantification (**B**) of the staining are shown. MDA in the skin tissue was measured by the TBARS assay (**C**). Oxidative stress in the blood was determined by the leukocyte comet assay and plasma glutathione concentration. DNA damage was detected by the tail DNA (%) (**D**) and tail length (μm) (**E**). Plasma glutathione (GSH) concentrations were compared (**F**). Nrf2 protein levels were assessed by Western blot and a representative image of the blot is shown (**G**). The mRNA expression of catalase (**H**) and SOD1 (**I**) are shown as assessed by q-PCR. Values are mean ± SE. Values with different letters (a, b, c, d) indicate statistical significance ($p < 0.05$), as analyzed by one-way ANOVA. * $p < 0.05$, ** $p < 0.01$, student t-test. Abbreviations: Normal group (NOR), UVB-irradiated group (UVB), UVB-irradiated and low (2 g/kg/day) CS-treated group (CSL), UVB-irradiated and high (4 g/kg/day) CS-treated group (CSH).

UVB irradiation decreased Nrf2 protein expression in liver tissue, but CSL significantly recovered the UVB-induced loss of Nrf2 levels (Figure 5H). In addition, catalase and SOD1 expression significantly increased in skin tissue CSH compared with the UVB group (Figure 5H,I). As a result, CS reduced UVB-induced oxidative stress in the mouse skin and liver tissues.

2.7. Effect of CS Extract on Skin Inflammatory Gene Expression in UVB-Irradiated Mice

Expression levels of NF-κB target inflammatory genes including iNOS, IL-1β, and COX-2 in UVB-irradiated mouse skin and liver tissue were examined (Figure 6A–D). In mouse skin, iNOS, IL-1β, and COX-2 levels increased in the UVB group compared with the NOR group and decreased in the CS groups compared with the UVB group (Figure 6A–C). In mouse liver, iNOS was decreased in CSL and CSH compared with the UVB group (Figure 6D). Therefore, CS decreased levels of inflammatory gene expression in UVB-irradiated skin and liver tissues.

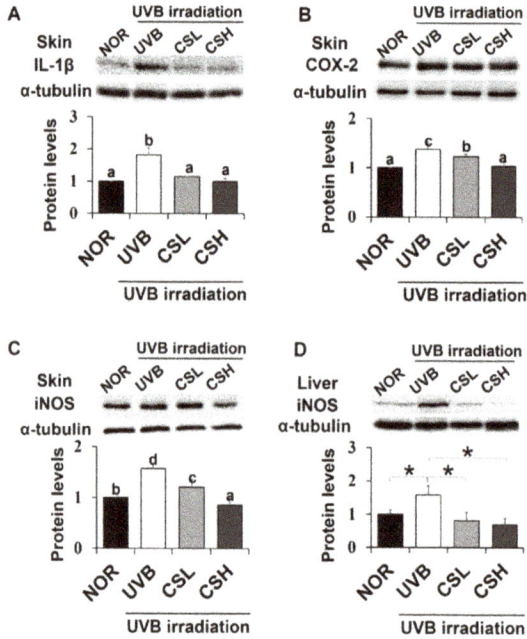

Figure 6. Effect of corn silk (CS) extract on inflammatory gene expressions in UVB-irradiated mice skin and liver. Protein expressions of IL-1β (**A**), COX-2 (**B**), and iNOS (**C**) in mouse skin, and iNOS in mouse liver (**D**) were assessed by Western blot analysis and their representative images of multiple independent experiments ($n = 3$) are presented. Protein results of iNOS in mouse liver is shown in (**F**) and its representative blot image is shown in (**E**). Results are expressed as mean ± SE. Mean values sharing different letters (a, b, c, d) over bars are significantly different ($p < 0.05$), as analyzed by ANOVA. * $p < 0.05$, student t-test.

2.8. Effect of CS Extract on UVB-Irradiated Human Keratinocytes

Additional experiments were carried out on the human HaCaT keratinocyte cell line to further examine the mechanism of the CS extract's photoprotective effect on skin. First, MTT assay was performed to investigate the cytotoxic effect of UVB and CS extract on HaCaT cells. A 24-h treatment of CS extract did not show cytotoxicity at concentrations up to 5 μg/mL (Figure 7A). UVB irradiation above 30 mJ/cm^2 significantly inhibited cell growth in a concentration-dependent manner (Figure 7B). Therefore, the UVB dose for cell experiments was set as 30 mJ/cm^2. In accordance with these results, CS treatment on 30 mJ/cm^2 UVB-irradiated cells did not show cytotoxicity up to 5 μg/mL (Figure 7C).

Based on this data, 5 μg/mL was defined as the higher concentration (CSH), and a ten-fold dilution of 0.5 μg/mL was determined as the lower concentration (CSL).

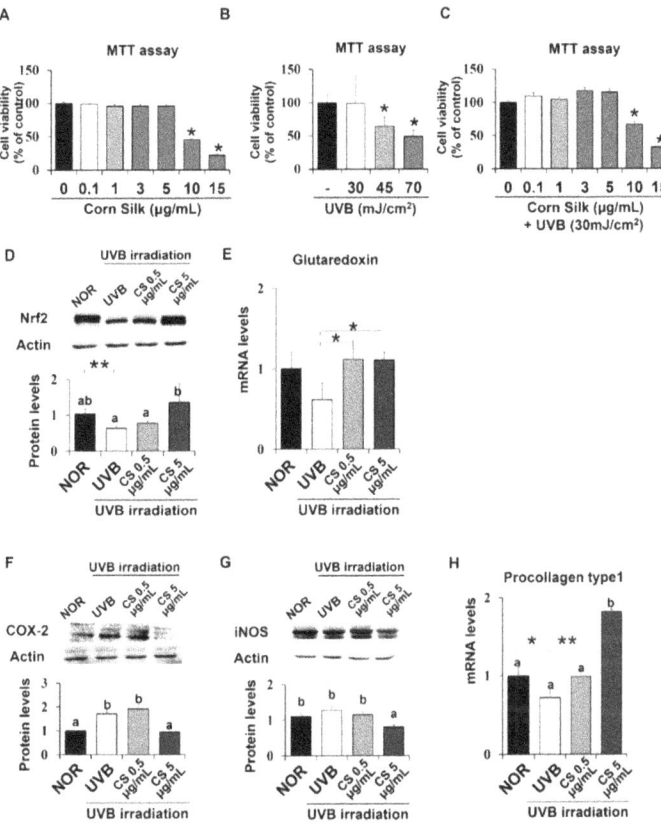

Figure 7. Viability of CS- or UVB treated HaCaT cells and CS effect on antioxidant and anti-inflammatory gene expressions in HaCaT cells. MTT assays showed the viability of HaCaT cells after exposure to either CS extract (**A**), only UVB (**B**), or both UVB and CS extract treatment (**C**). Protein levels of Nrf2 (**D**) were analyzed by Western blot and the representative images of the blot (three repetitions) are shown. Protein levels of COX-2 (**F**) and iNOS (**G**) were analyzed by Western blot and the blot images represent three repetitions. mRNA levels of Glutaredoxin (**E**), a target of Nrf2, and procollagen type 1 (**H**) was analyzed by qPCR and normalized to GAPDH. Results are mean ± SE. Different lowercase letters (a, b) represent statistical difference, as analyzed by ANOVA ($p < 0.05$). * $p < 0.05$, ** $p < 0.01$, student t-test.

Expression levels of Nrf2 were confirmed in human skin cells, which showed similar positive effects of CS extract as did in mice. Nrf2 protein level was significantly reduced by UVB irradiation but recovered by CS treatment at 5 μg/mL (Figure 7D). Nrf2 target gene, glutaredoxin, showed similar regulation by CS treatment at both 0.5 and 5 μg/mL (Figure 7E). NF-κB target inflammatory genes, including COX-2 and iNOS, were also examined in UVB-irradiated epithelial HaCaT cells. COX-2 and iNOS were significantly decreased in the UVB group treated with CS 5 ug/mL compared with the non-CS treated UVB group (Figure 7F,G). Procollagen type 1 mRNA level was significantly improved in both doses of CS extract compared with the UVB group (Figure 7H). Overall, the CS extract improved Nrf2 signaling and alleviated inflammatory gene expression levels in UVB-irradiated HaCaT cells.

2.9. Metabolite Identification in CS Using LC-MS/MS

LC-MS/MS analysis revealed putative detection of 6083 peaks in the CS extract, and the top 100 peaks in the order of peak intensities were listed in Supplementary Materials (Table S1). The peak numbers below in parentheses indicate the order of the metabolites detected in the CS extract from highest to lowest peak intensities. Out of the top 100 peaks in the CS extract, the top 30 metabolites were further identified whether they exhibit antioxidant and/or anti-inflammatory effects based on previous studies. Indole (1st peak), 3-(3-hydroxyphenyl)propanoic acid (2nd peak), and proline betaine (7th peak) were revealed as the three most abundant metabolites in the CS extract that exhibit antioxidant and/or anti-inflammatory effects (Table S1). This suggested that the CS contained antioxidant compounds might have contributed to the antioxidant effect in skin protection. In mice, skin metabolites were compared between NOR, UVB, CSL and CSH groups (Figure S1A). Five hundred eight metabolites were altered in the CS groups compared to the UVB group (Figure S1B). Metabolites found in the CS extract were also detected in among the 161 up-regulated metabolites in the skin of CS groups compared with the UVB group. These included proline betaine (7th peak), L-proline (in the form of L-phenylalanyl-L-proline, 11th peak), L-phenylalanine (in the form of L-Aspartyl-L-phenylalanine, 13th peak), phytosphingosine (14th peak), nicotinic acid (in the form of 6-Hydroxynicotinic acid, 23rd peak), ascorbic acid (in the form of dehydroascorbic acid, 28th peak), and vitamin A (29th peak) in the order of highest to lowest peak intensities. These seven metabolites were previously implicated in the antioxidant and/or anti-inflammatory roles.

3. Discussion

In the present study, we demonstrated that the CS water extract ameliorated the hyperproliferation of UVB-induced skin epithelial tissues and wrinkle formation in addition to preserving epidermal collagen content in UVB-irradiated SKH-1 hairless mice. CS extract was also effective in the alteration of Nrf2 and NF-κB target inflammatory genes, which are influenced by oxidative stress, in mouse skin and human skin cells. These anti-UVB effects appeared to be mediated by the antioxidant and anti-inflammatory effects of CS, as shown in mice and in HaCaT cells.

The UVB-induced skin changes, including skinfold thickness, wrinkle depression volume and epidermal thickness, were ameliorated conspicuously in the CS-treated groups. Reduction in skin photoaging in the CS groups appeared to be due to inhibition of aberrant UVB-induced hyper-proliferation because significant reductions in proliferation markers were detected in the skin of the CS groups. Moreover, prolonged UV exposure in the skin is known to trigger cell proliferation with damaged DNA [1]. However, oral administration of the CS markedly decreased hyperproliferation and DNA damage.

The collagen content in the dermis, which lies below the epidermis, confers resilience and strength to the skin [28]. Continuous UV exposure can lead to the loss of collagen through the reduction in the production of type 1 collagen and increased activities of MMP [28]. In our study, MT and VVG staining showed that collagen fiber was greatly reduced in mice exposed to UVB, but a significant recovery was observed after treatment with CS or its components. The impairment of collagen synthesis by UV irradiation occurs via interference in the TGF-β and Smad2/3 signaling pathway in the skin [3,29]. These aberrations result in a reduction in the phosphorylation of Smad2/3, which consequently decreases the transcription of type 1 procollagen [29]. Remarkable reactivation of TGF-β and Smad2/3 signaling pathway was achieved by the CS in UVB-irradiated mice, suggesting that the synthesis of type 1 procollagen might have been recovered by the CS. Similar results were shown in HaCaT cells, where the CS extract significantly increased the low mRNA levels of procollagen type 1 in UVB-irradiated cells. In addition, expression of MMP-9, which displays proteolytic activities and degrades the extracellular matrix containing collagen and elastin [4], was inhibited by the CS groups. As seen in the CSH group, reduction in TIMP-1, a major inhibitor of MMP-9 [30], might have reflected the condition of lowered MMP-9 to balance the activities of MMPs and TIMPs. Overall the CS prevented the UVB-induced loss of collagen fibers possibly by activating TGF-β and Smad2/3 signaling and inhibiting MMP-9 expression.

Chronic UVB radiation on skin causes accumulation of ROS, adjacent and tumoral oxidative stress, and oxidative damage [31]. As previously investigated by analytical methods, CS itself or its components exert antioxidant capacities [15–17,32]. Antioxidative effects of our CS water extract were in accordance with these studies, showing a dose-dependent increase in radical scavenging capacity. The effects were far lower than that of ascorbic acid, therefore the CS extract may not be considered as a direct antioxidant, but a potential material exerting positive effects on skin protection perhaps with the synergistic effects of various compounds identified in the literature [11–14]. The radical scavenging activities detected in the CS extract were in agreement with an increase in the murine blood levels of GSH, an antioxidant molecule. GSH acts as a direct scavenger of free radicals [33]. Oxidative stress levels in both blood and skin were lessened by the CS, as shown by the results of the skin 8OHdG, TBARS, and blood comet assays. These antioxidant effects seen in the skin were especially exciting considering that the CS extract was orally administered instead of being applied topically. The UV exposure is known to disturb the antioxidant systems in the body other than the skin and increase oxidative stress markers in the liver and blood [34]. The antioxidative effects observed in the skin tissue and blood might have indicated that the CS reached the skin and blood circulation system and played protective roles in the UVB-induced oxidative stress conditions. Similarly, other studies reported that the oral administration of polyphenol-rich plant extracts prevented UV-induced lipid peroxidation in skin and DNA damage in peripheral blood [35]. The administration of natural food extracts was able to restore the blood GSH concentration in a diabetic animal model [36].

Nrf2 is a major regulator of antioxidant responses in cellular level through antioxidant response element (ARE)-mediated transcriptional regulation [37]. Nrf2-deficient mice have shown accelerated oxidative skin damage and photoaging in response to UVB radiation but no difference in carcinogenesis, suggesting that Nrf2 system may play an essential role in relieving UVB-induced oxidative stress in skin [38,39]. Catalase and SOD1 are well known antioxidant enzymes that neutralize excess reactive oxygen species in cells [40]. SOD1 is a direct ROS quencher and its promoter is known to contain Nrf2-ARE binding site [41]. No ARE site has been found in catalase promoter region so direct binding of Nrf2 remains controversial [42], but Nrf2-dependent expression of catalase has been shown in mouse-derived cells [43,44]. We showed that CS extract increased Nrf2 protein in liver tissue and in HaCaT cells, suggesting a positive role of CS in the antioxidant pathway. In accordance with the activation of Nrf2 protein, catalase and SOD1 increased in skin tissue compared with the UVB group. Another Nrf2-regulated antioxidant, glutaredoxin, was reported to alleviate oxidative stress in human retinal pigment epithelial cells [45,46]. We showed that the CS extract significantly improved the mRNA levels compared with that of the UVB group in HaCaT cells. The Nrf2-mediated antioxidant enzyme regulation could have contributed to the photoprotective effect of the CS extract on UVB-irradiated skin. Although we expected CS dose-dependent increases in Nrf-2 protein levels in both animal and cell experiments, we only observed these effects in the cells. The reasons we observed no further increase in protein level of Nrf2 in CSH group could include possible toxic effects of a high dose of CSH itself or effects of negative feedback mechanism after CS intake. According to Heo et al., Nrf2 protein is degraded after antioxidant enzymes [47]. In another study, with increased UVB irradiation, HaCaT cells have been reported to exclude Nrf2 from the nucleus, compared with lower doses of UVB where nuclear translocation was increased [48]. Thus, the Nrf2 protein in the CSH group may have shown no increase due to tight regulation of this protein and possible negative feedback mechanism.

ROS induced by UVB radiation triggers signaling molecules such as NF-κB, a major regulator of pro-inflammatory genes including iNOS [49]. Inflammatory response caused by UVB-irradiated skin activates the transcription of MMPs, which degrade the dermal collagen and connective tissue in skin [3]. UVB irradiation significantly activated NF-κB signaling, which in turn was blocked only by the higher dose of CS. In contrast, IL-1β and iNOS, which are well-known NF-κB targets [50,51], were successfully downregulated by the CS regardless of the doses in skin and liver tissues. On the other hand COX-2, another NF-κB target [51], was only lowered by the higher dose of CS. In HaCaT cells iNOS was only decreased in the higher dose of CS extract. Collectively, the photoprotective effects of CS might have been involved in the inhibition of UVB-activated NF-κB signaling pathway, leading to the reduction in the expression of proinflammatory genes and MMP-9.

Metabolites both up-regulated in the skin of the CS group and found in the top 100 peaks in CS extract included proline betaine, L-proline, L-phenylalanine, phytosphingosine, nicotinic acid, ascorbic acid, and vitamin A, in the highest to lowest peak intensity order. Proline and glycine betaine are antioxidants that also protect plants from dehydration [52], salt stress, and cell death [53]. L-phenylalanine exerts lipophilic antioxidant capacity as tested by DPPH and ABTS assays [54] and anti-inflammatory effects on carrageenan-induced edema [55]. Phytosphingosine, an active lipid abundant in both plants and animals, constitutes the stratum corneum (outer layer of skin) and exhibits anti-inflammatory effect and defense against microbes [56]. Phytosphingosine-1-phosphate has been reported to promote epidermal growth factor in human dermal fibroblasts, and promotes anti-aging effects in human skin [57]. Nicotinic acid, known as vitamin B_3, stimulates keratinocyte differentiation, stabilizes epidermal barrier function, and benefits aging skin by reducing wrinkles and exerting anti-photocarcinogenesis effects [58]. In addition, nicotinic acid has shown anti-inflammatory effects in TNF-α-exposed mouse adipocytes ascorbic acid by suppressing inflammatory chemokines [59]. Ascorbic acid, known as vitamin C, also benefits the skin by promoting collagen formation, scavenging free radicals, and protecting from photoaging and UVB-induced lipid peroxidation [60]. Oral ingestion of vitamin C has been suggested to be more effective on the skin than topical administration [61]. Vitamin A has been effective in alleviating inflammation in skin disorders, broncho-pulmonary dysplasia, and pneumonia [62]. These substances in the CS might have attributed to the UVB protective effects on the skin.

There are some limitations regarding the measurements of candidate antioxidants in the skin of mice and its molecular relationship with CS's antioxidant effects. The inclusion of groups for bioactive constituents with the equivalent dose to their content in the CS extract would have provided further support to our study. Previous studies suggested that allantoin [63] and luteolin [64] are present in CS, and may exhibit anti-inflammatory or anti-oxidative effects [65–67]. However, allantoin and luteolin in our CS extract were present as the 58th and 3244th most abundant chemical according to our LC-MS/MS analysis and might have not significantly contributed to the CS effects. However, when a 15-fold lower dose of allantoin and a 15-fold higher dose of luteolin were provided to the UVB-irradiated animals, we observed significant improvements in UVB-induced skin damages along with oxidative stress and inflammatory markers (unpublished data). In addition, our CS metabolite analysis suggested other potential antioxidant and/or anti-inflammatory components. Further studies are warranted to identify bioactive constituents for the UVB protective effects of the CS.

In conclusion, our data demonstrated that the oral administration of the CS extract ameliorated UVB-induced skin photoaging by the prevention of aberrant cell proliferation and DNA damage, and that these effects might be mediated by antioxidant and anti-inflammatory gene pathways. Histological results of skin tissue showed that the CS extract effectively reduced UVB-induced wrinkle formation and cell proliferation, and increased collagen synthesis. Mediators of the antioxidant defense system such as Nrf2, catalase, SOD1, and glutaredoxin were elevated, and inflammation-related genes in the NF-κB signaling pathway, such as IL-1β, COX-2, and iNOS were reduced upon oral ingestion of dietary CS extract. In human cells, similar results were shown in the Nrf2 and NF-κB pathways. As revealed by the LC-MS/MS results, the chemical composition of the CS extract included potential antioxidants, which might have contributed to its anti-photoaging effects in animal tissue and in cells. The results indicate that the CS extract was effective in the prevention of UVB-induced skin damage through different signaling pathways. Further studies on the molecular level of the photoprotective effect of CS water extract on the skin are required.

4. Materials and Methods

4.1. Materials and Reagents

2,2-Diphenyl-1-picrylhydrazyl (DPPH) was purchased from Alfa Aesar (Haverhill, MA, USA). 2,2-azinobis(3-ethyl-benzothiazoline-6-sulfonic acid) (ABTS), dimethyl sulfoxide (DMSO), and sodium bicarbonate were purchased from Sigma-Aldrich Co. (St. Louis, MO, USA). Potassium persulfate was purchased from Duksan (Ansan-si, Gyeonggi-do, Korea). The assay kits for GSH analysis were purchased from BioVision Research Products (Mountain View, CA, USA). Other chemicals were commercially available and in analytical grade.

4.2. Preparation of CS Extract

Water extract of corn silk was prepared and supplied by Kwang Dong Pharmaceutical Co. Ltd. (Seoul, Korea), and stored at 4 °C until use. The corn silk was harvested from Jilin Province in China, sterilized at 125 °C for 30 min, extracted with water at 98 °C–100 °C for 1 h, filtered through microfilter paper, and concentrated under reduced pressure at 50 °C or lower (concentrated brix: 44–48 brix). After final sterilization at 95 °C–98 °C for 20 min, 1 L of corn silk extract was obtained from 4 kg of corn silk. The moisture content of corn silk extract was 64.98%. The extract consisted of 16.21% carbohydrate, 9.78% protein, 0.44% lipid, 5.54% dietary fiber, 0.06% crude fiber, and 8.59%. The nutritional composition of the corn silk extract was determined using the Association of Official Agricultural Chemists (AOAC) method (1996) established by the Korea Health Supplement Institute (Seongnam, Korea) [68]. Finally, lyophilization using a freeze-dryer (FD8512, ilShin BioBase Co. Ltd., Yangju, Korea) for a minimum of 72 h removed water from the extract. In total, 125 g of the freeze-dried corn silk extract (CS) was collected.

4.3. Measurement of Antioxidant Effects of CS Extract

To measure the DPPH radical scavenging activity of the CS water extract, 80 µL of DPPH solution (0.4 mM DPPH in ethanol) was vigorously mixed with 20 µL of CS solution (1.25, 2.5, 5, 10 mg/mL in water). For the control, 20 µL water was added to 80 µL DPPH After incubation for 10 min, the absorbance of the solution was measured at 492 nm. The standard content was calculated using the absorbance of L-Ascorbic acid (100 µg/mL) that were treated in the same way as the samples. The ABTS radical scavenging activity was determined by the modified method of Re et al. [69]. In brief, 7 mM ABTS in water was reacted with 2.45 mM potassium persulfate, allowed to stand in dark for 12–16 h to make ABTS•+. This was diluted with methanol (50%, v/v), to absorbance of 0.70 ± 0.02 at 734 nm, 30 °C, and 990 µL of this solution was added to 10 µL CS or water. Absorbance was measured at 734 nm after 1 min incubation. The free radical scavenging ability of DPPH and ABTS was calculated by the following equation: Percentage of inhibition of DPPH or ABTS (%) = (1 − O.D. of sample/O.D. of control) × 100. IC_{50} values of CS extract in relation to ABTS and DPPH free radicals was calculated and compared using L-ascorbic acid (0, 12.5, 25, 50, 100 µg/mL) as a positive control.

4.4. Experimental Animals

Fifty-six 6-week-old female SKH-1 hairless mice were obtained from Orient Bio Inc. (Seongnam, Korea). The animals were housed at 23 ± 2 °C, with a relative humidity of 55 ± 10%, in a 12 h light/dark cycle with free access to food (5L79, Orient Bio Inc., Seongnam, Korea) and water. After a one-week acclimatization, the mice were randomly allocated into six groups: (i) Vehicle (saline)-treated normal group (NOR, n = 10), (ii) UVB-irradiated group (UVB, n = 9), (iii) UVB-irradiated and 2 g/kg/day CS-treated group (CSL, n = 9), and (iv) UVB-irradiated and 4 g/kg/day CS-treated group (CSH, n = 10).

The oral dose of each sample was adapted from Guo et al. and Wang et al. at which CS administration did not induce weight loss, histopathological changes, or death [70,71]. The oral dose of the group was set at 4.0 g/kg/day. The oral dose of the low dose group was set at 2.0 g/kg/day.

Each sample was dissolved in saline and orally administered at a volume of 0.2 mL each. In the normal and control groups, saline was administered at a dose of 0.2 mL/day.

To observe the protective effects of the extract on mice before tumorigenesis, we defined 19 weeks as the endpoint of our study in reference to a report that UVB-induced tumor development time in 50% untreated hairless mice was 20 weeks [28]. The animals were monitored daily and weighed weekly. All experimental protocols were approved by the Institutional Animal Care and Use Committee (IACUC) of Yonsei University, Korea (Permit number: 201608-495-02).

Mouse dorsal skin was exposed to UVB three times per week using the Biolink crosslinker BLX-312 (Vilbert Lourmat; Marne-La Vallee, France). Fifteen-centimeter distance was maintained between the light source and mouse. The UVB source was 5 UVB lamps (5 × 8 W [8 J/s]) with a 312 nm peak emission. The minimal erythematous dose was 180 mJ/cm^2. The UVB radiation was 180 mJ/cm^2 in weeks 2–11 and increased to 360 mJ/cm^2 in weeks 12–19 by modified methods of Mantena et al. [72] and Record and Dreosti [73]. No UVB was radiated in the first week.

4.5. Assessment of Skin Thickness and Wrinkle Formation in Mice

Hairless mice were anesthetized, and their dorsal skin was photographed at the end of the study (19 weeks). The UV-induced skin fold thickness was measured at a point mid-way between the neck and hips by using an electronic digital micrometer caliper (Marathon Watch Company Ltd., Ontario, Canada). A replica of the mouse dorsal skin was obtained by using silicon rubber (Repliflo, CuDerm Corp., TX, USA). The skin impressions were photographed using an Antera 3D® camera (Miravex, Dublin, Ireland) and analyzed by Antera CS program (Miravex). The volume of the depression, the affected area of depression, maximum depth, and wrinkle length were measured on the surface of the replica (a circle with a 16.8 mm-diameter).

4.6. Histological and Immunohistochemical Analysis in Mice

The dorsal skin samples (1 × 1 cm^2) were fixed in 10% neutralized formalin for at least 24 h and embedded in paraffin. Prior to staining, 4 μm sections were deparaffinized in xylene, and rehydrated through a graded ethanol series (100%–70%). The sections were stained with hematoxylin and eosin (H&E), Masson's trichrome (MT), and Verhoeffe–Van Gieson (VVG). The immunohistochemical detection of proliferating cell nuclear antigen (PCNA), 8-hydroxy-2'-deoxyguanosine (8-OHdG), and Ki67 was performed in 4 μm thick deparaffinized sections. For antigen retrieval, the sections were incubated with Tris-EDTA buffer solution (pH 9.0) for PCNA or citrate buffer solution (pH 6.0) for 8-OHdG and Ki67 for 15 min in a decloaking chamber (Biocare Medical). The sections were treated with 3% H2O2 for 10 min to inhibit the endogenous peroxidase activity and rinsed in 0.1 M Tris-buffered saline (TBS) solution. Non-specific binding sites were blocked by the incubation of the sections with 5% BSA for 1 h. The sections were incubated with 1:100 diluted anti-8OHdG or anti-Ki67 primary antibody (Abcam, Cambridge, UK) overnight at 4 °C, followed by incubation with the secondary antibody (DAKO Envision+ System-HRP Labelled Polymer: Anti-mouse for PCNA and 8-OHdG, and anti-rabbit for Ki-67) for 1 h. The sections were washed in 0.1 M TBS, incubated with 3,3'-diaminobenzidine tetrahydrochloride peroxidase substrate solution (k-3468, DAKO Corp., CA, USA) for 1–3 min, counterstained with Mayer's hematoxylin solution, and dehydrated through a graded series of 70%–100% alcohol in xylene. Representative photomicrographs were taken by a light microscope (Eclipse Ti microscope; Nikon, Tokyo, Japan). The epidermal thickness and staining density of collagen were quantified using ImageJ software (National Institutes of Health, MD, USA).

4.7. Measurement of Reduced GSH Content in Mouse Plasma

The plasma GSH level was determined by using the Glutathione Fluorometric Assay Kit (BioVision, CA, USA) in accordance with the manufacturer's instructions. Each sample was added to a 96-well plate. Each well had a total volume of 100 μL containing 20 μL of the plasma from each mouse. Subsequently, 2 μL of GST reagent and 2 μL of monochlorobimane (MCB) was added. After incubation for 1 h at 37 °C, fluorescence was measured by using a GENios fluorescence plate reader at an excitation wavelength of 335 nm and an emission wavelength of 460 nm.

4.8. Comet Assay (Alkaline Single-Cell Gel Electrophoresis)

The alkaline comet assay was conducted in accordance with the method of Singh et al., with minor modifications [74]. Leukocytes were isolated from whole blood using Histopaque 1077 (Sigma Aldrich Co.), mixed with 0.7% low melting-point agarose and added to slides. The slides were immersed in cold lysing solution (2.5 M NaCl, 100 mM EDTA, 10 mM Tris, 1% sodium laurylsarcosine, pH 10, 1% Triton X-100, and 10% DMSO) at 4 °C for 1 h. After lysis, the slides were transferred to electrophoresis buffer (300 mM NaOH and 10 mM Na2EDTA, pH 13.0) at 4 °C for 40 min. For electrophoresis, an electric current of 25 V/300 ± 3 mA was applied at 4 °C for 20 min. The slides were washed three times with neutralizing buffer (0.4 M Tris, pH 7.5) at 4 °C and treated with ethanol for 5 min. All steps were conducted in the dark to prevent additional DNA damage. Fifty cells from two replicate slides each were analyzed using a fluorescence microscope (LEICA DM LB, Bensheim, Germany) and image analysis software (Komet 4.0; Kinetic Imaging, UK) to compute the tail intensity (equivalent to the percentage of DNA in the tail), tail length, and tail moment (tail length × tail intensity).

4.9. Determination of Lipid Peroxidation in Skin Tissue

Mouse skin tissue was homogenized in 1.15% KCl solution (30 mg/mL). After centrifugation (1,500 g, 15 min, 4 °C), 100 µL supernatant was reacted with 400 µL of TBARS reagent (0.8% TBA) and incubated at 95 °C for 1 h. To terminate the reaction, 250 µL of distilled water and 1.25 mL of n-butanol/pyridine (15:1, v/v) were added, and the solution was centrifuged again (1,500 g, 15 min). The absorbance of the supernatant was measured at 540 nm and the concentration of lipid peroxides was calculated based on the malondialdehyde (MDA) standard curve and normalized to the protein content of each sample by the bicinchoninic acid assay (BCA; Pierce, Rockford, USA).

4.10. Cell Culture

HaCaT cells (Item no. 300493, Cell Lines Service, Eppelheim, Germany) were cultured in Dulbecco's modified Eagle medium nutrient mixture F-12 (Ham) 1:1 (D-MEM/F-12, GibcoBRL, Braunschweig, Germany) powder medium supplemented with 10% fetal calf serum (FCS) (GibcoBRL, Grand Island, NY, USA), 1% antibiotic/antimycotic solution (Corning, NY, USA) and 1.2 g/L sodium bicarbonate (NaHCO3; Sigma-Aldrich, cat. No. S6014). Cells were incubated in 5% CO_2 at 37 °C.

Cells were irradiated with UVB in Chambres Noires darkrooms (Vilber, France) under a UVB light lamp (VL-6 MC; Vilber, France) emitting 315 nm. The UVB emission was calculated as 30 mJ/cm^2 = 580 µW/cm^2 × 52 s.

4.11. Cell Viability (MTT) Assay

Cytotoxicity of CS and UVB on HaCaT cells was measured by colorimetric MTT assay. Cells were seeded in 96-well plates to make 2×10^4 cells/well. After 24 h incubation in complete medium, water (control) or 0.1~15 µg/mL CS extract was added to each well. After 24 h incubation, cells were washed and either replaced with fresh complete medium or UVB-irradiated at 30, 45, and 70 mJ/cm^2 (52, 77, 120 s) in 200 µL PBS and then replaced with fresh complete medium with the same concentration of CS extract or water (control). After 5 h incubation, 1 mg/mL MTT solution was added to each well and allowed to react for 4 h. The supernatant was removed and 100 µL of isopropyl alcohol (Merck, Darmstadt, Germany) was added to dissolve the generated formazan crystals. The absorbance was measured at 570 nm using a microplate reader (Infinite® 200 PRO, Tecan, Switzerland).

4.12. Western Blot Analysis

The UVB-irradiated total dorsal skin was homogenized (Polytron System PT 1200 E, Luzernerstrasse, Switzerland) in RIPA lysis buffer with freshly added protease and phosphatase inhibitor cocktails. After centrifugation (4 °C, 12,500 g, 20 min), the supernatant protein concentration was determined by using the Bradford reagent (BioRad, CA, USA). Equal amounts of total protein were separated by SDS-PAGE and transferred to PVDF membranes (Millipore Corporation). Next, the membranes were blocked by incubation in 5% fat-free dry milk in 1× phosphate-buffered saline (PBS) for 1 h at room temperature. The membranes were then incubated overnight 4 °C with 1:1000 dilutions of the primary antibodies specific for α-tubulin, IL-1β, PCNA, MMP9, TIMP-1, Smad2, p-Smad2 (Santa Cruz Biotechnology, Dallas, TX, USA), iNOS, COX-2 (BD Biosciences, San Jose, CA, USA), TGF-β (R&D Systems Inc., Minneapolis, MN, USA), 8OHdG (Abcam, Cambridge, UK), Ki67 (Millipore Corporation, Billerica, MA, USA), and Nrf2 (Invitrogen, MA, USA). The membranes were rinsed with PBST and incubated with peroxidase-conjugated 1:5000 dilutions of the anti-mouse and anti-rabbit secondary antibodies (Millipore Corporation, Billerica, MA, USA). The antibody signals were visualized by a chemiluminescence detection system (GE Healthcare Life Sciences, Buckinghamshire, England) and photographed by an AE-9300 Ez-Capture system (ATTO, Tokyo, Japan). Band density was quantified using ImageJ software.

HaCaT cells were seeded in a 60 mm culture dish to make 8×10^5 cells/well and incubated in complete media for 24 h. Then, water (NOR, UVB), 0.5 μg/mL CS extract or 5 μg/mL CS extract was treated and incubated for 24 h. Then, cells were washed with PBS and replaced with fresh complete medium (NOR) or UVB-irradiated at 315 nm for 52 s at 30 mJ/cm^2 in 2 mL PBS, and then replaced with fresh complete medium with the same concentration of CS extract or water (control). After 5 h incubation, protein was extracted from the cells in RIPA lysis buffer for Western blot analysis.

4.13. Reverse Transcriptase (RT) and Quantitative Polymerase Chain Reaction (qPCR)

Skin tissue total RNA was extracted by homogenization in TRIzol reagent (MRC, Cincinnati, OH, USA. Cell total RNA was extracted by scrapping in TRIzol reagent (MRC, Cincinnati, OH, USA). The purity of the total RNA was measured with a spectrophotometer and reverse transcribed using ImProm II Reverse Transcriptase kit (Promega, Madison, Wis., USA). cDNA was synthesized according to the manufacturer's protocol. qPCR was performed in a Mic real-time PCR system (BMS, biomolecular systems, Australia) using 5× HOT FIREPOL® EvaGreen® qPCR Supermix (Solis biodyne, Tartu, Estonia) in a volume of 18 uL depending on the manufacturer's cycling conditions. Relative gene expression was measured using the comparative 2-($\Delta\Delta$Cq) method. Expression of housekeeping GAPDH mRNA was used for qPCR data standardization. The primers used are shown in Table 2.

Table 2. Primers used for quantitative polymerase chain reaction (qPCR).

Gene	Forward Sequence	Reverse Sequence	Product Size
m.Catalase	AACGCTGGATGGATTCTCCC	GCCCTAACCTTTCATTTCCCTTCAG	133
m.Procollagen type 1	CCCTAGCCTTTTCTCCGCC	TGGCAACTCCAAGTCCATCAT	238
m.Nrf2	GTGAGACGTGGAAACCCGAG	GCCATAGGACATCTGGGAAGC	347
m.TXN	GAGCAAGGAAGCTTTTCAGGAG	GTCCCGTTTTGGATCCGAGT	252
m.SOD1	ATGGCGACGAAGGCCGTGTG	GACCACCAGTGTGCGGCCAA	360
m.GAPDH	AAGGTCGGTGTGAACGGATTT	CAGAAGGGGCGGAGATGATG	364
h.Glutaredoxin	CATCGGCATGGCTCAAGAG	AATCTGCTTTAGCCGCGTCA	313
h.Procollagen type 1	AGGACAAGAGGCATGTCTGGTT	TTGCAGTGTAGGTGATGTTCTG	156
h.GAPDH	AAGGTCGGTGTGAACGGATTT	CAGAAGGGGCGGAGATGATG	364

4.14. Sample Preparation for Liquid Chromatography-Tandem Mass Spectrometer (LC-MS/MS) Analysis

Non-targeted LC-MS/MS was used to analyze the components present in the CS extract. The CS extract was diluted 10,000 times with deionized water and filtered 0.45 µm. CS extract samples were stored at −20 °C until LC-MS/MS analysis.

4.15. LC-MS/MS Analysis and Identification of Metabolites

Ultimate 3000 UHPLC and Q-Extractive Orbitrap Plus was equipped with an ACQUITY C18 column (10 cm × 2.1 mm, particle size 1.7 µm, Waters, USA). The injection volume for each sample was 5 µL. The column was eluted using the following binary gradient solutions: A (deionized water with 0.1% formic acid) and B (methanol, UPLC graded) with a flow rate of 0.4 mL/min, A: B = 100: 0 at 1 min, 0: 100 at 16 min, 0: 100 until 20 min, and 100: 0 at 22 min. The full scan/dd-MS2 system parameters were: FTMS, ESI-positive mode with mass resolution of 70,000, full scan range: 80~1000 m/z, dd-MS2 (Top 10) resolution of 17,500 with collision energy 30, flow rate of nitrogen sheath gas and auxiliary gas: 40 (arbitrary units) and 10 (arbitrary units), spray voltage: 3.5 kV, capillary temperature: 320 °C, S-lensRF level: 50, auxiliary gas heater temperature: 300 °C. Metabolomics analysis for mouse skin was carried out as outlined in the supplementary methods.

The original data from the UPLC-Orbitrap-MS2 analysis were extracted from the XCMS online platform (http://xcmsonline.scripps.edu/) for data alignment and peak detection. The parameters of the XCMS online were 10-sec bandwidth, 15 ppm tolerance for database research, and the rest were UPLC-orbitrap default values. The MS2 data for peak identification was extracted from the LC-raw file using Xcalibur 2.2 (Thermo Fisher Scientific, San Jose, CA, USA). The LC-MS/MS search function of the online database (MycompoundID (www.mycompoundid.org) and HMDB (www.hmdb.ca)) was used to perform metabolite identification using retention time, exact mass, and MS/MS peak intensities.

4.16. Statistical Analysis

The data are expressed as mean ± standard error (SE) or standard deviation (SD). The results were analyzed by one-way analysis of variance (ANOVA) and one tail t-test using SPSS software (SPSS, Version 23.0 IBM Inc., USA). The criterion for statistical significance was $p < 0.05$.

Supplementary Materials: The following are available online at http://www.mdpi.com/1420-3049/24/14/2587/s1, Table S1: Compounds identified in corn silk (CS) extract and mouse skin using LC-MS/MS; Figure S1: Heatmaps of UVB-irradiated and CS extract-administered mouse skin metabolites.

Author Contributions: Conceptualization, S.-M.L.; methodology, Y.-h.K., A.C., S.-A.K., H.H.; validation, E.-J.S., E.P.; formal analysis and investigation, Y.-h.K., A.C., S.-A.K., H.w.H, E.-J.S., E.P., S.-M.L.; data curation, Y.-h.K., A.C., S.A.K., M.K., H.w.H.; writing—original draft preparation, Y.-h.K., A.C., M.S.; writing—revising and editing, M.S., S.-M.L.; visualization, Y.-h.K., M.K.; supervision, S.-M.L.; project administration, S.-M.L., E.P.

Funding: This work was supported by the BK21 Plus Project for Bioactive Nutrition, Yonsei University, Seoul 03722, Republic of Korea.

Acknowledgments: The corn silk extract was provided by Kwang Dong Pharmaceutical, Seoul, Republic of Korea.

Conflicts of Interest: The authors declare no conflict of interest.

References

1. Nichols, J.A.; Katiyar, S.K. Skin photoprotection by natural polyphenols: Anti-inflammatory, antioxidant and DNA repair mechanisms. *Arch. Dermatol. Res.* **2010**, *302*, 71–83. [CrossRef] [PubMed]
2. Quan, T.; Qin, Z.; Xia, W.; Shao, Y.; Voorhees, J.J.; Fisher, G.J. Matrix-degrading metalloproteinases in photoaging. *J. Investig. Dermatol. Symp. Proc.* **2009**, *14*, 20–24. [CrossRef] [PubMed]
3. Natarajan, V.T.; Ganju, P.; Ramkumar, A.; Grover, R.; Gokhale, R.S. Multifaceted pathways protect human skin from UV radiation. *Nat. Chem. Biol.* **2014**, *10*, 542–551. [CrossRef] [PubMed]
4. Pillai, S.; Oresajo, C.; Hayward, J. Ultraviolet radiation and skin aging: Roles of reactive oxygen species, inflammation and protease activation, and strategies for prevention of inflammation-induced matrix degradation—A review. *Int. J. Cosmet. Sci.* **2005**, *27*, 17–34. [CrossRef] [PubMed]

5. Kammeyer, A.; Luiten, R. Oxidation events and skin aging. *Ageing Res. Rev.* **2015**, *21*, 16–29. [CrossRef] [PubMed]
6. Svobodová, A.; Psotová, J.; Walterová, D. Natural phenolics in the prevention of UV-induced skin damage. A review. *Biomed. Pap. Med Fac. Univ. Palackyolomouccechoslovakia* **2003**, *147*, 137–145. [CrossRef]
7. Quan, T.; He, T.; Kang, S.; Voorhees, J.J.; Fisher, G.J. Solar ultraviolet irradiation reduces collagen in photoaged human skin by blocking transforming growth factor-β type II receptor/Smad signaling. *Am. J. Pathol.* **2004**, *165*, 741–751. [CrossRef]
8. Fernández-García, E. Skin protection against UV light by dietary antioxidants. *Food Funct.* **2014**, *5*, 1994–2003. [CrossRef]
9. Ren, S.C.; Liu, Z.L.; Ding, X.L. Isolation and identification of two novel flavone glycosides from corn silk (Stigma maydis). *J. Med. Plants Res.* **2009**, *3*, 1009–1015.
10. Hasanudin, K.; Hashim, P.; Mustafa, S. Corn silk (Stigma maydis) in healthcare: A phytochemical and pharmacological review. *Molecules* **2012**, *17*, 9697–9715. [CrossRef]
11. Ku, K.M.; Kim, S.K.; Kang, Y.H. Antioxidant activity and functional components of corn silk (Zea mays L.). *Korean J. Plant Resour.* **2009**, *22*, 323–329.
12. Choi, S.Y.; Lee, Y.; Kim, S.S.; Ju, H.M.; Baek, J.H.; Park, C.S.; Lee, D.H. Inhibitory Effect of Corn Silk on Skin Pigmentation. *Molecules* **2014**, *19*, 2808–2818. [CrossRef]
13. Fossen, T.; Slimestad, R.; Andersen, Ø.M. Anthocyanins from maize (Zea mays) and reed canarygrass (Phalaris arundinacea). *J. Agric. Food Chem.* **2001**, *49*, 2318–2321. [CrossRef]
14. Hu, Q.; Deng, Z. Protective effects of flavonoids from corn silk on oxidative stress induced by exhaustive exercise in mice. *Afr. J. Biotechnol.* **2011**, *10*, 3163–3167.
15. Maksimović, Z.; Malenčić, Đ.; Kovačević, N. Polyphenol contents and antioxidant activity of Maydis stigma extracts. *Bioresour. Technol.* **2005**, *96*, 873–877. [CrossRef]
16. Liu, J.; Wang, C.; Wang, Z.; Zhang, C.; Lu, S.; Liu, J. The antioxidant and free-radical scavenging activities of extract and fractions from corn silk (Zea mays L.) and related flavone glycosides. *Food Chem.* **2011**, *126*, 261–269. [CrossRef]
17. Wang, K.-J.; Zhao, J.-L. Corn silk (Zea mays L.), a source of natural antioxidants with α-amylase, α-glucosidase, advanced glycation and diabetic nephropathy inhibitory activities. *Biomed. Pharmacother.* **2019**, *110*, 510–517. [CrossRef]
18. Tian, J.; Chen, H.; Chen, S.; Xing, L.; Wang, Y.; Wang, J. Comparative studies on the constituents, antioxidant and anticancer activities of extracts from different varieties of corn silk. *Food Funct.* **2013**, *4*, 1526–1534. [CrossRef]
19. Choi, D.J.; Kim, S.-L.; Choi, J.W.; Park, Y.I. Neuroprotective effects of corn silk maysin via inhibition of H2O2-induced apoptotic cell death in SK-N-MC cells. *Life Sci.* **2014**, *109*, 57–64. [CrossRef]
20. Chang, C.-C.; Yuan, W.; Roan, H.-Y.; Chang, J.-L.; Huang, H.-C.; Lee, Y.-C.; Tsay, H.J.; Liu, H.-K. The ethyl acetate fraction of corn silk exhibits dual antioxidant and anti-glycation activities and protects insulin-secreting cells from glucotoxicity. *Bmc Complementary Altern. Med.* **2016**, *16*, 432. [CrossRef]
21. Guo, Q.; Xu, L.; Chen, Y.; Ma, Q.; Santhanam, R.K.; Xue, Z.; Gao, X.; Chen, H. Structural characterization of corn silk polysaccharides and its effect in H2O2 induced oxidative damage in L6 skeletal muscle cells. *Carbohydr. Polym.* **2019**, *208*, 161–167. [CrossRef]
22. Vranješ, M.; Popović, B.M.; Štajner, D.; Ivetić, V.; Mandić, A.; Vranješ, D. Effects of bearberry, parsley and corn silk extracts on diuresis, electrolytes composition, antioxidant capacity and histopathological features in mice kidneys. *J. Funct. Foods* **2016**, *21*, 272–282. [CrossRef]
23. Oyabambi, A.O.; Areola, E.D.; Olatunji, L.A.; Soladoye, A.O. Uric acid is a key player in salt-induced endothelial dysfunction: The therapeutic role of stigma maydis (corn silk) extract. *Appl. Physiol. Nutr. Metab.* **2019**. [CrossRef]
24. Bai, H.; Hai, C.; Xi, M.; Liang, X.; Liu, R. Protective Effect of Maize Silks (Maydis stigma) Ethanol Extract on Radiation-Induced Oxidative Stress in Mice. *Plant Foods Hum. Nutr.* **2010**, *65*, 271–276. [CrossRef]
25. Zhang, Y.; Wu, L.; Ma, Z.; Cheng, J.; Liu, J. Anti-Diabetic, Anti-Oxidant and Anti-Hyperlipidemic Activities of Flavonoids from Corn Silk on STZ-Induced Diabetic Mice. *Molecules* **2016**, *21*, 7. [CrossRef]
26. Yang, B.; Ji, C.; Kang, J.; Chen, W.; Bi, Z.; Wan, Y. Trans-Zeatin inhibits UVB-induced matrix metalloproteinase-1 expression via MAP kinase signaling in human skin fibroblasts. *Int. J. Mol. Med.* **2009**, *23*, 555–560.

27. Byun, S.; Lee, K.W.; Jung, S.K.; Lee, E.J.; Hwang, M.K.; Lim, S.H.; Bode, A.M.; Lee, H.J.; Dong, Z. Luteolin inhibits protein kinase Cε and c-Src activities and UVB-induced skin cancer. *Cancer Res.* **2010**, *70*, 2415–2423. [CrossRef]
28. Fisher, G.J.; Wang, Z.Q.; Datta, S.C.; Varani, J.; Kang, S.; Voorhees, J.J. Pathophysiology of premature skin aging induced by ultraviolet light. *New Engl. J. Med.* **1997**, *337*, 1419–1428. [CrossRef]
29. Rittié, L.; Fisher, G.J. UV-light-induced signal cascades and skin aging. *Ageing Res. Rev.* **2002**, *1*, 705–720. [CrossRef]
30. Palei, A.C.; Sandrim, V.C.; Cavalli, R.C.; Tanus-Santos, J.E. Comparative assessment of matrix metalloproteinase (MMP)-2 and MMP-9, and their inhibitors, tissue inhibitors of metalloproteinase (TIMP)-1 and TIMP-2 in preeclampsia and gestational hypertension. *Clin. Biochem.* **2008**, *41*, 875–880. [CrossRef]
31. Carrara, I.M.; Melo, G.P.; Bernardes, S.S.; Neto, F.S.; Ramalho, L.N.Z.; Marinello, P.C.; Luiz, R.C.; Cecchini, R.; Cecchini, A.L. Looking beyond the skin: Cutaneous and systemic oxidative stress in UVB-induced squamous cell carcinoma in hairless mice. *J. Photochem. Photobiol. B: Biol.* **2019**, *195*, 17–26. [CrossRef]
32. Ebrahimzadeh, M.A.; Pourmorad, F.; Hafezi, S. Antioxidant activities of Iranian corn silk. *Turk. J. Biol.* **2008**, *32*, 43–49.
33. Divya, S.P.; Wang, X.; Pratheeshkumar, P.; Son, Y.O.; Roy, R.V.; Kim, D.; Dai, J.; Hitron, J.A.; Wang, L.; Asha, P. Blackberry extract inhibits UVB-induced oxidative damage and inflammation through MAP kinases and NF-κB signaling pathways in SKH-1 mice skin. *Toxicol. Appl. Pharmacol.* **2015**, *284*, 92–99. [CrossRef]
34. Svobodova, A.R.; Galandáková, A.; Šianská, J.; Doležal, D.; Ulrichová, J.; Vostálová, J. Acute exposure to solar simulated ultraviolet radiation affects oxidative stress-related biomarkers in skin, liver and blood of hairless mice. *Biol. Pharm. Bull.* **2011**, *34*, 471–479. [CrossRef]
35. Barg, M.; Rezin, G.T.; Leffa, D.D.; Balbinot, F.; Gomes, L.M.; Carvalho-Silva, M.; Vuolo, F.; Petronilho, F.; Dal-Pizzol, F.; Streck, E.L. Evaluation of the protective effect of Ilex paraguariensis and Camellia sinensis extracts on the prevention of oxidative damage caused by ultraviolet radiation. *Environ. Toxicol. Pharmacol.* **2014**, *37*, 195–201. [CrossRef]
36. Sathishsekar, D.; Subramanian, S. Beneficial effects of Momordica charantia seeds in the treatment of STZ-induced diabetes in experimental rats. *Biol. Pharm. Bull.* **2005**, *28*, 978–983. [CrossRef]
37. Huang, H.C.; Nguyen, T.; Pickett, C.B. Regulation of the antioxidant response element by protein kinase C-mediated phosphorylation of NF-E2-related factor 2. *Proc. Natl. Acad. Sci. USA* **2000**, *97*, 12475. [CrossRef]
38. Kawachi, Y.; Xu, X.; Taguchi, S.; Sakurai, H.; Nakamura, Y.; Ishii, Y.; Fujisawa, Y.; Furuta, J.; Takahashi, T.; Itoh, K. Attenuation of UVB-induced sunburn reaction and oxidative DNA damage with no alterations in UVB-induced skin carcinogenesis in Nrf2 gene-deficient mice. *J. Investig. Dermatol.* **2008**, *128*, 1773–1779. [CrossRef]
39. Hirota, A.; Kawachi, Y.; Yamamoto, M.; Koga, T.; Hamada, K.; Otsuka, F. Acceleration of UVB-induced photoageing in nrf2 gene-deficient mice. *Exp. Dermatol.* **2011**, *20*, 664–668. [CrossRef]
40. Ighodaro, O.M.; Akinloye, O.A. First line defence antioxidants-superoxide dismutase (SOD), catalase (CAT) and glutathione peroxidase (GPX): Their fundamental role in the entire antioxidant defence grid. *Alex. J. Med.* **2018**, *54*, 287–293. [CrossRef]
41. Dreger, H.; Westphal, K.; Weller, A.; Baumann, G.; Stangl, V.; Meiners, S.; Stangl, K. Nrf2-dependent upregulation of antioxidative enzymes: A novel pathway for proteasome inhibitor-mediated cardioprotection. *Cardiovasc. Res.* **2009**, *83*, 354–361. [CrossRef]
42. Glorieux, C.; Zamocky, M.; Sandoval, J.M.; Verrax, J.; Calderon, P.B. Regulation of catalase expression in healthy and cancerous cells. *Free Radic. Biol. Med.* **2015**, *87*, 84–97. [CrossRef]
43. Zhu, H.; Itoh, K.; Yamamoto, M.; Zweier, J.L.; Li, Y. Role of Nrf2 signaling in regulation of antioxidants and phase 2 enzymes in cardiac fibroblasts: Protection against reactive oxygen and nitrogen species-induced cell injury. *Febs Lett.* **2005**, *579*, 3029–3036. [CrossRef]
44. Zhu, H.; Jia, Z.; Zhang, L.; Yamamoto, M.; Misra, H.P.; Trush, M.A.; Li, Y. Antioxidants and phase 2 enzymes in macrophages: Regulation by Nrf2 signaling and protection against oxidative and electrophilic stress. *Exp. Biol. Med. (Maywoodn.J.)* **2008**, *233*, 463–474. [CrossRef]
45. Liu, X.; Jann, J.; Xavier, C.; Wu, H. Glutaredoxin 1 (Grx1) protects human retinal pigment epithelial cells from oxidative damage by preventing AKT glutathionylation. *Investig. Ophthalmol. Vis. Sci.* **2015**, *56*, 2821–2832. [CrossRef]

46. Batliwala, S.; Xavier, C.; Liu, Y.; Wu, H.; Pang, I.-H. Involvement of Nrf2 in ocular diseases. *Oxidative Med. Cell. Longev.* **2017**, *2017*. [CrossRef]
47. Heo, H.S.; Han, G.E.; Won, J.; Cho, Y.; Woo, H.; Lee, J.H. Pueraria montana var. lobata root extract inhibits photoaging on skin through Nrf2 pathway. *J. Microbiol. Biotechnol.* **2019**, *29*, 518–526. [CrossRef]
48. Kannan, S.; Jaiswal, A.K. Low and high dose UVB regulation of transcription factor NF-E2-related factor 2. *Cancer Res.* **2006**, *66*, 8421–8429. [CrossRef]
49. Chang, E.J.; Kundu, J.K.; Liu, L.; Shin, J.W.; Surh, Y.J. Ultraviolet B radiation activates NF-kappaB and induces iNOS expression in HR-1 hairless mouse skin: Role of IkappaB kinase-beta. *Mol. Carcinog.* **2011**, *50*, 310–317. [CrossRef]
50. Abeyama, K.; Eng, W.; Jester, J.V.; Vink, A.A.; Edelbaum, D.; Cockerell, C.J.; Bergstresser, P.R.; Takashima, A. A role for NF-kappaB-dependent gene transactivation in sunburn. *J. Clin. Investig.* **2000**, *105*, 1751–1759. [CrossRef]
51. Sharma, S.D.; Meeran, S.M.; Katiyar, S.K. Dietary grape seed proanthocyanidins inhibit UVB-induced oxidative stress and activation of mitogen-activated protein kinases and nuclear factor-κB signaling in in vivo SKH-1 hairless mice. *Mol. Cancer Ther.* **2007**, *6*, 995–1005. [CrossRef]
52. Bandurska, H.; Niedziela, J.; Chadzinikolau, T. Separate and combined responses to water deficit and UV-B radiation. *Plant Sci.* **2013**, *213*, 98–105. [CrossRef]
53. Banu, M.N.A.; Hoque, M.A.; Watanabe-Sugimoto, M.; Matsuoka, K.; Nakamura, Y.; Shimoishi, Y.; Murata, Y. Proline and glycinebetaine induce antioxidant defense gene expression and suppress cell death in cultured tobacco cells under salt stress. *J. Plant Physiol.* **2009**, *166*, 146–156. [CrossRef]
54. Nausheen, J.; Sabina Bibi Jhaumeer, L.; Prakashanand, C.; Prashant Suresh, K. Antioxidant, Antidiabetic and Anticancer Activities of L-Phenylalanine and L-Tyrosine Ester Surfactants: In vitro and In Silico Studies of their Interactions with Macromolecules as Plausible Mode of Action for their Biological Properties. *Curr. Bioact. Compd.* **2018**, *14*, 1–13. [CrossRef]
55. Saxena, R.; Pendse, V.; Khanna, N. Anti-inflammatory and analgesic properties of four amino-acids. *Indian J. Physiol. Pharmacol.* **1984**, *28*, 299–305.
56. Pavicic, T.; Wollenweber, U.; Farwick, M.; Korting, H. Anti-microbial and-inflammatory activity and efficacy of phytosphingosine: An in vitro and in vivo study addressing acne vulgaris. *Int. J. Cosmet. Sci.* **2007**, *29*, 181–190. [CrossRef]
57. Kwon, S.B.; An, S.; Kim, M.J.; Kim, K.R.; Choi, Y.M.; Ahn, K.J.; An, I.-S.; Cha, H.J. Phytosphingosine-1-phosphate and epidermal growth factor synergistically restore extracellular matrix in human dermal fibroblasts in vitro and in vivo. *Int. J. Mol. Med.* **2017**, *39*, 741–748. [CrossRef]
58. Gehring, W. Nicotinic acid/niacinamide and the skin. *J. Cosmet. Dermatol.* **2004**, *3*, 88–93. [CrossRef]
59. Digby, J.E.; McNeill, E.; Dyar, O.J.; Lam, V.; Greaves, D.R.; Choudhury, R.P. Anti-inflammatory effects of nicotinic acid in adipocytes demonstrated by suppression of fractalkine, RANTES, and MCP-1 and upregulation of adiponectin. *Atherosclerosis* **2010**, *209*, 89–95. [CrossRef]
60. Pullar, J.; Carr, A.; Vissers, M. The roles of vitamin C in skin health. *Nutrients* **2017**, *9*, 866. [CrossRef]
61. Marini, A. Beauty from the inside. Does it really work? *Der Hautarzt; Z. Fur Dermatol. Venerol. Und Verwandte Geb.* **2011**, *62*, 614–617. [CrossRef]
62. Reifen, R. Vitamin A as an anti-inflammatory agent. *Proc. Nutr. Soc.* **2002**, *61*, 397–400. [CrossRef]
63. Khanpour, E.; Modarresi, M. Quantitative analysis of allantoin in Iranian corn silk. *Res. J. Pharmacogn.* **2017**, *4*, 16.
64. Žilić, S.; Janković, M.; Basić, Z.; Vančetović, J.; Maksimović, V. Antioxidant activity, phenolic profile, chlorophyll and mineral matter content of corn silk (Zea mays L): Comparison with medicinal herbs. *J. Cereal Sci.* **2016**, *69*, 363–370. [CrossRef]
65. Seelinger, G.; Merfort, I.; Schempp, C.M. Anti-oxidant, anti-inflammatory and anti-allergic activities of luteolin. *Planta Med.* **2008**, *74*, 1667–1677. [CrossRef]
66. Ueda, H.; Yamazaki, C.; Yamazaki, M. Luteolin as an anti-inflammatory and anti-allergic constituent of Perilla frutescens. *Biol. Pharm. Bull.* **2002**, *25*, 1197–1202. [CrossRef]
67. Lee, M.Y.; Lee, N.H.; Jung, D.; Lee, J.A.; Seo, C.S.; Lee, H.; Kim, J.H.; Shin, H.K. Protective effects of allantoin against ovalbumin (OVA)-induced lung inflammation in a murine model of asthma. *Int. Immunopharmacol.* **2010**, *10*, 474–480. [CrossRef]

68. Cunniff, P.; Association of Official Agricultural, C. *Official Methods of Analysis of AOAC International*, 16th ed.; AOAC International: Gaithersburg, MA, USA, 1996.
69. Re, R.; Pellegrini, N.; Proteggente, A.; Pannala, A.; Yang, M.; Rice-Evans, C. Antioxidant activity applying an improved ABTS radical cation decolorization assay. *Free Radic. Biol. Med.* **1999**, *26*, 1231–1237. [CrossRef]
70. Guo, J.; Liu, T.; Han, L.; Liu, Y. The effects of corn silk on glycaemic metabolism. *Nutr Metab (Lond)* **2009**, *6*, 47. [CrossRef]
71. Wang, C.; Zhang, T.; Liu, J.; Lu, S.; Zhang, C.; Wang, E.; Wang, Z.; Zhang, Y.; Liu, J. Subchronic toxicity study of corn silk with rats. *J. Ethnopharmacol.* **2011**, *137*, 36–43. [CrossRef]
72. Mantena, S.K.; Meeran, S.M.; Elmets, C.A.; Katiyar, S.K. Orally administered green tea polyphenols prevent ultraviolet radiation-induced skin cancer in mice through activation of cytotoxic T cells and inhibition of angiogenesis in tumors. *J. Nutr.* **2005**, *135*, 2871–2877. [CrossRef]
73. Record, I.R.; Dreosti, I.E. Protection by black tea and green tea against UVB and UVA+B induced skin cancer in hairless mice. *Mutat. Res./Fundam. Mol. Mech. Mutagenesis* **1998**, *422*, 191–199. [CrossRef]
74. Singh, N.P.; McCoy, M.T.; Tice, R.R.; Schneider, E.L. A simple technique for quantitation of low levels of DNA damage in individual cells. *Exp. Cell Res.* **1988**, *175*, 184–191. [CrossRef]

Sample Availability: Samples of the compounds are not available from the authors.

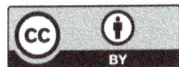 © 2019 by the authors. Licensee MDPI, Basel, Switzerland. This article is an open access article distributed under the terms and conditions of the Creative Commons Attribution (CC BY) license (http://creativecommons.org/licenses/by/4.0/).

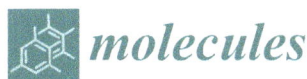

Article

Investigation of the Biological Activities and Characterization of Bioactive Constituents of *Ophiorrhiza rugosa* var. *prostrata* (D.Don) & Mondal Leaves through In Vivo, In Vitro, and In Silico Approaches

Md. Adnan [1,2,†], Md. Nazim Uddin Chy [3,4,†], A.T.M. Mostafa Kamal [3,*], Md Obyedul Kalam Azad [1,5], Arkajyoti Paul [4,6], Shaikh Bokhtear Uddin [7], James W. Barlow [8], Mohammad Omar Faruque [7], Cheol Ho Park [1] and Dong Ha Cho [1,*]

[1] Department of Bio-Health Technology, Kangwon National University, Chuncheon 24341, Korea; mdadnan1991.pharma@gmail.com (M.A.); azadokalam@gmail.com (M.O.K.A.); chpark@kangwon.ac.kr (C.H.P.)
[2] Senior Scientist, Rentia Plant Factory, Chuncheon 24341, Korea
[3] Department of Pharmacy, International Islamic University Chittagong, Chittagong 4318, Bangladesh; nazim107282@gmail.com
[4] Drug Discovery, GUSTO A Research Group, Chittagong 4000, Bangladesh; arka.bgctub@gmail.com
[5] Head of Research and Technology, Rentia Plant Factory, Chuncheon 24341, Korea
[6] Department of Microbiology, Jagannath University, Dhaka 1100, Bangladesh
[7] Ethnobotany and Pharmacognosy Lab, Department of Botany, University of Chittagong, Chittagong 4331, Bangladesh; bokhtear@cu.ac.bd (S.B.U.); omf@cu.ac.bd (M.O.F.)
[8] Department of Chemistry, Royal College of Surgeons in Ireland, D02YN77 Dublin, Ireland; jambarlow@rcsi.ie
* Correspondence: mostafa@pharm.iiuc.ac.bd (A.T.M.M.K.); chodh@kangwon.ac.kr (D.H.C.)
† These authors contributed equally to this work.

Academic Editors: Raffaele Capasso and Lorenzo Di Cesare Mannelli
Received: 13 March 2019; Accepted: 4 April 2019; Published: 8 April 2019

Abstract: *Ophiorrhiza rugosa* var. *prostrata* is one of the most frequently used ethnomedicinal plants by the indigenous communities of Bangladesh. This study was designed to investigate the antidiarrheal, anti-inflammatory, anthelmintic and antibacterial activities of the ethanol extract of *O. rugosa* leaves (EEOR). The leaves were extracted with ethanol and subjected to in vivo antidiarrheal screening using the castor oil-induced diarrhea, enteropooling, and gastrointestinal transit models. Anti-inflammatory efficacy was evaluated using the histamine-induced paw edema test. In parallel, in vitro anthelmintic and antibacterial activities were evaluated using the aquatic worm and disc diffusion assays respectively. In all three diarrheal models, EEOR (100, 200 and 400 mg/kg) showed obvious inhibition of diarrheal stool frequency, reduction of the volume and weight of the intestinal contents, and significant inhibition of intestinal motility. Also, EEOR manifested dose-dependent anti-inflammatory activity. Anthelmintic action was deemed significant ($P < 0.001$) with respect to the onset of paralysis and helminth death. EEOR also resulted in strong zones of inhibition when tested against both Gram-positive and Gram-negative bacteria. GC-MS analysis identified 30 compounds within EEOR, and of these, 13 compounds documented as bioactive showed good binding affinities to M3 muscarinic acetylcholine, 5-HT3, tubulin and GlcN-6-P synthase protein targets in molecular docking experiments. Additionally, ADME/T and PASS analyses revealed their drug-likeness, likely safety upon consumption and possible pharmacological activities. In conclusion, our findings scientifically support the ethnomedicinal use and value of this plant, which may provide a potential source for future development of medicines.

Keywords: *Ophiorrhiza rugosa*; Rubiaceae; antidiarrheal; anti-inflammatory; anthelmintic; antibacterial; in silico molecular docking; ADME/T and PASS

1. Introduction

Due to ongoing reports of antibiotic resistance by various pathogens, researchers have refocused their interest in the use of natural antimicrobial agents to treat infections instead of established antibiotics [1]. Although some conventional antibiotics may be bactericidal, they remain unable to inhibit the release of bacterial toxins which complicates the clinical picture [2]. Analogous to bacterial infections, helminths can persistently infect both humans and animals throughout their lifespan. Helminths exhibit greater complexity than other pathogens and are capable of producing chronic disease, yet these diseases are often neglected in developing regions [3]. The association of bacteria and parasites with gastrointestinal disorders is a common situation in developed and developing countries. Various etiological (*Salmonella*, *Campylobacter*, *Escherichia*, *Shigella*, *Yersinia enterocolitica*, parasites, and viruses) agents responsible for enteric infections may lead to dysentery-like chronic diarrhea [4]. Such infectious diseases cannot be cured easily at present, due to rapid resistance to available drugs; therefore screening of new therapeutic avenues such as plants may provide an alternate and effective approach for the development of novel agents.

Throughout the ages, plants have served humans for innumerable therapeutic interventions, ranging from the common cold to life-threatening conditions. The value of phytomedicinal approaches still resonates with the R&D departments of modern pharmaceutical giants [5]. The development of modern medicines has, in many instances, stemmed from ethnic medicinal uses, and meticulous investigation of naturally occurring bioactive compounds derived from plant screening programs assists the development of new synthetic drugs [6]. As plant-derived drugs contain a pool of metabolites with potential complementary pharmacological actions, their use in mitigating chronic diseases through synergism is an area of intense interest [7]. In this light, indigenous knowledge can help to contribute to the rational drug discovery and development of new drugs from medicinal plants [8]. While indigenous communities typically have a rich knowledge of ethnic medicines, these uses are based on empirical evidence, and proper mechanistic knowledge of biological or pharmacological properties necessitates a scientifically sound investigation, followed by the documentation and characterization of bioactive components of the studied species [9,10]. Hence, proper research on medicinal plants is invaluable in the search for novel bioactive agents for the management of the disease. Cognizant of these principles, we selected the ethnomedicinal plant *Ophiorrhiza rugosa* var. *prostrata* for the present study.

Ophiorrhiza rugosa var. *prostrata* (D.Don) Deb & Mondal (syn: *Ophiorrhiza harrisiana* B.Heyne ex Hook.f, *Ophiorrhiza prostrata* D.Don) is an annual herb belonging to the Rubiaceae family, which naturally grows in Chittagong and both the Chittagong Hill Tract and Sylhet regions of Bangladesh, where it is variously known as 'Jari' or 'kalashona' (Chakma), 'Jariphul' (Tanchangya) or 'Pahari mehedi' (Marma). *O. rugosa* var. *prostrata* is used by the Tanchangya, Marma, and Chakma indigenous communities for the treatment of different diseases. For example, a paste of the leaves is used for the treatment of skin infections (boils) by the Tanchangya people. The Marma community prepares a tea from the leaves, which is drunk daily for the treatment of body aches and chest pain, while the Chakma community applies sun-dried crushed leaves to the ears for the treatment of earache (personal communication). In addition, the crushed roots of the plant are used for the treatment of dysentery [11,12]. Juice from the leaves is drunk in the treatment of diarrhea within the Marma community (personal communication). However, despite such widespread use, there has been no scientific investigation to date on either pharmacological or phytochemical aspects of the plant to validate its traditional uses. Therefore, we aimed to investigate the bioactive components of *O. rugosa* var. *prostrata* leaves using gas chromatography-mass spectrometry (GC-MS). As plants contain a mixture of phytochemicals, robust separation and identification methods are important to elucidate potential bioactive and toxic constituents [13]. GC-MS, coupled with appropriate detection systems is an invaluable tool for the separation and identification of the components of complex, volatile mixtures [14]. Many plant secondary metabolites are sufficiently small, adequately volatile, and thermostable in the GC environment to be easily analyzed by GC-MS [15]. In addition to the phytochemical investigation, we aimed to investigate the known therapeutic applications of the plant through a combination of in vivo (antidiarrheal and anti-inflammatory), in vitro (anthelmintic and antibacterial) and in silico (molecular docking, ADME/T and PASS) analyses.

2. Results

2.1. GC-MS Analysis

The GC-MS analysis of EEOR revealed 30 compounds, which are listed in Table 1, along with their chemical composition, while the total ionic chromatogram (TIC) is shown in Figure 1. The most abundant component by peak area was shown to be phytol (15.50%), followed by γ-sitosterol (14.94%), stigmasterol (7.92%), erucamide (5.39%), squalene (4.83%), methyl palmitate (3.95%), methyl linoleate (2.96%), vitamin E (2.51%), methyl stearate (1.21%), ethyl linolenate (1.17%), loliolide (1.10%), 2-palmitoylglycerol (0.91%), and neophytadiene (0.86%). The structures of these compounds are presented in Figure 2.

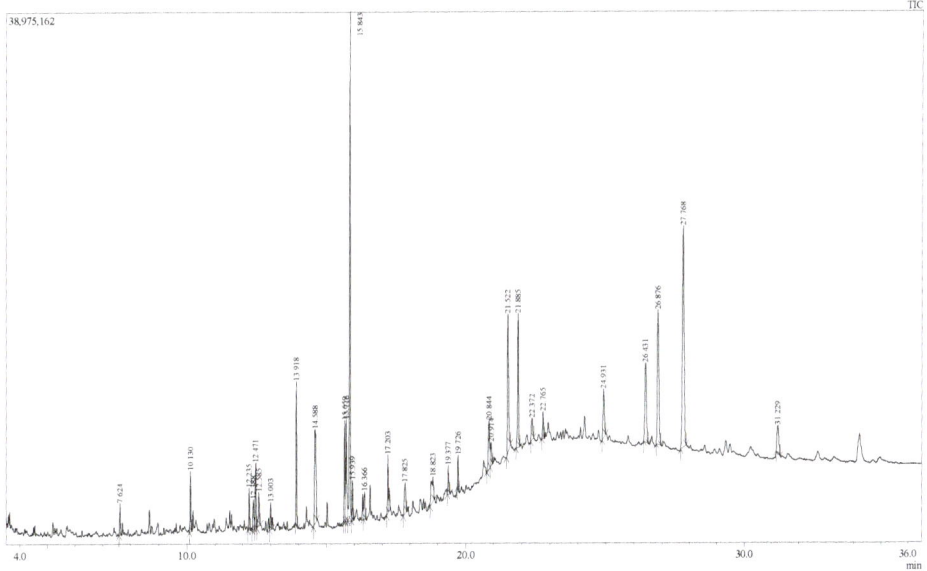

Figure 1. Total ionic chromatogram (TIC) of EEOR (GC-MS, 70eV).

Table 1. List of compounds identified in EEOR by GC-MS analysis.

S.N.	RT (min)	PA (%)	Name of Compound	Molecular Formula
1	7.624	0.92	Carbonic acid, hexadecyl methyl ester	$C_{18}H_{36}O_3$
2	10.130	1.77	1-Nonadecene	$C_{19}H_{38}$
3	12.235	1.29	Succinic acid, tridec-2-yn-1-yl trans-4-methylcyclohexyl ester	$C_{24}H_{40}O_4$
4	12.388	1.10	6-Hydroxy-4,4,7α-trimethyl-5,6,7,7α-tetrahydrobenzofuran-2(4H)-one, or Loliolide	$C_{11}H_{16}O_3$
5	12.471	1.97	1-Nonadecene	$C_{19}H_{38}$
6	12.585	1.38	2-Cyclohexen-1-one, 4-hydroxy-3,5,6-trimethyl-4-(3-oxo-1-butenyl)-	$C_{13}H_{18}O_3$
7	13.003	0.86	Neophytadiene	$C_{20}H_{38}$
8	13.918	3.95	Hexadecanoic acid, methyl ester or Methyl Palmitate	$C_{17}H_{34}O_2$
9	14.588	5.47	9H-Pyrido[3,4-b]indole, 1-methyl-	$C_{12}H_{10}N_2$
10	15.659	2.96	9,12-Octadecadienoic acid (Z,Z)-, methyl ester or Methyl linoleate	$C_{19}H_{34}O_2$
11	15.716	4.33	8,11,14-Docosatrienoic acid, methyl ester	$C_{23}H_{40}O_2$
12	15.843	15.50	Phytol	$C_{20}H_{40}O$
13	15.939	1.21	Methyl stearate	$C_{19}H_{38}O_2$
14	16.366	1.17	9,12,15-Octadecatrienoic acid, ethyl ester, (Z,Z,Z)- or Ethyl linolenate	$C_{20}H_{34}O_2$
15	17.203	1.92	Octadecanoic acid, 3-hydroxypropyl ester	$C_{21}H_{42}O_3$
16	17.825	1.61	1-Heptatriacotanol	$C_{37}H_{76}O$
17	18.823	2.21	6,9-Octadecadienoic acid, methyl ester	$C_{19}H_{34}O_2$
18	19.377	0.91	Hexadecanoic acid, 2-hydroxy-1-(hydroxymethyl)ethyl ester, or 2-Palmitoylglycerol	$C_{19}H_{38}O_4$
19	19.726	0.95	Diisooctyl phthalate	$C_{24}H_{38}O_4$
20	20.844	2.87	E,E,Z-1,3,12-Nonadecatriene-5,14-diol	$C_{19}H_{34}O_2$
21	20.914	1.10	Ethyl 9,12,15-octadecatrienoate	$C_{20}H_{34}O_2$
22	21.522	5.39	13-Docosenamide, (Z)- or Erucamide	$C_{22}H_{43}NO$
23	21.885	4.83	Squalene	$C_{30}H_{50}$
24	22.372	1.14	α-Tocospiro B	$C_{29}H_{50}O_4$
25	22.765	0.92	1,6,10,14,18,22-Tetracosahexaen-3-ol, 2,6,10,15,19,23-hexamethyl-, (all-E)-	$C_{30}H_{50}O$
26	24.931	2.51	Vitamin E	$C_{29}H_{50}O_2$
27	26.431	5.00	Campesterol	$C_{28}H_{48}O$
28	26.876	7.92	Stigmasterol	$C_{29}H_{48}O$
29	27.768	14.94	γ-Sitosterol	$C_{29}H_{50}O$
30	31.229	1.91	Lup-20(29)-en-3-ol, acetate, (3β)-	$C_{32}H_{52}O_2$

RT: Retention time; PA: Peak area.

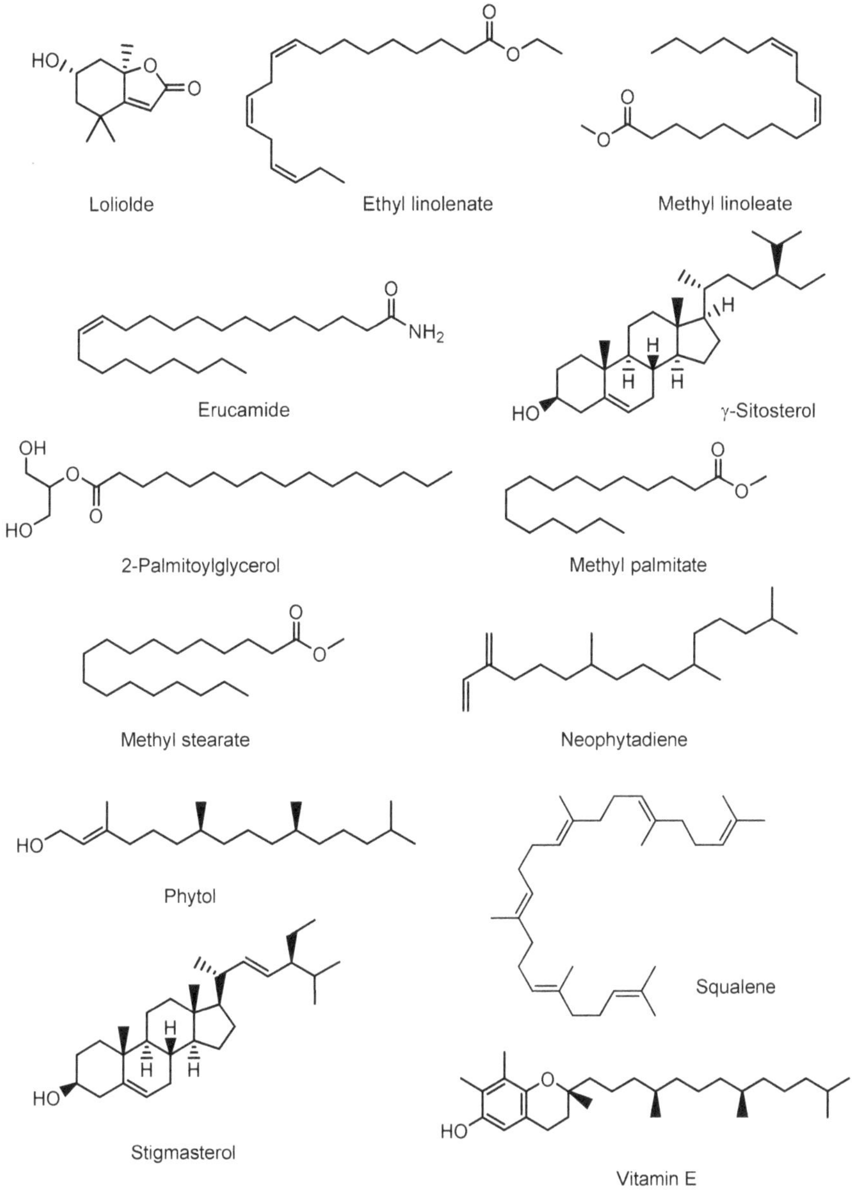

Figure 2. Chemical structures of the major bioactive compounds identified in the EEOR.

2.2. Acute Toxicity Test

The acute oral toxicity testing of EEOR did not show any particular evidence of toxicity or behavioral abnormalities at doses of 5, 50, 100, 200, 400, 1000 or 2000 mg/kg. During the 72 h inspection period, no mortality or physical changes such as allergic reactions, loss of body weight, etc. were observed at the specified doses (data not shown).

2.3. Qualitative Phytochemical Screening

Preliminary phytochemical screening of EEOR suggested the presence of alkaloids, carbohydrates, flavonoids, phenols, tannins, saponins, steroids, sterols, quinones, oxalate, coumarins, and terpenoids (data not shown).

2.4. Effects of EEOR on Castor Oil-Induced Diarrhea in Mice

The effects of EEOR administration on castor oil-induced diarrhea are summarized in Table 2. In this model, EEOR caused significant inhibition of diarrhea, in a dose-dependent manner. The maximum inhibitory effect was observed at a dose of 400 mg/kg (62.50%, $P < 0.001$), which is similar to the reference drug loperamide (65.62%, $P < 0.001$). In addition, EEOR caused a noticeable reduction in defecation numbers at doses of 100 mg/kg (45.20%, $P < 0.01$), 200 mg/kg (52.05%, $P < 0.001$) and 400 mg/kg (60.27%, $P < 0.001$) respectively, compared to the negative control. The reduction of diarrheal feces was also exhibited dose-dependently, with the best antidiarrheal effect observed at the higher dose of 400 mg/kg, compared to the standard drug.

Table 2. The effect of *Ophiorrhiza rugosa* extract on feces count in castor oil-induced diarrhea in mice.

Treatment (mg/kg)	Total Number of Feces	% Inhibition of Defecation	Total Number of Diarrheal Feces	% Inhibition of Diarrhea
Control (0.1 mL/mouse)	14.60 ± 0.74		6.40 ± 0.81	
Loperamide (5)	5.40 ± 0.24 ***	63.01	2.20 ± 0.20 ***	65.62
EEOR (100)	8.00 ± 0.44 **	45.20	5.00 ± 0.31 ***	21.87
EEOR (200)	7.00 ± 0.83 ***	52.05	3.80 ± 0.48 **	40.62
EEOR (400)	5.80 ± 0.20 ***	60.27	2.40 ± 0.24 ***	62.50

Significantly different when compared with that of the control group at ** $P < 0.01$, *** $P < 0.001$. Results are presented as mean ± SEM ($n = 6$).

2.4.1. Effects of EEOR on Castor Oil-Induced Enteropooling in Mice

The effect of EEOR on castor oil-induced enteropooling (Table 3) was a significant reduction in the volume and weight of the intestinal contents. In comparison to the negative control (0.51 ± 0.025), the mean volume of intestinal fluids decreased dose-dependently (0.440 ± 0.014, 0.40 ± 0.017 and 0.34 ± 0.063 at doses of 100, 200 and 400 mg/kg EEOR respectively). In addition, compared to the standard drug loperamide, the dose of 400 mg/kg showed a maximal inhibitory effect on both volume (32.29%, $P < 0.05$) and weight (49.57%, $P < 0.001$) of intestinal contents.

Table 3. The effect of *Ophiorrhiza rugosa* extract on castor oil-induced enteropooling in mice.

Treatment (mg/kg)	Volume of Intestinal Content (mL)	% Inhibition	Weight of Intestinal Content (gm)	% Inhibition
Control (0.1 mL/mouse)	0.51 ± 0.025		0.71±0.022	
Loperamide (5)	0.26 ± 0.013 ***	49.42	0.29±0.012 ***	58.87
EEOR (100)	0.44 ± 0.014 **	13.22	0.55±0.030 **	22.25
EEOR (200)	0.40 ± 0.017 ***	21.78	0.44±0.090 **	38.02
EEOR (400)	0.34 ± 0.063 *	32.29	0.35±0.047 ***	49.57

Significantly different when compared with that of the control group at * $P < 0.05$, ** $P < 0.01$, *** $P < 0.001$. Results are presented as mean ± SEM ($n = 6$).

2.4.2. Effects of EEOR on Charcoal-Induced Intestinal Transit in Mice

The outcomes following different doses of EEOR on intestinal transit are shown in Table 4. In contrast to the negative control, EEOR significantly ($P < 0.001$) reduced the peristalsis index at three different doses. Of these, the 400 mg/kg dose produced the most significant inhibition (58.33%) of intestinal motility, comparable to the standard drug loperamide (57.73%).

Table 4. The effect of *Ophiorrhiza rugosa* extracts on intestinal transit in mice using a charcoal meal as a marker.

Treatment (mg/kg)	Total Length of Intestine (cm)	Distance Travelled by Marker (cm)	Peristalsis Index (%)	% Inhibition Relative to Control
Control (0.1 mL/mouse)	48.60 ± 0.51	41.40 ± 0.93	85.19 ± 1.74	
Loperamide (5)	49.20 ± 0.58	20.80 ± 0.73	42.26 ± 1.32 ***	57.73
EEOR (100)	44.20 ± 0.37 **	29.20 ± 0.58 **	66.07 ± 1.32 ***	33.92
EEOR (200)	43.00 ± 0.44 **	24.80 ± 0.86 ***	57.69 ± 2.08 ***	42.30
EEOR (400)	48.30 ± 0.25 ***	20.10 ± 1.36 ***	41.66 ± 3.02 ***	58.33

Significantly different when compared with that of the control group at ** $P < 0.01$, *** $P < 0.001$. Results are presented as mean ± SEM ($n = 6$).

2.5. Effects of EEOR on Histamine-Induced Mouse Paw Edema

The anti-inflammatory activity of EEOR and diclofenac sodium against histamine-induced edema is shown in Table 5. The results show that the standard drug significantly ($P < 0.001$) inhibited the inflammatory response (42.42%, 60.29%, 66.66% and 78.57%, respectively, at 1 h intervals for 4 h) after sub-plantar injection of histamine, compared to the control group. On the other hand, oral administration of EEOR (100–400 mg/kg) significantly blocked the inflammatory response induced by histamine in a dose-dependent manner, with a dose of 400 mg/kg displaying statistically significant 38.38%, 42.64%, 54.76% and 57.14% ($P < 0.001$) reductions in paw edema at all hourly intervals over 4 h.

Table 5. Anti-inflammatory activity of *Ophiorrhiza rugosa* extract on histamine-induced paw edema.

Treatment (mg/kg)	Paw Volume (mm) (% Inhibition)			
	1 h	2 h	3 h	4 h
Control (0.1mL/mouse)	0.454 ± 0.010	0.392 ± 0.012	0.340 ± 0.007	0.312 ± 0.008
Diclofenac-Na (10)	0.350 ± 0.004 *** (42.42)	0.290 ± 0.007 *** (60.29)	0.264 ± 0.010 *** (66.66)	0.248 ± 0.012 *** (78.57)
EEOR (100)	0.422 ± 0.005 ** (11.11)	0.358 ± 0.015 *** (17.64)	0.310 ± 0.010 *** (23.8)	0.290 ± 0.004 ** (21.42)
EEOR (200)	0.398 ± 0.007 *** (20.20)	0.334 ± 0.009 *** (30.88)	0.294 ± 0.006 *** (35.71)	0.278 ± 0.006 *** (32.14)
EEOR (400)	0.344 ± 0.012 *** (38.38)	0.300 ± 0.006 *** (42.64)	0.260 ± 0.005 *** (54.76)	0.246 ± 0.005 *** (57.14)

Each value is expressed as mean ± SEM ($n = 6$). ** $P < 0.01$, *** $P < 0.001$ compared with the control group (Dunnett's test).

2.6. Anthelmintic Activity

Figure 3 represents the anthelmintic activity of EEOR. The degree of anthelmintic activity shown by the extract was found to be directly proportional to the concentration employed, ranging from the lowest to highest concentration (5, 8, and 10 mg/mL). At concentrations of 5, 8 and 10 mg/mL, EEOR showed significant ($P < 0.001$) paralysis times of (23.28 ± 1.07), (15.30 ± 0.72) and (10.67 ± 0.31) min, while times to death were (57.63 ± 4.42), (32.83 ± 1.95) and (24.59 ± 1.43) min respectively. In the experiment, the positive control (levamisole, 1 mg/mL) showed a paralysis time of (3.22 ± 0.08) min and time to death of (6.19 ± 0.61) min.

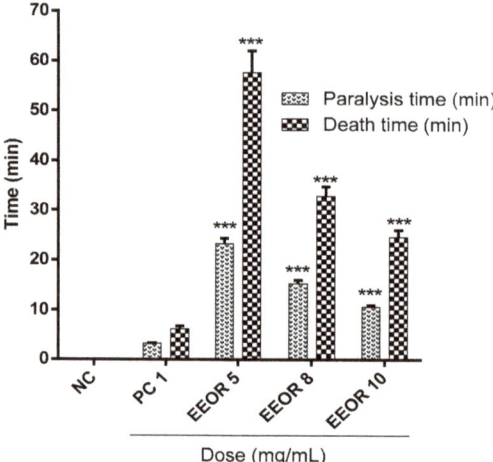

Figure 3. Anthelmintic activity of the ethanol extract of *Ophiorrhiza rugosa* leaves (EEOR). Each value in the table is represented as mean ± SEM (n = 3); NC: Negative control; PC: Positive control, Levamisole (1 mg/mL). *** P < 0.001 compared with PC (Dunnett's test).

2.7. Antibacterial Activity

The antibacterial activity of EEOR is presented in Table 6. The most potent inhibitory effects were exhibited against one Gram-positive (*Bacillus subtilis*), and two Gram-negative (*Salmonella typhi* and *Escherichia coli*) bacteria. The broadest zone of inhibition (16.23 ± 0.68 mm) was found against *Escherichia coli* at a concentration of 1000 µg/disc, followed by *Bacillus subtilis* (14.80 ± 0.72 mm) and *Salmonella typhi* (12.80 ± 0.34 mm). On the other hand, the extract showed no inhibitory effect against four bacteria, namely *Staphylococcus aureus*, *Bacillus cereus*, *Salmonella paratyphi*, and *Pseudomonas aeruginosa*.

Table 6. Antibacterial effects of the ethanol extract of *Ophiorrhiza rugosa* leaves.

Bacterial Strain	Name of the Bacteria	Zone of Inhibition (mm)			
		Concentration (µg/disc)			Kanamycin (30 µg/disc)
		EEOR 500	EEOR 800	EEOR 1000	
Gram-positive	*Staphylococcus aureus* (ATCC 6538)	-	-	-	29.30 ± 0.60
	Bacillus subtilis (ATCC 6633)	7.33 ± 0.57	11.70 ± 0.75	14.80 ± 0.72	32.81 ± 0.67
	Bacillus cereus (ATCC 14579)	-	-	-	27.50 ± 0.58
Gram-negative	*Salmonella typhi* (ATCC 29629)	-	7.33 ± 0.57	12.80 ± 0.34	28.218±0.81
	Salmonella paratyphi (ATCC 9150)	-	-	-	30.51 ± 0.50
	Escherichia coli (ATCC 8739)	8.20 ± 0.72	11.26 ± 1.16	16.23 ± 0.68	31.20 ± 0.82
	Pseudomonas aeruginosa (ATCC 9027)	-	-	-	26.28 ± 0.36

Values are presented as mean inhibition zone (mm) ± SD of three replicates; -: no activity.

2.8. Molecular Docking Study for Antidiarrheal Activity

Results of docking analyses for antidiarrheal activity are shown in Table 7, and the docking figures are shown in Figures S1–S5. In this study, two major receptors (M3 muscarinic acetylcholine receptor, PDB: 4U14; and 5-HT3 receptor, PDB: 5AIN) involved in intestinal motility were used to explore the possible antidiarrheal activity of EEOR. In the case of the M3 muscarinic acetylcholine receptor (PDB: 4U14), Vitamin E showed the highest docking score (−8.80 kcal/mol), better than the standard drug loperamide (−7.32 kcal/mol). On the other hand, for the 5-HT3 receptor (PDB: 5AIN), loliolide

(−5.47 kcal/mol) exhibited the highest docking score, followed by ethyl linolenate, phytol, methyl linoleate, neophytadiene, methyl palmitate, and methyl stearate.

Analysis of the docking fits of each compound suggested various interactions between the ligands and the target enzymes. Loliolide interacts with the M3 muscarinic receptor through one H-bond to Asn507 and two π-π stacking interactions with Tyr529 and Tyr533 (docking score −6.63 Kcal/mol). Ethyl linolenate interacts with the same enzyme through the formation of two H-bonds with Ile222 and Leu225 residues (docking score −6.76 kcal/mol), while methyl linoleate interacted with the enzymatic pocket by establishing one H-bond with Ile222 (docking score −3.26 kcal/mol). 2-Palmitoylglycerol interacted through two H-bonds with Asn152 and Ser151 (docking score −3.55 kcal/mol). Methyl palmitate (score: −2.00 kcal/mol), phytol (score: −3.62 kcal/mol), and vitamin E (score: −8.80 kcal/mol) each form one H-bond, with Tyr148, Ile222 and Ser151 residues respectively.

Table 7. Docking scores of the major bioactive compounds.

Compound Name	Docking Score [1]			
	4U14	5AIN	1SA0	1XFF
Loliolide	−6.63	**−5.47**	−4.49	**−4.88**
Ethyl linolenate	−6.76	−3.47	−5.36	−3.10
Methyl linoleate	−3.26	−1.65	−1.87	0.25
Erucamide	–	–	−2.35	−1.21
γ-Sitosterol	–	–	−7.00	–
2-Palmitoylglycerol	−3.55	–	–	−1.16
Methyl palmitate	−2.00	−0.25	−1.10	+1.81
Methyl stearate	–	+1.62	–	+2.76
Neophytadiene	−2.55	−0.69	−0.59	+1.18
Phytol	−3.62	−2.08	−2.30	−0.12
Squalene	–	–	–	–
Stigmasterol	–	–	−7.13	–
Vitamin E	**−8.80**	–	−6.65	–
Reference drugs (Loperamide/Levamisole/Kanamycin)	−7.32	–	−6.26	−2.73

[1] Docking scores in kcal/mol; Bold text indicates the highest score.

On the other hand, loliolide binds to the enzymatic pocket of the 5-HT3 receptor (PDB ID: 5AIN) by forming one hydrogen bond with Ile116 (docking score −5.47 kcal/mol). Ethyl linolenate (score: −3.47 kcal/mol) and methyl linoleate (score: −1.65 kcal/mol) interact with the same enzymatic pocket, via one H-bond with Glu191 and Arg57 respectively. Methyl stearate interacts with this same enzymatic pocket, by forming one H-bond with Arg57, with a docking score +1.62 kcal/mol. Phytol interacts with the same enzymatic pocket by stabilizing one H-bond with Thr34 (docking score −2.08 kcal/mol). However, methyl palmitate and neophytadiene did not show any interactions with 5AIN. The standard drug loperamide interacts with 4U14 by forming two π-π stacking interactions with Trp525, with a docking score of −7.32 kcal/mol Figure S10C,F.

2.9. Molecular Docking Study for Anthelmintic Activity

Results of docking analysis for anthelmintic activity are presented in Table 7. From the results, it is clear that stigmasterol showed the highest docking score against tubulin (−7.13 kcal/mol), followed by γ-sitosterol (−7.00 kcal/mol), vitamin E (−6.65 kcal/mol), ethyl linolenate (−5.36 kcal/mol), loliolide (−4.49 kcal/mol), erucamide (−2.35 kcal/mol), phytol (−2.30 kcal/mol), methyl linoleate (−1.87 kcal/mol), methyl palmitate (−1.10 kcal/mol), and neophytadiene (−0.59 kcal/mol). Among all compounds, three, namely stigmasterol (−7.13 kcal/mol), γ-sitosterol (−7.00 kcal/mol), and vitamin E (−6.65 kcal/mol) showed better docking scores in comparison to the standard levamisole (−6.26 kcal/mol). However, 2-palmitoylglycerol and squalene did not dock with tubulin (PDB: 1XFF). In this study, the best fits found for illustrating the interactions with tubulin are shown in Figures S6 and S7. Ethyl linolenate and methyl linoleate interact with tubulin by forming one H-bond with

Lys254, whereas erucamide interacted with the same pocket by establishing one H-bond with Asn101. Methyl palmitate and phytol instead form one H-bond with Lys254. Five compounds, namely loliolide, γ-sitosterol, neophytadiene, stigmasterol, and vitamin E did not show any interactions with tubulin. The docking figures of standard drugs are shown in Figure S10B,E.

2.10. Molecular Docking Study for Antibacterial Activity

Thirteen compounds of EEOR were docked with the GlcN-6-P synthase enzyme to assess possible antibacterial activity. Our results indicated that loliolide had the highest binding affinity with the GlcN-6-P synthase enzyme, with a docking score of −4.88 kcal/mol, followed by ethyl linolenate (−3.10), erucamide (−1.21), 2-palmitoylglycerol (−1.16), phytol (−0.12), methyl linoleate (0.25), neophytadiene (+1.18), methyl palmitate (+1.81) and methyl stearate (+2.76). Among all compounds, loliolide and ethyl linolenate showed the best binding affinity against 1XFF, with docking scores of −4.88 and −3.10 kcal/mol respectively, which also ranked better than the standard drug kanamycin (−2.73 kcal/mol). In the antibacterial docking study, the best fit found for loliolide in the enzymatic pocket of GlcN-6-P synthase involved stabilization through the formation of four H-bonds with Hie86, Cyt1, Trp74 and Gly99. The best-ranked fit of ethyl linolenate to the same enzyme was to the binding pocket of 1XFF through two H-bonds to Thr76, and one H-bond with each of Arg73, Asp123, and His77. Methyl linoleate interacts with 1XFF by forming three H-bonds with Arg73, Hie86, and Thr76. The best fit for erucamide in the same enzymatic pocket involved stabilization through the formation of four H-bonds, with Hie86, Arg73, His77, and Asp123. 2-Palmitoylglycerol interacts with the enzyme by forming two H-bonds with Thr76, and two H-bonds with Asp123 and His77. Methyl palmitate interacts with 1XFF via only one H-bond with Arg73, and methyl stearate by forming two H-bonds, with Hie86 and Arg73. Finally, phytol binds to the enzymatic pocket of 1XFF by forming two H-bonds with Asp123 and Thr76. On the other hand, neophytadiene did not show any interactions with 1XFF. The reference drug kanamycin interacts with GlcN-6-P synthase by forming three H-bonds with Trp74, Cyt1, and Gly99, with a docking score of −2.73 kcal/mol. The docking scores obtained for each compound are shown in Table 7, and the docking figures are shown in Figures S8 and S9. The docking figures of standard drugs are shown in Figure S10A,D.

2.11. ADME Analysis

According to Lipinski's rule of five, the compounds γ-sitosterol, squalene, stigmasterol, and vitamin E violated rules of lipophilicity and molecular refractivity. Conversely, loliolide and 2-palmitoylglycerol met Lipinski's conditions, which are considered to predict optimal drug-like character. All other compounds contravened no more than one rule (Table 8).

Table 8. ADME property prediction for the major compounds of EEOR, obtained using Swiss ADME.

Compound Name	MW [1] (g/mol)	HB Acceptor [2]	HB Donor [3]	Log $P_{o/w}$ [4]	Molar Refractivity [5]	Rule of Five [6]
Loliolide	196.24	3	1	1.53	52.51	0
Ethyl linolenate	306.48	2	0	5.82	98.12	1
Methyl linoleate	297.47	2	0	5.69	98.78	1
Erucamide	337.58	1	1	6.77	110.30	1
γ-Sitosterol	414.71	1	1	7.19	133.1	2
2-Palmitoylglycerol	330.50	4	2	4.72	97.06	0
Methyl palmitate	270.45	2	0	5.54	85.12	1
Methyl stearate	298.50	2	0	6.24	94.73	1
Neophytadiene	278.52	0	0	7.07	97.31	1
Phytol	296.53	1	1	6.22	98.94	1
Squalene	410.72	0	0	9.38	143.48	2
Stigmasterol	412.69	1	1	6.96	132.75	2
Vitamin E	430.71	2	1	8.27	139.27	2

[1] MW, Molecular weight (acceptable range: <500). [2] HB, Hydrogen bond acceptor (acceptable range: ≤10). [3] HB, Hydrogen bond donor (acceptable range: ≤5). [4] Lipophilicity (expressed as Log $P_{o/w}$, acceptable range: <5). [5] Molar refractivity should be between 40 and 130. [6] Rule of five: Number of violations of Lipinski's rule of five; recommended range: 0–4.

2.12. PASS Prediction

PASS analysis indicated possible targets and likely pharmacological activities of each of the major compounds within EEOR. We evaluated six biological properties for each compound, based on the values of Pa > Pi and Pa > 7. This prediction approach suggested several important activities of the compounds studied, including antibacterial, anthelmintic, anti-inflammatory, spasmolytic and antiprotozoal actions, which are relevant to our present study. The predicted pharmacological activity profiles of all major compounds are presented in Table 9.

Table 9. Biological activities predicted for *Ophiorrhiza rugosa* major compounds by PASS online.

Compound Name	Biological Properties Predicted by Pass Online	Pa	Pi
Loliolide	Sugar-phosphatase inhibitor	0.727	0.028
	Antibacterial	0.418	0.026
	Spasmolytic, urinary	0.454	0.062
	Anti-inflammatory	0.416	0.088
	Antiperistaltic	0.345	0.018
	Antihelmintic	0.345	0.071
Ethyl linolenate	Lipid metabolism regulator	0.951	0.003
	Anti-inflammatory	0.826	0.005
	Histamine release inhibitor	0.523	0.028
	Antiparasitic	0.489	0.017
	Antihelmintic	0.488	0.019
	Anti-inflammatory, intestinal	0.438	0.015
Methyl linoleate	Lipid metabolism regulator	0.881	0.004
	Antisecretoric	0.781	0.005
	Anti-inflammatory	0.727	0.013
	Reductant	0.637	0.009
	Antihelmintic (Nematodes)	0.500	0.017
	Anti-infective	0.424	0.038
Erucamide	Sugar-phosphatase inhibitor	0.828	0.012
	Anti-infective	0.501	0.022
	Prostaglandin E1 antagonist	0.470	0.005
	Anti-inflammatory, intestinal	0.444	0.014
	Albendazole monooxygenase inhibitor	0.450	0.026
	Antitoxic	0.387	0.025
γ-Sitosterol	Antihypercholesterolemic	0.977	0.001
	Antiviral (Influenza)	0.686	0.006
	Antiinflammatory	0.572	0.038
	Antiacne	0.529	0.005
	Antiprotozoal (*Leishmania*)	0.316	0.091
	Antibacterial	0.282	0.067
2-Palmitoylglycerol	Sugar-phosphatase inhibitor	0.927	0.003
	Lipid metabolism regulator	0.889	0.004
	Antiinfective	0.757	0.005
	Anti-inflammatory, intestinal	0.578	0.004
	Histamine release inhibitor	0.573	0.015
	Antiprotozoal (*Leishmania*)	0.560	0.018
Methyl palmitate	Anti-inflammatory, intestinal	0.758	0.002
	Calcium channel (voltage-sensitive) activator	0.637	0.014
	Antihelmintic (Nematodes)	0.619	0.005
	Reductant	0.523	0.020
	Antimutagenic	0.513	0.014
	Antiprotozoal (*Leishmania*)	0.442	0.035
Methyl stearate	GABA aminotransferase inhibitor	0.820	0.003
	Anti-inflammatory, intestinal	0.758	0.002
	Lipid metabolism regulator	0.740	0.009
	Gastrin inhibitor	0.716	0.004
	Antihelmintic (Nematodes)	0.619	0.005
	Antinociceptive	0.538	0.019

Table 9. Cont.

Compound Name	Biological Properties Predicted by Pass Online	Pa	Pi
Neophytadiene	Carminative	0.691	0.007
	Gastrin inhibitor	0.641	0.012
	Antiulcerative	0.585	0.012
	Histamine release inhibitor	0.506	0.034
	Antiprotozoal (*Leishmania*)	0.460	0.031
	Antiparasitic	0.395	0.032
Phytol	Lipid metabolism regulator	0.828	0.005
	Antiparasitic	0.615	0.008
	Antihelmintic	0.605	0.004
	Antiprotozoal (*Leishmania*)	0.601	0.014
	Histamine release inhibitor	0.526	0.027
	Spasmolytic	0.506	0.027
Squalene	Sugar-phosphatase inhibitor	0.854	0.009
	Gastrin inhibitor	0.743	0.003
	Anti-inflammatory	0.699	0.016
	Antiparasitic	0.555	0.011
	Histamine release inhibitor	0.558	0.018
	Antihelmintic	0.538	0.005
Stigmasterol	Dermatologic	0.809	0.004
	Antiacne	0.552	0.004
	Antiinflammatory	0.541	0.045
	Antiprotozoal (*Leishmania*)	0.403	0.047
	Antisecretoric	0.367	0.068
	Bone formation stimulant	0.306	0.020
Vitamin E	Lipid peroxidase inhibitor	0.978	0.002
	Anti-inflammatory	0.830	0.005
	Free radical scavenger	0.783	0.003
	Spasmolytic	0.525	0.024
	Histamine release inhibitor	0.396	0.093
	Anti-infective	0.277	0.122

Pa = Probable activity; Pi = Probable inactivity.

3. Discussion

Infectious and parasitic diseases continue to represent intimidating issues for developing countries, due to the lack of useful and safe drugs and the increasing resistance of pathogens to available antibiotics or anti-parasitic agents. A common manifestation of these issues is infectious diarrhea, attributable to both enteric bacterial pathogens and parasites [16]. Such infectious agents may evoke not only adverse effects on intestinal functions but also increase systemic risk via compromising host immunity, leading to increased morbidity and mortality [17]. To treat such infectious diseases, different plant parts, plant extracts, and plant-derived products have been used in traditional medicine. However, many of these traditional medicines have not been formally reported in the literature to date. Recent comprehensive reports on plants used for the treatment of infectious diseases, including diarrhea and dysentery have indicated their possible applications as alternative therapies [18]. In Ethiopia for example, a range of medicinal plants including *Calpurnia aurea*, *Croton marcostachyus*, and *Echinops kebercho* have been scientifically validated as anti-infective agents [19]. In addition, combined screening of anti-diarrheal and anti-infective properties of medicinal plants could prove a valid strategy to identify novel therapeutics. A study conducted by *Taylor* et al. 2013 suggested that plants demonstrating significant anti-bacterial activity against entero-pathogens could be considered as potential diarrheal treatments [20]. In vitro and in vivo investigation of *Rhus* plants including *Rhus semialata*, *Rhus javanica*, and *Rhus tripartitum* produced significant anti-bacterial and antidiarrheal effects and the authors concluded that the presence of antibacterial agents might mediate the diarrhea prevention [21,22]. However, to recognize the intrinsic value of plant extracts, the involvement of both in vitro and in vivo approaches is important in the clinically search for effective anti-infective agents. Studies of plants with established ethnomedicinal uses must consider ethnomedicinal preparation practices when evaluating materials scientifically in the laboratory environment. Thorough extraction protocols are important to completely evaluate both therapeutic and toxicological potential of medicinal plants. Typically, plant phytochemicals possess diverse chemical functionalities, yet most are readily soluble in methanol or ethanol, due to their high extractability and high polarity. Many nonpolar compounds are also soluble in this solvent [23,24]. Therefore methanol and ethanol are frequently used for extraction of medicinal plants prior to evaluation of their therapeutic potential, and we selected ethanol for our extraction of *O. rugosa* leaves, the most commonly used part of the plant. Our study identified potential novel active components from the ethanol extract of *Ophiorrhiza rugosa* leaves (EEOR), having antidiarrheal, anti-inflammatory, anthelmintic and antibacterial properties.

To verify the ethnomedicinal uses of *Ophiorrhiza rugosa*, we examined its antidiarrheal activity, as well as its possible mechanism(s) of action in different animal diarrheal models. In all diarrheal experiments, a high dose of the natural laxative castor oil (0.5 mL) was administered to each mouse. The active metabolite of the oil (ricinoleic acid) is liberated via the action of small intestinal lipases, thus altering the motility of gastrointestinal smooth muscle [25,26]. Upon binding of the metabolite with EP3 prostanoid receptors on smooth muscle cells, it inhibits water and electrolyte absorption from the intestine, resulting in accumulation of fluid and interruption of secretory functions, which in turn generates a deleterious effect in the intestine [27,28]. Apart from its laxative effect, ricinoleic acid causes intestinal dysfunction via local inflammation and stimulation of prostaglandin biosynthesis, which also inhibits reabsorption of ions and water [29]. In all antidiarrheal assays, loperamide was used as a standard drug, which enhances the rate of absorption by reducing the volume and movement of intestinal contents [30].

In castor oil-induced diarrhea, the ethanol extract of *O. rugosa* produced a remarkable inhibitory effect, in terms of both defecation rate and diarrhea. The extract, at all doses (100, 200, 400 mg/kg) decreased the total number of feces at 1h intervals over 4h, while diarrheal feces were reduced, indicating an alteration of defecation frequency and consistency. Among all three doses of EEOR, 200 and 400 mg/kg significantly ($P < 0.001$) reduced defecation numbers by 52.05% and 60.27% respectively, which indicates a dose-dependent antidiarrheal action. A dose of the extract with 400 mg/kg EEOR exhibited inhibition (62.50%) of diarrhea that was comparable to the standard drug loperamide (65.62%). This demonstrates that a relatively high dose of EEOR is required to evoke the desired response, and a similar phenomenon has been observed by similar studies on different plant species [31].

The anti-enteropooling potential of EEOR was investigated to explore its antidiarrheal efficacy further and to aid mechanistic interpretation. Our results show that the extract markedly inhibited castor oil-induced enteropooling into the small intestine, likely through suppressing castor oil stimulated prostaglandin biosynthesis. All tested doses significantly decreased intraluminal fluid compared to the control, with the highest dose of 400 mg/kg decreasing both the volume by 32.29% ($P < 0.05$) and weight of intestinal contents by 49.57% ($P < 0.001$). These results confirm the antidiarrheal efficiency of our extract and are comparable with an analogous study conducted by Agbon et al. [32].

To further characterize the effect of EEOR in reducing intestinal hypermotility, we investigated gastrointestinal motility using a charcoal meal tracer. We observed that the administration of the extract delayed the transit of the charcoal marker through the entire intestine. This inhibitory effect was seen with all doses employed and implies that an anti-motility action underlies the mechanism of action of the extract. Maximal inhibition of the peristaltic index was exhibited following a dose of 400 mg/kg (41.66%, $P < 0.001$), and was equipotent with the standard drug loperamide (42.26%, $P < 0.001$). Our findings suggest that the extract both decreases hypermotility and increases the transit time through the suppression of intestinal muscle spasm, thus extending the time for absorptive processes [33].

As aforementioned, castor oil promotes prostaglandin biosynthesis, which leads to the release of various pro-inflammatory mediators, leading to inflammation and irritation. Non-steroidal anti-inflammatory drugs (NSAIDs) may prevent diarrhea through inhibition of castor oil stimulated prostaglandin synthesis [34]. In this study, we assessed the anti-inflammatory activity of EEOR following histamine challenge. Histamine causes contraction of the smooth muscle of small intestine, uterus, bronchi, and bronchioles through activation of H1-receptors [35]. The mechanism of the local inflammatory response induced by histamine is through the activation of vasodilation, edema formation, vascular permeability, and cytokine release. [36]. Our results showed that EEOR significantly ($P < 0.001$) suppressed histamine-induced paw edema, which provides evidence of a potential anti-inflammatory effect. EEOR may thus ameliorate an acute inflammatory response via inhibition of prostaglandins or other inflammatory mediators.

In the anthelmintic study, we utilized the aquatic worm *Tubifex tubifex*, a species of aquatic oligochaete that is a suitable host for the *Myxobolus cerebralis* parasite, responsible for whirling disease in salmonid fish [37]. Our data revealed that exposure to EEOR dose-dependently reduced ($P < 0.001$) both paralysis and death times of the worm, indicating the presence of a potential anthelmintic compound(s). The reference drug levamisole (a nicotinic receptor agonist) activates excitatory nicotinic acetylcholine (nACh) receptors on the muscle of the worm, causing paralysis and death [38], and a similar mechanism may account for the anthelmintic action of EEOR.

We investigated the antimicrobial activity of EEOR through the disc diffusion method, and the extract induced a significant zone of inhibition against both *Bacillus subtilis* (a model Gram-positive microorganism) and *Escherichia coli* (Gram-negative microorganism) at concentrations of 500, 800 and 1000 µg/disc. The lowest concentration (500 µg/disc) failed to show activity against *Salmonella typhi* (Gram-negative microorganism), but the other two concentrations exhibited significant antibacterial activity. These results indicate the existence of a broad-spectrum antibiotic effect of the plant extract and represent the first such data on the extract. On the other hand, we did not find any noticeable effect of our extracts on the Gram-positive *Staphylococcus aureus* or *Bacillus cereus*, or on the Gram-negative organisms *Salmonella paratyphi* or *Pseudomonas aeruginosa*, even at 1000 µg/disc. Broadly, our results suggest that EEOR constituents may interrupt general cellular functions or disrupt bacterial membrane potential [39,40].

Generally, plants are rich in secondary metabolites with diverse biological actions, acting as natural defense mechanisms against bacteria, insects, viruses, and fungi. Our preliminary phytochemical evaluation suggested a distinct phytoconstituent profile in EEOR. Among these, alkaloids, flavonoids, phenols, tannins, terpenoids, and saponins are commonly reported to possess both antibacterial and anthelmintic activities [41,42]. Reports on various plant extracts suggest that antidiarrheal effects may also be mediated through the action of saponins, tannins, steroids flavonoids and alkaloids [43], whereas tannins and flavonoids are well known to aid reabsorption of intestinal fluids and electrolytes [44]. Additionally, tannins reduce intestinal motility by inhibiting bowel irritation, thereby exhibiting an antidiarrheal effect [45]. Various phytochemicals including flavonoids, steroids, and phenols have been ascribed anti-inflammatory actions [46]. As EEOR showed significant anthelmintic and antibacterial activity, especially on certain entero-pathogenic (*Bacillus subtilis*, *Salmonella typhi* and *Escherichia coli*) organisms, coupled with its observed effects on gut motility, this supports its possible utility in infectious diarrhea.

GC-MS analysis of EEOR identified a total of thirty different compounds. Based on the literature, thirteen of these have already been documented to be bioactive. Loliolide [47], ethyl linoleate [48], 2-palmitoylglycerol, and erucamide [49] have been shown to possess antibacterial activity, while γ-sitosterol, stigmasterol, vitamin E, and squalene [47] have both antibacterial and anti-inflammatory activities. Phytol and methyl palmitate have nematicidal, pesticidal, antibacterial, and anti-inflammatory activities. Notably, phytol is very active against *Salmonella typhi* [49]. Finally, neophytadiene [50] and methyl linoleate [47] have demonstrated anti-inflammatory activity.

Molecular docking studies have been widely used for the prediction of ligand-target interactions and to obtain better insights into the biological activity of natural products. It also gives additional clues about possible mechanisms of action and binding modes inside the binding pocket of various enzymes [51]. In order to obtain better insight into the observed biological activity (antidiarrheal, anthelmintic, and antibacterial) of EEOR constituents, thirteen representative compounds within EEOR were selected for docking analyses. These compounds were then docked against four targets, namely the M3 muscarinic acetylcholine receptor (PDB ID: 4U14), the 5-HT3 receptor (PDB ID: 5AIN), tubulin (PDB ID: 1SA0) and GlcN-6-P synthase (PDB: 1XFF).

Molecular docking studies with the M3 muscarinic acetylcholine receptor (PDB ID: 4U14) revealed that, among the thirteen compounds, seven interacted with several amino acid residues through hydrogen bonds and π-π stacking interactions (Tyr529, Tyr533, Ile222, Leu225, Asn152, Ser151, Tyr148), with docking scores ranging between −2.00 and −8.80 kcal/mol. On the other hand, five compounds interacted with a number of amino acid residues (Ile116, Glu191, Arg57, Arg57, and Thr34) within the 5-HT3 receptor (PDB ID: 5AIN) with docking scores ranging from −0.69 to −5.47 kcal/mol. From these results, we can conclude that the studied phytoconstituents may in part be responsible for the antidiarrheal activity of EEOR through interaction with these target proteins.

In the anthelmintic docking study, the thirteen compounds were docked with tubulin (PDB ID: 1SA0) and showed docking scores ranging from −0.59 to −7.13 kcal/mol. From the results, it is clear that the phytoconstituent stigmasterol displayed the highest score against tubulin, followed by γ-sitosterol, vitamin E, ethyl linolenate, loliolide, erucamide, phytol, methyl linoleate, methyl palmitate, and neophytadiene. It has been previously reported that phytol and methyl palmitate possess nematicidal and pesticidal activities [49], and the anthelmintic activity of EEOR may be related to these phytoconstituents. In the case of the antibacterial docking study, loliolide had the highest binding affinity towards the GlcN-6-P synthase enzyme (PDB: 1XFF), followed by ethyl linolenate, erucamide, 2-palmitoylglycerol, phytol, methyl linoleate, neophytadiene, methyl palmitate, and methyl stearate. The antibacterial activity of the EEOR may thus be explained by the presence of loliolide, ethyl linolenate, erucamide, 2-palmitoylglycerol, and phytol, which have good docking scores and for which bioactivity has previously been reported [47,48].

All bioactive compounds were further characterized using the online-based prediction program ADME analysis to explore their drug-likeness, pharmacokinetics and physiochemical characteristics. Almost all compounds, except for γ-sitosterol, squalene, stigmasterol and vitamin E exhibited orally active drug-likeness properties, according to Lipinski's rule. It is reported that compounds with lower molecular weight, lipophilicity, and hydrogen bond capacity have high permeability [52], good absorption and bioavailability [53,54]. However, this analysis does not assess if a compound has any particular pharmacological effect.

To predict a likely pharmacological profile of the compounds, we utilized the structure-based biological activity prediction program Prediction of Activity Spectra for Substances (PASS). The results suggested several activities, among these, we established probable activity values (Pa range 0.235–0.826) for all 13 compounds for anthelmintic, antibacterial, anti-inflammatory, spasmolytic and antiprotozoal actions, supporting our laboratory investigations of EEOR. Moreover, other activities were predicted, suggesting the broader potential of this species. In summary, our comprehensive analyses, utilizing complementary tools, support the traditional uses of EEOR. The observed effects may be due to the combined actions of several phytoconstituents, both those documented herein and potentially other as yet uncharacterized compounds.

4. Materials and Methods

4.1. Drugs and Chemicals

All drugs and chemicals used in this research were of analytical grade. Loperamide was obtained from Square Pharmaceuticals Ltd. (Dhaka, Bangladesh), levamisole from ACI Limited (Dhaka, Bangladesh), and castor oil from WELL's Health Care (Madrid, Spain). Ethanol (Merck, Darmstadt, Germany), Kanamycin (Sigma Chemical Co., St. Louis, MO, USA) and histamine (BDH Chemicals Ltd. Poole, UK) were procured from the mentioned sources.

4.2. Chemical Compounds Studied in This Article

Loliolide (PubChem CID: 100332); Ethyl linolenate (PubChem CID: 6371716); Methyl linoleate (PubChem CID: 5284421); Erucamide (PubChem CID: 5365371); γ-Sitosterol (PubChem CID: 457801); 2-Palmitoylglycerol (PubChem CID: 123409); Methyl Palmitate (PubChem CID: 8181); Methyl stearate (PubChem CID: 8201); Neophytadiene (PubChem CID: 10446); Phytol (PubChem CID: 5280435); Squalene (PubChem CID: 638072); Stigmasterol (PubChem CID: 5280794); Vitamin E (PubChem CID: 14985).

4.3. Plant Collection, Identification, and Extraction

The leaves of *Ophiorrhiza rugosa* var. *prostrata* (D.Don) Deb & Mondal were collected in September 2017 from Kaptai National Park (22°30'08"N 92°12'04"E), Rangamati District, Chittagong Division, Bangladesh. The plant was certified and authenticated by Dr. Shaikh Bokhtear Uddin, Professor, Ethno-botany and Pharmacognosy Lab, Department of Botany, University of Chittagong, Bangladesh, with a voucher specimen (accession no: 7609 CTGUH) deposited in the Herbarium of the University of Chittagong (CTGUH). After subsequent washing with normal and distilled water, the collected leaves were cut and oven-dried for a week at constant temperature (50 °C), before milling into a coarse powder using an automatic grinder. Then, the fine powder (350 g) was soaked in 850 mL of ethanol for seven days at room temperature, with regular shaking and stirring on a shaker machine (model VTRS-1, Nunes Instruments, Tamil Nadu, India). After 7 days, the macerate was filtered through a sterilized cotton plug followed by Whatman filter paper No. 1, and the eluting solvent evaporated on a rotary evaporator (RE 200, Sterling, Norman Way Industrial Estate, Cambridge, UK) at room temperature to afford a semisolid extract (EEOR: 10 g), which was kept in a refrigerator (-4 °C) until further use.

4.4. Animals and Ethical Statements

Adult Swiss albino mice (20–25 g) of both sexes were obtained from Jahangir Nagar University, Savar, Dhaka, Bangladesh. The animals were housed in polypropylene cages for adaptation, under standard laboratory conditions (room temperature 25 ± 2 °C; relative humidity 55–60%, 12 h light/dark cycle), with food pellets and water *ad libitum*. All animals were acclimatized for 2 weeks and fasted overnight before starting all experiments. This experiment was designed based on the Ethical Principles and Guidelines guided by The Swiss Academy of Medical Sciences and the Swiss Academy of Sciences. All tests were run in a remote and noiseless ambiance, between 9.00 a.m. and 5.00 p.m. The study protocol was approved by both the Ethical review committee and the P&D committee of the Department of Pharmacy, International Islamic University Chittagong, Bangladesh under the code Pharm-P&D-61/08'16-122.

4.5. GC-MS (Gas Chromatography-Mass Spectroscopy) Analysis of EEOR

GC-MS analysis of EEOR was evaluated using a model 7890A capillary gas chromatograph along with a mass spectrometer (Agilent Technologies, Santa Clara, CA, USA). The column was a fused silica capillary column of 95% dimethyl-poly-siloxane and 5% phenyl (HP-5MSI; length: 90 m, diameter: 0.250 mm and film: 0.25 μm). Parameters for GC-MS detection were an injector temperature of 250 °C, an initial oven temperature of 90 °C gradually raised to 200 °C at a speed of 3 °C/min for 2 min and with a final increase to 280 °C at 15 °C/min for 2 min. The total GC-MS run time was 36 min, using 99.999% helium as a carrier gas, at a column flow rate of 1 mL/min. The GC to MS interface temperature was fixed at 280 °C, and an electron ionization system was set on the MS in scan mode. The mass range evaluated was 50–550 *m/z*, where MS quad and source temperatures were maintained at 150 °C and 230 °C respectively. The NIST-MS Library 2009 was used to search and identify each component, and to measure the relative percentage of each compound, relative peak areas of the TIC (total ionic chromatogram) were used, with calculations performed automatically.

4.6. Acute Toxicity Testing of EEOR

Acute toxicity testing was assessed under standard laboratory conditions following OECD guidelines [55]. Animals ($n = 6$) of the control and test groups were each administered 1% Tween-80 or a single oral dose (5, 50, 100, 200, 400, 1000 and 2000 mg/kg body weight) of the test extract (EEOR). Before administration of extract, mice were kept fasting overnight, and food was also delayed for 3 to 4 h after receiving the extract. All experimental animals were observed individually, paying particular attention to any unexpected responses, including behavioral changes, allergic syndromes (itching, skin rash), and mortality over the next 72 h.

4.7. Qualitative Phytochemical Screening of EEOR

Qualitative phytochemical analysis of EEOR was carried out following standard procedures, as previously reported by Tiwari et al. [56].

4.8. Antidiarrheal Activity Evaluation of EEOR (In Vivo)

4.8.1. Castor Oil-Induced Diarrhea

The conditions of Awouters et al. [34] were followed with slight modifications. Mice were fasted overnight prior to the experiment. Experimental animals were separated randomly into control and test groups consisting of 6 mice in each category. Group-I served as a negative control, and received 1% Tween-80 in distilled water; group-II (positive control) received loperamide (5 mg/kg BW; p.o), while test groups III-V were treated with EEOR (100, 200 and 400mg/kg BW; p.o) respectively. After 1 h, each mouse was put into an individual cage and diarrhea induced (0.5 mL castor oil, p.o). Blotting paper on the floor of each cage was monitored to observe both the number and consistency of fecal droppings. Blotting papers were replaced every 60 min during the 4h observation period. The total numbers of both dry and wet feces excreted by the animals were counted. The following equation was used to calculate percent inhibition of diarrhea:

$$\text{percentage of inhibition of diarrhea} = \frac{\text{Total number of diarrheal faces} \times (\text{control} - \text{test groups})}{\text{Total number of diarrheal faces of the control}} \times 100, \quad (1)$$

4.8.2. Castor Oil-Induced Enteropooling

Intraluminal fluid accumulation was evaluated by the method described by Robert et al. [57]. Dosing treatments were as for castor oil-induced diarrheal testing, again with six animals per group. One hour post administrations of each test dose, animals were treated with castor oil (0.5 mL) to induce diarrhea. Two hours later, the mice were sacrificed, and the small intestine was isolated from pyloric sphincter to caecum. The small intestine was weighed (g) and the volume of intestinal contents (ml) was measured by milking into a graduated tube. The intestine was reweighed, and the differences between full and empty intestines were calculated. To calculate, the percentage volume and weight of intestinal contents were determined using the following formula:

$$\text{percentage of inhibition} = \frac{\text{Mean of intestinal content} \times (\text{control} - \text{test groups})}{\text{Mean of intestinal content of the control}} \times 100, \quad (2)$$

4.8.3. Gastrointestinal Motility

This experiment was performed based on the method of Mascolo et al. [58], with the treatment of animals of each group ($n = 6$) as described in the castor oil-induced diarrhea test. In brief, 0.5 mL of castor oil was administered to each animal to induce diarrhea. One hour after administration of each test dose, animals were treated orally with 1 mL of a charcoal meal (10% charcoal suspension in 5% gum acacia). After 1 h, animals were sacrificed and the distance traveled by the charcoal meal from the pylorus to caecum was measured (cm) and expressed as a percentage of the total distance of the intestine. The following formulae were used to express the percentage of inhibition and Peristalsis index:

$$\text{inhibition (\%)} = \frac{\text{Distance (cm) travel by the charcoal} \times (\text{control} - \text{test groups})}{\text{Distance travel by the charcoal in the control group}} \times 100, \quad (3)$$

$$\text{Peristalsis Index} = \frac{\text{Distance travel by the charcoal meal}}{\text{Total length of the small intestine}} \times 100, \quad (4)$$

4.9. Histamine-Induced Paw Edema

The anti-inflammatory activity of EEOR was evaluated following injection of histamine into the plantar surface of the mouse hind paw [59]. Animals were divided into four groups ($n = 6$); Group I (negative control) received 1% Tween-80 (2 mL/kg); Group II (Positive control) received diclofenac sodium (10 mg/kg BW; p.o); and Groups III and IV received EEOR (200 and 400 mg/kg BW; p.o) respectively. 30 min following treatment, 0.05 mL histamine (1 mg/kg, in 1% Tween-80 with D.W) was injected in the sub-plantar area of the right paw of each mouse to induce acute inflammation, and micrometer slide calipers were used to measure the paw volume at 1, 2, 3 and 4 h. The percentage inhibition of the inflammatory effect of the extract was calculated using the following expression:

$$\text{\% inhibition of inflammation} = \frac{\text{Mean degree of inflammation (control} - \text{test groups})}{\text{Mean degree of inflammation of control}} \times 100 \quad (5)$$

4.10. Anthelmintic Activity of EEOR (In Vitro)

Anthelmintic activity was assessed following the method of Ajaiyeoba et al. with slight modifications [60,61]. In this experiment, the sludge worm, or sewage worm (*Tubifex tubifex*, size: 2 to 2.5 cm in length), was used for its physiological and anatomical relevance to intestinal worms, e.g., Annelida. Testing was performed in triplicate. In brief, 5 to 10 worms were randomly placed in each Petri dish, divided into four groups (I, II, III and IV). To each, 3 mL of either EEOR at a specified concentration (5, 8 or 10 mg/mL) or the standard drug levamisole (1 mg/mL) added. Anthelmintic activity was calculated at two different stages, namely 'time of paralysis' and 'time of death' of the worms. Time to paralysis was counted as the time when worms lost their natural movement. The time of death was recorded after confirming that the worms moved neither when vigorously shaken nor when dipped in slightly warm water.

4.11. Antibacterial Activity of EEOR (In Vitro)

The antibacterial effect of EEOR was evaluated by the disc diffusion technique [62]. Prepared Nutrient agar was placed into Petri dishes under laminar airflow for solidification. Overnight cultures of Gram-positive *Bacillus subtilis* (ATCC 6633), *Staphylococcus aureus* (ATCC 6538) and *Bacillus cereus* (ATCC 14579) and Gram-negative *Salmonella typhi* (ATCC 29629), *Salmonella paratyphi* (ATCC 9150), *Escherichia coli* (ATCC 8739) and *Pseudomonas aeruginosa* (ATCC 9027) organisms were each prepared with 100 µL bacteria (bacterial inocula were adjusted to 10^8 CFU/mL), spread smoothly on the agar surface. Dry sterile discs (6mm diameter) were laid upon the seeded agar plate using a sterile forceps. Each desired concentration of EEOR (500, 800 or 1000 µg) was loaded on these discs and then incubated (at 37 °C for 24 h). The diameter of each zone of inhibition was recorded and measured in mm. As a positive control, kanamycin (30 µg/disc) was used.

4.12. In silico Molecular Docking

The major bioactive compounds of EEOR, as detected by GC-MS, were selected for molecular docking studies, to understand better possible molecular interactions based on their affinity to interact with different target proteins. Docking studies were performed using the Schrödinger suite-Maestro v10.1, LLC, New York, NY, USA, and Accelrys Discovery Studio 4.0 software (BIOVIA, San Diego, CA, USA) was used for visualization of 3D structures.

4.12.1. Ligand Preparation

The structures of thirteen major compounds were obtained from the PubChem compound repository, and the ligands prepared using the LigPrep tool embedded in Maestro v 10.1 (Schrödinger suite, LLC New York, NY, USA), neutralized at pH 7.0 ± 2.0 using Epik 2.2, and minimized by force field OPLS_2005.

4.12.2. Receptor Preparation

3D crystal structures of the proteins used for the test were downloaded from the Protein Data Bank; RCSB PDB [63], GlcN-6-P synthase (PDB ID: 1XFF) [64], tubulin (PDB ID: 1SA0) [65] 5-HT3 receptor (PDB ID: 5AIN) [66] and M3 muscarinic acetylcholine receptor (PDB ID: 4U14) [67]. The Protein Preparation Wizard of the Schrödinger suite-Maestro version 10.1 was used to prepare and refine the crystal structures. Charges and bond orders were assigned, hydrogens added to heavy atoms and selenomethionines and selenocysteines converted into methionines and cysteines respectively, followed by removing all water molecules. Using force field OPLS_2005, minimization was performed to set a maximum heavy atom RMSD to 0.30 Å.

4.12.3. Grid Generation and Molecular Docking

Receptor grid generation and molecular docking experiments were performed using Glide (Schrödinger suite-Maestro version 10.1) [68,69] For each protein, a grid was produced using the following default parameters: van der Waals scaling factor 1.00 and charge cut-off value 0.25, subjected to the OPLS_2005 force field. A cubic box of definite dimensions centered on the centroid of the active site residues was generated for the receptor, and the box size was set to 14 Å × 14 Å × 14 Å for docking. Docking experiments were carried out using the Standard Precision (SP) scoring function of Glide, and only the best scoring fit with docking score was noted for each ligand.

4.13. In Silico ADME Analysis

The pharmacokinetic properties of all major identified compounds were evaluated using Lipinski's rule of five [70]. Lipinski stated that a compound could show drug-like behavior if it does not fail more than one of the following criteria: (i) molecular weight not more than 500; (ii) H-bond donors ≤5; (iii) H-bond acceptors ≤10; (iv) Lipophilicity <5; and (v) molar refractivity between 40 and 130. The web tool Swiss ADME [71] was used to assess the ADME parameters of all compounds. Compounds which obey Lipinski rule are considered as ideal drug candidates.

4.14. In Silico PASS Prediction

Possible biological activities of identified major compounds were evaluated using the online computer program PASS (Prediction of Activity Spectra for Substances) [72]. This tool predicts up to 3750 biological properties of a compound, associated with an analysis of its chemical structure. The outcomes of this analysis were denoted as Pa (probable activity) and Pi (probable inactivity), where the values of both Pa and Pi may differ from 0.000 to 1.000. We considered values of $P_a > P_i$ and Pa > 0.700 to indicate biological activity for a compound [73].

5. Statistical Analysis

Data were analyzed using SPSS 20.0 statistical software (SPSS, IBM Corporation, Armonk, NY, USA). Results were presented as mean ± SEM (standard error of the mean), and one-way ANOVA followed by Dunnett's test was applied. A *p*-value of less than 0.05 was considered significant.

6. Conclusions

In summary, our study demonstrates that EEOR possesses significant and dose-dependent antidiarrheal activity in different models, which supports the traditional use of this plant in folk medicine. The study also provides further evidence of inhibition of inflammatory mediators, which rationalise the anti-inflammatory activity of the plant extract. The positive results regarding anthelmintic and antibacterial activities increase the value of this plant. Collectively, these outcomes support the ethnomedicinal use of *O. rugosa* for the management of various infectious diseases. Furthermore, various potential bioactive constituents identified by GC-MS analysis showed promising binding affinity toward different proteins in molecular docking experiments, and their drug-like characteristics were demonstrated through ADME/T analysis. PASS predictions of bioactive constituents were in agreement with our laboratory findings. Therefore, *O. rugosa* may represent a viable candidate for the treatment of infectious diseases. However, further studies are needed to identify and isolate the pure compounds responsible for the observed biological effects, and to characterize its toxicity profile and longer-term safety.

Supplementary Materials: The following are available online, Figure S1. 2D interactions of the best fit found for (A) Loliolide, (B) Ethyl linolenate, (C) Methyl linoleate, (D) 2-Palmitoylglycerol, (E) Methyl palmitate, (F) Neophytadiene, (G) Phytol, and (H) Vitamin E docked to the M3 muscarinic acetylcholine receptor (PDB ID: 4U14); Figure S2. Best ranked fit of (A) Loliolide, (B) Ethyl linolenate, (C) Methyl linoleate, (D) 2-Palmitoylglycerol, (E) Methyl palmitate, (F) Neophytadiene, (G) Phytol and (H) Vitamin E in the binding pocket of the M3 muscarinic acetylcholine receptor (PDB ID: 4U14); Figure S3. 2D interactions of the best fit found for (A) Loliolide, (B) Ethyl linolenate, (C) Methyl linoleate, (D) Methyl palmitate, (E) Methyl stearate and (F) Neophytadiene docked to the 5-HT3 receptor (PDB ID: 5AIN); Figure S4. Best ranked fit of (A) Loliolide, (B) Ethyl linolenate, (C) Methyl linoleate, (D) Methyl palmitate, (E) Methyl stearate and (F) Neophytadiene in the binding pocket of the 5-HT3 receptor (PDB ID: 5AIN); Figure S5. Best ranked fit of Phytol (A) in the binding pocket of 5-HT3 (PDB ID: 5AIN) and 2D representation of key interactions in the binding pocket for Phytol (B); Figure S6. 2D interactions of the best fit found for (A) Loliolide, (B) Ethyl linolenate, (C) Methyl linoleate, (D) Erucamide, (E) γ-Sitosterol, (F) Methyl palmitate, (G) Neophytadiene, (H) Phytol, (I) Stigmasterol and (J) Vitamin E docked to tubulin (PDB ID: 1SA0); Figure S7. Best ranked fit of (A) Loliolide, (B) Ethyl linolenate, (C) Methyl linoleate, (D) Erucamide, (E) γ-Sitosterol, (F) Methyl palmitate, (G) Neophytadiene, (H) Phytol, (I) Stigmasterol and (J) Vitamin E in the binding pocket of tubulin (PDB ID: 1SA0); Figure S8. 2D interactions of the best fit found for (A) Loliolide, (B) Ethyl linolenate, (C) Methyl linoleate, (D) Erucamide, (E) 2-Palmitoylglycerol, (F) Methyl palmitate, (G) Methyl stearate, (H) Neophytadiene and (I) Phytol docked to GlcN-6-P synthase (PDB ID: 1XFF); Figure S9. Best ranked fit of (A) Loliolide, (B) Ethyl linolenate, (C) Methyl linoleate, (D) Erucamide, (E) 2-Palmitoylglycerol, (F) Methyl palmitate, (G) Methyl stearate, (H) Neophytadiene and (I) Phytol in the binding pocket of GlcN-6-P synthase (PDB ID: 1XFF); Figure S10. (A) Best fit and (D) 2D interaction diagram of Kanamycin docked at the binding pocket of GlcN-6-P synthase (PDB ID: 1XFF). (B) Best fit and (E) 2D interaction diagram of Levamisole docked at the binding pocket of tubulin (PDB ID: 1SA0). (C) Best fit and (F) 2D interaction diagram of Loperamide docked at the binding pocket of M3 muscarinic acetylcholine receptor (PDB ID: 4U14).

Author Contributions: M.A. and M.N.U.C. conceived and designed the experiments, prepared the plant extract, carried out all the experimental works and collected and analyzed the data. M.A. drafted the final manuscript. M.O.K.A. helped to perform in vivo antidiarrheal experiments. M.N.U.C. and A.P. performed the in silico study. D.H.C., A.T.M.M.K., S.B.U., J.W.B., M.O.F., and C.H.P. supervised the study, evaluated the experimental data and reviewed the final manuscript. All authors read and approved the final manuscript.

Funding: This research received no external funding.

Acknowledgments: This research was supported by the Department of Pharmacy, International Islamic University Chittagong, Bangladesh, Kangwon National University, and Central Laboratory of Kangwon National University, Chuncheon, 24341, Korea.

Conflicts of Interest: The authors declare that they have no conflict of interest.

Abbreviations

EEOR	Ethanol extract of *Ophiorrhiza rugosa* leaves
p.o.	per oral
i.p.	Intraperitoneal
ANOVA	Analysis of variance
BW	body weight
SEM	standard error of mean

SPSS	statistical package for social science
ADME/T	Absorption, Distribution, Metabolism, Excretion, and Toxicity
PASS	Prediction of Activity Spectra for Substances

References

1. Saritha, K.; Rajesh, A.; Manjulatha, K.; Setty, O.H.; Yenugu, S. Mechanism of antibacterial action of the alcoholic extracts of *Hemidesmus indicus* (L.) R. Br. ex Schult, Leucas aspera (Wild.), *Plumbago zeylanica* L., and Tridax procumbens (L.) R. Br. ex Schult. *Front. Microbiol.* **2015**, *6*, 577. [CrossRef] [PubMed]
2. Clatworthy, A.E.; Pierson, E.; Hung, D.T. Targeting virulence: A new paradigm for antimicrobial therapy. *Nat. Chem. Biol.* **2007**, *3*, 541. [CrossRef] [PubMed]
3. Perry, B.D.; Randolph, T.F. Improving the assessment of the economic impact of parasitic diseases and of their control in production animals. *Vet. Parasitol.* **1999**, *84*, 145–168. [CrossRef]
4. Vasco, G.; Trueba, G.; Atherton, R.; Calvopina, M.; Cevallos, W.; Andrade, T.; Eguiguren, M.; Eisenberg, J.N.S. Identifying etiological agents causing diarrhea in low income Ecuadorian communities. *Am. J. Trop. Med. Hyg.* **2014**, *91*, 563–569. [CrossRef] [PubMed]
5. Hammer, K.A.; Carson, C.F.; Riley, T.V. Antimicrobial activity of essential oils and other plant extracts. *J. Appl. Microbiol.* **1999**, *86*, 985–990. [CrossRef]
6. Matthews, H.B.; Lucier, G.W.; Fisher, K.D. Medicinal herbs in the United States: Research needs. *Environ. Health Perspect.* **1999**, *107*, 773–778. [CrossRef]
7. Normile, D. The new face of traditional Chinese medicine. *Science* **2003**, *299*, 188–190. [CrossRef]
8. Wagner, H.; Ulrich-Merzenich, G. Synergy research: Approaching a new generation of phytopharmaceuticals. *Phytomedicine* **2009**, *16*, 97–110. [CrossRef]
9. Coan, K.E.D.; Ottl, J.; Klumpp, M. Non-stoichiometric inhibition in biochemical high-throughput screening. *Expert Opin. Drug Discov.* **2011**, *6*, 405–417. [CrossRef] [PubMed]
10. Sneader, W. *Drug Discovery: A History*; John Wiley & Sons: Hoboken, NJ, USA, 2005; ISBN 0471899798.
11. Bangladesh Ethnobotany Online Database. Ophiorrhiza Horrisiana Heyne. Available online: http://www.ebbd.info/ophiorrhiza-horrisiana.html (accessed on 4 December 2018).
12. Quattrocchi, U. *CRC World Dictionary of Medicinal and Poisonous Plants. Common Names, Scientific Names, Eponyms, Synonyms, and Etymology*; CRC Press: Boca Raton, FL, USA, 2012; ISBN 9788578110796.
13. Gherman, C.; Culea, M.; Cozar, O. Comparative analysis of some active principles of herb plants by GC/MS. *Talanta* **2000**, *53*, 253–262. [CrossRef]
14. Yi, T.; Li, S.-M.; Fan, J.-Y.; Fan, L.-L.; Zhang, Z.-F.; Luo, P.; Zhang, X.-J.; Wang, J.-G.; Zhu, L.; Zhao, Z.-Z. Comparative analysis of EPA and DHA in fish oil nutritional capsules by GC-MS. *Lipids Health Dis.* **2014**, *13*, 190. [CrossRef]
15. Huertas-Pérez, J.F.; Ernest, M.; Badoud, F. Quantification of folpet and phthalimide in tea and herbal infusions by LC-high-resolution MS and GC–MS/MS. *Food Addit. Contam. Part A* **2019**, *36*, 109–119. [CrossRef]
16. Hodges, K.; Gill, R. Infectious diarrhea: Cellular and molecular mechanisms. *Gut Microb.* **2010**, *1*, 4–21. [CrossRef]
17. Petri, W.A.; Miller, M.; Binder, H.J.; Levine, M.M.; Dillingham, R.; Guerrant, R.L. Enteric infections, diarrhea, and their impact on function and development. *J. Clin. Investig.* **2008**, *118*, 1277–1290. [CrossRef]
18. Dubreuil, J. Antibacterial and antidiarrheal activities of plant products against enterotoxinogenic Escherichia coli. *Toxins* **2013**, *5*, 2009–2041. [CrossRef]
19. Tadesse, E.; Engidawork, E.; Nedi, T.; Mengistu, G. Evaluation of the anti-diarrheal activity of the aqueous stem extract of Lantana camara Linn (Verbenaceae) in mice. *BMC Complement. Altern. Med.* **2017**, *17*, 190. [CrossRef]
20. Taylor, P.W. Alternative natural sources for a new generation of antibacterial agents. *Int. J. Antimicrob. Agents* **2013**, *42*, 195–201. [CrossRef]
21. Tangpu, V.; Yadav, A.K. Antidiarrhoeal activity of Rhus javanica ripen fruit extract in albino mice. *Fitoterapia* **2004**, *75*, 39–44. [CrossRef]
22. Bose, S.K.; Dewanjee, S.; Gupta, A.S.; Samanta, K.C.; Kundu, M.; Mandal, S.C. In vivo evaluation of antidiarrhoeal activity of Rhus semialata fruit extract in rats. *African J. Tradit. Complement. Altern. Med.* **2008**, *5*, 97–102. [CrossRef]

23. Boeing, J.S.; Barizão, É.O.; e Silva, B.C.; Montanher, P.F.; de Cinque Almeida, V.; Visentainer, J.V. Evaluation of solvent effect on the extraction of phenolic compounds and antioxidant capacities from the berries: Application of principal component analysis. *Chem. Cent. J.* **2014**, *8*, 48. [CrossRef]
24. Adnan, M.; Chy, M.N.U.; Kamal, A.T.M.M.; Barlow, J.W.; Faruque, M.O.; Yang, X.; Uddin, S.B. Evaluation of anti-nociceptive and anti-inflammatory activities of the methanol extract of Holigarna caustica (Dennst.) Oken leaves. *J. Ethnopharmacol.* **2019**, *236*, 401–411. [CrossRef]
25. Kulkarni, S.R.; Pandit, A.B. Enzymatic hydrolysis of castor oil: An approach for rate enhancement and enzyme economy. *Indian J. Biotechnol.* **2005**, *4*, 241–245.
26. Mathias, J.R.; Martin, J.L.; Burns, T.W.; Carlson, G.M.; Shields, R.P. Ricinoleic acid effect on the electrical activity of the small intestine in rabbits. *J. Clin. Investig.* **1978**, *61*, 640–644. [CrossRef]
27. Tunaru, S.; Althoff, T.F.; Nüsing, R.M.; Diener, M.; Offermanns, S. Castor oil induces laxation and uterus contraction via ricinoleic acid activating prostaglandin EP3 receptors. *Proc. Natl. Acad. Sci. USA* **2012**, *109*, 9179–9184. [CrossRef]
28. Racusen, L.C.; Binder, H.J. Ricinoleic acid stimulation of active anion secretion in colonic mucosa of the rat. *J. Clin. Investig.* **1979**, *63*, 743–749. [CrossRef]
29. Pierce, N.F.; Carpenter, C.C.J.; Elliott, H.L.; Greenough, W.B. Effects of prostaglandins, theophylline, and cholera exotoxin upon transmucosal water and electrolyte movement in the canine jejunum. *Gastroenterology* **1971**, *60*, 22–32.
30. Schiller, L.R.; Santa Ana, C.A.; Morawski, S.G.; Fordtran, J.S. Mechanism of the antidiarrheal effect of loperamide. *Gastroenterology* **1984**, *86*, 1475–1480.
31. Trease, G.E.; Evans, W.C. *Pharmacognosy*, 13th ed.; Bailliere Tindall Ltd.: London, UK, 1989.
32. Agbon, A.N.; Kwaneshie, H.O.; Hamman, W.O. Antidiarrheal activity of aqueous fruit extract of Phoenix dactylifera (DATE PALM) in Wistar rats. *Br. J. Pharmacol. Toxicol.* **2013**, *4*, 121–127. [CrossRef]
33. Islam, M.M.; Pia, R.S.; Sifath-E-Jahan, K.; Chowdhury, J.; Akter, F.; Parvin, N.; Akter, S. Antidiarrheal activity of Dillenia indica bark extract. *Int. J. Pharm. Sci. Res.* **2013**, *4*, 682.
34. Awouters, F.; Niemegeers, C.J.E.; Lenaerts, F.M.; Janssen, P.A.J. Delay of castor oil diarrhoea in rats: A new way to evaluate inhibitors of prostaglandin biosynthesis. *J. Pharm. Pharmacol.* **1978**, *30*, 41–45. [CrossRef]
35. Abbas, A.K.; Lichtman, A.H.; Pober, J.S. *Cellular and Molecular Immunology*; WB Saunders Company: Philadelphia, PA, USA, 1994.
36. Tamaddonfard, E.; Farshid, A.A.; Hosseini, L. Crocin alleviates the local paw edema induced by histamine in rats. *Avicenna J. Phytomed.* **2012**, *2*, 97.
37. Gilbert, M.A.; Granath, W.O., Jr. Whirling disease of salmonid fish: Life cycle, biology, and disease. *J. Parasitol.* **2003**, *89*, 658–667. [CrossRef]
38. Jamkhande, P.G.; Barde, S.R. Evaluation of anthelmintic activity and in silico PASS assisted prediction of Cordia dichotoma (Forst.) root extract. *Anc. Sci. Life* **2014**, *34*, 39–43. [CrossRef]
39. Patra, J.K.; Baek, K.-H. Antibacterial activity and action mechanism of the essential oil from Enteromorpha linza L. against foodborne pathogenic bacteria. *Molecules* **2016**, *21*, 388. [CrossRef]
40. Khan, R.; Islam, B.; Akram, M.; Shakil, S.; Ahmad, A.A.; Ali, S.M.; Siddiqui, M.; Khan, A.U. Antimicrobial activity of five herbal extracts against multi drug resistant (MDR) strains of bacteria and fungus of clinical origin. *Molecules* **2009**, *14*, 586–597. [CrossRef]
41. Okeke, M.I.; Iroegbu, C.U.; Eze, E.N.; Okoli, A.S.; Esimone, C.O. Evaluation of extracts of the root of Landolphia owerrience for antibacterial activity. *J. Ethnopharmacol.* **2001**, *78*, 119–127. [CrossRef]
42. Akter, K.N.; Karmakar, P.; Das, A.; Anonna, S.N. Evaluation of antibacterial and anthelmintic activities with total phenolic contents of Piper betel leaves. *Avicenna J. Phytomed.* **2014**, *4*, 320–329.
43. Macauder, P.J. Flavonoids affect acetylcholine, prostaglandin E and antigen mediated muscle contration. *Prog. Clin. Biol. Res.* **1986**, *231*, 489–492.
44. Carlo, G.D.; Mascolo, N.; Izzo, A.A.; Capasso, F. Effects of quercetin on the gastrointestinal tract in rats and mice. *Phyther. Res.* **1994**, *8*, 42–45. [CrossRef]
45. Daswani, P.G.; Brijesh, S.; Tatali, P.; Antia, N.H.; Birdi, T.J. Antidiarrhoeal activity of Zingiber officinale (Rosc.). *Curr. Sci.* **2010**, *98*, 222–229.
46. Bhaskar, V.H.; Balakrishnan, N. Analgesic, anti-inflammatory and antipyretic activities of Pergularia daemia and Carissa carandas. *Daru* **2009**, *17*, 168–174.

47. Duke, D. Dr. Duke's Phytochemical and Ethnobotanical Databases. Available online: https://phytochem.nal.usda.gov/phytochem/search/list (accessed on 17 January 2019).
48. Tyagia, T.; Argawak, M. Phytochemical screening and GC-MS analysis of bioactive constituents in the ethanolic extract of Pistia stratiotes L. and Eichhornia crassipes (Mart.) solms. *J. Pharmacogn. Phytochem.* **2017**, *6*, 195–206.
49. Rukshana, M.S.; Doss, A.; Kumari, P.R. Phytochemical screening and GC-MS ANALYSIS of leaf extract of Pergularia daemia (Forssk) Chiov. *Asian J. Plant Sci. Res.* **2017**, *7*, 9–15.
50. Mustapa, A.N.; Martin, Á.; Mato, R.B.; Cocero, M.J. Extraction of phytocompounds from the medicinal plant Clinacanthus nutans Lindau by microwave-assisted extraction and supercritical carbon dioxide extraction. *Ind. Crops Prod.* **2015**, *74*, 83–94. [CrossRef]
51. Khan, S.; Nazir, M.; Raiz, N.; Saleem, M.; Zengin, G.; Fazal, G.; Saleem, H.; Mukhtar, M.; Tousif, M.I.; Tareen, R.B. Phytochemical profiling, in vitro biological properties and in silico studies on Caragana ambigua stocks (Fabaceae): A comprehensive approach. *Ind. Crops Prod.* **2019**, *131*, 117–124. [CrossRef]
52. Duffy, F.J.; Devocelle, M.; Shields, D.C. Computational approaches to developing short cyclic peptide modulators of protein–protein interactions. In *Computational Peptidology*; Springer: Berlin, Germany, 2015; pp. 241–271.
53. Lipinski, C.A.; Lombardo, F.; Dominy, B.W.; Feeney, P.J. Experimental and computational approaches to estimate solubility and permeability in drug discovery and development settings. *Adv. Drug Deliv. Rev.* **1997**, *23*, 3–25. [CrossRef]
54. Daina, A.; Michielin, O.; Zoete, V. iLOGP: A simple, robust, and efficient description of n-octanol/water partition coefficient for drug design using the GB/SA approach. *J. Chem. Inf. Model.* **2014**, *54*, 3284–3301. [CrossRef]
55. Organisation for Economic Co-operation and Development. *Test No. 420: Acute Oral Toxicity—Fixed Dose Procedure*; OECD Publishing: Paris, France, 2002; ISBN 9789264070943.
56. Tiwari, P.; Kumar, B.; Kaur, M.; Kaur, G.; Kaur, H. Phytochemical screening and extraction: A review. *Int. Pharm. Sci.* **2011**, *1*, 98–106.
57. Robert, A.; Nezamis, J.E.; Lancaster, C.; Hanchar, A.J.; Klepper, M.S. Enteropooling assay: A test for diarrhea produced by prostaglandins. *Prostaglandins* **1976**, *11*, 809–828. [CrossRef]
58. Mascolo, N.; Izzo, A.A.; Autore, G.; Barbato, F.; Capasso, F. Nitric oxide and castor oil-induced diarrhea. *J. Pharmacol. Exp. Ther.* **1994**, *268*, 291–295.
59. Singh, S.; Majumdar, D.K.; Rehan, H.M.S. Evaluation of anti-inflammatory potential of fixed oil of *Ocimum sanctum* (Holybasil) and its possible mechanism of action. *J. Ethnopharmacol.* **1996**, *54*, 19–26. [CrossRef]
60. Ajaiyeoba, E.O.; Onocha, P.A.; Olarenwaju, O.T. In vitro anthelmintic properties of *Buchholzia coriaceae* and *Gynandropsis gynandra* extracts. *Pharm. Biol.* **2001**, *39*, 217–220. [CrossRef]
61. Adnan, M.; Chy, M.N.U.; Rudra, S.; Tahamina, A.; Das, R.; Tanim, M.A.H.; Siddique, T.I.; Hoque, A.; Tasnim, S.M.; Paul, A. Evaluation of *Bonamia semidigyna* (Roxb.) for antioxidant, antibacterial, anthelmintic and cytotoxic properties with the involvement of polyphenols. *Orient. Pharm. Exp. Med.* **2018**, 1–13. [CrossRef]
62. Bauer, A.W.; Kirby, W.M.M.; Sherris, J.C.; Turck, M. Antibiotic susceptibility testing by a standardized single disk method. *Am. J. Clin. Pathol.* **1966**, *45*, 493–496. [CrossRef]
63. Berman, H.M.; Battistuz, T.; Bhat, T.N.; Bluhm, W.F.; Bourne, P.E.; Burkhardt, K.; Feng, Z.; Gilliland, G.L.; Iype, L.; Jain, S. The protein data bank Acta Crystallogr. *D Biol. Crystallogr.* **2002**, *58*, 899–907. [CrossRef]
64. Isupov, M.N.; Obmolova, G.; Butterworth, S.; Badet-Denisot, M.-A.; Badet, B.; Polikarpov, I.; Littlechild, J.A.; Teplyakov, A. Substrate binding is required for assembly of the active conformation of the catalytic site in Ntn amidotransferases: Evidence from the 1.8 Å crystal structure of the glutaminase domain of glucosamine 6-phosphate synthase. *Structure* **1996**, *4*, 801–810. [CrossRef]
65. Ravelli, R.B.G.; Gigant, B.; Curmi, P.A.; Jourdain, I.; Lachkar, S.; Sobel, A.; Knossow, M. Insight into tubulin regulation from a complex with colchicine and a stathmin-like domain. *Nature* **2004**, *428*, 198. [CrossRef]
66. Price, K.L.; Lillestol, R.K.; Ulens, C.; Lummis, S.C.R. Varenicline interactions at the 5-HT3 receptor ligand binding site are revealed by 5-HTBP. *ACS Chem. Neurosci.* **2015**, *6*, 1151–1157. [CrossRef]
67. Thorsen, T.S.; Matt, R.; Weis, W.I.; Kobilka, B.K. Modified T4 lysozyme fusion proteins facilitate G protein-coupled receptor crystallogenesis. *Structure* **2014**, *22*, 1657–1664. [CrossRef]

68. Friesner, R.A.; Murphy, R.B.; Repasky, M.P.; Frye, L.L.; Greenwood, J.R.; Halgren, T.A.; Sanschagrin, P.C.; Mainz, D.T. Extra precision glide: Docking and scoring incorporating a model of hydrophobic enclosure for protein-ligand complexes. *J. Med. Chem.* **2006**, *49*, 6177–6196. [CrossRef]
69. Friesner, R.A.; Banks, J.L.; Murphy, R.B.; Halgren, T.A.; Klicic, J.J.; Mainz, D.T.; Repasky, M.P.; Knoll, E.H.; Shelley, M.; Perry, J.K. Glide: A new approach for rapid, accurate docking and scoring. 1. Method and assessment of docking accuracy. *J. Med. Chem.* **2004**, *47*, 1739–1749. [CrossRef]
70. Lipinski, C.A.; Lombardo, F.; Dominy, B.W.; Feeney, P.J. Experimental and computational approaches to estimate solubility and permeability in drug discovery and development settings. *Adv. Drug Deliv. Rev.* **2012**, *64*, 4–17. [CrossRef]
71. Swiss ADME. Available online: http://www.swissadme.ch/index.php (accessed on 17 January 2019).
72. Way2Drug—Main. Available online: http://www.pharmaexpert.ru/PASSonline/index.php (accessed on 17 January 2019).
73. Goel, R.K.; Singh, D.; Lagunin, A.; Poroikov, V. PASS-assisted exploration of new therapeutic potential of natural products. *Med. Chem. Res.* **2011**, *20*, 1509–1514. [CrossRef]

Sample Availability: Samples of the compounds are not available from the authors.

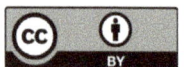

© 2019 by the authors. Licensee MDPI, Basel, Switzerland. This article is an open access article distributed under the terms and conditions of the Creative Commons Attribution (CC BY) license (http://creativecommons.org/licenses/by/4.0/).

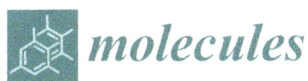

Review

Genus *Ophiorrhiza*: A Review of Its Distribution, Traditional Uses, Phytochemistry, Biological Activities and Propagation

Muhammad Taher [1,*], Siti Syazwani Shaari [1], Deny Susanti [2,*], Dayar Arbain [3,*] and Zainul Amiruddin Zakaria [4,*]

1. Department of Pharmaceutical Technology, Kulliyyah of Pharmacy, International Islamic University Malaysia, Kuantan 25200, Malaysia; syazwani1897@gmail.com
2. Department of Chemistry, Kulliyyah of Science, International Islamic University Malaysia, Kuantan 25200, Malaysia
3. Faculty of Pharmacy, Universitas 17 Agustus 1945, Jakarta 14350, Indonesia
4. Department of Biomedical Science, Faculty of Medicine and Health Sciences, Universiti Putra Malaysia, Serdang 43400, Selangor, Malaysia
* Correspondence: mtaher@iium.edu.my (M.T.); deny@iium.edu.my (D.S.); dayararbain@gmail.com (D.A.); zaz@upm.edu.my (Z.A.Z.); Tel.: +60-(09)-5704842 (M.T.)

Academic Editors: Raffaele Capasso and Lorenzo Di Cesare Mannelli
Received: 25 March 2020; Accepted: 15 April 2020; Published: 4 June 2020

Abstract: Almost 50 species of *Ophiorrhiza* plants were reviewed in this work and the main objective is to critically analyse their distribution, phytochemical content, biological activity, and propagation. Moreover, the information would be useful in promoting the relevant uses of the plant, especially in the medicinal fields based on in vitro and in vivo studies. To this end, scientific sources, including theses, PubMed, Google Scholar, International Islamic University Malaysia IIUM EBSCO, PubChem, and Elsevier, were accessed for publications regarding the *Ophiorrhiza* genus in this review. Scientific literature regarding the *Ophiorrhiza* plants revealed their wide distribution across Asia and the neighbouring countries, whereby they were utilised as traditional medicine to treat various diseases. In particular, various active compounds, such as alkaloids, flavonoids, and terpenoids, were reported in the plant. Furthermore, the *Ophiorrhiza* species showed highly diverse biological activities, such as anti-cancer, antiviral, antimicrobial, and more. The genus propagation reported could produce a high quality and quantity of potent anticancer compound, namely camptothecin (CPT). Hence, it is believed that the relevant uses of natural compounds present in the plants can replace the existing crop of synthetic anticancer drugs associated with a multitude of unbearable side effects. Additionally, more future studies on the *Ophiorrhiza* species should be undertaken to establish the links between its traditional uses, active compounds, and pharmacological activities reported.

Keywords: genus *Ophiorrhiza*; distribution; traditional uses; bioactive molecules; biological activity; propagation

1. Introduction

Genus *Ophiorrhiza* belongs to the Rubiaceae family, which is one of the Indo-Malaysian genera widely spread in the wet forests across tropical and subtropical Asia, Australia, New Guinea, and the Pacific Islands [1,2]. Most of the genera members are perennial herbs capable of growing from approximately 10 cm to 1 metre of height [2]. Normally, the *Ophiorrhiza* genus can be characterised by its succulent stems, five-petal flowers with slightly unequal opposite leaves, laterally compressed fruits, and numerous capsular seeds of small rhomboid shapes [3]. Currently, the *Ophiorrhiza* L. genus consists of 321 species, five varieties, and one subspecies. In particular, 46 species and five varieties are mainly distributed in the north-eastern states and Western Ghats of India [2], whereas 16 species and three varieties can be found in the state of Kerala, India [4].

2. Botany

For the past period of years, herbal medicines have been served as therapeutic agents and continue to be important lifesaving drugs for mankind. It is undeniable that plants can treat various forms of diseases including cancer. The demand for herbal drugs increases due to the increased awareness of the side effects and toxicity linked to synthetic drugs [5]. Plants from family Rubiaceae are known to contain several secondary metabolites like alkaloids, flavonoids, steroids, terpenoids, and fatty acids. Some of the compounds from this family, such as caffeine, quinine, emetine, and camptothecin, are of major pharmaceutical importance [6]. These metabolites can be utilized as natural medicines as they can inhibit the activity of DNA topoisomerase, which are the clinical targets for anticancer drugs [7]. Camptothecin (CPT) is a potent anti-cancer compound that has been widely isolated from *Ophiorrhiza* species (*O. mungos, O. mungos var. angustifolia, O. rugosa var. decumbens* and many others), after being first isolated from a Chinese tree, *Camptotheca acuminate,* in 1966 [6,8]. Later, many researchers extensively developed several other CPT analogues, and among them are topotecan and irinotecan, which showed better DNA-topoisomerase-1 inhibitor activity and are well-tolerated compared to natural CPT [9].

3. Methodology

In-depth information on the *Ophiorrhiza* genus was obtained via a literature search conducted for publications using various electronic databases, such as Google Scholar, International Islamic University Malaysia (IIUM), EBSCO, PubMed, PubChem, and Elsevier. Accordingly, ChemDraw software was employed to draw the bioactive molecules found in the *Ophiorrhiza* plants. In terms of the publications selected for review, no limitations for the range of years were subjected in this paper. The keyword 'genus *Ophiorrhiza*' was used for the primary searches, while the following terms were employed for secondary searches: 'Plant name', 'Phytochemicals', 'Biological activity', 'Pharmacological activity', and 'Propagation'. To highlight the therapeutic uses of genus throughout the medical field, not all of the identified plants were included in this paper. Only those subjected to in vitro and in vivo studies were presented in this review. Therefore, this review was not exhaustive for all *Ophiorrhiza* species typically utilised in traditional or modern medicines. The layout of the searching methodology is presented in Figure 1.

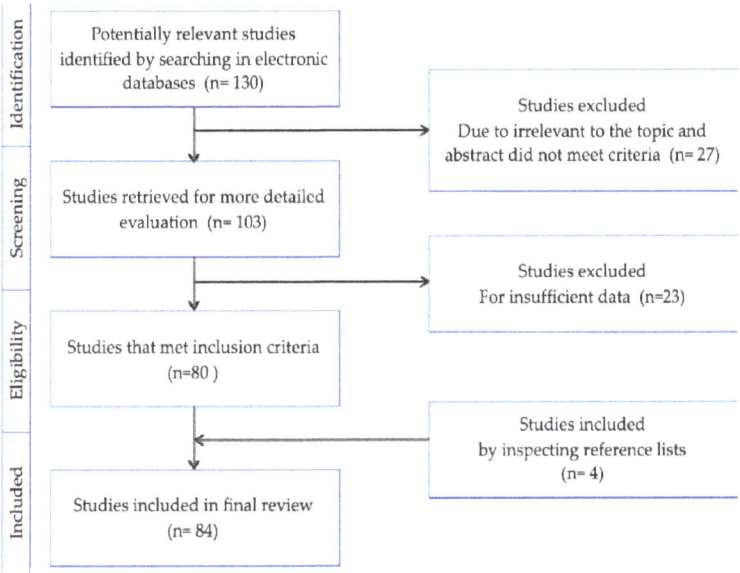

Figure 1. Methodology conducted.

4. Distribution

The Western Ghats are known as one of the diversity centres of *Ophiorrhiza* species following the Western Himalayas, which comprise of about 22 distributed taxa for the species [10]. Some of them that can be found in Andaman and the Nicobar islands of India include *O. infundibularis* Balakr, *O. mungos* L, *O. nicobarica* Balakr, and *O. trichocarpa* BL [11]. Meanwhile, about 30–35 species are documented in the shady and moist-to-wet areas in Thailand's lowland and mountain forests both [3], whereas Peninsular Malaysia is home to 21 species [6]. In contrast, 70 species of the *Ophiorrhiza* are distributed in China in which most of them are found in the southern area of Yangtze River, which traverses the provinces of Yunnan and Guangxi [12]. Figure 2 shows some of the *Ophiorrhiza* collections found in West Sumatra, while Table 1 shows the distribution of this species worldwide.

In general, most of the *Ophiorrhiza* species are widely discovered in the Asian regions, particularly India, Indonesia, and Malaysia. This suggests the highly suitable nature of the regional tropical and forest environments for the growth and distribution of these plants. Therefore, it is believed that newer *Ophiorrhiza* species can be discovered via the undertaking of extensive research in Asian countries.

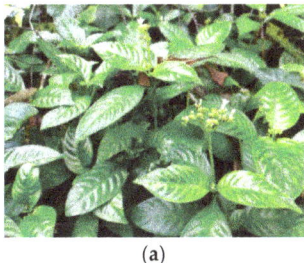
(a)

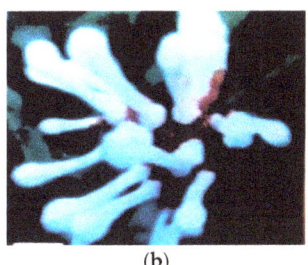
(b)

Figure 2. *Cont.*

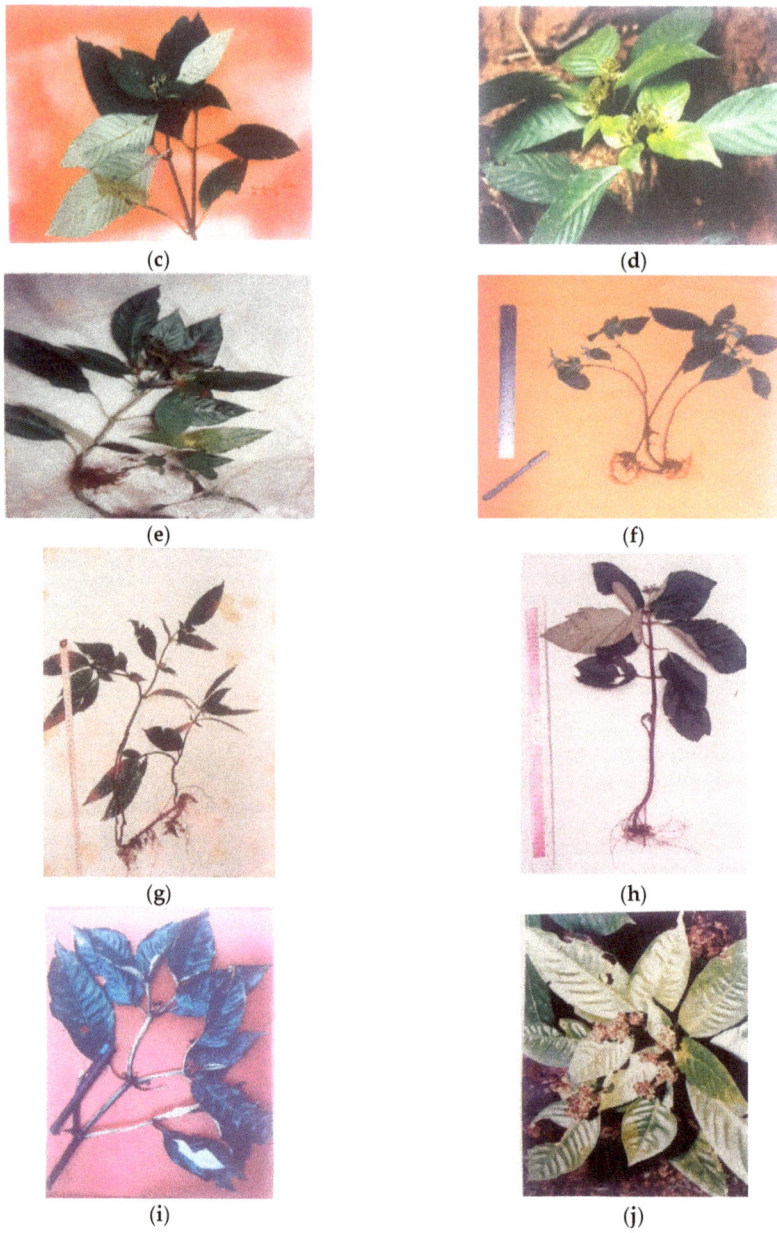

Figure 2. Photo collections of *Ophiorrhiza* species. (**a**) *Ophiorrhiza communis* [13]. (**b**) *Ophiorrhiza* sp. (*ex.* Gunung Singgalang) [14]. (**c**) *Ophiorrhiza* "Siberida DA-RT 6030" [15]. (**d**) *Ophiorrhiza* sp. (ex. Sako, TNKS) [16]. (**e**) *Ophiorrhiza longiflora* Bl. [17]. (**f**) *Ophiorrhiza* cf. *kunstlery* King. [18]. (**g**) *Ophiorrhiza* ex. Padang Panjang [19,20]. (**h**) *Ophiorrhiza* "DA-RT 7895" [21]. (**i**) *Ophiorrhiza* "Air Sirah DA-RT 6604" [22]. (**j**) *Ophiorrhiza* "Sako DA-RT 7577" [16].

Table 1. Distribution of *Ophiorrhiza* species around the world.

Species	Location	References
O. marginata	Mt Keronsong, Jambi, Indonesia	[23]
O. cf. *rosacea*	Solok, West Sumatra	[24]
O. communis	Ulu tembeling Malaysia Bungus, Padang, Indonesia	[6]
O. cf. *communis*	Sijunjung, West Sumatra	[13]
O. tomentosa	Cameron Highland, Malaysia	[6]
O. bracteata	Lubuk Alung West Sumatra	[25]
O. major	Anai Reserved Forest, West Sumatra	[26]
O. cf *ferruginea*	Anai forest, West Sumatra	[27]
O. rosacea	The Seven Mountain, Jambi	[28]
O. kunstlery	Pariaman, West Sumatra	[28]
O. cf. *kunstlery* King	Mount Letter W Kabupaten Padang Pariaman, Indonesia	[29]
O. filistipula	Pangian Lintau, West Sumatra	[30]
O. blumeana	Mount Tandikat, West Sumatra	[31]
O. trichocarpon Blume	Kerala, South India	[4]
O. pumila	Japan	[32]
O. pectinata	Tamil Nadu Kerala, India	[33]
O. radicans	Western Ghats Kerala, India	[34]
O. shendurunii	Kerala Western Ghast, India	[35]
O. prostrata	Agastyamala Hills of Western Ghats Thiruvananthapuram Kerala, India	[1]
O. rugosa	The northern part of Thailand	[3]
O. rugosa var. *prostrata (D.Don)* Deb & Mondal	Chittagong Hill Tract and Sylhet regions of Bangladesh	[36]
O. liukiunseis	Ishigaki Island of Okinawa, Japan, Taiwan, Philipines	[37]
O. kuroiwai	Ishigaki and other south-west islands of Okinawa	[38]
O. japonica	Ishigaki and other south-west islands of Okinawa	[38]
O. alata Craib	Chantaburi, Thailand	[39]
O. nicobarica Balakr.	Andaman and Nicobar Islands, India	[11]
O. infundibularis	Great Nicobar Island, India	[2]
O. jojui	Andaman Islands, India	[2]
O. shiqianensis	Guizhou Province, South-western China	[12]
O. neglecta BI. ex DC	Kabupaten 50 Kota, Indonesia	[40]
O. longiflora BL.	Tarok Lubuk Bonta, Indonesia	[17]
O. palidulla Ridl.	Tilatang Kamang, Indonesia	[41]
O. sp.	Kotamadya Padang Panjang, Indonesia	[19,20]
O. klosii Ridl.	Kabupaten Solok, Indonesia	[42]
O. ex. Simanau DA-RT 61, Solok	Kabupaten Solok, Indonesia	[43]
O. neglecta BI. Ex DC	Kabupaten 50 Kota, Indonesia	[40]
O. anonyma Val.	Silayang Kabupaten Agam, Indonesia	[44]
O. ex. Gunung Singgalang	Mount Singgalang Kabupaten Agam, Indonesia	[14]
O. "Air Sirah DA-RT 6604"	Air Sirah Kabupaten Solok Sumatera Barat, Indonesia	[22]
O. "Sako DA-RT 7577"	Sako Kabupaten Sumatera Barat, Indonesia	[16]
O. "Siberida DA-RT 6030"	National Park Siberida Rengat Riau, Indonesia	[15]
O. DA-RT 82 AT	Tes Lake Bengkulu, Indonesia	[45]
O. DA-RT 7895	Kerinci Seblat National Park (TSNK) Jambi, Indonesia	[21]

5. Traditional Uses

The plants species of *Ophiorrhiza* (Rubiaceae) genus have been associated to claims of various medicinal properties and wide-ranging applications in traditional and modern medicine alike [4,10,33]. Traditionally, the plants are used to treat inflammation, pain, cancer, and bacterial and viral-based infections. Furthermore, the *Ophiorrhiza* species are capable of healing snakebite, stomatitis, ulcers, and wounds [5,10,33], while also acting as an antioxidant [46], antitussive, and analgesic alternative [4]. They are also applied to tend to cases of gastropathy, leprosy, and amenorrhea, besides possessing sedative and laxative properties obtained from the extract of their root barks [33]. In fact, it interesting to note that *O. mungos* is specifically known as 'snakeroot' due to its known use as a treatment for snakebite [6].

In modern medicine, *Ophiorrhiza* plants are popular as a result of their constituent camptothecin's anti-cancer properties, which are attributable to its ability in inhibiting deoxyribonucleic acid (DNA) topoisomerase-1 [10]. However, their usage in treating different diseases may be dissimilar between varying tribes. For example, the Tanchangya people in Bangladesh uses the paste of *O. rugosa var. prostrata* (D.Don) Deb & Mondal in order to treat boils, those of the Mama tribe make tea from its leaves in tending to body aches or juices them for diarrhoea, whereas the Chakma tribe treats earache by applying sun-dried crushed leaves on the site of pain [36]. Regardless, various alternative traditional uses of this particular species have been detailed, which are shown in Table 2. The *Ophiorrhiza* species are evidently rich with bioactive molecules, offering superior pharmacological effects as they can be used to treat a multitude of diseases throughout mild to chronic stages.

In this review, all available information about *Ophiorrhiza* genus and its bioactive molecules linked with significant pharmacological properties are collected. This act is particularly crucial to promote the plants and their relevant applications in the medicinal fields according to pharmacological evidence obtained via in vitro and in vivo studies.

Table 2. Traditional uses of *Ophiorrhiza* species.

Ophiorrhiza Species	Traditional Uses	Hippocratic Screening	References
O. discolor Br.	Skin infections		[47]
O. filistipula Miq.	Skin infections and inflammation		[47]
O. cf. rosacea Ridl.		Vasodilator effect	[47]
Ophiorrhiza DART 6526		Analgesic and muscle relaxant	[47]
O. major Ridl.	Skin disorders like eczema		[25]
O. nicobarica	Herpetic lesions, skin infections, and irritation		[11]
O. mungos (root)	Cancer and snakebite, Sedative and laxative properties		[48]
O. communis	Poultice and treating cough		[6]
O. tomentosa	Poultice		[6]
O. rugosa var. prostrata (D. Don) & Mondal	Skin infections such as boils, body aches, and chest pain, earache, dysentery, diarrhea		[36]
O. singaporiensis	Snakebite		[17]

6. Phytochemistry

The Rubiaceae family is known with its capability of producing bioactive metabolites such as iridoids, indole alkaloids, anthraquinones, terpenoids (i.e., diterpenes and triterpenes), flavonoids, and many other derivatives of phenolic compounds, which result in their respective significant pharmacological activities [46]. The phytochemical analyses done for several species of *Ophiorrhiza* (Rubiaceae) have revealed the positive presence of alkaloids, flavonoids, and triterpenes, specifically in *O. radicans* [10], *O. mungos* [5], *O. liukiuensis* [37], and *O. nicobarica* [11]. Furthermore, some of the important phytochemicals found in most *Ophiorrhiza* species include camptothecin and its derivatives, namely pumiloside, luteolin, harman, tetrahydroalastonine, bracteatine, blumeanine, strictosidinic acid, and lyalosidic acid [49]. According to many studies, the therapeutic uses of these compounds can described by their anti-inflammatory, anticancer, antiviral, and antibacterial activities exhibited [46]. Therefore, the compounds derived from *Ophiorrhiza* species are perceived as useful as one of the natural alternative sources in drug development in order to replace chemically-synthesised medications associated with undesirable side effects such as dizziness, nausea, and vomiting.

6.1. Alkaloids

The *Ophiorrhiza* (Rubiaceae) species are highly prevalent among plant-rich indole alkaloids [24], which are characterised by a low molecular weight and contain at least one nitrogen atom in an amine-type structure. In their pure form, most of the alkaloids are colourless, non-volatile, and exist as crystalline solids [47]. They are typically useful due to their biological activities and defensive properties observed in plants, as well as for medicinal treatment purposes as they have excellent pharmacological properties [50].

One of the common alkaloids found in *Ophiorrhiza* species is harman (**1**). In particular, harman-2-oxide (**2**) generally found in *O. rosacea* is a crystalline alkaloid that can be reduced to harman (**1**) by reduction with zinc in acetic acid. Furthermore, strictosidinic acid (**3**) is another major bioactive molecule in *Ophiorrhiza* plants besides harman (**1**) [28]. Through Carbon-13 nuclear magnetic resonance (C-NMR), harman (**1**) can be characterised as a compound containing six non-substituted aromatics and one primary and three substituted aromatic carbons, whereas strictosidinic acid (**3**) consists of six quaternary, five methane, and 16 methylene carbons [6].

Next, palicoside (**4**) or *N*-methylstrictosidinic acid depicts a quite similar structure compared to strictosidine (**5**). However, the positioning of additional methyl groups at R^1 and R^2 differentiates them into two different structures. In particular, the formation of normalindine (**6**) and isonormalindine (**7**) can be derived from strictosidine (**5**) by introducing the β and α-configurations of a methyl group between N4 and C19, respectively [28]. Similarly, isomalindine-16-carboxylate (**8**) and malindine (**10**) display close spectroscopic data with isomalindine (**9**) at the C3,18 carbons and the N-Me group. However the difference between them is that there is a carboxylate group placed at C6 carbon of isomalindine-16-carboxylate (**8**), while in the case of malindine (**10**), there is a different orientation of the methyl group at C19 as compared to the other two compounds, namely isomalindine (**9**) and isomalindine-16-carboxylate (**8**) [13].

On top of this, camptothecin (**11**) is a modified monoterpene indole alkaloid having potent anti-cancer property has been reported to be found in abundance in *O. mungos* and *O. mungos* var. *angustifolia*, rendering them the main sources for its biomass production [8]. It consists of a pentacyclic ring structure, which includes a pyrrole (3,4β) quinoline moiety and an asymmetric centre within the α-hydroxyl lactone ring with 20S configuration [7]. Additionally, the pumiloside (**12**) and deoxypumiloside (**13**) found in *O. pumila* are further considered as the precursors for the biosynthesis of camptothecin (**11**). This is attributable towards their formation from the half structure of camptothecin (**11**) and half structure of strictosamide (**14**) accordingly [32].

Meanwhile, the two glucoalkaloids of lyalosidic acid (**15**) and 10-hydroxylyalosidic acid (**16**) have been found to coexist with their respective β-carbolines alkaloid counterparts, namely 6-hydroxyharman (**17**) and harman (**1**) in *O. japonica*. This suggests that these two constituents are closely correlated, whereby the hydrolysis of harman (**1**) at C6 will produce 6-hydroxyharman (**17**). Similarly, the diazomethane methylation of lyalosidic acid (**15**) and 10-hydroxylyalosidic (**16**) acid accordingly yields the two products of lyaloside (**18**) and 10-methoxylyaloside (**19**), respectively [51].

Moreover, the chemical structures of *ophiorrhizine* (**20**) isolated from *O. major* Ridl [25], *ophiorrine* A (**21**), and *ophiorrine* B (**22**) extracted from *O. japonica* [38], and six *ophiorrhisides*, namely *ophiorrhisides* A (**23**), B (**24**), C (**25**), D (**26**), E (**27**), and F (**28**) isolated from *O. trichocarpan* Blume [52] are quite similar. However, they are dissimilar regardless due to the differences in the additional groups and glucose orientation at a certain position of carbon atom. For example, the difference in stereochemistry configuration at C16 will thus differentiate *ophiorrine* A (**21**) and *ophiorrine* B (**22**) into two different betaine-type of indole alkaloids [38]. Accordingly, the chemical structures of the alkaloids under the umbrella of the *Ophiorrhiza* species are displayed in Figure 3.

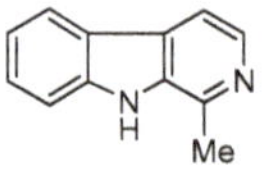

Harman (**1**)

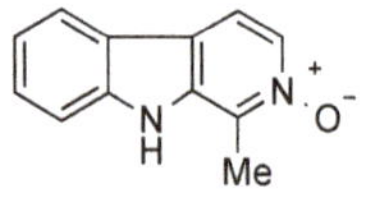

Harman-2-oxide (**2**)

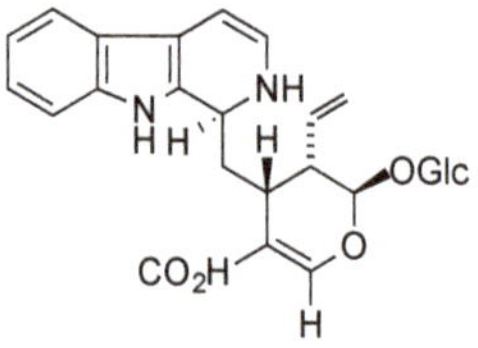

Strictosidinic acid (**3**)

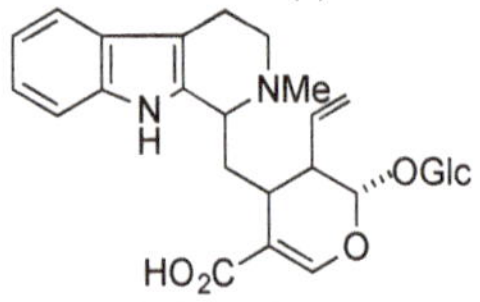

Palicoside (**4**)

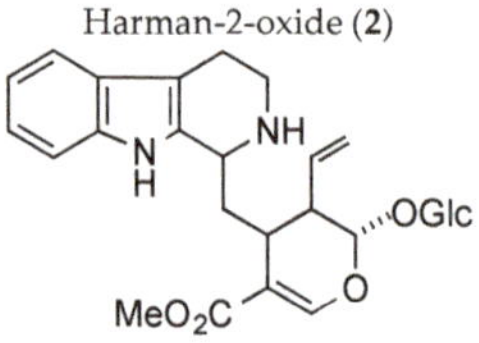

Strictosidine (**5**)

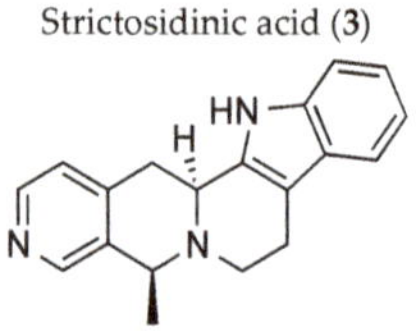

Normalindine (**6**)

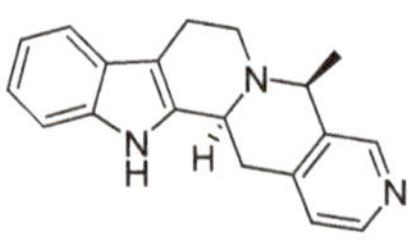

Isomalindine-16-carboxylate (**8**)

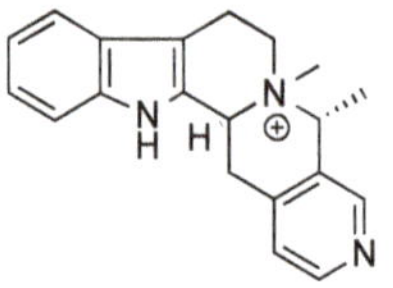

Isomalindine (**9**)

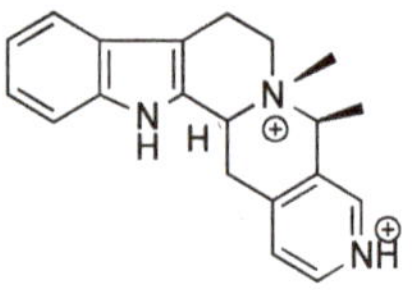

Malindine (**10**)

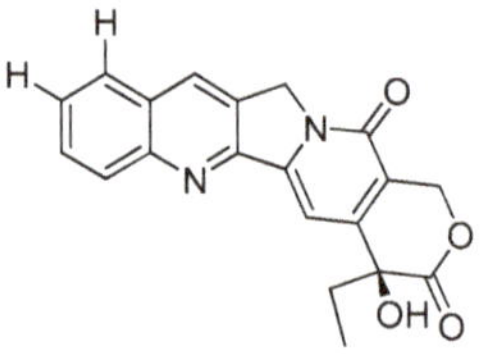

Camptothecin (**11**)

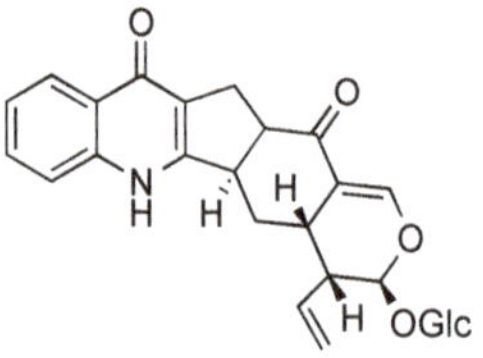

Deoxypumiloside (**13**)
3*H*-α: (3*S*)-Deoxypumiloside,
3*H*-β: (3*R*)-Deoxypumiloside

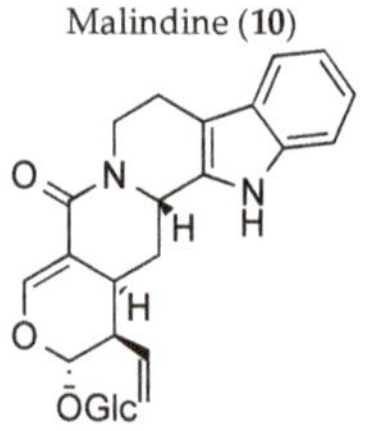

Strictosamide (**14**)

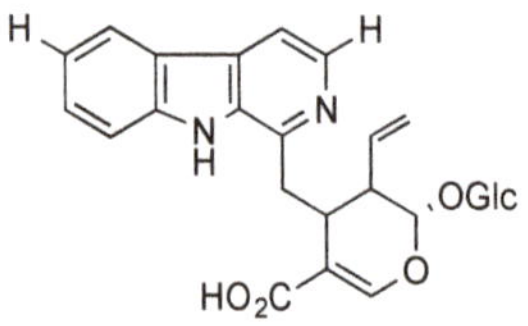

Lyalosidic acid (**15**)

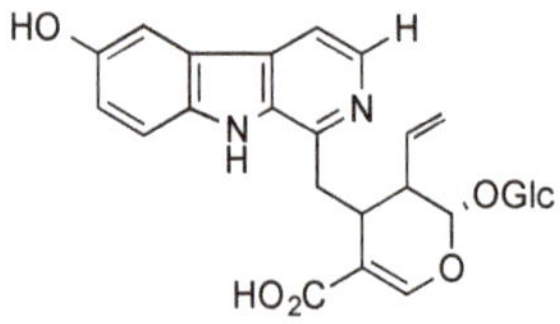

10-hydroxylyalosidic acid (**16**)

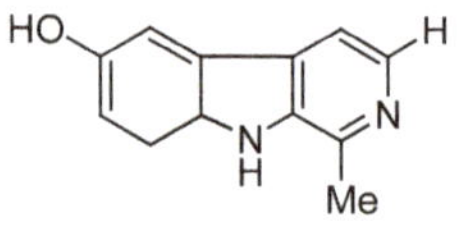

6-hydroxyharman (**17**)

Figure 3. *Cont.*

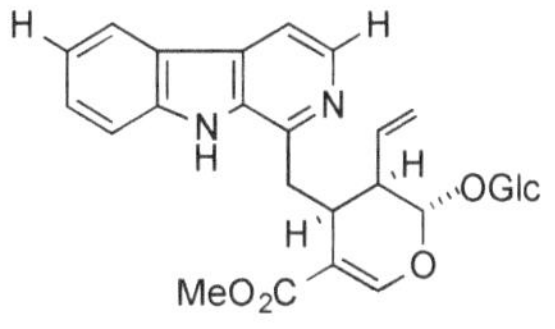

Lyaloside (**18**)

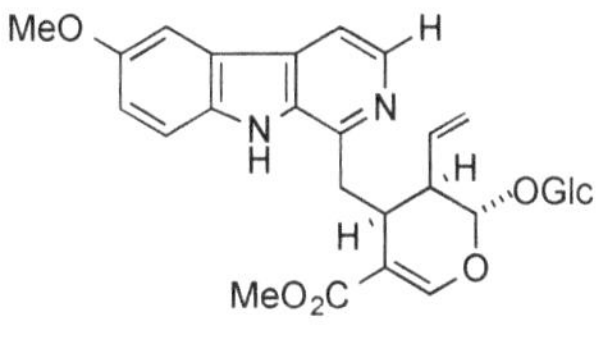

10-methoxylyaloside (**19**)

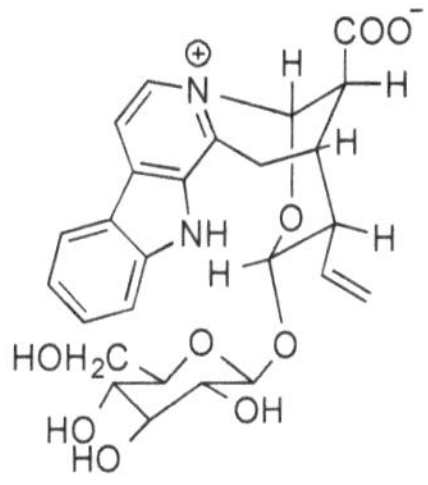

Ophiorrine A (**21**)

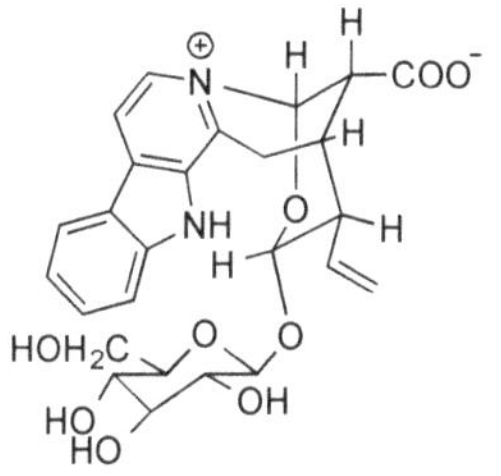

Ophiorrine B (**22**)

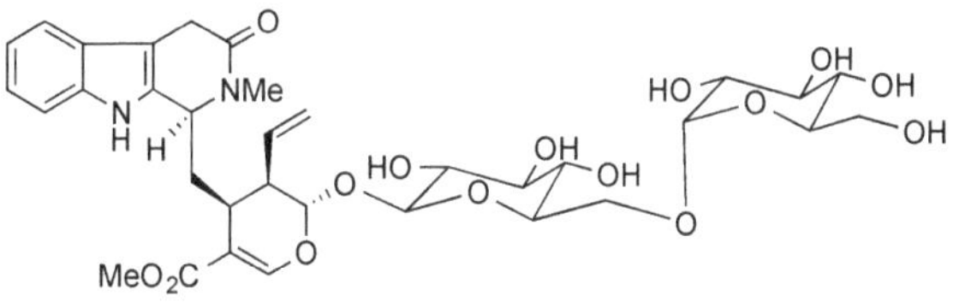

Ophiorrhiside A (**23**)

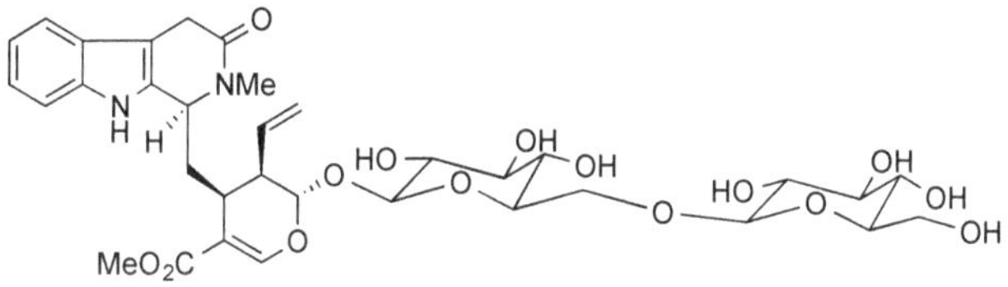

Ophiorrhiside B (**24**)

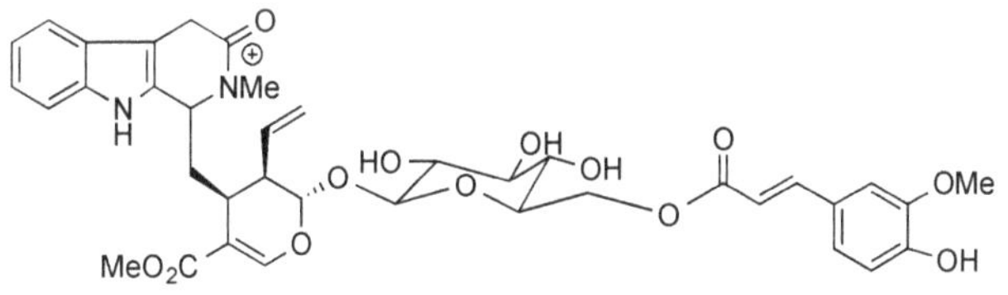

Ophiorrhiside C (**25**)

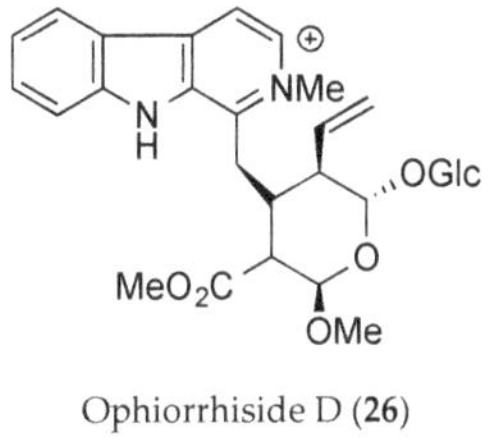

Ophiorrhiside D (**26**)

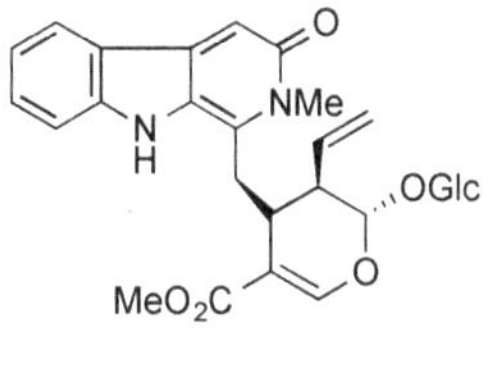

Ophiorrhiside E (**27**)

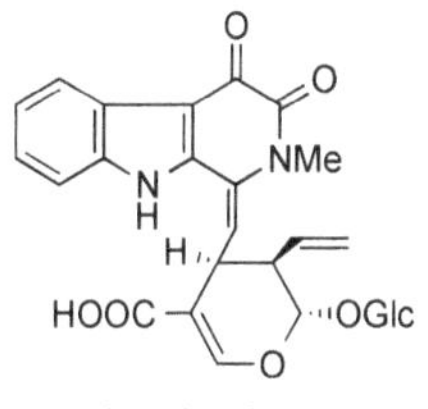

Ophiorrhiside F (**28**)

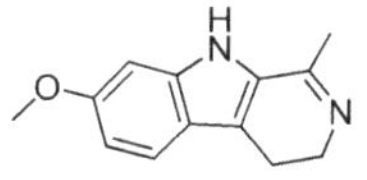

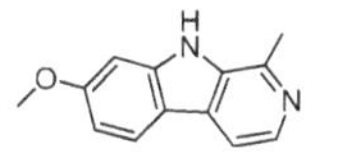

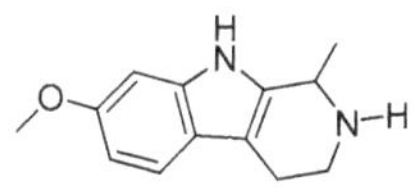

Figure 3. *Cont.*

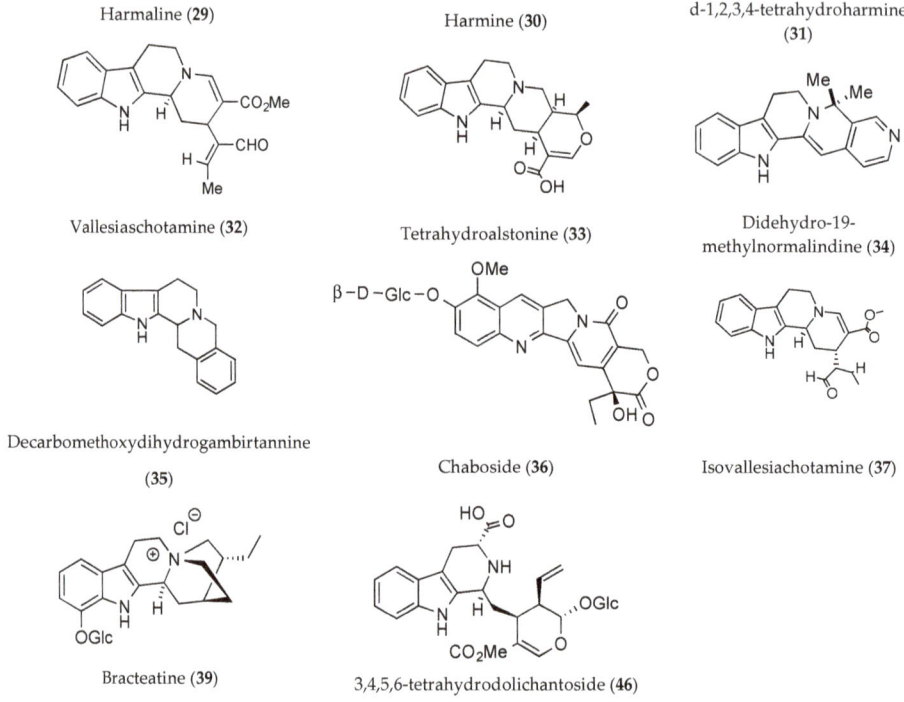

Figure 3. Alkaloids from the genus of *Ophiorrhiza*. *Glc = glucose molecule.

Furthermore, prior reports have detailed the pharmacological properties of some alkaloids, one of which is harmaline (**29**), also known as harmidine, which is found in *O. nicobarica*. When subjected to oxidation, it will be converted to a psychoactive substance known as harmine (**30**), whereas a reduction process will give rise to d-1,2,3,4-tetrahydroharmine (**31**) [11]. Similarly, compounds such as vallesiaschotamine (**32**), strictosidinic acid (**3**), and tetrahydroalstonine (**33**) have been proven to be capable of depressing the central nervous system, relaxing the muscles, and offering relief pain (i.e., tetrahydroalstonine only) when administered to mice, whereas lyalosidic acid (**15**) yields a vasodilator effect [24].

Various different alkaloids that can be found in *Ophiorrhiza* plants are summarised accordingly in Table 3. The most common types for this particular species consist of harman, ophiorrhine, and camptothecin as well as their respective derivatives. Most of these compounds display a pentacyclic amine-ring structure, which is an indication that they are of the alkaloid group. Therefore, it is undeniable that the *Ophiorrhiza* species is rife and abundant with alkaloid compounds, rendering them plants with a high potential of excellent therapeutic effects.

Table 3. Alkaloids contents in *Ophiorrhiza* species.

Species	Alkaloids Contents	Parts of Plant	References
O. rosacea	Harman (1), Harman-2-oxide (2)	Aerial part	[28]
O. kunstlery King	Palicoside (4), isomalindine (9), 3,14-didehydro-19-methylnormalindine (34)	Aerial part	[18,28,29]
O. communis	Harman (1)	Leaves	[53]
O. tomentosa	Harman (1), strictosidinic acid (3)	Leaves	[53]
O. japonica	Lyalosidic acid (15), 10-hydroxylyalosidic acid (16), 6-hydroxyharman (17)	Aerial part	[51]
O. japonica	Ophiorrine A (21), Ophiorrine B (22)	Leaves	[38]
O. kuroiwai Mak	Ophiorrine A (21), Ophiorrine B (22), lyasoside (18)	Aerial part	[38]
O. marginata	Decarbomethoxydihydrogambirtannine (35), strictosidinic acid (3)	Aerial part	[23]
O. cf. communis	Isomalindine-16-carboxylate (8)	Aerial part	[13]
O. liukiuensis	Camptothecin (11), 6-hydroxyharman (17)	Whole plant	[37]
O. pumila	Camptothecin (11), chaboside (36), pumiloside (12), deoxypumilosides (13)	Whole plant	[54]
O. nicobarica	Harmaline (29)	Whole plant	[11]
O. DA-RT 6526	Tetrahydroalstonine (33), Vallesiaschotamine (32), Isovallesiachotamine (37)	Aerial part	[47,55]
Ophiorrhiza DA-RT 6526b	Strictosidinic acid (3)	Aerial part	[24,56]
Ophiorrhiza DA-RT 82 A	Tetrahydroalstonine (33)	Aerial part	[45]
O. longiflora BL.	Tetrahydroalstonine (33)	Aerial part	[17]
O. cf. rosacea	Harman (1), lyalosidic acid (15)	Aerial part	[24]
O. mungos	Camptothecin (11)	Leaves	[57]
O. blumeana Korth	Ophiorrhizine-12-carboxylate (38), bracteatine (39), blumeanine (40)	Aerial part	[47]
O. bracteata Korth	Ophiorrhizine (20), bracteatine (39)	Aerial part	[47]
O. discolor Br.	Tetrahydroalstonine (33)	Aerial part	[47]
O. filistipula Miq.	7-methoxy-camptothecin (41), normalindine (6), strictosidinic acid (3)	Aerial part	[47]
O. cf. ferruginea Valeton	Dihydrocycloakagerine (42), mostuenein (43), tetrahydroakagerine (44), isomalindine (9)	Aerial part	[47]
O. major Bl.	Ophiorrhizine (20)	Aerial part	[47]
O. teysmaniana Miq.	Tetrahydroalstonine (33)	Aerial part	[47]
O. trichocarpon Blume	Ophiorrhiside A (23), Ophiorrhiside B (24), Ophiorrhiside C (25), Ophiorrhiside D (26), Ophiorrhiside E (27), Ophiorrhiside F (28), dolichantoside (45), 5-carboxystrictosidine (46), lyaloside (18), 3,4,5,6- Tetrahydrodolichantoside (47)	Whole part	[52]

6.2. Flavonoids

Flavonoids are the subgroups of phenolic compounds, which are characterised with at least one aromatic ring and one or more hydroxyl substituents [50]. Their basic structures consist of two benzene rings linked through a heterocyclic pyrane ring [58], whereupon the compounds can be classified into several subclasses, such as isoflavonoids, chalcones, flavanones, flavones, dihydroflavonols, flavonols, anthocyanidins, and catechins [7]. The presence of flavonoids in plants is responsible for providing an attractive colour in order to attract plant pollinators, protecting the leaves from fungal pathogens and UV-B radiation, and controlling normal physiological activities such as respiration and photosynthesis [58]. Furthermore, the compounds are linked to several pharmacological properties, such as anti-inflammatory, anti-platelet, anti-proliferative, anti-carcinogenic, and many others, as well as a minimal toxicity effect [59]. In fact, some of the flavonoids also possess anti-snake venom activity: they occur by inhibiting phospholipase A2, which is an essential constituent in snake venoms [5].

Various plants of the *Ophiorrhiza* species contain flavonoids, whereby *O. mungos* Linn. and *O. liukiuensis* have been specifically reported to have luteolin-7-O-glucosides (48) and hyperin (also known as quercetin-3-O-galactoside) (49) respectively (Figure 4). In particular, luteolin-7-O-glucosides (48) possess three aromatic ring structures with the characteristics of 5,7,3′,4 oxygenated flavones. Hydrolysis of luteolin-7-glycosides with acid will generate luteolin-7-O-β-glucosides [60].

Luteolin-7-O-glucosides (**48**) typically yield potent antioxidant, anti-inflammatory, and anti-cancer properties [60]. Additionally, it is newly reported that it can protect the gastrointestinal tract from ethanol and indomethacin-induced gastric ulcer upon its modelling in rats [59].

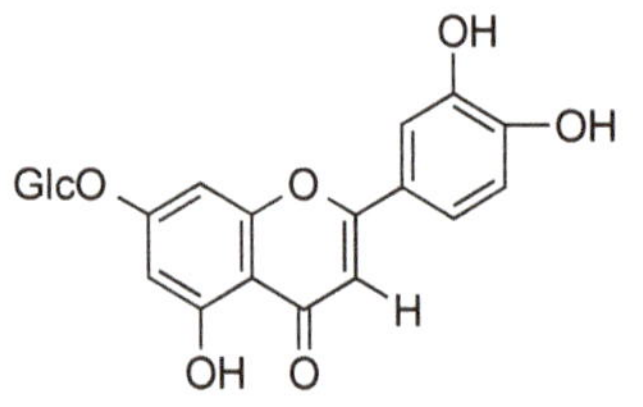

Luteolin-7-O-glucoside (**48**) 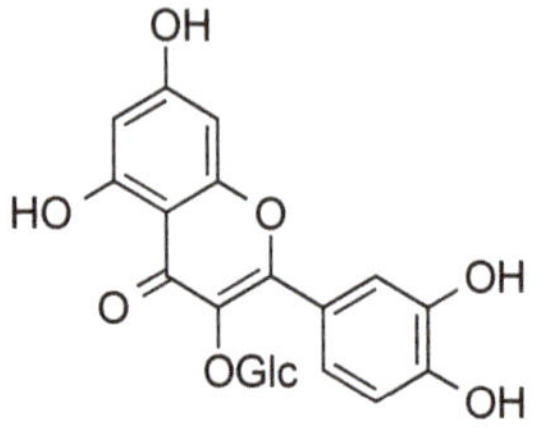   Hyperin (**49**)

Figure 4. Flavonoids from the genus of *Ophiorrhiza*. *Glc = glucose molecule.

Meanwhile, hyperin (**49**) is a tetrahydroxyflavone compound composed of quercetin and a beta-D-galactosyl residue attached at position 3 [61]. The butanol extract of *O. liukiuensis* whole plant has revealed the presence of hyperin (**49**) and other alkaloid compounds concomitantly [46]. Previously discovered in *Ericaceae, Guttifera,* and *Celastraceae*, the compound has been reported to produce anti-inflammatory effects. For example, it can the inhibit lipopolysaccharide (LPS)-induced inflammatory response by terminating the TLR4 and NLRP3 signalling pathways, which are generally associated with acute kidney injury [61]. This review thus reveals that flavonoid compounds are less abundant and present as much as alkaloids are in the *Ophiorrhiza* species. Regardless, several previous studies have shown that they are capable of providing a significant therapeutic effect to certain diseases in comparison with their alkaloid counterparts.

6.3. Terpenoids

Terpenoids, which are also known as isoprenoids, are derived from two precursors, namely isopentenyl diphosphate (IPP) and its isomer dimethyl allydiphosphate (DMAPP). Accordingly, they can be classified into monoterpenes (C_{10}), sesquiterpenes (C_{15}), diterpenes (C_{20}), sesterterpenes (C_{25}), triterpenes (C_{30}), tetraterpenes (C_{40}, carotenoids), and steroids (C_{18-30}) [50]. All terpenoids are derived from a repetitive fusion of branched five-carbon units based on the isopentane skeleton [62] and offer varying beneficial uses as flavourings and medicines alike [50].

In particular, ursolic acid (**50**) has been found together with camptothecin (**11**), 10-methoxy-camptothecin, and harman (**1**) from the chloroform extract of *O. liukuensis* whole plant [46]. It is a pentacyclic amphiphilic triterpene compound with a hydroxylated polycyclic structure, which is capable of exhibiting many functions. For example, it has selective induction of cell death properties with the help of caspase-3, may prevent the stimulation of lipoxygenase and cyclooxygenase, and selectively inhibits the cyclic AMP phosphotransferase and AMP-dependent protein kinase. Consequently, the metabolic activity of a cell, as well as its division, gene expression, and development, can be maintained accordingly [11], thereby collectively preventing the cell overgrowth that potentially leads to cancer.

In recent years, new triterpenoid fatty acid esters named lupan-20-ol-3(β)-yl hexadecanoate (**51**), lupan-20-ol-3(β)-yl acetate (**52**), and olean-18-en-3(β)-yl hexadecanoate (**53**) have been isolated from the hexane extract of *O. shendurunii*, which present as a white and waxy solid. These compounds manifest certain antimicrobial, antifungal, and anti-yeast activities through the diffusion disc method. In contrast, other compounds isolated from the hexane extract include doctriacontanoic acid (**54**) and stigmasterol (**55**), whereas rubiadin (**56**), nonadecanoic acid (**57**), hexadecanoic acid (**58**) (i.e., palmitic acid), and camptothecin (**11**) are obtained from the chloroform extract of *O. shendurunii* whole plant [35]. Figure 5 and Table 4 below show the terpenoid content in some of the *Ophiorrhiza* species accordingly.

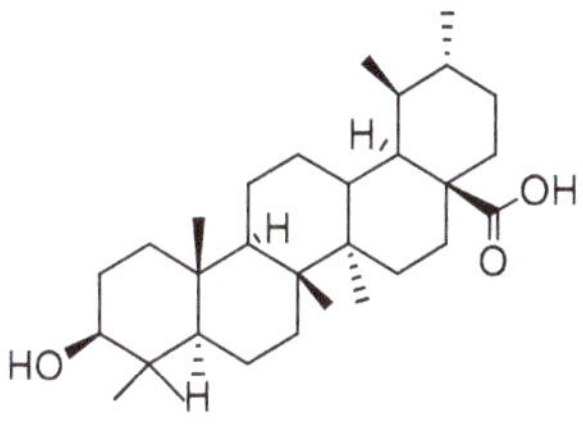

Ursolic acid (**50**)

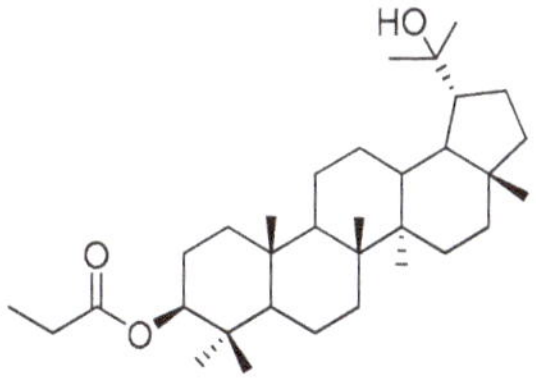

Lupan-20-ol-3 (β)-yl hexadecanoate (**51**)

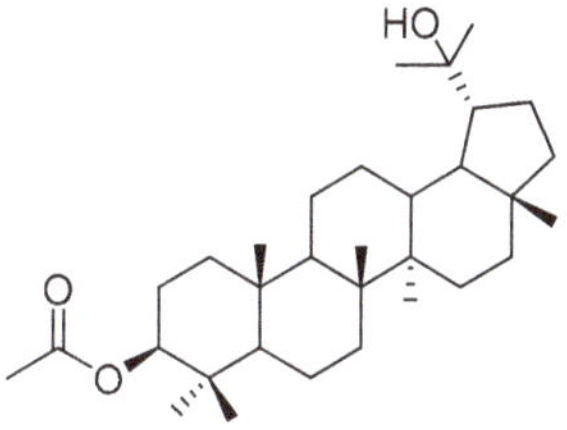

Lupan-20-ol-3(β)-yl acetate (**52**)

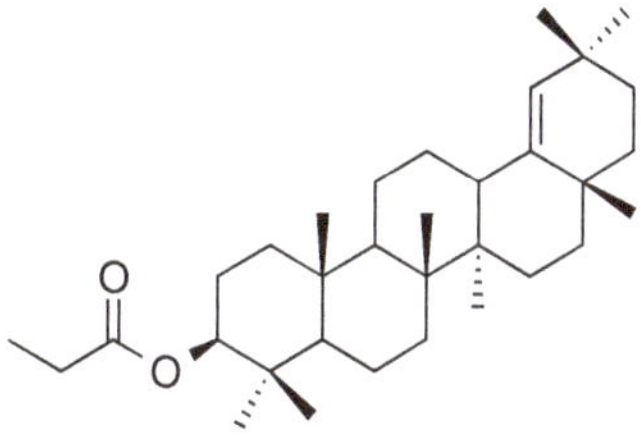

Olean-18-en-3(β)-yl hexadecanoate (**53**)

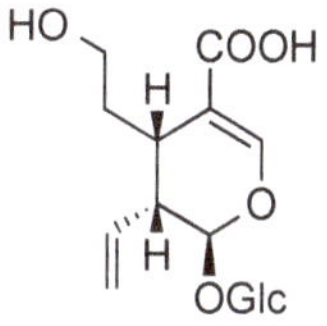

Demethylsecologanol (**59**)

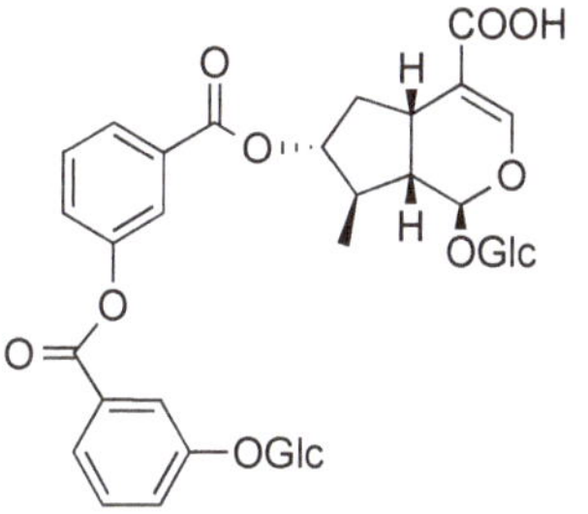

3-o-glucosylsenburiside II (**60**)

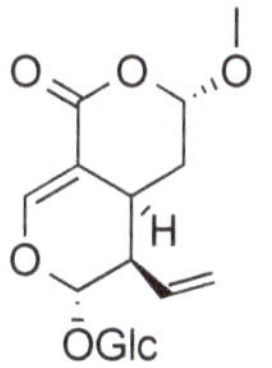

Epivogeloside (**61**)

Figure 5. Terpenoids from the genus of *Ophiorrhiza*. *Glc = glucose molecule.

Table 4. Terpenoids content in *Ophiorrhiza* species.

Species	Triterpenes	Parts of Plants	References
O. liukiuensis	Ursolic acid (**50**), demethylsecologanol (**59**), 3′′′-o-glucosylsenburiside II (**60**) (monoterpene), epivogeloside (**61**),	Whole plant	[37,46]
O. nicobarica	Ursolic acid (**50**)	Whole plant	[11]
O. shendurunii	Lupan-20-ol-3 (β)-yl hexadecanoate (**51**), lupan-20-ol-3(β)-yl acetate (**52**), olean-18-en-3(β)-yl hexadecanoate (**53**)	Whole plant	[8]

7. Biological Activity

7.1. Anticancer Activity

In general, normal cells will grow and divide themselves for some time before their growth stops, whereas reproduction will only occur in order to replace any damaged or dead cells. Therefore, cancer occurs in the presence of abnormal cell growth due to the altered gene expression of DNA in the affected cells, consequently resulting in their resistance to apoptosis and continuous division [63]. Moreover, the existence of reactive oxygen species (ROS) may further promote the development of these tumour cells as they directly alternate the cellular metabolic process. If the natural antioxidants found in the body cannot control the production of ROS or destroy them, severe damage to body tissues may be observed while the cancer cells continue to actively proliferate [60].

The conventional synthetic anticancer drugs have unbearable side effects such as fatigue, sleep disturbances, and hair loss, thereby rendering their substitution slowly with nature-derived alternatives [63]. In particular, the therapeutic effects of secondary metabolites possessed by alkaloids, flavonoids, terpenoids, polyphenols, and quinones may potentially inhibit the activity of DNA topoisomerase enzyme [62] and suppress the ROS activity, thus leading to fewer side effects [60].

The actions of the DNA topoisomerase enzyme causes DNA strands to be separated and re-joined, resulting in changes of the structure [62]. Accordingly, camptothecin (**11**) is one of the powerful alkaloids found in *Ophiorrhiza* plants in possession of excellent anticancer activity and acts as a potent inhibitor of DNA topoisomerase I [10,64]. The component is capable of preventing the enzymatic activity of DNA topoisomerase I specifically by trapping the reaction intermediate (i.e., the cleavable complex) during the breaking and re-joining process, causing disrupted cancer cell division [62]. Furthermore, it can bind to tubulin and inhibit microtubule formation in the dividing cells, subsequently enhancing the inhibition of the DNA topoisomerase [64]. Therefore, this review offers the notion that the development of novel anticancer drugs extracted from natural sources is possible due to the pharmacological effects of unique compounds present in the *Ophiorrhiza* plants.

Besides camptothecin (**11**), a multitude of phytochemicals show great anticancer properties as well, such as harmane (**1**) and harmaline (**29**)'s reported roles in scavenging the ROS and inhibiting thiol oxidation [65]. Accordingly, a comparative study has noted luteolin and quercetin's ability to inhibit topoisomerase II catalytic activity in Chinese hamster ovary AA8 cells, underlining them as a pioneering lead for cancer treatment [7]. Meanwhile, the UV filtering property of 11 natural plants including *O. mungos* has also been assessed in a preliminary study. Following this, the results suggest that secondary metabolites such as polyphenols and flavonoids can absorb UV radiation and scavenge the ROS produced from body cells [66]. This is an essential outcome as the free reactive atoms or molecules are harmful due to their ability to damage normal and key biological macromolecules in the body, such as lipid, protein, and DNA. In contrast, the anthraquinone fraction of *O. rugosa van decumbens* functions by causing cytotoxicity in cancer cells and increasing the intracellular ROS, thus leading to cell apoptosis [67].

Several works assessing the anti-inflammatory activities of the extracts obtained from *Ophiorrhiza* species have been conducted as they are highly beneficial in determining their respective anticancer properties. Inflammation is typically complicated, beyond one's control, and a continuous process that results in the progression of diseases such as atherosclerosis and cancer. Therefore, carrageen-induced inflammation is a commonly employed method in order to investigate the anti-inflammatory activity of certain compounds. To date, no exact mechanism of action for the anti-inflammatory activity of anthraquinone fraction from *O. rugosa* has been underlined. However, it is believed that inflammation reduction occurs via the inhibition of the lipid peroxidation and scavenging of hydroxyl radicals [67]. Table 5 shows the anticancer activities of certain *Ophiorrhiza* species based on previous studies.

Table 5. Anticancer activity.

Species	Phytochemicals	Extraction and Isolation	Biological Activity	Method (Dose/Concentration)	References
Ophiorrhiza mungos Linn.	Luteolin-7-O-glucosides (**48**)		Gastroprotective effect against ethanol-induced and indomethacin-induced gastric injury in rats	25 mg/kg b.w p.o	[59]
		Alcohol and aqueous extracts of *O. mungos* leaves	Anti-cancer property on Dalton's Ascites Lymphoma (DAL) in mice	Alcohol extract: 400 mg/kg b.w p.o (14 days) Aqueous extract: 800 mg/kg b.w. p.o (14 days)	[68]
	Luteolin-7-O-glucoside (**48**), camptothecin (**11**)	Methanolic extract of leaves and roots of the plant	Anti-cancer activity against COLO 320 DM, AGS, MCF-7, and A549 cancer cell lines in rats Notes: COLO 320 DM (human colon adenocarcinoma), AGS (human gastric cancer cell line), MCF-7 (human breast cancer cell line), A549 (human lung cancer cell lines) Suppressed β-catenin in COLO 320 DM	20 mg/kg b. w subcutaneously for 16 weeks and 120μM (Incubated for 24 h)	[60]
		Methanolic extract of leaves	UV filtering potential	1 mg/mL (The extract was exposed to direct sunlight for 21 days)	[66]
Ophiorrhiza rugosa van decumbens	Anthraquinones		Anti-cancer property in mice with: Ehrlich ascites carcinoma (EAC) Dalton's lymphoma ascites (DAL) Solid tumors	130 μg/mL b.w 160 μg/mL b.w 200 mg/kg b.w (p.o for 10 days)	[67]
Ophiorrhiza nicobarica	Major chemicals: ursolic acid (**50**), β-sitosterol, harmaline (**29**)	Alcoholic extract	Analgesic and anti-inflammatory activity in rats and mice	200 and 300 mg/kg b.w p.o Fractions: 50 mg/kg b.w p.o	[11]
Ophiorrhiza mungos	Presence of flavonoids, cardiac glycosides and phenolics		Prevention of hemorrhagic lesion induced by snake venom on the yolk sac membrane of the chick embryo.	10 μg/μL (Incubation of the venom with the extract before applying to the embryo for 30 min)	[5]

b.w = body weight; p.o = oral route.

7.2. Camptothecin Interest

Camptothecin (**11**) was first isolated via the extraction of the bark and stem of the Chinese tree *Camptotheca acuminata* in 1958 [8,69]. It was later found in *C. lowreyana, C. yunnanensis, Nothapodytes nimmoniana, Pyrenacantha klaineana, Merrilliodendron megacarpum, Ervatamia heyneana, Mostuea brunonis, O. mungos, O. pumila,* and *O. filistipula* as well [4,10,34,70]. Even though camptothecin is one of the potent topoisomerase-1 inhibitors, its usage and application in clinical trials and global market has been withdrawn as a result of its low aqueous solubility and severe toxicity during the S-phase of the cell cycle, which can lead to normal cell death [9]. In fact, the early 1970s yielded various camptothecin clinical trials in which the respective researchers had failed across several attempts in developing its sodium salt form to overcome its poor solubility characteristics. Following this, they had found that for camptothecin (**11**) to show its activity, the lactone ring moiety must remain intact. However, the ring was opened during the sodium salt preparation, thus resulting in its failure to show the anticipated activity [71].

Another earlier study has also suggested that a complete pentacyclic ring structure with the D ring pyrridone and E ring lactone formed via a 20S configuration is crucial towards the anticancer property of camptothecin (**11**) [7]. Scholarly interest in camptothecin molecules steadily increased in the mid-1980s in which two first-generation water-soluble camptothecin analogues with an intact lactone ring were developed, namely camptosar (irinotecan or CPT-11) (**62**) and hycamtin (topotecan) (**63**) (Figure 6). These two structures were obtained by modifying the A and B rings of camptothecin accordingly [7]. In 1996, the United State Food and Drug Administration (FDA) approved the use of these two analogues in the pharmaceutical industry, whereby they were marketed by Pharmacia (Pfizer) and GlaxoSmithKline for the treatment of metastatic colorectal, primary colon, and metastatic ovarian cancers [71].

Regardless, recent studies undertaken have shown that the isolated natural camptothecin derivatives such as 9-methoxycamptothecin and 10-hydroxy-camptothecin are water-soluble and possess antitumor activity [70]. Following this, more advanced therapeutic strategies by using target-oriented drug delivery systems have crowned camptothecin (**11**) as a major candidate for the treatment of multi-drug resistant cancers [8]. In fact, newer drug delivery via liposomal and copolymer vehicle-mediated systems are capable of significantly improving the safety and efficacy of CPT [9]. For example, its release mediated by pH-sensitive block copolymer is believed to enhance its subsequent delivery in the body, alongside better safety considerations [72]. Additionally, another new alternative strategy of stem cell-based research in the apoptogenic signalling of CPT is still in progress [73].

From these findings, clearly several approaches have been discovered by researchers in order to stimulate the application of CPT in regenerative medicine by using its chemical analogues. Among them, methods such as manipulating its ring structure, conjugating it with other molecules, developing its prodrug, and using specific protein-based drug delivery systems have been suggested to establish a better efficacy and safety of anticancer drugs. However, most of the analogues are still in the phase of clinical trials and their safety issues are attributed as the major reason why these compounds have yet to enter the market. Table 6 shows the camptothecin analogues that are still in the clinical trial phase in detail.

Table 6. Clinical trials of camptothecin analogues. Adapted from [9].

Camptothecin Analogues	Year Started	Clinical Trials/Progression	Indication	Company
9-aminocamptothecin	1993	Phase I/II	Ovarian and malignant lymphoma	
Karenitecin (BNP-1350)		Phase II	Malignant melanoma and brain tumor	
Diflomotecan (BN-80915)	2007	Phase II	Solid tumors and small cell lung cancer (SCLC)	Ipsen
Gimatecan (ST-1481)		Phase II	Advanced solid tumors and recurrent epithelial ovarian and fallopian tube cancers	
Elomotecan (BN-80927)		Phase I	Advanced solid tumors	Ipsen and Roche
DRF-1042		Phase I		Dr. Reddys Laboratories
Exatecan mesylate		Phase II	Gastric cancer and relapsed rhabdomyosarcoma 9 in children)	
Rubitecan		Phase II/III but already withdrawn due to unfavorable results	Pancreatic cancer	
CZ-48 *		Phase I	Solid tumors	
TP-300 *		Phase I	Advanced solid tumors	
EZN-2208 *		Phase I	Advanced malignancy	
MAG-CPT **		Discontinue after Phase I		Pharmacia and Upjohn
XMT-1001 **		Phase II	Lung cancer	
CRLX-101 **		Phase I/II	Advanced solid tumor	

* Conjugated form of camptothecin analogue; ** Prodrug form of camptothecin.

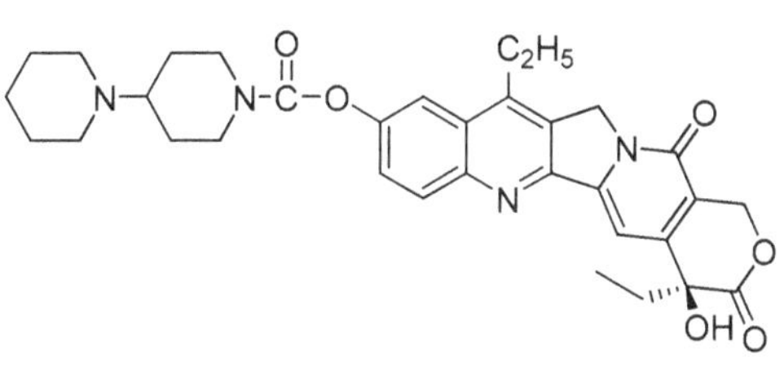

Irinotecan (**62**) 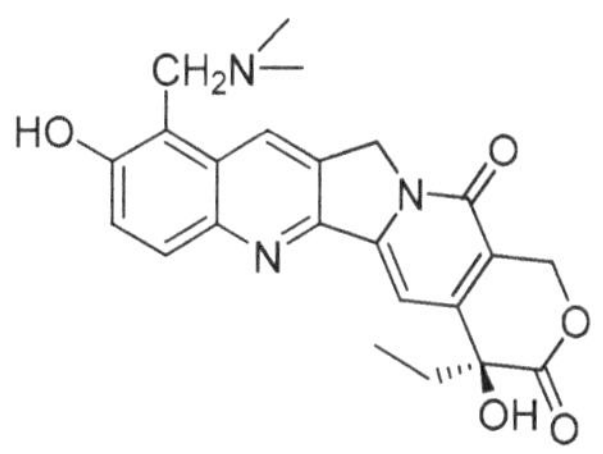 Topotecan (**63**)

Figure 6. Campthotechin analogues.

7.3. Antiviral Activity

Generally, flavonoids are one of the phytochemicals responsible for the activities against multiple viruses. For example, catechin can inhibit the property of viral infectivity of the respiratory syncytial virus (RSV) and herpes simplex virus-1 (HSV-1) but not their intracellular replication, whereas quercetin is capable of effectively reducing the infectivity of majority of viruses [74] and partially inhibiting DNA gyrase [58]. Meanwhile, coumarins may possess antiviral effects by stimulating the macrophages towards preventing infections and recurrence of cold sores caused by HSV-1 in humans, while terpenoids are active against yeasts such as *Candida albicans*. Similarly, harmane offers intercalating properties with the DNA of viruses [74] and has a strong activity against the intracellular amastigote of *Leishmania infantum*, which is partly due to its ability to inhibit the leishmanial protein kinase C (PKC) activity [75].

Furthermore, harmaline (**29**) or 7-methoxy-1-methyl-4,9-dihydro-3*H*-pyrido[3,4-β] indole alkaloid isolated from *O. nicobarica* is known for its potent antiviral activity against herpes simplex virus 1 (HSV-1. Rather than interfering with viral entry, it affects the recruitment of lysine-specific demethylase-1 (LSD1) and immediate-early (IE) complex binding on the promoter of ICP0. This will, in turn, contribute to the suppression of the viral IE gene synthesis, thereby causing a reduction of ICP4 and ICP27 expression [76]. Similarly, camptothecin (**11**) and 10-methoxycamptothecin previously isolated from the leaves of *O. mungos* have been noted to yield an active activity against the herpes virus [77]. Table 7 shows the antifungal, anti-yeast, and antiviral activities of five *Ophiorrhiza* species according to prior studies conducted on these plants.

Table 7. Antiviral activity.

Species	Phytochemicals	Extraction and Isolation	Biological Activity	Method (Dose/Concentration)	References
Ophiorrhiza trichocarpon Bl., Ophiorrhiza rugosa, and Ophiorrhiza aff. nutans Cl. ex Hk. f.	Alkaloid, coumarin, anthraquinone glycoside, scopoletin, saponins	Methanolic extract of the whole plant	Antifungal activity was determined by the agar-well diffusion method. Inhibition zone: Candida albicans (10 mm) Trichophyton mentagophyte (12 mm) Aspergillus flavus (12 mm)	50 mg/mL 30 mg/mL 75 mg/mL	[3]
Ophiorrhiza shenduruniii	Lupan-20-ol-3(β)-yl hexadecanoate (51), lupan-20-ol-3(β)-yl acetate (52), olean-18-en-3(β)-yl hexadecanoate (53)	Hexane and chloroform extract of the whole plant	Anti-yeast/antifungal activity of: The three compounds against: C. albicans (inhibition zone; 15, 10 and 16 mm respectively) Fusarium oxysporum (inhibition zone; 10, 8 and 8 mm respectively). Hexane extract: Candida albican (28/28 mm) Fusarium oxysporum (18/26 mm) Chloroform extract: Candida albican (28/28 mm) Fusarium oxysporum (24/26 mm)	100 µL	[35]
Ophiorrhiza nicobarica	harmaline (29)		Anti-HSV-1 activity in mice	0.25 and 0.5 mg/kg b.w p.o once daily (8 days)	[76]

7.4. Antimicrobial Activity

The components of alkaloids, carbohydrates, tannins, anthraquinones, hormones, terpenoids, saponins, flavonoids, essential oils, glycosides, and potassium are undeniably considered to have a curative effect against several pathogens [78]. Flavonoids, for example, can form a complex with extracellular bacterial soluble proteins and cell walls; those that are lipid-soluble may also disrupt the microbial membranes as they are lipophilic in nature. Meanwhile, coumarins and terpenoids are active against positive bacteria such as *Bacillus subtilis* and *Staphylococcus aureus*, despite the latter's lesser effect against gram-negative bacteria [74].

A majority of works assessing the antimicrobial activities of extracts from *Ophiorrhiza* species have been conducted using the diffusion assay method, namely by observing the inhibition zone of these extracts on certain microorganism growth. Different plant extracts will typically display distinct antibacterial activities, which are attributable to their varying phytochemical contents and properties. For instance, the ethyl acetate and methanol extracts have been underlined as the best options amongst other solvent extracts tested. Here, the lesser activity of other extracts is due to their inability to either extract the bioactive molecules with antimicrobial constituents or produce an effective concentration of antibacterial constituents [79]. Table 8 shows the antimicrobial activities of five *Ophiorrhiza* species, whereas their biological activities are summarised in Figure 7.

Table 8. Antimicrobial activity.

Species	Phytochemicals	Extraction and Isolation	Biological Activity	Method (Dose/Concentration)	References
Ophiorrhiza mungos	Presence of carbohydrates, proteins, phenolics, terpenoids, glycosides, reducing compounds and saponins	Hexane, chloroform, ethyl acetate, methanol and ethanol extracts of leaves and stem of the O. mungos.	Ethyl acetate and methanol extract showed potent antimicrobial activity against nine microorganisms (B. subtilis, L. lactis, S. aureus, M. luteus, P. aeruginosa, S. typhimurium, K. pneumonia, P. vulgaris, E. coli.). Inhibition zone: Ethyl acetate extract: 19–28 mm Methanol extract: 11–26 mm	500 µg/mL	[79]
	Carbohydrate, tannin, terpenoids, saponins, flavonoids, alkaloids and glycosides	Ethanolic extract of fresh flower	Antimicrobial activity against six pathogens with inhibition zone: B. subtilis (20 mm), K. pneumonia (19 mm), P. aeruginosa (14 mm), S. aureus (14 mm), S. mutans (11 mm) C. albicans (16 mm)	0.02 mL	[78]
Ophiorrhiza trichocarpon Bl., Ophiorrhiza rugosa and Ophiorrhiza aff. Nutans Cl. Ex Hk. f.	Alkaloids, coumarins, anthraquinone glycosides, scopoletin, saponins	Methanolic extract of the whole plant	Antibacterial activities of: Ophiorrhiza trichocarpon Bl. E.coli (10 mm) S.aureus (10.5 mm) Pseudomonas aeruginosa (10 mm) Ophiorrhiza rugosa E.coli (9.5 mm) S.aureus (10 mm) Pseudomonas aeruginosa (10 mm) Ophiorrhiza aff. Nutans Cl. Ex Hk. f. E.coli (10 mm) S.aureus (10.5 mm) Pseudomonas aeruginosa (10 mm)	75 mg/mL 10 mg/mL 10 mg/mL 100 mg/mL 10 mg/mL 50 mg/mL 100 mg/mL 10 mg/mL 10 mg/ml	[3]
Ophiorrhiza shendurunii	Lupan-20-ol-3(β)-yl hexadecanoate (51), lupan-20-ol-3(β)-yl acetate (52), olean-18-en-3(β)-yl hexadecanoate (53)	Hexane and chloroform extracts of the whole plant	Antibacterial activities of the chloroform extract using agar well diffusion assay are significant against: B. subtilis (22/18 mm), E. coli (19/23 mm). The hexane extract showed no antibacterial activity against Escherichia coli and Bacillus subtilis.	100 µL	[35]

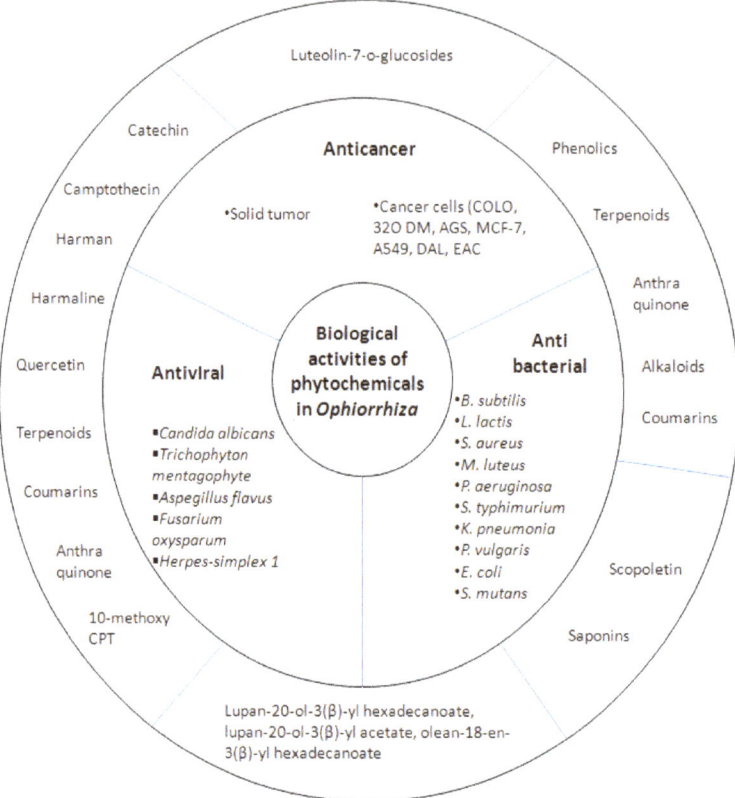

Figure 7. Summary of biological activity of phytochemicals in *Ophiorrhiza* species.

8. Propagation

Over time, several researchers have conducted biotechnology research on certain species of *Ophiorrhiza* in order to develop an efficient method for the development of camptothecin (**11**) and recognition of novel secondary metabolites from cultivated plants [32]. The high demand for camptothecin and other active pharmaceutical ingredients, as well as the overexploitation of *C. accumata* and *Nothapodytes foetida* as the main sources of this component have resulted in the development of various protocols for its in vitro cultivation and production by using *Ophiorrhiza* plants [1]. In fact, camptothecin is a highly valuable drug with market prices ranging from US$3500 to US$350,000 per kilogram. Therefore, it is considerably interesting for scholars to identify alternative ways of producing the component, such as by using plant cells and tissue cultures, as a result of its commercial value [64].

The successful regeneration of *O. pumila* from the callus tissue of its leaves and shoot has been reported, whereby a new glucosyloxy camptothecin (i.e., 9-β-glucosyloxycamptothecin) is isolated along with 15 metabolites, including six alkaloids linked to camptothecin (**11**). However, (3S)-deoxyppumiloside as one of camptothecin's possible biogenetic precursors has not been detected, whereas the (3R) epimer is isolated from regenerated plants. Accordingly, these well-developed callus cultures can also generate the anthraquinones which are not producible by non- culture *O. pumila* plants [54]. Therefore, a method for the micropropagation and generation of camptothecin from *O. mungos* via in vitro plants has been documented, whereas a protocol is also developed for rapid root and organogenesis proliferation. As a result, the high performance liquid chromatography

(HPLC) analysis of the method has proven that its in vitro production generates higher yields than natural-grown plants [80].

Moreover, a study on the effect of jasmonic acid in the cell suspension culture of *O. mungos* species has revealed the suspension's ability to increase the production of camptothecin significantly [81]. Similarly, another study has substantiated the effect of silver nitrate and yeast extract on the cell growth, camptothecin (**11**) accumulation, and cell viability, thereby leading to a significant increment in the production of biomass and camptothecin (**11**) alike [82]. In fact, a prolonged subculture of *O. trichocarpose* Blume by alternating the medium intensity in each subculture has resulted in a notable increment in the development of the plant's shoots and biomass [83].

In line with this, different concentrations of various auxins in *O. mungos* var. *angustifolia* culture have also been reported to influence the biomass camptothecin (**11**) production, whereby the result shows that both explants will not induce callus growth in the absence of exogenous hormones. In contrast, they will induce the growth of calli following their culture in the Murashige and Skoog (MS) medium at different strengths together with butyric acid (BA) and naphthalene acetic acid (NAA) solutions. The study underlined the ideal combination of solutions as half-strength MS solid medium with 10.74 μM NAA + 4.44 μM BA. Further, the scholars have discovered that the in vitro leaves are the best explants that can help to produce a higher content of camptothecin compared to their in vivo counterparts [69].

In contrast, an efficient plant regeneration system has been introduced in a study through somatic embryogenesis. Here, the embryogenic callus tissues extracted from aseptic leaf explants were used to induce the somatic embryos under callus tissues incubated across the different periods of 10 to 60 days. The outcomes showed that 40-day-long incubation in 0.5 mg/L 2,4-dichloro phenoxy acetic acid media was the optimum environment for the somatic embryogenesis in *O. pectinata*. Therefore, the study successfully substantiated the influence of callus tissue incubation period towards the differentiation of embryos in suspension cultures [33].

Moreover, a high production of camptothecin (**11**) has been obtained using the root cultures of both transformed and untransformed *O. mungos* [64] and *O. alata Craib* [39], respectively, thus promoting an alternative novel system in sustaining its bio-production as raw material for the pharmaceutical industry. The transformed hairy roots were obtained by infecting the node explants with *Agrobacterium rhizogenes* TISTR 1450 [39,64]: it was found that the CPT (**11**) concentration was consequently double the amount in the soil-growing plant [39].

In general, culture media containing ammonium as the nitrogen source is preferable, whereby nitrate is essential in regulating the pH value and promoting the growth of root and synthesis of camptothecin (**11**) [64]. The addition of polystyrene resin or Diaion HP-20 capable of absorbing camptothecin (**11**) has further led to its increased concentration in culture media, namely seven-fold higher compared to the control media [39]. Moreover, camptothecin (**11**) can be extracted more in root and hairy root cultures as they consist of differentiated tissues. Here, the secondary plant metabolite biosynthesis is still active and has not decreased in contrast to the cultures of undifferentiated callus or cell suspension [39,64].

Nevertheless, the accumulation of camptothecin (**11**) in the different parts of plants is identical [84], rendering it crucial for one to consider the specific selection and isolation of cells or organ lines in order to induce in vitro calli in biomass metabolite production. For example, undifferentiated callus and suspension cultures do not always produce the desired amount of compound of interest. In contrast, the shoot, root, and hairy root cultures will often generate the same compounds as in the appropriate organs [67]. Hence, the type of medium culture, suitable salt strength, nitrate level, phosphate level, and growth regulator level should be considered beforehand to obtain the desired metabolites at a high quantity and quality [84].

9. Conclusions

To conclude, compounds derived from *Ophiorrhiza* plants play an important role in treating diseases although they may not directly consider drugs. The compounds can be served as lead compounds that are beneficial for the development of potential anticancer drugs, particularly. This may help new researchers in understanding the diseases better, providing more efficient therapies with a new mechanism of action, increasing the patient compliance, reducing the synthetic anticancer drugs-related adverse effects as well as encouraging the development of future and novel anticancer drugs. The *Ophiorrhiza* species represent an enormous diversity throughout the world, yet not many have been explored. With the development of technology of apparatus and equipment nowadays, newly discovered bioactive compounds showing inhibition effects on cancer cells may rapidly be recognized. Thus, further extensive research and studies should be continued to discover more bioactive molecules in this species and their therapeutic effects to highlight the use of natural source-derived drugs in the medicinal field which are believed to be more well-tolerated and cost-effective.

Funding: This research was funded by INTERNATIONAL ISLAMIC UNIVERSITY MALAYSIA, grant number P-RIGS18-028-0028. The APC was funded by the Universiti Putra Malaysia.

Acknowledgments: The authors are thankful to the International Islamic University Malaysia for funding this work via Grant No. P-RIGS18-028-0028.

Conflicts of Interest: The authors declare no conflict of interest.

References

1. Gopalakrishnan, K.; Krishnan, S.; Narayanan, K.P. Tissue culture studies and estimation of camptothecin from *Ophiorrhiza* prostrata D. Don. *Indian J. Plant Physiol.* **2018**, *23*, 582–592. [CrossRef]
2. Hareesh, V.S.; Sabu, M. The genus *Ophiorrhiza* (Rubiaceae) in Andaman and Nicobar Islands, India with a new species. *Phytotaxa* **2018**, *383*, 259–272. [CrossRef]
3. Phoowiang, N.; Santiarworn, D.; Liawruangrath, B.; Takayama, H.; Liawruangrath, S. Phytochemical screening and antimicrobial activity of three *Ophiorrhiza* species from northern Thailand. *Naresuan Phayao* **2009**, *2*, 134–140.
4. Sibi, C.V.; Dintu, K.P.; Renjith, R.; Krishnaraj, M.V.; Roja, G.; Satheeshkumar, K. A new record of *Ophiorrhiza* trichocarpon Blume (Rubiaceae: Ophiorrhizeae) from Western Ghats, India: Another source plant of camptothecin. *J. Sci. Res.* **2012**, *4*, 529–532. [CrossRef]
5. Krishnan, S.A.; Dileepkumar, R.; Nair, A.S.; Oommen, O.V. Studies on neutralizing effect of *Ophiorrhiza* mungos root extract against *Daboia russelii* venom. *J. Ethnopharmacol.* **2014**, *151*, 543–547. [CrossRef]
6. Hamzah, A.S. Isolation, Characterization and Biological Activities of Chemical Constituents of *Ophiorrhiza* and *Hedyotis* Species. Master's Thesis, University Putra Malaysia, Serdang, Malaysia, 1994.
7. Supriya, B.; Nutan, M. Secondary metabolites as DNA topoisomerase inhibitors: A new era towards designing of anticancer drugs. *Pharmacogn. Rev.* **2010**, *4*, 12–26.
8. Rajan, R.; Varghese, S.C.; Kurup, R.; Gopalakrishnan, R.; Venkataraman, R.; Satheeshkumar, K.; Baby, S. HPTLC-based quantification of camptothecin in *Ophiorrhiza* species of the southern Western Ghats in India. *Cogent Chem.* **2016**, *2*, 1–9. [CrossRef]
9. Khazir, J.; Ahmad, B.; Pilcher, L.; Riley, D.L. Phytochemistry letters role of plants in anticancer drug discovery. *Phytochem. Lett.* **2014**, *7*, 173–181. [CrossRef]
10. Prabha, G.; Karuppusamy, S. Phytochemical profile and radical scavenging activity of alcoholic extract of *Ophiorrhiza* radicans Gardner (Rubiaceae)—A rare plant of Southern Western Ghats of India. *Trends Biosci.* **2018**, *11*, 1572–1576.
11. Chattopadhyay, D.; Das, S.; Mandal, A.B.; Arunachalam, G.; Bhattacharya, S. Evaluation of analgesic and antiinflammatory activity of *Ophiorrhiza* nicobarica, an ethnomedicine from Nicobar Islands, India. *Orient. Pharm. Exp. Med.* **2007**, *7*, 395–408. [CrossRef]
12. Duan, L.D.; Lin, Y.; Lu, Z. *Ophiorrhiza* shiqianensis (Rubiaceae), a new species from Guizhou, China. *PhytoKeys* **2019**, *121*, 43–51. [CrossRef] [PubMed]

13. Arbain, D.; Byrne, L.T.; Sargent, M.V. Isomalindine-16-carboxylate, a Zwitterionic Alkaloid from *Ophiorrhiza* cf. communis. *Aust. J. Chem.* **1997**, *50*, 1109–1110. [CrossRef]
14. Martono, R.A. Isolasi Senyawa Kimia Utama Dari Fraksi etil Asetat Ekstrak Metanol Batang *Ophiorrhiza* sp (ex. Gunung Singgalang). Master's Thesis, Andalas University, Padang, Indonesia, 2009.
15. Sofjeni, E. Isniyetti Isolasi Alkaloid Dari Tumbuhan *Ophiorrhiza* "Siberida DA-RT 6030,". Master's Thesis, Andalas University, Padang, Indonesia, 1997.
16. Teruna, H.H.Y. Isolasi Alkaloida Dari Herba *Ophiorrhiza* sp. "Sako DA-RT 7577,". Master's Thesis, Andalas University, Padang, Indonesia, 1997.
17. Roza, E. Isolasi Alkaloida Dari Tumbuhan *Ophiorrhiza* longiflora BL. Master's Thesis, Andalas University, Padang, Indonesia, 1992.
18. Susila, R. Isolasi Alkaloid Dari Tumbuhan *Ophiorrhiza* cf. kunstleri King. Master's Thesis, Andalas University, Padang, Indonesia, 1998.
19. Firmansyah, F. Isolasi Alkaloida Dari Tumbuhan *Ophiorrhiza* sp. Master's Thesis, Andalas University, Padang, Indonesia, 1994.
20. Gustampera, S. Isolasi Alkaloida Dari Tumbuhan *Ophiorrhiza* sp. Master's Thesis, Andalas University, Padang, Indonesia, 1993.
21. Yohannes, I. Isolasi Alkaloid Utama *Ophiorrhiza* "DA-RT 7895,". Master's Thesis, Andalas University, Padang, Indonesia, 1998.
22. Sofjeni, E. Isolasi Alkaloid Dari Daun *Ophiorrhiza* "Air Sirah DA-RT 6604,". Master's Thesis, Andalas University, Padang, Indonesia, 1997.
23. Arbain, D.; Handayani, D.; Yohannes, A.; Sargent, M.V. The alkaloids of *Ophiorrhiza* marginata. *ACGC Chem. Res. Commun.* **1998**, *7*, 38–40.
24. Arbain, D.; Susanti, D.; Gemala, S.; Taher, M.; Mukhtar, M.H.; Sargent, M.V. The alkaloids of three *Ophiorrhiza* species. *Asian Coord. Gr. Chem.* **1998**, *7*, 44–47.
25. Arbain, D.; Byrne, L.T.; Putra, D.P.; Sargent, M.V.; Skelton, B.W.; White, A.H. Ophiorrhizine, a new quaternary indole alkaloid related to Cinchonamine, from *Ophiorrhiza* major Ridl. *J. Chem. Soc. Perkin Trans.* **1992**, *1*, 663–664. [CrossRef]
26. Arbain, D.; Byrne, A.L.T.; Evrayoza, N.; Sargent, V.M. Bracteatine, a quaternary glucoalkaloid from *Ophiorrhiza* bracteata. *Aust. J. Chem.* **1997**, *50*, 1111–1112. [CrossRef]
27. Arbain, D.; Nordin, H.; Skeltonc, B.W.; Allan, H. The alkaloids of *Ophiorrhixa* cf. ferruginea. *Autralian J. Chem.* **1993**, *46*, 969–976. [CrossRef]
28. Arbain, D.; Deddi, P.P.; Sargent, M.V.; Revi, S.; Wahyuni, F.S. Indole alkaloids from two species of *Ophiorrhiza*. *Aust. J. Chem.* **2000**, *53*, 221–224.
29. Efdi, M. Isolasi Alkaloid Dari Daun Tumbuhan *Ophiorrhiza* cf. Kunstleri King. Master's Thesis, Andalas University, Padang, Indonesia, 1999.
30. Arbain, D.; Putra, D.P.; Sargent, M.V. The alkaloids of *Ophiorrhiza* filistipula. *Aust. J. Chem.* **1993**, *46*, 977–985. [CrossRef]
31. Arbain, D.; Sargent, M.V.; Dachriyanus, F.; Skelton, B.W.; White, A.H. Unusual indole alkaloids from *Ophiorrhiza* blumeana Korth. *J. Chem. Soc. Perkin Trans.* **1998**, *1*, 2537–2540. [CrossRef]
32. Kitajima, M. Chemical studies on monoterpenoid indole alkaloids from medicinal plant resources *Gelsemium* and *Ophiorrhiza*. *J. Nat. Med.* **2007**, *61*, 14–23. [CrossRef]
33. Midhu, C.K.; Hima, S.; Binoy, J.; Satheeshkumar, K. Influence of incubation period on callus tissues for plant regeneration in *Ophiorrhiza* pectinata Arn. through somatic embryogenesis. *Proc. Natl. Acad. Sci. USA* **2019**, *89*. [CrossRef]
34. Joseph, G.; Hareesh, V.S.; Sreekumar, V.B.; Hrideek, T.K. Rediscovery of *Ophiorrhiza* radicans (*Rubiaceae*) from the Western Ghats of Peninsular India. *Rheedea* **2013**, *23*, 19–21.
35. Rajan, R.; Venkataraman, R.; Baby, S. A new lupane-type triterpenoid fatty acid ester and other isolates from *Ophiorrhiza* shendurunii. *Nat. Prod. Res.* **2016**, *30*, 2197–2203. [CrossRef] [PubMed]
36. Adnan, M.; Chy, N.U.; Mostafa Kamal, A.T.M.; Azad, M.O.K.; Paul, A.; Uddin, S.B.; Barlow, J.W.; Faruque, M.O.; Park, C.H.; Cho, D.H. Investigation of the biological activities and characterization of bioactive constituents of ophiorrhiza rugosa var. prostrata (D.Don) & Mondal leaves through in vivo, in vitro, and in silico approaches. *Molecules* **2019**, *24*, 1367.

37. Kitajima, M.; Fujii, N.; Yoshino, F.; Sudo, H.; Saito, K.; Aimi, N.; Takayama, H. Camptothecins and two new monoterpene glucosides from *Ophiorrhiza liukiuensis*. *Chem. Pharm. Bull.* **2005**, *53*, 1355–1358. [CrossRef]
38. Aimi, N.; Tsuyuki, T.; Murakami, H.; Sakai, S.; Haginiwa, J. Structure of ophiorines A and B: Novel type glucoindole alkaloids isolated from *Ophiorrhiza* spp. *Tetrahedron Lett.* **1985**, *26*, 5299–5302. [CrossRef]
39. Ya-ut, P.; Chareonsap, P.; Sukrong, S. Micropropagation and hairy root culture of *Ophiorrhiza alata* Craib for camptothecin production. *Biotechnol. Lett.* **2011**, *33*, 2519–2526. [CrossRef]
40. Leonaldi, L. Isolasi Alkaloida Dari Tumbuhan *Ophiorrhiza* neglecta Bl. ex DC. Master's Thesis, Andalas University, Padang, Indonesia, 1995.
41. Yulian, F. Isolasi Alkaloida Dari Tumbuhan *Ophirrhiza* Palidulla Ridl. Master's Thesis, Andalas University, Padang, Indonesia, 2002.
42. Fitrya, F. Isolasi Alkaloida Dari Tumbuhan *Ophiorrhiza* klosii Ridl. Master's Thesis, Andalas University, Padang, Indonesia, 1996.
43. Alya, H. Isolasi Senyawa Kimia Utama Dari Daun *Ophiorrhiza* sp (ex. Simanau DA-RT61, Solok). Master's Thesis, Andalas University, Padang, Indonesia, 2009.
44. Yulyuswarni, Y. Isolasi Alkaloida Dari Tumbuhan *Ophiorrhiza* anonyma Val. Master's Thesis, Andalas University, Padang, Indonesia, 1995.
45. Aulia, D. Isolasi Alkaloid Dari Tumbuhan *Ophiorrhiza* sp "DA-RT 82 AT,". Master's Thesis, Andalas University, Padang, Indonesia, 2000.
46. Martins, D.; Nunez, C.V. Secondary metabolites from *Rubiaceae* species. *Molecules* **2015**, *20*, 13422–13495. [CrossRef]
47. Arbain, D. Inventory, constituents and conservation of biologically important *Sumatran* plants. *Nat. Prod. Commun.* **2012**, *7*, 799–806. [CrossRef]
48. Swamy, M.K.; Paramashivaiah, S.; Hiremath, L.; Akhtar, M.S.; Sinniah, U.R. Micropropagation and conservation of selected endangered anticancer medicinal plants from the Western Ghats of India. *Anticancer Plants Nat. Prod. Biotechnol. Implements* **2018**, *2*, 481–504.
49. Kumar, G.K.; Fayad, M.A.; Nair, A.J. *Ophiorrhiza mungos* var. angustifolia—Estimation of camptothecin and pharmacological screening. *Plant Sci. Today* **2018**, *5*, 113–120. [CrossRef]
50. Shitan, N. Secondary metabolites in plants: Transport and self-tolerance mechanisms. *Biosci. Biotechnol. Biochem.* **2016**, *80*, 1283–1293. [CrossRef] [PubMed]
51. Aimi, N.; Murakami, H.; Tsuyuki, T.; Nishiyama, T.; Sakai, S.; Haginiwa, J. Hydrolytic degradation of β-carboline-type monoterpenoid glucoindole alkaloids: A possible mechanism for harman formation in *Ophiorrhiza* and related *Rubiaceous* plants. *Chem. Pharm. Bull.* **1986**, *34*, 3064–3066. [CrossRef]
52. Kitajima, M.; Ohara, S.; Kogure, N.; Santiarworn, D. β-Carboline-type indole alkaloid glycosides from *Ophiorrhiza* trichocarpon. *Tetrahedron* **2013**, *69*, 9451–9456. [CrossRef]
53. Hamzah, A.S.; Arbain, D.; Sargent, M.V.; Lajis, N.H. The alkaloids of *Ophiorrhiza* communis and O. tomentosa. *Pertanika J. Sci. Technol.* **1994**, *2*, 33–38.
54. Kitajima, M.; Mio, N.; Hiromitsu, T.; Kazuki, S.; Joachim, S.; Norio, A. Constituents of regenertaed plants of *Ophiorrhiza pumila*; formation of a new glycocamptothecin and predominant formulation of (3R)-deoxypumiloside over (3S)-congener. *Tetrahedron Lett.* **1997**, *38*, 8997–9000. [CrossRef]
55. Khristine, N. Uji Aktivitas Alkaloida Hasil Isolasi Dari Daun Tumbuhan *Ophiorrhiza* "Air Sirah DA-RT 6526,". Master's Thesis, Andalas University, Padang, Indonesia, 1997.
56. Gemala, S. Isolasi Senyawa Alkaloida Dari Daun *Ophiorrhiza* "Air Sirah DA-RT 6526 B,". Master's Thesis, Andalas University, Padang, Indonesia, 1997.
57. Madhavan, V.; Yoganarasimhan, S.; Gurudeva, M.; John, C.; Deveswaran, R. Pharmacognostical studies on the leaves of *Ophiorrhiza mungos* Linn. (Rubiaceae). *Spat. DD* **2013**, *3*, 89–98. [CrossRef]
58. Cushnie, T.P.T.; Lamb, A.J. Antimicrobial activity of flavonoids. *Int. J. Antimicrob. Agents* **2005**, *26*, 343–356. [CrossRef]
59. Antonisamy, P.; Subash-Babu, P.; Albert-Baskar, A.; Alshatwi, A.A.; Aravinthan, A.; Ignacimuthu, S.; Choi, K.C.; Lee, S.C.; Kim, J.H. Experimental study on gastroprotective efficacy and mechanisms of luteolin-7-O-glucoside isolated from *Ophiorrhiza mungos* Linn. in different experimental models. *J. Funct. Foods* **2016**, *25*, 302–313. [CrossRef]

60. Baskar, A.A.; Ignacimuthu, S.; Michael, G.P.; Al Numair, K.S. Cancer chemopreventive potential of luteolin-7-O-glucoside isolated from *Ophiorrhiza mungos* linn. *Nutr. Cancer* **2011**, *63*, 130–138. [CrossRef] [PubMed]
61. Chunzhi, G.; Zunfeng, L.; Chengwei, Q.; Xiangmei, B.; Jingui, Y. Hyperin protects against LPS-induced acute kidney injury by inhibiting TLR4 and NLRP3 signaling pathways. *Oncotarget* **2016**, *7*, 82602. [CrossRef] [PubMed]
62. Viraporn, V.; Yamazaki, M.; Saito, K.; Denduangboripant, J.; Chayamarit, K.; Chuanasa, T.; Sukrong, S. Correlation of camptothecin-producing ability and phylogenetic relationship in the genus *Ophiorrhiza*. *Planta Med.* **2011**, *77*, 759–764. [CrossRef]
63. Jain, S.; Dwivedi, J.; Jain, P.K.; Satpathy, S.; Patra, A. Medicinal plants for treatment of cancer: A brief review. *Pharmacogn. J.* **2016**, *8*, 87–102. [CrossRef]
64. Wetterauer, B.; Wildi, E.; Wink, M. *Production of the Anticancer Compound Camptothecin in Root and Hairy Root Cultures of Ophiorrhiza mungos L.*; Springer: Singapore, 2018; pp. 303–341.
65. Kim, D.H.; Jang, Y.Y.; Han, E.S.; Lee, C.S. Protective effect of harmaline and harmalol against dopamine- and 6-hydroxydopamine-induced oxidative damage of brain mitochondria and synaptosomes, and viability loss of PC12 cells. *Eur. J. Neurosci.* **2001**, *13*, 1861–1872. [CrossRef] [PubMed]
66. Napagoda, M.T.; Malkanthi, B.M.A.S.; Abayawardana, S.A.K.; Qader, M.M.; Jayasinghe, L. Photoprotective potential in some medicinal plants used to treat skin diseases in Sri Lanka. *BMC Complement. Altern. Med.* **2016**, *16*, 1–6. [CrossRef] [PubMed]
67. Raveendran, V.V.; Vijayan, F.P.; Padikkala, J. Antitumor activities of an anthraquinone fraction isolated from in vitro cultures of *Ophiorrhiza rugosa var decumbens*. *Integr. Cancer Ther.* **2012**, *11*, 120–128. [CrossRef]
68. Madhavan, V.; Murali, A.; John, C.R. Anticancer activity of extracts of leaf of *Ophiorrhiza mungos* L. on Dalton's Ascitic lymphoma in mice. *MSRUAS-SASTech J.* **2007**, *14*, 29–32.
69. Krishnan, J.J.; Gangaprasad, A.; Satheeshkumar, K. Biosynthesis of camptothecin from callus and cell suspension cultures of *Ophiorrhiza mungos* L. var. angustifolia (Thw.) Hook. f. *Proc. Natl. Acad. Sci. USA* **2018**, *89*, 893–902. [CrossRef]
70. Lorence, A.; Nessler, C.L. Camptothecin, over four decades of surprising findings. *Phytochemistry* **2004**, *65*, 2735–2749. [CrossRef]
71. Oberlies, N.H.; Kroll, D.J. Camptothecin and taxol: Historic achievements in natural products research. *Nat. Prod.* **2004**, *67*, 129–135. [CrossRef]
72. Luo, Y.L.; Yang, X.L.; Xu, F.; Chen, Y.S.; Zhao, X. pH-triggered PMAA-b-HTPB-b-PMAA copolymer micelles: Physicochemical characterization and camptothecin release. *Colloid Polym. Sci.* **2014**, *292*, 1061–1072. [CrossRef]
73. García, C.P.; Videla Richardson, G.A.; Romorini, L.; Miriuka, S.G.; Sevlever, G.E.; Scassa, M.E. Topoisomerase I inhibitor, camptothecin, induces apoptogenic signaling in human embryonic stem cells. *Stem Cell Res.* **2014**, *12*, 400–414. [CrossRef] [PubMed]
74. Sher, A. Antimicrobial activity of natural products from medicinal plants: A review article. *Gomal J. Med. Sci.* **2009**, *7*, 72–78.
75. Di Giorgio, C.; Delmas, F.; Ollivier, E.; Elias, R.; Balansard, G.; Timon-David, P. In vitro activity of the β-carboline alkaloids harmane, harmine, and harmaline toward parasites of the species *Leishmania infantum*. *Exp. Parasitol.* **2004**, *106*, 67–74. [CrossRef]
76. Bag, P.; Ojha, D.; Mukherjee, H.; Halder, U.C.; Mondal, S.; Biswas, A.; Sharon, A.; Van Kaer, L.; Chakrabarty, S.; Das, G.; et al. A dihydro-pyrido-indole potently inhibits HSV-1 infection by interfering the viral immediate early transcriptional events. *Antiviral Res.* **2014**, *105*, 126–134. [CrossRef]
77. Perez, G.R.M. Antiviral activity of compounds isolated from plants. *Pharm. Biol.* **2003**, *41*, 107–157. [CrossRef]
78. Ganesan, S.; Manimegalai, K.; Latha, R. Antimicrobial activity of some flowers of Eastern Ghats, Tamil Nadu, India. *Glob. J. Bot. Sci.* **2014**, *2*, 26–31.
79. Jayadev, A.; Sari, S.; Nair, G.M. Phytochemical analysis and evaluation of antibacterial and antioxidant activities of *Vitex negundo* and *Ophiorrhiza mungos*. *Int. J. Pharmacogn. Phytochem. Res.* **2013**, *2*, 661–664.
80. Namdeo, A.G.; Priya, T.; Bhosale, B.B. Micropropagation and production of camptothecin form in vitro plants of *Ophiorrhiza mungos*. *Asian Pac. J. Trop. Biomed.* **2012**, *2*, S662–S666. [CrossRef]

81. Deepthi, S.; Satheeshkumar, K. Cell line selection combined with jasmonic acid elicitation enhance camptothecin production in cell suspension cultures of *Ophiorrhiza mungos* L. *Appl. Microbiol. Biotechnol.* **2017**, *101*, 545–558. [CrossRef] [PubMed]
82. Jaleel, A.; Velraj, K.M. Anti-cancer activity of *Ophiorrhiza* species endemic to Southern Western Ghats: A review. *J. Pharm. Sci. Res.* **2019**, *11*, 1156–1159.
83. Sibi, C.; Renjith, R.; Roja, G.; Ravichandran, P.; Satheeshkumar, K. A novel and efficient method for the enhanced production of multiple shoots and camptothecin from *Ophiorrhiza* trichocarpos blume through subculture passages in media of alternating strength. *Eur. J. Biotechnol. Biosci.* **2016**, *4*, 12–16.
84. Murthy, H.N.; Lee, E.J.; Paek, K.Y. Production of secondary metabolites from cell and organ cultures: Strategies and approaches for biomass improvement and metabolite accumulation. *Plant Cell. Tissue Organ Cult.* **2014**, *118*, 1–16. [CrossRef]

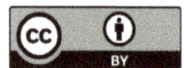

© 2020 by the authors. Licensee MDPI, Basel, Switzerland. This article is an open access article distributed under the terms and conditions of the Creative Commons Attribution (CC BY) license (http://creativecommons.org/licenses/by/4.0/).

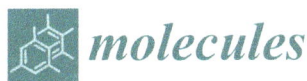

Review

Lamium Plants—A Comprehensive Review on Health Benefits and Biological Activities

Bahare Salehi [1], Lorene Armstrong [2], Antonio Rescigno [3,*], Balakyz Yeskaliyeva [4], Gulnaz Seitimova [4], Ahmet Beyatli [5], Jugreet Sharmeen [6], Mohamad Fawzi Mahomoodally [6,*], Farukh Sharopov [7,*], Alessandra Durazzo [8], Massimo Lucarini [8], Antonello Santini [9,*], Ludovico Abenavoli [10,*] and Javad Sharifi-Rad [12,*]

1. Student Research Committee, School of Medicine, Bam University of Medical Sciences, Bam 44340847, Iran; bahar.salehi007@gmail.com
2. Department of Pharmaceutical Sciences, State University of Ponta Grossa, Ponta Grossa, Paraná 84030900, Brasil; lorenearmstrong@hotmail.com
3. Department of Biomedical Sciences, University of Cagliari, s.s. 554 bivio Sestu, I-09042 Monserrato, CA, Italy
4. Faculty of Chemistry and Chemical Technology, Al-Farabi Kazakh National University, Almaty 480012, Kazakhstan; balakyz@mail.ru (B.Y.); sitigulnaz@mail.ru (G.S.)
5. Department of Medicinal and Aromatic Plants, University of Health Sciences, 34668 Istanbul, Turkey; ahmet.beyatli@sbu.edu.tr
6. Department of Health Sciences; Faculty of Science, University of Mauritius, Réduit 80837, Mauritius; sharmeenjugs@gmail.com
7. Department of Pharmaceutical Technology, Avicenna Tajik State Medical University, Rudaki 139, Dushanbe 734003, Tajikistan
8. CREA-Research Centre for Food and Nutrition, Via Ardeatina 546, 00178 Rome, Italy; alessandra.durazzo@crea.gov.it (A.D.); massimo.lucarini@crea.gov.it (M.L.)
9. Department of Pharmacy, University of Napoli Federico II, Via D. Montesano, 49-80131 Napoli, Italy
10. Department of Health Sciences, University Magna Graecia, viale Europa-Germaneto, 88100 Catanzaro, Italy
11. Department of Agricultural Sciences, University of Naples Federico II, 80055 Portici, Italy; rafcapas@unina.it
12. Zabol Medicinal Plants Research Center, Zabol University of Medical Sciences, Zabol 61615-585, Iran
* Correspondence: rescigno@unica.it (A.R.); f.mahomoodally@uom.ac.mu (M.F.M.); shfarukh@mail.ru (F.S.); asantini@unina.it (A.S.); l.abenavoli@unicz.it (L.A.); javad.sharifirad@gmail.com (J.S.-R.); Tel.: +39-0706754516 (A.R.); +23-057327341 (M.F.M.); +992-93-995-0370 (F.S.); +39-0812539317 (A.S.); +39-0961-3694387 (L.A.); +98-21-88200104 (J.S.-R.)

Academic Editor: Raphaël E. Duval
Received: 16 April 2019; Accepted: 14 May 2019; Published: 17 May 2019

Abstract: This work is an updated snapshot of *Lamium* plants and their biological activities. The main features of the plant are described and the components of its essential oils are summarized. The traditional medicinal uses of *Lamium* plants has been reported. The presence of these chemicals i.e., hydroxycinnamic acids, iridoids, secoiridoids, flavonoids, anthocyanins, phenylpropanoids, phytoecdysteroids, benzoxazinoids, betaine can provide biological activities. After the discussion of antioxidant properties documented for *Lamium* plants, the biological activities, studied using in vitro models, antimicrobial, antiviral, anti-inflammatory, anti-nociceptive activity, and pain therapy and cytotoxicity and cytoprotective activity are here described and discussed. Finally, targeted examples of in vivo studies are reported.

Keywords: *Lamium* plants; antiviral; antioxidant; anti-inflammatory; cytotoxicity

1. Introduction

Medicinal plants have been used since antiquity to treat illness and discomfort; their knowledge has been propagated from generation to generation by indigenous and local populations instigating the ethnobotanical study. Considering their global use, traditional, therapeutic and industrial value, many natural products are being investigated to lead the production of new drugs, wherefore, families and genera of plants with great potential are being researched for this purpose [1–3]. The recent review of Durazzo et al. [4] gives a current picture of main features of botanicals, by describing the strict relationship between the main plant biologically activity compounds and the nutraceutical role of botanicals [4–10].

Lamiaceae is a widespread family of flowering plants, also known as the mint family [11]. It is well distributed around the continents and, has about 250 genera described, which have 7,852 accepted species names [12]. The largest genera are *Salvia*, *Scutellaria*, *Stachys*, *Plectranthus*, *Hyptis*, *Teucrium*, *Vitex*, *Thymus* and *Nepeta* [3,11,13]. The plants of this family are normally shrubs or herbs with aromatic compounds in their leaves or flowers, such as essential oils. Many species are cultivated for their medicinal properties like antiseptic, antispasmodic, calmative, antimicrobials and, it is also used for culinary, fragrance, flavor and aromatherapy [11,14–16].

Within the family *Lamiaceae*, the genus *Lamium* is herbaceous and possess annuals or perennials forms, comprising around 40 species found in temperate and subtropical regions of Africa, Asia and Europe [16–19]. Regarding the botanical aspects, the leaves are cordate or reniform, ovate to lanceolate with an acute apex and cordate base, being petiolate on the lower nodes and sessile or uncommon amplexicaule at the upper nodes. It presents inflorescences with verticillasters in the axils of the floral leaves (2-12 flowered). The calyx is campanulate or tubular with subequal teeth. The corolla is bilabiate and shows a dark purple, yellowish green, white, yellow, etc. [17,19]. Species well studied of the genus are: *L. album* L., *L. purpureum* L., and *L. maculatum*. The popular name of "dead nettle" is due to the superficial similarity of the stinging nettles and, they do not have trichomes which can release toxic compounds [20].

The genus is used in folk medicine as antispasmodic, astringent, anti-proliferative, anti-inflammatory, antiviral, regulatory for sebaceous secretions and, also for the treatment of hypertension, scrofula, paralysis, prostate, menorrhagia, uterine hemorrhage, leucorrhea, trauma, fracture [19–22].

Ecologically this genus shows important characteristics such as self-pollination, being hosting for different insects species and they attract bumblebee queens and honeybees, which represents the entomophilous pollination [19]. This focused review wants to give an updated snapshot of main beneficial properties of *Lamium* plants, with a focus on antimicrobial, antiviral, anti-inflammatory, anti-nociceptive activity, and pain therapy and cytotoxicity and cytoprotective activity, in order to better address nutraceutical uses, formulations and applications; therefore, this review aims to bring information found in the literature data about different aspects of the *Lamium* genus and to demonstrate its importance regarding traditional, medicinal, chemical composition, biological and pharmacological activities, as well as industrial potential and economic use. The search was carried out using search engines Scopus, Science Direct, and PubMed and the following keywords were typed: *Lamium* and health benefits; *Lamium* and biological activities; *Lamium* and antioxidant properties; *Lamium* and antiviral activity; *Lamium* and anti-inflammatory activity; *Lamium* and antimicrobial activity; *Lamium* and antischistosomal activity; *Lamium* and antinociceptive activity; *Lamium* and pain therapy; *Lamium* and cytotoxicity; *Lamium* and cytoprotective activity; *Lamium* and anti-tyrosinase activity; *Lamium* and anticancer activity; *Lamium* and in vitro studies; *Lamium* and in vivo studies; *Lamium* and clinical studies.

2. A Shot on the Biologically Active Compounds in *Lamium* Plants

Chemically, *Lamium* is distinguished by the presence of different classes of chemical constituents, which we can mention hydroxycinnamic acids, terpenoids, among them iridoids and secoiridoids, flavonoids, anthocyanins, phenylpropanoids, phytoecdysteroids, benzoxazinoids, betaine [20–22]. Thus, the presence of these chemicals can provide biological activities tested in vitro and in vivo assays, such as antioxidant, anti-inflammatory, antimicrobial, antischistosomal, for pain relief in rheumatism and arthritis, a tonic for constipation, antinociceptive, anticancer [16,20–22]. Most of the bioactivities of *Lamium* species are linked to their principal constituents, that is, phenolics and essential oils [23–26]. Polyphenols, flavonoids, terpenes, steroidal derivatives, and ecdysteroids account for various biological activities of this species of *Lamium* [27–31]. In this regard, it is worth mentioning the review of Carović-Stanko et al. [32] focused on the *Lamiaceae* species and their secondary metabolites encompassing a wide array of beneficial functions and their applicability as sources of functional foods.

2.1. The Phenolic and Terpenoid Compounds of Lamium Plants

Here some studies showing the isolation of phenolic and terpenoid compounds are reported. For instance, Deng et al. [33], by studying constituents in the herb of *Lamium maculatum* L. var Kansuense, isolated and characterized ten compounds were obtained and they were identified as D-mannitol, beta-sitosterol, stigmasterol, rutin, 3'-methylquercetin-3-O-rutinoside, n-butyl-beta-D-fructopyranoside, daucosterol, acteoside, 20-hydroxyecdysone, allantoin. Nugroho et al. [34] isolated and characterized two new flavanol glycosides, together with other three just known using column chromatography from aerial parts of *L. amplexicaule*. The Czerwinska et al. [22] reported that the main constituents of the aerial part of *L. Album* were phenylpropanoids, iridoids, flavonoids and phenolic acids. Czerwinska et al. [35] in the herb of *L. album* underlined phenylpropanoid glycosides along with iridoids and flavonoids might be the valuable bioactive compounds present in these species. The peculiar constituents of *Lamium* plants are phenlypropanoids and iridoids. The phenylpropanoids consist in a group of compounds with a great diversity of structures including simple phenylpropanoids (i.e., derivatives of cinnamyl alcohols, cinnamic acids, phenylpropanes) and complex phenylpropanoids [36]. Generally they can occur rarely in the free form and are often present in bound form, linked to carbohydrates, as examples of main forms found in *Lamium* plants. Beside phenylpropanoids, another main constituent and potential chemotaxonomic marker of *Lamium* plants are iridoids: they are monoterpenes consisting of a cyclopenta[c]pyranoid skeleton (iridane skeleton) and mainly occurring as glycosides [37]. Molecules such as verbascoside, cis-acteoside, and lamalboside (lamiusides A), lamiusides B, C, and E, lamiridoside, lamiol, caryoptoside, alboside A and B are examples of phenylpropanoid glycosides, described *Lamium album* L. [21,27,35,38,39]. For instance, in the aerial parts of the *L. album* plant two phenylpropanoids glycosides, verbascoside and isoverbascoside (Figure 1), can make up 55% of the total phenolic compounds measured [40]. The iridoids found in the genus can work as markers of *L. album*, *L. amplexicaule*, *L. garganicum*, *L. maculatum*, and *L. purpureum* [20].

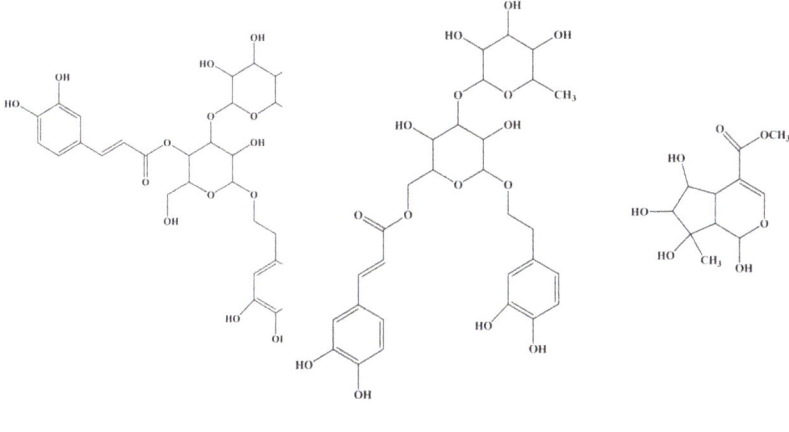

Verbascoside   isoverbascoside   lamiridosin

Figure 1. The chemical structure of some biologically active molecules from *Lamium* species.

2.2. Essential Oil Constituents of Lamium Plants

Considering how the therapeutic importance of *Lamiaceae* species is mostly based on their volatile oils [41], here essential oil constituents of *Lamium* plants are described. Even though plants belonging to the Lamiaceae family are recognized to contain an eminent amount of essential oils, the plants from the genus *Lamium* of the subfamily Lamioideae possess a small number of essential oils. The yields of the essential oils extracted from the fresh flowers of *Lamium* plants differ between 0.01–0.31% [42].

Numerous authors have studied the flavor composition from *Lamium* species [42–44]. However, the volatile components of only some species have been well studied so far, out of the 25 species of *Lamium* that are accepted [12]. Various studies have demonstrated that the biological and chemical activities of essentials oils from *Lamiaceae* plants, not merely varied within the species and its varieties but even amid the different agro-climatic and geographical regions [45–49]. Such variations in the composition of *Lamiaceae* plant essential oils can be essentially related to genetic as well as environmental factors that also define the genetic expressions and thereby influence the chemical constituents of the oils [50]. A study by Alipieva et al. [43] on the essential oils of four *Lamium* species from Bulgaria (namely, *L. album*, *L. purpureum*, *L. garganicum*, and *L. maculatum* flowers) collected from nine natural populations were analyzed by using GC-MS. Although a similarity of the volatile profiles of all samples was observed, quantitative and qualitative variations in oil composition of the plants obtained from different locations were also seen. For instance, hexahydrofarnesyl acetone was observed in *L. maculatum* (at Losen mountain: 1.9% while at Ljaskovetz: 1.2%), *L. purpureum* (at Vlado Trichkov: 1%) and *L. album* (at Vlado Trichkov: 0.2%) though not from all location sites. Besides, predominantly in *L. maculatum* and *L. garganicum* were identified other terpenoids, such as β-caryophyllene and α-humulene, found in highest concentrations in *L. maculatum* (at Losen mountain: 1.6% and 0.8%). Table 1 depicts more such examples where variations in the composition and percentages of main constituents of essential oils of *Lamium* species grown in different regions and/or countries.

Furthermore, the study of Flamini and workers [42] showed that the composition of essential oils varied, in different organs of *Lamium* species investigated. For instance, in *L. purpureum*, the content of α- and β-pinene was 35.7% in the leaves, 7.5% in the bracts while it was 75.3% in the flowers. In addition, in *L. bifidum*, bracts and leaves displayed a profile characterized by the common presence of germacrene D, β-caryophyllene, α-humulene, and β-elemene, while contrastingly, the flowers emitted profiles revealing high percentages of myrcene (47.2%), β-caryophyllene (11.8%) and sabinene (11.0%).

The previous work of Kapchina-Toteva et al. [51] also investigated the effect of micropropagation on the essential oil content in leaf extracts of *Lamium album* L. plants grown under in vitro and ex vitro conditions in contrast to in situ-grown plants. The in situ-grown plants were found to consist of 45 hydrocarbons, and as a result of micropropagation, the content of these compounds reduced about two-fold, reaching 24 during in vitro cultivation, and finally 19 after ex vitro acclimation. Moreover, while the in situ plants were characterized by the accumulation of long-chain alkanes (nonadecane; heneicosane; heptadecane; tricosane), both in vitro and ex vitro plants contained shorter hydrocarbons such as octane (3.9% and 1.1%, respectively) and undecane (3.0% in in vitro samples). Besides, certain alcohols such as phytol; octen-3-ol; 3-hexene-1-ol and acetate were observed to rise in micropropagated plants compared to in situ-grown ones. As for terpenes, 60 compounds were detected in the oil of in situ plants while it decreased in both in vitro and ex vitro ones—44 and 35 compounds. A variation in the terpene composition was also detected. The major sesquiterpenes in the in situ-grown plants were germacrene D (6.9%) and β-caryophyllene E (1.1%). In the course of micropropagation, elevated accumulation of these compounds was observed in both, in vitro- and ex vitro-grown plants [germacrene D (44.1% and 46.7%, correspondingly) and β-caryophyllene E (13.0% and 6.5%, correspondingly)]. Therefore, these results demonstrated the significance of growing conditions which were accountable for the variability in the level and composition of plant metabolites. The chemical structure of the main volatile secondary metabolites from *Lamium* species are represented in Figure 2.

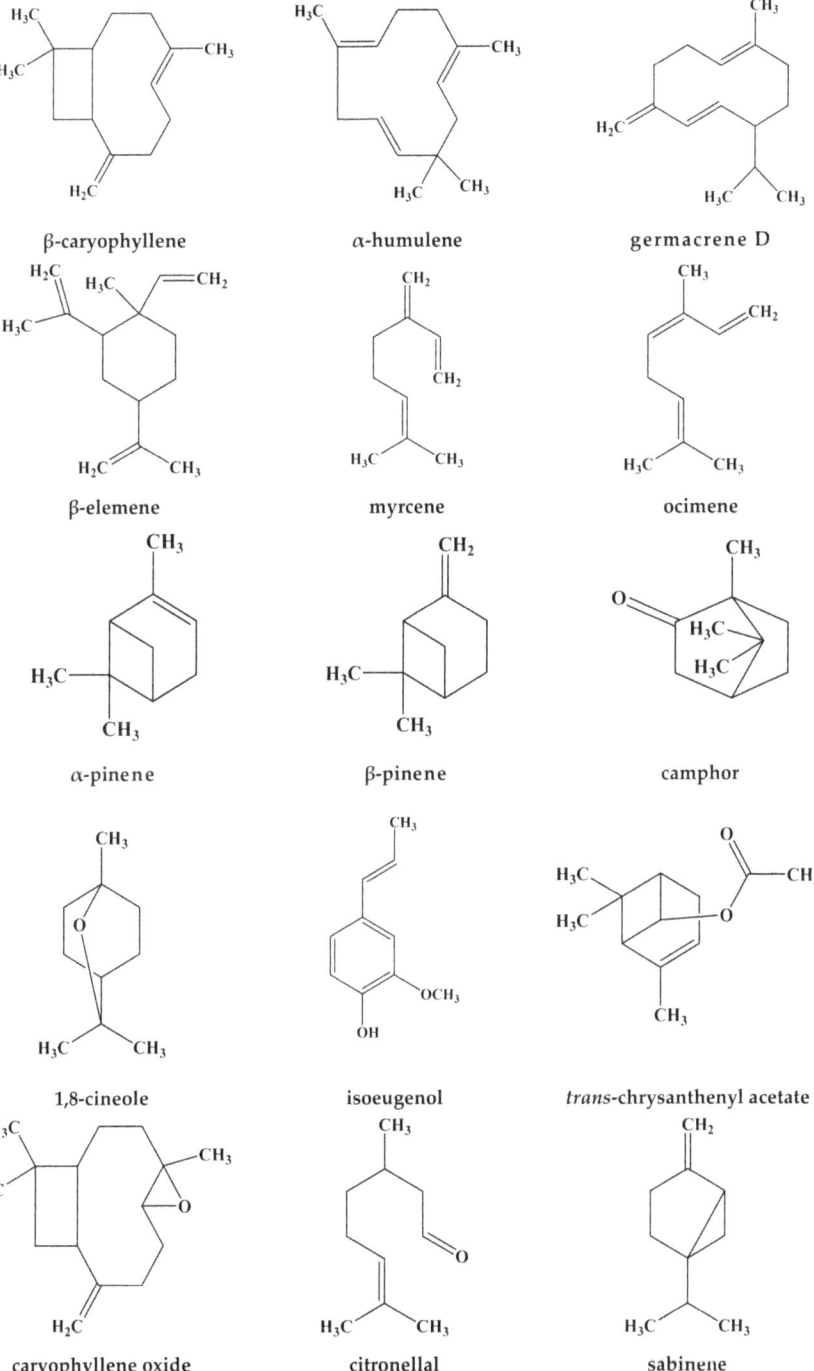

Figure 2. The chemical structure of the main volatile secondary metabolites from *Lamium* species.

Table 1. Main components of essential oil from *Lamium* species studied from the year 1976–2018.

Plant Name	Place/Country of Collection	Parts Used	Extraction Method Used	% Yield	Main Components	References
(1) *Lamium amplexicaule* L.	Khorassan-e Razavi province in northeastern Iran	aerial parts (flowers and leaves) *	Hydro-distillation	0.1 (w/w)	Trans-phytol (44.8%), octadecanol (12.0%), hexadecanoic acid (11.8%) and hexahydrofarnesyl acetone (10.6%)	[52]
	Huntsville, Alabama, USA	aerial parts **	Hydro-distillation	NA	Germacrene D (18.5–34.9%), (E)-caryophyllene (2.5–11.9%), α-pinene (2.2–16.2%), β-pinene (2.0–10.6%) and 1-octen-3-ol (3.5–8.0%)	[53]
	Pergole, Arcidosso Municipality, South Tuscany, Italy	Flowering aerial parts	Hydro-distillation	NA	Trans-chrysanthenyl acetate (41.1%), germacrene D (28.9%) and α-pinene (6.8%), ocimene (0.8%)	[42]
	Northeast of Tehran, Iran	aerial parts *	Hydro-distillation	0.1(v/w)	Germacrene-D (22.3%) and camphor (18.1%)	[54]
	El Dakahlyia governorate, Egypt	Leaves	NA	NA	Isophytol (14.8%), 9,12,15-octadecanoic acid methyl ester (19.2%), 6,10,14-trimethyl-2-pentadecanone (8.0%), dibutyl phathalate (6.1%), nonacosane (5.5%), hexadecanoic acid (3.4%) and nonyl phenol (3.2%)	[55]
	Syria	NA	Dry evaporation	NA	Imedazol and pyrimidene	[56]
	NA	NA	NA	0.09	NA	[57]
(2) *Lamium purpureum* L.	Huntsville, Alabama, USA	aerial parts **	Hydro-distillation	NA	Germacrene D (15.0–46.3%), α-pinene (4.1–15.3%), β-pinene (6.3–16.3%), and 1-octen-3-ol (4.2–15.3%), β-elemene (3.7–16.0%)	[53]
	Pergole (Arcidosso Municipality, South Tuscany, Italy	Flowering aerial parts	Hydro-distillation	NA	Germacrene D (35.4%), β-pinene (26.8%) and α-pinene (13.4%), ocimene (2.9%)	[42]
	Japan	Aerial parts	Steam distillation	NA	1-Octen-3-ol, cis-3-hexen-1-ol, phenethyl alcohol, benzyl alcohol, phenol, o-, m-, and p-cresols, guaiacol, eugenol	[44]
(3) *Lamium maculatum* L.	Experimental station of Faculty of Pharmacy, Zagazig University, Egypt	aerial parts **	Hydro-distillaion	0.35 (v/w)	β-caryophyllene (14.8%), caryophyllene oxide (13.8%), Z,E-α-farnesene (10.1%), dihydroedulan 1 (9.13%), α-humulene (6.1%), bornyl formate (6.0%) and α-bisabolene (5.3%)	[58]
	NA	Leaves	NA	NA	Hexahydrofarnesylactone (22%)	[59]
(4) *Lamium hybridum* Vill	Pergole (Arcidosso Municipality, South Tuscany, Italy	Flowering aerial parts	Hydro-distillation	NA	Germacrene D (39.0%), (Z)-ocimene (8.7%), methyl salicylate (7.5%) and β-caryophyllene (6.1%), ocimene (11.6%)	[42]
(5) *Lamium bifidum* Cyr.	Pergole (Arcidosso Municipality, South Tuscany, Italy	Flowering aerial parts	Hydro-distillation	NA	Germacrene D (34.9%), sabinene (12.4%), β-caryophyllene (11.5%), α-humulene (6.8%)	[42]
(6) *Lamium garganicum* L. subsp. *laevigatum* Arcangeli	Athens, Greece	aerial parts ***	Hydro-distillation	0.31	1,8-cineole (47.5%), citronellal (25.1%) and isoeugenol (11.8%)	[60]
(7) *Lamium album* L.	Behshahr, Mazandaran Province, North of Iran	Flowering aerial parts	Hydro-distillation	0.2 (w/w)	6,10,14-trimethyl-2-pentadecanone (10.2%) and 4-hydroxy-4-methyl-2-pentanone (9.1%)	[61]
	Experimental field of the Kaunas Botanical Garden of Vytautas Magnus University, Lithuania	Plants in the vegetation period	Supercritical carbon dioxide extraction method	NA	Prenol, farmesene-beta- E, tridecanol n, dodecanoic acid n, hexadecane-n, squalene, tetradecanol-n, undecane–n, benzoate-isopentyl, dodecanoate-butyl, phytone, neophytadiene	[62]
	NA	Aerial part	NA	0.04–0.46	NA	[57]
	NA	Flowers	NA	0.05	NA	[57]
	Kharkiv region, Ukraine	Leaves	NA	NA	α-Terpeniol, linalool, squalene, spatulenol, α-Bisabolol	[63]
(8) *Lamium moschatum* Mill.	NA	Flowers	Steam-washed	NA	Caryophyllene	[64]
(9) *Lamium striatum* Sibth. et. Smith		Flowers	Steam-washed	NA	Carboxylic acids	[64]

NA—Not Available/applicable; * Air-dried; ** fresh; *** fresh air-dried.

3. Traditional Medicinal Uses of *Lamium* Plants

Plants have been used by a human as food and medicine since ancient times. Examples of the traditional medicinal uses of *Lamium* plants are here described. White dead-nettle (*Lamium album* L.) used for decades in Europe, China, and Japan during times of famine [65]. Different aerial parts of this plant are edible and traditionally used as raw or cooked food in some countries. Especially in some dishes in Mediterranean and neighboring areas [66]. In addition, non-stinging nettle is considered a base component of some well-known vegetarian dishes and salads [40]. *L. album*, when added to food supplements, can prevent menstrual, musculoskeletal disorders and ameliorate fat metabolism [67,68]. *L. amplexicaule* is used in the preparation of Japanese traditional rice porridge which called "seven spring herbs" [69].

In traditional and folk medicine worldwide some *Lamium* species used in the treatment of fracture, hypertension, leucorrhoea, paralysis, putrescence, trauma and some gynecological diseases like menorrhagia, uterine hemorrhage, vaginal and cervical inflammation, bleeding after childbirth and believed to be a contraceptive, etc. [70–72]. Ethnobotanical studies indicate the use of aerial parts and floral branches of *L. album* for different kidney problems like the exertion of stones [73,74]. Leaves decoction and infusion for respiratory tract problems [75].

Moreover, there are many types of activities, e.g., antipyretic, astringent, bronchitis, diuretic, emollient, expectorant, insomnia, pains, sciatica, vasodilator, hemostatic, wound healing, antihypertensive, anti-inflammatory which recorded by literature [76–80]. *L. amplexicaule* used as anti-rheumatic, laxative and diaphoretic [81]. Sometimes fresh leaves of *L. amplexicaule* are crushed a paste formed used topically to joints swelling [82]. Aerial parts decoction of *L. galeobdolon* traditionally used for fever, malaria, warts, constipation, hair loss, rheumatism, dandruff, hemorrhage [83,84] depression, nerve tonic [85].

4. Biological Activities *Lamium* Plants

Our mental and physical well-being is directly related to what we introduce with the diet. In fact, the nutritional content of what we eat affects the composition of our cell membranes, blood, tissues, organs, skin, and so on. It has long been a common opinion, widely shared also by the scientific world, that diet and nutrition are also important factors that can, depending on the case, protect us or promote pathological conditions and chronic diseases. From this perspective, the great variety of biologically active molecules present in plants can offer a general condition of 'protection' and play an important role in maintaining a state of well-being of the individual.

In the years 1970–1980, scholars of popular culture and history of medicine began to record the traditional health habits of the peoples in the various countries, with an approach that tried to capture the full breadth without expressing value judgments. In this context, the notion of folk medicine has extended its meaning since the boundaries between popular traditions and scientific evidence present undeniable differences. Over time, therefore, the research has tried to find scientific evidence to validate or refute practices in the profane medical culture.

Folk medicine has made extensive use of plants of the *Lamium* genus over the centuries. The most common uses are described in the countries of the Mediterranean basin (Europe and North Africa) and in Western Asia. Buds, leaves, and flowers are also widely used in the kitchen for the preparation of various recipes of local tradition in many countries of the Mediterranean basin [21]. From health benefits, plants of the *Lamium* genus have found widespread applications in folk medicine thanks to the large presence of chemical compounds that constitute effective active ingredients in many situations of therapeutic interest.

4.1. In Vitro Studies

Most of the scientific evidence on the *Lamium* genus has been conducted through in vitro studies over the past 15–20 years. Extracts from the shoots, leaves, and flowers, have shown many biological activities. In this section, particularly, we will review the species of the *Lamium* genus used about various medicinal uses, highlighting those most promising studies given a possible use of the active ingredients extracted from these plants.

4.1.1. Antioxidant Activity

As is known, antioxidant molecules can be technically defined as agents that prevent or slow down the phenomenon of oxidation. Reactive oxygen species (ROS) are unavoidable sub-products of cellular aerobic metabolism [86]. However, free radicals can also originate from prolonged exposure to UV rays, cigarette smoke, and air pollution. The reactive oxygen molecules are capable of damaging the structures of the cell through the establishment of so-called oxidative stress, a situation that, if not kept under control, can lead or exacerbate many pathological states [87]. A large number of molecules, so-called antioxidants, can interrupt the chain of radical reactions and thus prevent damage to cells [88].

Our body can counteract the activity of free radicals through endogenous antioxidant mechanisms and the introduction through the diet of exogenous substances [89]. Among the endogenous factors are enzymes such as superoxide dismutase (SOD; EC 1.15.1.1) which catalyzes the dismutation of the superoxide radical (O_2^-) into either molecular oxygen (O_2) or hydrogen peroxide (H_2O_2), catalase (CAT; EC 1.11.1.6), which removes intracellular H_2O_2, and reduced glutathione (GSH) [90]. Among the non-exogenous non-enzymatic substances with antioxidant properties, we recall Vitamin E, Vitamin C, carotenoids, polyphenols, and anthocyanins instead.

While many foods have a protective effect on free radicals, on the other, improper eating habits can increase their activity, for example, a diet too rich in animal fats, excessive consumption of some vegetable oils and fatty fish, excess of iron, food intolerances.

The antioxidant properties are determined in vitro by common assays: the trolox equivalent antioxidant capacity (TEAC), oxygen radical absorbance capacity (ORAC), total radical-trapping antioxidant parameter (TRAP), ferric-reducing antioxidant power (FRAP) and 2,2-diphenyl-1-picrylhydrazyl (DPPH) radical scavenging activity assay [91,92]. They vary in their principles, mechanisms, and experimental condition, in the reference compounds used, i.e., trolox, gallic acid, or catechins and in how endpoints are measured [93–95].

These methods are based on the transfer of electrons (ET) or the transfer of hydrogen atoms (HAT) [96,97]. Another antioxidant mechanism is the transition metal chelation, (TMC): transition metals ions may be chelated by polyphenols, leading to stable complexed compounds [98]. The determination of the antioxidant power should be measured with at least two or three assays [99,100]. A more in-depth and correct investigation must also include the determination of the phenolic content and that of the flavonoids.

As marked by several authors [101–103] in the procedure of determination of antioxidant properties three critical elements should be taken into account: the extraction procedure, the antioxidant capacity measurements and the expression of results.

In this regard it is worth mentioning the point of view of Durazzo and Lucarini, [7] that well summarized the actual main strategies of research for evaluating antioxidant properties: the evaluation of bioactivities of pure compounds and/or their mixtures; the study of different biologically active compound-rich extracts and how these fractions contribute to the activity of total food extract; the isolation of extractable and non-extractable compounds.

The assessment of the interaction of bioactive compounds as antioxidant properties represents the first step for the evaluation of the health properties of medicinal plants [4]. Many species belonging to the *Lamium* genus have been studied to identify their antioxidant properties. Carović-Stanko et al. [32] pointed out that most of the *Lamiaceae* sources of antioxidants belong to the subfamily Nepetoideae, such as basil, lemon balm, marjoram, mint, oregano, rosemary, sage, etc [104]. *Lamium album* L. is absolutely the most studied species. Trouillas et al. [105] have studied and compared the water-soluble fraction of 16 plants, including *L. album*, typical of Limousin, a central-southern region of France. Presumably, the whole plant was used, whose main constituents are acid phenols, flavonoids, mucilage, iridoids. Water-soluble extracts have been tested for the ability to inhibit the DPPH radical, the superoxide radical generated by the xanthine/xanthine oxidase (X/XO) system, and the inhibition of the hydroxyl radical generated by the Fenton reaction. It is interesting to note that in the first two cases (DPPH and X/XO) the extracts of *L. album* (non-stinging nettle) showed to be very effective when compared with the other species studied; particularly, it was 12-16 times more effective than extracts of *Urtica dioica* (stinging nettle). This result diverged, significantly, from that obtained with a methanol extract of *L. album* that showed the same ability to inhibit the DPPH radical at an extract concentration about 140 times lower [106]. This discrepancy could be due to the better ability of methanol to extract flavonoids (≈193 mg of gallic acid equivalents per g of extract (mg GAE/g)). This higher extraction capacity was corroborated by the greater amounts of phenolic compounds extracted when compared to extraction in water. The content of phenolic compounds of the methanol extract was almost five times greater than the aqueous extract. This result was in agreement with the content of phenolic compounds found in methanol extracts of specimens of another species of the *Lamium* genus, *L. amplexicaule* L. collected during the flowering period in a region of south-eastern Anatolia, Turkey (≈184 mg GAE/g) [107]. The presence of polyphenols could, moreover, be the determining factor in explaining why the methanol extract and hexane of *L. amplexicaule* showed a significant reduction in the formation of nicked DNA and increased the native form of plasmid DNA pBR322.

Hydroxyl radicals generated by the Fenton reaction are known to cause oxidatively induced breaks in DNA strands via the subsequent free radical-induced reaction on plasmid DNA. Hydroxyl radicals can react with nitrogenous bases of DNA producing base radicals and sugar radicals. Polyphenols are potential protecting agents against the lethal effects of oxidative stress and offer protection to DNA by chelating redox-active transition metal ions [108,109]. For instance, Yumrutas et al. [107] showed that *L. amplexicaule* hexane extract seemed to possess a greater ability to protect DNA than the methanol extract. Hence, it might be said that available non-polar compounds in the hexane extracts might be contributing to phenolic compounds for protecting DNA.

As another example, the antioxidant effect of butanol extracts from wild specimens *L. album* and *L. purpureum* L. (red dead nettle) collected in Romania were compared for DPPH and chemiluminescence activity. A possible correlation between the chemical composition, especially for the amount of total phenols, and the antioxidant activity of the extracts was found [110]. In both cases, the extracts possessed dose-dependent scavenger activity evaluated after 30 min. Incubation with extracts, in all dose levels tested, whereas, the *L. purpureum* extract (1% concentration) exhibited the highest scavenging activity compared with *L. album* extract.

Vladimir-Knežević et al. [111], by studying different medicinal plants of the Lamiaceae family such as *Salvia officinalis*, *Mentha longifolia*, *Melissa officinalis*, *Lavandula angustifolia*, *Satureja montana* concluded that *Lamiaceae* species are a rich source of various natural AChE inhibitors and antioxidants.

Danila et al. [112] aimed at assessing the phenolic content of *L. album* and *L. maculatum* methanolic extracts, and their antioxidant capacity: for the DPPH assay the EC_{50} (µg/mL) values were 32.3 ± 0.1 for *L. maculatum* extract and 63.5 ± 0.7 for *L. album* extract, while in the ABTS assay EC50 (µg/mL) values were 13.2 ± 0.1 for *L. maculatum* extract and 19.9 ± 0.5 for *L. album* extract.

On the other hand, many studies have proven that some natural antioxidants are a double-edged sword. They can, under certain conditions, act as pro-oxidants in vitro, triggering lipid peroxidation, DNA damage and apoptotic phenomena [113]. Phenolics and carotenoids can also exhibit prooxidant activities, mainly in the presence of redox-active transition metal ions [114–116].

4.1.2. Antiviral Activity

As is known, viruses can replicate only within a host cell, exploiting their metabolic apparatus and using their own genetic information; however, multiplication occurs only in cells susceptible to the virus, that is, provided with specific superficial receptors and able to perform the replicative phases of its genome.

The search for an antiviral compound must be based on the interaction of the drug with specific stages of viral replication; for example, it can act on cellular penetration of the virus, on the replication of its genome, on protein synthesis or on the release of new viruses from the host cell. Herbal medicines and purified natural products provide a rich resource for novel antiviral drugs [117].

Some chemical compounds have been isolated in plants of the *Lamium* genus having interesting antiviral activities that are here reported. It is worth mentioning a phytochemical study of the aqueous extract of the flowering tops of *L. album*, a component herb in a commercial liver health herbal formula, that led to the identification of the antiviral activity of some iridoids [118]. Isomers lamiridosins A and B were found to significantly inhibit hepatitis C virus entry in vitro showing an IC_{50} 2.31 µM. Interestingly, the parent iridoid glucosides demonstrated no anti-HCV entry activity.

4.1.3. Antimicrobial Activity

Generally, the term 'natural antibiotics' refers to those substances endowed with antibacterial activity deriving from plants. In fact, antibiotics of natural origin do not derive only from plants, but also from fungi, bacteria, and animals. Antibiotics are substances used to fight bacterial infections and may have bacteriostatic action (i.e., inhibit bacterial growth) or bactericidal (i.e., they can kill bacteria). A similar argument can be made for the antimycotics that are used to counteract the development of pathogenic fungi.

Some types of plants can produce antibacterial and antifungal substances, even if they present an activity, usually, much lower than that possessed by antibiotics deriving from fungi and bacteria [119]. Furthermore, it is good to remember that the antibacterial or antifungal substances contained in these plants can interfere with possible pharmacological treatments already in place. Plants also contain other compounds that could potentially be hazardous to health. However, in the popular medicine of emerging countries, the use of plant preparations to counteract the growth of pathogenic microorganisms is often described.

Antifungal activity of *L. tenuiflorum* Fisch and Mey against some medical yeast species was described by Dulger et al. [120]. The ethanol extracts obtained from the leaves, rootstock, and the combined formulation of Turkish endemic specimens have been investigated for their antifungal activities against medical yeast *Candida* and *Cryptococcus* species. The extract (in the form of sticky black substances) was dissolved in DMSO before testing. The combination of plant extracts (1:1 ratio) was used in this test. Comparing the obtained result with those of the antifungal drug ketoconazole used as a reference, it was noted that the combination of plant extracts (both leaves and rootstock) exhibited greater antifungal effect against *Candida albicans* and that *Candida* spp. was more susceptible than *Cryptococcus* spp. Unfortunately, in that study, there is no correlation between quantity and type of polyphenols present in the extract of *L. tenuiflorum* and the antimycotic activity found. Conversely, none of the extracts obtained from *L. galactophyllum* Boiss and Reuter, *L. macrodon* Boiss and Huet and *L. amplexicaule* displayed activity towards *Candida albicans* ATCC 10231 [121]. Lacking such an antimycotic power could be due to the different quantity of polyphenols contained in these species, ranging between 94 and 112 mg GAE/g in respect to higher values found for *L. album* and *L. amplexicaule* which extracts ranged between 184 and 193 mg GAE/g [106,107].

The great variety of species of the *Lamium* genus present in Turkey [121] has meant that traditional folk medicine made extensive use of *Lamium* herbs. On the contrary, *L. album* extracts possess little antifungal activity as found by Chipeva et al. [122] who evaluate the antimicrobial activity of *L. album* plants. The extracts, obtained from leaves and flowers, were harvested either in the wild or from in vitro propagated plants. Four solvents (chloroform, methanol, ethanol, and water) and two methods of extraction (Soxhlet, thermostat) were used. The different combinations of extraction solvent and extraction method led to results that also varied due to the origin of the plant, i.e., wild or in vitro propagated. In conclusion, *L. album* extracts possessed a broad spectrum of antibacterial activity with greater efficacy towards Gram-positive bacteria. However, as the extracts have not been chemically characterized it is impossible to determine which molecule may be more responsible for such an antibacterial activity.

4.1.4. Anti-Inflammatory, Anti-Nociceptive Activity, and Pain Therapy

Arachidonic acid is the main precursor of eicosanoids, substances involved in the body's inflammatory response. In the presence of tissue damage, enzymes belonging to the phospholipase class A2 release the arachidonic acid from the membrane phospholipids. From this, two different molecular types can be obtained: the series 2 of prostaglandins and thromboxanes (from the cyclooxygenase pathway) and the series of leukotrienes (from the lipoxygenase pathway). The synthesis of the series 2 of prostaglandins (PG2) and thromboxanes is mediated by the enzyme cyclooxygenase, which is present in the human organism in the form of COX1 and COX2. The synthesis of leukotrienes is linked to the activity of the enzyme 5-lipoxygenase. From these observations, pharmacological research on molecules able to counteract the effects of arachidonic acid derivatives by inhibiting the enzymes involved in the inflammatory cascade has started. To this end, enzymes extracted from both animal and vegetable sources used as enzymatic model systems to evaluate the anti-inflammatory effect of plant extracts and active ingredients are also used.

Aqueous extracts of *L. album* have been shown to inhibit lipoxygenase activity in vitro [105], at relatively low concentrations of extract ($IC_{50} \approx 1.5$ mg/mL). As these extracts have not been further characterized, it is not possible to attribute this inhibition activity of lipoxygenase to a specific molecule. It is very likely that this effect is due to more than one molecule and through several mechanisms. In fact, many studies have established that free oxygen radicals are implicated in inflammatory processes [123] and that phenolic compounds can block lipoxygenase activity, or they can function as scavengers of free radicals which are released during the inflammatory cascade of arachidonic acid [124]. Anti-inflammatory bioactivity of compounds was also proved with aqueous-methanolic extract of *L. album* herb in human neutrophils as recently showed by Czerwinska [35]. This effect appears to be due to the inhibition of the release of some inflammation mediators, such as the IL-8 and 3 TNF cytokines, by neutrophil granulocytes.

Rheumatoid arthritis is a multifactorial chronic, systemic and disabling inflammatory disease with an undefined etiology, but probably of autoimmune origin. It mainly affects the symmetrical joints, but also tendons, synovium, muscles, bags and other tissues of the organism. Rheumatoid arthritis develops because, in a genetically predisposed subject, an environmental triggering event activates an auto-immune response; there is thus an abnormal activation of the immune system, which affects the joints causing chronic inflammation and consequent joint damage.

Rheumatoid arthritis can also be fought with plants [125] whose extracts can be used at least to reduce the quantities of methotrexate, one of the elective drugs used in the treatment of this pathology. As for the *Lamium* genus, the evidence that some species can provide benefits in the treatment of rheumatoid arthritis is quite weak [126] and are mostly speculative and based on the antioxidant and anti-inflammatory properties of *L. album* extracts.

About the inflammatory activity of *L. album* extracts, cannot be ignored a study in which the leaves of this herb have been used as a placebo to test the anti-inflammatory activity of *U. dioica* (stinging nettle) [127]. That study prompted from the observation that the sting of the common stinging nettle has long been used for self-treatment of arthritic pain. A randomized controlled double-blind crossover study in twenty-seven patients with osteoarthritic pain at the base of the thumb or index finger was performed to ascertain if the daily application of nettle leaves in the painful area brought relief. *L. album* leaves were chosen as a placebo since leaves are almost indistinguishable from stinging nettle leaves. It was remarkable that after a week of treatment the score reduction with *U. dioica* leaves was significantly greater than that with placebo (*L. album* leaves).

Pain therapy aims to recognize, evaluate and treat chronic pain in the most appropriate way. There are several classes of drugs that can be used for the treatment of pain. The type of drug to be used can vary depending on the origin, the nature and the intensity of the painful stimulus that is intended to be treated. Depending on the circumstances can be used: non-steroidal anti-inflammatory drugs (e.g., ketoprofen, diclofenac, naproxen and nimesulide), opioid analgesics (e.g., codeine, tramadol, buprenorphine, fentanyl, oxycodone, methadone, hydromorphone and morphine), antidepressants, very useful in the treatment of neuropathic pain (e.g., amitriptyline, clomipramine, duloxetine); anticonvulsants, also useful in the treatment of neuropathic pain (e.g., gabapentin, pregabalin); local anesthetics (e.g., lidocaine). Unfortunately, the use of such drugs is often accompanied by sometimes serious side effects, which may sometimes outweigh the benefits of the drug. For this reason, over the past few years, general attention has shifted to non-pharmacological therapies (e.g., radiotherapy, cryotherapy, thermotherapy, massages, physiotherapy, relaxation techniques). Increasing attention has also concerned the active ingredients from medicinal plants. Although widely used in traditional folk medicine, there are only a few studies investigating the potential analgesic effects of the *Lamium* genus. Most of the studies have been carried out concerning different genera of the *Lamiaceae* family, but very few are those concerning the *Lamium* genus [128].

4.1.5. Cytotoxicity and Cytoprotective Activity

Cytotoxicity is the measurement of how much a substance can damage or kill cells. This measurement can be performed both in vitro and in vivo, and this difference is significant, since it is one thing to measure the cytotoxic activity of a chemical agent on a cell culture in a homogeneous medium (e.g., a fibroblast layer on a medium of culture) and the measurement of cell *viability* in vivo is very different, where many biochemical and other factors are involved. Most of the cytotoxicity studies of plant extracts have been conducted in vitro because it is the simplest method. In vitro studies, in turn, offer several advantages; e.g., they are highly reproducible simplified systems, they allow to analyze the cellular and molecular mechanisms of toxicity, the identification of early damages and allow to contain costs and get rapid responses concerning animal experimentation. The main criticism that can be found in systems for measuring cytotoxicity in vitro concerns the excessive simplification of such methods concerning a multicellular organism. Nevertheless, in vitro tests are widely used; the cytotoxicity can be carried out and evaluated with different essays. The most used is the MTT assay, the SRB assay (with Sulforhodamine B), the TB assay (with Trypan blue). In the study of cytotoxicity mechanism, the choice of the cellular model should respond to the need to study in detail the organ-specific effects of certain compounds or mechanisms of action in specific cell types. Unfortunately, most often the cellular model is chosen independently of the needs mentioned above; for this reason, the results obtained in the different studies are hardly comparable.

As instance, Veleva et al. [129] studied the changes in the functional characteristics of tumor and normal cells after treatment with extracts of white dead-nettle, by adhesion test, MTT (3-(4,5-dimethylthiazol-2-yl)-2-5-diphenyl tetrazolium bromide), transepithelial resistance (TER), immunofluorescence staining and trypan blue exclusion test: extracts from *L. album* L. change TER and actin filaments, and somehow may block cell mechanisms, leading to the polarization of MDCK II cells (Madin-Darby canine kidney cells II).

From another work [105], aqueous extracts of the whole *L. album* plant have been shown to induce cytotoxicity in the mouse tumor cell line, the B16 mouse melanoma cells at relatively low concentrations. It is difficult to determine what may be the causes of this cytotoxicity although it could be related to the content of phenolic compounds of the extract [105].

Polyphenols can act as antioxidants through various mechanisms, including hydrogen donating reactions, metal chelation, inhibition of cytochrome P450 isoforms and up-regulation or protection of antioxidant defenses (e.g., intracellular glutathione levels) [130]. In particular, the possible cytotoxicity of these phenylpropanoids has long been debated. For instance, verbascoside has shown increased chromosome aberrations and in vitro sister chromatid exchanges in human lymphocyte cultures [131]. However, the results may be due to instability and degradation of verbascoside in caffeic acid and 3,4-dihydroxyphenyl ethanol [131]. The genotoxicity of verbascoside seems to have been ruled out entirely by a recent study [132]. This study clearly demonstrates that diets rich in verbascoside do not give rise to any mutagenic activity, resulting in non-cytotoxic to animals and suggesting its possible use in both animal and human diets.

In fact, products based on dried leaves and flowers of *L. album* are already on the market. *L. album* is numbered among dermatological plants with anti-inflammatory activity, and this plant is also used in wound healing [21]. Skin fibroblasts proliferation is considered as the most important initial stage of tissue repair. Thus, Paduch et al. [133] analyzed the plant extracts activity on human skin fibroblasts (HSF) proliferation and viability in order to add information on the effectiveness of these products. The sensitivity of HSF cells in culture to methanol, ethyl acetate, and heptane extracts of *Lamii albi flos* were investigated. Extracts with methanol, ethyl acetate and heptane of *Lamii albi flos* were prepared by heating 20 g of plant material with 300 mL of the appropriate solvent for 5 h at a temperature of 60 °C at reflux. Each of these extracts was subsequently concentrated under reduced pressure at 30 °C up to a volume of 100 mL. The extracts thus obtained were used for the determination of flavonoids, pentacyclic triterpenes, and iridoids. The triterpene component seemed to be responsible for the absence of cytotoxicity of the heptane extracts even at high concentrations and, indeed, triterpenes can exert stimulatory effects on the proliferative capacity of HSF cells.

When a model of chemical stress induced by potassium dichromate in human hepatoblastoma HepG2 cells was used, ethanolic extracts of *L. album* showed a cytoprotective effect in vitro [40]. Purified extract counteracted ROS formation in oxidative stress conditions in tested cells. The cytoprotective effect of 50 µg/mL *L. album* purified ethanolic extract seems related to the presence of verbascoside, which exhibited the highest cytoprotective action from all the polyphenols identified in the ethanolic extract.

It is interesting to reiterate that solvent extracts of the same species, *L. album*, can exert cytoprotective or cytotoxic effects according to the methods of extraction, application of the extract and the tested cell lines. Moscova-Doumanova et al. [134] investigated the effect of methanol, and chloroform extracts, obtained from in vivo and in vitro cultivated plants of *L. album*, on the cell viability, adhesion, and cell cycle of the type A549 human lung cell line. Different combinations of methanol and chloroform extracts were tested. Preliminary results showed that both the extracts have a cytotoxic effect on lung cancer cells. They caused a reduction in the adhesion properties of the cells with a stronger effect by extracts from in vivo plants. After 48 h of incubation time, all extracts cause retention in the G2 phase while a mixture of them leads to the apoptosis. However, without characterization of the extracts, it is not possible to hypothesize the molecular mechanism of the observed phenomena.

Other applications on corneal disease are described as follows. The cornea is the membrane that covers the front of the eye, through which it is possible to glimpse the iris and the pupil. Transparent and avascular, this structure represents the first 'lens' that the light encounters in its path to the brain. The cornea is, in fact, an essential element of the ocular dioptric system: it allows the passage of light rays towards the internal structures of the eye and helps to focus the images on the retina. The cornea's optical function is carried out thanks to its perfect transparency and the regularity of the contact surface with the air. Therefore, any inflammation and damage to the corneal epithelial should be quickly eliminated to maintain corneal transparency. In this context, the powerful antioxidant and anti-inflammatory properties of *L. album* extracts above described could make, in perspective, this medical herb a promising candidate in the formulation of natural remedies for topical use in corneal diseases.

This prompted Paduch et al. [135] to evaluate the effect of *L. album* extract on human corneal epithelial cells (10.014 pRSV-T cell line) cultured in vitro. In that study, the first goal achieved was to ascertain the ethanol extract of *L. album* was non-toxic to human corneal epithelial cells at concentrations up to 125 µg/mL. Ethanol extract contained polar compounds which contribute to maintaining cells intact, or even, stimulate cellular mitochondrial metabolism as verified by MTT assay. Besides, flavonoids and polyphenolic compounds, better represented in ethanol extracts, also contributed to the reduction of inflammatory phenomena and ROS scavenging. Therefore, it cannot be excluded that soon, after further in vivo experiments, supplements for the treatment of mild eye diseases based on extracts of *L. album* herb may be used.

At this point, it is worth mention *L. galeobdolon* L., commonly known as the 'yellow archangel, that has good potential as an ingredient for the preparation of functional foods. This species is a wildflower widespread in Europe and has been introduced elsewhere as a garden plant. An ethnobotanical study carried out on 49 edible wild plants traditionally harvested and consumed in a region of the Basque Country, Northern Spain, described the recreational use by children of nectar sucked from the base of *L. galeobdolon* flowers. Different benzoxazinoids (BXs), present as glucosides (Figure 3), have been identified in the yellow archangel.

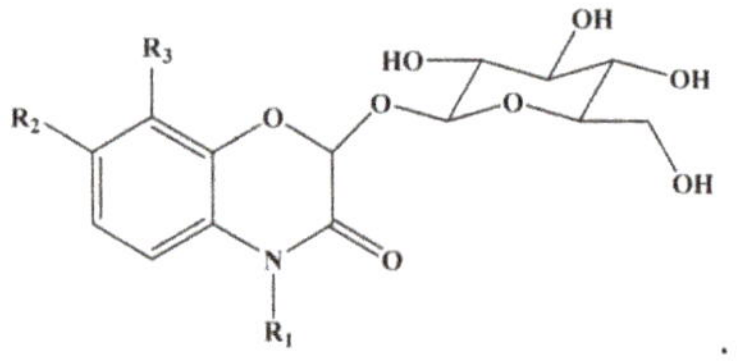

Figure 3. Benzoxazinone glucoside skeleton.

These compounds represent a class of indole-derived plant metabolites that work in defense against numerous parasites and pathogens [136]. Many recent studies have reported antimicrobial, anticancer, reproductive stimulatory effects, system stimulators central nervous system, and reduction of appetite and weight of BXs derivatives and their derivatives [137].

4.1.6. Antityrosinase Activity

Tyrosinase (EC 1.14.18.1) is a ubiquitous enzyme containing two copper ions. The dinuclear copper center of tyrosinase catalyzes the o-hydroxylation of monophenols, oxidation of catechols [138,139], quinonization of dihydroxycoumarins [140], o-aminophenols and aromatic o-diamines [141]. Tyrosinase is also one of the key enzymes in melanin biosynthesis. In animals, as the enzyme catalyzes the first two main steps of the melanogenesis. Overproduction of melanin can result in various hyperpigmentation disorders including melasma and age spots. Thus the discovery of new tyrosinase inhibitors has been since many years the main goal of numerous investigations [142,143]. Many studies deal with chemical compounds extracted from plants. Even though the presence of phenolic compounds in plants of the genus *Lamium* is abundant, and potentially there are many phenolic compounds able to influence the activity of tyrosinase, there are very few studies that describe such an influence on the tyrosinase enzyme.

Nugroho et al. [34] reported how two flavanol glycosides in methanol extracts of *L. amplexicaule* showed in vitro inhibitory activity against the mushroom tyrosinase. The tyrosinase inhibition mechanism and related kinetics have not been studied in detail. In the study, it is hypothesized that the high group of hydroxyl groups present on the isolated flavonoid molecule may be responsible for binding to the catalytic site of tyrosinase, and result in an inhibition phenomenon according to previous studies [144,145].

The current study of Etsassala et al. [146] applied a fast screening method using a cyclic voltammetry technique for evaluating anti-tyrosinase activity of twenty-five species of plants from the *Lamiaceae* family: among these, those that showed a fast current inhibition rate at a minimum concentration when compared to a kojic acid standard were classified as having the greatest anti-tyrosinase activity such as *Salvia chamelaeagnea*, *S. dolomitica*, *Plectranthus ecklonii*, *P. namaensis*, and *P. zuluensis*.

4.2. In Vivo Studies

The observation of in vivo phenomena is often considered more relevant to factual reality than in vitro reproductions, although the latter is equally useful because they allow analyzing a single phenomenon, isolating it from the context that could create a background noise that is too high to be able to distinguish the phenomenon clearly.

Unfortunately, in vivo studies using plants of the *Lamium* genus are very few compared to in vitro studies.

An in-depth study evaluated the anti-inflammatory and antinociceptive activities of various extracts prepared with methanol, dichloromethane, n-butanol, and water from the aerial parts of some species of the *Lamium* genus [25]. In this study, conducted on male Swiss albino mice, extracts of *L. eriocephalum* subsp. *eriocephalum*, *L. garganicum* subsp. *laevigatum*, *L. garganicum* subsp. *pulchrum* and *L. purpureum* var. *purpureum* were administered to the animals to alleviate inflammatory pain in a model of ear edema and in carrageenan-induced and Prostaglandin E_2-induced hind paw edema. The experimental data demonstrated that *L. garganicum* subsp. *laevigatum* and *L. garganicum* subsp. *pulchrum* displayed remarkable anti-inflammatory and antinociceptive activities in mice at 200 mg/kg dose without inducing any gastric damage.

The biological activities of the herbal extracts of the genus *Lamium* described up to now have concerned organic solvent extracts or water extracts. These extracts allowed to obtain concentrated solutions of phenolic compounds, flavonoids, iridoids, terpenes, steroidal derivatives, enriched with the various components depending on the polarity of the extracting mixture.

An unusual extraction procedure has been described in a study of the biological activity of an *L. album* oil extract [147] by using a biphasic solvent system consisting of 70% ethanol and sunflower oil at a ratio of 1:1, after the maceration of above-ground of *L. album* in water. The oil extract (OE) was then studied in models of hemolytic anemia (HA) induced with intramuscular (IM) administration of phenylhydrazide chloride to white mongrel male rats. Three groups of animals were formed: (i) intact animals, (ii) negative control group (with induced hemolytic anemia but untreated, (iii) OE treated (with induced hemolytic anemia and treated). The results showed that the administration of extract had anti-anemic effects since all blood parameters (e.g., number of erythrocytes, hemoglobin levels, hematocrit, and red blood cell indices) were significantly better throughout the twelve weeks of the experiment. The authors suggested that the anti-anemic effect of OE may be due to the antioxidant action of chlorophyll preparation. This explanation is not fully convincing since the sunflower oil used to obtain OE contains on average 59% of linoleic acid [148]. Recently, linoleic acid has been proved to induce red blood cells and hemoglobin damage via an oxidative mechanism, eventually leading to partial acute anemia [149]. In other words, if chlorophyll had effectively carried out anti-anemic action, such an action would be even stronger as it would have contrasted not only the anemic effect due to the administration of phenylhydrazide chloride, but also that induced by the linoleic acid contained in OE. It would have been interesting to know the effect of the administration of the extractor oil only in a further control group, but this eventuality has not been taken into consideration by the authors of this study.

An interesting in vivo use of *L. amplexicaule* has been described in Punjab, a region of southern Pakistan. In this region, the leaves of *L. amplexicaule* are administered orally to ruminants affected by helminth infections, at a rate of 250 g at a time [150]. The duration of treatment is not standardized and is not performed by veterinary staff but by local pastors. The efficacy of the treatment, therefore, is not certified by veterinarians and needs further investigation carried out with criteria and procedures of the veterinary medicine. However, the wide use of *L. amplexicaule* as an anthelmintic in ruminants suggests that there are concrete possibilities for effective action by substances contained in the plant.

4.3. Clinical Studies

Randomized controlled trial (RCT) is a study in which people are allocated at random (by chance alone) to receive one of several clinical interventions. If the in vivo studies conducted with herbs belonging to the *Lamium* genus are few, the RCTs studies are even less. Below we give an account of the few RCTs we have come to know.

Atopic dermatitis (AD) is a pruritic, chronic and inflammatory skin disease, the onset of which often coincides with the pediatric age. The 'atopic' appellation, attributed to dermatitis, underlines the absence of a skin location. Shapira et al. [151] describe a brief report about forty-nine patients who were recruited for a two weeks treatment to test the efficacy of tri-herbal combination on AD in a randomized, placebo-controlled trial. *L. album* was one of these three herbs. The medication was taken orally three times daily for two weeks. That study found that tri-herbal combination induced a highly significant improvement in both objective and subjective parameters of AD. However, placebo treatment induced equally positive results in all measured aspects, so it is not possible to attribute any therapeutic effect to the medicament *L. album* containing.

5. Conclusions and Future Perspectives

Beside specific aspects of plant biochemistry, this review underlined the use of *Lamiun* plants (some species) in the formulation of natural remedies for topical use, preparation of functional foods, possible action as tyrosinase inhibitors, among others. Lamiaceae is one of the most extensive and diverse plant families about their ethnomedicinal properties. Besides the great representativity of species, chemotaxonomic markers are individuated as well as targeted biological functions.

Generally, the ancient science of phytotherapy study represents a great challenge for future research in pharmacological and medical fields: from the exploitation of chemistry of plants to intervention studies until clinical trials in humans. New frontiers should be based on an integrated and multidisciplinary approach of research, in terms of health benefits and sustainable health applications and addressed towards advanced technologies such as the nanotechnologies and chemometrics.

Author Contributions: All authors contributed equally to this work. B.S., A.R., M.F.M., F.S., A.S., L.A. and J.S.-R. critically reviewed the manuscript. All the Authors read and approved the final manuscript.

Funding: This research received no external funding.

Conflicts of Interest: The authors declare no conflict of interest.

References

1. Sen, T.; Samanta, S.K. Medicinal plants, human health and biodiversity: A broad review. *Adv. Biochem. Eng. Biotechnol.* **2015**, *147*, 59–110. [PubMed]
2. Salehi, B.; Stojanović-Radić, Z.; Matejić, J.; Sharopov, F.; Antolak, H.; Kręgiel, D.; Sen, S.; Sharifi-Rad, M.; Acharya, K.; Sharifi-Rad, R.; et al. Plants of genus *Mentha*: From farm to food factory. *Plants* **2018**, *7*, 70. [CrossRef]
3. Sharifi-Rad, M.; Ozcelik, B.; Altın, G.; Daşkaya-Dikmen, C.; Martorell, M.; Ramírez-Alarcón, K.; Alarcón-Zapata, P.; Morais-Braga, M.F.B.; Carneiro, J.N.P.; Alves Borges Leal, A.L.; et al. *Salvia* spp. Plants-from farm to food applications and phytopharmacotherapy. *Trends Food Sci. Technol.* **2018**, *80*, 242–263. [CrossRef]
4. Durazzo, A.; D'Addezio, L.; Camilli, E.; Piccinelli, R.; Turrini, A.; Marletta, L.; Marconi, S.; Lucarini, M.; Lisciani, S.; Gabrielli, P.; et al. From plant compounds to botanicals and back: A current snapshot. *Molecules* **2018**, *23*, 1844. [CrossRef] [PubMed]
5. Durazzo, A. Extractable and Non-extractable polyphenols: An overview. In *Non-Extractable Polyphenols and Carotenoids: Importance in Human Nutrition and Health*; Saura-Calixto, F., Pérez-Jiménez, J., Eds.; Royal Society of Chemistry: London, UK, 2018; pp. 1–37.
6. Daliu, P.; Santini, A.; Novellino, E. From pharmaceuticals to nutraceuticals: Bridging disease prevention and management. *Expert Rev. Clin. Pharmacol.* **2019**, *12*, 1–7. [CrossRef] [PubMed]
7. Durazzo, A.; Lucarini, M. A current shot and re-thinking of antioxidant research strategy. *Braz. J. Anal. Chem.* **2018**, *5*, 9–11. [CrossRef]
8. Santini, A.; Tenore, G.C.; Novellino, E. Nutraceuticals: A paradigm of proactive medicine. *Eur. J. Pharm. Sci.* **2017**, *96*, 53–61. [CrossRef]
9. Santini, A.; Novellino, E. Nutraceuticals-Shedding Light on the Grey Area between Pharmaceuticals and Food. *Expert. Rev. Clin. Pharmacol.* **2018**, *11*, 545–547. [CrossRef]

10. Santini, A.; Cammarata, S.M.; Capone, G.; Ianaro, A.; Tenore, G.C.; Pani, L.; Novellino, E. Nutraceuticals: Opening the debate for a regulatory framework. *Br. J. Clin. Pharmacol.* **2018**, *84*, 659–672. [CrossRef]
11. Raja, R.R. Medicinally potential plants of labiatae (lamiaceae) family, an overview. *Res. J. Med. Plant.* **2012**, *6*, 203–213. [CrossRef]
12. The Plant List. Version 1.1. Available online: http://www.theplantlist.org/ (accessed on 29 April 2019).
13. Tamokou, J.D.D.; Mbaveng, A.T.; Kuete, V. Antimicrobial activities of african medicinal spices and vegetables. In *Medicinal Spices and Vegetables from Africa. Therapeutic Potential against Metabolic, Inflammatory, Infectious and Systemic Diseases*; Kuete, V., Ed.; Academic Press: New York, NY, USA, 2017; p. 694.
14. Lesjak, M.; Simin, N.; Orcic, D.; Franciskovic, M.; Knezevic, P.; Beara, I.; Aleksic, V.; Svircev, E.; Buzas, K.; Mimica-Dukic, N. Binary and tertiary mixtures of *Satureja hortensis* and *Origanum vulgare* essential oils as potent antimicrobial agents against *Helicobacter pylori*. *Phytother. Res.* **2016**, *30*, 476–484. [CrossRef] [PubMed]
15. Waller, S.B.; Cleff, M.B.; Serra, E.F.; Silva, A.L.; Gomes, A.D.; de Mello, J.R.; de Faria, R.O.; Meireles, M.C. Plants from lamiaceae family as source of antifungal molecules in humane and veterinary medicine. *Microb. Pathog.* **2017**, *104*, 232–237. [CrossRef]
16. Ghoneim, M.; Musa, A.; El-Hela, A.; Elokely, K. Evaluation and understanding the molecular basis of the antimethicillin-resistant *Staphylococcus aureus* activity of secondary metabolites isolated from *Lamium amplexicaule*. *Pharmacogn. Mag.* **2018**, *14*, 3–7.
17. Bendiksby, M.; Brysting, A.K.; Thorbek, L.; Gussarova, G.; Ryding, O. Molecular phylogeny and taxonomy of the genus *Lamium* L. (lamiaceae): Disentangling origins of presumed allotetraploids. *Taxon* **2011**, *60*, 986–1000. [CrossRef]
18. Mennema, J. *A Taxonomic Revision of Lamium (Lamiaceae)*; Brill Archive: Leiden, The Netherlands, 1989.
19. Baran, P.; Özdemdr, C. Morphological, anatomical and cytological studies on endemic *Lamium pisidicum*. *Pak. J. Bot.* **2013**, *45*, 73–85.
20. Yalcin, F.N.; Kaya, D. Ethnobotany, pharmacology and phytochemistry of the genus *Lamium* (lamiaceae). *FABAD J. Pharm. Sci.* **2006**, *31*, 43–52.
21. Yordanova, Z.P.; Zhiponova, M.K.; Iakimova, E.T.; Dimitrova, M.A.; Kapchina-Toteva, V.M. Revealing the reviving secret of the white dead nettle (*Lamium album* L.). *Phytochem. Rev.* **2014**, *13*, 375–389. [CrossRef]
22. Czerwińska, M.E.; Swierczewska, A.; Wozniak, M.; Kiss, A.K. Bioassay-guided iisolation of iridoids and phenylpropanoids from aerial parts of *Lamium album* and their anti-inflammatory activity in human neutrophils. *Planta Med.* **2017**, *83*, 1011–1019.
23. Zargari, A. *Medicinal Plants*; Tehran University Publications: Tehran, Iran, 1990; Volume 4.
24. Matkowski, A.; Tasarz, P.; Szypula, E. Antioxidant activity of herb extracts from five medicinal plants from lamiaceae, subfamily lamioideae. *J. Med. Plants Res.* **2008**, *2*, 321–330.
25. Akkol, E.K.; Yalçin, F.N.; Kaya, D.; Çalış, I.; Yesilada, E.; Ersöz, T. In vivo anti-inflammatory and antinociceptive actions of some lamium species. *J. Ethnopharmacol.* **2008**, *118*, 166–172. [CrossRef] [PubMed]
26. Yalcin, F.N.; Kaya, D.; Kilic, E.; Ozalp, M.; Erspz, T.; Calis, I. Antimicrobial and free radical scavenging activities of some *Lamium* species from turkey. *Hacet. Univ. J. Fac. Pharm.* **2007**, *27*, 11–22.
27. Alipieva, K.I.; Taskova, R.M.; Evstatieva, L.N.; Handjieva, N.V.; Popov, S.S. Benzoxazinoids and iridoid glucosides from four lamium species. *Phytochemistry* **2003**, *64*, 1413–1417. [CrossRef] [PubMed]
28. Budzianowski, J.; Skrzypczak, L. Phenylpropanoid esters from lamium album flowers. *Phytochemistry* **1995**, *38*, 997–1001. [CrossRef]
29. Damtoft, S. Iridoid glucosides from lamium album. *Phytochemistry* **1991**, *31*, 175–178. [CrossRef]
30. Damtoft, S.; Jensen, S.R. Hemialboside, a hemiterpene glucoside from lamium album. *Phytochemistry* **1995**, *39*, 923–924. [CrossRef]
31. Savchenko, T.; Blackford, M.; Sarker, S.D.; Dinan, L. Phytoecdysteroids from *Lamium* spp: Identification and distribution within plants. *Biochem. Syst. Ecol.* **2001**, *29*, 891–900. [CrossRef]
32. Carović-StanKo, K.; PeteK, M.; Martina, G.; Pintar, J.; Bedeković, D.; Ćustić, M.H.; Šatović, Z. Medicinal plants of the family lamiaceaeas functional foods—A review. *Czech J. Food Sci.* **2016**, *34*, 377. [CrossRef]
33. Deng, Y.R.; He, L.; Li, W.Q.; Wang, H.Q. Studies on chemical constituents in herb of *Lamium maculatum* L. var Kansuense. *Zhongguo Zhong Yao Za Zhi* **2003**, *28*, 730–732.

34. Nugroho, A.; Choi, J.K.; Park, J.H.; Lee, K.T.; Cha, B.C.; Park, H.J. Two new flavonol glycosides from *Lamium amplexicaule* L. And their in vitro free radical scavenging and tyrosinase inhibitory activities. *Planta Med.* **2009**, *75*, 364–366.
35. Czerwinska, M.E.; Swierczewska, A.; Granica, S. Bioactive constituents of *Lamium album* L. As inhibitors of cytokine secretion in human neutrophils. *Molecules* **2018**, *23*, 2770. [CrossRef]
36. Kurkin, V. Phenylpropanoids from medicinal plants: Distribution, classification, structural analysis, and biological activity. *Chem. Nat. Comp.* **2003**, *39*, 123–153. [CrossRef]
37. Cao, J.; Yu, H.; Wu, Y.; Wang, X. Occurrence and Biological Activities of Phenylpropionyl Iridoids. *Mini Rev. Med. Chem.* **2019**, *19*, 292–309. [CrossRef]
38. Damtoft, S.; Jensen, S.R.; Nielsen, B.J. Biosynthesis of iridoid glucosides in *Lamium album*. *Phytochemistry* **1991**, *31*, 135–137. [CrossRef]
39. Alipieva, K.I.; Taskova, R.M.; Jensen, S.R.; Handjieva, N.V. Iridoid glucosides from *Lamium album* and *Lamium maculatum* (Lamiaceae). *Biochem. Syst. Ecol.* **2006**, *34*, 88–91. [CrossRef]
40. Pereira, O.R.; Domingues, M.R.M.; Silva, A.M.S.; Cardoso, S.M. Phenolic constituents of lamium album: Focus on isoscutellarein derivatives. *Food Res. Int.* **2012**, *48*, 330–335. [CrossRef]
41. Moerman, D.E. The medicinal flora of native north america: An analysis. *J. Ethnopharmacol.* **1991**, *31*, 1–42. [CrossRef]
42. Flamini, G.; Cioni, P.L.; Morelli, I. Composition of the essential oils and in vivo emission of volatiles of four lamium species from italy: *L. purpureum*, *L. hybridum*, *L. bifidum* and *L. amplexicaule*. *Food Chem.* **2005**, *91*, 63–68. [CrossRef]
43. Alipieva, K.; Evstatieva, L.; Handjieva, N.; Popov, S. Comparative analysis of the composition of flower volatiles from *Lamium* L. Species and *Lamiastrum galeobdolon* heist. Ex fabr. *Z. Nat. C* **2003**, *58*, 779–782. [CrossRef]
44. Kurihara, F.; Kikuchi, M. On the constituents of the essential oil component from *Lamium purpureum* L. *Yakugaku Zasshi* **1976**, *96*, 1348–1351. [CrossRef]
45. Hussain, A.I.; Anvar, F.; Sherazi, S.T.H.; Przybylski, R. Chemical composition, antioxidant and antimicrobial activities of basil (*Ocimum basilicum*) essential oils depends on seasonal variations. *Food Chem.* **2008**, *108*, 986–995. [CrossRef]
46. Hussain, A.I.; Anvar, F.; Nigam, P.S.; Ashraf, M.; Gilani, A.H. Seasonal variation in content, chemical composition and antimicrobial and cytotoxic activities of essential oils from four *mentha* species. *J. Sci. Food Agric.* **2010**, *90*, 1827–1836. [CrossRef] [PubMed]
47. Celiktas, O.Y.; Kocabas, E.E.H.; Bedir, E.; Sukan, F.V.; Ozek, T.; Baser, K.H.C. Antimicrobial activities of methanol extracts and essential oils of rosmarinus officinalis, depending on location and seasonal variations. *Food Chem.* **2007**, *100*, 553–559. [CrossRef]
48. Ahmad, I.; Ahmad, M.S.A.; Ashraf, M.; Hussain, M.; Ashraf, M.Y. Seasonal variation in some medicinal and biochemical ingredients in *Mentha longifolia* (L.) huds. *Pak. J. Bot.* **2011**, *43*, 69–77.
49. Singh, M.; Guleria, N. Influence of harvesting stage and inorganic and organic fertilizers on yield and oil composition of rosemary (*Rosmarinus officinalis* L.) in a semi-arid tropical climate. *Ind. Crop. Prod.* **2013**, *42*, 37–40. [CrossRef]
50. Salman, M.; Abdel-Hameed, E.S.S.; Bazaid, S.A.; Dadi, M.M. Chemical composition for hydrodistillation essential oil of *Mentha longifolia* by gas chromatography-mass spectrometry from north regions in kingdom of saudi arabia. *Pharma Chem.* **2015**, *7*, 34–40.
51. Kapchina-Toteva, V.; Dimitrova, M.A.; Stefanova, M.; Koleva, D.; Kostov, K.; Yordanova, Z.P.; Stefanov, D.; Zhiponova, M.K. Adaptive changes in photosynthetic performance and secondary metabolites during white dead nettle micropropagation. *J. Plant Physiol.* **2014**, *171*, 1344–1353. [CrossRef] [PubMed]
52. Sajjadi, S.E.; Ghannadi, A. Analysis of the essential oil of *Lamium amplexicaule* L. from northeastern iran. *J. Essent. Oil Bear. Plants* **2012**, *15*, 577–581. [CrossRef]
53. Jones, C.D.; Woods, K.E.; Setzer, W.N. A chemical ecological investigation of the allelopathic potential of *Lamium amplexicaule* and *Lamium purpureum*. *Open J. Ecol.* **2012**, *2*, 167–177. [CrossRef]
54. Nickavar, B.; Mojab, F.; Bamasian, S. Volatile components from aerial parts of *Lamium amplexicaule* from Iran. *J. Essent. Oil-Bear. Plants* **2013**, *11*, 36–40. [CrossRef]
55. Abu-ziada, M.E.A.; Mashaly, I.A.; Abdelgawed, A.M.; Asmeda, A.A. Ecology and phytochemistry of *Lamium amplexicaule* L. *J. Environ. Sci.* **2014**, *43*, 311–327.

56. Layka, S.; Kara-Ali, A.; Sultan, A. A morphological, anatomical and chemical study on *Lamium amplexicaule* L. (lamiaceae). *Tishreen Univ. J. Res. Sci. Stud.* **2011**, *33*, 176–194.
57. *Rastitelnye Resursy Sssr*; Nauka: St. Petersburg, FL, USA, 1991; Volume 6.
58. El-Sayed, Z.I.A. Chemical composition, antimicrobial and insecticidal activities of the essential oil of *Lamium maculatum* L. Grown in egypt. *Biosci. Biotechnol. Res. Asia* **2008**, *5*, 65–72.
59. El-Sattar, A.; Handjieva, N.; Popov, S.; Evstatieva, L. Volatile constituents from *Lamium maculatum* leaves and *Nepeta mussini* roots. *C. R. Acad. Bulg. Sci.* **1993**, *46*, 37–39.
60. Roussis, V.; Chinou, I.; Perdetzoglou, D.; Loukis, A. Identification and bacteriostatic activity of the essential oil of *Lamium garganicum* L. ssp. *Laevigatum arcangeli. J. Essent. Oil Res.* **1996**, *8*, 291–293. [CrossRef]
61. Morteza-Semnani, K.; Saeedi, M.; Akbarzadeh, M. Chemical composition of the essential oil of the flowering aerial parts of *Lamium album* L. *J. Essent. Oil Bear. Plants* **2016**, *19*, 773–777. [CrossRef]
62. Mickene, R.; Bakutis, B.; Maruska, A.; Ragazinskiene, O.; Kaskoniene, V. Effect of volatile secondary metabolites of *Monarda didyma* L., *Lamium album* L. And *Myrrhis odorata* L. Plants against micromycetes of indoor environments of animals. *Veterinariia* **2014**, *68*, 48–54.
63. Kovalvoya, A.; Ilyina, T.; Kolesnik, Y. Study of component composition of the essential oil of leaves *Lamium album. Pharmacology* **2013**, *1*, 80–82.
64. Layka, S.; Kara-Ali, A.; Sultan, A. A morphological and chemical study of two species of *Lamium* L.: *Lamium moschatum* mill. And *Lamium striatum* sibth. Et smith. Belonging to lamiaceae family. *Tishreen Univ. Off. Website* **2009**, *31*, 133–147.
65. Turner, N.J.; Luczaj, L.J.; Migliorini, P.; Pieroni, A.; Dreon, A.L.; Sacchetti, L.E. Edible and tended wild plants, traditional ecological knowledge and agroecology. *Crit. Rev. Plant Sci.* **2011**, *30*, 198–225. [CrossRef]
66. Heinrich, M.; Müller, W.E.; Galli, C. *Local Mediterranean Food Plants and Nutraceuticals*; Karger: Basel, Switzerland, 2006; Volume 59, p. 186.
67. Ninomiya, K.; Nishida, S.; Matsura, Y.; Asada, M.; Kawahara, Y.; Yoshikawa, M.; Nishida, N.; Matsuura, Y. *Fat-Metabolism Improving Agent for Use in Food/Drink for Improving Fat Metabolism and Preventing/Treating Lifestyle Related Disease e.g. Diabetes, Contains Polar Solvent Extract of Herb e.g. Rose Hip Fruit, Mugwort or Safflower*; MORI-Non-Standard, Morishita Jintan KK; China, 2006; p. 19.
68. Xu, F. *Chinese Medicine e.g. for Treating Arthropathy, Comprises Broad Cocklebur, Vervain, Condyle Grass, Motherwort, Saxifrage, Cactus, Mulberry Branch, White Dead Nettle, Boston Ivy, Folium Photiniae, Water Pepper and Chinese Fever Vine*; XUFF-Individual; 2008; p. 10.
69. Picuric-Jovanovic, K.; Milovanovic, M.; Budincevic, M.; Vrbaski, Z. Antioxydative wirkung von lamium purpureum als nahrungsmittelzusatzstoff. In *Acta of the 6th Symposium "Vitamine und Zusatzstoffe in der Ernahrung von Mensch und Tier"*; Friedrich-Schiller Universitat: Jena, Germany, 1997.
70. Bremness, L. *The Complete Book of Herbs*; Dorling Kindersley: London, UK, 1995.
71. Cui, S.Y.; Chen, X.G.; Hu, Z. Identification and determination of ecdysone and phenylpropanoid glucoside and flavonoids in *Lamium maculatum* by capillary zone electrophoresis. *Biomed. Chromatogr.* **2003**, *17*, 477–482.
72. Malik, Z.A.; Bhat, J.A.; Ballabha, R.; Bussmann, R.W.; Bhatt, A.B. Ethnomedicinal plants traditionally used in health care practices by inhabitants of western himalaya. *J. Ethnopharmacol.* **2015**, *172*, 133–144. [CrossRef] [PubMed]
73. Bahmani, M.; Zargaran, A. Ethno-botanical medicines used for urinary stones in the Urmia, Northwest Iran. *Eur. J. Integr. Med.* **2015**, *7*, 657–662. [CrossRef]
74. Pieroni, A.; Sõukand, R.; Quave, C.L.; Hajdari, A.; Mustafa, B. Traditional food uses of wild plants among the gorani of south kosovo. *Appetite* **2017**, *108*, 83–92. [CrossRef] [PubMed]
75. Tetik, F.; Civelek, S.; Cakilcioglu, U. Traditional uses of some medicinal plants in malatya (Turkey). *J. Ethnopharmacol.* **2013**, *146*, 331–346. [CrossRef]
76. De Feo, V.; Aquino, R.; Menghini, A.; Ramundo, E.; Senatore, F. Traditional phytotherapy in the Peninsula Sorrentina, Campania, Southern Italy. *J. Ethnopharmacol.* **1992**, *36*, 113–125. [CrossRef]
77. Vokou, D.; Katradi, K.; Kokkini, S. Ethnobotanical survey of zagori (epirus, greece), a renowned centre of folk medicine in the past. *J. Ethnopharmacol.* **1993**, *39*, 187–196. [CrossRef]
78. Ugulu, I.; Baslar, S.; Yorek, N.; Dogan, Y. The investigation and quantitative ethnobotanical evaluation of medicinal plants used around Izmir province, Turkey. *J. Med. Plants Res.* **2009**, *3*, 345–367.
79. Grudzinskaya, L.M.; Gemedzhieva, N.G.; Nelina, N.B.; Karzhaubekova, Z.Z. *Annotated List of Medicinal Plants of Kazakhstan*; Almaty, Kazakhstan, 2014; Volume 20, p. 91.

80. Sokolov, P.D. *Plant. Resources of the USSR: Flowering Plants, Their Chemical Composition, Use. (Family. Hippuridaceae-Lobeliaceae)*; Nauka: St. Petersburg, Russia, 1991; pp. 38–39.
81. Rehman, K.; Mashwani, Z.U.; Khan, M.A.; Ullah, Z.; Chaudhary, H.J. An ethnobotanical perspective of traditional medicinal plants from the khattak tribe of chonthra karak, pakistan. *J. Ethnopharmacol.* **2015**, *165*, 251–259. [CrossRef]
82. Jan, H.A.; Ahmad, S.W.L.; Jan, S.; Ahmad, N.; Ullah, N. Ethnomedicinal survey of medicinal plants of chinglai valley, buner district, pakistan. *Eur. J. Integr. Med.* **2017**, *13*, 64–74.
83. Naghibi, F.; Mosaddegh, M.; Motamed, S.M.; Ghorbani, A. Labiatae family in folk medicine in iran: From ethnobotany to pharmacology. *Iran. J. Pharm. Res.* **2005**, *2*, 63–79.
84. Tomas-Barberan, F.A.; Gil, M.L. *Chemistry and Natural Distribution of Flavonoids in the Labiatae*; Royal Botanical Gardens: London, UK, 1992.
85. Offiah, V.N.; Chikwendu, U.A. Antidiarrhoeal effects of *Ocimum gratissimum* leaf extract in experimental animals. *J. Ethnopharmacol.* **1999**, *68*, 327–330. [CrossRef]
86. Birben, E.; Sahiner, U.M.; Sackesen, C.; Erzurum, S.; Kalayci, O. Oxidative stress and antioxidant defense. *World Allergy Organ. J.* **2012**, *5*, 9. [CrossRef]
87. Gülçin, I. Antioxidant activity of food constituents: An overview. *Arch. Toxicol.* **2012**, *86*, 345–391. [CrossRef]
88. Zucca, P.; Sanjust, E.; Trogu, E.; Sollai, F.; Rescigno, A. Evaluation of antioxidant capacity of antioxidant-declared beverages marketed in italy. *Ital. J. Food Sci.* **2010**, *22*, 313–319.
89. Belkhir, M.; Dhaouadi, K.; Rosa, A.; Atzeri, A.; Nieddu, M.; Tuberoso, C.I.G.; Rescigno, A.; Amri, M.; Fattouch, S. Protective effects of azarole polyphenolic extracts against oxidative damage using in vitro biomolecular and cellular models. *Ind. Crop. Prod.* **2016**, *86*, 239–250. [CrossRef]
90. Orrù, R.; Zucca, P.; Falzoi, M.; Atzori, E.; Rescigno, A.; Padiglia, A. First step towards the biomolecular characterization of pompia, an endemic citrus-like fruit from sardinia (italy). *Plant Biosyst.* **2017**, *151*, 464–473. [CrossRef]
91. Apak, R.A.; Özyürek, M.; Güçlü, K.; Çapanoğlu, E. Antioxidant activity/capacity measurement. 2. Hydrogen atom transfer (hat)-based, mixed-mode (electron transfer (et)/hat), and lipid peroxidation assays. *J. Agric. Food Chem.* **2016**, *64*, 1028–1045. [CrossRef]
92. Apak, R.a.; Özyürek, M.; Güçlü, K.; Çapanoğlu, E. Antioxidant activity/capacity measurement. 1. Classification, physicochemical principles, mechanisms, and electron transfer (et)-based assays. *J. Agric. Food Chem.* **2016**, *64*, 997–1027. [CrossRef] [PubMed]
93. Apak, R.; Capanoglu, E.; Shahidi, F. *Measurement of Antioxidant Activity and Capacity: Recent Trends and Applications*; John Wiley & Sons: New York, NY, USA, 2017.
94. Tabart, J.; Kevers, C.; Pincemail, J.; Defraigne, J.-O.; Dommes, J. Comparative antioxidant capacities of phenolic compounds measured by various tests. *Food Chem.* **2009**, *113*, 1226–1233. [CrossRef]
95. Tirzitis, G.; Bartosz, G. Determination of antiradical and antioxidant activity: Basic principles and new insights. *Acta Biochim. Pol.* **2010**, *57*, 139–142. [CrossRef]
96. Leopoldini, M.; Marino, T.; Russo, N.; Toscano, M. Antioxidant properties of phenolic compounds: H-atom versus electron transfer mechanism. *J. Phys. Chem. A* **2004**, *108*, 4916–4922. [CrossRef]
97. Leopoldini, M.; Marino, T.; Russo, N.; Toscano, M. Density functional computations of the energetic and spectroscopic parameters of quercetin and its radicals in the gas phase and in solvent. *Theor. Chem. Acc.* **2004**, *111*, 210–216. [CrossRef]
98. Ahmed, J.K.; Salih, H.A.; Hadi, A. Anthocyanins in red beet juice act as scavengers for heavy metals ions such as lead and cadmium. *Int. J. Sci. Technol.* **2013**, *2*, 269–274.
99. Rosa, A.; Nieddu, M.; Piras, A.; Atzeri, A.; Putzu, D.; Rescigno, A. Maltese mushroom (*Cynomorium coccineum* L.) as source of oil with potential anticancer activity. *Nutrients* **2015**, *7*, 849–864. [CrossRef] [PubMed]
100. Zucca, P.; Rosa, A.; Tuberoso, C.I.G.; Piras, A.; Rinaldi, A.C.; Sanjust, E.; Dessì, M.A.; Rescigno, A. Evaluation of antioxidant potential of "maltese mushroom" (*Cynomorium coccineum*) by means of multiple chemical and biological assays. *Nutrients* **2013**, *5*, 149–161. [CrossRef] [PubMed]
101. Apak, R.; Gorinstein, S.; Böhm, V.; Schaich, K.M.; Özyürek, M.; Güçlü, K. Methods of measurement and evaluation of natural antioxidant capacity/activity (iupac technical report). *Pure Appl. Chem.* **2013**, *85*, 957–998. [CrossRef]
102. Luthria, D.L. Significance of sample preparation in developing analytical methodologies for accurate estimation of bioactive compounds in functional foods. *J. Sci. Food Agric.* **2006**, *86*, 2266–2272. [CrossRef]

103. Durazzo, A. Study approach of antioxidant properties in foods: Update and considerations. *Foods* **2017**, *6*, 17. [CrossRef] [PubMed]
104. Lagouri, V.; Alexandri, G. Antioxidant properties of greek *O. dictamnus* and *R. officinalis* methanol and aqueous extracts—HPLC determination of phenolic acids. *Int. J. Food Prop.* **2013**, *16*, 549–562. [CrossRef]
105. Trouillas, P.; Calliste, C.A.; Allais, D.P.; Simon, A.; Marfak, A.; Delage, C.; Duroux, J.L. Antioxidant, anti-inflammatory and antiproliferative properties of sixteen water plant extracts used in the limousin countryside as herbal teas. *Food Chem.* **2003**, *80*, 399–407. [CrossRef]
106. Matkowski, A.; Piotrowska, M. Antioxidant and free radical scavenging activities of some medicinal plants from the lamiaceae. *Fitoterapia* **2006**, *77*, 346–353. [CrossRef]
107. Yumrutas, O.; Saygideger, S.D. Determination of in vitro antioxidant activities of different extracts of marrubium parviflorum fish et mey. and *Lamium amplexicaule* L. From south east of turkey. *J. Med. Plants Res.* **2010**, *4*, 2164–2172.
108. Li, A.S.H.; Bandy, B.; Tsang, S.S.; Davison, A.J. DNA-breaking versus DNA-protecting activity of four phenolic compounds in vitro. *Free Radic. Res.* **2000**, *33*, 551–566. [CrossRef]
109. Mira, L.; Fernandez, M.T.; Santos, M.; Rocha, R.; Florêncio, M.H.; Jennings, K.R. Interactions of flavonoids with iron and copper ions: A mechanism for their antioxidant activity. *Free Radic. Res.* **2002**, *36*, 1199–1208. [CrossRef]
110. Bubueanu, C.; Gheorghe, C.; Pirvu, L.; Bubueanu, G. Antioxidant activity of butanolic extracts of Romanian native species—*Lamium album* and *Lamium purpureum*. *Rom. Biotechnol. Lett.* **2013**, *18*, 7255–7262.
111. Vladimir-Knežević, S.; Blažeković, B.; Kindl, M.; Vladić, J.; Lower-Nedza, A.; Brantner, A. Acetylcholinesterase inhibitory, antioxidant and phytochemical properties of selected medicinal plants of the lamiaceae family. *Molecules* **2014**, *19*, 767–782. [CrossRef] [PubMed]
112. Danila, D.; Adriana, T.; Camelia, S.; Valentin, G.; Anca, M. Antioxidant activity of methanolic extracts of *Lamium album* and *Lamium maculatum* species from wild populations in the Romanian eastern Carpathians. *Planta Med.* **2015**, *81*. [CrossRef]
113. Eghbaliferiz, S.; Iranshahi, M. Prooxidant activity of polyphenols, flavonoids, anthocyanins and carotenoids: Updated review of mechanisms and catalyzing metals. *Phytother. Res.* **2016**, *30*, 1379–1391. [CrossRef]
114. Bhat, S.H.; Azmi, A.S.; Hadi, S.M. Prooxidant DNA breakage induced by caffeic acid in human peripheral lymphocytes: Involvement of endogenous copper and a putative mechanism for anticancer properties. *Toxicol. Appl. Pharmacol.* **2007**, *218*, 249–255. [CrossRef] [PubMed]
115. Cao, G.; Sofic, E.; Prior, R.L. Antioxidant and prooxidant behavior of flavonoids: Structure-activity relationships. *Free Radic. Boil. Med.* **1997**, *22*, 749–760. [CrossRef]
116. Procházková, D.; Boušová, I.; Wilhelmová, N. Antioxidant and prooxidant properties of flavonoids. *Fitoterapia* **2011**, *82*, 513–523. [CrossRef]
117. Lin, L.T.; Hsu, W.C.; Lin, C.C. Antiviral natural products and herbal medicines. *J. Tradit. Complement. Med.* **2014**, *4*, 24–35. [CrossRef]
118. Zhang, H.; Rothwangl, K.; Mesecar, A.D.; Sabahi, A.; Rong, L.; Fong, H.H.S. Lamiridosins, hepatitis c virus entry inhibitors from *Lamium album*. *J. Nat. Prod.* **2009**, *72*, 2158–2162. [CrossRef] [PubMed]
119. Gonçalves, M.J.; Piras, A.; Porcedda, S.; Marongiu, B.; Falconieri, D.; Cavaleiro, C.; Rescigno, A.; Rosa, A.; Salgueiro, L. Antifungal activity of extracts from *Cynomorium coccineum* growing wild in sardinia island (Italy). *Nat. Prod. Res.* **2015**, *29*, 2247–2250. [CrossRef]
120. Dulger, B. Antifungal activity of lamium tenuiflorum against some medical yeast candida and cryptococcus species. *Pharm. Biol.* **2009**, *47*, 467–470. [CrossRef]
121. Erbil, N.; Alan, Y.; Digrak, M. Antimicrobial and antioxidant properties of *Lamium galactophyllum* boiss & reuter, *L. macrodon* boiss & huet and *L. amplexicaule* from Turkish Flora. *Asian J. Chem.* **2014**, *26*, 549–554.
122. Chipeva, V.A.; Petrova, D.C.; Geneva, M.E.; Dimitrova, M.A.; Moncheva, P.A.; Kapchina-Toteva, V.M. Antimicrobial activity of extracts from in vivo and in vitro propagated *Lamium album* L. Plants. *Afr. J. Tradit. Complement. Altern. Med.* **2013**, *10*, 559–562. [CrossRef]
123. Kvietys, P.R.; Granger, D.N. Role of reactive oxygen and nitrogen species in the vascular responses to inflammation. *Free Radic. Boil. Med.* **2012**, *52*, 556–592. [CrossRef]
124. Mitjavila, M.T.; Moreno, J.J. The effects of polyphenols on oxidative stress and the arachidonic acid cascade. Implications for the prevention/treatment of high prevalence diseases. *Biochem. Pharmacol.* **2012**, *84*, 1113–1122. [CrossRef]

125. Lv, Q.W.; Zhang, W.; Shi, Q.; Zheng, W.J.; Li, X.; Chen, H.; Wu, Q.J.; Jiang, W.L.; Li, H.B.; Gong, L.; et al. Comparison of tripterygium wilfordii hook f with methotrexate in the treatment of active rheumatoid arthritis (Trifra): A randomised, controlled clinical trial. *Ann. Rheum. Dis.* **2015**, *74*, 1078–1086. [CrossRef] [PubMed]
126. Zarei, L.; Naji-Haddadi, S.; Pourjabali, M.; Naghdi, N.; Tasbih-Forosh, M.; Shahsavari, S. Systematic review of anti-rheumatic medicinal plants: An overview of the effectiveness of articular tissues and joint pain associated with rheumatoid arthritis. *J. Pharm. Sci. Res.* **2017**, *9*, 547–551.
127. Randall, C.; Randall, H.; Dobbs, F.; Hutton, C.; Sanders, H. Randomized controlled trial of nettle sting for treatment of base-of-thumb pain. *J. R. Soc. Med.* **2000**, *93*, 305–309. [CrossRef] [PubMed]
128. Uritu, C.M.; Mihai, C.T.; Stanciu, G.D.; Dodi, G.; Alexa-Stratulat, T.; Luca, A.; Leon-Constantin, M.M.; Stefanescu, R.; Bild, V.; Melnic, S.; et al. Medicinal plants of the family lamiaceae in pain therapy: A review. *Pain Res. Manag.* **2018**, *2018*, 7801543. [CrossRef] [PubMed]
129. Veleva, R.; Petkova, B.; Moskova-Doumanova, V.; Doumanov, J.; Dimitrova, M.; Koleva, P.; Mladenova, K.; Petrova, S.; Yordanova, Z.; Kapchina-Toteva, V. Changes in the functional characteristics of tumor and normal cells after treatment with extracts of white dead-nettle. *Biotechnol. Biotechnol. Equip.* **2015**, *29*, 181–188. [CrossRef] [PubMed]
130. Krishnaiah, D.; Sarbatly, R.; Nithyanandam, R. A review of the antioxidant potential of medicinal plant species. *Food Bioprod. Process.* **2011**, *89*, 217–233. [CrossRef]
131. Santoro, A.; Bianco, G.; Picerno, P.; Aquino, R.P.; Autore, G.; Marzocco, S.; Gazzerro, P.; Lioi, M.B.; Bifulco, M. Verminoside- and verbascoside-induced genotoxicity on human lymphocytes: Involvement of parp-1 and p53 proteins. *Toxicol. Lett.* **2008**, *178*, 71–76. [CrossRef] [PubMed]
132. Perucatti, A.; Genualdo, V.; Pauciullo, A.; Iorio, C.; Incarnato, D.; Rossetti, C.; Vizzarri, F.; Palazzo, M.; Casamassima, D.; Iannuzzi, L.; et al. Cytogenetic tests reveal no toxicity in lymphocytes of rabbit (*Oryctolagus cuniculus*, 2n = 44) feed in presence of verbascoside and/or lycopene. *Food Chem. Toxicol.* **2018**, *114*, 311–315. [CrossRef]
133. Paduch, R.; Wójciak-Kosior, M.; Matysik, G. Investigation of biological activity of lamii albi flos extracts. *J. Ethnopharmacol.* **2007**, *110*, 69–75. [CrossRef]
134. Moskova-Doumanova, V.; Miteva, G.; Dimitrova, M.; Topouzova-Hristova, T.; Kapchina, V. Methanol and chloroform extracts from *Lamium album* L. Affect cell properties of a549 cancer lung cell line. *Biotechnol. Biotechnol. Equip.* **2014**, *26*, 120–125. [CrossRef]
135. Paduch, R.; Woźniak, A. The effect of *Lamium album* extract on cultivated human corneal epithelial cells (10.014 prsv-t). *J. Ophthalmic Vis. Res.* **2015**, *10*, 229–237. [CrossRef] [PubMed]
136. Zhou, S.; Richter, A.; Jander, G. Beyond defense: Multiple functions of benzoxazinoids in maize metabolism. *Plant Cell Physiol.* **2018**, *59*, 1528–1533. [CrossRef] [PubMed]
137. Adhikari, K.B.; Tanwir, F.; Gregersen, P.L.; Steffensen, S.K.; Jensen, B.M.; Poulsen, L.K.; Nielsen, C.H.; Høyer, S.; Borre, M.; Fomsgaard, I.S. Benzoxazinoids: Cereal phytochemicals with putative therapeutic and health-protecting properties. *Mol. Nutr. Food Res.* **2015**, *59*, 1324–1338. [CrossRef] [PubMed]
138. Rescigno, A.; Sollai, F.; Rinaldi, A.C.; Soddu, G.; Sanjust, E. Polyphenol oxidase activity staining in polyacrylamide electrophoresis gels. *J. Biochem. Biophys. Methods* **1997**, *34*, 155–159. [CrossRef]
139. Rescigno, A.; Sanjust, E.; Pedulli, G.F.; Valgimigli, L. Spectrophotometric method for the determination of polyphenol oxidase activity by coupling of 4-*tert*-butyl-*O*-benzoquinone and 4-amino-*N*,*N*-diethylaniline. *Anal. Lett.* **1999**, *32*, 2007–2017. [CrossRef]
140. Asthana, S.; Zucca, P.; Vargiu, A.V.; Sanjust, E.; Ruggerone, P.; Rescigno, A. Structure-activity relationship study of hydroxycoumarins and mushroom tyrosinase. *J. Agric. Food Chem.* **2015**, *63*, 7236–7244. [CrossRef]
141. Rescigno, A.; Sanjust, E.; Soddu, G.; Rinaldi, A.C.; Sollai, F.; Curreli, N.; Rinaldi, A. Effect of 3-hydroxyanthranilic acid on mushroom tyrosinase activity. *Biochim. Biophys. Acta-Protein Struct. Mol.* **1998**, *1384*, 268–276. [CrossRef]
142. Rescigno, A.; Casañola-Martin, G.M.; Sanjust, E.; Zucca, P.; Marrero-Ponce, Y. Vanilloid derivatives as tyrosinase inhibitors driven by virtual screening-based QSAR models. *Drug Test. Anal.* **2011**, *3*, 176–181. [CrossRef]
143. Schlich, M.; Fornasier, M.; Nieddu, M.; Sinico, C.; Murgia, S.; Rescigno, A. 3-hydroxycoumarin loaded vesicles for recombinant human tyrosinase inhibition in topical applications. *Colloids Surf. B Biointerfaces* **2018**, *171*, 675–681. [CrossRef]

144. Kim, D.; Park, J.; Kim, J.; Han, C.; Yoon, J.; Kim, N.; Seo, J.; Lee, C. Flavonoids as mushroom tyrosinase inhibitors: A fluorescence quenching study. *J. Agric. Food Chem.* **2006**, *54*, 935–941. [CrossRef]
145. Xie, L.P.; Chen, Q.X.; Huang, H.; Wang, H.Z.; Zhang, R.Q. Inhibitory effects of some flavonoids on the activity of mushroom tyrosinase. *Biochemistry (Moscow)* **2003**, *68*, 487–491. [CrossRef]
146. Etsassala, N.G.; Waryo, T.; Popoola, O.K.; Adeloye, A.O.; Iwuoha, E.I.; Hussein, A.A. Electrochemical screening and evaluation of lamiaceae plant species from South Africa with potential tyrosinase activity. *Sensors* **2019**, *19*, 1035. [CrossRef] [PubMed]
147. Petukhova, N.M.; Buryakina, A.V.; Avenirova, E.L.; Burakova, M.A.; Drozhzhina, E.V. Studies of the biological activity of an oil extract of the snakeflower *Lamium album*. *Pharm. Chem. J.* **2008**, *42*, 354–356. [CrossRef]
148. National Sunflower Association (N.S.A.). Four Types of Sunflower Oil. Available online: https://www.sunflowernsa.com/oil/Four-Types-of-Sunflower-Oil/ (accessed on 29 April 2019).
149. Yuan, T.; Fan, W.B.; Cong, Y.; Xu, H.D.; Li, C.J.; Meng, J.; Bao, N.R.; Zhao, J.N. Linoleic acid induces red blood cells and hemoglobin damage via oxidative mechanism. *Int. J. Clin. Exp. Pathol.* **2015**, *8*, 5044–5052. [PubMed]
150. Jabbar, A.; Raza, M.A.; Iqbal, Z.; Khan, M.N. An inventory of the ethnobotanicals used as anthelmintics in the Southern Punjab (Pakistan). *J. Ethnopharmacol.* **2006**, *108*, 152–154. [CrossRef] [PubMed]
151. Shapira, M.Y.; Raphaelovich, Y.; Gilad, L.; Or, R.; Dumb, A.J.; Ingber, A. Treatment of atopic dermatitis with herbal combination of eleutherococcus, *Achillea millefolium*, and *Lamium album* has no advantage over placebo: A double blind, placebo-controlled, randomized trial. *J. Am. Acad. Dermatol.* **2005**, *52*, 691–693. [CrossRef]

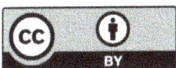

© 2019 by the authors. Licensee MDPI, Basel, Switzerland. This article is an open access article distributed under the terms and conditions of the Creative Commons Attribution (CC BY) license (http://creativecommons.org/licenses/by/4.0/).

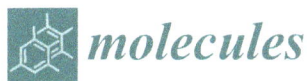

Review

Cucurbits Plants: A Key Emphasis to Its Pharmacological Potential

Bahare Salehi [1], Esra Capanoglu [2], Nabil Adrar [3], Gizem Catalkaya [2], Shabnum Shaheen [4], Mehwish Jaffer [4], Lalit Giri [5], Renu Suyal [5], Arun K Jugran [6], Daniela Calina [7], Anca Oana Docea [8], Senem Kamiloglu [9], Dorota Kregiel [10], Hubert Antolak [10], Ewelina Pawlikowska [10], Surjit Sen [11,12], Krishnendu Acharya [11], Zeliha Selamoglu [13], Javad Sharifi-Rad [14,*], Miquel Martorell [15,*], Célia F. Rodrigues [16], Farukh Sharopov [17], Natália Martins [18,19,*] and Raffaele Capasso [20,*]

1. Student Research Committee, School of Medicine, Bam University of Medical Sciences, Bam 44340847, Iran; bahar.salehi007@gmail.com
2. Faculty of Chemical & Metallurgical Engineering, Food Engineering Department, Istanbul Technical University, 34469 Maslak, Turkey; capanogl@itu.edu.tr (E.C.); catalkaya.gizem@gmail.com (G.C.)
3. Laboratoire de Biotechnologie Végétale et d'Ethnobotanique, Faculté des Sciences de la Nature et de la Vie, Université de Bejaia, Bejaia 06000, Algérie; n.adrar@hotmail.fr
4. Department of Plant Sciences, LCWU, Lahore 54000, Pakistan; shabnum_shaheen78@hotmail.com (S.S.); meh.jaffer@gmail.com (M.J.)
5. G.B. Pant National Institute of Himalayan Environment & Sustainable Development Kosi-Katarmal, Almora 263 643, India; lalitorchid@gmail.com (L.G.); renusuyal04@gmail.com (R.S.)
6. G.B. Pant National Institute of Himalayan Environment & Sustainable Development Garhwal Regional Centre, Srinagar 246174, India; arunjugran@gbpihed.nic.in
7. Department of Clinical Pharmacy, University of Medicine and Pharmacy of Craiova, 200349 Craiova, Romania; calinadaniela@gmail.com
8. Department of Toxicology, University of Medicine and Pharmacy of Craiova, 200349 Craiova, Romania; daoana00@gmail.com
9. Mevsim Gida Sanayi ve Soguk Depo Ticaret A.S. (MVSM Foods), Turankoy, Kestel, 16540 Bursa, Turkey; senemkamiloglu87@gmail.com
10. Institute of Fermentation Technology and Microbiology, Lodz University of Technology, Wolczanska 171/3, 90-924 Lodz, Poland; dorota.kregiel@p.lodz.pl (D.K.); hubert.antolak@p.lodz.pl (H.A.); ewelina.pawlikowska@edu.p.lodz.pl (E.P.)
11. Molecular and Applied Mycology and Plant Pathology Laboratory, Department of Botany, University of Calcutta, Kolkata 700019, India; surjitsen09@gmail.com (S.S.); krish_paper@yahoo.com (K.A.)
12. Department of Botany, Fakir Chand College, Diamond Harbour, West Bengal 743331, India
13. Department of Medical Biology, Faculty of Medicine, Nigde Ömer Halisdemir University, Campus, 51240 Nigde, Turkey; zselamoglu@ohu.edu.tr
14. Zabol Medicinal Plants Research Center, Zabol University of Medical Sciences, Zabol 61615-585, Iran
15. Department of Pharmacy, Faculty of Pharmacy, University of Concepcion, Concepcion 4070386, Chile
16. LEPABE, Department of Chemical Engineering, Faculty of Engineering, University of Porto, Rua Dr. Roberto Frias, s/n, 4200-465 Porto, Portugal; c.fortunae@gmail.com
17. Department of Pharmaceutical Technology, Avicenna Tajik State Medical University, Rudaki 139, Dushanbe 734003, Tajikistan; shfarukh@mail.ru
18. Faculty of Medicine, University of Porto, Alameda Prof. Hernâni Monteiro, 4200-319 Porto, Portugal
19. Institute for Research and Innovation in Health (i3S), University of Porto, 4200-135 Porto, Portugal
20. Department of Agricultural Sciences, University of Naples Federico II, 80055 Portici, Italy
* Correspondence: javad.sharifirad@gmail.com (J.S.-R.); martorellpons@gmail.com (M.M.); ncmartins@med.up.pt (N.M.); rafcapas@unina.it (R.C.); Tel.: +98-21-88200104 (J.S.-R.); +56-41-266-1671 (M.M.); +351-22-5512100 (N.M.); +39-081-678664 (R.C.)

Received: 2 April 2019; Accepted: 13 May 2019; Published: 14 May 2019

Abstract: *Cucurbita* genus has received a renowned interest in the last years. This plant species, native to the Americas, has served worldwide folk medicine for treating gastrointestinal diseases and intestinal parasites, among other clinical conditions. These pharmacological effects have been increasingly correlated with their nutritional and phytochemical composition. Among those chemical constituents, carotenoids, tocopherols, phenols, terpenoids, saponins, sterols, fatty acids, and functional carbohydrates and polysaccharides are those occurring in higher abundance. However, more recently, a huge interest in a class of triterpenoids, cucurbitacins, has been stated, given its renowned biological attributes. In this sense, the present review aims to provide a detailed overview to the folk medicinal uses of *Cucurbita* plants, and even an in-depth insight on the latest advances with regards to its antimicrobial, antioxidant and anticancer effects. A special emphasis was also given to its clinical effectiveness in humans, specifically in blood glucose levels control in diabetic patients and pharmacotherapeutic effects in low urinary tract diseases.

Keywords: cucurbits; pumpkin; squash; antimicrobial; antioxidant; anticancer; traditional medicine

1. Introduction

Cucurbita plants have been applied in different cultures as traditional medication. For instance, Native Americans have used pumpkins for the treatment of intestinal worms and urinary ailments, this therapeutic strategy being approved by American doctors in the early nineteenth century as an anthelmintic for worms annihilating [1]. Seeds are used as an anthelmintic, to treat issues of the urinary framework, high blood pressure, to prevent the development of kidney stones, to ease prostate disorders and even to improve the erysipelas skin contamination [2]. In southeastern Europe, *Cucurbita pepo* L. (pumpkin) seeds have been applied to heal irritable bladder and prostate enlargement. Specifically, in Germany, the use of pumpkin seeds was adopted for application by the authority for irritated bladder conditions and micturition problems of prostate enlargement, although the monograph written in 1985 noted a lack of pharmacological studies that could confirm its effective clinical effects. On the other hand, in the USA, the purchase of all such non-prescription medications for the therapy of prostate enlargement was banned in 1990. In traditional Chinese medicine, *Cucurbita moschata* Duchesne seeds were also applied for handling the parasitic diseases caused by worms, while Mexican herbalists have used *Cucurbita ficifolia* Bouché as a remedy for reducing blood sugar levels [3–7].

Indeed, increasing evidence has shown that cucurbits' medicinal properties depend upon the chemical compounds present, which produce a specific physiological effect in the human body [8–10]. Specifically, cucurbits fruits are found to be beneficial in blood cleansing, purification of toxic substances and good for digestion, besides giving the required energy to improve human health. These species possess a higher amount of proteins, phytosterols [11,12], unsaturated fatty acids [13,14], vitamins (like carotenoids, tocopherols) [15] and microelements (e.g., zinc) [16]. Fruits, seeds and leaves from various *Cucurbita* members (pumpkin, watermelon, melon, cucumber squash, gourds, etc.) possess different pharmacological effects [17,18], such as antidiabetic [19–21], antiulcer, analgesic, nephroprotective [22] and anticancer activities [18]. In this sense, this review provides a detailed overview to the folk medicinal uses of *Cucurbita* plants, an in-depth insight on the latest advances regarding its antimicrobial, antioxidant and anticancer effects, and lastly, a special emphasis to its clinical effectiveness in humans, specifically in blood glucose levels control and low urinary tract diseases (Figure 1).

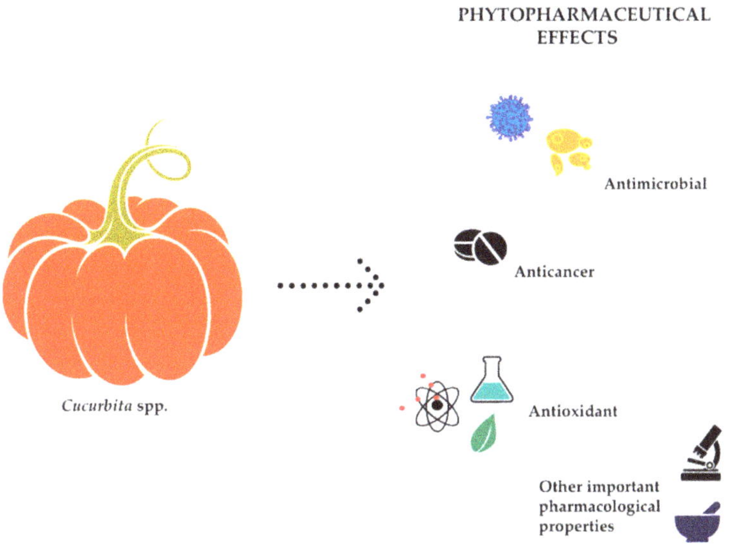

Figure 1. Most pronounced and investigated biological effects of *Cucurbita* spp.

2. *Cucurbita* Plants: A Brief Overview to Its Ethnopharmacological Uses

Recent ethnopharmacological studies showed that *C. pepo* and *Cucurbita maxima* Duchesne are among the most commonly used *Cucurbita* plants for traditional medicinal treatments. As shown in Table 1, many different components of *Cucurbita* plants are applied in diverse regions of the globe for handling different diseases.

Table 1. *Cucurbita* plants traditionally applied in the cures of different diseases in diverse regions of the world.

Scientific Name (Common Name)	Location	Local Name	Parts Used	Administration	Disease(s) Treatment	References
Cucurbita maxima Duchesne (Squash)	Basque Country, Iberian Peninsula	Kalabazea	Seeds	Oral	Digestive (Intestinal worms, Constipation)	[23]
	Mkuranga District, Tanzania	Maboga	Leaves	Oral	Anemia	[24]
	Polish people in Misiones, Argentina	Zapallo	Seeds	Oral	Intestinal parasites	[25]
	Nelliyampathy hills of Kerala, India	Parangi	Seeds	Oral	Vomiting blood, Blood bile	[26]
			Fruits	Oral	Urinal disorders	
			Flowers	Dermal	Cataract	
	Mauritius	Giromon	Seeds	Oral	Renal failure	[27]
			Fruits	Dermal	Wound	
	Agro Nocerino Sarnese, Campania, Southern Italy	Cocozza	Seeds	Oral	Prostatitis	[28]
	India	UNSP	Flowers	UNSP	Osteosarcoma	[29]
	Pakistani descent in Copenhagen, Denmark	Kadoo	Fruits	Oral	Blood pressure, constipation	[30]
	Ashanti region, Ghana	UNSP	Leaves	Oral	Cancer (lung, head)	[31]

Table 1. *Cont.*

Scientific Name (Common Name)	Location	Local Name	Parts Used	Administration	Disease(s) Treatment	References
Cucurbita pepo L. (Pumpkin)	Ghimbi District, Southwest Ethiopia	Buqqee	Seeds	Oral	Gonorrhea	[32]
	Mexico, Central America, Caribbean	Calabaza	Whole plant	Oral	Obesity	[33]
	Ripollès district, Pyrenees, Catalonia, Iberian Peninsula	Carbassa	Flowers	Dermal	Acne, Dermatitis, Ecchymosis, Fever, Toxicity, Wound Infection	[34]
			Fruits	Dermal		
	Nkonkobe Municipality, Eastern Cape, South Africa	Imithwane	Leaves	Oral	Arthritis, Blood booster	[35]
	West Bank, Palestine	Kare'a	Seeds	Oral	Breast cancer	[36]
	Delanta, Northwestern Wello, Northern Ethiopia	UNSP	Fruits	Oral	Gastritis, Stomachache	[37]
			Leaves	Dermal	Dandruff	
	Local Government Area, south-eastern Nigeria	Okeugu	Leaves	Oral	Malaria	[38]
Cucurbita galeottii Cogn. (Pumpkin)	Mauritius	Giraumon	Seeds	Oral	Mucous discharge	[39]

UNSP: Unspecified.

In particular, the positive health effects of *C. maxima* seeds are well-documented [23,25–28]. Raw *C. maxima* seeds are orally administered for the treatment of digestive disorders, such as intestinal worms [23,25], constipation [23] and vomiting blood and blood bile [26] by the local people in the Iberian Peninsula, Argentina and India, respectively. Also, sun-dried seeds of *C. maxima* are ingested in Mauritius for the treatment of renal failure [27], whereas raw seeds are consumed to treat prostatitis in the Agro Nocerino Sarnese in Campania, Southern Italy [28]. *C. maxima* seeds, fruits, flowers and leaves are also used as traditional medicine [24,26,27,29–31], where the treatment of urinary disorders, blood pressure regulation and prevention of constipation can be achieved with oral consumption of *C. maxima* fruits, and the wound healing with dermal application [26,27,30]. In Mkuranga district in Tanzania, *C. maxima* leaves are used for healing anemia [24], and in the Ashanti region in Ghana, this plant part is orally consumed for lung and head cancer treatment [31]. Furthermore, in Mauritius, *C. maxima* fruits are compressed externally on eyes against cataract [27], while in India the same petals are used to treat osteosarcoma [29]. Nonetheless, and to the authors knowledge, much is needed to support both the in vitro and in vivo biological effects of this plant, since most of the efforts has been made towards its agro-industrial applications.

With regards to *C. pepo* seeds, they are mainly regarded as agro-industrial wastes, while in some parts of the globe they are used raw, roasted or cooked, at a domestic scale [40]. Accordingly, in a study carried out in Ghimbi District in Southwest Ethiopia [32], it was reported that oral administration of cultivated seed of *C. pepo* is used as a gonorrhea therapy. Moreover, *C. pepo* seeds are also used as an herbal remedy by breast cancer patients in West Bank in Palestine [36]. In another study, conducted in Nkonkobe municipality in Eastern Cape, South Africa [35], it was indicated that arthritis and blood booster are treated with orally taken *C. pepo* leaves. *C. pepo* leaves are also used for the treatment of malaria and dandruff in the local government area in south-eastern Nigeria and Ghimbi District in Southwest Ethiopia, respectively [37,38]. In the latter study, it was also pointed out that the fruits of *C. pepo* are consumed to treat gastritis and stomachache [37]. Topical use of *C. pepo* fruit as an external antiseptic was reported in Ripollès district, the Pyrenees in Catalonia and Iberian Peninsula, whereas in the same location the flowers of this plant are used for antigenic, antidermatitic, antiecchymotic, antiophidian, antipyretic and anti-toxic purposes [34]. *C. pepo*, as the whole plant, is also applied in the folk medicine of Mesoamerica and Caribbean for the therapy of fitness due to its pancreatic lipase inhibition activity [33]. In addition to the above, the decoction prepared from the *Cucurbita galeottii* Cogn. seeds is used against mucous discharge in Mauritius [39].

3. *Cucurbita* Plants Phytochemical Composition

Carotenoids are highly present in the fruit of these plants, namely α-carotene, β-carotene, ζ-carotene, neoxanthin, violaxanthin, lutein, zeaxanthin, taraxanthin, luteoxanthin, auroxanthine, neurosporene, flavoxanthin, 5,6,5′,6′-diepoxy-β-carotene, phytofluene, α-cryptoxanthin and β-cryptoxanthin [41]. Total carotenoid content varied between 234.21 µg/g to 404.98 µg/g in *C. moschata* fruit [42], and 171.9 µg/g to 461.9 µg/g in *C. pepo* fruit [43]. There are also several publications on the carotenoid content of a number of *Cucurbita* plants such as *C. moschata*, *C. pepo* [42] and *C. maxima* [44]. Edible *Cucurbita* seeds are also rich in vitamin E (49.49 µg/g to 92.59 µg/g), γ-tocopherol is more abundant than α-tocopherol and the fruit contains less [45].

The study of Yang et al. [46] showed no flavonoid content (below detection limit: 0.05 mg/100 g) in either the immature or the mature fruit of *C. maxima*. Only the shoots and buds showed positive results. Sreeramulu and Raghunath [47] reported that average total phenolic content of *C. maxima* was 46.43 mg gallic acid equivalent (GAE)/100 g. In another study, *C. maxima* was analyzed for its flavonoid content and kaempferol was found to be the only flavonoid in this species at a concentration of 371.0 mg/kg of dry weight [48].

C. pepo was found to be very weak in polyphenol content. Only 0.02 mg GAE/100 mg sample has been found in its fresh fruit by Mongkolsilp et al. [49]. However, Iswaldi et al. [50] have reported for the first time a list of 34 polyphenols including a variety of flavonoids in the fruit of *C. pepo.*, in addition to other unknown polar compounds. Besides, the flowers of *C. pepo* may contain considerable amount of phenolic compounds. Andjelkovic et al. [51] studied the phenolic content of six pumpkin (*C. pepo*) seed oils and identified the following compounds: Tyrosol, vanillic acid, vanillin, ferulic acid and luteolin. Among them, tyrosol was the most abundant compound ranging from 1.6 mg/kg to 17.7 mg/kg.

Peričin et al. [52] studied the phenolic acid content of *C. pepo* seeds. *p*-Hydroxybenzoic acid was found to be the prevailing phenolic acid, with 34.72%, 67.38% and 51.80% of the total phenolic acid content in whole dehulled seed, kernels and hulls, respectively. Aside from p-hydroxybenzoic acid, the most dominant phenolic compounds can be listed in a decreasing order of quantity as follows: Caffeic, ferulic and vanillic acids in whole dehulled seeds. *Trans*-synapic and protocatechuic acids, and *p*-hydroxybenzaldehyde were the abundant phenolic acids presented in the kernels of hulled pumpkin variety; the hulls comprised p-hydroxybenzaldehyde, vanillic and protocatechuic acids with considerable amounts. Table 2 presents the main phenolic compounds found in the *Cucurbita* spp. and their structures.

Table 2. Main chemical structures of the phenolic compounds found in the *Cucurbita* spp.*.

Compound Name	Synonym(s)	Empirical Formula	Structure	References
Protocatechuic acid	3,4-Dihydroxybenzoic acid	$C_7H_6O_4$		[52] http://phenol-explorer.eu/compounds/412
***p*-Hydroxybenzoic acid**	4-Hydroxybenzoic acid	$C_7H_6O_3$		[52] http://phenol-explorer.eu/compounds/418
***p*-Hydroxybenzaldehyde**	4-Hydroxybenzaldehyde	$C_7H_6O_2$		[52] http://phenol-explorer.eu/compounds/725
Vanillic acid	4-Hydroxy-3-methoxybenzoic acid; *p*-Vanillic acid	$C_8H_8O_4$		[52] http://phenol-explorer.eu/compounds/414

Table 2. Cont.

Compound Name	Synonym(s)	Empirical Formula	Structure	References
Caffeic acid	3,4-Dihydroxycinnamic acid	$C_9H_8O_4$		[52] http://phenol-explorer.eu/compounds/457
Syringic acid	3,5-Dimethoxy-4-hydroxybenzoic acid	$C_9H_{10}O_5$		[52] http://phenol-explorer.eu/metabolites/420
trans-p-coumaric acid	trans-4-Hydroxycinnamic acid	$C_9H_8O_3$		[52] http://phenol-explorer.eu/compounds/454
Ferulic acid	3-Methoxy-4-Hydroxycinnamic acid; 3-Methylcaffeic acid; Coniferic acid	$C_{10}H_{10}O_4$		[52] http://phenol-explorer.eu/compounds/459

Table 2. Cont.

Compound Name	Synonym(s)	Empirical Formula	Structure	References
trans-sinapic acid	*trans*-4-Hydroxy-3,5-dimethoxy-cinnamic acid; *trans*-Sinapinic acid	$C_{11}H_{12}O_5$		[52] http://phenol-explorer.eu/compounds/464
Tyrosol	*p*-HPEA; 4-(2-Hydroxyethyl)phenol; 2-(4-Hydroxyphenyl)ethanol; 2,4-Hydroxyphenyl-ethyl-alcohol; 4-Hydroxyphenylethanol	$C_8H_{10}O_2$		[52] http://phenol-explorer.eu/compounds/673
Vanillin	4-Hydroxy-3-methoxy-benzoic aldehyde; Methylprotocatechuic aldehyde; Vanillic aldehyde; *p*-Vanillin	$C_8H_8O_3$		[52] http://phenol-explorer.eu/compounds/724

Table 2. Cont.

Compound Name	Synonym(s)	Empirical Formula	Structure	References
Luteolin	5,7,3′,4′-Tetrahydroxyflavone	$C_{15}H_{10}O_6$		[52] http://phenol-explorer.eu/compounds/229
Kaempferol	3,5,7,4′-Tetrahydroxyflavone	$C_{15}H_{10}O_6$		[52] http://phenol-explorer.eu/compounds/290

* The data were collected from the Phenol-Explorer database, which is an online comprehensive database on polyphenol contents in foods, http://phenol-explorer.eu (Accessed on 09.12.2018).

4. Looking at Cucurbita Plants Biological Activity

4.1. Antimicrobial Activity of Cucurbita Plants

4.1.1. In Vitro Studies

Pumpkin extracts showed a positive activity towards bacterial and fungal infections. They were effective against gram-positive: *Staphylococcus aureus, Bacillus subtilis,* as well as gram-negative bacterium: *Escherichia coli, Proteus vulgaris, Pseudomonas aeruginosa, Salmonella* spp. or *Klebsiella* spp. Pumpkin extracts also showed antibacterial activity against water borne bacteria *Vibrio cholerae* as well as intestinal flagellated parasite *Giardia lamblia*, often isolated from surface water. Other studies documented that pumpkin extracts showed a wide range of antifungal activity against species from the *Fusarium, Trichoderma, Aspergillus, Verticillium, Phytophora, Botrytis, Candida* and *Saccharomyces* genera (Table 3). However, the mechanisms of antimicrobial activity of pumpkin extracts are still unknown, although it seems to exist a synergistic action between all extracted bioactive substances. It is well known that plant extracts exert biological effects more prominent than their isolated compounds. In fact, recent evidence has established that, in whole matrices, the major compounds interact with those in trace amounts to potentiate their own potential, to provide additional properties other than those often recommended and even to help counterbalance the side effects of these isolated compounds. In addition, and not the least important to emphasize, is that such minor compounds by strengthening the biological effects of a specific bioactive also reduces the dose required to achieve a similar effect.

Table 3. Antimicrobial activity of *Cucurbita* spp. extracts evaluated in vitro.

Cucurbita spp./Plant Part	Extract	Microbial	References
Cucurbita pepo L. fruits	Water	*Escherichia coli*	[53]
Cucurbita pepo L. fruits	Methanol	*Bacillus cereus* *Bacillus subtilis* *Escherichia coli* *Enterobacter aerogenes* *Enterobacter agglomerans* *Salmonella enteritidis* *Salmonella choleraesuis* *Staphylococcus aureus* *Pseudomonas aeruginosa* *Enterobacter faecalis* *Klebsiella pneumoniae* *Bacillus sphericus* *Bacillus thruengenesis* *Cryptococcus meningitis* *Penicillium chrysogenum*	[54]
Cucurbita pepo L.	Phosphate buffered saline (PBS)	*Serratia marcescens* *Escherichia coli* *Streptococcus thermophilous* *Fusarium oxysporium* *Trichoderma reesei* *Aspergillus niger*	[55]
Cucurbita pepo L. fruits	Ethanol extract	*Heligmosoides bakeri* (worm)	[56]
Cucurbita pepo L. cortex	Water, methanol	*Staphylococcus aureus* *Escherichia coli* *Proteus mirabilis* *Klebsiella pneumoniae*	[57]

Table 3. Cont.

Cucurbita spp./Plant Part	Extract	Microbial	References
Cucurbita pepo L. seeds, backpeel	Methanol, ethanol	Staphylococcus aureus Salmonella typhi	[58]
Cucurbita pepo L. leaves	Ethanol	Serratia sp. Escherichia coli Klebsiella pneumoniae Bacillus subtilis	[59]
Cucurbita pepo L. leaves	Methanol	Providencia stuartii Pseudomonas aeruginosa Klebsiella pneumoniae Escherichia coli Enterobacter aerogenes Enterobacter cloacae	[60]
Cucurbita pepo L. leaves	Ethyl acetate, n-butanol, water	Bacillus subtilis Pseudomonas aeruginosa Staphylococcus aureus Candida albicans	[61]
Cucurbita moschata Duchesne seeds oil extract	Methanol	Rhodotorula rubra Trichoderma viride Penicillium chrysogenum Rhizopus oligosporus	[62]
Cucurbita moschata Duchesne crude protein from rinds, seeds and pulp	Acetone	Aspergillus fumigatus Aspergillus parasiticus Aspergillus niger Staphylococcus aureus Bacillus subtilis Klebsiella pneumoniae Pseudomonas aeruginosa Escherichia coli	[62]
Cucurbita maxima Duchesne fruit	Petroleum ether and methanol	Salmonella typhi, Giardia lamblia	[63]
Cucurbita maxima Duchesne flowers	Alcohol	Escherichia coli, Enterobacter faecalis, Bacillus cereus Curvularia lunata Candida albicans	[64]
Cucurbita maxima Duchesne peels	Water	Escherichia coli Pseudomonas sp. Vibrio cholerae Entamoeba histolytica	[65]
Cucurbita maxima Duchesne seeds	Ethanol	Staphylococcus aureus Bacillus subtilis Pseudomonas aeruginosa Escherichia coli Candida albicans Aspergillus niger	[66]
Cucurbita maxima Duchesne seeds	Ethanol	Staphylococcus aureus Bacillus subtilis Staphylococcus werneri Pseudomonas putida Pseudomonas aeruginosa Proteus mirabilis Escherichia coli Klebsiella pneumoniae	[67]

4.1.2. In Vivo Studies

Not only pumpkin extracts, but also proteins and peptides isolated from *Cucurbita* spp. were identified and characterized in terms of antimicrobial activity. Three pumpkin proteins inhibited the growth of fungi *Fusarium oxysporum*, *Verticillium dahliae* and *Saccharomyces cerevisiae* [68]. The antifungal peptide—cucurmoschin—isolated from black pumpkin seeds also demonstrated inhibitory activity against mold growth: *Botrytis cinerea*, *F. oxysporum* and *Mycosphaerella oxysporum* [69]. The ribosome-inactivating protein extracted from *C. moschata* showed an antimicrobial effect towards phytopathogenic fungi *Phytophora infestans* as well as against bacteria *Pseudomonas solanacearum* and *Erwinia amylovora* [70]. Additionally, PR-5 protein isolated from leaves of pumpkin, demonstrated synergism with combination of nikkomycin, a chitin synthase inhibitor, towards to *Candida albicans* [71]. Protein Pr-1 isolated from pumpkin rind inhibited the growth of plant pathogenic fungi, namely *B. cinerea*, *F. oxysporum*, *F. solani* and *Rhizoctonia solani*, as well as the opportunistic pathogenic yeast *C. albicans* [72]. These results demonstrate that the proteins from pumpkin may be of importance to clinical microbiology with a wide range of therapeutic applications (Table 4). As the most prominent ones, and given the current evidence, namely regarding its ability to trigger fungal membranes damages and to improve the plasma membranes permeability, they can be effectively used to combat fungal infections and even to use in combination with current antifungal agents, both to improve its effectiveness and even to reduce its side effects.

Table 4. In vitro antimicrobial activity of *Cucurbita* spp. proteins.

Cucurbita spp. Proteins	Microbial	References
Cucurbita maxima Duchesne seeds proteins	*Fusarium oxysporum*, *Verticillium dahliae* *Saccharomyces cerevisiae*	[68]
Cucurbita maxima Duchesne seeds protein RIP	*Phytophora infestans*, *Erwinia amylovora*, *Pseudomonas solanacearum*	[70]
Pumpkin leaves protein PR-5	*Candida albicans*	[71]
Pumpkin rind protein Pr-1	*Botrytis cinerea*, *Fusarium oxysporum*, *Fusarium solani*, *Rhizoctonia solani*, *Candida albicans*	[72]
Black pumpkin seeds protein cucurmoschin	*Botrytis cinerea*, *Fusarium oxysporum*, *Mycosphaerella oxysporum*	[69]

Pumpkin pulp, due to its antimicrobial properties, is widely used to relieve intestinal inflammation or stomach disorders [73] (Table 5). Pumpkin and its seeds, in the traditional world medicine, are often employed as an anti-helminthic remedy and for supportive therapy in functional diseases of the bladder as well as in the case of digestion problems. The usage of an extract of *C. pepo* cortex towards urinary tract infections may correspond to a new source of antibiotics against bacterial urinary tract infections [57]. Other studies represented the importance of oil from seeds of a pumpkin as a hopeful drug for treating wounds in vivo [74]. The researchers demonstrated a premium quality of pumpkin oil with a high quantity of polyunsaturated fatty acids, tocopherols that were able to perform efficient wound healing [74]. Morphometric evaluation and histological evidence in rats showed healed biopsies from pumpkin oil and a complete re-epithelialization with a recurrence of skin appendages and well re-growing collagen fibers out of cells inflammation.

Pumpkin-based foodstuff is well recognized as a source of anti-inflammatory remedies, which can be useful in arthritis treatment [75]. Pumpkin seed oil notably prevent adjuvant-induced arthritis in rats, similar to indomethacin, a well-known anti-inflammatory substance. Its clinical applicability as an antioxidant was also assessed on rheumatoid arthritis [76] and recently confirmed by Dixon [77].

Table 5. Antimicrobial property of *Cucurbita* spp. and its importance in vivo.

	Antimicrobial Property	References
Cucurbita pepo L. seeds	Wounds healing	[74]
Pumpkin seeds	Anthelmintic, treatment of bladder functional disorders	[78]
Pumpkin seed oil	Arthritis prevention	[75]
Pumpkin fruits	Control of gastrointestinal nematode infections	[56]
Cucurbita pepo L. cortex extract	Effective treatment of bacterial urinary tract infections	[57]

4.2. Anticancer Activities of Cucurbita Plants

Cucurbitacins are a unique gathering of triterpenoids that containing a cucurbitane basic structure skeleton, and an extensive variety of natural exercises is related with their substance basic multifaceted nature. Cucurbitacins have been accounted for the most secondary metabolites in the Cucurbitaceae. They have the biogenetically 10α-cucurbit-5-ene [19(10→19β) abeo-10α-lanostane skeleton, which is related to their cytotoxicity. A few reports credited in vitro and in vivo cytotoxic exercises to the cucurbitacins [79,80]. Jayaprakasam et al. [81] exhibited the anticancer properties of cucurbitacins B, D, E and I, confined from the products of *Cucurbita andreana* Naudin, towards colon, bosom, lung and focal sensory system disease cell lines. Cucurbitacin B is the most considered and keeping in mind that few investigations exhibited its viability in various models of malignant growth, incorporating into vivo tumor xenografts [82–85], there is a contradiction concerning the components hidden its anticancer action. Concealment of the oncogene STAT 3 (signal transducer and activator of transcription 3) has all the earmarks of being identified with tumor restraint [86], which does not prohibit elective. A malignant growth is in charge of 12% of the global impermanence. Medications incorporate chemotherapy medical procedure and radiation therapy. Be that as it may, chemotherapy endures constraints of medication obstruction, poisonous quality, reactions and lacking explicitness toward tumor cells [87]. Consequently, there is a solid enthusiasm for the utilization of plants as a promising wellspring of increasingly productive anticancer medications.

In Vitro Anticancer/Antitumor Effects

Presently over forty cucurbitacins have been isolated from the Cucurbitaceae family and different types of the herbs. The apoptotic impacts of cucurbitacins are expected of their capacity to change the qualities, transcriptional exercises using atomic components and mitochondrial trans-film potential and their ability to initiate or hinder ace or hostile to apoptotic proteins. Cucurbitacins are specific inhibitors of the JAK/STAT pathways; likewise, different instruments are involved in their apoptotic impacts, for example, PARP cleavage, MAPK pathway, articulation of dynamic caspase-3, diminished JAK3 and pSTAT3 levels and also diminishes in different downstream STAT3 targets, for example, Bcl-2, Mcl-1, cyclin D3 and Bclxl, which are all embroiled in the cell cycle control [88]. *C. pepo* alcohol extract demonstrated cytotoxicity towards HepG2 and CT26 cell lines with IC_{50} values 132.6 μg/mL and 167.2 μg/mL, individually. The ethanol extract of *C. pepo* was displayed a huge portion subordinate inhibitory impact towards HeLa cell development [89].

Cucurbita glycosides A and B isolated from *C. pepo* ethanol extract demonstrated cytotoxic action in vitro towards HeLa cells with IC_{50} 17.2 μg/mL and 28.5 μg/mL, individually [90]. Cucurbitacin B and E isolated from *C. pepo* cv *dayangua* demonstrated an antiproliferative in MCF-7, HCT-116, SF-268, A549 and NCI-H460 cell lines [81].

The antiproliferative impact of 23,24-dihydrocucurbitacin F, on human PCa cells may jump out at the enlistment of the cofilin-actin pole development and actin collection delivering to cell cytokinesis disappointment, hindered cell development cycle capture at G2/M stage and apoptosis [91]. Likewise, 23,24-dihydrocucurbitacin F has an inhibitory effect on Epstein-Barr infection actuation initiated by the tumor advertiser, 12-O-tetradecanoyl-phorbol-13-acetic acid derivation and furthermore, shows altogether hostile to tumor-advancement action on mouse skin tumor advancement [88].

Treatment with cucurbitacins B and E resulted in apoptosis and cell cycle capture of MDAMB-231 and MCF-7 breast cancer cell lines. Additionally, they tweaked the outflow of proteins associated with cell-cycle control in both of the estrogen-autonomous (MDA-MB-231) and estrogen-subordinate (MCF-7) in human bosom malignant growth cell lines. Growth hindrance and cytotoxic impact of cucurbitacin B on bosom disease cell lines SKBR-3 and MCF-7 were credited to G2/M stage capture and apoptosis. Cucurbitacin B treatment repressed Cyclin D1, c-Myc and β-catenin articulation levels, translocation to the core of β-catenin and galectin-3. Western smear investigation demonstrated expanded PARP cleavage proposing actuated caspase action and diminished mitogenic Wnt-related flagging particles galectin-3, β-catenin, c-Myc and cyclin D1 with changes in phosphorylated GSK-3β levels [92].

Cucurbitacin E caused disturbance of the cytoskeleton structure of actin and vimentin inhibiting the multiplication of prostate disease cells. Cucurbitacins also additionally hindered the expansion of endothelial cells joined by an interruption of the F-actin and tubulin microfilaments cytoskeleton, typical mitogen-prompted T-lymphocytes and lessened cell motility recommend an enemy of angiogenesis and hostile to the metastasis job for cucurbitacins. It is also fit for instigating and keeping up high multiplication rates in lymphocytes [93].

The literature has indicated that secondary metabolites of *C. pepo* have the potential anticancer activity, which represents great interest for the development of new chemotherapeutic agents for preventive growth of the tumor.

5. Clinical Effectiveness of *Cucurbita* Plants in Humans

5.1. Control of Blood Glucose Level in Diabetic Patients

Diabetes mellitus is a chronic disease characterized by changes in saccharide, lipid and protein metabolism resulting from a deficiency in insulin secretion from the pancreas, insulin resistance or both. The main clinical symptom is represented by increased blood sugar levels (hyperglycemia) that unconfrolled lead in time to a wide spectrum of complications [94]. Natural therapeutic alternatives to allopathic treatment always attracted the researchers to the intention of finding new drugs with fewer side effects [95–100]. Thus, the hypoglycemic effect of *Cucurbita* species (Table 6) is known and used for long traditional medicine in many countries, like China, India, Iran and Mexico [101–104].

Table 6. Pharmacotherapeutic effects of *Cucurbita* plants in human clinical studies.

	Part of the Plant with Active Compounds	*Cucurbita* spp.	References
Hypoglycemic	Polysaccharides from pulp fruit	*Cucurbita maxima* Duchesne *Cucurbita ficifolia* Bouché	[105,106]
	Non-pectines polysaccharides and pectines from pulp; proteins and oil from seeds	*Cucurbita ficifolia* Bouché	[107–109]
Reduced clinical symptoms of benign prostatic hyperplasia	Δ5-Δ7-Δ8-Phytosterols, unsaturated fatty acids from seeds extracts, lignans	*Cucurbita pepo* L.	[110–113]
Positive effects in stress urinary incontinence in female	Oil, sterols from seeds	*Cucurbita pepo* L.	[114,115]
Improved urinary symptoms in human overactive bladder	Seeds oil (sterols) blended with soy germ extract (phenols, isoflavones)	*Cucurbita pepo* L.	[116]
		Cucurbita maxima Duchesne	[117]

Mahmoodpoor et al. [106] in a recent study performed on patients with severe diabetes from the Intensive Care Unit showed the hypoglycemic effect of *C. maxima* pulp. The subjects received five grams of *C. maxima* powder per 12 h for three consecutive days. After the treatment, it was observed a decrease of serum glucose levels from 214.9 mg/dL to 214.9 mg/dL associated with a reduction of insulin doses from 48.05 IU to 39.5 IU [106]. *C. ficifolia* also showed a good hypoglycemic effect when the extract was administered in doses of 4 mL/kg to patients with type 2 diabetes and moderately elevated blood glucose level [105]. Five hours after administration, the mean of serum glucose level decreased from 217.2 mg/dL to 150.8 mg/dL [105].

The most important hypoglycemic active substances in pumpkin are non-pectines polysaccharides and pectines from pulp, proteins and oil obtained from seeds [107–109]. Alenazi et al. [118] reported a clinical case of a 12-year-old Asian diabetic patient that ate every day for four months 200 g of pumpkin. After two months of daily pumpkin consumption, a decrease of glycosylated hemoglobin (HbA1C) from 10.8% to 8.5% was observed [118]. The same positive hypoglycemic effect was also revealed in another study by Jain et al. [119]. Fourteen patients diagnosed with type 2 diabetes received *C. ficifolia* juice for 40 days, and glycosylated hemoglobin decreased with 22.5% [119]. Shi et al. [120] investigated the antidiabetic activity of pumpkin carbohydrate granules in patients with type 2 diabetes compared to a control placebo group. After one month of treatment, both blood and urine glucose levels were significantly decreased compared with the placebo control group [120]. The results of a randomized, placebo-controlled trial conducted showed that a rich diet in pumpkin (*C. maxima*) seeds significantly reduced postprandial blood glucose of adults with normal glycaemia [121]. This study included 25 normoglycemic adults who consumed daily 65 g of pumpkin seeds [121]. Possible mechanisms of antihyperglycemic action of *Cucurbita* species are not fully understood but several studies investigated this subject in the last decades. Zhang et al. [122] demonstrated that *C. moschata* heteropolysaccharides regenerate pancreatic islets by stimulating proliferation of pancreatic β-cells. Quanhong et al. [123] showed that polysaccharides bounded by protein (polysaccharide 41.21% and protein 10.13%) increase glucose tolerance level and reduce hyperglycemia. In the light of these results, supplements with natural extracts from *Cucurbita* plants can be considered as alternative hypoglycemic products and further multicenter randomized studies can confirm these results.

5.2. Pharmacotherapeutic Effects in Low Urinary Tract Diseases

Benign prostatic hyperplasia (BPH) represents an increase in the volume of the prostate under the influence of androgenic hormones, and 70% of aging men suffer from this condition. Since clinical evolution of urinary signs is slow, prevention of BPH is useful, phytotherapy being an alternative way [124]. For example, oil obtained from *C. pepo* seeds is traditionally used to treat urinary symptoms in BPH as the daily frequency of urination, nycturia, time of the bladder emptying and residual volume [110,111]. The main mechanism through which these effects are obtained is represented by the inhibition of 5-α-reductase. This enzyme is required to convert testosterone to dihydrotestosterone, which has a higher affinity than testosterone for androgen receptors. As a result, protein synthesis increases the volume of the prostate implicitly [113].

In a multicenter clinical trial, thousands of patients diagnosed with BPH were treated with capsules containing 500 mg of *C. pepo* seeds extracts. Their quality of life has been significantly improved by reducing the urinary symptoms of BPH [125].

Other modern studies have shown pharmacotherapeutic synergism in BPH when *C. Pepo* is administrated simultaneously with other plants. Thus, the combination with *Serenoa repens* (W. Bartram) Small significantly improved the urinary symptoms of BPH and decreased blood dihydrotestosterone levels [111]. Hong et al. [112] obtained similar results on urinary symptoms in Korean men with BPH treated with 320 mg of *C. pepo* plus 320 mg of *S. repens*. They also observed a decrease in prostatic antigen levels after the treatment, but without changes in prostate volume [112]. In a randomized Phase II clinical trial carried out by Coulson et al. [126] the efficacy of the ProstateEZE Max formulation obtained from a mixture of plants traditionally used in treating BPH was evaluated. ProstateEZE is a natural formulation containing *C. pepo*, *S. repens*, *Pygeum africanum* Hook.f., *E. parviflorum* Schreb. and lycopene. Fifty-seven male patients diagnosed with BPH were selected in the study. Thirty-two of them received a capsule of ProstateEZE Max daily for three consecutive months, and 25 patients were treated with a placebo. In patients treated with Prostate EZE, the clinical symptoms of BPH decreased by 35.9% compared with only 8.3% for the placebo. The frequency of nocturnal urination was reduced with 39.3% in subjects treated for three months with ProstateEZE compared to the placebo group [126].

Due to these beneficial therapeutic effects of *Cucurbita* plants in BPH, the European Medicines Agency approved the use of *C. pepo* for both BPH and other bladder disorders, such as urinary stress incontinence in women [127].

Urinary stress incontinence occurs when pelvic muscles that support the bladder and the sphincter muscle, which controls the urinary flow, are weakened. This disorder is associated with aging in women. The main symptom is urinary incontinence [115]. The seeds extract of *C. pepo* have a therapeutic effect in this condition through a double mechanism. Directly by relaxing the bladder muscles leading to a decrease in nycturia and indirectly through a hormonal mechanism by inhibiting 5-α reductase. This inhibition determines the anabolic effects that strengthen the bladder sphincter muscles [115,127]. The main chemical compounds in the pumpkin seeds that explain these effects are sterols (sitosterol, spinasterol) and fatty oil, which contain oleic, linoleic, palmitic acids and tocopherol) [114]. Gažová et al. [128] demonstrated these effects in a study of 86 women with urinary incontinence stress who were treated for twelve weeks with the preparation of a plant mix: *C. pepo*, *Equisetum arvense* L. and *Linum usitatissimum* L. Episodes of urinary incontinence during the day were reduced to 35% and nocturnal urinary frequency to 54% [128].

Overactive bladder syndrome (OAB) is characterized by the frequent urge to urinate during the day and night, followed by an involuntary loss of urine [116]. A human clinical trial conducted by Shim et al. (2014) investigated the efficacy and utility of Cucuflavone (tablets with a mixture of plant extracts 87.5% *C. pepo* seeds and 12.5% soy) in reducing OAB symptoms [116]. The active compounds of Cucuflavone are phenols (pyrogallol) and isoflavones (genistein, daidzin). One hundred and twenty patients were included in the study, divided into two groups: The Cucuflavone group and the placebo group. Patients from Cucuflavone group received two tablets twice a day (a total of 875 mg of *C. pepo* seed extract and 125 mg of soy extract daily) for twelve weeks. The final results of the investigation showed that urinary incontinence, the frequency of daily and nocturnal urination was statistically significantly reduced compared to the initial parameters [116]. In a recent investigation, Nishimura et al. obtained similar results. They confirmed the efficacy of *C. maxima* seeds oil on urinary disorders in OAB. Forty-five subjects with OAB were included and treated daily with 10 g of *C. maxima* seed oil for twelve weeks. At the end of the investigation, the frequency of average daily urination was reduced from 10.96 to 8.00 [117].

6. Conclusions and Future Perspectives

In short, the use of *Cucurbita* species and their active constituents in various clinical and pharmacological studies revealed the presence of multiple, effective and useful compounds, which provide the opportunity for further production of antidiabetic, analgesic, anti-inflammatory and cardioprotective drugs and foods. Indeed, the use of *Cucurbita* plants in the treatment of several diseases, including gastrointestinal disorders, intestinal parasites and hypertension, dates from a long time ago. The antimicrobial and antioxidant properties of these species have triggered a huge interest for multiple applications. First of all, free radicals are generated through various metabolic activities in the body, ultimately resulting in various deleterious diseases [99]. These diseases can be treated by supplementation of cucurbits as activities of some cucurbits are comparable with commercially available antibiotics. The present review markedly highlights that *Cucurbita* species have preventive and therapeutic abilities for treatment of different diseases. The presence of active phytochemicals in *Cucurbita* species further strengthens the opportunity for their application as an upcoming anticancer, antidiabetic, analgesic, anti-inflammatory and cardioprotective drugs, as well as foods. Finally, and not the least important, the application of Cucurbitaceae members in public health, as nutraceuticals is associated with great availability and a good safety profile.

Author Contributions: All authors contributed equally to this work. J.S.-R., M.M., N.M., and R.C., critically reviewed the manuscript. All the authors read and approved the final manuscript.

Funding: This research received no external funding.

Acknowledgments: This work was supported by CONICYT PIA/APOYO CCTE AFB170007. N. Martins would like to thank the Portuguese Foundation for Science and Technology (FCT-Portugal) for the Strategic project ref. UID/BIM/04293/2013 and "NORTE2020—Northern Regional Operational Program" (NORTE-01-0145-FEDER-000012) and C.F.R. for the project UID/EQU/00511/2019—Laboratory for Process Engineering, Environment, Biotechnology, and Energy—LEPABE funded by national funds through FCT/MCTES (PIDDAC).

Conflicts of Interest: The authors declare no conflict of interest.

References

1. Marie-Magdeleine, C.; Hoste, H.; Mahieu, M.; Varo, H.; Archimede, H. In vitro effects of *Cucurbita moschata* seed extracts on *Haemonchus contortus*. *Vet. Parasitol.* **2009**, *161*, 99–105. [CrossRef] [PubMed]
2. Yang, B.M.; Yang, S.T. A preliminary study on the cultivating technique of *Cucurbita pepo* cv Dayangua. *Spec. Econ. Amin. Plant* **2000**, *3*, 28–34.
3. Adnan, M.; Gul, S.; Batool, S.; Fatima, B.; Rehman, A.; Yaqoob, S.; Shabir, H.; Yousaf, T.; Mussarat, S.; Ali, N.; et al. A review on the ethnobotany, phytochemistry, pharmacology and nutritional composition of *Cucurbita pepo* L. *J. Phytopharm.* **2017**, *6*, 133–139.
4. Andolfo, G.; Di Donato, A.; Darrudi, R.; Errico, A.; Aiese Cigliano, R.; Ercolano, M.R. Draft of Zucchini (Cucurbita pepo L.) Proteome: A Resource for Genetic and Genomic Studies. *Front. Genet.* **2017**, *8*, 181. [CrossRef] [PubMed]
5. Dubey, S.D. Overview on Cucurbita maxima. *Int. J. Phytopharm.* **2012**, *2*, 68–71. [CrossRef]
6. Paris, H.S. Historical records, origins, and development of the edible cultivar groups of *Cucurbita pepo* (Cucurbitaceae). *Econ. Bot.* **1989**, *43*, 423–443. [CrossRef]
7. Ratnam, N. A review on Cucurbita pepo. *Int. J. Pharm. Phytochem. Res.* **2017**, *9*, 1190–1194. [CrossRef]
8. Salehi, B.; Valussi, M.; Jugran, A.K.; Martorell, M.; Ramírez-Alarcón, K.; Stojanović-Radić, Z.Z.; Antolak, H.; Kręgiel, D.; Mileski, K.S.; Sharifi-Rad, M.; et al. *Nepeta* species: From farm to food applications and phytotherapy. *Trends Food Sci. Technol.* **2018**, *80*, 104–122. [CrossRef]
9. Mishra, A.P.; Sharifi-Rad, M.; Shariati, M.A.; Mabkhot, Y.N.; Al-Showiman, S.S.; Rauf, A.; Salehi, B.; Župunski, M.; Sharifi-Rad, J.; Gusain, P.; et al. Bioactive compounds and health benefits of edible *Rumex* species-A review. *Cell. Mol. Biol.* **2018**, *64*, 27–34. [CrossRef]
10. Fapohunda, S.; Adewumi, A.; Jegede, D. Cucurbitaceae - the family that nourishes and heals. *MicroMedicine* **2018**, *6*, 85–93.
11. Phillips, K.M.; Ruggio, D.M.; Ashraf-Khorassani, M. Phytosterol composition of nuts and seeds commonly consumed in the United States. *J. Agric. Food Chem.* **2005**, *53*, 9436–9445. [CrossRef] [PubMed]
12. Ryan, E.; Galvin, K.; O'Connor, T.P.; Maguire, A.R.; O'Brien, N.M. Phytosterol, squalene, tocopherol content and fatty acid profile of selected seeds, grains, and legumes. *Plant Foods Hum. Nutr.* **2007**, *62*, 85–91. [CrossRef] [PubMed]
13. Applequist, W.L.; Avula, B.; Schaneberg, B.T.; Wang, Y.H.; Khan, I.A. Comparative fatty acid content of seeds of four *Cucurbita* species grown in a common (shared) garden. *J. Food Compos. Anal.* **2006**, *19*, 606–611. [CrossRef]
14. Sabudak, T. Fatty acid composition of seed and leaf oils of pumpkin, walnut, almond, maize, sunflower and melon. *Chem. Nat. Compd.* **2007**, *43*, 465–467. [CrossRef]
15. Stevenson, D.G.; Eller, F.J.; Wang, L.; Jane, J.L.; Wang, T.; Inglett, G.E. Oil and tocopherol content and composition of pumpkin seed oil in 12 cultivars. *J. Agric. Food Chem.* **2007**, *55*, 4005–4013. [CrossRef] [PubMed]
16. Glew, R.H.; Glew, R.S.; Chuang, L.T.; Huang, Y.S.; Millson, M.; Constans, D.; Vanderjagt, D.J. Amino acid, mineral and fatty acid content of pumpkin seeds (*Cucurbita* spp) and *Cyperus esculentus* nuts in the Republic of Niger. *Plant Foods Hum. Nutr.* **2006**, *61*, 49–54. [CrossRef]

17. Talukdar, S.N.; Hossain, M.N. Phytochemical, Phytotherapeutical and Pharmacological Study of *Momordica dioica*. *Evid.-Based Complement. Altern. Med.* **2014**, *2014*, 806082. [CrossRef]
18. Vijayakumar, M.; Eswaran, M.B.; Ojha, S.K.; Rao, C.V.; Rawat, A.K.S. Antiulcer activity of hydroalcohol extract of *Momordica dioica* roxb. Fruit. *Indian J. Pharm. Sci.* **2011**, *73*, 572–577. [CrossRef]
19. Chandrasekar, B.; Mukherjee, B.; Mukherjee, S.K. Blood sugar lowering potentiality of selected Cucurbitaceae plants of Indian origin. *Indian J. Med Res.* **1989**, *90*, 300–305. [PubMed]
20. Huseini, H.F.; Darvishzadeh, F.; Heshmat, R.; Jafariazar, Z.; Raza, M.; Larijani, B. The clinical investigation of *Citrullus colocynthis* (L.) schrad fruit in treatment of type II diabetic patients: A randomized, double blind, placebo-controlled clinical trial. *Phytother. Res.* **2009**, *23*, 1186–1189. [CrossRef]
21. Rashidi, A.A.; Mirhashemi, S.M.; Taghizadeh, M.; Sarkhail, P. Iranian medicinal plants for diabetes mellitus: A systematic review. *Pak. J. Biol. Sci.* **2013**, *16*, 401–411.
22. Jain, A.; Singhai, A.K. Effect of *Momordica dioica* Roxb on gentamicin model of acute renal failure. *Nat. Prod. Res.* **2010**, *24*, 1379–1389. [CrossRef]
23. Menendez-Baceta, G.; Aceituno-Mata, L.; Molina, M.; Reyes-García, V.; Tardío, J.; Pardo-De-Santayana, M. Medicinal plants traditionally used in the northwest of the Basque Country (Biscay and Alava), Iberian Peninsula. *J. Ethnopharmacol.* **2014**, *152*, 113–134. [CrossRef]
24. Peter, E.L.; Rumisha, S.F.; Mashoto, K.O.; Malebo, H.M. Ethno-medicinal knowledge and plants traditionally used to treat anemia in Tanzania: A cross sectional survey. *J. Ethnopharmacol.* **2014**, *154*, 767–773. [CrossRef]
25. Kujawska, M.; Pieroni, A. Plants used as food and medicine by polish migrants in Misiones, Argentina. *Ecol. Food Nutr.* **2015**, *54*, 255–279. [CrossRef]
26. Vijayakumar, S.; Morvin Yabesh, J.E.; Prabhu, S.; Manikandan, R.; Muralidharan, B. Quantitative ethnomedicinal study of plants used in the Nelliyampathy hills of Kerala, India. *J. Ethnopharmacol.* **2015**, *161*, 238–254. [CrossRef] [PubMed]
27. Mahomoodally, M.F.; Mootoosamy, A.; Wambugu, S. Traditional therapies used to manage diabetes and related complications in Mauritius: A comparative ethnoreligious study. *Evid.-Based Complement. Altern. Med.* **2016**, *2016*, 1–25. [CrossRef] [PubMed]
28. Motti, R.; Motti, P. An ethnobotanical survey of useful plants in the agro Nocerino Sarnese (Campania, southern Italy). *Hum. Ecol.* **2017**, *45*, 865–878. [CrossRef]
29. Nayak, D.; Ashe, S.; Rauta, P.R.; Nayak, B. Assessment of antioxidant, antimicrobial and anti-osteosarcoma potential of four traditionally used Indian medicinal plants. *J. Appl. Biomed.* **2017**, *15*, 119–132. [CrossRef]
30. Ramzan, S.; Soelberg, J.; Jäger, A.K.; Cantarero-Arévalo, L. Traditional medicine among people of Pakistani descent in the capital region of Copenhagen. *J. Ethnopharmacol.* **2017**, *196*, 267–280. [CrossRef] [PubMed]
31. Agyare, C.; Spiegler, V.; Asase, A.; Scholz, M.; Hempel, G.; Hensel, A. An ethnopharmacological survey of medicinal plants traditionally used for cancer treatment in the Ashanti region, Ghana. *J. Ethnopharmacol.* **2018**, *212*, 137–152. [CrossRef] [PubMed]
32. Balcha, A. Medicinal plants used in traditional medicine by Oromo people, Ghimbi District, Southwest Ethiopia. *J. Ethnobiol. Ethnomed.* **2014**, *10*, 1–15.
33. Alonso-Castro, A.J.; Dominguez, F.; Zapata-Morales, J.R.; Carranza-Alvarez, C. Plants used in the traditional medicine of Mesoamerica (Mexico and Central America) and the Caribbean for the treatment of obesity. *J. Ethnopharmacol.* **2015**, *175*, 335–345. [CrossRef] [PubMed]
34. Rigat, M.; Vallès, J.; Dambrosio, U.; Gras, A.; Iglésias, J.; Garnatje, T. Plants with topical uses in the Ripollès district (Pyrenees, Catalonia, Iberian Peninsula): Ethnobotanical survey and pharmacological validation in the literature. *J. Ethnopharmacol.* **2015**, *164*, 162–179. [CrossRef] [PubMed]
35. Asowata-Ayodele, A.M.; Afolayan, A.J.; Otunola, G.A. Ethnobotanical survey of culinary herbs and spices used in the traditional medicinal system of Nkonkobe Municipality, Eastern Cape, South Africa. *South Afr. J. Bot.* **2016**, *104*, 69–75. [CrossRef]
36. Jaradat, N.A.; Shawahna, R.; Eid, A.M.; Al-Ramahi, R.; Asma, M.K.; Zaid, A.N. Herbal remedies use by breast cancer patients in the West Bank of Palestine. *J. Ethnopharmacol.* **2016**, *178*, 1–8. [CrossRef]
37. Meragiaw, M.; Asfaw, Z.; Argaw, M. The Status of Ethnobotanical Knowledge of Medicinal Plants and the Impacts of Resettlement in Delanta, Northwestern Wello, Northern Ethiopia. *Evid.-Based Complement. Altern. Med.* **2016**, *2016*, 5060247. [CrossRef]

38. Odoh, U.E.; Uzor, P.F.; Eze, C.L.; Akunne, T.C.; Onyegbulam, C.M.; Osadebe, P.O. Medicinal plants used by the people of Nsukka Local Government Area, south-eastern Nigeria for the treatment of malaria: An ethnobotanical survey. *J. Ethnopharmacol.* **2018**, *218*, 1–15. [CrossRef]
39. Suroowan, S.; Mahomoodally, M.F. A comparative ethnopharmacological analysis of traditional medicine used against respiratory tract diseases in Mauritius. *J. Ethnopharmacol.* **2016**, *177*, 61–80. [CrossRef]
40. Peiretti, P.G.; Meineri, G.; Gai, F.; Longato, E.; Amarowicz, R. Antioxidative activities and phenolic compounds of pumpkin (*Cucurbita pepo*) seeds and amaranth (*Amaranthus caudatus*) grain extracts. *Nat. Prod. Res.* **2017**, *31*, 2178–2182. [CrossRef] [PubMed]
41. Azevedo-Meleiro, C.H.; Rodriguez-Amaya, D.B. Qualitative and quantitative differences in carotenoid composition among Cucurbita moschata, Cucurbita maxima, and Cucurbita pepo. *J. Agric. Food Chem.* **2007**, *55*, 4027–4033. [CrossRef] [PubMed]
42. Maria, L.; Carvalho, J.D.; Barros, P.; Luiz, R.; Godoy, D.O.; Pacheco, S.; Henrique, P.; Luiz, J.; Carvalho, V.D.; Regini, M.; et al. Total carotenoid content, α-carotene and β-carotene, of landrace pumpkins (*Cucurbita moschata* Duch): A preliminary study. *Food Res. Int.* **2012**, *47*, 337–340.
43. Perez Gutierrez, R.M. Review of Cucurbita pepo (Pumpkin) its Phytochemistry and Pharmacology. *Med. Chem.* **2016**, *6*, 12–21. [CrossRef]
44. Chandrika, U.G.; Basnayake, B.M.L.B.; Athukorala, I.; Colombagama, P.W.N.M.; Goonetilleke, A. Carotenoid Content and In Vitro Bioaccessibility of Lutein in Some Leafy Vegetables Popular in Sri Lanka. *J. Nutr. Sci. Vitaminol.* **2010**, *56*, 203–207. [CrossRef]
45. Mi, Y.K.; Eun, J.K.; Young-Nam, K.; Changsun, C.; Bo-Hieu, L. Comparison of the chemical compositions and nutritive values of various pumpkin (Cucurbitaceae) species and parts. *Nutr. Res. Pract.* **2012**, *6*, 21–27. [CrossRef]
46. Yang, R.Y.; Lin, S.; Kuo, G. Content and distribution of flavonoids among 91 edible plant species. *Asia Pac. J. Clin. Nutr.* **2008**, *17*, 275–279.
47. Sreeramulu, D.; Raghunath, M. Antioxidant activity and phenolic content of roots, tubers and vegetables commonly consumed in India. *Food Res. Int.* **2010**, *43*, 1017–1020. [CrossRef]
48. Koo, M.H.; Suhaila, M. Flavonoid (Myricetin, Quercetin, Kaempferol, Luteolin and Apigenin) Content of Edible Tropical Plants. *J. Agric. Food Chem.* **2001**, *49*, 3106–3112.
49. Mongkolsilp, S.; Pongbupakit, I.; Sae-Lee, N.; Sitthihaworm, W.; Article, O. Radical Scavenging Activity and Total Phenolic Content of Medicinal Plants Used in Primary Health Care Savitree Mongkolsilp, Isara Pongbupakit, Nittaya Sae-Lee and Worapan Sitthithaworn. *Swu J. Pharm. Sci.* **2004**, *9*, 32–35.
50. Iswaldi, I.; Gómez-Caravaca, A.M.; Lozano-Sánchez, J.; Arráez-Román, D.; Segura-Carretero, A.; Fernández-Gutiérrez, A. Profiling of phenolic and other polar compounds in zucchini (Cucurbita pepo L.) by reverse-phase high-performance liquid chromatography coupled to quadrupole time-of-flight mass spectrometry. *Food Res. Int.* **2013**, *50*, 77–84. [CrossRef]
51. Andjelkovic, M.; Van Camp, J.; Trawka, A.; Verhé, R. Phenolic compounds and some quality parameters of pumpkin seed oil. *Eur. J. Lipid Sci. Technol.* **2010**, *112*, 208–217. [CrossRef]
52. Peričin, D.; Krimer, V.; Trivić, S.; Radulović, L. The distribution of phenolic acids in pumpkin's hull-less seed, skin, oil cake meal, dehulled kernel and hull. *Food Chem.* **2009**, *113*, 450–456. [CrossRef]
53. El-Kamali, H.H.; Mahjoub, S.A.T. Antibacterial activity of Francoeuria crispa, Pulicaria undulata, Ziziphus spina-christi and Cucurbita pepo against seven standard pathogenic bacteria. *Ethnobot. Leafl.* **2009**, *13*, 722–733.
54. Dubey, A.; Mishra, N.; Singh, N. Antimicrobial activity of some selected vegetables. *Int. J. Appl. Biol. Pharm. Technol.* **2010**, *1*, 994–999.
55. Sood, A.; Kaur, P.; Gupta, R. Phytochemical screening and antimicrobial assay of various seeds extract of Cucurbitaceae family. *Int. J. Appl. Biol. Pharm. Technol.* **2012**, *3*, 401–409.
56. Grzybek, M.; Kukula-Koch, W.; Strachecka, A.; Jaworska, A.; Phiri, A.M.; Paleolog, J.; Tomczuk, K. Evaluation of anthelmintic activity and composition of pumpkin (*Cucurbita pepo* L.) seed extracts—in vitro and in vivo studies. *Int. J. Mol. Sci.* **2016**, *17*, 1456. [CrossRef]
57. Al-Ghazal, A.T. Evaluation of Antibacterial Effect of *Cucurbita pepo* (Yakten) Extracts on Multi-antibiotic Resistance Bacterial Strains Isolated From Human Urinary Tract Infections. *Rafidain J. Sci.* **2012**, *23*, 1–7.
58. Chonoko, U.G.; Rufai, A.B. Phytochemical screening and antibacterial activity of *Curbita pepo* (Pumpkin) against *Staphylococcus aureus* and *Salmonella typhi*. *J. Pure Appl. Sci.* **2011**, *4*, 145–147.

59. Jasim, S.; Alwan, A.N.; Altimimi, H.W.; Kareem, K.H. Evaluation of antimicrobial activity of flavonoids extract from *Cucurbita pepo* leaves. *Bas. J. Vet. Res.* **2010**, *9*, 10–17.
60. Noumedem, J.A.K.; Mihasan, M.; Lacmata, S.T.; Stefan, M.; Kuiate, J.R.; Kuete, V. Antibacterial activities of the methanol extracts of ten Cameroonian vegetables against Gram-negative multidrug-resistant bacteria. *BMC Complement. Altern. Med.* **2013**, *13*, 26. [CrossRef]
61. Dar, A.H.; Sofi, S.A. Pumpkin the functional and therapeutic ingredient: A review. *Int. J. Food Sci. Nutr.* **2017**, *2*, 165–170.
62. Abed El-Aziz, A.; Abed El-Aziz, H. Antimicrobial proteins and oil seeds from pumpkin. *Nat. Sci.* **2011**, *9*, 105–119.
63. Elhadi, I.M.; Koko, S.W.; Dahab, M.M.; El Imam, J.M.; El Mageed, M.A.E. Antigiardial activity of some *Cucurbita* species and *Lagenaria siceraria*. *J. For. Prod. Ind.* **2013**, *2*, 43–47.
64. Muruganantham, N.; Solomon, S.; Senthamilselvi, M.M. Anti-cancer activity of *Cucumis sativus* (cucumber) flowers against human liver cancer. *Int. J. Pharm. Clin. Res.* **2016**, *8*, 39–41.
65. Geetha, S. Antimicrobial activity of selected vegetable peels against water borne pathogens. *Int. J. Adv. Pharm. Biol. Chem.* **2014**, *3*, 937–940.
66. Kabbashi, A.S.; Koko, W.S.; Mohammed, S.E.A.; Musa, N.; Elbadri, E.; Dahab, M.M.; Mohammed, A.K. In vitro a moebicidal, antimicrobial and antioxidant activities of the plants *Adansonia digitata* and *Cucurbit maxima*. *Adv. Med. Plant Res.* **2014**, *2*, 50–57.
67. Ravishankar, K.; Kiranmayi, G.V.N.; Appa Reddy, G.V.; Sowjanya, V.V.L.; Baba Sainadh, V.; Lakshmi, V.G.; Prasad, T. Preliminary phytochemical screening and *In-vitro* antibacterial activity of *Cucurbita maxima* seed extract. *Int. J. Res. Pharm. Chem.* **2012**, *2*, 86–91.
68. Cassel, C.K. Policy challenges and clinical practices. *Hosp. Pract.* **1993**, *28*, 9–10. [CrossRef]
69. Wang, H.X.; Ng, T.B. Isolation of cucurmoschin, a novel antifungal peptide abundant in arginine, glutamate and glycine residues from black pumpkin seeds. *Peptides* **2003**, *24*, 969–972. [CrossRef]
70. Barbieri, L.; Polito, L.; Bolognesi, A.; Ciani, M.; Pelosi, E.; Farini, V.; Stirpe, F. Ribosome-inactivating proteins in edible plants and purification and characterization of a new ribosome-inactivating protein from *Cucurbita moschata*. *Biochim. Biophys. Acta* **2006**, *760*, 783–792. [CrossRef]
71. Cheong, N.E.; Choi, Y.O.; Kim, W.Y.; Bae, I.S.; Cho, M.J.; Hwang, I.; Lee, S.Y. Purification and characterization of an antifungal PR-5 protein from pumpkin leaves. *Mol. Cells* **1997**, *7*, 214–219.
72. Park, S.C.; Lee, J.R.; Kim, J.Y.; Hwang, I.; Nah, J.W.; Cheong, H.; Hahm, K.S. Pr-1, a novel antifungal protein from pumpkin rinds. *Biotechnol. Lett.* **2009**, *32*, 125–130. [CrossRef] [PubMed]
73. Karanja, J.; Mugendi, J.; Muchugi, A.; Karanja, J.K.; Mugendi, B.J.; Khamis, F.M.; Muchugi, A.N. Nutritional evaluation of some kenyan pumpkins (*Cucurbita* spp.). *Int. J. Agric. For.* **2016**, *4*, 195–200.
74. Bardaa, S.; Ben Halima, N.; Aloui, F.; Ben Mansour, R.; Jabeur, H.; Bouaziz, M.; Sahnoun, Z. Oil from pumpkin (*Cucurbita pepo* L.) seeds: Evaluation of its functional properties on wound healing in rats. *Lipids Health Dis.* **2016**, *15*, 783–792. [CrossRef]
75. Seo, J.S.; Burri, B.J.; Quan, Z.; Neidlinger, T.R. Extraction and chromatography of carotenoids from pumpkin. *J. Chromatogr. A* **2005**, *1073*, 371–375. [CrossRef] [PubMed]
76. van Vugt, R.M.; Rijken, P.J.; Rietveld, A.G.; van Vugt, A.C.; Dijkmans, B.A.C. Antioxidant intervention in rheumatoid arthritis: Results of an open pilot study. *Clin. Rheumatol.* **2008**, *27*, 771–775. [CrossRef]
77. Dixon, W.G. Rheumatoid arthritis: Biological drugs and risk of infection. *Lancet* **2015**, *386*, 224–225. [CrossRef]
78. Fokou, E.A.M. Preliminary nutritional evaluation of five species of egusi seeds in Cameroon. *Afr. J. Food Agric. Nutr. Dev.* **2004**, *4*, 1–11. [CrossRef]
79. Duncan, K.L.K.; Duncan, M.D.; Alley, M.C.; Sausville, E.A. Cucurbitacin E-induced disruption of the actin and vimentin cytoskeleton in prostate carcinoma cells. *Biochem. Pharmacol.* **1996**, *52*, 1553–1560. [CrossRef]
80. Fang, X.; Phoebe, C.H.; Pezzuto, J.M.; Fong, H.H.; Farnsworth, N.R.; Yellin, B.; Hecht, S.M. Plant anticancer agents, XXXIV. Cucurbitacins from *Elaeocarpus dolichostylus*. *J. Nat. Prod.* **1984**, *47*, 988–993. [CrossRef] [PubMed]
81. Jayaprakasam, B.; Seeram, N.P.; Nair, M.G. Anticancer and antiinflammatory activities of cucurbitacins from *Cucurbita andreana*. *Cancer Lett.* **2003**, *189*, 11–16. [CrossRef]
82. Chan, K.T.; Meng, F.Y.; Li, Q.; Ho, C.Y.; Lam, T.S.; To, Y.; Toh, M. Cucurbitacin B induces apoptosis and S phase cell cycle arrest in BEL-7402 human hepatocellular carcinoma cells and is effective via oral administration. *Cancer Lett.* **2010**, *294*, 118–124. [CrossRef] [PubMed]

83. Liu, T.; Zhang, M.; Zhang, H.; Sun, C.; Deng, Y. Inhibitory effects of cucurbitacin B on laryngeal squamous cell carcinoma. *Eur. Arch. Oto-Rhino-Laryngol.* **2008**, *265*, 1225–1232. [CrossRef]
84. Wakimoto, N.; Yin, D.; O'Kelly, J.; Haritunians, T.; Karlan, B.; Said, J.; Koeffler, H.P. Cucurbitacin B has a potent antiproliferative effect on breast cancer cells in vitro and in vivo. *Cancer Sci.* **2008**, *99*, 1793–1797. [CrossRef]
85. Zhang, M.; Zhang, H.; Sun, C.; Shan, X.; Yang, X.; Li-Ling, J.; Deng, Y. Targeted constitutive activation of signal transducer and activator of transcription 3 in human hepatocellular carcinoma cells by cucurbitacin B. *Cancer Chemother. Pharmacol.* **2009**, *63*, 635–642. [CrossRef] [PubMed]
86. Chan, K.T.; Li, K.; Liu, S.L.; Chu, K.H.; Toh, M.; Xie, W.D. Cucurbitacin B inhibits STAT3 and the Raf/MEK/ERK pathway in leukemia cell line K562. *Cancer Lett.* **2010**, *289*, 46–52. [CrossRef] [PubMed]
87. Carvalho, L.J.; Smiderle, L.A.S.; Carvalho, J.L.V.; Cardoso, F.S.N.; Koblitz, M.G.B. Assessment of carotenoids in pumpkins after different home cooking conditions. *Food Sci. Technol.* **2014**, *34*, 365–370. [CrossRef]
88. Konoshima, T.; Takasaki, M.; Kozuka, M.; Nagao, T.; Okabe, H.; Irino, N.; Nishino, H. Inhibitory effects of cucurbitane triterpenoids on Epstein-Barr virus activation and two-stage carcinogenesis of skin tumor. *Biol. Pharm. Bull.* **1994**, *18*, 284–287. [CrossRef]
89. Shokrzadeh, M.; Azadbakht, M.; Ahangar, N.; Hashemi, A.; Saravi, S. Cytotoxicity of hydro-alcoholic extracts of *Cucurbita pepo* and *Solanum nigrum* on HepG2 and CT26 cancer cell lines. *Pharmacogn. Mag.* **2010**, *6*, 176. [CrossRef]
90. Wang, D.C.; Xiang, H.; Li, D.; Gao, H.; Cai, H.; Wu, L.J.; Deng, X.M. Purine-containing cucurbitane triterpenoids from *Cucurbita pepo* cv dayangua. *Phytochemistry* **2008**, *69*, 1434–1438. [CrossRef]
91. Ren, S.; Ouyang, D.Y.; Saltis, M.; Xu, L.H.; Zha, Q.B.; Cai, J.Y.; He, X.H. Anti-proliferative effect of 23,24-dihydrocucurbitacin F on human prostate cancer cells through induction of actin aggregation and cofilin-actin rod formation. *Cancer Chemother. Pharmacol.* **2012**, *70*, 415–424. [CrossRef]
92. Dakeng, S.; Duangmano, S.; Jiratchariyakul, W.; U-Pratya, Y.; Bögler, O.; Patmasiriwat, P. Inhibition of Wnt signaling by cucurbitacin B in breast cancer cells: Reduction of Wnt-associated proteins and reduced translocation of galectin-3-mediated β-catenin to the nucleus. *J. Cell. Biochem.* **2012**, *113*, 49–60. [CrossRef]
93. Attard, E.; Cuschieri, A.; Scicluna-Spiteri, A.; Brincat, M.P. The effects of cucurbitacin E on two lymphocyte models. *Pharm. Biol.* **2004**, *42*, 170–175. [CrossRef]
94. Alam, U.; Asghar, O.; Azmi, S.; Malik, R.A. General aspects of diabetes mellitus. *Handb. Clin. Neurol.* **2014**, *126*, 211–222. [PubMed]
95. Sharifi-Rad, M.; Fokou, P.V.T.; Sharopov, F.; Martorell, M.; Ademiluyi, A.O.; Rajkovic, J.; Salehi, B.; Martins, N.; Iriti, M.; Sharifi-Rad, J. Antiulcer agents: From plant extracts to phytochemicals in healing promotion. *Molecules* **2018**, *23*, 1751. [CrossRef] [PubMed]
96. Mishra, A.P.; Saklani, S.; Salehi, B.; Parcha, V.; Sharifi-Rad, M.; Milella, L.; Iriti, M.; Sharifi-Rad, J.; Srivastava, M. *Satyrium nepalense*, a high altitude medicinal orchid of Indian Himalayan region: Chemical profile and biological activities of tuber extracts. *Cell. Mol. Biol.* **2018**, *64*, 35–43. [CrossRef]
97. Sharifi-Rad, M.; Nazaruk, J.; Polito, L.; Morais-Braga, M.F.B.; Rocha, J.E.; Coutinho, H.D.M.; Salehi, B.; Tabanelli, G.; Montanari, C.; del Mar Contreras, M.; et al. *Matricaria* genus as a source of antimicrobial agents: From farm to pharmacy and food applications. *Microbiol. Res.* **2018**, *215*, 76–88. [CrossRef]
98. Sharifi-Rad, J.; Tayeboon, G.S.; Niknam, F.; Sharifi-Rad, M.; Mohajeri, M.; Salehi, B.; Iriti, M.; Sharifi-Rad, M. *Veronica persica* Poir. extract - antibacterial, antifungal and scolicidal activities, and inhibitory potential on acetylcholinesterase, tyrosinase, lipoxygenase and xanthine oxidase. *Cell. Mol. Biol.* **2018**, *64*, 50–56. [CrossRef] [PubMed]
99. Sharifi-Rad, M.; Ozcelik, B.; Altın, G.; Daşkaya-Dikmen, C.; Martorell, M.; Ramírez-Alarcón, K.; Alarcón-Zapata, P.; Morais-Braga, M.F.B.; Carneiro, J.N.P.; Alves Borges Leal, A.L.; et al. *Salvia* spp. plants-from farm to food applications and phytopharmacotherapy. *Trends Food Sci. Technol.* **2018**, *80*, 242–263. [CrossRef]
100. Salehi, B.; Sharopov, F.; Martorell, M.; Rajkovic, J.; Ademiluyi, A.O.; Sharifi-Rad, M.; Fokou, P.V.T.; Martins, N.; Iriti, M.; Sharifi-Rad, J. Phytochemicals in Helicobacter pylori infections: What are we doing now? *Int. J. Mol. Sci.* **2018**, *19*. [CrossRef] [PubMed]
101. Caili, F.; Huan, S.; Quanhong, L. A review on pharmacological activities and utilization technologies of pumpkin. *Plant Foods Hum. Nutr.* **2006**, *61*, 73–80. [CrossRef] [PubMed]

102. Andrade-Cetto, A.; Heinrich, M. Mexican plants with hypoglycaemic effect used in the treatment of diabetes. *J. Ethnopharmacol.* **2005**, *99*, 325–348. [CrossRef]
103. Jia, W.; Gao, W.; Tang, L. Antidiabetic herbal drugs officially approved in China. *Phytother. Res.* **2003**, *17*, 1127–1134. [CrossRef] [PubMed]
104. Mukherjee, P.K.; Maiti, K.; Mukherjee, K.; Houghton, P.J. Leads from Indian medicinal plants with hypoglycemic potentials. *J. Ethnopharmacol.* **2006**, *106*, 1–28. [CrossRef]
105. Acosta-Patiño, J.L.; Jiménez-Balderas, E.; Juárez-Oropeza, M.A.; Díaz-Zagoya, J.C. Hypoglycemic action of *Cucurbita ficifolia* on Type 2 diabetic patients with moderately high blood glucose levels. *J. Ethnopharmacol.* **2001**, *77*, 99–101. [CrossRef]
106. Mahmoodpoor, A.; Medghalchi, M.; Nazemiyeh, H.; Asgharian, P.; Shadvar, K.; Hamishehkar, H. Effect of *Cucurbita maxima* on control of blood glucose in diabetic critically ill patients. *Adv. Pharm. Bull.* **2018**, *8*, 347–351. [CrossRef]
107. Adams, G.G.; Imran, S.; Wang, S.; Mohammad, A.; Kok, S.; Gray, D.A.; Harding, S.E. The hypoglycaemic effect of pumpkins as anti-diabetic and functional medicines. *Food Res. Int.* **2011**, *44*, 862–867. [CrossRef]
108. Cai, T.; Li, Q.; Yan, H.; Li, N. Study on the hypoglycemic action of pumpkin seed protein. *J. Chin. Inst. Food Sci. Technol.* **2003**, *3*, 7–11.
109. Xiong, X.; Cao, J. Study of extraction and isolation of effective pumpkin polysaccharide component and its reducing glycemia function. *Chin. J. Mod. Appl. Pharm.* **2001**, *18*, 662–664.
110. Gossell-Williams, M.; Davis, A.; O'Connor, N. Inhibition of testosterone-induced hyperplasia of the prostate of sprague-dawley rats by pumpkin seed oil. *J. Med. Food* **2006**, *9*, 284–286. [CrossRef]
111. *PDR for Herbal Medicines*, 4th ed.; Thomson Healthcare: Montvale, NJ, USA, 2007.
112. Hong, H.; Kim, C.S.; Maeng, S. Effects of pumpkin seed oil and saw palmetto oil in Korean men with symptomatic benign prostatic hyperplasia. *Nutr. Res. Pract.* **2009**, *3*, 323. [CrossRef] [PubMed]
113. Ramak, P.; Mahboubi, M. The beneficial effects of pumpkin (*Cucurbita pepo* L.) seed oil for health condition of men. *Food Rev. Int.* **2018**, 1–11. [CrossRef]
114. Rezig, L.; Chouaibi, M.; Msaada, K.; Hamdi, S. Chemical composition and profile characterisation of pumpkin (*Cucurbita maxima*) seed oil. *Ind. Crop. Prod.* **2012**, *37*, 82–87. [CrossRef]
115. Sogabe, H.; Terado, T. Open clinical study of effects of pumpkin seed extract/soybean germ extract vixture-containing processed food on nocturia. *Jpn. J. Med. Pharm. Sci.* **2001**, *46*, 727–737.
116. Shim, B.; Jeong, H.; Lee, S.; Hwang, S.; Moon, B.; Storni, C. A randomized double-blind placebo-controlled clinical trial of a product containing pumpkin seed extract and soy germ extract to improve overactive bladder-related voiding dysfunction and quality of life. *J. Funct. Foods* **2014**, *8*, 111–117. [CrossRef]
117. Nishimura, M.; Ohkawara, T.; Sato, H.; Takeda, H.; Nishihira, J. Pumpkin seed oil extracted from *Cucurbita maxima* improves urinary disorder in human overactive bladder. *J. Tradit. Complement. Med.* **2014**, *4*, 72–74. [CrossRef] [PubMed]
118. Alenazi, B.; Deeb, A.; Alrowaili, A.; Alkhaldi, A.; Alanazi, A. Does pumpkin affect glycemic control in diabetic patient. Case report and literature review. *Eur. J. Pharm. Med. Res.* **2017**, *4*, 42–45.
119. Jain, A.; Mishra, M.; Yadav, D.; Khatarker, D.; Jadaun, P.; Tiwari, A.; Prasad, G. Evaluation of the antihyperglycemic, antilipidemic and antioxidant potential of *Cucurbita ficifolia* in human type 2 diabetes. *Prog. Nutr.* **2018**, *20*, 191–198.
120. Shi, Y.; Xiong, X.; Cao, J.; Kang, M. Effect of pumpkin polysaccharide granules on glycemic control in type 2 diabetes. *Cent. South Pharm.* **2003**, *1*, 275–276.
121. Cândido, F.G.; de Oliveira, F.C.E.; Lima, M.F.C.; Pinto, C.A.; da Silva, L.L.; Martino, H.S.D.; Alfenas, R.C.G. Addition of pooled pumpkin seed to mixed meals reduced postprandial glycemia: A randomized placebo-controlled clinical trial. *Nutr. Res.* **2018**, *56*, 90–97. [CrossRef]
122. Zhang, Y.; Chen, P.; Zhang, Y.; Jin, H.; Zhu, L.; Li, J.; Yao, H. Effects of polysaccharide from pumpkin on biochemical indicator and pancreatic tissue of the diabetic rabbits. *Int. J. Biol. Macromol.* **2013**, *62*, 574–581. [CrossRef]
123. Li, Q.; Fu, C.; Rui, Y.; Hu, G.; Cai, T. Effects of protein-bound polysaccharide isolated from pumpkin on insulin in diabetic rats. *Plant Foods Hum. Nutr.* **2005**, *60*, 13–16.
124. Allkanjari, O.; Vitalone, A. What do we know about phytotherapy of benign prostatic hyperplasia? *Life Sci.* **2015**, *126*, 42–56. [CrossRef] [PubMed]

125. Schiebel-Schlosser, G.; Friederich, M. Phytotherapy of BPH with pumpkin seeds-a multicenter clinical trial. *Phytotherapy* **1998**, *19*, 71–76.
126. Coulson, S.; Rao, A.; Beck, S.L.; Steels, E.; Gramotnev, H.; Vitetta, L. A phase II randomised double-blind placebo-controlled clinical trial investigating the efficacy and safety of ProstateEZE Max: A herbal medicine preparation for the management of symptoms of benign prostatic hypertrophy. *Complementary Ther. Med.* **2013**, *21*, 172–179. [CrossRef]
127. *Assessment Report on Cucurbita pepo L. Semen*; European Medicines Agency: Amsterdam, The Netherlands, 2013.
128. Gažová, A.; Valášková, S.; Žufková, V.; Castejon, A.M.; Kyselovič, J. Clinical study of effectiveness and safety of CELcomplex®containing *Cucurbita pepo* seed extract and flax and casuarina on stress urinary incontinence in women. *J. Tradit. Complement. Med.* **2018**, *9*, 138–142. [CrossRef]

© 2019 by the authors. Licensee MDPI, Basel, Switzerland. This article is an open access article distributed under the terms and conditions of the Creative Commons Attribution (CC BY) license (http://creativecommons.org/licenses/by/4.0/).

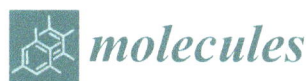

Review

Fragaria Genus: Chemical Composition and Biological Activities

Radu Claudiu Fierascu [1,2], Georgeta Temocico [1,*], Irina Fierascu [1,2,*], Alina Ortan [1] and Narcisa Elena Babeanu [1]

1. University of Agronomic Sciences and Veterinary Medicine of Bucharest, 59 Mărăști Blvd., 011464 Bucharest, Romania; radu_claudiu_fierascu@yahoo.com (R.C.F.); alina_ortan@hotmail.com (A.O.); narcisa.babeanu@gmail.com (N.E.B.)
2. Emerging Nanotechnologies Group, National Institute for Research & Development in Chemistry and Petrochemistry—ICECHIM Bucharest, 202 Spl. Independentei, 060021 Bucharest, Romania
* Correspondence: gtemocico@gmail.com (G.T.); dumitriu.irina@yahoo.com (I.F.)

Academic Editors: Raffaele Capasso, Lorenzo Di Cesare Mannelli and Nicola Volpi
Received: 23 December 2019; Accepted: 22 January 2020; Published: 23 January 2020

Abstract: The strawberries represent in our days one of the main fresh fruits consumed globally, inevitably leading to large amounts of by-products and wastes. Usually appreciated because of their specific flavor, the strawberries also possess biological properties, including antioxidant, antimicrobial, or anti-inflammatory effects. In spite of the wide spread of the *Fragaria* genus, few species represent the subject of the last decade scientific research. The main components identified in the *Fragaria* species are presented, as well as several biological properties, as emerging from the scientific papers published in the last decade.

Keywords: *Fragaria* genus; chemical composition; biological properties

1. Introduction

The production of different fruits all around the world exceeds millions of tons, depending on geographical zones, consumption, and growing traditions, inevitably leading to large amounts of by-products and wastes. *Fragaria* genus (*Rosaceae*), commonly known as strawberry, represents one of the most important food plants all over the world, with a double global production compared with all other fruit berries combined [1]. Their widespread use, primarily because of their flavor, can also lead to considerable benefits to human health. Among other characteristics, nonvisual properties like taste, nutritional values, or aroma make these fruits to be in the top of consumer preferences [2].

Known and consumed for thousands of years, *Fragaria* species are encountered throughout the northern hemisphere, as well as in some areas of South America [1]. Several authors present the historical consumption of strawberries in pre-Columbian sites, Picunche and Mapuche people (Chile), Romans or ancient China. [1,3–5] The exact number of accepted species of the genus remains a subject of debate, ranging from 22 [6] to 16 [7]. In addition, there are many hybrids and cultivars representing ploidy levels ranging from diploid ($2n = 2x = 14$) to decaploid ($2n = 10x = 70$), influencing the size of the fruits. Most of the research regarding the genus can be traced to the extraordinary work of Antoine Nicolas Duchesne, that offered botanical description, details on the history, cultivation, sex, and polyploidy of different species [5]. Generally speaking, all *Fragaria* species share some common characteristics: are low-growing perennials, with usually evergreen and trifoliolate leaves, insect-pollinated, with white actinomorphic flowers (usually 5-petalled). The main difference between species is represented by the animal-dispersed accessory aggregate fruits, in terms of color, shape, and achene (the 1-seeded simple fruits) and calyx positions at maturity. From the different composition and other characteristics of those fruits, also arise the potential commercial value of the species. Many cultivars are perennials that vary in their photoperiod needs, leading to varying harvesting times (June-bearers, ever-bearers, day-neutral) [8].

Among the 247 varieties known and listed, only few present commercial interest: *Fragaria x ananassa* Duchesne (octoploid hybrid-containing 56 chromosomes, known as garden strawberry, native to northern America, cultivated all over the world), and, to a lesser extent, *Fragaria vesca* L. (diploid species, known as wild strawberry, native to Northern hemisphere) and *Fragaria chiloensis* (L.) Mill. (octoploid species, known as Chilean strawberry, native to northern, pacific and southern America) [1].

As previously mentioned, the strawberries represent one of the most important fruit plants. Their production reached 9.22 million tones (world level) in 2017, the major producers being China (40.3% of total world production), United States (15.7%), Mexico (7.14%), Egypt (4.42%), Turkey (4.34%), Spain (3.9%), Republic of Korea (2.28%), Poland, Russian Federation, Morocco, Japan, Germany, United Kingdom, and Italy (between 1 and 2%) [9]. This mass-production invariably leads to large amounts of wastes, that can be further exploited in multiple areas, including medicine, cosmetics, and food industry [10]. The wastes are generated throughout the growth cycle (maturation, multiplication, and expansion), while the large-scale methods of cultivation (e.g., in fields, plastic tunnels., etc.) leads to large amounts of wastes from leaves, stolons, fruits, etc.

The present review paper aims to present the identified components in different species of the *Fragaria* genus, as well as their potential biological activities, as emerging from the scientific papers published in the past decade. The selection of the articles to be included in the present review was performed using the well-known data-bases (Scopus, Web of Science, ScienceDirect, and PubMed), using specific keywords ("composition", "therapeutic", "cytotoxic", "anti*"—returning results for "antimicrobial", "antifungal", "anti-inflammatory", etc.). The validation of the articles was performed manually (by reading the entire article) and in the present review were inserted only articles with significant contribution to the field of research.

2. Composition of *Fragaria* L. Genus

Giampieri et al. [11] reviewed the composition of the strawberry (*Fragaria x ananassa*), while Morales-Quintana and Ramos [12] reviewed the composition and potential applications of the Chilean strawberry (*Fragaria chiloensis* (L.) Mill.), while the functional properties of the berries, in general, and of the strawberries, in particular, were reviewed by Jimenez-Garcia et al. [13]. As resulting from various literature studies [11–15], the general composition of the strawberries (in terms of major components) can be summarized in Table 1 (with a general image provided in Figure 1).

Table 1. Major (common) components in *Fragaria* L. aggregate fruits (adapted from [11–15]).

Class	Compound	Ref.
Anthocyanins	Pelargonidin 3-glucoside, cyanidin 3-glucoside, cyanidin 3-rutinoside, pelargonidin 3-galactoside, pelargonidin 3-rutinoside, pelargonidin 3-arabinoside, pelargonidin 3-malylglucoside	[11–13]
Flavonols	Quercetin, kaempferol, fisetin, their glucuronides, and glycosides	[11–13,16]
Flavanols	Catechin, proanthocyanidin B1, proanthocyanidin trimer, proanthocyanidin B3	[11]
Ellagitannins	Sanguiin H-6, ellagitannin, ellagic acid, lambertianin C, galloylbis-hexahydroxydiphenoyl-glucose	[11]
Phenolic acids	4-coumaric acid, p-hydroxybenzoic acid, ferulic acid, vanillic acid, sinapic acid	[15]
Vitamins	Vitamin C, vitamin B9	[14]
Minerals	Mn, K, mg, P, Ca	[11]
Others	Sugars (glucose, fructose, and sucrose), fibers	[11]

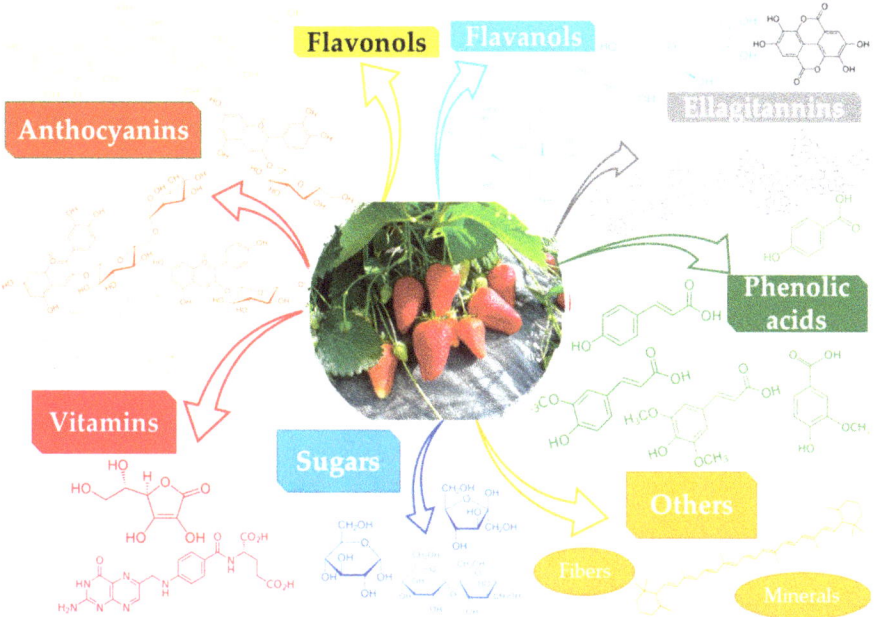

Figure 1. Main components *Fragaria* species identified according literature data.

The presented composition varies with a series of factors, including the value of the cultivar, seasonal variation, and the degree of fruit ripeness. In the reviewed time period, several studies presented the evaluation of species belonging to *Fragaria* genus. Their main findings are presented in Table 2, while relevant studies are presented in the following paragraphs.

As the major bioactive constituents of *Fragaria* fruits are represented by anthocyanins, most of the literature studies are focused on their identification/quantification. Cerezo et al. [17] identified multiple anthocyanins and other phenolic compounds present in *Fragaria x ananassa* (*Camarosa* variety) puree, among which three of them (delphinidin-3-glucoside, peonidin-3-glucoside, cyanidin-3-galactoside) were proposed for the first time in the literature. A correlation between the cultivation system (classic/organic) and the composition of the strawberries was established by Crecente-Campo et al. [18]. The authors observed higher values of the identified anthocyanins and ascorbic acid (accompanied by a darker, redder color and a superior nutritional value) in the case of organic cultivated strawberries. The differences in terms of volatile esters composition between wild and cultivated strawberries were presented by Dong et al. [19]. The authors suggested that the composition in volatile esters (dominated in the case of *F. vesca* by acetate esters, and by ethyl hexanoate, in the case of *Fragaria x ananassa*) is the key factor in the differences in terms of aroma patterns between the two species. Yang et al. [20] evaluated the phenolic compounds present in *Fragaria x ananassa* Duch. cv. *Falandi* fruits, identifying flavone glucuronides, lignan glycosides, and other compounds. The authors also isolated, for the first time in the literature, three phenolic glucosides (2,3''-epoxy-4-(butan-2-one-3-yl)-5,7,40-trihydroxy flavane 3-glucoside, kaempferol 3-(6-butylglucuronide), benzyl 2-glucosyl-6-rhamnosylbenzoate), offering their spectroscopic characteristics in support of the suggested structures. Roy et al. [21] studied comparatively the polyphenolic composition of *Fragaria x ananassa* and *Fragaria vesca* mutant fruits (white-colored) with regular fruits. Their study revealed the presence of 22 compounds belonging to different groups, as anthocyanins (cyanidin-3-glucoside, pelargonidin-3-glucoside, peonidin-3-glucoside, pelargonidin malonyl-glucoside, peonidin-malonyl-glucoside, and cyanidin-malonyl-glucoside) flavonols (quercetin, quercetin-3-glucoside, kaempferol-3-glucoside, kaempferol-acetyl glucoside, and kaempferol-coumaroyl hexoside), flavan-3-ols (proanthocyanidin dimers, catechin and epicatechin), hydroxycinnamic acids (caffeic acid, chlorogenic acid, and p-coumaroyl hexose), and ellagic acid-derived compounds (ellagic acid deoxyhexoside, methyl ellagic acid pentoside, and dimethyl ellagic acid pentoside). The major difference recorded between the white and red fruits (for both species) was the anthocyanins content. The white fruits had much lower total anthocyanin levels (0.11–0.35 for *F. vesca* and 0.89 mg/100 g fresh fruits for *Fragaria x ananassa*), compared with the red fruits (8.36, respectively 15.20 mg/100 g fresh fruits). Another major difference was recorded in terms of free ellagic acid and its derivatives (higher for *F. vesca* white fruits compared with the red fruits). Although the study was focused on the identification of specific mutations in different white-fruited genotypes, the article offers a very good insight on the variation of the phenolic composition, both with species and genotype. This could be further useful for the selection of the phenotype for separation of bioactive compounds for targeted applications. Two different compounds (a protease enzyme with molecular weight 65.8 kDa, stable at high temperatures and over a wide pH range, with specificity toward hemoglobin, respectively a cysteine protease inhibitor cystatin FchCYS1) were isolated in 2018 from *Fragaria x ananassa* [22], respectively *Fragaria chiloensis* [23], while a new ellagitannin (a galloylated derivative of agrimoniin, with molecular weight 2038) named fragariin A was isolated in 2019 by Karlińska et al. from strawberry fruits (*Fragaria x ananassa* Duch.) [24]. The distribution of the active compounds found in *Fragaria x ananassa* Duch. fruits was elucidated in 2019 by Nizioł et al. [25], by applying mass spectrometry imaging with ^{109}Ag nanoparticle enhanced target. The authors studied thirty-two known metabolites and reached the conclusion that γ-aminobutyric acid, quinic acid, vitamin C, catechin, xylose, 4-hydroxy-2,5-dimethyl-3(2H)-furanone and nonanal are located under the fruit's skin, aldehydes (hexanal, benzaldehyde) and ketones (1-penten-3-one, geranylacetone) are distributed throughout the fruits (in the inner core and in the cortex layer), while asparagine, lysine, gambriin C, oxalic acid and 2-methylbutanoic acid are found on/around the surface of the achenes. The authors suggested that their distribution is strongly connected with both the sites of their biosynthesis and to their function.

Table 2. Composition of *Fragaria* species (as presented by original works published in the reviewed period; references presented in chronological order).

Species	Plant Part, Other Variables	Identified Compounds and Main Findings	Identification Method	Ref.
F. chiloensis	Ripe fruits	Anthocyanins (cyanidin 3-O-glucoside, pelargonidin 3-O-glucoside cyanidin-malonyl-glucoside and pelargonidin-malonyl-glucoside); procyanidins, ellagitannins, ellagic acid and flavonol derivatives	HPLC-DAD, LC-ESI-MS	[26]
F. chiloensis	Leaves	Procyanidins, ellagitannins, ellagic acid and flavonol derivatives	HPLC-DAD, LC-ESI-MS	[26]
F. chiloensis	Rhizomes	Procyanidins, ellagitannins, ellagic acid and flavonol derivatives	HPLC-DAD, LC-ESI-MS	[26]
Fragaria × *ananassa*	Fruits	Anthocyanins (pelargonidin-3-glucoside, pelargonidin-3-rutinoside, cyanidin-3-rutinoside, pelargonidin-3,5-diglucoside, pelargonidin-3(6-acetyl)-glucoside, 5-carboxypyranopelargonidin-3-glucoside, delphinidin-3-glucoside, peonidin-3-glucoside, cyanidin-3-galactoside), p-hydroxybenzoic acid, (+)-catechin, ellagic acid, p-coumaric acid, quercetin glucoside	LC-MS/MS, HPLC-UV/Vis	[17]
Fragaria × *ananassa*	Fruits, cultivar and seasonal variations	Vitamin C, β-carotene; total phenolics, total anthocyanins; genotype influence is stronger than the environmental influence	Colorimetric	[27]
Fragaria × *ananassa*	Fruits, different cultivars on different ripeness stage	Total vitamin C, total phenolics, total anthocyanins, total ellagic acid/pelargonidin-3-glucoside and cyanidin-3-glucoside; higher amounts in pink fruits compared with fully ripped fruits	Colorimetric/HPLC-DAD	[28]
Fragaria × *ananassa*	Fruits, different farming methods	Total phenolics/pelargonidin-3-glucoside and cyanidin-3-glucoside, vitamin C, higher in organic farming fruits	Colorimetric/HPLC-DAD	[18]
Fragaria × *ananassa*	Fruits, different cultivars (27) and ripening stages	Phenolic compounds (multiple classes, including anthocyanins, flavanols and ellagitannins); composition dependent on cultivar, cinnamic acid conjugates and anthocyanins levels increased with the ripening stage	HPLC-DAD-MS	[29]
Fragaria × *ananassa*, *F. vesca*	Fruits	Quercetin and isorhamnetin glycosides (higher levels in wild strawberry)	HPLC-DAD, LC-ESI-MS	[34]
Fragaria × *ananassa*, *F. vesca*	Fruits, different cultivars	Volatile esters (including ethyl acetate, hexyl acetate, methyl butanoate, ethyl butanoate, hexyl butanoate, methyl hexanoate, ethyl hexanoate, hexyl hexanoate); higher levels in cultivated strawberries.	GC-MS	[19]
F. vesca	Fruits, two different cultivars	Anthocyanins (cyanidin 3-O-glucoside, pelargonidin 3-O-glucoside, peonidin 3-O-glucoside, cyanidin 3-O-malonylglucoside, pelargonidin 3-O-malonylglucoside, peonidin 3-O-malonylglucoside), dihydroflavonol and flavonols (taxifolin 3-O-arabinoside, kaempferol 3-O-glucoside, quercetin 3-O-glucoside, quercetin-acetylhexoside, kaempferol 3-O-acetylhexosides), flavan-3-ols and proanthocyanidins (catechin, B type proanthocyanidin dimers, trimers, and tetramers), ellagic acid and derivatives (glycosylated, methyl pentoside, methylellagic acid methyl pentoside, ellagitannins), other compounds (benzoic acid, ferulic acid hexose derivative, citric acid, furaneol glucoside)	HPLC-DAD	[31]
Fragaria × *ananassa*, *F. vesca*	Fruits	Anthocyanins (cyanidin, pelargonidin), cyanidin 3-glucosides (cyanidin 3-glucoside, cyanidin 3-arabinoside, cyanidin 3-sambubioside, delphinidin 3-galactoside, delphinidin 3-glucoside, delphinidin 3-malonylglucoside); higher levels of cyanidin glycosides in wild species	HPLC-DAD	[12]
F. vesca	Leaves	Ellagitannins (sanguiin H-2 isomer, sanguiin H-10 isomer, sanguiin H-6/agrimoniin/lambertianin A isomer, castalagin/vescalagin isomer, sanguiin H-10 isomer, sanguiin H-2 isomer, casuarictin/potentillin isomer	LC-PDA-ESI-MS	[13]
Fragaria × *ananassa*	Fruits, different cultivars and production years	Vitamin C, anthocyanins (pelargonidin 3-glucoside, cyanidin 3-glucoside, pelargonidin 3-rutinoside), ellagic acid; strongly dependent on the cultivar and production year	HPLC-UV/Vis	[34]
Fragaria × *ananassa*	Fruits, at different ripening stage	Vitamin C, pelargonidin-3-rutinoside, ellagic acid, catechin, ellagic acid-3-glucoside, quercetin (red fruits), neochlorogenic, pelargonidin-3-glucoside, pelargonidin-3-rutinoside, epicatechin, quercetin-3-β-D-glucoside, ellagic acid (green fruits)	LC-ESI-TOF	[35]
Fragaria × *ananassa*	Calyx (red and green)	Quercetin-3-β-D-glucoside, ellagic acid, kaempferol-3-O-glucoside, vitamin C (red), catechin, quercetin-3-β-D-glucoside, ellagic acid (green)	LC-ESI-TOF	[35]
Fragaria × *ananassa*	Flower	Catechin, quercetin, quercetin-3-β-D-glucoside, ellagic acid, kaempferol-3-O-glucoside, vitamin C	LC-ESI-TOF	[35]
Fragaria × *ananassa*	Leaf	Procyanidin dimer and trimer, catechin, quercetin-3-β-D-glucoside, quercetin 3-O-glucoside (derivative), vitamin C, ellagic acid	LC-ESI-TOF	[35]
Fragaria × *ananassa*	Stolon	Neochlorogenic, procyanidin dimer, catechin, quercetin-3-β-D-glucoside, ellagic acid, vitamin C, kaempferol-3-O-glucoside	LC-ESI-TOF	[35]
Fragaria × *ananassa*	Stem	Procyanidin dimer, catechin, ferulic acid, quercetin-3-β-D-glucoside, ellagic acid	LC-ESI-TOF	[35]
Fragaria × *ananassa*	Crown	Procyanidin dimer and trimer, catechin, propelargonidin dimer, ellagic acid	LC-ESI-TOF	[35]
Fragaria × *ananassa*	Root	Procyanidin dimer and trimer, catechin, neochlorogenic, propelargonidin dimer	LC-ESI-TOF	[35]
Fragaria × *ananassa*	Fruits, different novel cultivars	Phenolic acids (p-coumaric acid, ellagic acid, ferulic acid derivative, p-coumaric acid derivatives), monomeric flavanols ((+)-catechin), flavonols (quercetin 3-O-glucoside, fisetin, quercetin 3-O-glucoside derivative), anthocyanins (cyanidin 3-glucoside, cyanidin 3-rutinoside, cyanidin pentoside, pelargonidin 3-glucoside, pelargonidin 3-galactoside, pelargonidin 3,5-diglucoside, pelargonidin 3-glucoside, pelargonidin 3-rutinoside, cyanidin 3-Oacetylglucoside, cyanidin hexoside, pelargonidin 3-O-monoglucuronide, pelargonidin derivatives)	HPLC-DAD, LC-ESI-QTOF	[36]

Table 2. *Cont.*

Species	Plant Part, Other Variables	Identified Compounds and Main Findings	Identification Method	Ref.
Fragaria × ananassa	Fruits, grown on different altitudes, on consecutive years	Hydroxybenzoic acid, *p*-coumaric acid, other hydroxycinnamic acids, (+)-catechin, (−)-epicatechin, procyanidins, flavonols, anthocyanins (cyanidin 3-glucoside, pelargonidin 3-glucoside, pelargonidin derivative); higher levels recorded at lower altitudes.	HPLC-DAD	[37]
Fragaria × ananassa	Fruits	Kaempferol 3-(6-methylglucuronide), quercetin 3-(6-methylglucuronide), isorhamnetin 3-(6-methylglucuronide), trichocarpin, 2-*p*-hydroxybenzoyl-2,4,6-tri hydroxyphenylacetate, 2-*p*-hydroxyphene thyl-6-caffeoylglucoside, zingerone 4-glucoside, b-hydroxypropiovanillone 3-glucoside, (+)-isolariciresinol 9O-glucoside, (+)-isolariciresinol 9O-glucoside, aviculin, (−)-seccoisolariciresinol 4-glucoside, cupressoside A, cedrusin, icariside E4, dihydrodehydrodiconiferyl alcohol 9O-glucoside, massonianoside A, uroliguoside, (−)-pinoresinol 4-glucoside, 2,3″-epoxy-4-(butan-2-one-3-yl)-5,7,4O-trihydroxy flavane 3-glucoside, kaempferol 3-(6-butylglucuronide), benzyl 2-glucosyl-6-rhamnosylbenzoate	^{1}H NMR, ^{13}C NMR, HMBC, HPLC-UV/Vis, LC-MS/MS, HR-ESI-MS,	[20]
F. vesca	Fruits, wild and cultivated, from different geographical areas	39 phenolic compounds (including cyanidin 3-O-glucoside, delphinidin-3-O-glucoside, pelargonidin-3-O-glucoside, pelargonidin-3-O-rutinoside, (+) catechin, (−) epicatechin, procyanidin B1 and B2, isoquercetin, gallic acid, *p*-coumaric acid, phloridzin); composition dependent on the geographical area	LC-ESI-Orbitrap-MS, LC-ESI-QTrap-MS, LC-ESI-QTrap-MS/MS	[38]
Fragaria × ananassa	Fruits, different cultivars	Cyanidin 3-O-glucoside, pelargonidin-3-O-glucoside, pelargonidin-O-rutinoside, total anthocyanins content, dependent on the cultivar	UPLC-PDA-ESI-MS, HPLC-DAD	[39]
F. vesca	Fruits	Volatile composition—one hundred compounds (including esters, aldehydes, ketones, alcohols, terpenoids, furans and lactones).	GS-MS	[40]
F. vesca	Leaves	27 metabolites (organic acids, flavonoids, catechin and its oligomers, ellagitannins), including quinic acid, chelidonic acid, quercetin derivatives, catechin and procyanidins, phloridzin, pedunculagin, methyl ellagic acid glucuronide.	LC-ESI-Orbitrap-MS	[41]
Fragaria × ananassa, *F. vesca*	White-fruited mutants, different genotypes	Anthocyanins, flavonols, flavan-3-ols, hydroxycinnamic acids, and ellagic acid—content compounds, dependent on genotype	LC-ESI-MS/MS	[21]
F. chilensis	Fruits	Anthocyanins (cyanidin-3-O-glucoside, pelargonidin hexoside, cyanidin manlonyl hexoside, pelargonidin-malonyl hexoside), ellagitannins (ellagic acid hexoside, pentoside, rhamnoside), proanthocyanidin dimers, epicatechin, flavonols (quercetin pentoside, glucuronide)	HPLC-DAD, LC-ESI-MS	[42]
Fragaria × ananassa	Fruits, different cultivars	Anthocyanins, flavonoids, cinnamic acid derivatives, tannins and related compounds, triterpenoids; concentration dependent on the cultivar	UPLC-ESI-QTOF-MS/MS, HPLC-DAD	[43]

where: ^{13}C NMR—Carbon-13 nuclear magnetic resonance; GC-MS—gas chromatography–mass spectrometry; ^{1}H NMR—proton nuclear magnetic resonance; HMBC—heteronuclear multiple bond correlation; HPLC-DAD—high-performance liquid chromatography with diode array detector; HPLC-UV/Vis—high-performance liquid chromatography equipped with UV/vis detector; HR-ESI-MS—high-resolution electrospray ionization mass spectrometry analysis; LC-ESI-MS(MS)—liquid chromatography electrospray ionization (tandem) mass spectrometry analysis; LC-ESI-Orbitrap-MS—liquid chromatography electrospray ionization Orbitrap mass spectrometry; LC-ESI-QTrap-MS(MS)—liquid chromatography electrospray ionization quadrupole ion trap mass spectrometry; LC-ESI-(Q)TOF—liquid chromatography electrospray ionization with (quadrupole) time-of-flight; LC-MS/MS—liquid chromatography-tandem mass spectrometry; LC-PDA-ESI-MS—liquid chromatography equipped with photodiode array detector coupled to mass spectrometry using the electrospray ionization interface; UPLC-ESI-QTOF-MS/MS—ultra-performance liquid chromatography equipped quadrupole time of flight coupled to tandem mass spectrometry using the electrospray ionization interface; UPLC-PDA-ESI-MS—ultra-performance liquid chromatography equipped with photodiode array detector coupled to mass spectrometry using the electrospray ionization interface.

The composition of the fruits, although representing a characteristic of each species, can be influenced by a number of factors (as presented in Table 2), including the characteristics of the cultivar [21,27,29,31,34,39,43–46], cultivation factors, and the environmental conditions [18,27,37,38,47–50], ripening stage [28,29,35,51], or by biotechnological approaches [52–54]. For example, the variation in composition of a large number of *Fragaria × ananassa* Duch. cultivars was presented in 2019 by Nowicka et al. [43]. The authors identified as main components in the strawberry fruits the anthocyanins (pelargonidin-3-O-β-glucoside, cyanidin-3-O-β-glucoside, pelargonidin-3-O-rutinoside, cyaniding-3-O-(6″malonyl)glucoside, pelargonidin-3-O-(6″malonyl)glucoside)), flavonoids (derivatives of quercetin, kaempferol and isorhamnetin), cinnamic acid derivatives (isomers of 1-O-p-coumaroylhexose, 1-O-feruloylhexose, 1-O-p-coumaroyl-β-glucose, 1-O-trans-cinnamoyl-β-glucose), tannins and related compounds (gallotannins, glycosides of ellagic acid and methylellagic acid, free ellagic acid, flavan-3-ol derivatives), and triterpenoids (methyl or hydroxyl derivatives of tormentic or dihydrotormentic acid). More importantly, using the variation of the analyzed compounds allowed the authors to propose some of the cultivars for future studies and biomedical uses. Another interesting study was presented in 2011 by Pineli et al. who studied the compositional differences between two *Fragaria x ananassa* cultivars (*Osogrande* and *Camino Real*) in different ripening stages. Interestingly, the authors observed higher amounts of total phenolics, total ellagic acid, and vitamin C in the pink strawberries (3/4 ripe, as defined by the authors), compared with the green and fully ripe ones [28]. The differences recorded between the cited literature studies can be thus explained by the influence of those factors, as well as by the extraction procedure followed (which also have a strong influence on the final composition of the extracts), as demonstrated by Pawlaczyk-Graja et al. on the structure of polyphenolic-polysaccharide conjugates obtained from the leaves of *Fragaria vesca* using different classical and modern methods [55].

As the primary economic importance of the *Fragaria* genus is related to their fruits, it must be stated that, besides the previously presented factors, their composition (and finally, their health benefits) is correlated with the applied processing methods. The most encountered forms of products (besides fresh fruits) are represented by the dried fruits and puree. Méndez-Lagunas et al. [56] studied the influence of the thermal drying on the anthocyanins and total phenolic content of *Fragaria × ananassa* Duch. fruits. The study revealed a 26% loss of anthocyanins content when drying at 50 °C, respectively a 45% loss upon drying at 60 °C. The total phenolic content was even more seriously affected by the thermal process, with 60.9% loss associated with 50 °C, and 78.1% for the 60 °C treatment, respectively. Thus, the importance of fresh fruits consumption and when not possible, application of appropriate drying methods was emphasized; the authors propose the 50 °C treatment as suitable for preserving the bioactive compounds found in the strawberries (particularly anthocyanins). Álvarez-Fernández et al. [57] evaluated the variation in non-anthocyanin phenolic composition (hydrolyzed tannins, flavanols and condensed tannins, ellagic acid and derivatives, hydroxycinnamic acids, flavonol glycosides and stilbenes) of strawberry puree in different production stages. If mashing process affected the content of some phenolics (gallic acid, monogalloylglucoside and ellagic acid), the pasteurization process induced the decrease of all the compounds' concentration. However, the non-anthocyanin phenolic profile was not significantly affected, suggesting that the strawberry puree represents a good source of phenolic compounds.

The strawberry "seeds" (achenes) were proven to be a valuable source of unsaturated fatty acids. Thus, several studies revealed that commercially available achenes oil contained high amounts of linoleic and α-linoleic acids (over 70%), with a total content of over 90% unsaturated fatty acids (also including oleic and traces of palmitoleic acid), while the saturated fatty acids were mainly represented by palmitic and stearic acids [58,59]. In the same time, the seeds could also be considered a source of dietary fibers, proteins, polyphenols (mainly ellagitannins), and vitamins [60]. Figure 1 summarizes the main classes of constituents found in *Fragaria* genus.

3. Biological Activities of *Fragaria* Genus

3.1. Antioxidant Properties

Traditionally consumed in the form of fruits (as previously presented), *Fragaria* species have also found application in traditional medicine. For example, *Fragaria vesca* leaves and fruits were traditionally used for the treatment of external rashes, as well as internally, as blood purification and roborontarium, for the treatment of diarrhea [61], as macerate for renal stones, or as tea (together with other medicinal plants) for treating stomach inflammations, sedation, or regulation of digestion [62]. The following paragraphs presents the main biological properties of different *Fragaria* species, as emerging from the literature data published in the past decade. Particularly, the anthocyanins family represent the subject of several review papers published in the last years, dealing with their bioavailability and potential health benefits [63–65]. The following chapters includes only the studies regarding the biological activity of compounds or extracts obtained from *Fragaria* species (not studies presenting the activity of compounds that are found in those plants).

The major classes of compounds found in the Fragaria species (anthocyanins and non-anthocyanin phenolic compounds) are known for their antioxidant properties [65,66]. As can be expected, the vast majority of the literature presenting the biological activities of species belonging to Fragaria genus present their antioxidant activity. However, the studies that will be presented should be carefully considered, as many are performed using assays predisposed to positive results in the presence of oxygenated functions on aromatic rings (thus being considered more "class-related" than as specific molecular targeting) [67]. Thus, those studies, although useful as screening tools, should be confirmed by more specific assays, such as in vivo or cell-based models [66,67].

Pineli et al. [28] performed a study on two Fragaria × ananassa Duch. cultivars (Osogrande and Camino Real), regarding the correlation between composition and the antioxidant activity (established using 2,2-Diphenyl-1-picrylhydrazyl radical-scavenging activity—DPPH and ferric reducing antioxidant power—FRAP assays) of acetone extracts obtained from fruits at different ripening stages. Very interestingly, although, as expected, the anthocyanins levels were higher in the red fruits (full ripe), the best antioxidant activities, for both cultivars and both assays were obtained for the pink fruits. The only exception is represented by the DPPH assay results for Osogrande cultivar (for which the best results were obtained for the red fruits); however, the differences between the results of the DPPH assay for the cultivar at the three ripening stages were not statistically significant. The differences between the results can be explained by the different mechanisms of the assays (as previously described by our group) [66]. A much better correlation was observed by the authors with the total phenolic and vitamin C content. Finally, the Osogrande cultivar presented superior antioxidant properties (associated with higher levels of the total phenolic and total ellagic acid content, especially in pink and red fruits). Zhu et al. [35] evaluated the influence of the solvent used for room-temperature extraction (water/ethanol) and of the extracted Fragaria × ananassa var. Amaou parts (red fruit, green fruit, red calyx, green calyx, flower, leaf, stolon, stolon leaf, stem, crown, and root) on the antioxidant properties of the extract. Their conclusion was that the ethanol was the solvent of choice (because of different polarities of the phenolic compounds found in the plant) and, among the plant parts, best results (presented as Trolox equivalents—TE per gram or extract and per 100 g of plant fresh weight—FW) were obtained for flower extracts (1460.1 μMol TE/g extract), respectively for crown (6212.3 μMol TE/100g FW), when reported to a fresh weight basis. Stolon leaves (1456.7 μMol TE/g extract, respectively 5244.2 μMol TE/100g FW) also exhibited a very good antioxidant activity.

Individual compounds (including phenolic glucosides, flavone glucuronides, and lignan glycosides) were isolated from the Fragaria x ananassa Duch. cv. Falandi fruits by Yang et al. [20] and tested for antioxidant properties. The best results were obtained for flavone glucuronides (in the ABTS and DPPH assays), and a lignan glycoside (in the FRAP assay), respectively. Considering the results obtained for the positive control used in the antioxidant assays (ascorbic acid), the authors suggested that the investigated phenolic compounds play an important role in the overall antioxidant property of the plant. Contrary to other studies, Chaves et al. [39] demonstrated a correlation between the total anthocyanin content and the antioxidant potential of strawberry fruits, in a study over seven cultivars. The antioxidant potential of plants, as it results from literature studies, seems to be correlated with total anthocyanins and not with total phenolic content.

In 2019, Nowicka et al. [43] published a study regarding the variation in composition and antioxidant properties of 90 cultivars of Fragaria × ananassa Duch. fruits over two years of production. The results (average values presented in Table 3) revealed not only that some cultivars can be considered as having superior antioxidant properties (Roxana, Gigaline, Selvik, Thuriga ISK, Eratina, Siria, Dagol, Plarionfre, Grenadier, and Kimberly), but also, considering the phytochemical profile, that the main compounds responsible for the activity are the tannins, especially ellagitannins and procyanidins.

As previously stated, because of the increasing request, strawberries are often commercialized as processed products. The effect of fruit drying on the antioxidant potential of the Fragaria × ananassa Duch., Diamante var. fruits was presented by Méndez-Lagunas et al. [56]. The antioxidant assay performed on the processed fruits (DPPH) revealed 74.7% loss of antioxidant activity for the thermal treatment at 50 °C, while the 60 °C treatment led to a 66.2% loss of the activity. The results suggested that, beyond temperature, heat treatment time has a stronger effect on the antioxidant activity (as at higher temperature, shorter periods are necessary). Similar, several researches were performed regarding the changes of antioxidant activity (determined using ORAC and DPPH assays) during different stages of puree production [57]. Although slight reduction of the antioxidant properties was recorded (statistically significant only for the pasteurization step), the authors recommended the strawberry puree as an excellent source of antioxidants. The same group [68] observed no effect of the gluconic fermentation of strawberry puree (applied for the production of beverages) on the antioxidant activity (determined using the DPPH assay); the authors even reported an increase of the antioxidant potential after the pasteurization step, which was correlated with an increase in the gallic acid and hydroxycinnamic derivatives content. The results would suggest that the gluconic fermentation could maintain the antioxidant potential of the fresh products upon processing.

The antioxidant potential of strawberries could rapidly find industrial applications, as was the case for other plant-derived antioxidants [69,70] in, for example, meat industry, as recently reviewed by Lorenzo et al. [71], for increasing the shelf-life of different products (as sausages or raw, cooked, and cooked-chilled porcine patties).

Table 3 summarizes the main findings regarding the antioxidant potential of Fragaria species, as well as the responsible classes of compounds (as presented by the authors).

As a general remark, it can be observed that most authors assign the antioxidant potential to the total phenolic content in general, and in particular to some classes of compounds, such as anthocyanins, flavan-3-ols or tannins. Considering the individual species, Fragaria x ananassa fruits presented antioxidant properties in the DPPH assay (the assays with the widest application) between 76.73–100 mg/mL (IC_{50}) for various cultivars (the best results being obtained for the Camarosa cultivar) [39] or between 300 and 1300 µMol trolox/100 g fresh weight, for a larger survey (comprising 90 cultivars) [43]. Also, regarding the differences between the antioxidant potential of different plant parts, for F. chiloensis methanolic extracts the best activity was observed for fruits [26], while for Fragaria × ananassa for the crown ethanolic extract (6213.3 µMol trolox/100 g fresh weight). Fragaria vesca was mainly evaluated in terms of leaves, roots, or vegetative parts antioxidant activity, with antioxidant potential ranging from 13.46 mg/L to approx. 140 mg/L (IC_{50}), strongly dependent on the source of vegetal material and applied extraction technique [72,73].

Table 3. Antioxidant properties of different extracts obtained from *Fragaria* species (references presented in chronological order).

Species	Extraction Method	Antioxidant Assay	Antioxidant Potential	Responsible Compounds	Ref.
Fragaria × ananassa, Camarosa var. fruits	Anthocyanins isolated using CCC	ORAC, FRAP	ORAC: 2.7–24.46 mmol Trolox/g; FRAP: 2.75–12.5 mmol Fe^{2+}/g (depending on the fraction)	Anthocyanins	[17]
Fragaria chiloensis spp. *chiloensis* form *chiloensis* fruits	Methanol: formic acid (99:1 v/v) extraction	DPPH, SAS	DPPH assay: IC_{50} = 38.7 mg/L; SAS: 79.3%	Aglycone and glycosylated ellagic acid and flavonoids	[26]
Fragaria chiloensis spp. *chiloensis* form *chiloensis* leaves	Methanol: formic acid (99:1 v/v) extraction	DPPH, SAS	DPPH assay: IC_{50} = 49.4 mg/L; SAS: 67.60%	Aglycone and glycosylated ellagic acid and flavonoids	[26]
Fragaria chiloensis spp. *chiloensis* form *chiloensis* rhizomes	Methanol: formic acid (99:1 v/v) extraction	DPPH, SAS	DPPH assay: IC_{50} = 64.8 mg/L; SAS: 55%	Aglycone and glycosylated ellagic acid and flavonoids	[26]
Fragaria × ananassa Oso grande var. frozen fruits	Acetone (80%) extraction	DPPH, FRAP	DPPH: 11.91–12.83 µMol BHT eq/g FW; best results for ripe fruits FRAP: 27.37–36.75 µMol FS eq./g FW; best results for green fruits	Total phenolic content, vitamin C	[38]
Fragaria × ananassa Camino Real var. frozen fruits	Acetone (80%) extraction	DPPH, FRAP	DPPH: 9.75–12.01 µMol BHT eq/g FW, FRAP: 24.13–28.49 µMol FS eq/g FW (best results for pink fruits)	Total phenolic content, vitamin C	[28]
F. vesca leaves	Methanol, ultrasounds extraction	DPPH, FRAP	DPPH: IC_{50} = 13.46 mg/L; FRAP: 0.878 mmol Fe^{2+}/g DW	Total phenolics, total tannins	[72]
F. vesca roots, wild-growing	Hydromethanolic extraction, infusion, decoction	DPPH, FRAP, β-Carotene bleaching inhibition, TBARS	IC_{50}, mg/L: DPPH—50.03/50.56/50.62; FRAP—40.98/44.78/49.23; β-C bleaching—116.26/44.88/66.10; TBARS—35.76/4.76/6.14	Total phenolics, total flavan-3-ols, total dihydroflavonols	[73]
F. vesca roots, commercial	Hydromethanolic extraction, infusion, decoction	DPPH, FRAP, β-Carotene bleaching inhibition, TBARS	IC_{50}, mg/L: DPPH—68.89/255.81/51.32; FRAP—327.75/78.99/67.92; β-C bleaching—68.34/23.44/114.67; TBARS—6.69/24.25/10.62	Total phenolics, total flavan-3-ols, total dihydroflavonols	[73]
Fragaria × ananassa var. *Amaou*, fruits, at different ripening stage	Ethanol or water room temperature extraction	Modified ABTS assay	Ethanol: 150.5/151.9; water: 227.2/189.4 (red/green fruits) µMol TE/100 g FW	Total phenolic content	[35]
Fragaria × ananassa var. *Amaou* calyx (red and green)	Ethanol or water room temperature extraction	Modified ABTS assay	Ethanol: 241.1/1239.9; water: 1716.6/577.7 µMol TE/100 g FW (red/green calyx)	Total phenolic content	[35]
Fragaria × ananassa var. *Amaou* flower	Ethanol or water room temperature extraction	Modified ABTS assay	4234.4/3875 µMol TE/100 g FW (ethanol/water)	Total phenolic content	[35]
Fragaria × ananassa var. *Amaou* leaves	Ethanol or water room temperature extraction	Modified ABTS assay	2401.7/241.1 µMol TE/100 g FW (ethanol/water)	Total phenolic content	[35]
Fragaria × ananassa var. *Amaou* stolon	Ethanol or water room temperature extraction	Modified ABTS assay	1089.4/1856.7 µMol TE/100 g FW (ethanol/water)	Total phenolic content	[35]
Fragaria × ananassa var. *Amaou* stem	Ethanol or water room temperature extraction	Modified ABTS assay	1338.6/1123.1 µMol TE/100 g FW (ethanol/water)	Total phenolic content	[35]
Fragaria × ananassa var. *Amaou* crown	Ethanol or water room temperature extraction	Modified ABTS assay	6213.3/128.7 µMol TE/100 g FW (ethanol/water)	Total phenolic content	[35]
Fragaria × ananassa var. *Amaou* root	Ethanol or water room temperature extraction	Modified ABTS assay	253.1/69.2 µMol TE/100 g FW (ethanol/water)	Total phenolic content	[35]
F. vesca vegetative parts (leaves and stems), wild-growing	Hydromethanolic and aqueous extracts; wild-growing infusion microencapsulated in alginate and incorporated in k-carrageenan gelatine	DPPH, FRAP, β-Carotene bleaching inhibition, TBARS	IC_{50}, mg/L: DPPH—56.71/12.34/13.40; TBARS—12.63/3.12/5.03 (hydromethanolic/infusion/decoction); FRAP—81.40/62.36/77.28; β-C bleaching—56.71/12.34/13.40; TBARS—12.63/3.12/5.03 (hydromethanolic/infusion/decoction); Final formulation (mg/mL): DPPH—2.74; FRAP = 1.23	Total phenolics, total flavan-3-ols, total dihydroflavonols	[74]
F. vesca vegetative parts (leaves and stems), commercial	Hydromethanolic and aqueous extracts	DPPH, FRAP, β-Carotene bleaching inhibition, TBARS	IC_{50}, mg/L: DPPH—139.33/121.94/118.89; FRAP—324.49/91.88/88.20; β-C bleaching—388.90/76.41/69.98; TBARS—24.36/23.07/17.52 (hydromethanolic/infusion/decoction)	Total phenolics, total flavan-3-ols, total dihydroflavonols	[74]
Fragaria × ananassa cv. *Falandi* fruit	22 compounds isolated from ethanolic extracts	ABTS, DPPH, FRAP	Best results (IC_{50}): ABTS—4.42 µM kaempferol 3-(6-methylglucuronide); DPPH—32.12 µM quercetin 3-(6-methylglucuronide); FRAP—0.05 nmnol/g—urolignoside.	Individual compounds	[20]
Fragaria × ananassa cv. *Albion, Aromas, Camarosa, Camino Real, Monte Rey, Portola,* and *San Andreas* fruits	Ultrasonic extraction with acidified methanol	DPPH	IC_{50} (mg/mL) ranging from 7673 (*Camarosa*)—100 (*Camino Real*)	Total anthocyanin content	[39]
F. vesca leaves native to Italy	Ultrasonic extraction with ethanol: water solvent (70:30, v/v)	TEAC	0.34–0.35 mg/mL Trolox eq., compared with quercetin (0.40)	Condensed tannins and flavonoid derivatives	[41]
Fragaria × ananassa cv. *Tochiotome* leaves	Supercritical CO_2 extraction with different entrainers	DPPH	0.07 (simple supercritical extraction)—5.82 µMol BHT/g sample (with ethanol, dried at 40 °C)	Phenolic compounds	[10]
Fragaria × ananassa fruits (90 cultivars)	Ultrasonic aqueous methanol (70%) acidified with 1.5% formic acid, at room temperature	DPPH, ABTS	Average values (µmol Trolox/100 g):765.06 (DPPH), 1637.96 (ABTS)	Tannin-based compounds.	[43]

where: ABTS—2,2′-azino-bis(3-ethylbenzothiazoline-6-sulfonic acid) assay; BHT—butylated hydroxytoluene; DPPH—reduction of 2,2-diphenyl-1-picrylhydrazyl; DW—dry weight; eq.—equivalents; FRAP—ferric reducing ability of plasma; FS—ferrous sulphate; FW—fresh weight; IC_{50}—half maximal inhibitory concentration; ORAC—oxygen radical absorbance capacity; SAS—superoxide anion assay; TBARS—thiobarbituric acid reactive substances assay; TEAC—Trolox equivalent antioxidant capacity.

3.2. Anti-Inflammatory Properties

As previously stated, one of the traditional uses of *Fragaria* is as an *anti-inflammatory agent* [61,62]. Most of the authors assign the anti-inflammatory properties to the presence of anthocyanins (the most representative being pelargonidin and cyanidin derivatives) [75], molecules with known anti-inflammatory potential [76,77], demonstrated both in vitro and in vivo [78,79]. Similar to the other biomedical potential, the anti-inflammatory action is also correlated with the composition of different *Fragaria* species. The traditional use of *F. vesca* as an anti-inflammatory agent was supported by the study of Liberal et al. [80]. The authors observed the decrease of a relevant mediator of the inflammatory response (nitric oxide) produced by macrophages, cultured in the presence of a NO-production inducing bacterial endotoxin (LPS). The ethanolic extract obtained from *Fragaria vesca* leaves, used at non-cytotoxic concentrations (80 and 160 mg/L), induced a 31%, and 40% inhibition, respectively. The authors assigned the NO decrease to a direct scavenging effect (as demonstrated by a 23% inhibition of the nitrite content in the culture media, correlated with the absence of a significant effect when quantifying the inducible nitric oxide synthase—iNOS and the pro-inflammatory cytokine IL-1β). The authors also observed a statistically insignificant increase in the phosphorylated IκBα (nuclear factor of kappa light polypeptide gene enhancer in B-cells inhibitor, alpha) content, suggesting either an increase of its expression or a decrease in its degradation. More than that, the authors observed an increased conversion of the microtubule-associated protein light chain LC3-I to LC3-II (a marker of autophagy), suggesting further anti-cancer properties. Methanolic extracts of *Fragaria x ananassa,* var. *Alba* fruits were also confirmed by Gasparrini et al. [81] to lower the intracellular levels of reactive oxygen species (ROS), decrease apoptotic rate and improve antioxidant defenses and mitochondria functionality in *E. Coli* induced inflammation in human dermal fibroblast cells. Their results showed significant decrease of TNF-α (tumor necrosis factor alpha), IL-1β and IL-6 (interleukin 6) levels. The authors proposed as responsible mechanism the action on AMPK (5′ AMP-activated protein kinase) related pathways (increment in phosphorylated AMPK expression). Between the two presented studies there are several experimental design/inputs differences that can explain the different obtained results (including the species and the solvent used for extraction). Thus, the higher levels of bioactive molecules in the *Fragaria x ananassa* fruits (compared with the *F. vesca* leaves, as previously presented) can explain the differences observed by the authors in terms of anti-inflammatory action. Similar observations were made by Molinett et al. [82] who proved the anti-inflammatory and hepatoprotective effect of aqueous *F. chiloensis* fruits extracts on LPS-inducted liver injury on rats. The anti-inflammatory effect of the *Fragaria x ananassa var. Camarosa* fruits was also in vivo evaluated on female mice by Duarte et al. [83], who assigned the activity to the presence of anthocyanins. Moreover, the authors performed in vitro experiments using pelargonidin-3-*O*-glucoside (the major anthocyanin in *Fragaria*) in order to establish its molecular mechanism of action. Regarding the in vivo experiments the authors noticed the inhibition of the carrageenan-induced leukocyte influx to the pleural cavity upon crude extract treatment, due to the reduction in neutrophil migration. The extract also induced a reduction of myeloperoxidase activity and reduced the exudate concentration in the pleural cavity and NO levels. The pure compound pelargonidin-3-*O*-glucoside produced similar results, inhibiting IkBα, also reducing the phosphorylation of p65 NF-kB (nuclear factor kappa-light-chain-enhancer of activated B cells) subunit. The authors proposed as mechanism of the anthocyanin the mitogen-activated protein kinase (MAPK) pathways, leading to the decrease in NF-kB and activated protein 1 (AP-1) translocation. In 2019, Van de Velde et al. [84] supported the previously reported anti-inflammation properties of strawberry extracts, also proposing another possible application, by evaluating the wound-healing effects. The extract and polyphenolics/anthocyanins-enriched fractions influenced the skin fibroblast migration (45% of the migration registered for the positive control—fetal bovine serum, for the crude extract, 50% of the positive control for the anthocyanins enriched fraction at 1 mg/L, 30% of the positive control for the polyphenolics enriched fraction), suggesting that the wound-healing properties are strongly associated with the anthocyanins presence. The dietary use of strawberry achenes commercial oil has also been proven to reduce the activity of superoxide dismutase

(SOD) and glutathione peroxidase (cGPx) in rats (38.73, respectively 10.5 international units/gram of hemoglobin—U/g Hb, compared with the control group—67.33, and 22.9 U/g Hb, respectively), thus being qualified as a potential nutraceutical reducing oxidative stress [58].

3.3. Other Potential Applications

The *anti-microbial properties* were evaluated within the reviewed time period, especially for *F. vesca*. Hydromethanolic extracts obtained from leaves and roots of *Fragaria vesca* L. were evaluated by Gomes et al. [85] as antimicrobial agents a series of *S. aureus* strains. The results suggested a weak antimicrobial potential of the extracts (5–9 mm inhibition halos in the qualitative assays), which did not qualify the extracts for quantitative determinations. Superior results in terms of antimicrobial properties were obtained by Cardoso et al. [86]. Using hydroalcoholic extracts, the authors observed good antimicrobial properties of the crude extract against a series of *Helicobacter pylori* isolates (inhibition zones ≥ 15 mm) at a 25 mg/mL concentration. The ellagitannin-enriched fraction was efficient against all isolates at lower concentrations (7.5 mg/mL), which led the authors to assume that the ellagitannins were the main class of compounds responsible for the anti-microbial properties. As the *H. pylori* represents a pathogen involved in several gastric pathologies (including gastritis, gastroduodenal ulcer disease, gastric adenocarcinoma and mucosa-associated lymphoid tissue lymphoma), the authors proposed the wild strawberry extract as a potential candidate for human health applications.

The *anti-allergenic* potential of several compounds (linocinnamarin, 1-*O*-trans-cinnamoyl-b-D-glucopyranose, *p*-coumaric acid, cinnamic acid, chrysin, kaempferol, catechin, and trans-tiliroside) isolated from *Fragaria x ananassa* var. *Minomusume* fruits were evaluated by Ninomiya et al. [87], through the determination of their inhibitory effects on antigen-stimulated degranulation in rat basophilic leukemia RBL-2H3 cells. Among the studied compounds, linocinnamarin (95% inhibition of control at 100 μM) and cinnamic acid (approx. 80% of control at 100 μM) were the most efficient in degranulation suppression (through direct inactivation of spleen tyrosine kinase), being proposed as promising tools for alleviating symptoms of type I allergy.

The commercially-available strawberry freeze-dried powder was demonstrated by Abdulazeez [88] to reverse alloxan-induced diabetes (results not presented in Table 4 as authors used commercial powder product); in a similar study, Yang et al. [12] evaluated the potential *anti-diabetic application* of new and known compounds isolated from strawberry fruits (as presented in Section 2) by determining the α-glucosidase inhibitory activity. The best results were obtained for cupressoside A (IC_{50} = 25.39 μM), kaempferol 3-(6-methylglucuronide) (IC_{50} = 65.22 μM), and 2-*p*-hydroxybenzoyl-2,4,6-*tri* hydroxyphenylacetate (IC_{50} = 97.81 μM), with very good results obtained for a newly proposed structure (kaempferol 3-(6-butylglucuronide)-IC_{50} = 107.52 μM); results superior to the positive control (acarbose-IC_{50} = 619.94 μM) were also obtained for five other compounds.

Another interesting study is represented by the one performed by Zhu et al. [35]. Besides the phytochemical and anti-oxidant studies (previously presented), the authors also evaluated the anti-obesity, anti-allergy, and skin-lightening effects of extracts obtained from different parts of strawberry in different ripening stages. The extracts exhibited anti-obesity activity (the water extract of unripe fruit and the ethanol extracts of the stem, stolon leaf, and crown ripe fruits exhibiting anti-lipase activity, as well as inhibitory effect on adipocyte differentiation), anti-allergy function (the ethanol extracts of flower, stolon leaf and red calyx showing strong suppression effect on the release of β-hexosaminidase), and skin-lightening potential (ethanol extracts of ripe fruits, unripe fruit and the crown exhibiting melanogenesis inhibitory action, correlated with the tyrosinase-inhibitory activities).

The *cytotoxic potential* of the *Fragaria* species was demonstrated in several studies. Somasagara et al. [89] evaluated the potential application of methanolic strawberry extract in leukemia (CEM) and breast cancer (T47D) cell lines ex vivo, as well as its therapeutic and chemopreventive potential in vivo. The MTT, trypan blue and LDH assays revealed the cytotoxicity of the extract on cancer cells, in a concentration-dependent manner, while the in vivo studies revealed the anti-proliferative action on tumor cells. Forni et al. [90] investigated the antiproliferative and differentiation potential of an anthocyanin-rich strawberry fruit extract on B16-F10 murine melanoma cells. Their results showed the reduction of cell proliferation (30% after 48 h), accompanied by the lowering of the intracellular levels of polyamines (63.8% decrease of spermidine, 52.9% decrease of spermine, after 72 h), and the enhancement of tissue transglutaminase (172% increase after 48 h). The used extract also down-regulated p53 and p21 expression (47.2%, and 32.6%, respectively). Liberal et al. [33] presented the cytotoxic potential of an ellagitannin-enriched fraction from *Fragaria vesca* leaves on human hepatic carcinoma cell line (HepG2). Their results showed that the crude extract and, more pronounced, the ellagitannin-enriched fraction, were able to interfere with cell cycle distribution. The ellagitannin-enriched fraction also induced necrosis and apoptosis in the threated cells, decreased chymotrypsin-like activity of the 26S proteasome, impaired autophagic flux, promoted the accumulation of ubiquitinated proteins, and decreased the expression of several proteasome subunits. Lucioli et al. [91] evaluated the influence of hydroalcoholic extracts (methanol, ethanol, isopropanol) from in vitro cell suspension on the proliferation of several cancer cells (neuroblastoma, colon, and cervix carcinoma cell lines). The extracts induced a statistically significant reduction of cell growth but did not affect the human fibroblasts from healthy donors. The chemoprotective action of strawberries was also studied by Casto et al. [92] (results not presented in Table 4 as authors used commercial strawberry powder). The chemoprotective role of strawberries on colorectal cancer in inflammatory bowel disease was recently reviewed by Chen et al. [93], who proposed a mechanism of action involving the suppression of cytokines release, decrease of oxidative stress, reduction of genomic instability, and inhibition of NFκB (nuclear factor kappa-light-chain-enhancer of activated B cells) and related signalling pathways. Table 4 summarizes the main biological activities (except anti-oxidant properties, presented in Table 3), as emerging from the literature survey, considering the main constituents of the tested extracts.

Table 4. Main biological activities presented in the literature (references listed in chronological order).

Action	Plant	Extraction Method	Assay	Results	Responsible Compounds	Ref.
Anti-inflammatory on inflammatory bowel disease	*Fragaria vesca* leaves	Eth. extraction	MPO activity, GSH, SOD and CAT levels	Prevention of increase in colon weight and disease activity index, decrease in macroscopic and microscopic lesion score; significant improvement of MPO, CAT and SOD levels at 500 mg/kg 5 days oral treatment	Phenolic acids, flavonoids	[34]
Anti-inflammatory	*Fragaria vesca* leaves	Eth. extraction at room temperature, infusion	Nitric oxide production, western blot analysis (expression of pro-inflammatory proteins in lipopolysaccharide-triggered macrophages); nitric oxide scavenger activity	Inhibition of nitrite production on pre-treated cells (at 80 and 160 mg/L—31%/40%); 23% inhibition in culture media, at 160 mg/L	Phenolic content	[80]
Anti-inflammatory	*Fragaria x ananassa*, var. *Alba* fruits	Meth. extraction at room temperature, infusion	Determination of ROS intracellular levels, apoptosis detection, antioxidant enzyme activities, immunoblotting analysis, determination of mitochondrial respiration and extracellular acidification rate in cells	Reduction of intracellular ROS levels (significant at 100 mg/L), decreased apoptotic rate (significant at 50 and 100 mg/L); Increased ARE-antioxidant enzymes expression, reduced NO and inflammatory cytokines production (at 50 and 100 mg/L) to control levels	Vitamin C, anthocyanins, flavonoids	[81]
Anti-inflammatory, hepatoprotective	*Fragaria chiloensissp. Chiloensis* fruits	Aq. extracts	Histological analyses, determination of transaminases, cytokines, F2-isoprostanes, and glutathione assays	maintained hepatocellular membrane, structural integrity, attenuated hepatic oxidative stress, and inhibited inflammatory response in LPS-induced liver injury; downregulation of cytokines (TNFα, IL-1β, and IL-6)	Phenolic content	[82]
Anti-inflammatory	*Fragaria x ananassa* var. *Camarosa* fruits	Ultrasonic-assisted, acidified meth. extraction, separation	*In vivo*: quantification of the leukocyte content, exudate concentration, MPO and ADA activities, nitric oxide products, TNF-α and IL-6 levels; *in vitro*: MTT assay, measurement of nitric oxide products, TNF-α and IL-6 levels, western blot analysis	Inhibition of the carrageenan-induced leukocyte influx to the pleural cavity; reduction of myeloperoxidase activity, exudate concentration, NO levels.	Phenolic compounds, anthocyanins (particularly pelargonidin-3-O-glucoside)	[83]
Anti-inflammatory, wound healing	*Fragaria x ananassa* var. *San Andreas* fruits	Ultrasound-assisted extraction, acidified meth.: aq. (80:20); separation of different fractions	MTT assay, ROS, NO levels, effects on inflammatory markers and on skin fibroblast migration	ROS reduction, suppression of IL-1β, IL-6 and iNOS gene expressions; enhanced skin fibroblast migration	Polyphenolic compounds, especially anthocyanins	[84]
Anti-microbial	*Fragaria vesca* leaves and roots	Centrifugation extraction with meth.: aq. (80:20)	Disc diffusion assay	6-9 mm inhibition zones for leaves, 5-9 mm for roots (depending on *S. aureus* strain)	Phenolic compounds	[85]
Anti-microbial	*Fragaria vesca* leaves	Hydroalcoholic extraction, separation	Disc diffusion assay	Good inhibition potential at 25 mg/mL, better effect for the ellagitannin-enriched fraction	Ellagitannins	[86]
Anti-allergenic	*Fragaria x ananassa* var. *Minomusume* fruits	Methanol fraction of fruits juice (obtained by squeezing)	Antigen-stimulated degranulation in RBL-2H3 cells	degranulation suppression (95-60% inhibition for linocinamarin, cinnamic acid, chrysin, kaempferol, trans-tiliroside)	Best results - phenylpropanoid glycoside	[87]
Anti-diabetic	*Fragaria x ananassa* var. *Falandi* fruits	Compounds isolated from eth. extracts	α-glucosidase inhibitory activity	IC$_{50}$ values better than the positive control (acarbose) for nine compounds (537.43 to 25.39 μM)	Individual compounds	[21]
Anti-obesity, anti-allergy, skin-lightening	*Fragaria Xananassa* var. *Amaou*, entire plant (red fruit, green fruit, red calyx, green calyx, flower, leaf, stolon, stolon leaf, stem, crown and root)	Eth. or aq. room temperature extraction	Anti-lipase assay, adipocyte differentiation inhibition assay, melanogenesis inhibition assay, β-hexosaminidase inhibition assay, tyrosinase inhibition assay	Crown, stolon leaf and flowers extracts exhibited the highest effects	Total phenolic content	[35]
Antihyperuricemic	*Fragaria x ananassa* cv. *Tochiotome* leaves	Supercritical CO$_2$ extraction with different entrainers	Uric acid production in AML12 hepatocytes	Reduction of uric acid at 100 mg/mL (96 mmol/2 h/mg protein), compared with the control (16,096 mmol/2 h/mg protein)	Kaempferol, quercetin	[10]
Cytotoxic, anti-proliferative	*Fragaria x ananassa* fruits	Meth. extraction	Ex vivo: cell viability assay; in vivo: developing tumor size determination	Cytotoxic on cancer cells, blocked the proliferation of tumor cells	Phenolic compounds	[88]

Table 4. Cont.

Action	Plant	Extraction Method	Assay	Results	Responsible Compounds	Ref.
Antineoplastic	*Fragaria x ananassa* var. *Pajaro* fruits	Acidified hydro-eth. extraction	Transglutaminase assay and polyamine detection, immunoblot analysis	reduction of cell proliferation, lowering of the intracellular levels of polyamine, enhancement of tissue transglutaminase activity	Anthocyanins	[94]
Cytotoxic	*Fragaria vesca* L. leaves	Hydroalcoholic extract at room temperature, ellagitannins-enriched fraction	Effects on HepG2 cells—cell viability assessment, cell proliferation, cell cycle and cell death analysis, Western blot analysis, proteasome chymotrypsin-like activity	Inhibition of HepG2 cell viability IC$_{50}$ = 690 mg/L (extract)/113 mg/L (fraction); fraction induced necrosis and apoptosis, influenced the cellular proteolytic mechanisms	Ellagitannins	[33]
Chemopreventive	Lyophilized *Fragaria x ananassa* fruits	Ultrasound-assisted extraction with acidified acetone	Histological studies, Western blot analysis, PGE$_2$ measurement, and nitrate/nitrite colorimetric assay	Decreased tumor incidence, decreased levels of TNF-α, IL-1β, IL-6, COX-2 and iNOS, inhibition of the phosphorylation of PI3K, Akt, ERK, and NFκB	anthocyanins, ellagitannin/ellagic acid/ellagic acid derivatives flavonols	[95]
Cytotoxic	*Fragaria x ananassa* leaves	Hydroalcoholic extracts (meth., eth., isopropanol) from in vitro cell suspension	Cell proliferation, cell viability	Under 50% viable cells for colorectal adenocarcinoma and colon adenocarcinoma upon treatment with extracts containing 0.29 mM ethoxy-dihydrofuro-furan	Polyphenols	[91]

where: ADA—adenosine-deaminase; Akt—Protein Kinase B; aq.—water (aqueous); CAT—catalase; COX-2—cyclooxygenase-2 enzyme; ERK—extracellular signal-regulated kinase; eth—ethanol; GSH—glutathione; HepG2—human liver cancer cell line; IC$_{50}$—half maximal inhibitory concentration; IL-1β—Interleukin 1 beta cytokine protein; IL-6—interleukin 6; iNOS—inducible nitric oxide synthase; meth.—methanol; MPO—myeloperoxidase; MTT—3-(4,5-dimethylthiazol-2-yl)-2,5-diphenyltetrazolium bromide; NFκB—nuclear factor kappa-light-chain-enhancer of activated B cells; NO—nitric oxide; PGE$_2$—Prostaglandin E$_2$; PI3K—phosphatidylinositol 3-kinase; RBL—rat basophilic leukemia cells; ROS—reactive oxygen species; SOD—superoxide dismutase; TNF-α—tumor necrosis factor alpha.

4. Current Limitations and Future Perspectives

In spite of the wide spread of the *Fragaria* genus, few species represent the subject of the last decade scientific research, with many works focused on the composition and bioactivities of wild and garden species. Although those species, with certain commercial value, represent a very valuable source of different classes of polyphenols (including proanthocyanidins, anthocyanins, ellagitannins, flavonoids, phenylpropanoids, stilbenes, phenol glycosides, and dihydrochalcones) and thus possessing important nutritional value [96], the researchers should also focus on less-studied species, native to different parts of the world. This could represent an important opportunity for future studies. Also, the evaluation of other possible application (such as cosmetic products) could represent an interesting area of research. As an example, Sikora et al. [59] used supercritical CO_2 extraction for obtaining strawberry seeds (achenes) oil and applied it (in varying concentration from 0.5–2%) for the development of shower/bath cosmetics with good skin-moisturizing properties, without influencing the stability of the products.

A drawback that limits the potential beneficial effects of the strawberries' consumption is represented by their processing. As previously mentioned, the thermal treatment reduces both the bioactive compounds and their biological activities. In this area, new protective coatings obtained using nanotechnological approaches were proposed for increasing their shelf-lives [97], or as post-harvest treatments, alternatives to the classical thermal treatments currently applied [98,99].

As emerging from the literature study, most of the research is performed via classical extraction methods in order to align with traditional uses of the species (infusion, decoction), and only few are including modern extraction and separation techniques (such as countercurrent chromatography). In this area, would be beneficial to evaluate the use of modern methods of extraction/separation of biological active compounds [100].

The rich anthocyanin content of the genus seems to offer promising compounds for very important applications, such as anti-cancer or chemoprotective agents. Another surprising aspect emerging from the reviewed works is the relatively few studies concerning the potential of *Fragaria* species towards anti-microbial applications. Although the literature abounds in examples regarding the anti-microbial potential of different plants extracts, it appears that the *Fragaria* could still offer some surprising results in this domain (considering its rich composition). Also, the application of *Fragaria* extracts in other areas, such as nanotechnology, is only "surface-scratched" at this moment. For example, Demirbas et al. [101] evaluated anthocyanins-rich berry extracts (including strawberry) for the phytosynthesis of silver nanoparticles and evaluated their antioxidant and anti-microbial potential. Although the results of the phytosynthesis process were promising (smallest dimensions, compared with the blackberry or raspberry extracts (35 nm), and with less aggregation, the antimicrobial effect was relatively poor (and only on *B. cereus*). The field of nanotechnology in general, and of nanoparticles phytosynthesis in special, represents a continuously increasing domain, so the extracts obtained from different species of the genus could demonstrate their usefulness in this area [102]. Other different nanoparticles could be obtained using the extracts, as well with tuned properties, using enrichment of the extracts [103]. Correlated with the anti-microbial properties, the potential toward nanotechnology could also lead to the development of other materials (such as polymeric encapsulated nanoparticles or even natural extracts) for different anti-microbial applications or for wider applications in increasing the quality of food products [104,105].

Finally, as a more general remark, the absence of standardized methods for the evaluation of different potential applications represents a major draw-back in the comparison of the results presented by different authors.

5. Conclusions

Fragaria represents a widely spread genus, with species encountered all over the world. The current study aimed to present the progress made in the last decade in the study of the composition and potential applications of the species belonging to the *Fragaria* genus. However, in spite the wide spread of its species, only a few represents the subject of current research. The literature study revealed that three species represent the major subject of research, respectively the wild, garden and beach strawberry.

Used in traditional medicine especially as an anti-inflammatory adjuvant, the scientific research supports this application, as well as several other potentially important uses, for example as a chemoprotective agent.

The composition of the genus, rich in polyphenolic compounds in general, and in anthocyanins in particular, suggests its possible application in multiple other areas. The relatively under-study of the genus (and the severe lack of literature for some of the species) offers in turn an opportunity for future research. At the same time, elucidation of the composition and properties of the commercially valuable products represents a very important aspect, as the characteristics of such a widely consumed product should be thoroughly elucidated.

Author Contributions: R.C.F., A.O., N.E.B., G.T., and I.F. contributed to data collection and analysis, and manuscript design. R.C.F., G.T., and I.F. prepared and revised the manuscript, and are the main authors of the study. All authors have read and agreed to the published version of the manuscript.

Funding: The authors gratefully acknowledge the support obtained through the project SusMAPWaste, SMIS 104323, Contract No. 89/09.09.2016, from the Operational Program Competitiveness 2014-2020, project co-financed from the European Regional Development Fund.

Conflicts of Interest: The authors declare no conflict of interest.

References

1. Liston, A.; Cronn, R.; Ashman, T.L. *Fragaria*: A genus with deep historical roots and ripe for evolutionary and ecological insights. *Am. J. Bot.* **2014**, *101*, 1686–1699. [CrossRef]
2. Awad, M.A.; De Jager, A. Influences of air and controlled atmosphere storage on the concentration of potentially healthful phenolics in apples and other fruits. *Postharv. Biol. Technol.* **2003**, *27*, 53–58. [CrossRef]
3. Pauketat, T.R.; Kelly, L.S.; Fritz, G.J.; Lopinot, N.H.; Elias, S.; Hargrave, E. The residues of feasting and public ritual at Early Cahokia. *Amer. Antiq.* **2002**, *67*, 257–279. [CrossRef]
4. Finn, C.E.; Retamales, J.B.; Lobos, G.A.; Hancock, J.F. The Chilean strawberry (Fragaria chiloensis): Over 1000 years of domestication. *HortScience* **2013**, *48*, 418–421. [CrossRef]
5. Duchesne, A.N. *Histoire Naturelle des Fraisiers Contenant les Vues d'économie Réunies à la Botanique et Suivie de Remarques Particulières sur Plusieurs Points qui ont Rapport à l'Histoire Naturelle Générale*; Didot le Jeune: Paris, France, 1766.
6. Plants of the World Online: *Fragaria* L. Available online: http://powo.science.kew.org/taxon/urn:lsid:ipni.org:names:30014957-2 (accessed on 3 January 2020).
7. The Plant List: Fragaria. Available online: http://www.theplantlist.org/1.1/browse/A/Rosaceae/Fragaria/ (accessed on 3 January 2020).
8. Petran, A.J. Performance and impact of strawberry (Fragaria x ananassa) season extension in the United States Upper Midwest using organic practices. Ph.D. Thesis, University of Minnesota, Minneapolis, MN, USA, April 2016.
9. Food and Agriculture Organization of the United Nations (FAO). 2017. Available online: http://www.fao.org/faostat/en/#data/QC (accessed on 3 January 2020).
10. Sato, T.; Ikeya, Y.; Adachi, S.I.; Yagasaki, K.; Nihei, K.I.; Itoh, N. Extraction of strawberry leaves with supercritical carbon dioxide and entrainers: Antioxidant capacity, total phenolic content, and inhibitory effect on uric acid production of the extract. *Food Bioprod. Process* **2019**, *117*, 160–169. [CrossRef]
11. Giampieri, F.; Tulipani, S.; Alvarez-Suarez, J.M.; Quiles, J.L.; Mezzetti, B.; Battino, M. The strawberry: Composition, nutritional quality, and impact on human health. *Nutrition* **2012**, *28*, 9–19. [CrossRef]
12. Morales-Quintana, L.; Ramos, P. Chilean strawberry (*Fragaria chiloensis*): An integrative and comprehensive review. *Food Res. Int.* **2019**, *119*, 769–776. [CrossRef]
13. Jimenez-Garcia, S.N.; Guevara-Gonzalez, R.G.; Miranda-Lopez, R.; Feregrino-Perez, A.A.; Torres-Pacheco, I.; Vazquez-Cruz, M.A. Functional properties and quality characteristics of bioactive compounds in berries: Biochemistry, biotechnology, and genomics. *Food Res. Int.* **2013**, *54*, 1195–1207. [CrossRef]

14. Nile, S.H.; Park, S.W. Edible berries: Bioactive components and their effect on human health. *Nutrition* **2014**, *30*, 134–144. [CrossRef]
15. Vuong, Q.V.; Hirun, S.; Phillips, P.A.; Chuen, T.L.; Bowyer, M.C.; Goldsmith, C.D.; Scarlett, C.J. Fruit-derived phenolic compounds and pancreatic cancer: Perspectives from Australian native fruits. *J. Ethnopharmacol.* **2014**, *152*, 227–242. [CrossRef]
16. Khan, N.; Syed, D.N.; Ahmad, N.; Mukhtar, H. Fisetin: A dietary antioxidant for health promotion. *Antioxid. Redox Signal.* **2013**, *2*, 151–162. [CrossRef] [PubMed]
17. Cerezo, A.B.; Cuevas, E.; Winterhalter, P.; Garcia-Parrilla, M.C.; Troncoso, A.M. Isolation, identification, and antioxidant activity of anthocyanin compounds in Camarosa strawberry. *Food Chem.* **2010**, *123*, 574–582. [CrossRef]
18. Crecente-Campo, J.; Nunes-Damaceno, M.; Romero-Rodrıguez, M.A.; Vazquez-Oderiz, M.L. Color, anthocyanin pigment, ascorbic acid and total phenolic compound determination in organic versus conventional strawberries (*Fragaria x ananassa* Duch, cv Selva). *J. Food Compos. Anal.* **2012**, *28*, 23–30. [CrossRef]
19. Dong, J.; Zhang, Y.; Tang, X.; Jin, W.; Han, Z. Differences in volatile ester composition between *Fragaria×ananassa* and *F. vesca* and implications for strawberry aroma patterns. *Sci. Horticult.* **2013**, *150*, 47–53. [CrossRef]
20. Yang, D.; Xie, H.; Jiang, Y.; Wei, X. Phenolics from strawberry cv. *Falandi* and their antioxidant and α-glucosidase inhibitory activities. *Food Chem.* **2016**, *194*, 857–863. [CrossRef] [PubMed]
21. Roy, S.; Wu, B.; Liu, W.; Archbold, D.D. Comparative analyses of polyphenolic composition of *Fragaria* spp. Color mutants. *Plant Physiol. Biochem.* **2018**, *125*, 255–261. [CrossRef] [PubMed]
22. Alici, E.H.; Arabaci, G. A novel serine protease from strawberry (*Fragaria ananassa*): Purification and biochemical characterization. *Int. J. Biol. Macromol.* **2018**, *114*, 1295–1304. [CrossRef]
23. Aceituno-Valenzuela, U.; Covarrubias, M.P.; Aguayo, M.F.; Valenzuela-Riffo, F.; Espinoza, A.; Gaete-Eastman, C.; Herrera, R.; Handford, M.; Norambuena, L. Identification of a type II cystatin in *Fragaria chiloensis*: A proteinase inhibitor differentially regulated during achene development and in response to biotic stress-related stimuli. *Plant Physiol. Biochem.* **2018**, *129*, 158–167. [CrossRef]
24. Karlińska, E.; Pecio, L.; Macierzyński, J.; Stochmal, A.; Kosmala, M. Structural elucidation of the ellagitannin with a molecular weight of 2038 isolated from strawberry fruit (*Fragaria ananassa* Duch.) and named fragariin A. *Food Chem.* **2019**, *296*, 109–115. [CrossRef]
25. Nizioł, J.; Misiorek, M.; Ruman, T. Mass spectrometry imaging of low molecular weight metabolites in strawberry fruit (*Fragaria x ananassa* Duch.) cv. Primoris with 109Ag nanoparticle enhanced target. *Phytochemistry* **2019**, *159*, 11–19.
26. Simirgiotis, M.J.; Schmeda-Hirschmann, G. Determination of phenolic composition and antioxidant activity in fruits, rhizomes and leaves of the white strawberry (*Fragaria chiloensis* spp. Chiloensis form chiloensis) using HPLC-DAD–ESI-MS and free radical quenching techniques. *J. Food Compos. Anal.* **2010**, *23*, 545–553. [CrossRef]
27. Singh, A.; Singh, B.K.; Deka, B.C.; Sanwal, S.K.; Patel, R.K.; Verma, M.R. The genetic variability, inheritance and inter-relationships of ascorbic acid, β-carotene, phenol and anthocyanin content in strawberry (*Fragaria×ananassa* Duch.). *Sci. Horticult.* **2011**, *129*, 86–90. [CrossRef]
28. Pineli, L.L.O.; Moretti, C.L.; dos Santos, M.S.; Campos, A.B.; Brasileiro, A.V.; Cordova, A.C.; Chiarello, M.D. Antioxidants and other chemical and physical characteristics of two strawberry cultivars at different ripeness stages. *J. Food Compos. Anal.* **2011**, *24*, 11–16. [CrossRef]
29. Aaby, K.; Mazur, S.; Nes, A.; Skrede, G. Phenolic compounds in strawberry (*Fragaria x ananassa* Duch.) fruits: Composition in 27 cultivars and changes during ripening. *Food Chem.* **2012**, *132*, 86–97. [CrossRef] [PubMed]
30. Mikulic-Petkovsek, M.; Slatnar, A.; Stampar, F.; Veberic, R. HPLC-MS^n identification and quantification of flavonol glycosides in 28 wild and cultivated berry species. *Food Chem.* **2012**, *135*, 2138–2146. [CrossRef] [PubMed]
31. Sun, J.; Liu, X.; Yang, T.; Slovin, J.; Chen, P. Profiling polyphenols of two diploid strawberry (*Fragaria vesca*) inbred lines using UHPLC-HRMSn. *Food Chem.* **2014**, *146*, 289–298. [CrossRef] [PubMed]
32. Veberic, R.; Slatnar, A.; Bizjak, J.; Stampar, F.; Mikulic-Petkovsek, M. Anthocyanin composition of different wild and cultivated berry species. *LWT Food Sci. Technol.* **2015**, *60*, 509–517. [CrossRef]

33. Liberal, J.; Costa, G.; Carmo, A.; Vitorino, R.; Marques, C.; Domingues, M.R.; Domingues, P.; Goncalves, A.C.; Alves, R.; Sarmento-Ribeiro, A.B.; et al. Chemical characterization and cytotoxic potential of an ellagitannin-enriched fraction from *Fragaria vesca* leaves. *Arab. J. Chem.* **2015**. [CrossRef]
34. Kim, S.K.; Kim, D.S.; Kim, D.Y.; Chun, C. Variation of bioactive compounds content of 14 oriental strawberry cultivars. *Food Chem.* **2015**, *184*, 196–202. [CrossRef]
35. Zhu, Q.; Nakagawa, T.; Kishikawa, A.; Ohnuki, K.; Shimizu, K. In vitro bioactivities and phytochemical profile of various parts of the strawberry (*Fragaria × ananassa* var. Amaou). *J. Funct. Food* **2015**, *13*, 38–49. [CrossRef]
36. Fernández-Lara, R.; Gordillo, B.; Rodríguez-Pulido, F.J.; González-Miret, M.L.; del Villar-Martínez, A.A.; Dávila-Ortiz, G.; Heredia, F.J. Assessment of the differences in the phenolic composition and color characteristics of new strawberry (*Fragaria x ananassa* Duch.) cultivars by HPLC-MS and Imaging Tristimulus Colorimetry. *Food Res. Int.* **2015**, *76*, 645–653. [CrossRef] [PubMed]
37. Guerrero-Chavez, G.; Scampicchio, M.; Andreotti, C. Influence of the site altitude on strawberry phenolic composition and quality. *Sci. Horticult.* **2015**, *192*, 21–28. [CrossRef]
38. D'Urso, G.; Maldini, M.; Pintore, G.; d'Aquino, L.; Montoro, P.; Pizza, C. Characterisation of *Fragaria vesca* fruit from Italy following a metabolomics approach through integrated mass spectrometry techniques. *LWT Food Sci. Technol.* **2016**, *74*, 387–395. [CrossRef]
39. Chaves, V.C.; Calvete, E.; Reginatto, F.H. Quality properties and antioxidant activity of seven strawberry (*Fragaria x ananassa* Duch) cultivars. *Sci. Horticult.* **2017**, *225*, 293–298. [CrossRef]
40. Urrutia, M.; Rambla, J.L.; Alexiou, K.G.; Granell, A.; Monfort, A. Genetic analysis of the wild strawberry (*Fragaria vesca*) volatile composition. *Plant Physiol. Biochem.* **2017**, *121*, 99–117. [CrossRef]
41. D'Urso, G.; Pizza, C.; Piacente, S.; Montoro, P. Combination of LC–MS based metabolomics and antioxidant activity for evaluation of bioactive compounds in *Fragaria vesca* leaves from Italy. *J. Pharmaceut. Biomed. Anal.* **2018**, *150*, 233–240. [CrossRef]
42. Chamorro, M.F.; Reiner, G.; Theoduloz, C.; Ladio, A.; Schmeda-Hirschmann, G.; Gómez-Alonso, S.; Jiménez-Aspee, F. Polyphenol composition and (bio)activity of berberis species and wild strawberry from the Argentinean Patagonia. *Molecules* **2019**, *24*, 3331. [CrossRef]
43. Nowicka, A.; Kucharska, A.Z.; Sokół-Łętowska, A.; Fecka, I. Comparison of polyphenol content and antioxidant capacity of strawberry fruit from 90 cultivars of *Fragaria × ananassa* Duch. *Food Chem.* **2019**, *270*, 32–46. [CrossRef]
44. Vandendriessche, T.; Vermeir, S.; Mayayo Martinez, C.; Hendrickx, Y.; Lammertyn, J.; Nicolaï, B.M.; Hertog, M.L.A.T.M. Effect of ripening and inter-cultivar differences on strawberry quality. *LWT Food Sci. Technol.* **2013**, *52*, 62–70. [CrossRef]
45. Mazur, S.P.; Nes, A.; Wold, A.B.; Remberg, S.F.; Martinsen, B.K.; Aaby, K. Effects of ripeness and cultivar on chemical composition of strawberry (*Fragaria x ananassa* Duch.) fruits and their suitability for jam production as a stable product at different storage temperatures. *Food Chem.* **2014**, *146*, 412–422. [CrossRef]
46. Akšic, M.F.; Zagorac, D.D.; Sredojevic, M.; Milivojevic, J.; Gašic, U.; Meland, M.; Nati, M. Chemometric characterization of strawberries and blueberries according to their phenolic profile: Combined effect of cultivar and cultivation system. *Molecules* **2019**, *24*, 4310. [CrossRef] [PubMed]
47. Moshiur Rahman, M.; Rahman, M.M.; Hossain, M.M.; Khaliq, Q.A.; Moniruzzaman, M. Effect of planting time and genotypes growth, yield and quality of strawberry (*Fragaria x ananassa* Duch.). *Sci. Horticult.* **2014**, *167*, 56–62. [CrossRef]
48. Zhang, Y.; Jiang, L.; Li, Y.; Chen, Q.; Ye, Y.; Zhang, Y.; Luo, Y.; Sun, B.; Wang, X.; Tang, H. Effect of red and blue light on anthocyanin accumulation and differential gene expression in strawberry (*Fragaria x ananassa*). *Molecules* **2018**, *23*, 820. [CrossRef] [PubMed]
49. Ferreira, J.F.S.; Liu, X.; Suarez, D.L. Fruit yield and survival of five commercial strawberry cultivars under field cultivation and salinity stress. *Sci. Horticult.* **2019**, *243*, 401–410. [CrossRef]
50. Mozafari, A.A.; Ghaderi, N.; Havas, F.; Dedejani, S. Comparative investigation of structural relationships among morphophysiological and biochemical properties of strawberry (*Fragaria × ananassa* Duch.) under drought and salinity stresses: A study based on in vitro culture. *Sci. Horticult.* **2019**, *256*, 108601. [CrossRef]
51. Voća, S.; Žlabur, J.S.; Dobričević, N.; Jakobek, L.; Šeruga, M.; Galić, A.; Pliestić, S. Variation in the bioactive compound content at three ripening stages of strawberry fruit. *Molecules* **2014**, *19*, 10370–10385. [CrossRef]

52. Salvatierra, A.; Pimentel, P.; Moya-León, M.A.; Herrera, R. Increased accumulation of anthocyanins in *Fragaria chiloensis* fruits by transient suppression of FcMYB1 gene. *Phytochemistry* **2013**, *290*, 25–36. [CrossRef]
53. Dias, M.I.; Barros, L.; Sousa, M.J.; Oliveira, M.B.P.P.; Santos-Buelga, C.; Ferreira, I.C.F.R. Enhancement of nutritional and bioactive compounds by in vitro culture of wild *Fragaria vesca* L. vegetative parts. *Food Chem.* **2017**, *235*, 212–219. [CrossRef]
54. Delgado, L.D.; Zúñiga, P.E.; Figueroa, N.E.; Pastene, E.; Escobar-Sepúlveda, H.F.; Figueroa, P.M.; Garrido-Bigotes, A.; Figueroa, C.R. Application of a JA-Ile biosynthesis inhibitor to methyl jasmonate-treated strawberry fruit induces upregulation of specific MBW complex-related genes and accumulation of proanthocyanidins. *Molecules* **2018**, *23*, 1433. [CrossRef]
55. Pawlaczyk-Graja, I.; Balicki, S.; Wilk, K.A. Effect of various extraction methods on the structure of polyphenolic-polysaccharide conjugates from *Fragaria vesca* L. leaf. *Int. J. Biol. Macromol.* **2019**, *130*, 664–674. [CrossRef]
56. Méndez-Lagunas, L.; Rodríguez-Ramírez, J.; Cruz-Gracida, M.; Sandoval-Torres, S.; Barriada-Bernal, G. Convective drying kinetics of strawberry (*Fragaria ananassa*): Effects on antioxidant activity, anthocyanins and total phenolic content. *Food Chem.* **2017**, *230*, 174–181. [CrossRef] [PubMed]
57. Álvarez-Fernández, M.A.; Hornedo-Ortega, R.; Cerezo, A.B.; Troncoso, A.M.; García-Parrilla, M.C. Effects of the strawberry (*Fragaria ananassa*) purée elaboration process on non-anthocyanin phenolic composition and antioxidant activity. *Food Chem.* **2014**, *164*, 104–112. [CrossRef] [PubMed]
58. Pieszka, M.; Tombarkiewicz, B.; Roman, A.; Migdał, W.; Niedziółka, J. Effect of bioactive substances found in rapeseed, raspberry and strawberry seed oils on blood lipid profile and selected parameters of oxidative status in rats. *Environ. Toxicol. Pharmacol.* **2013**, *36*, 1055–1062. [CrossRef] [PubMed]
59. Sikora, E.; Michorczyk, P.; Olszanska, M.; Ogonowsk, J. Supercritical CO_2 extract from strawberry seeds as a valuable component of mild cleansing compositions. *Int. J. Cosmet. Sci.* **2015**, *37*, 574–578. [CrossRef]
60. Grzelak-Błaszczyk, K.; Karlińska, E.; Grzęda, K.; Rój, E.; Kołodziejczyk, K. Defatted strawberry seeds as a source of phenolics, dietary fiber and minerals. *LWT Food Sci. Technol.* **2017**, *84*, 18–22. [CrossRef]
61. Wichtl, M. Herbal drugs and phytopharmaceuticals. In *A Handbook of Practice on a Scientific Basis*; Brinckmann, J.A., Lindenmaier, M.P., Eds.; CRC Press: Boca Raton, FL, USA, 2004; pp. 220–221.
62. Saric-Kundalic, B.; Dobes, C.; Klatte-Asselmeyer, V.; Saukel, J. Ethnobotanical study on medicinal use of wild and cultivated plants in middle, south and west Bosnia and Herzegovina. *J. Ethnopharmacol.* **2010**, *131*, 33–55. [CrossRef]
63. Zhu, F. Anthocyanins in cereals: Composition and health effects. *Food Res. Int.* **2018**, *109*, 232–249. [CrossRef]
64. Sinopoli, A.; Calogero, G.; Bartolotta, A. Computational aspects of anthocyanidins and anthocyanins: A review. *Food Chem.* **2019**, *297*, 124898. [CrossRef]
65. Braga, A.R.C.; Murador, D.C.; de Souza Mesquita, L.M.; Rosso, V.V. Bioavailability of anthocyanins: Gaps in knowledge, challenges and future research. *J. Food Compos. Anal.* **2018**, *68*, 31–40. [CrossRef]
66. Fierascu, R.C.; Ortan, A.; Fierascu, I.C.; Fierascu, I. In vitro and in vivo evaluation of antioxidant properties of wild-growing plants. A short review. *Curr. Opin. Food Sci.* **2018**, *24*, 1–8. [CrossRef]
67. Heinrich, M.; Appendino, G.; Efferth, T.; Fürst, R.; Izzo, A.A.; Kayser, O.; Pezzuto, J.M.; Viljoen, A. Best practice in research–Overcoming common challenges in phytopharmacological research. *J. Ethnopharmacol.* **2020**, *246*, 112230. [CrossRef] [PubMed]
68. Álvarez-Fernández, M.A.; Hornedo-Ortega, R.; Cerezo, A.B.; Troncoso, A.M.; García-Parrilla, M.C. Non-anthocyanin phenolic compounds and antioxidant activity of beverages obtained by gluconic fermentation of strawberry. *Innov. Food Emerg. Technol.* **2014**, *26*, 469–481. [CrossRef]
69. Kebede, M.; Admassu, S. Application of antioxidants in food processing industry: Options to improve the extraction yields and market value of natural products. *Adv. Food. Technol. Nutr. Sci. Open J.* **2019**, *5*, 38–49. [CrossRef]
70. Lourenço, S.C.; Moldão-Martins, M.; Alves, V.D. Antioxidants of natural plant origins: From sources to food industry applications. *Molecules* **2019**, *24*, 4132. [CrossRef] [PubMed]
71. Lorenzo, J.M.; Pateiro, M.; Domínguez, R.; Barba, F.J.; Putnik, P.; Bursać Kovačević, D.; Shpigelman, A.; Granato, D.; Franco, D. Berries extracts as natural antioxidants in meat products: A review. *Food Res. Int.* **2018**, *106*, 1095–1104. [CrossRef]

72. Zugic, A.; Đordevic, S.; Arsic, I.; Markovic, G.; Zivkovic, J.; Jovanovic, S.; Tadi, V. Antioxidant activity and phenolic compounds in 10 selected herbs from Vrujci Spa, Serbia. *Ind. Crop Prod.* **2014**, *52*, 519–527. [CrossRef]

73. Dias, M.I.; Barros, L.; Oliveira, M.B.P.P.; Santos-Buelga, C.; Ferreira, I.C.F.R. Phenolic profile and antioxidant properties of commercial and wild *Fragaria vesca* L. roots: A comparison between hydromethanolic and aqueous extracts. *Ind. Crop Prod.* **2015**, *63*, 125–132. [CrossRef]

74. Dias, M.I.; Barros, L.; Fernandes, I.P.; Ruphuy, G.; Oliveira, M.B.P.P.; Santos-Buelga, C.; Barreiro, M.F.; Ferreira, I.C.F.R. A bioactive formulation based on *Fragaria vesca* L. vegetative parts: Chemical characterization and application in κ-carrageenan gelatin. *J. Funct. Food.* **2015**, *16*, 243–255. [CrossRef]

75. Giampieri, F.; Alvarez-Suarez, J.M.; Battino, M. Strawberry and human health: Effects beyond antioxidant activity. *J. Agricult. Food Chem.* **2014**, *62*, 3867–3876. [CrossRef]

76. Vendrame, S.; Klimis-Zacas, D.J. Anti-inflammatory effect of anthocyanins via modulation of nuclear factor-κB and mitogen-activated protein kinase signaling cascades. *Nutr. Rev.* **2015**, *73*, 348–358. [CrossRef]

77. Li, S.; Wu, B.; Fu, W.; Reddivari, L. The anti-inflammatory effects of dietary anthocyanins against ulcerative colitis. *Int. J. Mol. Sci.* **2019**, *20*, 2588. [CrossRef] [PubMed]

78. Szymanowska, U.; Złotek, U.; Karaś, M.; Baraniak, B. Anti-inflammatory and antioxidative activity of anthocyanins from purple basil leaves induced by selected abiotic elicitors. *Food Chem.* **2015**, *172*, 71–77. [CrossRef] [PubMed]

79. Peng, Y.; Yan, Y.; Wan, P.; Chen, D.; Ding, Y.; Ran, L.; Mi, J.; Lu, L.; Zhang, Z.; Li, X.; et al. Gut microbiota modulation and anti-inflammatory properties of anthocyanins from the fruits of *Lycium ruthenicum* Murray in dextran sodium sulfate-induced colitis in mice. *Free Radic. Biol. Med.* **2019**, *136*, 96–108. [CrossRef] [PubMed]

80. Liberal, J.; Francisco, V.; Costa, G.; Figueirinha, A.; Amaral, M.T.; Marques, C.; Girão, H.; Lopes, M.C.; Cruz, M.T.; Batista, M.T. Bioactivity of *Fragaria vesca* leaves through inflammation, proteasome and autophagy modulation. *J. Ethnopharmacol.* **2014**, *158*, 113–122. [CrossRef]

81. Gasparrini, M.; Giampieri, F.; Forbes-Hernandez, T.Y.; Afrin, S.; Cianciosi, D.; Reboredo-Rodriguez, P.; Varela-Lopez, A.; Zhang, J.; Quiles, J.L.; Mezzetti, B.; et al. Strawberry extracts efficiently counteract inflammatory stress induced by the endotoxin lipopolysaccharide in Human Dermal Fibroblast. *Food Chem. Toxicol.* **2018**, *114*, 128–140. [CrossRef]

82. Molinett, S.; Nuñez, F.; Moya-León, M.A.; Zúñiga-Hernández, J. Chilean strawberry consumption protects against LPS-induced liver injury by anti-inflammatory and antioxidant capability in Sprague-Dawley rats. *Evid.-Based Compl. Alt. Med.* **2015**, *2015*, 320136. [CrossRef]

83. Duarte, L.J.; Chaves, V.C.; dos Santos Nascimento, M.V.P.; Calvete, E.; Li, M.; Ciraolo, E.; Ghigo, A.; Hirsch, E.; Simões, C.M.O.; Reginatto, F.H.; et al. Molecular mechanism of action of Pelargonidin-3-O-glucoside, the main anthocyanin responsible for the anti-inflammatory effect of strawberry fruits. *Food Chem.* **2018**, *247*, 56–65. [CrossRef]

84. Van de Velde, F.; Esposito, D.; Grace, M.H.; Pirovani, M.E.; Lila, M.A. Anti-inflammatory and wound healing properties of polyphenolic extracts from strawberry and blackberry fruits. *Food Res. Int.* **2019**, *121*, 453–462. [CrossRef]

85. Gomes, F.; Martins, N.; Barros, L.; Rodrigues, M.E.; Oliveira, M.B.P.P.; Henriques, M.; Ferreira, I.C.F.R. Plant phenolic extracts as an effective strategy to control *Staphylococcus aureus*, the dairy industry pathogen. *Ind. Crop. Prod.* **2018**, *112*, 515–520. [CrossRef]

86. Cardoso, O.; Donato, M.M.; Luxo, C.; Almeida, N.; Liberal, J.; Figueirinha, A.; Batista, M.T. Anti-*Helicobacter pylori* potential of *Agrimonia eupatoria* L. and *Fragaria vesca*. *J. Funct. Food.* **2018**, *44*, 299–303. [CrossRef]

87. Ninomiya, M.; Itoh, T.; Ishikawa, S.; Saiki, M.; Narumiya, K.; Yasuda, M.; Koshikawa, K.; Nozawa, Y.; Koketsu, M. Phenolic constituents isolated from *Fragaria ananassa* Duch. Inhibit antigen-stimulated degranulation through direct inhibition of spleen tyrosine kinase activation. *Bioorg. Med. Chem.* **2010**, *18*, 5932–5937. [CrossRef] [PubMed]

88. Abdulazeez, S.S. Effects of freeze-dried *Fragaria x ananassa* powder on alloxan-induced diabetic complications in Wistar rats. *J. Taibah Univ. Med. Sci.* **2014**, *9*, 268–273. [CrossRef]

89. Somasagara, R.R.; Hegde, M.; Chiruvella, K.K.; Musini, A.; Choudhary, B.; Raghavan, S.C. Extracts of strawberry fruits induce intrinsic pathway of apoptosis in breast cancer cells and inhibits tumor progression in mice. *PLoS ONE* **2012**, *7*, 47021. [CrossRef] [PubMed]

90. Forni, C.; Braglia, R.; Mulinacci, N.; Urbani, A.; Ronci, M.; Gismondi, A.; Tabolacci, C.; Provenzano, B.; Lentini, A.; Beninati, S. Antineoplastic activity of strawberry (*Fragaria x ananassa* Duch.) crude extracts on B16-F10 melanoma cells. *Mol. Biosyst.* **2014**, *10*, 1255–1263. [CrossRef] [PubMed]
91. Lucioli, S.; Pastorino, F.; Nota, P.; Ballan, G.; Frattarelli, A.; Fabbri, A.; Forni, C.; Caboni, E. Extracts from cell suspension cultures of strawberry (*Fragaria x ananassa* Duch): Cytotoxic effects on human cancer cells. *Molecules* **2019**, *24*, 1738. [CrossRef] [PubMed]
92. Casto, B.C.; Knobloch, T.J.; Galioto, R.L.; Yu, Z.; Accurso, B.T.; Warner, B.M. Chemoprevention of oral cancer by lyophilized strawberries. *Anticancer Res.* **2013**, *33*, 4757–4766.
93. Chen, T.; Shi, N.; Afzali, A. Chemopreventive effects of strawberry and black raspberry on colorectal cancer in inflammatory bowel disease. *Nutrients* **2019**, *11*, 1261. [CrossRef]
94. Kanodia, L.; Borgohain, M.; Das, S. Effect of fruit extract of Fragaria vesca L. on experimentally induced inflammatory bowel disease in albino rats. *Indian. J. Pharmacol.* **2011**, *43*, 18–21. [CrossRef]
95. Shi, N.; Clinton, S.K.; Liu, Z.; Wang, Y.; Riedl, K.M.; Schwartz, S.J.; Zhang, X.; Pan, Z.; Chen, T. Strawberry phytochemicals inhibit azoxymethane/dextran sodium sulfate-induced colorectal carcinogenesis in Crj: CD-1 mice. *Nutrients* **2015**, *7*, 1696–1715. [CrossRef]
96. Gasperotti, M.; Masuero, D.; Mattivi, F.; Vrhovsek, U. Overall dietary polyphenol intake in a bowl of strawberries: The influence of *Fragaria* spp. in nutritional studies. *J. Funct. Foods* **2015**, *18*, 1057–1070. [CrossRef]
97. Valenzuela, C.; Tapia, C.; López, L.; Bunger, A.; Escalona, V.; Abugoch, L. Effect of edible quinoa protein-chitosan based films on refrigerated strawberry (Fragaria × ananassa) quality. *Electron. J. Biotechnol.* **2015**, *18*, 406–411. [CrossRef]
98. Shin, Y.J.; Song, H.Y.; Song, K.B. Effect of a combined treatment of rice bran protein film packaging with aqueous chlorine dioxide washing and ultraviolet-C irradiation on the postharvest quality of 'Goha' strawberries. *J. Food. Eng.* **2012**, *113*, 374–379. [CrossRef]
99. Weisany, W.; Amini, J.; Samadi, S.; Hossaini, S.; Yousefi, S.; Struik, P.C. Nano silver-encapsulation of *Thymus daenensis* and *Anethum graveolens* essential oils enhances antifungal potential against strawberry anthracnose. *Ind. Crop. Prod.* **2019**, *141*, 111808. [CrossRef]
100. Fierascu, R.C.; Fierascu, I.; Avramescu, S.M.; Sieniawska, E. Recovery of natural antioxidants from agro-industrial side streams through advanced extraction techniques. *Molecules* **2019**, *24*, 4212. [CrossRef]
101. Demirbas, A.; Yilmaz, V.; Ildiz, N.; Baldemir, A.; Ocsoy, I. Anthocyanins-rich berry extracts directed formation of Ag NPs with the investigation of their antioxidant and antimicrobial activities. *J. Molec. Liq.* **2017**, *248*, 1044–1049. [CrossRef]
102. Fierascu, I.; Georgiev, M.I.; Ortan, A.; Fierascu, R.C.; Avramescu, S.M.; Ionescu, D.; Sutan, A.; Brinzan, A.; Ditu, L.M. Phyto-mediated metallic nanoarchitectures via *Melissa officinalis* L.: Synthesis, characterization and biological properties. *Sci. Rep.* **2017**, *7*, 12428. [CrossRef]
103. Sutan, N.A.; Manolescu, D.S.; Fierascu, I.; Neblea, A.M.; Sutan, C.; Ducu, C.; Soare, L.C.; Negrea, D.; Avramescu, S.M.; Fierascu, R.C. Phytosynthesis of gold and silver nanoparticles enhance in vitro antioxidant and mitostimulatory activity of *Aconitum toxicum* Reichenb. rhizomes alcoholic extracts. *Mat. Sci. Eng. C* **2018**, *93*, 746–758. [CrossRef]
104. Fierascu, I.; Fierascu, I.C.; Dinu-Pirvu, C.E.; Fierascu, R.C.; Anuta, V.; Velescu, B.S.; Jinga, M.; Jinga, V. A short overview of recent developments on antimicrobial coatings based on phytosynthesized metal nanoparticles. *Coatings* **2019**, *9*, 787. [CrossRef]
105. Fierascu, R.C.; Ortan, A.; Avramescu, S.M.; Fierascu, I. Phyto-nanocatalysts: Green synthesis, characterization, and applications. *Molecules* **2019**, *24*, 3418. [CrossRef]

Sample Availability: Not available..

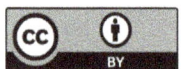

© 2020 by the authors. Licensee MDPI, Basel, Switzerland. This article is an open access article distributed under the terms and conditions of the Creative Commons Attribution (CC BY) license (http://creativecommons.org/licenses/by/4.0/).

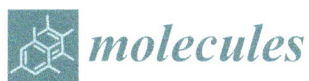

Article

In Vitro and In Situ Characterization of the Intestinal Absorption of Capilliposide B and Capilliposide C from *Lysimachia capillipes* Hemsl

Xu Zhang [1], Xiao Cheng [2], Yali Wu [1], Di Feng [1], Yifan Qian [1], Liping Chen [1], Bo Yang [1] and Mancang Gu [1,*]

1. College of Pharmacy, Zhejiang Chinese Medical University, Hangzhou 311402, China; zhangxu@zcmu.edu.cn (X.Z.); wuyali@zcmu.edu.cn (Y.W.); fengdi@zcmu.edu.cn (D.F.); qianyifan@zcmu.edu.cn (Y.Q.); LipingChen@zcmu.edu.cn (L.C.); Yangbo@zcmu.edu.cn (B.Y.)
2. Huzhou Institute for Food and Drug Control, Huzhou 313000, China; cheng_xiao1981@163.com
* Correspondence: gmancang@zcmu.edu.cn; Tel.: +86-571-617-68158; Fax: +86-571-866-13606

Academic Editor: Raffaele Capasso
Received: 27 February 2019; Accepted: 26 March 2019; Published: 28 March 2019

Abstract: The goal of this investigation was to determine the processes and mechanism of intestinal absorption for capilliposide B (CAPB) and capilliposide C (CAPC) from the Chinese herb, *Lysimachia capillipes* Hemsl. An analysis of basic parameters, such as drug concentrations, time, and behavior in different intestinal segments was analyzed by liquid chromatography-tandem mass spectrometry (LC-MS). The susceptibility of CAPB and CAPC to various inhibitors such as P-glycoprotein (P-gp) inhibitor (verapamil); multidrug resistance-associated protein 2 (MRP2) inhibitor (indomethacin); cytochrome P450 protein 3A4 (CYP3A4) inhibitor (ketoconazole); and the co-inhibitor of P-gp, MRP2 and CYP3A4 (cyclosporine A) were assessed using both caco-2 cell monolayer and single-pass intestinal perfusion (SPIP) models. As a result, CAPB and CAPC are both poorly absorbed in the intestines and exhibited segment-dependent permeability. The intestinal permeability of CAPB and CAPC were significantly increased by the co-treatment of verapamil, indomethacin. In addition, the intestinal permeability of CAPB was also enhanced by ketoconazole and cyclosporine A. It can be concluded that the intestinal absorption mechanisms of CAPB and CAPC involve processes such as facilitated passive diffusion, efflux transporters, and enzyme-mediated metabolism. Both CAPB and CAPC are suggested to be substrates of P-gp and MRP2. However, CAPB may interact with the CYP3A4 system.

Keywords: capilliposide B; capilliposide C; intestinal absorption; caco-2 cell; single-pass intestinal perfusion; liquid chromatography-tandem mass spectrometry

1. Introduction

The oral delivery route for the therapeutic administration of drugs remains one of the most desirable and important routes in drug delivery. With a combination of increased patient compliance, safety and ease of administration, orally-delivered drugs often offer greater clinical efficacy than other options, particularly in minimizing potential infections [1]. However, many therapeutics are unable to utilize this sought-after delivery route due to the poor solubility and instability of many compounds in gastrointestinal fluids. Furthermore, properties such as rapid metabolic elimination, low intestinal permeability, and efflux by protein transporters are major obstacles to the oral delivery of various compounds [2]. In recent years, there have been many attempts to overcome these hurdles described by the aforementioned limitations on oral administration.

The efflux transporters, such as the adenosine triphosphate-binding cassette transporters (ABC transporters), play a critical role in the absorption and distribution of drugs in the intestinal organs. These transporters are important factors dictating the bioavailability of the administered drug in addition to the enzymes responsible for drug metabolism [3,4]. ABC transporters such as, P-glycoprotein (P-gp), multidrug resistance-associated proteins (MRPs) and breast cancer resistance protein (BCRP) are capable of excreting drugs in the cellular compartment into the interstitial compartment, decreasing bioavailability [5]. Many active components of traditional Chinese medicine (TCM), such as saponins (akebia saponin D, ginsenoside Rh2, araloside A, the total saponins of Mao-Dong-Qing), flavones (apigenin, epimedins) and alkaloids (reserpine, vincristine, vinblastine) [6–12] have been shown to be substrates of efflux transporters, which negatively affect the absorption of drugs in the intestine and result in poor bioavailability.

Aside from ABC transporters, drug metabolism enzymes are also critical factors in determining the bioavailability of drugs, among which the cytochrome P450 enzyme (CYP450) plays a major role [13]. The CYP3A4 subset of CYP450 accounts for 30% of the total CYP450 enzyme system [14,15] and is responsible for the bio-transformation of several drugs with a key role in pharmacological effects.

Several permeability models have been employed to understand mechanisms of intestinal absorption, including an in vitro epithelial cell monolayer model such as caco-2 monolayer model and MDCK-MDRI epithelial cell monolayer model [16,17], in vitro everted intestinal sac [18], in vivo or in situ intestinal perfusion models [19], and in vivo pharmacokinetic models. Among these permeability models, the caco-2 cell monolayer model and in situ intestinal perfusion (SPIP) technique are considered as the gold standard in intestinal permeability research and have been wildly utilized to predict intestinal permeability [20,21]. Caco-2 cells express active transport systems, such as P-gp and MRPs [5,22]. However, because of its low expression levels of P450 enzymes and the absence of a protective mucus layer, the cell lines cannot be used for studying the interaction of transporters with underlying metabolic actions.

Lysimachia capillipes Hemsl, a Chinese herb and medicinal plant, is widely used as a remedy for the treatment of colds and arthritis as observed for Cannabis sativa extracts [23,24]. Recently, pharmacological investigations revealed that capilliposide B (CAPB) and capilliposide C (CAPC), the major components of saponins isolated from the Lysimachia genus [25], exhibit an inhibitory effect on cell proliferation in various cancers, such as esophageal cancer [26], human non-small cell lung cancer [27], prostate cancer [28], and nasopharyngeal cancer [29]. Although CAPB and CAPC possess anticancer activity, their poor intestinal absorption obstructs further applications. This poor performance may be attributed to two key factors. On one hand, systemic exposure of CAPB and CAPC was low with significant variation among individuals after oral administration. This is likely a result of its extensive biotransformation in the gastrointestinal tract [30]. On the other hand, the low intestinal permeability of CAPB and CAPC may also serve as a critical barrier, resulting in poor bioavailability and low exposure in tissues after oral administration [31]. However, the specific mechanisms which affect the permeability of CAPB and CAPC through the intestinal epithelium are unknown. Thus, a systemic study is required to investigate the intestinal absorption of CAPB and CAPC.

Therefore, the primary aim of this study was to investigate the process and mechanisms by which CAPB and CAPC are absorbed by intestinal cells using caco-2 cell monolayer and in situ intestinal perfusion models. The effect of parameters such as drug concentration, transport time and behavior in different intestinal segments were analyzed. Furthermore, the susceptibility of CAPB and CAPC absorption to treatment with various inhibitors, such as P-gp inhibitor (verapamil), MRP2 inhibitor (indomethacin); CYP3A4 inhibitor (ketoconazole); and the co-inhibitor of P-gp, MRP2 and CYP3A4 (cyclosporine A) were also assessed.

2. Results

2.1. Liquid Chromatography-Tandem Mass Spectrometry Analysis Method Validation

The concentration of CAPB and CAPC across caco-2 cell monolayer was detected by liquid chromatography-tandem mass spectrometry (LC-MSn). The total ion chromatogram and product ion mass spectra of CAPB, CAPC and dioscin (IS) are shown in Figure 1, while the standard curves of CAPB and CAPC over the concentrate range of 1.0–5000 ng/mL are shown in Figure S1. The equations of the regression line were y = 40.84x − 8.1502 (r^2 = 0.998) for CAPB (over 1–250 ng/mL), y = 64.736x − 147.9 (r^2 = 0.998) for CAPB (over 250–5000 ng/mL), y = 38.961x − 11.532 (r^2 = 0.987) for CAPC (over 1–250 ng/mL), and y = 68.756x − 104.59 (r^2 = 0.994) for CAPC (1–5000 ng/mL). Extraction recoveries at concentrations of 10, 150 and 3000 ng/mL were determined to be 91.6%, 98.41% and 98.44% for CAPB; and 82.05%, 96.65% and 81.65% for CAPC, respectively. The matrix effect of CAPB and CAPC was between 1.01 and 1.11 (RSD < 3.3%) as evaluated internally by a standard-normalized matrix factor. Intra-day and Inter-day variations were both less than 4%.

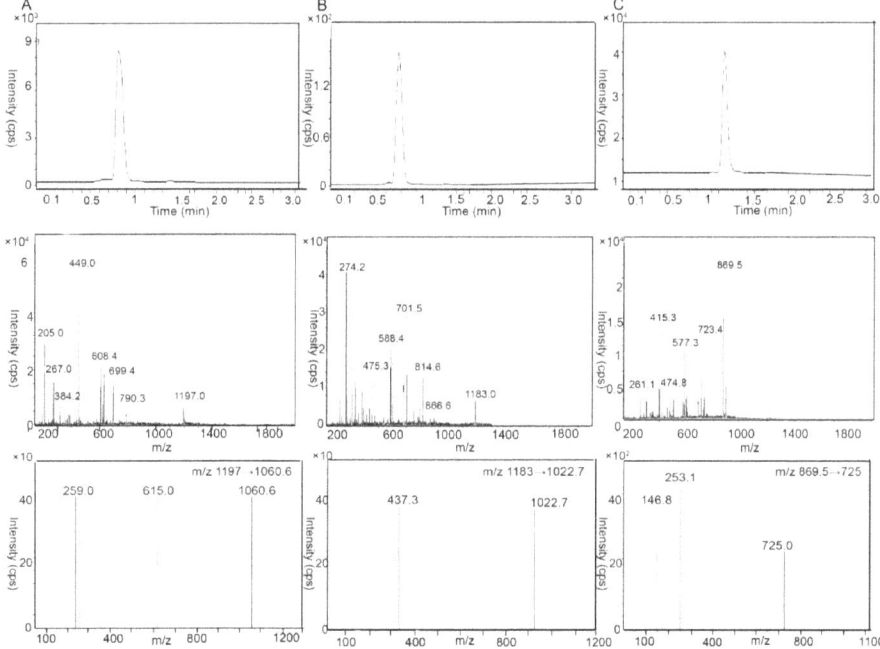

Figure 1. Total ion chromatogram (top panel), product ion mass spectra (middle panel) and the multiple reaction monitoring (MRM) transitions of the deprotonated molecular ions mass spectrogram (bottom panel) of capilliposide B (CAPB, **A**), capilliposide C (CAPC, **B**) and dioscin (IS, **C**). The chromatograms monitoring of CAPB was at m/z 1197.0→1060.6, CAPC at m/z 1183.0→1022.7 and IS at m/z 869.5→725.0.

2.2. The Characterization of Caco-2 Cell Monolayer

The integrity of the monolayer was evaluated by measuring the trans-epithelial electrical resistance (TEER) and phenol red permeability studies. In our data, the monolayer displayed a TEER values >300 Ωcm² andthe apparent permeability (P_{app}, cm/s) values of Phenol <10^5 cm/s after growing for 20 days. These results indicate that caco-2 cell monolayer may be used for permeability studies. In addition, cell viability was verified by MTT assay. As shown in Figure S2, CAPB and CAPC less than 40 μg/mL did not inhibit cell growth significantly. However, a concentration of CAPB and CAPC over 40 μg/mL resulted in significantly decreased cell viability. Hence, 10, 20 and 40 μg/mL of CAPB and CAPC was selected as the testing concentrations for the drug transport study.

2.3. The Characterization of the Intestinal Permeability Features of CAPB and CAPC In a Caco-2 Cell monolayer

A caco-2 cell monolayer model was used to explore the intestinal permeability features of CAPB and CAPC. Firstly, the P_{app} values were measured at different drug concentrations (10, 20, 40 µg/mL), and the P_{app} of CAPB and CAPC were all found to be less than 2×10^{-6} cm/s, as shown in Figure 2A,B. Our data also showed that P_{app} values increased as the CAPB and CAPC concentration increased to high and medium concentrations. Both CAPB and CAPC displayed a significant increase in permeability compared to lower concentrations ($p < 0.05$). However, no significant difference was found between high concentrations and medium concentrations of CAPB and CAPC ($p > 0.05$). Furthermore, the P_{app} values obtained after incubation with CAPB and CAPC for 45, 60 and 90 min across caco-2 cell monolayer in the AP-BL and BL-AP direction is presented in Figure 2C. It was found that P_{app} values showed an upward trend over time. As shown in Figure 2D, the P_{app} (BA)/P_{app} (AB) values (efflux ratio values, ER values) of CAPB and CAPC at different initial drug concentrations (10, 20, 40 µg/mL) were more than 1.0 and less than 1.5.

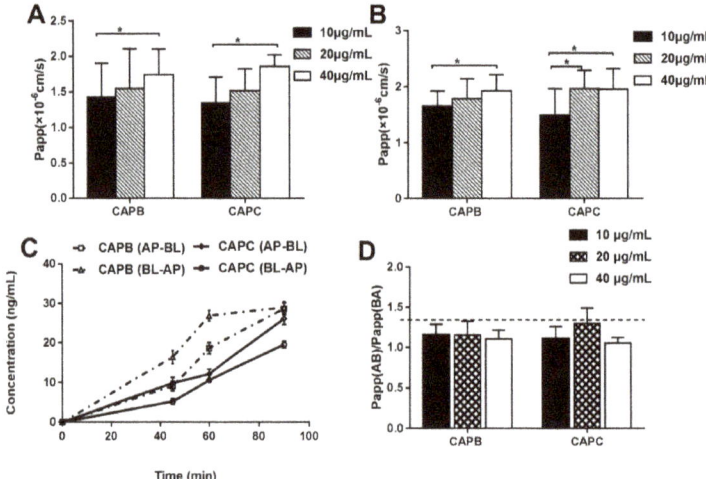

Figure 2. Bidirectional transport studies of capilliposide B (CAPB, **A**), capilliposide C (CAPC, **B**) at different initial drug concentrations (10, 20 and 40 µg/mL). $p < 0.05$ (*), comparison with the 10 µg/mL capilliposides (CAPs) group. The apparent permeability (P_{app}, cm/s) values of CAPB and CAPC at 0, 45, 60 and 90 min (**C**). The P_{app} (BA)/P_{app} (AB) values of CAPB and CAPC were at different initial drug concentrations (10, 20 and 40 µg/mL) (**D**). All results are expressed as mean ± S.D. (n = 3).

2.4. The Role of P-gp, MRP2 and CYP3A4 on CAPB and CAPC Transport Across Caco-2 Cell Monolayer

It was also speculated that the efflux transporter and metabolism enzyme plays an important role in the permeability of CAPB and CAPC across caco-2 cell monolayer as shown in Figure 3. Compared with treatment using CAPs alone, for the co-treatment with either P-gp inhibitor (verapamil); MRP2 inhibitor (indomethacin); or the co-inhibitor of P-gp, MRP2 and CYP3A4 (cyclosporine A), the P_{app} values of CAPB increased about 25 times ($p < 0.01$), 11 times ($p < 0.05$) and 10 times ($p < 0.05$), respectively, on the AP-BL side and around 30 times ($p < 0.01$), 10 times ($p < 0.05$) and 10 times ($p < 0.05$), respectively on the BL-AP side. The P_{app} values of CAPC on the AP-BL side were also significantly increased up to 11 times ($p < 0.05$) and 16 times ($p < 0.01$) in the presence of verapamil and indomethacin, respectively. However, in the presence of cyclosporin A, the permeability of CAPC showed only a small increase ($p > 0.05$), while CAPB showed a 10-fold increase ($p < 0.05$). Therefore, the in vitro transport data indicates that CAPB and CAPC may be the substrate of the efflux protein P-gp and MRP2; moreover CAPB may also be affected by CYP3A4.

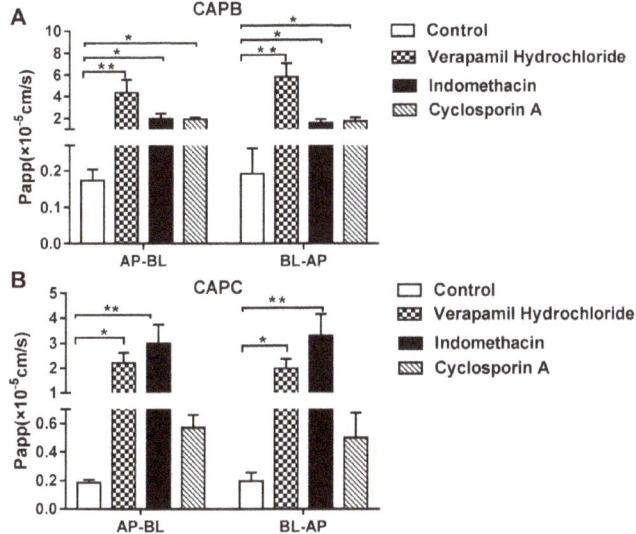

Figure 3. The effect of different factors on the transportation of capilliposide B (CAPB) and capilliposide C (CAPC) across caco-2 cell monolayer. The data are presented as the apparent permeability (P_{app}, cm/s). Effect of P-glycoprotein (P-gp) inhibitor (verapamil hydrochloride); multidrug resistance-associated protein 2 (MRP2) inhibitor (indomethacin); and the co-inhibitor of P-gp, MRP2 and cytochrome P450 protein 3A4 (CYP3A4) on caco-2 cell monolayer for CAPB (**A**) and CAPC (**B**). $p < 0.05$ (*), $p < 0.01$ (**), comparison with control. All results are expressed as mean ± S.D. (n = 3).

2.5. The Characterization of the Intestinal Permeability of CAPB and CAPC In Rats

The SPIP model was used to further explore the intestinal permeability features of CAPB and CAPC in rats. Firstly, we determined the stability of CAPB and CAPC in the Krebsringer buffer (K-R buffer) across different pH values. As shown in Figure 4A, CAPB and CAPC were more stable at pH 5.0 and pH 6.55 than pH 7.43. In other words, CAPB and CAPC were stable in a weakly acidic environment. Because the pH of intestinal juice was close to 6.55, we used a K-R buffer at pH 6.55 as the perfusion solution.

The effective permeability (P_{eff}, cm/s) and absorption rate constants (ka, s^{-1}) values of CAPB and CAPC were measured at different drug concentrations (20, 50 and 80 μg/mL). As shown in Figure 4B, the P_{eff} and Ka values of CAPB showed a slight decline between 20 and 50 μg/mL. However, a significant increase was seen at 80 μg/mL of drug concentration. However, the P_{eff} and Ka values of CAPC showed a slight increase between 20 to 50 μg/mL followed by a significant decrease ($p < 0.05$) as drug concentration increased.

Subsequently, the P_{eff} and Ka values of CAPB and CAPC in the different intestinal segments including duodenum, jejunum and ileum were assessed. As shown in Figure 4C, the order of P_{eff} and Ka values of CAPB in three different intestinal segments was duodenum > jejunum > ileum. The order of CAPC followed the same pattern as CAPB. The permeability in the duodenum was significantly greater than that in jejunum and ileum, respectively ($p < 0.05$). Our data demonstrated that CAPB and CAPC may exhibit segmental-dependent permeability and were best absorbed in the duodenum.

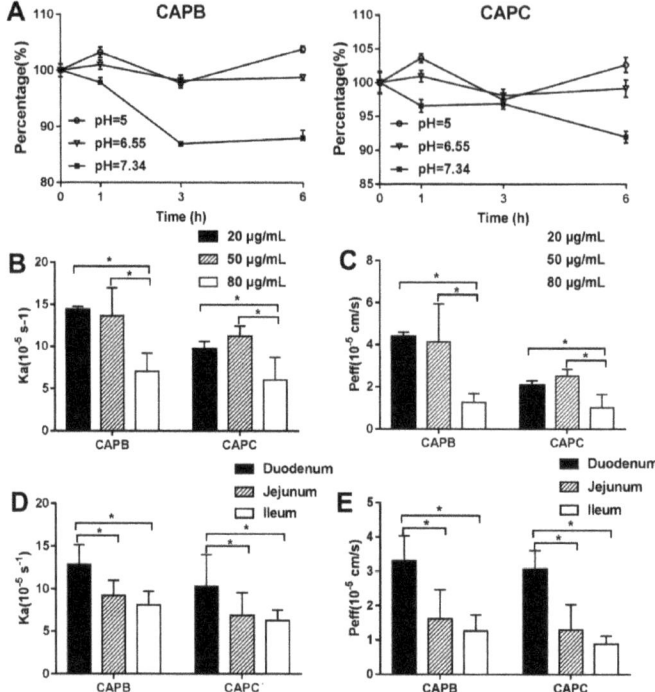

Figure 4. The characterization of the intestinal permeability of capilliposide B (CAPB) and capilliposide C (CAPC) in single-pass intestinal perfusion (SPIP) model. The stability of CAPB and CAPC were measured at different pH values (pH 5, pH 6.55, and pH 7.34, respectively) (**A**). The absorption rate constants (ka, s^{-1}) values (**B**) and effective permeability (P_{eff}, cm/s) values (**C**) for CAPB and CAPC at different initial drug concentrations (20 μg/mL, 50 μg/mL, and 80 μg/mL, respectively). $p < 0.05$ (*) compared with with the group at 80 μg/mL. The Ka values (**D**) and P_{eff} values (**E**) of CAPB and CAPC obtained from the duodenum, jejunum, and ileum in SPIP models. $p < 0.05$ (*) compared with the duodenum. All the results are expressed as mean ± S.D. (n = 3).

2.6. The Role of P-gp, MRP2, and CYP3A4 on Intestinal Permeability of CAPB and CAPC

To further confirm the role of P-gp, MRP2 and CYP3A4 on the intestinal permeability of CAPB and CAPC, the P_{eff} and Ka values were measured in the presence of verapamil, indomethacin, ketoconazole, and cyclosporine A. As the findings in Figure 5 indicate, The P-gp inhibitor, verapamil, resulted in a 1.5-fold increase ($p < 0.05$) on the intestinal transport of CAPB and CAPC. In the presence of indomethacin, the Ka and P_{eff} values increased significantly ($p < 0.05$). The P_{eff} value of CAPB showed an even more significant increase at 4.2 fold while the P_{eff} of CAPC only increased 2 fold. It is worth noting that the P_{eff} values of CAPB and CAPC are equal in the absence of an inhibitor. Therefore it is indicated that the affinity between CAPB and MRP2 is stronger than that of CAPC.

In the presence of the CYP3A4 inhibitor, ketoconazole, CAPB showed a two-fold higher permeability than CAPB alone ($p < 0.05$). However, CAPC exhibited minimal alteration of permeability in the presence of ketoconazole ($p > 0.05$). The substrate of CYP3A4 protein is therefore elucidated to be CAPC over CAPB. In the presence of cyclosporin A, a co-inhibitor of P-gp, MRP2, and CYP3A4, the permeability of CAPC increased slightly ($p > 0.05$), while CAPB increased around two-fold ($p < 0.05$).

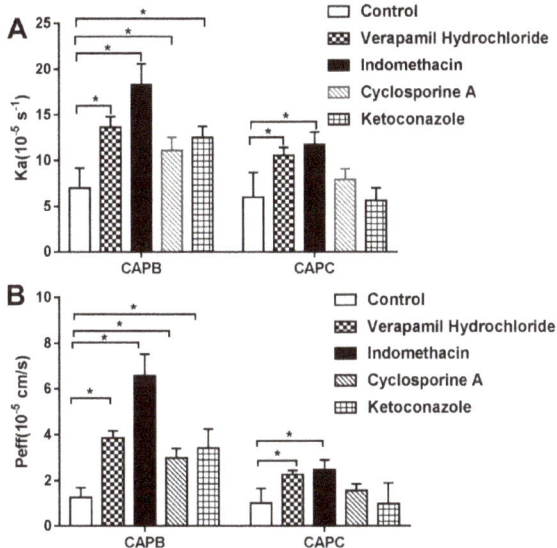

Figure 5. The effect of different factors on intestinal absorption of capilliposide B (CAPB) and capilliposide C (CAPC). The data are presented as absorption rate constants (ka, s^{-1}) values (B) and effective permeability (P_{eff}, cm/s). P-glycoprotein (P-gp) inhibitor (verapamil hydrochloride); multidrug resistance-associated protein 2 (MRP2) inhibitor (indomethacin); and the co-inhibitor of P-gp, MRP2 and cytochrome P450 protein 3A4 (CYP3A4) (cyclosporine A); and CYP3A4 inhibitor (ketoconazole) on small intestinal absorption of CAPB (**A**) and CAPC (**B**). $p < 0.05$ (*), in comparison with control. All the results are expressed as mean ± S.D. (n = 3).

3. Discussion

CAPB and CAPC, two major compounds of *L. capillipes* Hemsl, exhibit significant cytotoxicity against many human cancer cell lines, including prostate cancer cell PC3 and DU145, along with nasopharyngeal cancer CNE-2 cells; ovarian cancer SK-OV-3 and A2780 subtypes; and lung cancer PC-9, A549, H1299, and H460 cells [25–30]. Moreover, CAPB and CAPC were found to inhibit tumor growth without inducing significant toxicity to hepatic or renal tissues in a mouse model [26,27,32]. Previously, studies have evaluated the pharmacokinetics, tissue distribution, and excretion of CAPB and CAPC systematically [31,33,34]. Both compounds showed poor bioavailability and low exposure in tissues after oral administration [31]. However, the intestinal absorption mechanics and underline transport systems of CAPB and CPAC were still unclear. In this study, we revealed that both CAPB and CAPC showed low permeability across intestinal epithelial cells. However, the intestinal absorption of CAPB and CAPC may involve facilitated passive diffusion, and may be affected by efflux transporters and metabolic enzymes.

In a caco-2 cell model, our data showed that the P_{app} of CAPB and CAPC were both less than 2×10^{-6} cm/s, which represents a low permeability of compounds in vitro. The amount of CAPB and CAPC across the cell monolayer accumulated as concentration and time increased. Meanwhile, the ER values of CAPB and CAPC were between 1.00 and 1.50, indicating that facilitated diffusion and efflux mechanisms may be involved in the intestinal epithelium transportation of CAPB and CAPC [22,35]. On the other hand, P_{eff} values of CAPB and CAPC were both much less than 0.2×10^{-4} cm/s in a single-pass intestinal perfusion model, which confirmed the in vitro transportation results. Interestingly, we found that the P_{eff} of CAPB and CAPC fluctuated only slightly from 20 to 50 μg/mL but were drastically restrained at 80 μg/mL in an in situ intestinal infusion model. A possible explanation was that the facilitated passive diffusion may involve intestinal transport, similar to the transport mechanism of sodium taurocholate [36]. However, we did not assess the transportation features of CAPB and CAPC at 80 µg/mL in the caco-2 monolayers model, as the drug showed cytotoxicity when the concentration of CAPB and CAPC was above 40 µg/mL. Because the P_{app} of CAPB and CAPC increased linearly from 10µg/mL to 40 µg/mL in the caco-2 monolayer model, we wanted to further characterize the intestinal permeability of compounds at higher concentrations in the SPIP model. In addition, this data showed that P_{eff} and Ka values of CAPB and CAPC in the duodenum were significantly higher than that in the jejunum and ileum. This may be related to pKa of the drug, the degree of dissociation, the pH in the four intestinal segments, the relative abundance of microvilli and villi, and the distribution of efflux transporters and uptake transporters [37].

The P-gp and MRP2 proteins are two major efflux transporters which affect the absorption of drugs in the intestines [38,39] and are shown to be highly expressed in intestinal epithelium as well as on the membranes of caco-2 cells [4]. Numerous studies have shown that active components of traditional Chinese medicine are the substrates of P-gp and MRP2 proteins, which are likely explanations for the reduced intestinal absorption of oral ginsenoside Rh2, a member of the saponins [40]. As examples, akebia saponin D demonstrates poor intestinal absorption as a result of MRPs in the intestine [41]. Ginsenoside Rh2 [42,43] and araloside A [22] have poor intestinal absorption, because they are both substrates of P-gp.

This in vitro transport data and in situ intestinal infusion data showed that the inhibition of P-gp and MRP2 activity could significantly enhance the permeability of CAPB and CAPC across intestinal epithelia. These results indicated that CAPB and CAPC, also members of the saponins family, may be substrates for the efflux protein P-gp and MRP2. The intestinal permeability of CAPB and CAPC may, at least partly, be limited by P-gp and MRP2.

In addition to the ABC transport protein, metabolic enzymes play a critical role in the intestinal absorption of drugs [44]. For example, CYP3A4 was shown to also influence ginsenoside Rh2 intestinal absorption as it was the predominant enzyme responsible for the oxidation of ginsenoside Rh2 [43,45]. The best example perhaps, is with paclitaxel, whose poor bioavailability is caused by a combination of poor water solubility, P-gp efflux, and CYP3A4 metabolism. In an excretion study of CAPB, it was proven that CAPB experienced extensive metabolism prior to excretion [34]. Likewise, CAPC also demonstrated extensive metabolism in rat intestinal microflora and a strong anticancer activity [46]. Prior studies also systematically characterized 19 metabolites of CAPB and CAPC in mice and proposed a major metabolic pathway (deglycosylation and esterolysis) following oral dosing [32]. However, caco-2 cells do not always express the appropriate amount of metabolic enzymes, such as P450 enzymes, which can affect the uptake of certain drugs that are transported through metabolic-specific pathways [4,47]. Because of its low expression levels of P450 enzymes, the role of CYP3A4 was investigated primarily by adding the co-inhibitor of P-gp, MRP2 and CYP3A4 (cyclosporin A) in the caco-2 cells and SPIP model. Furthermore, the inhibitor of CYP3A4 (ketoconazole) was added to the SPIP model only for the reasons mentioned above. Our in vitro transport data and in situ intestinal infusion data showed that the inhibition of CYP3A4 could significantly enhance the permeability of CAPB across the intestinal epithelia. It was found that CAPB may be the substrate of CYP3A4, but CAPC may not.

While the results are promising, the current study still suffers from certain limitations. The intestinal absorption of drugs was affected by numerous factors, such as transporters, and intestinal microflora [37]. However, the scope of this study sought to focus on the permeability features of CAPB and CAPC, along with the major transporters and metabolic enzymes in intestinal epithelium including P-gp, MRP2 and CYP3A4 [5,13]. While previous studies have already evaluated the pharmacokinetics, distribution, intestinal metabolism, and excretion of CAPB and CAPC [31–34], the absorption characteristics of CAPB and CAPC in the intestinal tract were largely unknown. Additionally, classical inhibitors were used to test the possible drug transport mechanisms instead of a knockout cell or mouse model. This was chosen to make the study more straightforward. In future studies, our group seeks to focus on the effects of intestinal microflora, along with other transporters and metabolic enzymes on the intestinal absorption mechanisms of CAPB and CAPC. A gene-editing protocol may also be employed to further investigate the transport mechanisms of CAPB and CAPC.

4. Materials and Methods

4.1. Materials

Capilliposide B ($C_{58}H_{96}O_{24}$, CAPB), capilliposide C ($C_{57}H_{94}O_{24}$, CAPC) and *Lysimachia capillipes* Hemsl API (more than 70% total of CAPB and CAPC) were obtained from Professor Tian Jingkui, College of Biomedical Engineering and Instrument Science, Zhejiang University (Zhejiang, China). Dioscin (Internal standard, IS, purity $\geq$ 98%) and Verapamil Hydrochloride were obtained from National Institutes for Food and Drug Control (Beijing, China). Phenol Red, Ketoconazole, Novobiocin and Cyclosporin (purity $\geq$ 98%) were purchased from Shanghai Yuanye Biotechnology Co., Ltd. (Shanghai, China). The caco-2 human cell line was obtained from the Shanghai Cell Bank of The Chinese Academy of Sciences. HPLC-grade methanol and acetonitrile and other chemicals were of analytical grade.

4.2. Liquid Chromatography-Tandem Mass Spectrometry (LC-MS) Analysis

The liquid chromatography system used in this study was an Agilent Technologies model 1290 Infinity (Agilent Technologies, Santa Clara, CA, USA). Separations were carried out using a UItimate XB-C18 column (250 × 4.6 mm, 5 µm, Phenomenex, Toran, CA, USA) at 40 °C. The mobile phase was composed of 0.3% formic acid in water as mobile phase A (MA) and acetonitrile as mobile phase B (MB) using a gradient elution of 49% MB (0–10 min) and 49% to 90% MB from 10–25 min. Separation was carried out at a flow rate of 1.0 mL/min. The sample injection volume was 10 µL.

An Agilent 6460 Triple Quad mass separometer (Agilent Technologies) equipped with a Turboionspray source (TIS) was operated in the positive ionization mode with multiple reaction monitoring (MRM) for LC-MS analysis. The MS parameter was optimized as follows: TIS temperature, 600 °C; ionspray voltage, −4500 V; curtain gas, nitrogen, 30 psi; nebulizing gas, 50 psi; declustering potential, 135 V for CAPB, 135 V for CAPC and 90 V for dioscin (IS); entrance potential, 10 V; collision energy 10 eV for CAPB, CAPC and dioscin (IS); collision cell exit potential, 15 V. The following MRM transition was used: m/z 1197→1060.6 for CAPB, 1182.8→1022.0 for CAPC, 869.5→725.6 for dioscin.

4.3. Caco-2 Cell Culture

Caco-2 cells were routinely cultured in high glucose Dulbecco's modified Eagle's medium (DMEM) containing 10% fetal bovine serum (FBS), 1% nonessential amino acids, and 1% penicillin/streptomycin. Cells were kept at 37 °C in a 90% relative humidity atmosphere containing 5% CO_2. Cells were seeded onto transwells purchased from Corning Costar Co. (New York, NY, USA) on 12-well plates for transport studies and uptake studies at 5×10^4 cells per insert. Cells were grown for 20 days. The integrity of monolayer was evaluated by measuring the trans-epithelial electrical resistance (TEER) and by phenol red permeability studies.

The effects of CAPs on caco-2 cell viability were checked by 3-(4,5-dimethyl-2-thiazolyl)-2,5-diphenyl-2-H-tetrazolium bromide (MTT) colorimetric assay [12], which is adapted to analyze cell proliferation and drug cytotoxicity. Cells with decreased viability are considered to be less metabolically active and hence will reduce less MTT. In brief, caco-2 cells were seeded at 4×10^3 cells/well into 96-well culture plates and were incubated at 37 °C for 24 h before the assay. The cells were treated with different concentrations (0, 10, 20, 40, 80, 120, 160 and 240 µg/mL) of CAPs. After 24 h of incubation, 20 µL of MTT (5 mg/mL) was added to each well and the cells were incubated for another 4 h. After removing the culture medium, 100 µL of dimethyl sulfoxide was added to dissolve the contents in the plate. Then, the absorbance was measured at 570 and 630 nm (reference wavelength) using a microplate reader (Multiskan MK3; Thermo Fisher Scientific, Waltham, MA, USA).

4.4. Permeability Studies Using Caco-2 Cells

DMEM was removed and the monolayer was washed with Hank's Balanced Salt Solution (HBSS). The blank HBSS was replaced by 0.4 mL of HBSS containing 40, 20 and 10 μg/mL of drug on the apical (AP) side and 2.1 mL of HBSS on the basolateral (BL) side. In the AP-BL direction studies, 0.4 mL of HBSS containing 40 μg/mL drug and P-gp inhibitor (53 μg/mL verapamil); MRP2 inhibitor (17.9 μg/mL indomethacin); or the co-inhibitor of P-gp, MRP2 and CYP3A4 (10 μg/mL cyclosporin A) were added to the AP side; 2.1 mL of HBSS was added to the BL side. In the BL-AP direction studies, 0.4 mL of HBSS containing 40 μg/mL drug and different inhibitors were added to the BL side, and 2.1 mL of HBSS was added to AP side. Samples (0.4 mL) were taken from the BL or AP side after 45, 60 and 90 min incubation at 37 °C. An additional 0.4 mL of HBSS was added at the same time. The concentrations of samples were analyzed by LC-MS.

4.5. In Situ Single-Pass Intestinal Perfusion (SPIP) Studies In Rats

Male Sprague–Dawley (SD) rats (280 ± 30 g) were supplied by the Laboratory Animal Center, Zhejiang Chinese Medical University (Zhejiang, China). All animals were fasted overnight (12–18 h) with free access to water before experiments. All experiments were performed in accordance with the guidelines for the care and use of animals as established by the Laboratory Animal Centre, Zhejiang Chinese Medical University (Zhejiang, China) (approval number: ACXK20150016).

The perfusion experiment was performed as previously reported. In brief, rats were fasted overnight but permitted to drink water freely the day before the experiments. After being anesthetized, the rats were placed on the surface of a thermostatic device and maintained at 37 °C. An incision of approximately 3 cm was made along the midline of the abdominal cavity to expose the contents of the abdomen. Perfusate entered the duodenum (1 cm below pylorus) and exited from the jejunum (15 cm from the pylorus). Then the incision was made at both sides of the segment. The intestinal contents were rinsed with saline preheated at 37 °C, drained with air, and connected to the perfusion system with the catheter.

One-hundred millitlers of pre-prepared perfusate was taken and preheated at 37 °C. The perfusion was started at a circulation speed of 1.0 mL/min for 10 min. The flow rate was subsequently increased to 0.2 mL/min for 30 min to ensure steady-state conditions. Samples were collected in glass tubes (2 mL/per) at 10-min intervals for 90 min. The samples were filtered through a membrane filter (0.45 μm) and the concentration of CAPB, CAPC and phenol red were measured by LC-MS. The rest of the samples were stored at −20 °C for further studies.

4.6. Data Analysis

The apparent permeability (P_{app}, cm/s) across caco-2 cell monolayer was calculated from the linear plot of drugs accumulated in the receiver side versus time using Equation (1):

$$P_{app} = \left(\frac{1}{C_0 A}\right)\left(\frac{dQ}{dt}\right) \qquad (1)$$

where dQ/dt represents the steady-state flux of the drug on the receiver (serosal in the case of AP-BL studies or mucosal in the case of BL-AP studies) side, C_0 is the initial concentration of the drug in the donor side, and A is the monolayer growth surface area (4.67 cm^2). Linear regression was carried out to obtain the steady-state appearance rate of the drug on the receiver side.

Effective permeability (P_{eff}) and absorption rate constants (Ka) were calculated using the following Equations (2), (3) and (4), respectively

$$\frac{C'_{out}}{C'_{in}} = \frac{C_{out}}{C_{in}} \times \frac{C_{in,phenolred}}{C_{out,phenolred}}, \qquad (2)$$

$$P_{eff}(m/s) = \frac{-Q\ln(C'_{out}/C'_{in})}{2\pi RL}, \quad (3)$$

$$Ka = Q(1 - \frac{C'_{out}}{C'_{in}})\pi R^2 L, \quad (4)$$

where C_{in} phenol red and C_{out} phenol red is equal to the concentrations of phenol red in the inlet and outlet samples, respectively; C'_{out}/C'_{in} is the ratio of the outlet and inlet concentration of the tested drug that has been adjusted for water transport, Q is the perfusion buffer flow rate (0.2 and 0.1 mL/min for rats and mice, respectively), R is the radius of the intestinal segment (set to 0.2 and 0.1 cm for rats and mice, respectively), and L is the length of the intestinal segment.

4.7. Statistical Analysis

All experiments were performed in triplicate (minimum) and results were expressed as mean values ± standard deviation (SD). Statistical comparisons were performed by Student's t-tests or one-way analysis of variance (ANOVA) using the SPSS version 22 software. Comparisons between two groups were analyzed using Student's t-tests. When a *p*-value was smaller than 0.05, it was considered statistically significant. All data were represented for at least three independent experiments.

5. Conclusions

The present study has revealed that CAPB and CAPC are poorly absorbed in the intestines and likely exhibited segmental-dependent permeability; it can also be found that the intestinal absorption mechanism of CAPB and CAPC may involve facilitated passive diffusion associated with the efflux transporters P-gp and MRP2, along with the metabolic enzyme CYP3A4. As a whole, CAPB may be the substrate of the P-gp, MRP2 and CYP3A4, while CAPC may be the substrate of the P-gp and MRP2, but not of the CYP3A4. In conjunction with results from previous studies along the direction of CAPB and CAPC, these results provide updated information concerning the intestinal absorption process and the possible mechanism of these two compounds.

Supplementary Materials: The following are available online at http://www.mdpi.com/1420-3049/24/7/1227/s1, Figure S1: The standard curve of CAPB and CAPC across caco-2 cell monolayer was detected by LC-MS. Figure S2: CAPs inhibited the proliferation of caco-2 cells.

Author Contributions: X.Z. and X.C. wrote and substantively revised the manuscript. X.Z., Y.W. and D.F. performed the experiments. Y.Q., L.C. and B.Y. analyzed the data. M.G. acted as a supervisor.

Acknowledgments: The work was supported by National Natural Science Foundation of China grants (Grant No. 81673607, 81303235, 81774011, 81473434); Natural Science Foundation of Zhejiang Province grants (Grant No. Y19H280009, LY17A040010); as well as the Public Welfare Research Project of Huzhou Science and Technology Grant (Grant No. 2018GZ24). We appreciate Tian Jinkui from Zhejiang University for giving the Capilliposide B, capilliposide C and *Lysimachia capillipes* Hemsl API as kindly gifts.

Conflicts of Interest: The authors report no conflicts of interest.

References

1. Tang, L.; Fu, L.L.; Zhu, Z.F.; Yang, Y.; Sun, B.X.; Shan, W.G.; Zhang, Z.H. Modified mixed nanomicelles with collagen peptides enhanced oral absorption of Cucurbitacin B: preparation and evaluation. *Drug Deliv.* **2018**, *25*, 862–871. [CrossRef]
2. Yun, Y.; Cho, Y.W.; Park, K. Nanoparticles for oral delivery: Targeted nanoparticles with peptidic ligands for oral protein delivery. *Adv. Drug Deliv. Rev.* **2013**, *65*, 822–832. [CrossRef]
3. Porat, D.; Dahan, A. Active intestinal drug absorption and the solubility-permeability interplay. *Int. J. Pharm.* **2018**, *537*, 84–93. [CrossRef] [PubMed]
4. Estudante, M.; Morais, J.G.; Soveral, G.; Benet, L.Z. Intestinal drug transporters: An overview. *Adv. Drug Deliv. Rev.* **2013**, *65*, 1340–1356. [CrossRef]

5. Li, M.; de Graaf, I.A.M.; van de Steeg, E.; de Jager, M.H.; Groothuis, G.M.M. The consequence of regional gradients of P-gp and CYP3A4 for drug-drug interactions by P-gp inhibitors and the P-gp/CYP3A4 interplay in the human intestine ex vivo. *Toxicol. In Vitro* **2017**, *40*, 26–33. [CrossRef]
6. Del Hierro, J.N.; Herrera, T.; Fornari, T.; Reglero, G.; Martin, D. The gastrointestinal behavior of saponins and its significance for their bioavailability and bioactivities. *J. Funct. Foods* **2018**, *40*, 484–497. [CrossRef]
7. Yang, Z.; Wang, J.R.; Niu, T.; Gao, S.; Yin, T.J.; You, M.; Jiang, Z.H.; Hu, M. Inhibition of P-Glycoprotein Leads to Improved Oral Bioavailability of Compound K, an Anticancer Metabolite of Red Ginseng Extract Produced by Gut Microflora. *Drug Metab. Dispos.* **2012**, *40*, 1538–1544. [CrossRef] [PubMed]
8. Lee, J.A.; Ha, S.K.; Kim, Y.C.; Choi, I. Effects of friedelin on the intestinal permeability and bioavailability of apigenin. *Pharmacol. Rep.* **2017**, *69*, 1044–1048. [CrossRef]
9. Liu, L.; Sun, S.; Li, X.H. In vitro Characterization of the Intestinal Absorption Mechanism of Dihydromyricetin in Caco-2 Cell Model. *Lat. Am. J. Pharm.* **2018**, *37*, 908–913.
10. Xi, G.M.; Sun, B.; Jiang, H.H.; Kong, F.; Yuan, H.Q.; Lou, H.X. Bisbibenzyl derivatives sensitize vincristine-resistant KB/VCR cells to chemotherapeutic agents by retarding P-gp activity. *Bioorgan. Med. Chem.* **2010**, *18*, 6725–6733. [CrossRef] [PubMed]
11. Kuang, G.J.; Yi, H.; Zhu, M.J.; Zhou, J.; Shang, X.Y.; Zhao, Z.X.; Zhu, C.C.; Liao, Q.F.; Guan, S.X.; Zhang, L. Study of Absorption Characteristics of the Total Saponins from Radix Ilicis Pubescentis in an In Situ Single-Pass Intestinal Perfusion (SPIP) Rat Model by Using Ultra Performance Liquid Chromatography (UPLC). *Molecules* **2017**, *22*, 1867. [CrossRef] [PubMed]
12. Chen, Y.; Wang, Y.; Zhou, J.; Gao, X.; Qu, D.; Liu, C.Y. Study on the Mechanism of Intestinal Absorption of Epimedins A, B and C in the Caco-2 Cell Model. *Molecules* **2014**, *19*, 686–698. [CrossRef] [PubMed]
13. Sun, X.Y.; Duan, Z.J.; Liu, Z.; Tang, S.X.; Li, Y.; He, S.C.; Wang, Q.M.; Chang, Q.Y. Inhibition of P-glycoprotein, multidrug resistance-associated protein 2 and cytochrome P450 3A4 improves the oral absorption of octreotide in rats with portal hypertension. *Exp. Ther. Med.* **2016**, *12*, 3716–3722. [CrossRef]
14. Tang, L.; Ye, L.; Lv, C.; Zheng, Z.J.; Gong, Y.; Liu, Z.Q. Involvement of CYP3A4/5 and CYP2D6 in the metabolism of aconitine using human liver microsomes and recombinant CYP450 enzymes. *Toxicol. Lett.* **2011**, *20*, 47–54. [CrossRef]
15. Chen, J.; Liu, D.Y.; Zheng, X.; Zhao, Q.; Jiang, J.; Hu, P. Relative contributions of the major human CYP450 to the metabolism of icotinib and its implication in prediction of drug-drug interaction between icotinib and CYP3A4 inhibitors/inducers using physiologically based pharmacokinetic modeling. *Expert. Opin. Drug Met.* **2015**, *11*, 857–868. [CrossRef] [PubMed]
16. Wang, X.X.; Liu, G.Y.; Yang, Y.F.; Wu, X.W.; Xu, W.; Yang, X.W. Intestinal Absorption of Triterpenoids and Flavonoids from Glycyrrhizae radix et rhizoma in the Human Caco-2 Monolayer Cell Model. *Molecules* **2017**, *22*, 1627. [CrossRef]
17. Chen, Z.L.; Ma, T.T.; Huang, C.; Zhang, L.; Zhong, J.; Han, J.W.; Hu, T.T.; Li, J. Efficiency of transcellular transport and efflux of flavonoids with different glycosidic units from flavonoids of Litsea coreana L. in a MDCK epithelial cell monolayer model. *Eur. J. Pharm. Sci.* **2014**, *53*, 69–76. [CrossRef]
18. Gurunath, S.; Nanjwade, B.K.; Patila, P.A. Enhanced solubility and intestinal absorption of candesartan cilexetil solid dispersions using everted rat intestinal sacs. *Saudi Pharm. J.* **2014**, *22*, 246–257. [CrossRef] [PubMed]
19. Xin, L.; Liu, X.H.; Yang, J.; Shen, H.Y.; Ji, G.; Shi, X.F.; Xie, Y. The intestinal absorption properties of flavonoids in Hippophae rhamnoides extracts by an in situ single-pass intestinal perfusion model. *J. Asian Nat. Prod. Res.* **2017**, *10*, 1–14. [CrossRef]
20. Stappaerts, J.; Brouwers, J.; Annaert, P.; Augustijns, P. In situ perfusion in rodents to explore intestinal drug absorption: challenges and opportunities. *Int. J. Pharm.* **2015**, *478*, 665–681. [CrossRef]
21. Zhang, D.D.; Lei, T.L.; Lv, C.N.; Zhao, H.M.; Xu, H.Y.; Lu, J.C. Pharmacokinetic studies of active triterpenoid saponins and the total secondary saponin from Anemone raddeana Regel. *J. Chromatogr. B* **2017**, *1044*, 54–62. [CrossRef] [PubMed]
22. Yang, H.; Zhai, B.T.; Fan, Y.; Wang, J.; Sun, J.; Shi, Y.J.; Guo, D.Y. Intestinal absorption mechanisms of araloside A in situ single-pass intestinal perfusion and in vitro Caco-2 cell model. *Biomed. Pharmacother.* **2018**, *106*, 1563–1569. [CrossRef]
23. Tian, J.K.; Xu, L.Z.; Zou, Z.M.; Yang, S.L. Two new triterpene saponins from Lysimachia capillipes. *J. Asian Nat. Prod. Res.* **2006**, *8*, 439–444. [CrossRef]

24. Bonini, S.A.; Premoli, M.; Tambaro, S.; Kumar, A.; Maccarinelli, G.; Memo, M.; Mastinu, A. Cannabis sativa: A comprehensive ethnopharmacological review of a medicinal plant with a long history. *J. Ethnopharmacol.* **2018**, *227*, 300–315. [CrossRef]
25. Tian, J.K.; Xu, L.Z.; Zou, Z.M.; Yang, S.L. Three novel triterpenoid saponins from Lysimachia capillipes and their cytotoxic activities. *Chem. Pharm. Bull. (Tokyo)* **2006**, *54*, 567–569. [CrossRef]
26. Shen, Z.; Xu, L.; Li, J.; Zhang, N. Capilliposide C Sensitizes Esophageal Squamous Carcinoma Cells to Oxaliplatin by Inducing Apoptosis Through the PI3K/Akt/mTOR Pathway. *Med. Sci. Monit.* **2017**, *23*, 2096–2103. [CrossRef]
27. Fei, Z.H.; Wu, K.; Chen, Y.L.; Wang, B.; Zhang, S.R.; Ma, S.L. Capilliposide Isolated from Lysimachia capillipes Hemsl. Induces ROS Generation, Cell Cycle Arrest, and Apoptosis in Human Nonsmall Cell Lung Cancer Cell Lines. *Evid. Based Complement Alternat. Med.* **2014**, *2014*. [CrossRef] [PubMed]
28. Li, R.; Zhang, L.; Zhang, L.; Chen, D.; Tian, J.; Cao, L.; Zhang, L. Capilliposide C derived from Lysimachia capillipes Hemsl inhibits growth of human prostate cancer PC3 cells by targeting caspase and MAPK pathways. *Int. Urol. Nephrol.* **2014**, *46*, 1335–1344. [CrossRef] [PubMed]
29. Hua, Y.; Hu, Q.; Piao, Y.; Tang, Q.; Feng, J. Effect of capilliposide for induction apoptosis in human nasopharyngeal cancer CNE-2 cells through up-regulating PUMA expression. *J. Cancer Res. Ther.* **2015**, *11*, C239–C243.
30. Zhang, S.R.; Xu, Y.S.; Jin, E.; Zhu, L.C.; Xia, B.; Chen, X.F.; Li, F.Z.; Ma, S.L. Capilliposide from Lysimachia capillipes inhibits AKT activation and restores gefitinib sensitivity in human non-small cell lung cancer cells with acquired gefitinib resistance. *Acta Pharmacol. Sin.* **2017**, *38*, 100–109. [CrossRef]
31. Cheng, Z.; Zhang, L.; Zhang, Y.; Chen, G.; Jiang, H. Simultaneous determination of capilliposide B and capilliposide C in rat plasma by LC-MS/MS and its application to a PK study. *Bioanalysis* **2014**, *6*, 935–945. [CrossRef]
32. Cheng, Z.; Zhou, X.; Du, Z.; Li, W.; Hu, B.; Tian, J.; Zhang, L.; Huang, J.; Jiang, H. Metabolic Stability and Metabolite Characterization of Capilliposide B and Capilliposide C by LC(-)QTRAP(-)MS/MS. *Pharmaceutics* **2018**, *10*, 178. [CrossRef]
33. Cheng, Z.; Zhou, X.; Hu, B.; Li, W.; Chen, G.; Zhang, Y.; Tian, J.; Zhang, L.; Li, M.; Jiang, H. Tissue distribution of capilliposide B, capilliposide C and their bioactive metabolite in mice using liquid -tandem mass spectrometry. *Biomed. Chromatogr.* **2017**, *31*. [CrossRef]
34. Cheng, Z.; Zhou, X.; Li, W.; Hu, B.; Zhang, Y.; Xu, Y.; Zhang, L.; Jiang, H. Optimization of solid-phase extraction and liquid chromatography-tandem mass spectrometry for simultaneous determination of capilliposide B and its active metabolite in rat urine and feces: Overcoming nonspecific binding. *J. Pharm. Biomed. Anal.* **2016**, *131*, 6–12. [CrossRef]
35. Sun, H.D.; Pang, K.S. Permeability, transport, and metabolism of solutes in caco-2 cell monolayers: A theoretical study. *Drug Metab. Dispos.* **2008**, *36*, 102–123. [CrossRef] [PubMed]
36. Gao, H.; Wang, M.; Sun, D.D.; Sun, S.L.; Sun, C.; Liu, J.G.; Guan, Q.X. Evaluation of the cytotoxicity and intestinal absorption of a self-emulsifying drug delivery system containing sodium taurocholate. *Eur. J. Pharm. Sci.* **2017**, *106*, 212–219. [CrossRef] [PubMed]
37. Pang, K.S. Modeling of intestinal drug absorption: roles of transporters and metabolic enzymes. *Drug Metab. Dispos.* **2003**, *31*, 1507–1519. [CrossRef] [PubMed]
38. Zakeri-Milani, P.; Valizadeh, H. Intestinal transporters: enhanced absorption through P-glycoprotein-related drug interactions. *Expert Opin. Drug Met.* **2014**, *10*, 859–871. [CrossRef] [PubMed]
39. Vaessen, S.F.C.; van Lipzig, M.M.H.; Pieters, R.H.H.; Krul, C.A.M.; Wortelboer, H.M.; van de Steeg, E. Regional Expression Levels of Drug Transporters and Metabolizing Enzymes along the Pig and Human Intestinal Tract and Comparison with Caco-2 Cells. *Drug Metab. Dispos.* **2017**, *45*, 353–360. [CrossRef]
40. Zhang, B.; Ye, H.; Zhu, X.M.; Hu, J.N.; Li, H.Y.; Tsao, R.; Deng, Z.Y.; Zheng, Y.N.; Li, W. Esterification enhanced intestinal absorption of ginsenoside Rh2 in Caco-2 cells without impacts on its protective effects against H(2)O(2)-induced cell injury in human umbilical vein endothelial cells (HUVECs). *J. Agric. Food Chem.* **2014**, *62*, 2096–2103. [CrossRef]
41. Zhou, Y.Q.; Li, W.Z.; Chen, L.Y.; Ma, S.W.; Ping, L.; Yang, Z.L. Enhancement of intestinal absorption of akebia saponin D by borneol and probenecid in situ and in vitro. *Environ. Toxicol. Phar.* **2010**, *29*, 229–234. [CrossRef] [PubMed]

42. Yang, Z.; Gao, S.; Wang, J.R.; Yin, T.J.; Teng, Y.; Wu, B.J.; You, M.; Jiang, Z.H.; Hu, M. Enhancement of Oral Bioavailability of 20(S)-Ginsenoside Rh2 through Improved Understanding of Its Absorption and Efflux Mechanisms. *Drug Metab. Dispos.* **2011**, *39*, 1866–1872. [CrossRef] [PubMed]
43. Jin, Z.H.; Qiu, W.; Liu, H.; Jiang, X.H.; Wang, L. Enhancement of oral bioavailability and immune response of Ginsenoside Rh2 by co-administration with piperine. *Chin. J. Nat. Medicines* **2018**, *16*, 143–149. [CrossRef]
44. Ahmmed, S.M.; Mukherjee, P.K.; Bahadur, S.; Harwansh, R.K.; Kar, A.; Bandyopadhyay, A.; Al-Dhabi, N.A.; Duraipandiyan, V. CYP450 mediated inhibition potential of Swertia chirata: An herb from Indian traditional medicine. *J. Ethnopharmacol.* **2016**, *178*, 34–39. [CrossRef] [PubMed]
45. Li, L.; Chen, X.Y.; Zhou, J.L.; Zhong, D.F. In Vitro Studies on the Oxidative Metabolism of 20(S)-Ginsenoside Rh2 in Human, Monkey, Dog, Rat, and Mouse Liver Microsomes, and Human Liver S9. *Drug Metab. Dispos.* **2012**, *40*, 2041–2053. [CrossRef] [PubMed]
46. Cheng, Z.; Huang, M.; Chen, G.; Yang, G.; Zhou, X.; Chen, C.; Zhang, Y.; Xu, Y.; Feng, Y.; Zhang, L.; et al. Cell-based assays in combination with ultra-high performance liquid chromatography-quadrupole time of flight tandem mass spectrometry for screening bioactive capilliposide C metabolites generated by rat intestinal microflora. *J. Pharm. Biomed. Anal.* **2016**, *119*, 130–138. [CrossRef] [PubMed]
47. Zhou, W.; Di, L.Q.; Wang, J.; Shan, J.J.; Liu, S.J.; Ju, W.Z.; Cai, B.C. Intestinal absorption of forsythoside A in in situ single-pass intestinal perfusion and in vitro Caco-2 cell models. *Acta Pharmacol. Sin.* **2012**, *33*, 1069–1079. [CrossRef] [PubMed]

Sample Availability: Samples of the compounds are not available from the authors.

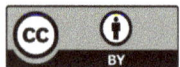

© 2019 by the authors. Licensee MDPI, Basel, Switzerland. This article is an open access article distributed under the terms and conditions of the Creative Commons Attribution (CC BY) license (http://creativecommons.org/licenses/by/4.0/).

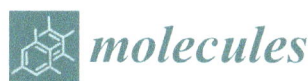

Article

Solvent Fractionation and Acetone Precipitation for Crude Saponins from *Eurycoma longifolia* Extract

Lee Suan Chua [1,2,*], Cher Haan Lau [1], Chee Yung Chew [2] and Dawood Ali Salim Dawood [1]

[1] Metabolites Profiling Laboratory, Institute of Bioproduct Development, Universiti Teknologi Malaysia, Skudai, Johor Bahru 81310 UTM, Johor, Malaysia; cherhaan@gmail.com (C.H.L.); alisalim883@yahoo.com (D.A.S.D.)

[2] Department of Bioprocess and Polymer Engineering, School of Chemical and Energy Engineering, Faculty of Engineering, Universiti Teknologi Malaysia, Skudai, Johor Bahru 81310 UTM, Johor, Malaysia; chee_yung@live.com.my

* Correspondence: chualeesuan@utm.my; Tel.: +607-5531566

Academic Editors: Raffaele Capasso and Lorenzo Di Cesare Mannelli
Received: 22 March 2019; Accepted: 2 April 2019; Published: 10 April 2019

Abstract: *Eurycoma longifolia* is a popular folk medicine in South East Asia. This study was focused on saccharide-containing compounds including saponins, mainly because of their medical potentials. Different organic solvents such as ethyl acetate, butanol, and chloroform were used to fractionate the phytochemical groups, which were consequently precipitated in cold acetone. Solvent fractionation was found to increase the total saponin content based on colorimetric assay using vanillin and sulfuric acid. Ethyl acetate fraction and its precipitate were showed to have the highest crude saponins after acetone precipitation. The samples were shown to have anti-proliferative activity comparable with tamoxifen (IC_{50} = 110.6 μg/mL) against human breast cancer cells. The anti-proliferative activities of the samples were significantly improved from crude extract (IC_{50} = 616.3 μg/mL) to ethyl acetate fraction (IC_{50} = 185.4 μg/mL) and its precipitate (IC_{50} = 153.4 μg/mL). LC-DAD-MS/MS analysis revealed that the saccharide-containing compounds such as m/z 497, 610, 723, 836, and 949 were abundant in the samples, and they could be ionized in negative ion mode. The compounds consisted of 226 amu monomers with UV-absorbing property at 254 nm, and were tentatively identified as formylated hexoses. To conclude, solvent fractionation and acetone precipitation could produce saccharide-containing compounds including saponins with higher anti-proliferative activity than crude extract against MCF-7 cells. This is the first study to use non-toxic solvents for fractionation of bioactive compounds from highly complex plant extract of *E. longifolia*.

Keywords: *Eurycoma longifolia*; Simaroubaceae; solvent fractionation; acetone precipitation; saponins; LC-DAD-MS/MS.

---

1. Introduction

Eurycoma longifolia has traditionally been used as ethnomedicine by indigenous people from ASEAN (Association of Southeast Asian Nations) countries to treat many illnesses, such as tertian malaria, ulcer, syphilis, gonorrhea, and dysentery, as well as to relieve headache, stomachache, and insect bites [1]. The roots of the plant, which is locally known as Malaysian Ginseng, are popular mainly because of its aphrodisiac effects [2–4]. Quassinoids are the most extensively studied phytochemicals from the roots of the plant, mostly C18-20 quassinoids [5]. They are degraded and highly oxygenated triterpenes, which mainly contribute to the bitter taste of plants of the Simaroubaceae family. Saponins are another important class of bioactive phytochemicals, but they are relatively limited in literature for this plant. This could be due to the difficulties in separating and identifying saponins.

Recently, spectrophotometric techniques have been widely applied to estimate total saponin content, based on the method proposed by Hiai et al. [6] for plant samples. This method uses strong acids such as sulfuric acid and perchloric acid to oxidize triterpene saponins and react with vanillin to give a distinctive red-purple colored complex, which can be measured at the visible range of wavelengths ranging from 473 to 560 nm. The reaction is also dependent upon the structure of ring A in triterpenes [7]. Although it is a simple assay to estimate total saponins, specific saponin compounds need to be identified by chromatographic technique. Generally, saponins do not have a chromophore for ultraviolet absorbance in liquid chromatography. Moreover, saponins exhibit low sensitivity in detectors like refractive index and evaporative light scattering, partly due to the restriction in solvent of choice and gradient condition. Although derivatization using 4-bromophenacyl bromide prior to HPLC analysis was proposed by Slacanin et al. [8], Oleszek et al. [9] and Nowacka and Oleszek [10] found that the derivatized standards decomposed in a short period of time (48 h) at room temperature. Therefore, liquid chromatography coupled with mass spectrometry has been the method of choice in the detection and identification of saponins in recent years. Previously, this combined technique has been used to chemically characterize saponins from *Pulsatilla chinensis* [11], *Paris polyphylla* [12], *Chenopodium quinoa* [13], *Tribulus terrestris*, and *Panax ginseng* [14], and *Quillaja saponaria* bark extract [15].

Saponin consists of triterpenoid or steroidal aglycones that are substituted with different number of sugar moieties or organic acids. Saponins are sometimes called glycosaponins, and the unsubstituted aglycones are classified as sapogenins, which are usually nonpolar. Sapogenins could be either triterpenoid (C30) or steroid (C27) aglycones. The hydrophilic sugar moiety and hydrophobic aglycone of saponins make them act as biological detergents. Sawai and Saito [16] reported that plants often accumulate triterpenoids, including steroids in their glycosylated form, saponins. Indeed, glycosylation could stabilize the compounds against thermal degradation during heat processing, and result in greater bioactivities than their aglycones [17].

According to the Malaysian Standard (MS 2409: 2011) [18], the total glycosaponins of the plant could make up more than 40% w/v in the freeze dried water extract. This yield is significantly higher than that value recorded for *Panax ginseng*, which is only up to 15% of total saponins [19]. Saponins have been associated with various biological activities, such as anti-inflammatory, cholesterol lowering and anti-cancer properties [20–22]. Therefore, it is important to investigate saponins in *E. longifolia* extract in order to explain its enthopharmacological properties scientifically.

The present study investigated total saponin content in *E. longifolia* extract, and in its fractions and precipitates. Because of the complex phytochemicals present in the plant extract, liquid–liquid extraction was used to partition the target compounds, using different solvents such as ethyl acetate, butanol, and chloroform. Subsequently, the organic fractions were precipitated in cold acetone to further recover the compounds. Saponins can be precipitated by lowering the dielectric constant of medium using acetone. Therefore, this work compared the estimated total saponin in different organic fractions and their precipitates, as well as highlighting the fragmentation patterns of the identified saccharide-containing compounds from the fractions and precipitates. The anti-proliferative activities of ethyl acetate fraction and precipitate were also examined, using human breast cancer for comparison.

2. Results and Discussion

2.1. Effect of Ethanol Concentration on Saponin Content

Different concentrations of ethanol (0–100%) were used to extract phytochemicals from the roots of *E. longifolia*. In the present study, aqueous ethanol was selected as the solvent of choice, mainly due to the low toxicity and high solubility for terpenes and saponins [23]. The yield of crude extract was around 3.5% using aqueous ethanol ranged from 0–70% (Figure 1). The yield was significantly decreased when the concentration of ethanol was more than 80%. The reduction of solvent polarity by increasing ethanol content showed most saponins in the plant extract to have low solubility.

Hence, *E. longifolia* roots might have a high content of polar to semi-polar saponins. The diverse characteristics of saponins are attributed to different functional groups attached to the triterpenoid (pentacyclic structure) or steroidal (tetracyclic structure) aglycones.

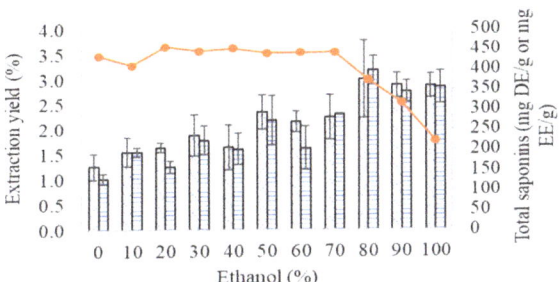

Figure 1. Yield of extraction (line) and total saponins using diosgenin (dot bar) and escin (line bar) as standard chemicals.

The saponin assay showed that the total saponins of *E. longifolia* extracts increased proportionally with the increase of ethanol concentration in the solvent system used for reflux extraction. This also indicates higher solubility of saponins in ethanol than in water. The results expressed as escin equivalent or diosgenin equivalent are almost similar. The ratio of both results is near 1 at different ethanol concentrations. Although diosgenin is not a saponin, the hydroxyl group at C-3 and double bond at C-5 could react with acidic vanillin under oxidization of sulfuric acid to form chromogen. The assay involves the condensation reaction of the aldehyde group of vanillin with the hydroxyl group of triterpenic acid to form red condensates for detection.

2.2. Fractionation by Liquid–Liquid Extraction

Organic solvents such as ethyl acetate, butanol, and chloroform were used to partition crude extract using the technique of liquid–liquid extraction. The highly polar substances, such as organic acid, polysaccharides, and proteins, may stay in the aqueous phase, while the other relatively less polar compounds, including terpenoids and saponins, are partitioned into the organic phase. This explains the increment of total saponin content after fractionation (Figure 2). Ethyl acetate fraction was found to have the highest total saponin content among the organic fractions.

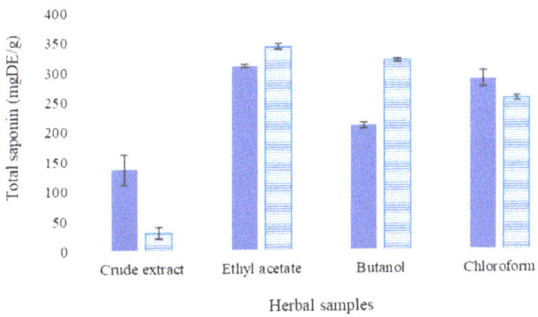

Figure 2. Total saponins of organic fractions (solid bar) and precipitates (line bar) expressed as mg DE/g in different solvent systems.

The chromatograms shown in Figure 3 show the peaks detected at 254 nm after fractionation. The chromatographic profiles of the organic fractions are almost similar, but their mass spectra are significantly different. The chromatographic profiles display the compounds with UV-absorbing property, whereas compounds like terpenoids and saponins mostly do not have such a property. On the other hand, the mass analyzer will only detect ionizable compounds in the samples. Ethyl acetate and butanol fractions were found to have less polar compounds, whereas chloroform seemed to partition more polar compounds from crude extract. The difference between the organic fractions can also be seen from the results of colorimetric assays. In line with the colorimetric assay, the butanol fraction exhibited the lowest peak area.

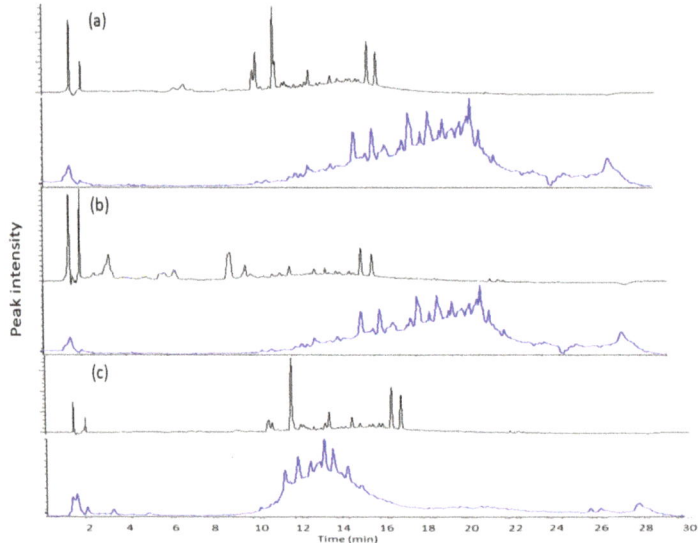

Figure 3. Chromatograms (black line) and total ion chromatograms (blue line) of mass spectrometer for organic fractions from ethyl acetate (**a**), butanol (**b**), and chloroform (**c**).

2.3. Cold Acetone Precipitation

Cold acetone precipitation appeared to slightly increase the total saponin content from the organic fractions. The increment was more significant for butanol fraction. Again, ethyl acetate precipitate could obtain the highest total saponin content. The fractions were added dropwise into cold acetone, and precipitate was formed due to the sudden drop of dielectric constant of media. The dielectric constant (ε) of acetone is 20.7, which is about half the dielectric constant of 70% ethanol (ε = 41.1). Precipitation occurred, most probably because of the steric hindrance of lipophilic terpenoidal skeleton, limiting its solubility in acetone. Usually, glycosylated terpenoids or steroids were precipitated in acetone, thus contributing to higher saponin content.

The chromatograms of the precipitates show peak 1 (10.6 min), peak 2 (10.9 min), peak 3 (11.1 min), and peak 4 (12.2 min), as illustrated in Figure 4. They are tentatively identified as m/z 427, m/z 239 (β-carboline-1-propionic acid), m/z 497, and m/z 723, respectively. The mass spectra at those retention times revealed the presence of m/z 497 [2M + HCOOH − H]$^-$, m/z 610 [2M + HCOOH + 113 − H]$^-$, m/z 723 [3M + HCOOH − H]$^-$, m/z 836 [3M + HCOOH + 113 − H]$^-$, and m/z 949 [4M + HCOOH − H]$^-$. In the present study, M was found to be the monomer of 226 amu, which is formylated hexose. Most probably, the neutral loss of 113 is acylglycerol. The formylated saccharides have the same fragmentation patterns as the compounds detected in *Rhamnus davurica* Pall [24] and *Rubia cordifolia* L. [25] extracts. Hence, cold acetone was likely to precipitate saccharide-containing compounds, as presented in Table S1 (Supplementary Materials). The table lists the product ions and neutral losses attributed to sugar moieties. The neutral loss of the peaks revealed that the precipitated compounds were saccharide-containing compounds, including saponins. Since saponins do not have chromophores for UV detection, their mass spectra are presented in Figure 5. The mass spectra of the precipitates clearly show the fragment ions, which were mostly ionized saccharides, as intense peaks. The common sugar fragment ions in the figure are m/z 179 (hexose − H), 225 (hexose + HCOOH − H), 341 (dihexose − H_2O − H), 377 (dihexose + H_2O − H), and 387 (dihexose − H_2O + HCOOH − H). Negative ionization was also found to be more preferable for the precipitated compounds in this study.

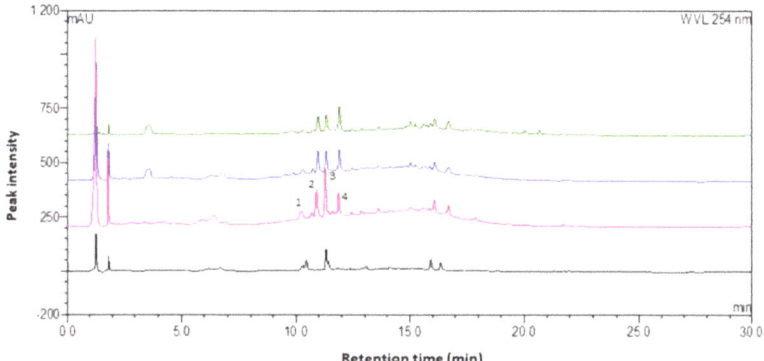

Figure 4. Chromatograms of precipitates in acetone using different organic fractions.

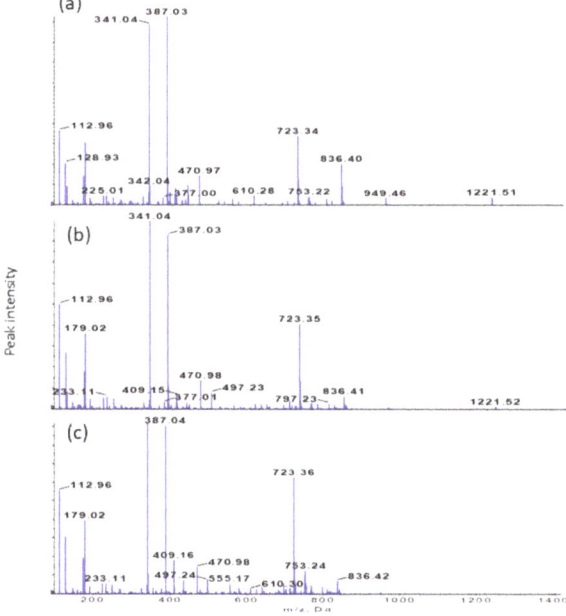

Figure 5. Mass spectra of ethyl acetate (**a**), butanol (**b**), and chloroform (**c**) precipitates.

High performance unsupervised statistical techniques, namely heat mapping and principal component analysis, were used to classify the huge datasets. The heat map explains that the number of metabolites precipitated from butanol fraction was less than the other two organic fractions (Figure 6a).

The butanol precipitate contained higher masses of compounds, mostly higher than 600 Da, while the ethyl acetate precipitate was found to have a wide range of compounds. The mass profile of the ethyl acetate precipitate was close to the mass profile of the chloroform precipitate based on the dendogram. In line with the dendrogram, ethyl acetate and chloroform precipitates showed closer metabolite profiles, as explained by the first principal component (PC1) in Figure 6c. The first two principal components explain 84.6% of the total variance for the precipitates. Hence, different organic solvents extracted different metabolites from the crude extract of *E. longifolia*, subsequently contributing to different profiles of metabolites in those precipitates.

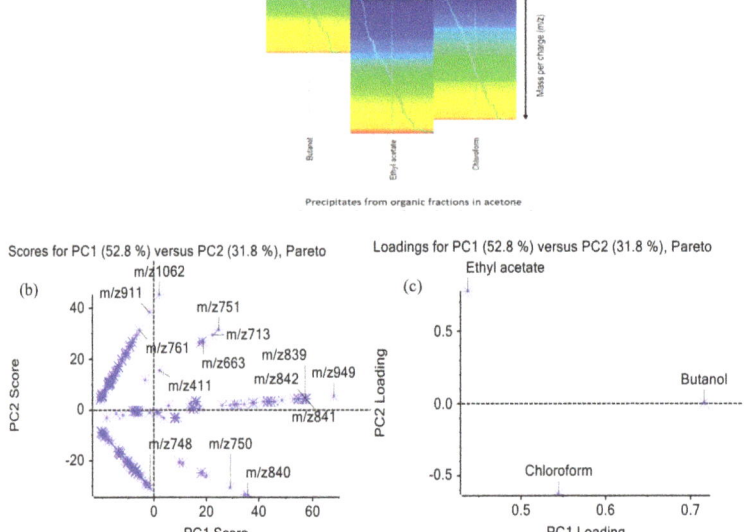

Figure 6. Heat mapping (**a**) and principal component analysis with score (**b**) and loading (**c**) plots.

2.4. Phytopharmacological Significance of Bioactive Precipitate

Ethyl acetate fraction and its precipitate were found to exhibit the highest total saponin content. Therefore, the anti-proliferative activities of ethyl acetate fraction and its precipitate were tested on a human breast cancer cell line in the subsequent experiments. The results found that the inhibitory action of the samples was improved from crude extract (IC_{50} = 616.3 µg/mL) to ethyl acetate fraction (IC_{50} = 185.4 µg/mL) and its precipitate (IC_{50} = 153.4 µg/mL). The IC_{50} of ethyl acetate precipitate was close to the value of tamoxifen, 110.6 µg/mL (Figure 7). Tamoxifen is the most common drug used to treat breast cancer patients [26]. Previous studies also reported that saponins could be potential anticancer agents [21,27]. Hence, the processing technology to concentrate terpenoids and their glycosylated derivatives could increase the performance of herbal samples in suppressing MCF-7 cell proliferation. This can also be seen from the high IC_{50} (733.7 µg/mL) of ethyl acetate filtrate, which means a high concentration of sample is required to exhibit its anti-proliferative activity. Direct precipitation using crude extract seemed to be less cytotoxic against MCF-7 cells. The combination of solvent fractionation and acetone precipitation could increase the biological activity of the plant extract. This technique should be recommended, as previous researchers used toxic solvents such as methanol and chloroform to get bioactive fraction in their pharmacological studies [28,29]. The presence of solvent residues in the plant extracts make them unsuitable for product formulation, particularly products for human consumption. Therefore, food grade solvents such as ethanol, acetone, and ethyl acetate are the primary choice of consumers.

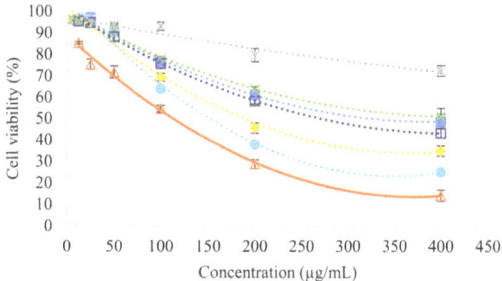

Figure 7. MCF-7 cell viability after treated with tamoxifen (Δ), crude extract (■), crude precipitate (x), crude filtrate (□), ethyl acetate fraction (♦), ethyl acetate precipitate (●), and ethyl acetate filtrate (✱).

3. Materials and Methods

3.1. Chemicals and Plant Material

The roots of *Eurycoma longifolia* (SK 3317/18) were harvested from Bentong, Pahang, Malaysia. The samples were then dried and shredded into chip form, about 1 cm in size. Human breast cancer cell line (MCF-7) was obtained from the American Type Culture Collection (ATCC, Manassas, VA, USA) and maintained in Dulbecco's Modified Eagle Medium. Dimethyl sulfoxide (DMSO, 99.9%), vanillin (≥97%), oleanolic acid (≥97%), and escin (≥95%) were purchased from Sigma-Aldrich, St. Louis, MO, USA. Ethanol, acetic acid, perchloric acid, sulfuric acid, formic acid, ethyl acetate, butanol, chloroform, acetonitrile, and acetone were sourced from Merck, Darmstadt, Germany.

3.2. Heat Reflux Extraction

The dried *E. longifolia* chips were then finely ground into powder (~2 mm) by a grinder. The samples (25 g) were extracted with different concentrations of ethanol (250 mL) in a heat reflux system for 2 h. After extraction, the solution was cooled and filtered for drying using a rotary evaporator. The extraction yield was recorded for each solvent system.

3.3. Liquid-Liquid Extraction

The crude extract of 70% ethanol was used in the fractionation process. The fractionation was carried out using the technique of liquid–liquid extraction. Three types of organic solvents, namely ethyl acetate, butanol, and chloroform were selected to partition crude extract into individual fractions. Crude extract (0.5 g) was reconstituted in water (10 mL) and vigorously extracted by ethyl acetate (20 mL) in a 100 mL separating funnel. The solution was left for phase separation after extraction. The organic phase was withdrawn, and another 20 mL ethyl acetate was added into the remaining aqueous solution for extraction again. This fractionation process was repeated in triplicate. The organic fraction of ethyl acetate was combined and dried by a rotary evaporator. A similar fractionation process was also carried out to prepare butanol and chloroform fractions.

3.4. Cold Acetone Precipitation

The fractions of ethyl acetate, butanol, and chloroform were then reconstituted in 70% ethanol (5 mL) and added dropwise into cold acetone (20 mL). Phytochemicals with poor solubility in cold acetone were precipitated. The precipitated phytochemicals were filtered and dissolved in 50% methanol for LC-DAD-MS/MS analysis, and dissolved in 50% ethanol for total saponin assay.

3.5. Total Saponin Content

The total saponin content was determined colorimetrically according to the procedures described by Makkar et al. [30]. A 250 µL sample (1 mg/mL) was mixed with 250 µL vanillin (8g/100 mL ethanol) and topped up with 2.5 mL sulfuric acid (72%). The mixture was heated for 10 min at 60 °C, and then cooled in an ice-water bath for 5 min. The absorbance of the mixture was recorded by a UV-vis spectrophotometer (UV-1800, Shimadzu, Japan) at 544 nm. Escin (5.7–71.4 mg/L) was used as the standard chemical to build a calibration curve. The results are expressed as mg escin equivalent per g sample (mg EE/g), or mg diosgenin equivalent per g sample (mg DE/g).

3.6. Cell Proliferation Using MTT Assay

MTT assay was performed to determine the viability of MCF-7 cells treated with samples (crude extract, ethyl acetate fraction, and its precipitate). Standard chemicals, namely escin and tamoxifen were used as positive controls in the experiments, whereas DMSO was used as a negative control. Tumor cells (1×10^5 cell/mL) were seeded in 96 flat well microtiter plates, with 200 µL culture medium in each well. The microplate was covered by sterilized parafilm and shaken gently before incubation at 37 °C, in 5% CO_2 for 24 h. After incubation, the medium was removed and two-fold serial dilutions of samples were added to the wells for 24 h treatment at 37 °C with 5 % CO_2. A 10 µL MTT solution was added to each well and further incubated at 37 °C for 4 h. The media solution was carefully removed and 100 µL of solubilization solution was added into each well. The absorbance was determined using an ELISA reader at a wavelength of 575 nm. Each concentration of samples was assayed in triplicate. The growth of MCF-7 cells treated with herbal samples was determined based on their viability after treatment. The results are expressed in effective concentration required to inhibit 50% of viable cells (IC_{50}).

3.7. LC-DAD-MS/MS

A liquid chromatograph (Dionex Corporation Ultimate 3000; Sunnyvale, CA, USA) integrated with a diode array detector (Dionex Ultimate 3000) and a quadrupole and time-of-flight (QTOF) mass spectrometer (AB SCIEX QSTAR Elite; Foster City, CA, USA) was used to screen phytochemicals. A C18 reversed phase XSelect HSS T3 column (2.1 × 100 mm, 2.5 µm) with a flow rate of 150 µL/min was used for separation, and compound peaks were detected at 254 nm. A binary gradient system consisting of solvent A (water with 0.1% formic acid) and solvent B (acetonitrile) was programmed as: 0–10 min, 10% B; 10–20 min, 10–85% B; 20–25 min, 85% B; 25–25.1 min, 85–10% B; 25.1–30 min, 10% B. The injection volume was 5 µL. All samples were filtered with 0.2 mm nylon membrane filter prior to injection.

The QTOF mass spectrometer was used for phytochemical screening from m/z 100–2000. A single information dependent acquisition (IDA) method was created to acquire both TOF MS and two dependent runs of product ion scan with rolling collision energy. Nitrogen gas was used for nebulizing (40 psi) and curtain gas (20 psi). Collision gas was set at 3, the accumulation time was 1 s for TOF MS and 2 s for each product ion scan. The voltage of ion spray was 4500 V for negative ion mode. The declustering potential was 40 V and the focusing potential was set at 300 V.

3.8. Statistical Analysis

Heat-map and cluster analysis were used to visually classify the detected ions in precipitates using R version 2.11.1. Principal component analysis was carried out using Pareto scaling in the data processing software MarkerView 1.1 (Applied Biosystems/MDSSciex, Foster City, CA, USA).

4. Conclusions

The technique of solvent fractionation, followed by acetone precipitation seems to be able to recover saccharide-containing compounds from the highly complex crude extract of *E. longifolia*.

Usually, large molecules like triterpenoids and saponins which have intermediate polarity would be recovered and then further precipitated in a highly polar acetone. Ethyl acetate appears to be more effective to recover saccharide-containing compounds. This is the first study to concentrate saccharide-containing compounds for MCF-7 cell inhibition. Further investigation will be carried out to identify the recovered saccharide-containing compounds.

Supplementary Materials: The following are available online, Table S1: Precipitated compounds in cold acetone from organic fractions of *Eurycoma longifolia*.

Author Contributions: Conceptualization, L.S.C.; methodology, L.S.C.; data curation, C.H.L., C.Y.C. and D.A.S.D.; writing, L.S.C.; supervision, L.S.C.; funding acquisition, L.S.C.

Funding: This research was funded by the Ministry of Higher Education, Malaysia, grant number HICoE 4J263 and The APC was funded by the Ministry of Higher Education, Malaysia.

Acknowledgments: The authors would like to thank the assistance of internship students in the laboratory.

Conflicts of Interest: The authors declare no conflict of interest.

References

1. Kuo, P.C.; Damu, A.G.; Lee, K.H.; Wu, T.S. Cytotoxic and antimalarial constituents from the roots of *Eurycoma longifolia*. *Bioorg. Med. Chem.* **2004**, *12*, 537–544. [PubMed]
2. Gimlette, J.D.; Thomson, H.W. *A Dictionary of Malayan Medicine*; Oxford University Press: Kuala Lumpur, Malaysia, 1977; p. 183.
3. Ang, H.H.; Ngai, T.H. Aphrodisiac evaluation in non-copulator male rats after chronic administration of *Eurycoma longifolia* Jack. *Fundam. Clin. Pharmacol.* **2001**, *15*, 265–268. [CrossRef]
4. Ang, H.H.; Ngai, T.H.; Tan, T.H. Effects of Eurycoma longifolia Jack on sexual qualities in middle aged male rats. *Phytomedicine* **2003**, *10*, 590–593. [CrossRef]
5. Chua, L.S.; Mohd Amin, N.A.; Neo, J.C.H.; Lee, T.H.; Lee, C.T.; Sarmidi, M.R.; Aziz, R.A. LC–MS/MS-based metabolites of *Eurycoma longifolia* (Tongkat Ali) in Malaysia (Perak and Pahang). *J. Chromatogr. B* **2011**, *879*, 3909–3919. [CrossRef] [PubMed]
6. Hiai, S.; Oura, H.; Nakajima, T. Color reaction of some sapogenins and saponins with vanillin and sulfuric acid. *Planta Med.* **1976**, *29*, 116–122. [CrossRef] [PubMed]
7. Polonsky, J. Chemistry and Biogenesis of the Quassinoids (Simaruobolides). In *Terpenoids: Structure, Biogenesis, and Distribution: Recent Advances in Phytochemistry*; Runeckles, V.C., Mabry, T.J., Eds.; Academic Press, Inc.: New York, NY, USA, 1973; p. 43.
8. Slacanin, I.; Marston, A.; Hostettmann, K. Quantitative HPLC analysis of molluscicidal saponins from *Phytolacca dodecandra*. *Planta Med.* **1988**, *54*, 581. [CrossRef]
9. Oleszek, W.; Price, K.R.; Colquhoun, I.J.; Jurzysta, M.; Ploszynski, M.; Fenwick, G.R. Isolation and identification of alfalfa (*Medicago sativa* L.) root saponins: Their activity in relation to a fungal bioassay. *J. Agric. Food Chem.* **1990**, *38*, 1810–1817. [CrossRef]
10. Nowacka, J.; Oleszek, W. High performance liquid chromatography of zanhic acid glycoside in alfalfa (*Medicago sativa*). *Phytochem. Anal.* **1992**, *3*, 227–230. [CrossRef]
11. Ouyang, H.; Guo, Y.; He, M.; Zhang, J.; Huang, X.; Zhou, X.; Jiang, H.; Feng, Y.; Yang, S. A rapid and sensitive LC-MS/MS method for the determination of Pulsatilla saponin D in rat plasma and its application in a rat pharmacokinetic and bioavailability study. *Biomed. Chromatogr.* **2015**, *29*, 373–378. [CrossRef]
12. Yang, G.; Lu, W.; Pan, M.; Zhang, C.; Zhou, Y.; Hu, P.; Hu, M.; Song, G. An LC–MS/MS method for simultaneous determination of nine steroidal saponins from *Paris polyphylla* var. in rat plasma and its application to pharmacokinetic study. *J. Pharm. Biomed. Anal.* **2017**, *145*, 675–681. [CrossRef]
13. Madl, T.; Sterk, H.; Mittelbach, M.; Rechberger, G.N. Tandem mass spectrometric analysis of a complex triterpene saponin mixture of *Chenopodium quinoa*. *J. Am. Soc. Mass Spec.* **2006**, *17*, 795–806.
14. Liu, S.; Liu, M.; Liu, Z.; Song, F.; Mo, W. Structural analysis of saponins from medicinal herbs using electrospray ionization tandem mass spectrometry. *J. Am. Soc. Mass Spec.* **2004**, *15*, 133–141. [CrossRef] [PubMed]

15. Van Setten, D.C.; Zomer, G.; van de Werken, G.; Wiertz, E.J.H.J.; Leeflang, B.R.; Kamerling, J.P. Ion trap multiple-stage tandem mass spectrometry as a pre-NMR tool in the structure elucidation of saponins. *Phytochem. Anal.* **2000**, *11*, 190–198. [CrossRef]
16. Sawai, S.; Saito, K. Triterpenoid biosynthesis and engineering in plants. *Front. Plant Sci.* **2011**, *2*, 25. [CrossRef] [PubMed]
17. Moses, T.; Papadopoulou, K.K.; Osbourn, A. Metabolic and functional diversity of saponins, biosynthetic intermediates and semi-synthetic derivatives. *Crit. Rev. Biochem. Mol. Biol.* **2014**, *49*, 439–462. [CrossRef] [PubMed]
18. *Phytopharmaceutical Aspect of Freeze Dried Water Extract from Tongkat Ali Roots—Specification*; Department of Standards Malaysia: Cyberjaya, SGR, Malaysia, 2011.
19. Hou, J.P.; Jin, Y. Chapter 5: Miraculous Tonic Herbs: Strengthening the First Line of Defense and Fortifying the Immune System. In *The Healing Power of Chinese Herbs and Medicinal Recipes*; The Haworth Integrative Healing Press: New York, NY, USA, 2004; pp. 81–135.
20. Xiang, L.; Yi, X.; Wang, Y.; He, X. Antiproliferative and anti-inflammatory polyhydroxylated spirostanol saponins from *Tupistra chinensis*. *Sci. Rep.* **2016**, *6*, 31633. [CrossRef] [PubMed]
21. Xu, X.H.; Li, T.; Fong, C.M.V.; Chen, X.; Chen, X.J.; Wang, Y.T.; Huang, M.Q.; Lu, J.J. Saponins from Chinese medicines as anticancer agents. *Molecules* **2016**, *21*, 1326. [CrossRef]
22. Milgate, J.; Roberts, D.C.K. The nutritional & biological significance of saponins. *Nutr. Res.* **1995**, *15*, 1223–1249.
23. Gafner, S.; Bergeron, C.; McCollom, M.M.; Cooper, L.M.; McPhail, K.L.; Gerwick, W.H.; Angerhofer, C.K. Evaluation of the efficiency of three different solvent systems to extract triterpene saponins from roots of *Panax quinquefolius* using high-performance liquid chromatography. *J. Agric. Food Chem.* **2004**, *52*, 1546–1550. [CrossRef]
24. Chen, G.; Li, X.; Saleri, F.; Guo, M. Analysis of flavonoids in *Rhamnus davurica* and its antiproliferative activities. *Molecules* **2016**, *21*, 1275. [CrossRef]
25. Zheng, Z.; Li, S.; Zhong, Y.; Zhan, R.; Yan, Y.; Pan, H.; Yan, P. UPLC-QTOF-MS identification of the chemical constituents in rat plasma and urine after oral administration of *Rubia cordifolia* L. extract. *Molecules* **2017**, *22*, 1327. [CrossRef]
26. Villegas, V.E.; Rondón-Lagos, M.; Annaratone, L.; Castellano, I.; Grismaldo, A.; Sapino, A.; Zaphiropoulos, P.G. Tamoxifen treatment of breast cancer cells: Impact on Hedgehog/GLI1 signaling. *Int. J. Mol. Sci.* **2016**, *17*, 308. [CrossRef]
27. Man, S.; Gao, W.; Zhang, Y.; Huang, L.; Liu, C. Chemical study and medical application of saponins as anti-cancer agents. *Fitoterapia* **2010**, *81*, 703–714. [CrossRef]
28. Tee, T.T.; Azimahtol, H.L.P. Induction of apoptosis by *Eurycoma longifolia* Jack extracts. *Anticancer Res.* **2005**, *25*, 2205–2214.
29. Hussain, Z.; Mohamad, I.N.; Shuid, A.Z. *Eurycoma longifolia*, a potential phytomedicine for the treatment of cancer: Evidence of p53-mediated apoptosis in cancerous cells. *Curr. Drug Targets* **2019**, *19*, 1109–1126. [CrossRef]
30. Makkar, H.P.S.; Siddhuraju, P.; Becker, K. Saponins, Plant Secondary Metabolites. In *Methods in Molecular Biology*; Humana Press: Clifton, NJ, USA, 2007; Volume 393, pp. 93–100.

Sample Availability: Samples of the compounds are not available from the authors.

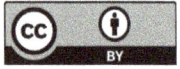 © 2019 by the authors. Licensee MDPI, Basel, Switzerland. This article is an open access article distributed under the terms and conditions of the Creative Commons Attribution (CC BY) license (http://creativecommons.org/licenses/by/4.0/).

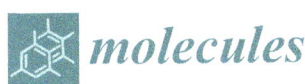

Article

Inhibitory Effect of Osthole from *Cnidium monnieri* on Tobacco Mosaic Virus (TMV) Infection in *Nicotiana glutinosa*

Ya-Han Chen [1,2], Dong-Sheng Guo [2], Mei-Huan Lu [2,3], Jian-Ying Yue [1], Yan Liu [4], Chun-Ming Shang [4], De-Rong An [2,*] and Ming-Min Zhao [1,*]

1. College of Horticulture and Plant Protection, Inner Mongolia Agricultural University, Hohhot 010019, China; yhchen1018@nwafu.edu.cn (Y.-H.C.); yuejianying2018@163.com (J.-Y.Y.)
2. College of Plant Protection and State Key Laboratory of Crop Stress Biology for Arid Areas, Northwest A&F University, Yangling 712100, China; gds1995908@163.com (D.-S.G.); lu_meihuan@sina.com (M.-H.L.)
3. Microbial Resources of Research Center, Microbiology Institute of Shaanxi, Xi'an 710043, China
4. Academy of Agriculture science in Baotou, Baotou 014010, China; liuyanww@126.com (Y.L.); chunmingsh@163.com (C.-M.S.)
* Correspondence: anderong323@163.com (D.-R.A.); Mingminzh@163.com (M.-M.Z.); Tel.: +86-158-2909-7529 (D.-R.A.); +86-157-7136-0659 (M.-M.Z.); Fax: +86-029-8708-2710 (D.-R.A.); +86-0471-638-5801 (M.-M.Z.)

Academic Editor: Raffaele Capasso
Received: 3 December 2019; Accepted: 18 December 2019; Published: 24 December 2019

Abstract: The coumarin compound of osthole was extracted from *Cnidium monnieri* and identified by LC-MS and ^{1}H- and ^{13}C-NMR. Osthole was tested for anti-virus activity against tobacco mosaic virus (TMV) using the half-leaf method. The results showed that stronger antiviral activity on TMV infection appeared in *Nicotiana glutinosa* than that of eugenol and ningnanmycin, with inhibitory, protective, and curative effects of 72.57%, 70.26%, and 61.97%, respectively. Through observation of the TMV particles, we found that osthole could directly affect the viral particles. Correspondingly, the level of coat protein detected by Western blot was significantly reduced when the concentrations of osthole increased in tested plants compared to that of the control. These results suggest that osthole has anti-TMV activity and may be used as a biological reagent to control the plant virus in the half-leaf method.

Keywords: *Cnidium monnieri*; osthole; tobacco mosaic virus; half-leaf method; inhibitory

1. Introduction

Tobacco mosaic virus (TMV) belongs to the genus *Tobamovirus* and is transmitted by mechanical inoculation and insects with chewing mouthparts in a propagative manner [1,2]. TMV is an economically and destructively important plant virus with a wide host range, infecting more than 400 plant species from 36 families [3]. Recently, a survey of plant viruses was collected from 31 provinces in mainland China over a period from 2013 to 2017, which included over 41,000 vegetable crop samples from the *Solanaceae, Cucurbitaceae, Leguminosae,* and *Cruciferae* families. The results showed that TMV is distributed in all the surveyed provinces and is one of the most dominant viruses among 63 virus species detected in these four families [4]. TMV leads to one hundred million dollars losses in crops around the world in a year [5]. TMV is dependent on the plant cell to replicate and infect, which causes extreme difficulty for antiviral therapies to inhibit only the virus without damaging the host [6,7]. Therefore, the chemical method was not effective in controlling plant viruses in crop fields.

The use of pesticides has brought with it a host of issues, like the increase in drug resistance of plant pathogens, environmental pollution, and health risks to animals and humans [8,9]. In recent years, more and more people have begun to focus on the use of botanical pesticides, which display great development potential for controlling plant viral diseases, because they have low reside and are environmentally safe, biodegradable, and safe to non-target organisms [10,11]. Up until now, many kinds of plant compounds have already been demonstrated to have anti-viral ability, such as *Amaranthaceae, Nyctaginaceae, Asteraceae, Chenopodiaceae, Asclepiadaceae, Polygonaceae, Simaroubaceae, Acanthaceae, Liliaceae, Cruciferae, Leguminosae sp., Boraginaceae, Oleaceae, Taxaceae, Ranunculaceae, Juglandaceae, Saxifragaceae, Theaceae, Schisandraceae, Cupressaceae, Labiatae*, and *Caryophyllaceae* [12–15].

Among these plants, the effective antiviral compounds are mainly proteins, alkaloids, flavonoids, phenols, essential oils, and polysaccharides. In China, four reported plant-derived ingredients have been widely used in viral disease control, including oligosaccharides, rhyscion, matrine, and fatty acids [10]. Many studies have reported the inhibitory effects of plant-derived antiviral pesticides on TMV. Tagitinin C (Ses-2) and 1β-methoxydiversifolin-3-0-methyl ether (Ses-5), two sesquiterpenoids isolated from *Tithonia diversiflia*, were found to have higher inhibitory activities than the control agent ningnanmycin [16]. Wang et al. found that sulfated lentinan induced systemic and long-term protection against TMV in tobacco [17].

Cnidium monnieri (L.) Cusson is a traditional Chinese medicine that is widely distributed throughout China. Many studies have suggested that it has pharmacological functions, such as anti-allergic, antipruritic, antibacterial, antidermatophytic, anti-osteoporotic, and antifungal activities [18–22]. *C. monnieri* was reported to contain a number of biologically active compounds such as osthole, imperatorin, bergapten, isopimpinellin, xanthotoxol, xanthotoxin, cnidimonal and cnidimarin, glucosides, sesquiterpenes, etc. [23–25]. The anti-viral activity of ethanol extracted from *C. monnieri* in plants remains unknown.

In this study, we performed the osthole isolation from *C. monnieri*. We investigated whether the exogenous application of osthole is able to induce anti-viral activity in the tobacco plant when infected with TMV. The inhibitory, protective, and curative effects on TMV infection were measured. Furthermore, we observed whether osthole could affect the TMV particles and coat protein (CP) accumulation.

2. Results

2.1. Compound Structure of Osthole

Osthole (7-methoxy-8-isopentenylcoumarin): is a white solid with the molecular formula $C_{15}H_{17}O_3$, as identified by high-performance liquid chromatography (HPLC) (Figure 1), proton nuclear magnetic resonance (^{1}H-NMR), carbon-13 nuclear magnetic resonance (^{13}C-NMR) (Figure 2), and high-resolution mass spectrometry (HR-MS) spectra (Figure 3). As indicated by Figure 1, the purity was greater than 98%. The spectral data was identical to that previously reported in the literature [26].

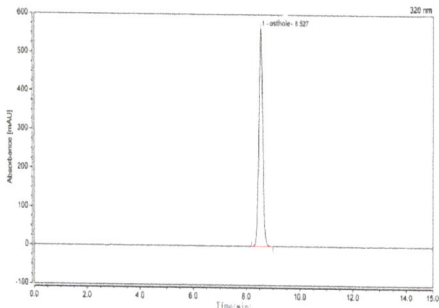

Figure 1. The HPLC chromatogram of osthole.

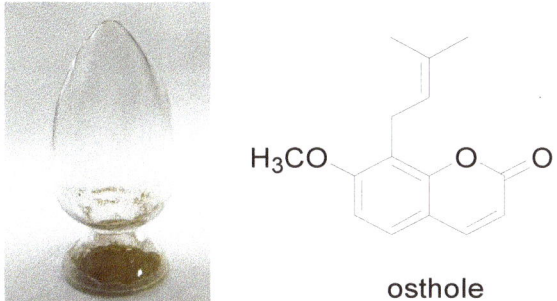

Figure 2. Samples and structure of the compound identified from osthole.

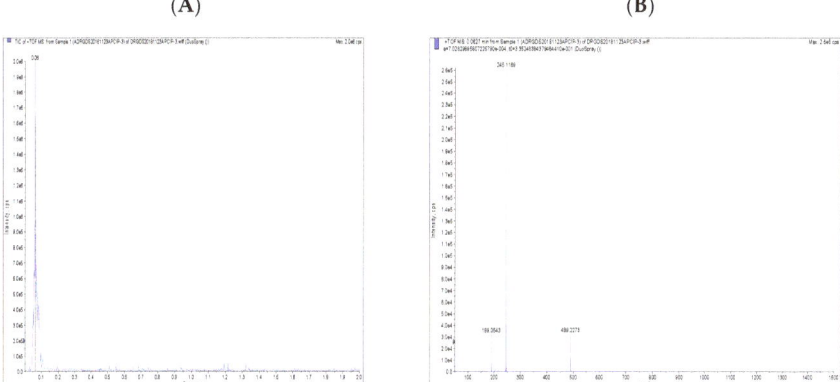

Figure 3. The high-performance liquid chromatography/mass spectrometry (HPLC/MS) chromatogram of osthole. (**A**) The HPLC/MS of chromatogram of osthole. (**B**) The MS of chromatogram of osthole.

1H-NMR (500 MHz, DMSO-$d6$): δ (ppm) 1.61 (s, 3H), 1.71 (s, 3H), 3.40 (d, J = 7.2 Hz, ^{2}H), 3.89 (s, 3H), 5.11–5.14 (m, ^{1}H), 6.26 (d, J = 9.6 Hz, ^{1}H), 7.05 (d, J = 8.4 Hz, ^{1}H), 7.55 (d, J = 8.4 Hz, ^{1}H), 7.96 (d, J = 9.6 Hz, ^{1}H); ^{13}C-NMR (125 MHz, DMSO-$d6$): δ (ppm) 18.1, 21.9, 25.9, 56.7, 108.5, 112.7, 113.1, 116.6, 121.7, 127.6, 132.2, 145.1, 152.6, 160.2, 160.7; HR-MS (ESI): m/z calculated for $C_{15}H_{17}O_3$ ([M + H]$^+$) 245.1170, found 245.1169. For the NMR data please see the Supplementary Figures S1 and S2.

2.2. Anti-TMV Activities of Osthole

The anti-TMV activity of osthole from *C. monnieri* (L.) Cusson was tested at a concentration of 5 mg/mL in *N. glutinosa* using the half-leaf method. Based on the inhibition rates of local lesions on the leaves of *N. glutinosa* (Figure 4), the antiviral activity of osthole was shown to be superior to that of eugenol and ningnanmycin (Table 1), with an inhibitory effect of 72.57%, protective effect of 70.26%, and curative effect of 61.97%.

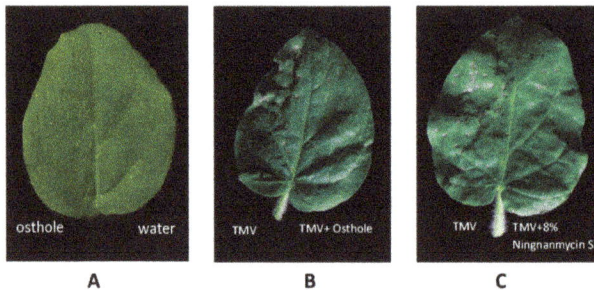

Figure 4. Anti-tobacco mosaic virus (TMV) activities of osthole in *N. glutinosa*. The half-leaf was smeared with osthole extract mixed with TMV at the same volume, and the right half-leaf was smeared with 40 µL of TMV. (**A**) Osthole extract (5 mg/mL) and water. (**B**) Osthole extract (5 mg/mL) and TMV. (**C**) Ningnanmycin SL (8%; 1000-X dilution) and TMV.

Table 1. The anti-viral activity of osthole against TMV.

Drug	Inhibitory Effect (%)	Protective Effect (%)	Curative Effect (%)
Osthole	72.57 ± 9.24 [aA]	70.26 ± 10.49 [aA]	61.97 ± 7.84 [aA]
Eugenol	60.39 ± 5.48 [aA]	56.04 ± 4.98 [aA]	60.83 ± 4.49 [bB]
8% Ningnanmycin SL (1000-X dilution)	64.11 ± 2.43 [aA]	60.57 ± 7.24 [aA]	55.45 ± 10.96 [aA]

Values are presented as the mean ± SE. Different upper and lower letters in the same column indicate significant difference at $p < 0.01$ or $p < 0.05$ level by Duncan's new multiple range test.

2.3. The Effect of Osthole on Viral Particles

In order to determine whether osthole could directly affect the viral particle, TMV particles were mixed with the osthole at 3 mg/mL and 5 mg/mL with an equal volume for 45 min at room temperature. We found that non-treated TMV particles as observed by a Hitachi H-600 Electron Microscope appeared normal and baculiform (Figure 5A). In contrast, those treated with osthole presented with a strong detrimental effect on the virus particles (Figure 5B,C). The virus particles were gradually destroyed: as the concentration of osthole increased, the more severely the virus particles were damaged.

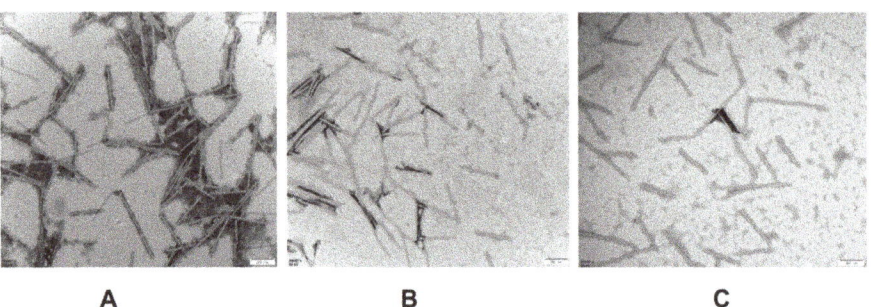

Figure 5. Electron microscopic observation of TMV particles after treatment with osthole for 45 min. The concentration of the purified TMV was 0.60 mg/mL. The sample was observed under 49,000× magnifications using a Hitachi H-600 Electron Microscope. (**A**) Normal TMV particles. (**B**) TMV treated with osthole at 3 mg/mL for 45 min. (**C**) TMV treated with osthole at 5 mg/mL for 45 min.

2.4. Kinetic Analysis of the Effect of Osthole Against TMV Infection

To examine which concentration of osthole could be most effective against TMV infection, a kinetic analysis was performed. The level of CP was detected by Western blot. We found that the CP level was significantly reduced when the concentration of osthole increased from 1 to 7 mg/mL in treated plants, as compared to that of the control (Figure 6). Osthole at 7 mg/mL could completely inhibit CP accumulation in TMV. This result indicates that osthole may inhibit the replication of TMV in plants. As shown in Table 2, we found that there was a significant positive correlation between the concentration of osthole and inhibitory effects on TMV infection.

Table 2. The anti-viral activity of osthole against TMV at varying concentrations.

Concentration (mg/mL)	Inhibitory Effect (%)
1	34.46 ± 5.19 [cC]
3	53.23 ± 3.13 [bB]
5	72.57 ± 9.24 [aA]
7	83.22 ± 3.68 [aA]

Data in the table are mean ± SD. Different upper and lower letters in the same column indicate significant difference at $p < 0.01$ or $p < 0.05$ level by Duncan's new multiple range test.

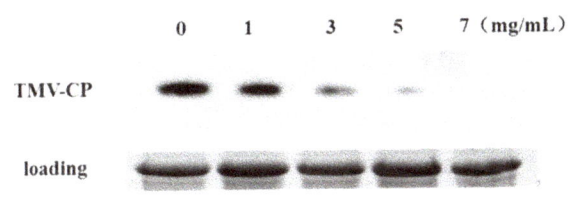

Figure 6. TMV coat protein (CP) accumulation detected by Western blot analysis.

3. Discussion

In this study, osthole was isolated from *C. monnieri* with 98% purity. Osthole is a coumarin compound, a kind of secondary metabolite in plants, which has been shown to play an important role in plant defense responses [27]. Additional properties of osthole include antibacterial, antifungal, and pesticidal functions [28]. It was reported that osthole exhibits a wide range of inhibition in mycelial growth against many fungal diseases (*Rhizoctonia solani*, *Macrophoma kawatsukai*, and *Fusarium graminearum*) [28]. However, its anti-viral activity against plant viruses has not been reported. In this study, we found that osthole has stronger anti-viral activity than eugenol and ningnanmycin.

Furthermore, we evaluated whether osthole could directly inhibit viral particles. Through observation of TMV particles using a Hitachi H-600 Electron Microscope, we found that the compound could directly affect the particles; TMV particles were gradually destroyed. When the osthole concentration increased, the more severely the viral particles were damaged. Many reports have indicated that many changes occur in the morphology of TMV particles after treatment with plant extracts. Wang et al. found that TMV particles treated with eugenol showed ruptures and abnormality [29]. Particles were destroyed and shortened by treated with *Eupatorium adenophorum* leaf extract as reported by Jin et al. (2014) [30]. These results suggest that the method underlying viral particle destruction is a common mechanism by which plant-derived reagents act on viral infection.

CP is critical for systemic infection and viral replication, protecting nucleic acid from enzymatic degradation, which is related to the long-distance movement of TMV and the expression of host symptoms [31–33]. In this study, we found the level of CP was significantly reduced to varying degrees when the concentration of osthole increased in treated plants, as compared to that of the control. Osthole at a concentration of 7 mg/mL completely inhibited expression of the TMV CP. The present results are in agreement with those reported by Li et al. (2007), Wang et al. (2014), and Chen et al.

(2018) [7,11,17]. However, it remains to be further studied whether the function of osthole is through inhibiting CP synthesis or the stereoscopic assembly of the virus.

In conclusion, osthole was isolated and purified from *C. monnieri*, and identified by ^{1}H- and ^{13}C-NMR and HR-MS. Osthole showed potent inhibitory activity against TMV infection. However, the antiviral mechanism of osthole on plant viruses remains unclear. In the future, we will examine whether osthole exerts its effect on CP synthesis or the stereoscopic assembly of TMV. This is the first published report on the anti-TMV activities of osthole.

4. Materials and Methods

4.1. Chemicals and Materials

Ningnanmycin AS (8%) was obtained from Deqiang Biology Co., Ltd. (Harbin, China.). Eugenol was purchased from Mckuin biological Co. LTD (Shanghai, China)

C. monnieri (L.) Cusson was purchased from the Jihetang Pharmacy (Yangling, China), and was identified by Professor Xiaoqian Mu at Northwest A&F University (Yangling, China).

TMV isolates were provided by the Laboratory of Molecular Plant Pathology, Southwest University (Chongqing, China) in the form of virus infected plants of *N. benthamiana*.

The seeds of *N. glutinosa* were provided by the Laboratory of Plant Virus, Inner Mongolia Agricultural University (Hohhot, China), and cultivated in an insect-free greenhouse at 24 ± 1 °C. The experiments were conducted when the plant had grown 5–6 leaves.

4.2. Virus Purification

The Gooding method [34] was used for the purification of TMV-inoculated *N. benthamiana*, and the isolates were stored at −20 °C and diluted to 50 µg/mL with 0.01 M PBS (phosphate-buffered saline) before use. Absorbance values were estimated at 260 nm by using an ultraviolet spectrophotometer Tu-1901 (Beijing General Instrument co. LTD, Beijing, China). To calculate the concentration of virus, the following formula was used (Equation (1)):

$$\text{Virus concentration} = (A_{260} \times \text{dilution ratio}) / E_{1\,cm}^{0.1\%,260\,nm} \tag{1}$$

4.3. Isolation and Purification of Active Compounds and Structure Analysis

The *C. monnieri* (100 g) was powdered and extracted with 500 mL 90% methanol by reflux three times (1.5 h each). The combined methanol extract was concentrated (50 g) and incubated with quicklime (100 g) for 24 h. Subsequently, it was washed three times using five times diluted hydrochloric acid and concentrated, suspended in chloroform (90 mL), and isolated with alkaline water (0.5% NaOH solution). The crystal was filtered from the solution by adjusting the pH value to 7. After drying at a low temperature, the solution that was filtered from the crystal with petroleum for 1 h was naturally cooled to room temperature, and the final product was analyzed by liquid chromatography-mass spectrometry (LC-MS). The structure was identified by ^{1}H- and ^{13}C-NMR spectra.

4.4. Inhibitory Effect of Osthole on TMV Infection

The compounds of osthole and eugenol were dissolved in DMSO (dimethyl sulfoxide) (1000 mg/mL) and diluted to the required concentration with Tween-20 and distilled water (1:1000 *v/v*). Ningnanmycin (8%) was diluted with water to a concentration of 500 µg/mL and used for the following experiment. The inhibitory, protective, and curative effects were examined using the half-leaf method.

Osthole, eugenol, and ningnanmycin were mixed with the virus (TMV at 6 × 10^{-3} mg/mL) at the same volume or concentration for 10 min, and then were smeared with a cotton swab onto the left leaves of tobacco (*N. glutinosa*) along the main vein, whereas the virus sap and the DMSO solvent in the right half of the leaves were inoculated in each of the three treatment groups (total of 12 leaves). Each half of the leaf was smeared with 40 µL of TMV extract, and each inoculated leaf was washed with water after 10 min. The local lesion numbers were recorded for 3–4 days after inoculation and each compound and control agent was repeated three times.

The inhibition rates of osthole, magnolol, honokiol, and ningnanmycin were recorded and calculated according to the following formula (Equation (2)):

$$\text{Inhibition rate (\%)} = [(C - T)/C] \times 100\% \tag{2}$$

where C is average lesion number of the control halves and T is the average mean lesion number on the drug-treated half-leaves.

4.5. Protective Effect of Osthole on TMV Infection

Osthole, eugenol, and ningnanmycin were gently smeared with cotton swabs on the left side of the leaves. The DMSO solution was spread as a negative control in the right lobe of tobacco leaves of the same ages. After 24 h, 40 µL of TMV (50 µL/mL) was inoculated onto whole leaves of *N. glutinosa*, each dealing with three treatment groups repeated in triplicate (total of 12 leaves were recorded), and each inoculated leaf was washed with water after 10 min. The number of lesions on tested leaves was investigated for 3–4 days.

4.6. Curative Effect of Osthole on TMV Infection

TMV (6×10^{-3} mg/mL) was inoculated on the whole leaves of *N. glutinosa* by cotton swabs. Then, the leaves were washed with water and dried. After 24 h, osthole, eugenol, and ningnanmycin were smeared onto the left leaf side, while the DMSO solution was smeared onto the right side for the control. The local lesion numbers were recorded for 3–4 days after viral inoculation. Each experiment was repeated three times.

4.7. Viral Particle Observation by Transmission Electron Microscope (TEM)

TMV particles were mixed with the osthole at 3 and 5 mg/mL with an equal volume for 60 min at room temperature [30]. Then, samples were placed on a carbon-coated grid, and negatively stained with a few drops of 2% phosphotungstic acid for 1 min at room temperature. They were then washed and the excess fluid was absorbed on filter paper. The samples were observed with an electron microscope (H-500, Hitachi Co. Ltd., Tokyo, Japan). An untreated virus sample served as a negative control.

4.8. Western Blot Analysis to Detect the CP of TMV

The levels of the TMV CP were analyzed by Western blotting. Total protein was extracted from leaves of *N. glutinosa* (0.1 g, fresh weight), that were treated by water, and 1, 3, 5, and 7 mg/mL of osthole. Samples were ground in liquid nitrogen and dissolved in 200 µL extraction buffer (125 mM Tris-HCl, pH 7.5, 2% SDS, 6 M UREA, 5% β-mercaptoethanol and bromophenol blue). The extracts were then heated at 95 °C for 10 min and centrifuged at $12,000 \times g$ at 4 °C for 10 min. Equal sample volumes (5 µL) were loaded on a 12% polyacrylamide gel, and proteins were separated by electrophoresis at 120 V for 70 min. After being transferred to a PVDF membrane, CP was detected using a primary antibody (1:800) and was subsequently probed with AP-coupled goat anti-rabbit IgG (1:5000; Abcam, Cambridge, UK). The signals on the membrane were visualized using Clarity Western ECL Substrate (Bio-Rad Company, Hercules, CA, USA).

4.9. Statistical Analysis

All data were expressed as the mean ± SD by measuring three independent replicates. The Data Processing System 15.10 (Hefei, China) was used to perform the statistical analysis. The significance of the statistical differences between three means was determined using Duncan's new complex range method at the 5% level.

Supplementary Materials: The following are available online, Figure S1: H-NMR of osthole, Figure S2: C-NMR of osthole.

Author Contributions: Y.-H.C., D.-S.G. and M.-H.L. isolated and purified of active compounds and analyzed the structure. Y.-H.C. tested anti-TMV activities of osthole. D.-S.G. tested Transmission Electron Microscope (TEM). J.-Y.Y., C.-M.S. and Y.L. analyzed the kinetic analysis of the osthole effect against TMV infection. D.-R.A. and M.-M.Z. designed the experiments and supervised the study. M.-M.Z. and Y.-H.C. wrote the manuscript. All authors have read and agreed to the published version of the manuscript.

Funding: The study was supported by Start-up Funding of High-level Talent Researcher in Inner Mongolia Agricultural University (No. NDGCC2016-23) to Mingmin Zhao. Science and Technology Major Project of Inner Mongolia (2018) to Chunming Shang, and the Demonstration and Application of Control Technology of Plant Pests and Diseases in Shaanxi Province (No. K4030218261) to Derong An.

Acknowledgments: We thank Xian-Chao Sun (Southwest University, the People's Republic of China) for providing the primary antibody of TMV. We thank the Life Science Research Core Services (LSRCS) of Northwest A&F University, the People's Republic of China, for their help collecting the LC-MS and NMR data.

Conflicts of Interest: The authors declare no conflicts of interest.

References

1. Hong, J.; Li, D.B.; Zhou, X.P. *The Classification of Plant Viruses*, 1st ed.; Beijing Science Press: Beijing, China, 2001; p. 189.
2. Wu, Y.F. *Principles and Methods of Plant Virology*, 1st ed.; Xi'an Cartographic Publishing House: Xi'an, China, 1999; pp. 26–30.
3. Liu, L.R. *The Control of Tobacco Diseases and Pests*, 1st ed.; Beijing Science Press: Beijing, China, 1998; pp. 10–12.
4. Liu, Y.; Li, F.; Zhang, S.; Gao, X.; Xie, Y.; Zhang, A.; Dai, L.; Cheng, Z.; Ding, M.; Niu, Y.; et al. Identifcation, distribution and occurrence of viruses in the main vegetables of China. *Sci. Agric. Sin.* **2019**, *52*, 239–261.
5. Wu, Y.F.; Cao, R.; Wei, N.S.; Zhou, G.H. Screening and application of biological virus pesticides. *World Pestic.* **1995**, *5*, 35–36.
6. Fan, H.; Song, B.; Bhadury, P.S.; Jin, L.H.; Hu, D.Y.; Yang, S. Antiviral Activity and Mechanism of Action of Novel Thiourea Containing Chiral Phosphonate on Tobacco Mosaic Virus. *Int. J. Mol. Sci.* **2011**, *12*, 4522–4535. [CrossRef] [PubMed]
7. Li, Y.M.; Wang, L.H.; Li, S.L.; Chen, X.Y.; Shen, Y.M.; Zhang, Z.K.; He, H.P.; Xu, W.B.; Shu, Y.L.; Liang, G.D.; et al. Seco-pregnane steroids target the subgenomic RNA of alphavirus-like RNA viruses. *Proc. Natl. Acad. Sci. USA* **2007**, *104*, 8083–8088. [CrossRef] [PubMed]
8. Pimentel, D. Environmental and economic costs of the application of pesticides primarily in the United States. *Environ. Dev. Sustain.* **2005**, *7*, 229–252. [CrossRef]
9. Yoon, M.Y.; Cha, B.; Kim, J.C. Recent trends in studies on botanical fungicides in Agriculture. *Plant Pathol. J.* **2013**, *29*, 1–9. [CrossRef] [PubMed]
10. Zhao, L.; Feng, C.; Wu, K.; Chen, W.B.; Chen, Y.J.; Hao, X.A.; Wu, Y.F. Advances and prospects in biogenic substances against plant virus: A review. *Pestic. Biochem. Phys.* **2016**, *135*, 15–26. [CrossRef]
11. Chen, Y.H.; Ru, B.L.; Zhai, Y.Y.; Li, J.; Cheng, J.L.; Zhang, Q.; An, D.R. Screening of antiviral activity of extracts from medicinal plants against Tobacco mosaic virus (TMV). *Acta Phytophy. Sin.* **2018**, *45*, 463–469.
12. Grange, M.; Ahmed, S. *Handbook of Plants with Pest-Control Properties*, 1st ed.; Miss University Press: New York, NY, USA, 1988; p. 470.
13. Zhu, S.F.; Qiu, W.F. A primary study of the therapeutic effects of some medicinal herb extracts on the pepper mosaic caused by CMV. *Acta Phytopathol. Sin.* **1989**, *19*, 123–128.
14. Jing, B.N.; Ma, Z.Q.; Feng, J.T.; Liang, H.Y.; Li, C.; Zhang, X. Evaluation of the antiviral activity of extracts from plants grown in the Qinling region of China against infection by tobacco mosaic virus (TMV). *J. Phytopathol.* **2012**, *160*, 181–186. [CrossRef]
15. Esam, K.F.E.; Ehab, M.R.M.; Omar, A.A. Antiviral activity of Thuja orientalis extracts against watermelon mosaic virus (WMV) on *Citrullus lanatus*. *Saudi J. Biol. Sci.* **2015**, *22*, 211–219.
16. Zhao, L.H.; Dong, J.H.; Hu, Z.H.; Li, S.L.; Su, X.X.; Zhang, J.; Yin, Y.Y.; Xu, T.; Zhang, Z.K.; Chen, H.R. Anti-TMV activity and functional mechanisms of two sesquiterpenoids isolated from, *Tithonia diversifolia*. *Pestic. Biochem. Phys.* **2017**, *140*, 24–29. [CrossRef] [PubMed]

17. Wang, J.; Yu, G.H.; Li, Y.H.; Shen, L.L.; Qian, Y.M.; Yang, J.G.; Wang, F.L. Inhibitory effects of sulfated lentinan with different degree of sulfation against tobacco mosaic virus (TMV) in tobacco seedlings. *Pestic. Biochem. Phys.* **2015**, *122*, 38–43. [CrossRef] [PubMed]
18. Basnet, P.; Yasuda, I.; Kumagai, N.; Tohda, C.; Nojima, H.; Kuraishi, Y.; Komatsu, K. Inhibition of itch-scratch response by fruits of *Cnidium monnieri* in mice. *Biol. Pharm. Bull.* **2001**, *24*, 1012–1015. [CrossRef] [PubMed]
19. Bao, J.J.; Xie, M.L.; Zhu, L.J. Treatment of osthol on osteoporosis in ovariectomized rats. *Chin. Pharm. Bull.* **2011**, *27*, 591–592.
20. Matsuda, H.; Ido, Y.; Hirata, A.; Ino, Y.; Naruto, S.; Amamiya, T.; Kubo, M. Antipruritic effect of *Cnidii monnieri* Fructus (fruits of *Cnidium monnieri* Cusson). *Biol. Pharm. Bull.* **2002**, *25*, 260–263. [CrossRef]
21. Matsuda, H.; Tomohiro, N.; Ido, Y.; Kubo, M. Anti-allergic effects of *Cnidii monnieri* fructus (dried fruits of *Cnidium monnieri*) and its major component, osthol. *Biol. Pharm. Bull.* **2002**, *25*, 809–812. [CrossRef]
22. Li, Y.M.; Jia, M.; Li, H.Q.; Zhang, N.D.; Wen, X.; Rahman, K.; Zhang, Q.Y.; Qin, L.P. *Cnidium monnieri*: A Review of Traditional Uses, Phytochemical and Ethnopharmacological Properties. *Am. Chin. Med.* **2015**, *43*, 835–877. [CrossRef]
23. Kitajima, J.; Aoki, Y.; Ishikawa, T.; Tanaka, Y. Monoterpenoid glucosides of *Cnidium monnieri* fruit. *Chem. Pharm. Bull.* **1999**, *47*, 639–642. [CrossRef]
24. Oh, H.; Kim, J.S.; Song, E.K.; Cho, H.; Kim, D.H.; Park, S.E.; Lee, H.S.; Kim, Y.C. Sesquiterpenes with hepatoprotective activity from *Cnidium monnieri* on tacrine-induced cytotoxicity in Hep G2 cells. *Planta Med.* **2002**, *68*, 748–749. [CrossRef]
25. Zhao, J.Y.; Zhou, M.; Liu, Y.; Zhang, G.L.; Luo, Y.G. Chromones and coumarins from the dried fructus of *Cnidium monnieri*. *Fitoterapia* **2011**, *82*, 767–771. [CrossRef] [PubMed]
26. Li, K.P.; Gao, C.K.; Li, W.M. Analysis of coumarins in cnidium extracts by UPLC/ESI-TOF-MS/MS. *Chin. Pat. Med.* **2009**, *31*, 584–587.
27. Chappell, J. The biochemistry and molecular biology of isoprenoid metabolism. *Plant Physiol.* **1995**, *107*, 1–6. [CrossRef] [PubMed]
28. Shi, Z.Q.; Shen, S.G.; Xu, L.L.; Fan, Y.J. Preliminary study on the inhibitory mechanism of osthol on plant pathogenic fungi. *Chin. J. Pestic. Sci.* **2004**, *4*, 28–32.
29. Wang, C.M.; Su, H.; Chen, H.; Shi, Z.Q.; Fan, Y.J. Mode of action of natural compound eugenol on Tobacco mosaic virus disease. *Agrochemicals* **2012**, *1*, 32–34, 39.
30. Jin, Y.; Hou, L.Y.; Zhang, M.Z.; Tian, Z.F.; Cao, A.C.; Xie, X.M. Antiviral activity of Eupatorium adenophorum leaf extract against tobacco mosaic virus. *Crop Prot.* **2014**, *60*, 28–33. [CrossRef]
31. Hilf, M.E.; Dawson, W.O. The tobamovirus capsid protein functions as a host-specific determinant of long-distance movement. *Virology* **1993**, *193*, 106–114. [CrossRef]
32. Asurmendi, S.; Berg, R.H.; Koo, J.C.; Beachy, R.N. Coat protein regulates formation of replication complexes during tobacco mosaic virus infection. *Proc. Natl. Acad. Sci. USA* **2004**, *101*, 1415–1420. [CrossRef]
33. Siddiqui, S.A.; Sarmiento, C.; Valkonen, S.; Truve, E.; Lehto, K. Suppression of infectious TMV genomes expressed in young transgenic tobacco plants. *Mol. Plant-Microbe Interact.* **1489**, *20*, 1489–1494. [CrossRef]
34. Gooding, G.V.; Hebert, T.A. A simple technique for purification of tobacco mosaic virus in large quantities. *Phytopathology* **1967**, *57*, 1285–1289.

Sample Availability: Samples of the compounds are not available from the authors.

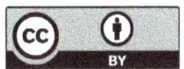

© 2019 by the authors. Licensee MDPI, Basel, Switzerland. This article is an open access article distributed under the terms and conditions of the Creative Commons Attribution (CC BY) license (http://creativecommons.org/licenses/by/4.0/).

MDPI
St. Alban-Anlage 66
4052 Basel
Switzerland
Tel. +41 61 683 77 34
Fax +41 61 302 89 18
www.mdpi.com

Molecules Editorial Office
E-mail: molecules@mdpi.com
www.mdpi.com/journal/molecules

www.ingramcontent.com/pod-product-compliance
Lightning Source LLC
Chambersburg PA
CBHW051618020226
39067CB00061B/126